DUNS SCOTU
LOURDES COLLEGE
SYLVANIA, OHIO

3 0379

D0945104

Brain
Peptides

Brain Peptides

Edited by

DOROTHY T. KRIEGER
MICHAEL J. BROWNSTEIN
JOSEPH B. MARTIN

A Wiley-Interscience Publication
JOHN WILEY & SONS
New York · Chichester · Brisbane · Toronto · Singapore

065229

Copyright © 1983 by John Wiley & Sons, Inc.

All rights reserved. Published simultaneously in Canada.

Reproduction or translation of any part of this work
beyond that permitted by Section 107 or 108 of the
1976 United States Copyright Act without the permission
of the copyright owner is unlawful. Requests for
permission or further information should be addressed to
the Permissions Department, John Wiley & Sons, Inc.

Library of Congress Cataloging in Publication Data:

Main entry under title:

Brain peptides.

"A Wiley-Interscience publication."
Includes index.
1. Brain chemistry. 2. Peptides. I. Krieger,
Dorothy T. II. Brownstein, Michael, 1943- .
III. Martin, Joseph B. (DNLM: 1. Brain—Physiology.
2. Peptides—Physiology. WL 300 B81375)
QP430.B7   1983   591.1'88   83-6761
ISBN 0-471-09433-1

Printed in the United States of America

10 9 8 7 6 5 4 3

Preface

From time to time there occurs in the general field of biology an explosion of information that serves as a catapult to open entire new vistas of discovery and interdisciplinary study. The discovery of the brain peptides incited such an explosion. The identification of more than thirty potential new peptide neurotransmitters in the brain and the recognition that similar groups of small molecular peptides, often derived from a common precursor, are contained within nerve cells, endocrine cells, and within the body fluids (blood and cerebrospinal fluid) have required the complete restructuring of old ideas and the development of new hypotheses. Many of the distinctions of phylogeny and ontogeny are now blurred. Some of these brain peptides appear to be present in organisms that lack a defined nervous system. Ontogenetic studies indicate that cells may change their neurotransmitter production and release, switching from one type to another during normal development. And it is now common to find that nerve cells, and in some cases hormone-producing cells, contain two or three separate transmitter candidates derived from different biosynthetic pathways.

It can be anticipated that the equally expanding fields of molecular biology, biochemistry, and developmental biology will further add to the growth of the field of brain peptides by identifying precursor molecules for known peptides, by delineating alternative modes of mRNA splicing of such precursors to yield heretofore unknown peptides, and by characterizing the factors involved in peptide expression. For example, the identity of the precursor for the enkephalins in adrenal tissue, if found applicable also to brain, will add strength to the emerging hypothesis that individual nerve cells produce families of neuroactive substances, all of which are presumably released at synaptic sites or into extracellular spaces of the brain, including the cerebrospinal fluid.

We still have only a primitive understanding of how peptides, produced in various tissues and perhaps under separate gene regulation, participate in the overall integration of neuronal, neuroendocrine, and hormonal functions. There is little question that peptides reside in selected and heretofore undefined neuroanatomic pathways in the central and peripheral nervous system and within cells of the hypothalamus important for neuroendocrine regulation. The administration of peptides to animals induces highly specific endocrine and behavioral responses, although in many instances the physiologic significance of the observed effect can only be surmised. Potential implications of endogenous disorders of peptide function in human neurological and psychiatric disease have been speculated upon but to date no specific disease caused by a peptide defect has been described.

Many books have been published on the brain peptides, primarily as the permanent records of meetings held throughout the world to share information in this exploding area. No attempt has been made to bring together in a single volume the entire subject, carefully edited and reviewed for the purpose of making a critical statement of the current status of the field. This volume was proposed to accomplish that end. Authors were invited to participate not only on the basis of their contributions to the area of investigation but also because they were considered able to assess critically the meaning and interpretations of the available information. The editors have carefully reviewed the chapters and worked closely with the authors to produce a uniformity of depth, discussion, and interpretation.

To provide coherence to the volume, the chapters are organized into four parts. Part 1 gives an overview of the broad biological implications of the brain peptides with reference to evolutionary, embryological, and interspecies comparisons and to the development of systems of intercellular communication. Part 2 examines the role of multiple peptides as they interact to influence major homeostastic systems. Part 3 probes the strengths and limitations of the current methodologies applicable to the study of brain peptides. Part 4 provides, for those peptides best characterized, a summary of the present state of knowledge peptide by peptide. We hope that this organization will make the volume useful to basic neurobiologists, to endocrinologists, and to clinicians dealing in the neurosciences.

DOROTHY T. KRIEGER
MICHAEL J. BROWNSTEIN
JOSEPH B. MARTIN

New York, New York
Bethesda, Maryland
Boston, Massachusetts
September 1983

Contents

CHAPTER

CHAPTER

CHAPTER

PART 4   SPECIFIC NEUROPEPTIDES

CHAPTER

Brain
Peptides

1

Introduction

DOROTHY T. KRIEGER
*Department of Medicine
Mount Sinai School of Medicine
New York, New York*

MICHAEL J. BROWNSTEIN
*Laboratory of Cell Biology
National Institute of Mental Health
Bethesda, Maryland*

JOSEPH B. MARTIN
*Department of Neurology
Massachusetts General Hospital
Harvard Medical School
Boston, Massachusetts*

1 HISTORICAL PERSPECTIVE

It is now widely acknowledged that cell-to-cell communication in diverse organisms is mediated primarily by chemical messengers. These molecules take many forms; they range from amino acids such as gamma-aminobutyric acid (GABA) or glycine to biogenic amines, peptides, and small proteins. In the nervous system such intercellular communication occurs predominantly at synapses via release of neurotransmitters (see refs. 1–3). In the past decade an increasing number of peptides have been added to the list of putative neurotransmitters. The elucidation of their role in neural function will constitute a quantum leap forward in our understanding of brain function.

It was principally the Scharrers (4) who promulgated the concept that nerves can secrete hormones into the bloodstream as well as into the synaptic cleft, although they did not originate the concept of the "glandular neuron." As early as 1919, Carl Speidel (5) had noted that giant neurons in the posterior spinal cord of elasmobranch fish have anatomical features associated with secretory activity. Subsequently, Ernst Scharrer found similar cells in vertebrate brains—initially in fish hypothalamus. By the late 1940s, Palay and Bargmann (6, 7) had shown that secretory neurons in the vertebrate hypothalamus were the source of axons that projected to the neurohypophysis, and that such axons and their terminals were also rich in secretory material. They inferred that posterior pituitary hormones were synthesized in the neurons of this hypothalamo-neurohypophyseal system and were released from its terminals. This concept slowly gained acceptance over the then-prevailing notion that the posterior pituitary hormones were made in the pituicytes of the posterior lobe that were in turn only regulated by the innervation arising from central neurons. It was not until the 1950s, however, that Du Vigneaud and his colleagues (8) succeeded in isolating and chemically characterizing two neurohypophyseal hormones, vasopressin and oxytocin. Since then, a number of related slightly chemically modified molecules, the neurophypophyseal nonapeptides, have been isolated from diverse species (see Chapter 5). It is possible that over the course of evolution these molecules have acquired different functions.

A number of analogs to the hypothalamo-neurohypophyseal system are known to exist in invertebrates: among them are the corpus cardiacum/corpus allatum in insects and the eyestalk X-organ/sinus gland complex in crustaceans. Knowles coined the term "neurohemal organ" to describe those areas of the nervous system wherein axon terminals of neurosecretory cells make contact with blood vessels and release their secretory products into the bloodstream (9).

It next became evident that neuropeptides were not only destined for secretion into the vascular system, with resultant action on target tissues, but that such peptides also had local neural actions. Many years after the Scharrers' initial studies, it has become evident that projections from vasopressinergic and oxytocinergic neurons exist elsewhere in the central nervous system than in the neurohypophyseal tract, and that such projections may mediate various behavioral responses; see Chapters 16 and 25.

In contrast to vasopressin and oxytocin, substance P—the doyenne of biologically active peptides—was first isolated from intestine, not brain (10). This presaged the large number of other peptides subsequently described as being present in both gastrointestinal tract and brain. Some of these peptides were initially characterized in brain and then in gastrointestinal tissue; others, like substance P, were first characterized in the gastrointestinal tract. It is now evident that other kinds of peptides coexist in the anterior pituitary and central nervous system. Whether all the cells that make and release a particular peptide form a "system" and coordinate events in the brain and periphery remains to be seen.

Substance P defied purification until the early 1970s. Chang et al. (11) noticed that bovine hypothalamic extracts were rich in an agent that provoked intense salivation. They identified this sialogogic factor as Arg-Pro-Lys-Pro-Gln-Gln-Phe-Phe-Gly-Leu-Met-NH$_2$ and recognized that its amino acid composition was similar to that of the best available preparations of substance P. They therefore suggested, and Studer et al. (12) later demonstrated conclusively, that the sialogogic factor and substance P were one and the same. Since then, a number of closely related molecules—tachykinins—have been isolated from the skin of amphibians (physalaemin, Lys^5-Thr^6-physalaemin, uperolein, phyllomedusin, kassinin, Glu^2-Pro^5-kassinin, and hylambitin) and from the salivary glands of a mollusc, the Mediterranean octopus (eledoisin, 13). Indeed, many of these latter substances were chemically characterized well before substance P was finally isolated.

2 PEPTIDE FAMILIES

The families of neurohypophyseal hormones and tachykinins already noted are illustrative of molecules that have evolved in different species, each family member arising as a modification from a common ancestral peptide (see Chapter 5). Genetic reduplication provides a different mechanism for the generation of other kinds of peptide "families." In these, closely related amino acid sequences are found to be represented several times within the same precursor molecule in the same species. Such sequences are subsequently enzymatically released from this precursor molecule and exist as separate moieties. The nature of such enzymatic processing, however, may differ in two given tissues in which a common precursor molecule is present. Examples of such repeated sequences can be found in the pro-opiomelanocortin precursor, which contains the three similar amino acid sequences of α-, β-, and α-melanocyte-stimulating hormone (MSH). In like manner, the proenkephalin molecule contains six Met-enkephalins (Try-Gly-Gly-Phe-Met) and one Leu-enkephalin sequence (Try-Gly-Gly-Phe-Leu); the dynorphin precursor contains the three active components α-neoendorphin, dynorphin A, and dynorphin B, each one of which has Tyr-Gly-Gly-Phe-Leu at its N-terminus (14–16). The significance of the presence of these multiple copies of structurally related molecules (e.g., the opioid peptides) remains to be determined. Just as there are several opioid peptides, there are also several distinct opioid receptors that appear to be specific for different opiate ligands. It is not unreasonable, therefore, to suppose that a variety of distinct physiological roles are effected by the individual opioid peptides and mediated by their respective receptors.

Another type of peptide family is exemplified by sequences arising from the calcitonin gene (17). It appears that alternative processing of RNA transcripts from this gene results in the production of distinct small mRNAs encoding either the hormone calcitonin or a product referred to as "calcitonin gene-regulated peptide" (CGRP). In the thyroid, processing of the calcitonin gene leads to a predominance of calcitonin mRNA, whereas in the hypothalamus (Figure 1) the CGRP-specific mRNA appears to predominate.

3 METHODOLOGIES FOR DELINEATING CURRENTLY "UNKNOWN" PEPTIDES

The number of brain peptides reported has increased since this book was first outlined. In addition to the peptides cited in Chapters 25–39, a number of "new peptides" have been reported to be present in brain, for example Hydra head-budding factor, PHI, PYY, FmRF amide, phoriscotrophic hormone (PTTH), and CGRP. Some of these have been visualized immunohistochemically but have not been measured in brain extracts; others have been detected by means of radioimmunoassay but have not been further characterized. Some of the newer methodologic strategies being employed offer promise that numerous other brain peptides will be delineated (1). Viktor Mutt and his coworkers (18) have described a strategy for looking for new active peptides in brain (and in gastrointestinal extracts). Based on the reasoning that any molecule with a C-terminal amide is likely to be biologically important, they devised a method for removing amino acid amides from peptides and delineating the structures of the parent molecules. On the basis of their work to date, they are confident that several uncharacterized amidated peptides are present in brain in relatively high concentrations, as high as those for peptides already described (18). Another approach is through the use of techniques that characterize peptide precursor mRNAs or the genes that encode them. Characterization of such peptide

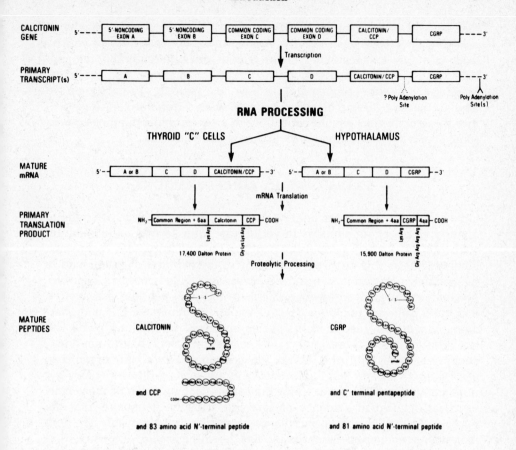

Figure 1. A model to describe the tissue-specific expression of the calcitonin (Cal) gene during peptide-switching events. The 5' and 3' termini are indicated as dashed lines because their structural organization remains unknown. The structural organization of coding blocks A and B, and the presence of A within CGRP mRNSs, are not unequivocally indicated. The forked arrow indicates tissues in which pCal reactiv e RNAs predominate (thyroid) or pCGRP reactive RNAs predominate (hy pothalamus). The predicted proteolytic products of the primary translation product directed by Cal mRNA are established, those of CGRP mRNA predicted. Reproduced with permission from Amara et al. (17).

precursors will delineate other potential sequences contained therein (e.g., the structure of γ-MSH was inferred from the predicted amino acid sequence of pro-opiomelanocortin, and the two dynorphins, A and B, were revealed to be present when the precursor molecule was identified based on recombinant technology). It is obvious that in the future the other peptides predicted to be present in such precursors will have to be isolated and their structures determined (3). It is also anticipated that several other peptides will undoubtedly be isolated by means of assaying their biological activity. Among those of great interest will be trophic factors that regulate cellular growth and differentiation, the peptide that prescribes the structure of the motor endplate, and the phospholipase inhibitor (lipomodulin) that has recently been shown to mediate certain effects of steroids on cellular differentiation. Research into these molecules should contribute to a better understanding of neuronal specialization, axonal growth, and synaptogenesis.

4 EVOLUTIONARY CONSIDERATIONS

Other leads in characterizing new peptides will derive from attempts to identify invertebrate peptides in vertebrate brain as well as the characterization of known vertebrate peptides in invertebrates. From such studies to date, it is apparent that many of the peptides characterized in mammalian nervous tissue, for which specific functions have been delineated, are present in lower forms in which such peptides presumably had quite different functions. (For example, hypothalamic releasing hormones have been identified in species in which the pituitary gland has not differentiated. There have also been reports that "neural peptides" such as somatostatin and ACTH are present in unicellular organisms; see Chapters 26 and 36.) Phylogenetically, neurons with elementary synaptic contacts first appear in the coelenterates, and some of these cells manifest cytological evidence of secretory activity. It appears that the nervous system in such primitive invertebrates is responsible for both neural and endocrine functions. It has been suggested, therefore, that the neurosecretory neuron of higher vertebrates retains more of the ancient characteristics of this nerve cell precursor than either the conventional neuron or the endocrine cell, both of which may be derived from such a precursor. It is not surprising, therefore, that the peptide products of neural and endocrine cells are similar, though it is apparent that changes in processing of a precursor molecule can also occur with evolution. Many of these peptides may have arisen with a neurocrine or paracrine function, only later in evolution acquiring roles that required more widespread distribution.

5 POSSIBLE FUNCTIONS OF BRAIN PEPTIDES

It is difficult to make meaningful general statements about the functions of various brain peptides. The "hypothalamic" hormones, for example, were isolated on the basis of their action on cells of the anterior pituitary, but soon after their characterization it was shown that these releasing or release-inhibiting factors were not confined to the hypothalamus or even to the brain. Consequently, it became clear that they must have roles separate from those exerted at the level of the median eminence in the control of anterior pituitary function.

Although we are at a very early stage in understanding the function of these peptides in the central nervous system, studies to date indicate that they are involved in the regulation of the major bodily homeostatic systems; have local effects on cerebral circulation and on neuronal firing; are involved in developmental structure-function relations and the acquisition of neuronal plasticity; and are implicated in behavioral expression. Whether loss of specific peptide function may become manifest as neurological disease, similar to the documented loss of dopaminergic cells in Parkinson's disease, remains to be determined. Although individual peptide concentrations have been found to be abnormal in some of the neural-degenerative diseases, the cause-and-effect nature of these findings is unclear.

Functions of peptides have typically been defined in terms of the distance over which they exert their effects. Thus, a given peptide can act as a neurotransmitter (or neuromodulator), a neurohormone, a paracrine mediator, or a hormone. For example, luteinizing hormone releasing hormone (LHRH), in addition to effecting the release of LH from the pituitary, has also been shown to be released from synaptic nerve endings onto ganglionic neurons, that is, acting like a neurotransmitter. Allusion has also been made to vasopressin, considered to be a neurohormone when released from nerve endings in the posterior pituitary into the systemic circulation to act on the kidney, but which acts as a neurotransmitter within the central nervous system. Somatostatin, another hypothalamic releasing factor considered to be a neurohormone when inhibiting the release of growth hormone, also acts as a paracrine mediator when it is released by cells within the pancreatic islets to inhibit glucagon and/or insulin release by neighboring cells. Adrenocorticotrophic hormone (ACTH), considered a "classical" hormone released by corticotrophs of the anterior pituitary into the systemic circulation, thereby stimulating steroid production and release by the adrenal cortex, also exists (and to a greater extent fragments derived from it exist) within the central nervous system, where it is postulated to have a neurotransmitter or neuromodulatory role.

6 RECENT ADVANCES IN CHARACTERIZING BRAIN PEPTIDES

The criteria that must be satisfied by a molecule if it is to be called a chemical mediator are essentially the same regardless of its role. It is useful to enumerate these criteria, because many studies outlined in the following chapters are devoted to providing data to meet them; this is done in Table 1.

TABLE 1   Criteria that Must Be Met in Order to Call a Molecule a Chemical Mediator

1. The substance must be present in the effector cell.
2. It must be synthesized by the effector cell.
3. It must be released by the effector cell in response to appropriate stimuli.
4. Exogenously administered material must act on the follower cell in a manner that is qualitatively and quantitatively to the actions of the substance released from the effector cell. (Some equate this to demonstration of the existence of a specific, saturable, high-affinity receptor, but see Chapter 24).
5. There must be a mechanism for rapidly terminating the actions of the substance.
6. Drugs that affect the actions of the substance released from the effector cell (e.g., antagonists, inhibitors of degradation) should have a similar effect on exogenously administered material.

For technical reasons it has been easier to prove conclusively that an agent is a neurotransmitter in the peripheral nervous system than to do so in the central nervous system. Technical advances in the last decade, however, have made possible experiments that were only dreamed of earlier. Combinations of these techniques should facilitate the characterization of such mediators.

6.1   Peptide Isolation and Characterization

Attempts to purify many peptides, including the releasing factors, failed until recently because of the methods employed. Classical methods including organic solvent extraction and precipitation were augmented by countercurrent, molecular sieving and ion exchange chromatography, and high-voltage electrophoresis. Very large amounts of starting material were required in order to recover enough material for analysis at the end of the preparative steps. Now, amino acid analysis can be performed on as little as 5–10 pmol of pure peptide. Given a 10 pmol sample, fast atom bombardment mass spectroscopy can be used to determine the molecular weight of a peptide and subnanomole amounts of peptide can be sequenced with modified Edman degradation methodology. This has resulted in the characterization of peptides that are present in very low levels in brain extracts and has allowed the use of scaled-down preparative procedures. The most important of these is high performance liquid chromatography (HPLC), a method that has come into its own in the past five years. The commercial availability of reliable and easy-to-use instruments and high-resolution columns has made it possible for workers in many laboratories to exploit this technique. The method is fast, results in excellent recovery of submicrogram amounts of peptide, and can be used either preparatively or analytically. Initially, reversed phase (i.e., hydrophobic) columns were employed almost exclusively for peptide separations, but recently excellent columns have been introduced for molecular sieving, ion exchange, and chromato-focusing applications.

6.2 Localizing Peptidergic Neurons

Neuroanatomists have played a particularly important role in winning converts to the field of peptide research. This was based on their dem-onstration of discrete populations of peptide-containing neurons, the mapping of their projections, and on the development of relatively straightforward methods for removing discrete brain nuclei for biochem-ical analysis. The former demonstrations, of course, were based on immunohistochemistry—the use of antipeptide antibodies as histochem-ical reagents (see Chapter 21). While technical difficulties remain to be resolved, the method is being broadly applied at the light and electron microscopic levels. Biochemical, physiological, and pharmacological studies have quickly followed the anatomical advances. A useful ad-junct to immunocytochemistry is the combination of brain microdissec-tion and microassay. This combination provides quantitative estimates of peptide levels in selected brain areas, allows biochemical analysis of the immunoreactive species that have been visualized, and (used with lesions) provides information about the location of cells that provide a particular nucleus its complement of peptide. In addition, the "micropunch method" (see Chapter 22) can be employed for pulse-chase or recombinant DNA–based studies.

A particularly promising method for evaluating the development, structure, and function of peptidergic cells is *in situ* hybridization cyto-chemistry. This technique is conceptually similar to immunocytochemis-try, except that complementary DNA is used to visualize mRNA instead of using an antibody to detect a peptide. It should be especially power-ful for evaluating the switching on or off of genes in the course of devel-opment.

6.3 Peptide Biosynthesis

Members of several laboratories have already begun to apply methods developed by molecular geneticists to answer questions about neuro-peptide biosynthesis. By sequencing cloned DNA complementary to mRNAs that encode peptide precursors, these investigators have deduced the structures of prepro-enkephalin, -dynorphin, -opiomelanocortin, -somatostatin, and -vasopressin. On the basis of these structural analy-ses, certain rules about precursor processing have been inferred; these are outlined in Chapter 3. It is evident that at least three types of en-zymes are involved in liberating active peptides from their precursors: trypsin-like and carboxypeptidase B-like enzymes, and an amidating en-zyme recently described by Smythe and his coworkers.

6.4 Physiological Studies

New methods to insure the viability of neurons in culture have resulted in the use of new physiological preparations. Brain slices and dissociated cell cultures are particularly promising. The former allows cells to be studied in a nearly intact milieu; the latter allows them to be investigated in the absence of confounding inputs. Furthermore, new electronic developments, including the single-electrode and patch clamp, allow the mechanism of action of peptides on single small cells to be evaluated. One hopes that in simple systems it will be possible to determine the effects of two transmitters applied simultaneously and to better understand why transmitters coexist in certain neurons (Chapter 22). In addition, one hopes that ultimately it will be possible to grasp the significance of temporal patterning of neuronal inputs and outputs on performance of the brain.

6.5 Receptors

In the past few years a number of peptide agonists and antagonists have been radiolabeled to high specific activity. This has resulted in the identification of binding sites for particular peptides. Students of the opioid peptides have led the way in this field because of the rich library of pharmacological probes already available at the time that the opioid peptides were discovered. Just as there is more than one receptor for norepinephrine, there seems to be more than one receptor for each peptide thus far studied. Binding assays should prove especially useful to pharmacologists for screening large numbers of peptide derivatives to detect agonist or antagonist activity. The proof, however, that a peptide derivative is biologically important still depends on bioassays, and more time needs to be spent in developing fast, reliable, and specific assays for the central actions of peptides. Indeed, the central actions of some of the agents reported to be present in the brain remain to be uncovered.

Many of the chapters in this volume are intended to provide background data and strategies for studies of peptides in the central nervous system. In this regard, if peptides are administered peripherally, special attention must be paid to answering the following questions: Can the effects observed be peripheral in origin? Does the peptide escape being degraded for a reasonable period of time and does it enter the brain in significant amounts?

6.6 Metabolism of Peptides

Although it is possible to predict some of the features of enzymes involved in processing peptide precursors, it is harder to establish criteria for identifying the enzymes responsible for terminating the action of peptides. If one assumes that the metabolizing enzymes function in a similar manner to acetylcholinesterase, then they might have the following properties:

1. They should reside near the pre- or post-synaptic peptide receptors, and should probably be membrane bound.

2 Since they should degrade peptides released into the synaptic space, they should be active at near neutral pH.

3. Since many neuropeptides have blocked (i.e., derivatized) N- and C-termini [see the structures of LHRH and thyrotropin releasing hormone (TRH) for example], they should be, and indeed seem to be, metabolized by endopeptidases.

4. It is not yet clear whether there is one specific peptidase to degrade each peptide or whether several peptides can be degraded by single peptidases. Nor is it clear that all the peptidases belong to a class of structurally and functionally similar enzymes. These questions are especially important to pharmacologists; the more different the peptidases are, the more likely it is that inhibitors will be found that act specifically on one or another of them.

7 OVERVIEW

The composition of this book reflects the rapid growth of interest in brain peptides. Our hope is to provide a thorough but not overly specialized volume summing up the current state of the art in this field as of the time of writing, and to provide a critical assessment of the data accumulated to date. It is also our hope, and that of the other contributors, that we have conveyed some of the excitement that discoveries in this field have generated with regard to the existence of such peptides, their distribution, function, and the insights they have provided into developmental biology and evolution.

REFERENCES

1. W. E. Dixon, *Med. Mag. (London)* **16**, 454 (1907).
2. T. R. Elliott, *J. Physiol. (London)* **32**, 401 (1905).
3. O. Loewi, *Arch Ges. Physiol.* **189**, 239 (1921).
4. E. Scharrer and B. Scharrer, *Res. Publ. Assoc. Res. Nerv. Mental Dis.* **20**, 170 (1940).
5. C. G. Speidel, *Carnegie Inst. Wash. Publ.* **13**, 1 (1919).
6. S. L. Palay, *J. Comp. Neurol.* **82**, 129 (1945).
7. W. Bargmann, *Endeavor* **19**, 125 (1945).
8. V. duVigneaud, *Harvey Lectures* **40**, 1 (1956).
9. D. B. Carlisle and F. G. W. Knowles, *Endocrine Control in Crustaceans*, Cambridge University Press (1959).
10. U. S. vonEuler and J. H. Gaddum, *J. Physiol. (London)* **72**, 74 (1931).

11.   M. M. Chang, S. E. Leeman, and H. D. Niall, *Nature* **232**, 86 (1971).
12.   R. O. Studer, H. Trzeciak, and W. Lergier, *Helv. Chim. Acta* **56**, 860 (1973).
13.   V. Erspamer, *Trends Neurosci.* **4**, 267 (1973).
14.   S. Nakanishi, A. Inoue, T. Kita, M. Nakamura, A. C. Y. Chang, S. N. Cohen, and S. Numa, *Nature* **278**, 423 (1979).
15.   M. Comb, P. H. Seeburg, J. Adelman, L. Eiden, and E. Herbert, *Nature* **295**, 663, (1982).
16.   Y. Morimoto, T. Hirose, M. Asai, S. Inayama, S. Nakanishi, and S. Numa, *Nature* **298**, 245 (1982).
17.   S. G. Amara, V. Jonas, M. G. Rosenfeld, E. S. Ong, and R. M. Evans, *Nature* **298**, 240 (1982).
18.   K. Tatemoto, M. Carlquist, and V. Mutt, *Nature* **296**, 659 (1982).

PART

1

Cell Biology, Evolutionary, and Embryological Aspects of Peptide Hormones

2

Peptide Hormone Genes: Structure and Evolution

WALTER L. MILLER

JOHN D. BAXTER

NORMAN L. EBERHARDT

Departments of Pediatrics, Medicine, and Biochemistry and Biophysics
Howard Hughes Medical Institute Laboratories
and the Metabolic Research Unit
University of California, San Francisco

1 INTRODUCTION

Remarkable progress has been achieved in the field of molecular biology, largely due to advances in recombinant DNA technology. These techniques permit the isolation, purification (cloning), and determination of the precise structures (nucleotide sequences) of both the genes and the messenger RNAs (mRNAs), which direct the synthesis of proteins. Several polypeptide hormone genes have been cloned in bacteria and their nucleotide sequences have been determined. This information has greatly advanced our understanding of the mechanisms and patterns of gene evolution and regulation. In this chapter we review recently accumulated knowledge and theories germane to the evolution of hormone genes.

1.1 Polypeptide Hormone Synthesis and Secretion

A polypeptide hormone is often the product of a single gene and may be synthesized as an intact hormone such as growth hormone (GH) or prolactin (Prl) or as a prohormone such as proinsulin, proparathyroid hormone (pro-PTH), pro-opiomelanocortin (POMC), and procalcitonin. In the latter case the prohormone is converted by posttranslational modification to the intact hormone. In the case of insulin and relaxin, this modification includes the covalent linkage of the A and B chains by disulfide bridges and the proteolytic excision of the connecting C peptide. The processing of ACTH requires the proteolytic cleavage of pro-opiomelanocortin, which is also the precursor of β-endorphin and α- and β-melanocyte-stimulating hormone (MSH). In some cases the hormones may be glycosylated before secretion; examples are thyroid stimulating hormone (TSH), luteinizing hormone (LH), chorionic gonadotropin (CG), and follicle stimulating hormone (FSH). In addition, these hormones consist of two subunits (encoded by different genes) that associate with each other after their synthesis.

In all cases the polypeptide hormones or prohormones, like other secreted proteins (for reviews, see refs. 1 and 2), are synthesized as larger precursor forms (prehormones) by direct translation of the mRNA. The prehormone contains an NH_2-terminal signal peptide sequence that functions in the transfer of the protein from polyribosomes on the rough endoplasmic reticulum (RER) into the RER itself. The signal peptide is subsequently cleaved by a specific protease (signal peptidase) concomitant with vesiculation of the hormone or prohormone within the RER, which occurs before further processing and secretion.

1.2   Application of Recombinant DNA Techniques to the Study of Hormone Structure and Evolution

Recombinant DNA technology permits the detailed examination of polypeptide hormone gene structure. Some of the basic methods summarized below are reviewed elsewhere (3–5). DNA fragments containing polypeptide hormone gene sequences linked to "vector" DNA can be replicated in bacteria or mammalian cells and in this way are amplified so that they can be obtained in sufficient quantities for nucleotide sequence analysis and other uses.

Small, naturally occurring DNA molecules are used as vectors to introduce recombinant DNA molecules into a cell. Most recombinant experiments use *Escherichia coli* or other bacteria as hosts; hence, two types of vectors are available: plasmids and bacteriophages (6). Plasmids are small, circular DNA molecules that replicate independently of the host cell DNA. They are familiar to clinicians as resistance-transfer factors, often conveying resistance to antibiotics not previously encountered by the bacteria. The ability of plasmids to confer antibiotic resistance to their host is useful for DNA cloning, since this provides a selection mechanism for obtaining the desired clones. Free plasmids may be assimilated from the surrounding medium, or certain plasmids containing sexual factors may be actively transferred between bacteria by conjugation. Bacteriophages, or phages, are bacterial viruses that consist of DNA and a surrounding protein coat. The bacteriophages infect certain bacteria and utilize the host cell's metabolism for replication. The phage DNA is copied and enveloped in new phage protein, which is specified by genes contained in the phage DNA. In many cases phage replications cause the lysis and death of the bacterium. When such a vector containing foreign DNA sequences replicates in a host cell, the host synthesizes many identical copies of it; hence this process is referred to as the "cloning" of DNA.

The introduction of DNA into a vector in a specific manner was made possible by the discovery of enzymes called restriction endonucleases (for a review, see ref. 7). These enzymes cleave DNA at specific sequences of nucleotides which are generally four to six base pairs long. Each enzyme is absolutely specific for the sequence of nucleotides it recognizes; hence, the resulting pieces of DNA, often termed "restriction fragments," are precisely defined and can be generated reproducibly. Many of these enzymes make symmetrical but staggered cuts in the DNA (Figure 1) and produce short single-stranded regions of DNA at the end of the restriction fragment. Since the hydrogen bond base pairing of the individual nucleotides is highly specific—adenosine (A) binds to thymidine (T) or uridine (U), and guanosine (G) binds to cytosine (C)—such single-stranded regions will hybridize only to single-

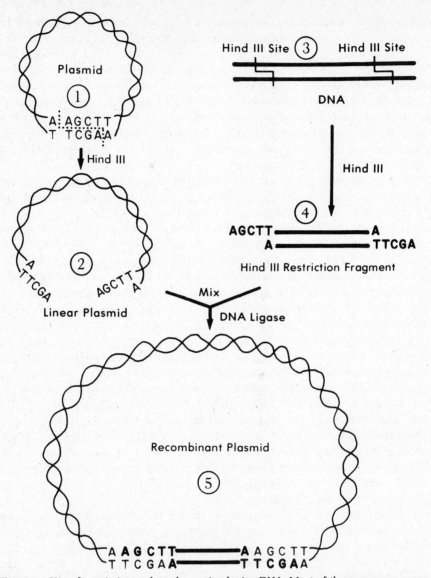

Figure 1. Use of restriction endonucleases in cloning DNA. Most of these enzymes recognize 4 to 6 bases of DNA, which form the same sequence when read in either direction; such sequences are often called palindromes. The experiment shown uses the enzyme Hind III, which recognizes and cuts DNA of the sequence

$$5' \ldots \text{AAGCTT} \ldots 3' \; 3' \ldots \text{TTCGAA} \ldots 5'$$

Note that the sequence of bases on the two strands is identical when read in the 5' to 3' direction. A plasmid (cloning vehicle) is selected that has only a single site recognized by Hind III (1). This enzyme cuts between the two A residues on each strand, as shown by the dotted line (1). Cutting the plasmid with Hind III will result in a single piece of DNA, a linear plasmid. Each end of the plasmid will have identical single-stranded projections of DNA having the sequence 3' . . . TCGA 5' remaining from the digestion with Hind III stranded ends of other DNA fragments containing "complementary" nucleotides, and hence they are often identified as "sticky ends." This permits the planned assembly of pieces of DNA like the assembly of the uniquely interlocking pieces of a jigsaw puzzle.

1.2.1 Complementary DNA Cloning

Complementary DNA (cDNA) is obtained by copying mRNA into DNA with the enzyme called reverse transcriptase, found in RNA tumor viruses (8, 9), and then copying the single-stranded cDNA into a double-stranded form with the use of DNA polymerase (Figure 2). In order to clone this double-stranded cDNA, sticky ends must be created so that the cDNA may be inserted into a plasmid, as shown in Figure 1. The most widely used procedure for adding sticky ends to double-stranded cDNA is called tailing (10; Figure 3). This technique is usually applied with the plasmid called pBR322, which has been designed and built for recombinant DNA experiments (11). Only a single site in this plasmid is recognized by the restriction endonuclease Pst I, which cleaves between the fifth and sixth bases of the sequence 5'-CTGCAG-3'.* By cutting pBR322 with this enzyme and adding a tail of deoxyguanosine residues, the recognition site for the endonuclease Pst I is preserved, permitting the cloned cDNA to be recovered from the plasmid.

Since cDNA is a copy of mRNA, cDNA contains sequences corresponding to the gene's coding sequences but does not contain DNA corresponding to intervening sequences or flanking regions (discussed below). This is more informative than amino acid sequence data because it includes the structure of the leader peptide and untranslated regions of the mRNAs. The codons of the mRNA then indicate the primary structure of the protein. The genetic code is redundant, that is, all but two of the amino acids may be encoded by more than one triplet of nucleotides (codons). Thus, whereas knowledge of the codons provides an unambiguous assessment of the primary amino acid sequence of the protein, the amino acid sequence does not provide an unambiguous assignment of the mRNA nucleotide sequence.

---

*The designations 5' and 3' refer to the positions on the sugar to which the phosphate groups are linked and thus indicate the orientation of the fragment.

---

(2). These single-stranded projections are "sticky ends." If other DNA is also cut with Hind III (3), it will also have sticky ends identical to those of the linear plasmid (4). When the linear plasmid and restriction fragment are mixed under proper conditions, the sticky ends of the plasmid and of the restriction fragment hybridize by hydrogen-bond base pairing, so that the restriction fragment and plasmid combine to form a recombinant plasmid (5). The recombinant plasmid now has two Hind III sites; the nucleotides in each site that came from the restriction fragment are shown in heavier print. The process is completed by recreating the broken phosphodiester bonds with DNA ligase.

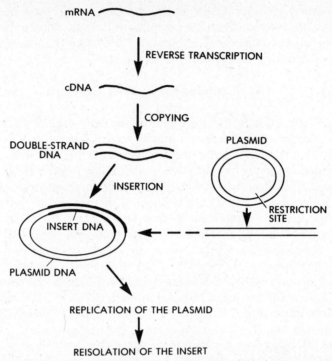

Figure 2. Synthesis and cloning of complementary DNA (cDNA). Messenger RNA is copied into cDNA with the enzyme reverse transcriptase. The heteroduplex of mRNA and
cDNA is digested with alkali, leaving single-stranded cDNA. The single-stranded material
is copied with either reverse transcriptase or DNA polymerase I to yield double-stranded
cDNA. The double-stranded cDNA is then inserted into a plasmid that has been
previously linearized by cleavage with a restriction endonuclease. The insertion is generally done as shown in Figures 1 or 3. The recombinant plasmid with its inserted DNA is
then used to transform (infect) bacteria, which replicate the plasmid. In this fashion an
unlimited number of copies of a single DNA molecule can be produced, hence the molecule is said to be "cloned." Plasmid DNA may then be prepared from a clonal strain of
bacteria and the cloned cDNA insert may be isolated.

1.2.2 Genomic DNA Cloning

Genomic DNA refers to the nucleotides of the genes as they exist in the
chromosome. The principles of genomic DNA cloning are analogous to
those described for cDNA cloning. However, since the relative amounts
of DNA to be cloned are generally greater, different vectors have been
developed. The most common vectors are derivatives of bacteriophages,
which can accommodate DNA fragments up to 20,000 bases (20
kilobases, kb) in length (12, 13). More recently, cosmid vectors, which
are hybrids of bacteriophages and plasmids, have been developed (14).

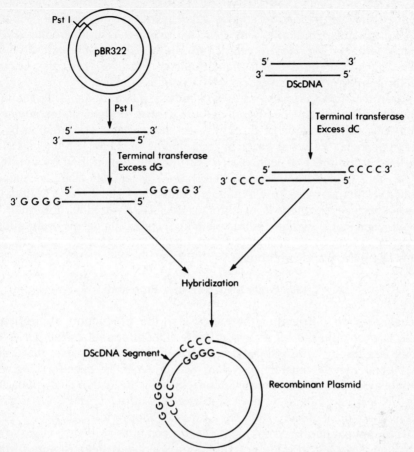

Figure 3. Cloning of cDNA by tailing. A bacterial plasmid such as pBR322 is cleaved with a restriction endonuclease such as Pst I. Since there is only one Pst I site in pBR322, the cleavage results in a linear plasmid having short, single-stranded 3' ends as a result of the cleavage. A polymeric chain ("tail") of deoxyguanosine residues is added to these 3' ends by terminal transferase, an enzyme that extends single-stranded 3' ends. Deoxycytosine residues are added to linear double-stranded cDNA (DScDNA) in the same manner. The tailed cDNA and tailed plasmid are mixed, and the 3' ends of poly(G) and poly(C) hybridize by base pairing, forming a stable, circular, recombinant plasmid. In practice, the tails of dC and dG are 15 to 30 nucleotides in length, forming very stable hybrids that do not need to be sealed by DNA ligase (as in Figure 1).

The average length of DNA successfully cloned in cosmid vectors is about 35 kb.

The most common strategy for genomic cloning is to generate random fragments of total, unsheared DNA that have the appropriate size for the particular cloning vector. Usually this is accomplished by limited digestion of the DNA with one or two restriction endonucleases that cleave the DNA frequently and by subsequent size fractionation of the DNA on sucrose gradients. This DNA is then ligated to the vector DNA, which contains appropriate restriction sites. This recombinant DNA is then "packaged" into viable bacteriophage particles with the use of bacteriophage proteins so that bacteria can be infected.

Cosmids can be propagated as plasmids or bacteriophages. In the latter case, recombinant bacteriophage are grown on agar plates covered with susceptible strains of *E. coli*; when the bacteria are infected by a phage particle, the lysed bacteria form visible plaques. The phage DNA containing the piece of human DNA of interest is identified by hybridization to a cloned cDNA probe. "Libraries" of genomic DNA fragments cloned in this way are now available for human beings and a variety of other species. An analysis of chromosomal DNA provides information about gene copy number, chromosomal localization, gene orientation, and the existence of associated structures that may be important for their expression and evolution.

1.3   Gene Structure and Function

Genes provide information necessary for the production of proteins. This is accomplished by a flow of molecular information from DNA to RNA and finally to protein. According to the simplest tenets, three deoxyribonucleotides specify a codon, whose sequence specifies a given amino acid. The DNA is transcribed, yielding RNA complementary to the DNA from which it was synthesized (pre-mRNA). The RNA is processed and subsequently translated into the appropriate protein.

The application of recombinant DNA techniques to higher eukaryotic organisms has led to a more detailed knowledge of the structure of the eukaryotic gene. From analyses of a relatively larger number of genes, a significant number of nearly universal features have emerged. A gene may be functionally divided into three basic parts: a 5'-flanking region, the structure transcribed into pre-mRNA, and a 3'-flanking region (Figure 4). The structure that is transcribed into pre-mRNA contains, in the order in which it is transcribed, a 5' untranslated portion of the mRNA, the codons of the protein, and the 3' untranslated portion of the mRNA. These structures can be interrupted by intervening sequences whose RNA transcripts are removed in the processing of the pre-mRNA. Each of these basic structures is described below.

1.3.1   Introns and Exons

One of the most remarkable discoveries afforded by recombinant DNA technology was the finding that higher eukaryotic gene structure is considerably more complex than previously envisioned. For most eukaryotic genes, including all of the polypeptide hormone genes studied to date,

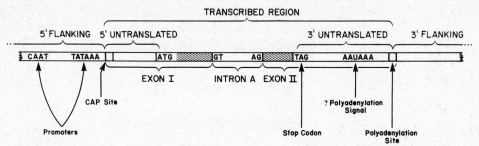

Figure 4. Schematic representation of the structure of a eukaryotic gene. The putative promoter structure, containing CAAT (or CATAAA) and TATAAA sequences, and the putative polyadenylation signal, AATAAA, are shown in the 5'-flanking region and the 3' untranslated region, respectively. The transcription initiation site (CAP) and stop site (polyadenylation site) are designated. Introns generally interrupt the coding sequences of most eukaryotic genes; the intron splice signals GT and AG are designated. Hatched regions refer to coding sequences of the gene, which are translated. Details are discussed in the text.

the nucleotide sequences that encode the mature mRNA, called exons, are interrupted by intervening, noncoding nucleotide sequences, called introns (for reviews, see 15–17). The introns are initially transcribed in a colinear fashion along with the exons, resulting in the synthesis of heterogenous nuclear RNA (hnRNA) or pre-mRNA (Figure 5). The RNA regions corresponding to the introns are subsequently excised and the ends of the RNA pieces corresponding to the exons are ligated together. Polyadenylation at the 3' end and modification of the 5' end of this RNA results in a mature mRNA that serves as a template for the synthesis of protein.

The function and significance of the intervening sequences has not been established; however, it has been proposed that introns may divide the exonic gene regions into functional domains. Subsequent shuffling of these domains during evolution may account in part for the very rapid evolution and diversification of higher eukaryotes (15). These concepts are discussed in more detail below (Section 1.4). The existence of introns and consequent mRNA processing also affords the possibility of forming multiple gene products from a single gene by alternate processing pathways. Specific examples are discussed below in the case of growth hormone and calcitonin.

The sequences at the junction of introns and exons (splice sites) have been found to be remarkably constant, suggesting a common splicing mechanism for all eukaryotic pre-mRNAs (18, 19). The consensus sequences for the 5'-splice "donor" and the 3'-splice "acceptor" are: AG| GT(A/G)AG and (T/C)X(T/C)(T/C)(T/C)XCAG|, respectively (18). In the notation, the symbols (T/C) and (A/G) designate that (T or C) or (A or G) occurs at the position, the X represents any nucleotide, and the splice occurs at the vertical lines. The predominant occurrence of GT

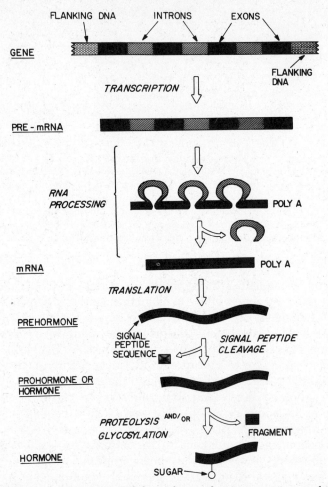

Figure 5. Schematic representation of the pathway of gene expression resulting in poly-peptide hormone synthesis. The gene is transcribed, producing a pre-mRNA containing intron DNA sequences. RNA processing of this pre-mRNA includes the removal of introns and the addition of a poly(A) tail, resulting in a mature mRNA. The mRNA is translated on polyribosomes; the signal sequence is involved in translocation of the newly synthe-sized polypeptide into the endoplasmic reticulum. Subsequent posttranslational process-ing, which may include proteolysis and/or glycosylation steps, results in the mature hormone.

after the 5′-splice site and AG before the 3′-splice site has led to the general rule that each intron begins with the dinucleotide GT and ends with the dinucleotide AG. This is often referred to as the GT-AG pair. The exact mechanism of the splicing reaction is not known. In many in-stances these processing reactions are required to produce translatable cytoplasmic mRNAs (20). These studies have suggested that mRNA processing may be associated with the transport of a functional mRNA into the cytoplasm. Evidence has also accumulated that small ribonucleoprotein particles (snRNPs) containing the small nuclear U1 RNA may be involved in processing hnRNA (21–25). Thus splicing of adenoviral early RNA sequences is inhibited by antibodies from lupus erythymatosus patients that react with snRNPs (24). In addition, the intron 5'- and 3'- splice junctions share nucleotide sequence complementarity with U1 RNA (22, 23, 25). The enzymes involved in splicing pre-tRNA have been localized to the nucleus (26); however, the detailed mechanisms involved in hnRNA processing remain to be elucidated.

The division of the polypeptide coding regions by introns is unique to eukaryotic genes. In prokaryotes the structure of the genes, transcribed mRNAs, and encoded proteins are colinear. The presence of introns in eukaryotic DNA accounts in part for the greater DNA content in eukaryotes. In addition, prokaryotic genes are often concatenated, forming a closely linked gene family the transcription of which is often regulated by a single operon, whereas eukaryotic genes are usually regulated individually and are often separated from one another by several thousand bases. These two factors probably account for the fact that eukaryotes possess 100 times as much DNA as prokaryotes, although they contain only about 10 times as many genes. The compact organization of prokaryotic genes may also account for their evolutionary rigidity relative to eukaryotes.

1.3.2   5' and 3' Untranslated Regions

The mature messenger RNA is flanked on the 5' and 3' ends by regions of RNA that are not translated into protein (Figure 4). These regions may contain structures that are involved in the initiation and regulation of translation as well as signals for the final processing of the mRNA itself.

The 5' terminus of the mRNA contains a 5'-5'-pyrophosphate linkage to one, two, or three nucleotides that are methylated to varying degrees (27–29). This structure is referred to as the CAP, and the nucleotide immediately adjacent to the CAP structure defines the transcription initiation site. The exact function of the CAP is unknown; however, such structures may serve to prevent mRNA degradation or provide a recognition signal for ribosome binding, or they may function in the transport of the mRNA into the cytoplasm. Evidence indicates that the CAP is more important for ribosome binding (30–32). Eukaryotic mRNAs also contain structures in the 5' untranslated region that are analogous to the Shine-Dalgarno sequence in prokaryotes (33; for a review see ref. 34). This latter sequence is complementary to a part of the 3'-terminal sequence of prokaryotic 16S rRNA, providing a mechanism for the base pairing observed between the mRNA and rRNA (35). These complemen-

065229

tary structures may promote binding of the mRNA to ribosomes in addition to the binding provided by the CAP structures.

The function of the 3' untranslated region is less well defined than
that of the 5' untranslated region. Most eukaryotic mRNAs are terminated by a sequence of polyadenylic acid, called poly(A), that is added after transcription and before translocation of the mRNA to the
cytoplasm. This polyadenylation appears to be associated with transport of the mRNA from the nucleus; however, this cannot be a universal
obligatory function since some mRNAs lack poly(A). Alternatively,
polyadenylation may also provide increased stability to the mRNA or
may function in the attachment of mRNA to membranes. A large number of eukaryotic mRNAs contain the sequence AAUAAA just "upstream" from the polyadenylation site (36, 36a). This sequence may
function as a polyadenylation recognition signal; however, definitive
data regarding this function are lacking. Several genes also contain sequences related to the sequence UUUCACUGC, which is also located
upstream from the polyadenylation site (37). The function of this sequence is currently unknown.

1.3.3   5'-Flanking and 3'-Flanking Regions

The DNA regions which lie proximal to the 5' and 3' untranslated regions and which are not transcribed are referred to as the 5'-flanking
and 3'-flanking regions, respectively (Figure 4). The function, if any, of
the 3'-flanking region is at present completely unknown, nor is it known
whether this structure contains information relevant to the expression
or regulation of gene expression. Some information is available concerning the 5'-flanking region. This region contains a structure (promoter) that is required for the efficient initiation of transcription, and it
probably contains information required for the regulation of gene transcription by hormones and other effector molecules. Information relevant to the tissue-specific expression of particular genes may also
reside in this region.

The structure of the promoter for genes that direct protein synthesis
is just beginning to be understood. The structure TATAAA (the Gold-
berg-Hogness box), or a somewhat similar sequence, is located 31 ± 2
nucleotides upstream from the transcription initiation site (38). This
structure appears to be important for specifying the location of the start
of transcription, although its presence does not appear to improve the
overall extent of initiation. Other upstream structures are also important for this function. Some (but not all) eukaryotic genes contain a
sequence related to GG(C/T)CAATCT, located approximately 40 nucleotides upstream from the TATAAA sequence (37). The function of this
sequence is unknown. In addition, some eukaryotic promoters have regions of dyad symmetry upstream from the transcription initiation site

(37, 39, 40). The function of these regions is not known; however, since these dyads form intrastrand complementary base pairs, these regions might form secondary structures important for transcription initiation or regulation.

The structures that may be involved in the hormonal regulation of transcription in eukaryotic genes have not been localized or defined at the present time. Evidence from gene transfer experiments suggests that such structures do exist on the 5'-flanking regions of hormone-responsive genes (41–45). The structures responsible for glucocorticoid regulation of the human growth hormone gene may reside on a fragment of DNA extending approximately 500 base 5' pairs to the CAP site (45). At present there is no information about any DNA structures involved in the tissue-specific regulation of gene expression.

1.4 Molecular Evolution

Darwinian natural selection described slowly occurring, spontaneous phenotypic changes that made the organism either more or less "fit," leading to its "selection." The discovery of the genetic code led to speculation about the molecular basis of natural selection. In 1959, Ingram showed that a single amino acid change resulted in the significantly altered phenotype of persons with the disease sickle-cell anemia (46). It was quickly deduced that this amino acid change was caused by the change of a single base in the DNA, a "point mutation." Point mutations remained the dominant mechanisms envisioned for molecular evolution until very recently. Other mechanisms, such as unequal crossover, DNA transposition, and reverse transcription, are discussed below.

1.4.1 Mechanisms of Point Mutation

Point mutations are mutations that affect a single base pair in the DNA, either by adding, deleting, or changing the base. These may occur in several ways (47).

1. Base removal: When purines are destroyed by acid or heat, base removal is possible even under physiologic conditions. Alkylating agents (or other nucleophilic compounds) or ionizing radiation may chemically modify bases. Depurinated or modified bases may then be excised by enzymes. Intercalating agents such as acridine dyes can induce replication errors leading to either the omission or addition of a base.

2. Base addition: Intercalating agents may also lead to unequal crossover events that add (or delete) bases.

3. Base change: Deamination may spontaneously change cytosine to uracil or adenine to hypoxanthine (this may also be induced by

nitrous acid). Incorrect bases in structural genes may also result from mutations in DNA polymerases or enzymes involved in "proofreading" DNA. Ionizing radiation and alkylating agents may also cause changes that are not removed.

4. Other changes: Ultraviolet light may cause formation of thymidine dimers. A failure to excise and repair such dimers causes the disease xeroderma pigmentosa. DNA strand breaks may occur directly from radiation or chemical agents, or they may be due to base removal and incomplete repair. Failure to repair strand breaks may be involved in the etiology of Bloom's Syndrome, a heritable disorder characterized by chromosome breaks, sister chromatid exchanges, and malignancies. Psoralen, mitomycin C, and bifunctional alkylating agents may also cause DNA crosslinking.

This wealth of mechanisms that cause point mutations, all of which were proved by laboratory studies with bacteria, led to the evolutionary clock hypothesis. This hypothesis tacitly assumes that (i) *transitions* (changes of one purine to another or one pyrimidine to another) are as likely as *transversions* (a change of a purine to pyrimidine or vice versa); (ii) point mutations are the predominant mechanism of evolution; and (iii) the rate of fixation of mutations in the genomes of a population is constant in evolutionary time, that is, there are no cataclysmic events.

1.4.2   The Evolutionary Clock Hypothesis

Zuckerkandl and Pauling were the first to notice that proteins generally appear to evolve at a constant rate (48, 49). This was taken to indicate that mutations occur at a roughly constant rate, permitting the use of amino acid or nucleotide sequence homology data as an evolutionary clock. The classic way of comparing apparently related proteins is by aligning the amino acids and quantifying the number of amino acid differences. If mutations occur at an approximately constant rate in evolution, then the number of amino acids that are different in two related proteins will serve as an index of the elapsed evolutionary time since the genes for the two proteins diverged. Several procedures have been devised for comparing such amino acid homologies (50, 51). The most widely used system is the Unit Evolutionary Period (UEP), which directly incorporates the concept of the evolutionary clock. The Unit Evolutionary Period is simply the length of time (in millions of years) required for 1% of the amino acids to change in two related proteins. Some proteins appear to evolve more slowly than others. Comparison of amino acid homology data to paleontologically determined times of species divergence indicates that a 1% amino acid difference accumulates in the protein cytochrome c every 15 million years (hence its UEP is 15), whereas 400 million years are required for a 1% change in histone H4. Thus the evolutionary clock runs much faster for cytochrome c than for histones.

If the evolutionary date of divergence of two peptides can be calculated by comparing the amino acid sequences in various species, that is, if it is possible to generate an evolutionary clock, then it must be possible to calculate the time of evolutionary divergence of various species based on known amino acid sequences of common peptides of known UEP. In other words, the clock must apply to both the peptides and the species. Therefore, a valid evolutionary clock should be able to determine either the divergence pattern of the species (by comparing one gene or protein in several animals) or the divergence patterns of the genes (by comparing related genes or proteins in a single species).

1.4.3 Comparison of Sequences

To compare the nucleotide or amino acid sequences of related sequences, gaps must be introduced in some sequences to compensate for deletions and insertions so that homologous regions can be aligned. Inspection of related sequences usually identifies certain areas of homology but does not reveal where the required gaps in the various sequences should lie. Some investigators have introduced gaps with computer programs designed to maximize nucleotide sequence homologies (52–54). However, if evolutionary selective pressure acts primarily to choose favorable protein hormones rather than favorable nucleotide sequences, evolutionary drift in nonexpressed sites (i.e., those changes that do not result in amino acid differences) might induce a computer program to assign gaps too arbitrarily, without considering the impact of amino acid changes on protein configuration. Therefore, we introduce gaps in sequences by estimating the "acceptability" of possible amino acid pairings. To do this, we compare the relative frequency with which any given amino acid will replace a homologous amino acid in two related peptides. These relative frequencies have been determined empirically by the examination of 250 amino acid replacements in various proteins (55). These relative frequencies correlate closely with amino acid pair distances based on comparisons of amino acid volume and polarity (56). The details of our procedure have been published (57, 58). Using this procedure, our alignments of human growth hormone and prolactin and of rat growth hormone and prolactin result in an alignment of the sites where intervening sequences occur in the native genes, suggesting the alignments are consistent with the structures of the genes.

Although evolutionary clocks that run on point mutations can be very useful, they cannot be relied upon if mechanisms other than point mutation have played a major role in the evolution of a particular gene.

Among the other mechanisms of molecular evolution, the most important are gene duplication, unequal crossover events, and DNA transposition.

1.4.4 Gene Duplication

Gene duplication is a common phenomenon in eukaryotic genomes. Many related proteins are encoded by related genes that appear to have evolved from a single evolutionary ancestor gene following an event of gene duplication. The best-studied model of gene duplication concerns the globin genes. The α and β chains of hemoglobin are encoded by separate clusters of genes, located on chromosomes 16 and 11 respectively (59, 60). The α locus contains four nonallelic genes ($\xi 2$, $\xi 1$, $\alpha 2$, and $\alpha 1$). The β locus contains five functional genes (ϵ, $^G\gamma$, $^A\gamma$, δ and β) plus two pseudogenes. (Pseudogenes are stretches of DNA which are highly homologous to a functional gene, but which cannot themselves encode protein due to deleted or mutant regulatory regions, frame-shifts, etc.) All of these genes are structurally related, suggesting they arose through gene duplication. Gene duplications of this sort can become fixed in a population rapidly. For example, sarcoma cells exposed *in vitro* to methotrexate respond by duplicating the gene for dihydrofolate reductase, resulting in increased resistance to methotrexate. Given such a powerful selective pressure, the dihydrofolate reductase gene can be duplicated to 200 copies per cell in only a few hundred cell generations (61).

The means by which genes are duplicated are not yet known in molecular detail, but they certainly entail two well-established mechanisms. The first is the classic genetic process of unequal crossover events, and the second concerns transposable elements called transposons.

1.4.5 Unequal Crossovers

The crossover of sister chromatids, entailing the breaking and rejoining of genetic material, has been studied throughout this century, primarily in drosophila and yeast. It is now known that chromatid crossover entails the scission and ligation of the DNA in the sister chromatids in homologous regions. Unequal crossovers occur when regions of internal homology exist in one chromatid, permitting the choice of which of these regions might align with the sister chromatid. As a result of an unequal crossover, one chromatid will be left with less DNA while the other will have acquired more.

A considerable portion of the genomes of all eukaryotic organisms consists of DNA that is present in multiple copies. An extreme example of this is the so-called "satellite DNA," which in *Drosophila virilis* contains about 10 million copies of a repeated heptanucleotide sequence.

Such multicopy sequences were first identified by nucleic acid hybridization, which permitted fractionation of the genome into "highly repetitive" DNA, "middle-repetitive" DNA, and "unique-sequence" DNA (62). In the human genome, these three categories represent about 10, 25, and 65% of total DNA, respectively (63, 64). In general, genes encoding proteins are "unique" even though they may exist in several copies, in distinction to ribosomal RNA genes which exist in hundreds of copies and are in the "middle-repeat" class. Mathematical models (65) and computer simulations (66) indicate that random crossover events will lead to a high degree of repetitive periodicity in DNA sequences not maintained by selective pressures. Such models help to explain the presence in the genome of vast quantities of DNA that serve no known function. It has been proposed that such DNA poses no burden to the organism even though it serves no function, and hence it is termed "selfish DNA" (67, 68). In this view of molecular evolution, DNA does not exist solely to provide a selective advantage to the organism—rather, the organism is DNA's way of making more DNA.

Unequal crossover events also clearly affect genes encoding proteins. The abnormal hemoglobin Lepore (69) contains "hybrid" β chains in which the amino end of the protein is part of a δ chain while the carboxy end is part of a β chain. Hemoglobin Lepore is one of nine hemoglobinopathies caused by deletions of DNA ranging from 1 to 40 kb long (70). Thus, unequal crossover events are known to result in duplications of repetitive DNA and in deletions of gene segments bounded by homologous regions. Hence it is widely believed that the corollary to these genomic deletions is gene duplications, which probably are usually phenotypically silent and hence cannot be readily identified and studied.

In most known families of duplicated genes, such as immunoglobulin genes, β-globin genes, and growth hormone genes, the duplicated genes lie relatively close to one another on the same strand of DNA on the same chromosome. However, β globin genes on chromosome 11 (60) are clearly related to α globin genes on chromosome 16 (59) and growth hormone genes on chromosome 17 (71) are related to the prolactin gene on chromosome 6 (72). Hence duplicated gene families may extend beyond the immediately contiguous DNA to other chromosomes. Such interchromosomal exchanges of genetic material may occur either by unequal crossover between chromatids of different chromosomes or by direct DNA transposition.

1.4.6 DNA Transposition

The transposition of large pieces of DNA from one genetic locus to another may occur in at least three ways. First, genomic DNA may be incorporated into a retrovirus and transmitted to other individuals or species. Second, it may be mobilized within a genome as part of a transposon. Third, a messenger RNA molecule might be reverse-transcribed into DNA by viral enzymes and reinserted into the genome.

Retroviruses are RNA viruses that cause tumors in certain species. These viruses carry RNA copies of cancer-causing genes termed oncogenes. Oncogenes are themselves part of the normal genome of the organism serving as the viral host (73, 74). Retroviruses deficient in their oncogene will still infect the host and acquire the oncogene from the host (75). While such events are not proved to occur with other genes, the transportation of genetic elements from one animal to another by viral vectors is now a proven fact. Hence animal viruses may mediate the acquisition of new genetic information in a manner analogous to the prophage state of certain bacteriophages.

"Transposons," or transposable DNA elements, are sequences of DNA of defined lengths having the ability to become inserted into or deleted from other DNA. They may themselves contain intact genes or DNA regions that initiate or terminate transcription. Furthermore, they may induce deletion, inversion, or fusion of nearby DNA. Such elements have been found in bacteria, yeast, maize, and drosophila, and they probably exist in higher organisms as well (76). Transposons contain "insertion sequences" which are believed to encode small proteins responsible for linking nonhomologous DNA sequences together. Transposons themselves appear to have arisen as insertion sequences that now contain accompanying DNA. Such elements permit advantageous genes to proliferate in a population very rapidly, essentially as a form of Lamarckian inheritance where postnatally acquired characteristics may be passed on to progeny via the germ line. A relationship of transposons to retroviruses is suggested by the characteristic presence of short-terminal repeated sequences in each.

It has recently been suggested that a certain group of repetitive DNA sequences called the Alu family (because all contain the restriction endonuclease cleavage site recognized by the enzyme Alu I) are transposable DNA elements created by reverse transcription (77). Such a process would entail copying the DNA into RNA, which is then reverse-transcribed back into DNA and inserted elsewhere in the genome. Recent observations that certain genes appear to have lost intervening sequences with precisely the correct boundaries are consistent with this mechanism but do not prove it. Other genes, such as those encoding interferon, have no intervening sequences at all, again suggesting they might have arisen by reverse transcription.

1.4.7 Origins of Hormone Genes

Since large pieces of DNA may be exchanged so readily among organisms, we might ask if these genes arose spontaneously in higher eukaryotes or if they arose in lower organisms. The ultimate evolutionary origins of the polypeptide hormones have been a subject of increasing interest in recent years. Stimulated by the detection of molecules similar to human chorionic gonadotropin in bacteria (78, 79), recent studies have focused on the determination of other polypeptide hormones in unicellular organisms (for a review, see ref. 80). Table 1 summarizes the types of polypeptide hormones and the unicellular organisms in which similar substances have been identified. Insulin-like substances have been detected in three strains of *Escherichia coli*, two species of fungi, and a species of protozoa (81, 82). Materials similar to somatostatin, ACTH, and β-endorphin have been detected in protozoa (83, 84). The protozoan forms of both ACTH and β-endorphin can be detected immunologically on single, high-molecular-weight macromolecules, suggesting that these molecules are synthesized as a single precursor that is subsequently processed, as is the case in higher eukaryotes (Section 4). These findings suggest that structures similar to those contained within the polypeptide hormones existed in prokaryotes and other unicellular organisms. These could be the precursors to the polypeptide hormones; unfortunately nothing is yet known about the structures of the genes that encode such hormone-related peptides in these unicellular organisms.

In addition to the findings of polypeptide hormone-like effector substances in unicellular organisms, limited evidence suggests that receptors for these effectors are also present. For example, epinephrine stimulates adenylate cyclase in protozoa, an effect that is blocked by propanolol, the specific receptor antagonist (80, 85). In amoebas, opioid peptides and alkaloids alter feeding behavior, and this effect is inhibited by naloxone, the receptor antagonist (80, 86). Thus, unicellular organisms appear to contain effectors and receptors, the necessary components required to complete a hormonal communication system. Nevertheless, it has not been established that any of these effector–receptor systems actually has a biological function in a unicellular organism. The

TABLE 1   Hormone-like Substances Found in Unicellular Organisms

Hormone-like Substance	Source	References
ACTH	Protozoa	84
β-Endorphin	Protozoa	84
Insulin	Protozoa	81
	Fungi (2 species)	81
	E. coli (3 strains)	82
Arginine vasotocin	Protozoa	80
Cholecystokinin-pancreozymin	Protozoa	80
Glucagon	Protozoa	80
Calcitonin (salmon type)	Protozoa	80
Chorionic gonadotropin	Bacteria	78, 79
Somatostatin	Protozoa	83

finding that these hormone-like counterparts retain immunological and biological activity indicates that certain structural features have been conserved, thereby implying that selective pressure operates to preserve some important function. Taken together these data suggest that the progenitors of the endocrine effector–receptor systems originated in unicellular organisms, possibly prokaryotes. Further studies will be required to assess the significance of these findings.

Knowledge about the structure and behavior of the eukaryotic genome is expanding very rapidly. With the exception of point mutation, crossover, and gene duplication events, the mechanisms for altering the genome outlined here were unknown 10 years ago. As our knowledge of genetic rearrangement mechanisms expands, so will our knowledge of how genomes and organisms evolve and are selected. The information already available, however, clearly indicates that evolution need not always be a slow, gradual process. Large amounts of "alien" DNA can enter the genetic baggage of a species in an extremely short time. Hence molecular biology now tells us that evolution can move in quantum leaps as well as gradually.

2   THE GROWTH HORMONE FAMILY OF GENES

Prolactin (Prl), growth hormone (GH), and chorionic somatomammotropin (CS, placental lactogen) form a set of related polypeptide hormones that appear to have derived from a common evolutionary ancestor protein (87–90). They are related by function, immunochemistry, and structure. All are lactogenic and growth-promoting, they are all of similar size (190 to 199 amino acids among various species), and they all have similar protein structures. Each hormone has a single homologous tryptophan residue at about locus 85 (GH and CS) or 91 (Prl) and two homologous disulfide bonds. Each of the three hormones also contains four internal regions of homology that are themselves homologous among the three hormones. Based on these observations from the amino acid sequencing data available in 1971, Niall et al. postulated (90) that the three hormones had arisen by duplication of an ancestral hormone gene. Recombinant DNA technology now permits the detailed analysis of the gene sequences encoding these hormones, permitting reevaluation of this hypothesis from data describing the gene sequences themselves.

To examine the evolution of this related set of genes one can make two types of comparison: comparing the genes for a single hormone in several species, and comparing the genes for the three related hormones in a single species. At present, complete cDNA sequence data exist for bovine (91), human (92, 93), and rat (94) growth hormone (bGH, hGH, and rGH); bovine (57, 95), human (54), and rat (96, 97) prolactin (bPrl, hPrl, and rPrl); and human chorionic somatomammotropin (hCS) (98,

99). Comparison of cDNA sequences is useful for examining rates of nucleotide changes that cause one amino acid to be replaced by another (replacement mutations) and for examining nucleotide changes that cause no amino acid change (silent changes). A second useful procedure entails examining the structure and organization of the genes themselves. Cloned genomic DNA reveals information about gene size, arrangement, and origins, providing a macroscopic counterpoint that reveals earlier evolutionary events, in contrast with the detailed analysis generally done with cDNA.

2.1   Structure of the Cloned cDNAs

All but two of the amino acids may be encoded by more than one codon. Where redundancy exists in the genetic code, it is usually the identity of the third nucleotide in the codon that varies. Commonly there is a choice between A and T or C and G. A simple way of quantifying codon choice is simply to count the number of codons ending in G or C as opposed to those ending in A or T. Because of the specifics of the genetic code and the fact that certain amino acids are rarely used, random codon selection would result in 42% of codons ending in G or C. All of the growth hormone and prolactin genes, however, have a preference for codons ending in G or C, ranging from 50 to 82%. Codon choice does not appear to be a species-related phenomenon (57). All three GH mRNAs and hCS mRNA exhibit a strong preference for G and C (74–82%), and the three Prl mRNAs have a lesser preference (50–63%). Codon choice may be determined by the need to establish or prohibit the formation of secondary structures, but this is unproved (57).

The sequence of a cDNA may also reveal the structure of the untranslated portions of the mRNA. Upon examining the available sequences of the 5' untranslated regions of the seven cloned cDNAs in the growth hormone family (Figure 6; 54, 91–98), obvious homologies are not apparent except between hGH and hCS, where 26 of the distal 29 nucleotides are identical. Examination of the 3' untranslated regions is more rewarding. The three prolactin mRNAs appear to form a group different from the GH and CS mRNAs based on the structure of their 3' untranslated regions as well as on their codon choice (57). Hence, on the basis of codon use and the structures of the untranslated regions of the mRNAs, it appears that the prolactin and growth hormone constitute different groups and that hCS appears to be a variant of hGH.

2.2   Application of the "Evolutionary Clock"

To apply the evolutionary clock hypothesis to the GH/CS/Prl system, we first introduced gaps in the various sequences to align regions of obvious homology (57, 58). The alignments of the three growth hormone

5' UNTRANSLATED REGIONS

bGH: ACGGCUCAGGUGGUGCAGCUCACCACCU   AUG
              ** **   *   **

rGH: GUGGACAGAUCACUGAGUGGCG   AUG
              *   *   **

hGH: GGAUCCUGUGCACAGCUCACUAGCUUGCA   AUG
              ** **   * *

hCS: UCUUUGCCACACUUGCCUUGAUCCCUUGGUCCUUGGACAGCUCACCUAGUGGCA   AUG

bPrl: UFCUUCCUGAGCAGCCAUAGEAGAGAGCUUCCUGUGAACUGUUCUUCUGAAAUCAUCACCACC   AUG
              * *   *   *

rPrl: AGUGGUUCUCUCUUAGGACUUCUUGGGGAAGUGUGUCCCAGUGGUCAUCACC   AUG
                                              * *

hPrl: AAAC   AUG

3' UNTRANSLATED REGIONS

bGH: UUGCCAGCCAUCUGUUUGUUGCCC::CUCCCCCGUUGCCUUCCUUG:ACCCUGGAAGGUGCCACUCCCCACUG:::::UCCUUUCCUAAUAAAUGAGGAAAUUGCAUGCC
              * *****   * ** ** **   **********   *

rGH: GCACACCACUCGGUCUGCGGCA::CUCCCCCCGUUACCCCCCCUGUACUCUUG:CAACUGCCACCCCUACAC:::::::UUUGUCCUAAUAAAUGAUGAGCAUCAUCAUC
              *** *****   *   ** ** ** **   **********   *

hGH: CUGCCCCCGGCUGGCAUCCUUGGACCCUCUGACCCCCAGUCCCCCUCCUGGCCCUGGAAGUUGCCACUCCAGUGCCCACCAGCCUUGUCCUAAUAAAUUAAGUUGCAUC
              *   * ** ** **   **   **********   *

hCS: GUGCCCCGGAGUAGCCAUCCCUCCUCCCUCCCUGGCC
              *   * ** **

bPrl: GCCCACAUUCCAUCCUAUCCAUUCUGAGAUCCAUUCGUUCUUAAUGAUCCUCCGCAAACUCCUCGGCCUUUAACCUUAGAUCCUUUGUAUUACCUUAUUACCAUCGU
              *** ****   ***   ***   *

rPrl: GCCUACAUUCAUUCC:AUGUACAUCCGGAUCUUCUUAAAAGUCUAUUCUCAAAAGUCUAUUGCAUUGCAUUACAAACUUCAGCAUUCCAGCAUCUAAGA
              *** *****   *   ***   ** *

hPrl: GCCCACAUCCAUGUC:AUCUAUUUCUGAGAGAACGUUUCUUUGUAUUCAAGAUCGGUCCAUUCAAGCUCAUUGAUCGGUUUUGAAUCCCUUUGAAUCCAUCGU
              **** ****   **   ***   *

bPrl: :CGCCUCUAAUGGUUCAUCUU:::AAAUAAAAACAGACUCUGUAGGGAUGUCAAAAUCUpolyA
              ** * **** *** ****   ***** ***** ** **

hPrl: UGGGUGUAACAGGUCUCCUCUUAAAAAAUAAAAAUAGACUCGUAGACGACAUCpolyA

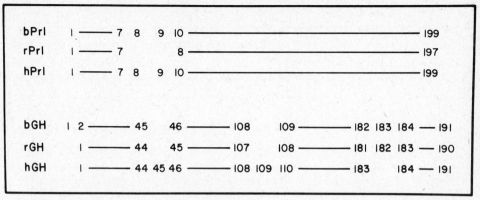

Figure 7. (Top) Alignment of the amino acid and nucleotide sequences of bovine, rat, and human prolactins. (Bottom) Alignment of bovine, rat, and human growth hormone sequences. Numbers refer to amino acid residues.

sequences and the three prolactin sequences are shown in Figure 7, and the paired alignments of the growth hormone and prolactin sequences from each species are shown in Figure 8. We then used these alignments to compare the amino acid sequences by the UEP method (51) and to compare the nucleotide sequences by three different procedures. Wilson et al. estimate the UEP values for prolactin and growth hormone as 5.0 and 4.0 respectively (51). We concur with the hypothesis that growth hormone and prolactin arose from a common evolutionary ancestor (87–90), and because comparisons between the two hormones are facilitated by identical UEP values, we use the value 4.5. This is also the value calculated for growth hormone and prolactin by Cooke et al. (54) using the procedure of Perler et al. (52).

We used both the amino acid and nucleotide comparisons to compare the evolution of the hormones and the evolution of the species. Comparison of the amino acid sequences of GH and Prl in cattle, rats, and humans gives consistent results. Using the alignments shown in Figures 9 and 10, we counted the number of amino acids that are identical

---

Figure 6. Known 5' and 3' untranslated regions of mRNA's related to growth hormone as revealed by cDNA sequencing. (Top) 5' untranslated regions of bovine, rat, and human GH, human CS, and bovine, rat, and human Prl. Nucleotides that are homologous among all established sequences are indicated by asterisks between the sequences. The AUG codon for the N-terminal methionine residue of each prehormone is shown for orientation. (Bottom) 3' untranslated regions of bovine, rat, and human GH; human CS; and bovine, rat, and human Prl. The UAG stop codons of the GH's and CS and the UAA stop codons of the Prl's are not shown. Gaps were introduced by inspection to align regions of obvious homology. Asterisks indicate bases that are homologous among all known sequences. The brackets enclose the palindromic regions and the overlining indicates the AAUAAA sequences of each mRNA.

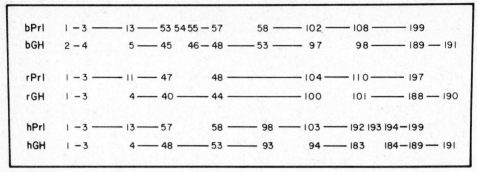

Figure 8. Alignment of prolactin and growth hormone sequences from (top) bovine, (middle) rat, and (bottom) human species. The locations of gaps were assigned by the procedure described previously (57, 58).

or replaced. The number of amino acids that are different between GH and Prl ranges from 79.6% in humans to 76.5% in cattle. Using a UEP figure of 4.5, the calculated divergence times are 344 to 357 million years ago (57). When the calculation is made comparing pre-GH to pre-Prl, similar values of about 350 million years are obtained. These calculations suggest that the gene duplication that led to the evolution of separate GH and Prl genes had to become fixed in a wide variety of species more than 350 million years ago. This is consistent with the observation that all vertebrates have both types of hormones in their pituitaries, and that amphibians diverged from fish about 400 million years ago. Although fish prolactin is obviously not engaged in the control of lactation, it is apparently involved in the maintenance of intracellular osmotic tonicity and control of salt and water flux across membranes, roles that may well be related to the secretion of a hyperosmolar fluid such as milk.

A similar comparison of the sequences of human GH and human CS indicates that the ancestral genes for these two modern hormones duplicated about 61 to 64 million years ago. Thus it would appear that GH and Prl diverged in distant evolutionary time, and that GH and CS diverged as the result of a much more recent gene duplication. The hGH and hCS genes indeed are closely linked (N. L. Eberhardt, unpublished results) on chromosome 17 (71), whereas the hPrl gene is on chromosome 6 (72), in good agreement with this hypothesis. But there is a problem with this simplistic analysis. The paleontological record is quite

Figure 9. Complete cDNA sequences of bovine, rat, and human growth hormone and human chorionic somatomammotropin. The sequences are aligned as diagrammed in Figure 7, with identical hGH and hCS alignments. Amino acids enclosed in boxes are identical in all four sequences.

```
                              -26        -20                                    -10
Bovine Growth Hormone    Met Met Ala Ala Gly Pro Ala Arg Thr Ser Leu Leu Leu Ala Phe Ala Leu Leu Cys Leu Pro Trp Thr
ACGGCUCAGGGUCCGUGACAGCCUCACCAGCU  AUG AUG GCU GCA GGC CCC AGG ACC UCC CUG CUC CUG GCU UUC GCC CUG CUC UGC CUG CCC UGG ACU

                              -26        -20                                    -10
Rat Growth Hormone       Met Ala Ala Asp Ser Gln Thr Pro Trp Leu Leu Thr Phe Ser Leu Leu Cys Leu Leu Trp Pro
GACAGAUCACUGAGUGGCG  AUG GCU GCA GAC UCU CAG ACC CCC UGG CUC CUC ACC UUC AGC CUG CUC UGC CUG CUC UGG CCU

                              -26        -20                                    -10
Human Growth Hormone     Met Ala Thr Gly Ser Arg Thr Ser Leu Leu Leu Ala Phe Gly Leu Leu Cys Leu Pro Trp Leu
GGAUCCUGUGGACAGCUCACCUAGUUGCA  AUG GCU ACA GGC UCC CGA ACG UCC CUG CUC CUG GCU UUU GGC CUG CUC UGC CUG CCU UGG CUU

                              -26        -20                                    -10
Human Chorionic Somatomammotropin   Met Ala Pro Gly Ser Arg Thr Ser Leu Leu Leu Ala Phe Ala Leu Leu Cys Leu Pro Trp Leu
CCCCUUGGGUCCUGUGGGACAGCUCACCUAGUGGCA  AUG GCU CCA GGC UCC CGG ACG UCC CUG CUC CUG GCU UUU GCC CUG CUC UGC CUG CCC UGG CUU
```

```
          1                            10                            20
tGH:  Gln Val Val Gly Ala Phe Pro Ala Met Ser Leu Ser Gly Leu Phe Ala Asn Ala Val Leu Arg Ala Gln His Leu His Gln Leu Ala Ala
      CAG GUG GUG GGC GCC UUC CCA GCC AUG UCC UUG UCC GGC CUG UUU GCC AAC GCU GUG CUC CGG GCU CAG CAC CUG CAC CAG CUG GCU GCU
          1                            10                            20
rGH:  Gln Glu Ala Gly Ala Leu Pro Ala Met Pro Leu Ser Ser Leu Phe Ala Asn Ala Val Leu Arg Ala Gln His Leu His Gln Leu Ala Ala
      CAA GAG GCG GGA GCU UUA CCU GCC AUG CCC UUG UCC AGU CUG UUU GCA AAU GCU GUG CUC CGA GCA CAG CAC CUG CAU CAG CUG GCU GCU
          1                            10                            20
hGH:  Gln Tyr Ser Phe Pro Phe Pro Thr Ile Pro Leu Ser Arg Leu Phe Asp Asn Ala Met Leu Arg Ala His Arg Leu His Gln Leu Ala Phe
      CAA UAU UCA GGA CCU UUC CCA ACC AUU CCA UUA UCC AGA CUU UUU GAC AAC GCU AUG CUC CGC GCC CAU CGU CUG CAU CAG CUG GCC UUU
          1                            10                            20
hCS:  Gln Ala Ala Gly Ala Val Gln Thr Val Pro Leu Ser Arg Leu Phe Asp His Ala Met Leu Gln Ala His Arg Ala His Gln Leu Ala Ile
      CAA GAG GCG GGU GCA GUC CAA ACC GUU CCG UUA UCC ACG CUU UUU GAC CAC GCU AUG CUC CAA GCU CAU CGU GCA CAC CAG CUG GCC AUU
```

```
          30                           40                              50
tGH:  Asp Thr Phe Lys Glu Phe Glu Arg Thr Tyr Ile Pro Glu Gly Gln Arg Tyr Ser Ile     Gln Asn Thr Gln Val Ala Phe Cys Phe Ser
      GAC ACC UUC AAA GAG UUU GAG CGU ACC UAC AUC CCG GAG GGA CAG AGA UAC UCC AUC :::  CAG AAC ACC CAG GUU GCC UUC UGC UUC UCC
          30                           40                              50
rGH:  Asp Thr Tyr Lys Glu Phe Glu Arg Ala Tyr Ile Pro Glu Gly Gln Arg Tyr Ser Ile     Gln Asn Ala Gln Ala Ala Phe Cys Phe Ser
      GAC ACC UAC AAA GAG UUU GAG CGU GCC UAC AUU CCC GAG GGA CAG AGA UAC UCC AUU :::  CAG AAU GCC CAG GCG GCG UUC UGC UUC UCA
          30                           40                              50
hGH:  Asp Thr Tyr Gln Glu Phe Glu Glu Ala Tyr Ile Pro Lys Glu Gln Lys Tyr Ser Phe Leu Gln Asn Pro Gln Thr Ser Leu Cys Phe Ser
      GAC ACC UAC CAG GAG UUU GAA GAA GCC UAU AUC CCA AAG GAA CAG AAG UAU UCA UUC CUG CAG AAC CCA CAG ACC UCU CUG UGC UUC UCA
          30                           40                              50
hCS:  Asp Thr Tyr Gln Glu Phe Glu Glu Thr Tyr Ile Pro Lys Asp Gln Lys Tyr Ser Phe Leu His Asp Ser Gln Thr Ser Phe Cys Phe Ser
      GAC ACC UAC CAG GAG UUU GAA GAA ACC UAU AUC CCA AAG GAC CAG AAG UAU UCG UUC CUG CAU GAC UCC CAG ACC UCC UUC UGC UUC UCA
```

```
          60                           70                           80
tGH:  Glu Thr Ile Pro Ala Pro Thr Gly Lys Asn Glu Ala Gln Gln Lys Ser Asp Leu Glu Leu Leu Arg Ile Ser Leu Leu Leu Ile Gln Ser
      GAA ACC AUC CCG GCC CCC ACG GGC AAG AAU GAG GCC CAG CAG AAA UCA GAC UUG GAG CUG CUU CGC AUC UCA CUG CUC CUC AUC CAG UCG
          60                           70                           80
rGH:  Glu Thr Ile Pro Ala Pro Thr Gly Lys Glu Glu Ala Gln Gln Arg Thr Asp Met Glu Leu Leu Arg Phe Ser Leu Leu Leu Ile Gln Ser
      GAG ACC AUC CCA GCC CCC ACC GGC AAG GAG GAA GCU CAG CAG AGA ACU GAC AUG GAA CUG CUU CGC UUC UCG CUG CUG CUC AUC CAG UCA
          60                           70                           80
hGH:  Glu Ser Ile Pro Thr Pro Ser Asn Arg Glu Glu Thr Gln Gln Lys Ser Asn Leu Glu Leu Leu Arg Ile Ser Leu Leu Leu Ile Gln Ser
      GAG UCU AUU CCG ACA CCC UCC AAC AGG GAG GAA ACA CAA CAG AAA UCC AAC CUA GAG CUG CUC CGC AUC UCC CUG CUG CUC AUC CAG UCG
          60                           70                           80
hCS:  Asp Ser Ile Pro Thr Pro Ser Asn Met Glu Glu Thr Gln Gln Lys Ser Asn Leu Glu Leu Leu Arg Ile Ser Leu Leu Leu Ile Glu Ser
      GAC UCU AUU CCU ACA CCC UCC AAC AUG GAG GAA ACG CAA CAG AAA UCC AAU CUA GAG CUG CUC CGC AUC UCC CUG CUG CUC AUC GAG UCG
```

```
          90                           100                          110
tGH:  Trp Leu Gly Pro Leu Gln Phe Leu Ser Arg Val Phe Thr Asn Ser Leu Val Phe Gly Thr Ser Asp Arg     Val Tyr Glu Lys Leu Lys
      UGG CUU GGG CCC CUG CAG UUU CUC AGC AGG GUC UUC ACC AAC AGC CUG GUU UUC GGC ACC UCG GAC AGG :::  GUC UAU GAG AAG CUG AAG
          90                           100                          110
rGH:  Trp Leu Gly Pro Val Gln Phe Leu Ser Arg Ile Phe Thr Asn Ser Leu Met Phe Gly Thr Ser Asp Arg     Val Tyr Glu Lys Leu Lys
      UGG CUG GGG CCU GUG CAG UUC CUC AGC AGG AUC UUU ACC AAC AGC CUG AUG UUU GGU ACC UCG GAC CGC :::  GUC UAU GAG AAA CUG AAG
          90                           100                          110
hGH:  Trp Leu Glu Pro Val Gln Phe Leu Arg Ser Val Phe Ala Asn Ser Leu Val Tyr Gly Ala Ser Asp Ser Asn Val Tyr Asp Leu Leu Lys
      UGG CUG GAG CCC GUG CAG UUC CUC AGG AGU GUC UUC GCC AAC AGC CUG GUG UAC GGC GCC UCU GAC AGC AAC GUC UAU GAC CUC CUA AAG
          90                           100                          110
hCS:  Trp Leu Glu Pro Val Arg Phe Leu Arg Ser Met Phe Ala Asn Asn Leu Val Tyr Asp Thr Ser Asp Ser Asp Asp Tyr His Leu Leu Lys
      UGG CUG GAG CCC GUG CGG UUC CUC AGG AGU AUG UUC GCC AAC AAC CUG GUG UAU GAC ACC UCG GAC AGC GAU GAC UAU CAC CUC CUA AAG
```

```
          120                          130                          140
tGH:  Asp Leu Glu Glu Gly Ile Leu Ala Leu Met Arg Glu Leu Glu Asp Gly Thr Pro Arg Ala Gly Gln Ile Leu Lys Gln Thr Tyr Asp Lys
      GAC CUG GAG GAA GGC AUC UUG GCC CUG AUG CGG GAG CUG GAA GAU GGC ACC CCC CGG GCU GGG CAG AUC CUC AAG CAG ACC UAU GAC AAA
          120                          130                          140
rGH:  Asp Leu Glu Glu Gly Ile Gln Ala Leu Met Gln Glu Leu Glu Asp Gly Ser Pro Arg Ile Gly Gln Ile Leu Lys Gln Thr Tyr Asp Lys
      GAC CUG GAG GAG GGC AUC CAG GCA CUG AUG CAG GAA CUG GAA GAU GGC AGC CCC CGU AUU GGG CAG AUC CUC AAG CAA ACA UAU GAC AAG
          120                          130                          140
hGH:  Asp Leu Glu Glu Gly Ile Gln Thr Leu Met Gly Arg Leu Glu Asp Gly Ser Pro Arg Thr Gly Gln Ile Phe Lys Gln Thr Tyr Ser Lys
      GAC CUA GAG GAA GGC AUC CAA ACG CUG AUG GGG AGG CUG GAA GAU GGC AGC CCC CGG ACU GGG CAG AUC UUC AAG CAG ACC UAC AGC AAG
          120                          130                          140
hCS:  Asp Leu Glu Glu Gly Ile Gln Thr Leu Met Gly Arg Leu Glu Asp Gly Ser Arg Arg Thr Gly Gln Ile Leu Lys Gln Thr Tyr Ser Lys
      GAC CUA GAG GAA GGC AUC CAA ACG CUG AUG GGG AGG CUG GAA GAU GGC AGC CGC CGG ACU GGG CAG AUC CUC AAG CAG ACC UAC AGC AAG
```

```
          150                          160                          170
tGH:  Phe Asp Thr Asn Met Arg Ser Asp Asp Ala Leu Leu Lys Asn Tyr Gly Leu Leu Ser Cys Phe Arg Lys Asp Leu His Lys Thr Glu Thr
      UUU GAC ACA AAC AUG CGC AGU GAU GAC GCA CUG CUC AAG AAC UAC GGU CUG CUC UCC UGC UUC CGG AAG GAC CUG CAU ACG GAG ACG
          150                          160                          170
rGH:  Phe Asp Ala Asn Met Arg Ser Asp Asp Ala Leu Leu Lys Asn Tyr Gly Leu Leu Ser Cys Phe Lys Lys Asp Leu His Lys Ala Glu Thr
      UUU GAC GCC AAC AUG CGC AGC GAU GAC GCU CUG CUC AAA AAC UAU GGG CUG CUC UCC UGC UUC AAG AAG GAC CUG CAU AAG GCA GAG ACC
          150                          160                          170
hGH:  Phe Asp Thr Asn Ser His Asn Asp Asp Ala Leu Leu Lys Asn Tyr Gly Leu Leu Tyr Cys Phe Arg Lys Asp Met Asp Lys Val Asp Thr
      UUC GAC ACC AAC UCA CAC AAC GAU GAC GCA CUA CUC AAG AAC UAC GGG CUG CUC UAC UGC UUC AGG AAG GAC AUG GAC AAG GUC GAC ACA
          150                          160                          170
hCS:  Phe Asp Thr Asn Ser His Asn His Asp Ala Leu Leu Lys Asn Tyr Gly Leu Leu Tyr Cys Phe Arg Lys Asp Met Asp Lys Val Glu Thr
      UUU GAC ACA AAC UCC CAC AAC CAU GAC GCA CUG CUC AAG AAC UAC GGG CUG CUC UAC UGC UUC AGG AAG GAC AUG GAC AAG GUG GAA ACA
```

```
          180                      190 191
tGH:  Tyr Leu Arg Val Met Lys Cys Arg Arg Phe Gly Glu Ala Ser Cys Ala Phe AM
      UAC CUG AGG GUC AUG AAG UGC CGC CGC UUC GGG GAG GCC AGC UGU GCC UUC UAG   UUGCCAGCCAUCUGUUGUUGGGCUCCCCGGGUGUGCCUUCCUUGACCCU
          180                      190
rGH:  Tyr Leu Arg Val Met Lys Cys Arg Arg Phe Ala Glu Ser Ser Cys Ala Phe AM
      UAC CUG AGG GUC AUG AAG UGC CGC CGC UUC GCC GAG AGC UCC UGC GCU UUC GCA   GCACACUGGGUGUCUGGCGCACUCCCCGGUUACCCCCUCGUGACU
          180                      190 191
hGH:  Phe Leu Arg Ile Val Gln Cys Arg     Ser Val Glu Gly Ser Cys Gly Phe AM
      UUC CUG CGC AUC GUG CAG UGC CGC :::  UCU GUG GAG GGC AGC UGU GGC UUC UAG   CUGCCCGGGUGGCAUCCCUGUGACCCCUCCCCAGUGCCUCUCCUGGCC
          180                      190 191
hCS:  Phe Leu Arg Met Val Gln Cys Arg     Ser Val Glu Gly Ser Cys Gly Phe AM
      UUC CUG CGC AUG GUG CAG UGC CGC :::  UCU GUG GAG GGC AGC UGU GGC UUC UAG   GUGCCCGAGUAGCAUCCCUGUGACCCCUCCCCAGUGCCUCUCCUGGCC
```

tGH: CCGAAGUGCCACCCCCACUGUCCCUUUCCUAAUAAAGGGAAAUUGCAUCGCpolyA

rGH: CUGGCCAACUGCCACCCCCACCCCCUACACUUUGUCCUAAUUAAAUUAAUUGAUGCAUCACAUCpolyA

hGH: CUGGAAGUUGCCACUCCAGUGCCCACCAGCCUUGUCCUAAUAAAUUAAUUAAAUUGCAUCpolyA

hCS: . . .

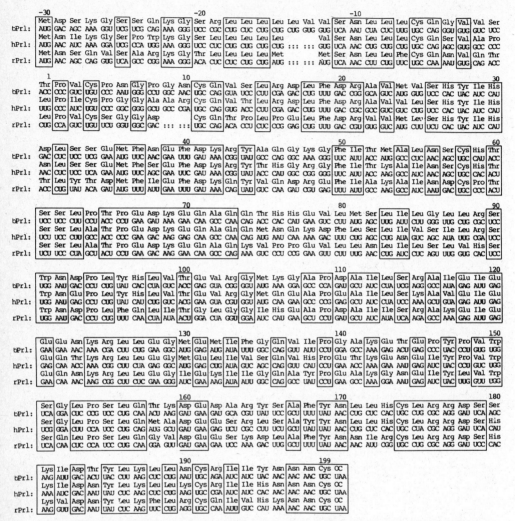

Figure 10. Complete cDNA sequences of bovine, human, and rat prolactin. The sequences are aligned as diagrammed in Figure 7. Amino acids enclosed in boxes are identical in all three sequences.

detailed and accurate for mammalian speciation, fixing the "mammalian radiation" at 85–100 million years ago. If the evolutionary precursors to various modern mammalian species diverged from one another about 85 million years ago and the GH and CS gene duplicated only 60 million years ago, then such a gene duplication would have to have occurred separately in each mammalian species, since all placental mammals appear to have a separate GH and CS. This seems highly unlikely.

Another way of using an evolutionary clock is to examine a single gene or protein in a variety of animals. This should tell us when the evolutionary precursors to the modern species diverged from each other, just as comparing related genes in one species tells us when the species diverged. If we compare the amino acid sequences of growth hormone from cattle, rats, and humans and apply the published UEP of 4.0 for GH (51) we determine that our evolutionary ancestors diverged from the ancestors of cattle and rats 140 million years ago and that the ancestors of cattle and rats diverged 65 million years ago (91). If we compare prolactin in the same three species, using a UEP of 4.5, we conclude that humans and cattle diverged from rats 170 million years ago and that humans and cattle subsequently diverged 120 million years ago (57). Although these figures can be changed slightly by using different UEP values or by including or excluding the leader peptides of these secreted hormones, the general pattern is always the same: The patterns of mammalian speciation revealed by the GH and Prl sequences are inconsistent with one another, and both are inconsistent with the fossil record (Figure 11). Thus two different types of inconsistencies are found when the evolutionary clock hypothesis is applied to the GH/CS/Prl system. First, the calculated time of the GH/CS duplication is unrealistically recent; second, the predicted patterns of mammalian speciation are inconsistent with the well-established fossil record.

It has been suggested that the use of nucleotide sequences for calculating and calibrating evolutionary clocks might be a more accurate and informative procedure for comparing related sequences than the use of amino acid sequences. The availability of nucleotide sequences of cloned cDNAs for GH and Prl from cattle, rats, and humans now permits us to test this hypothesis in the growth hormone/prolactin system. Efstratiadis and colleagues calculated the percent sequence divergence for nucleotide changes resulting in new amino acids (replacement

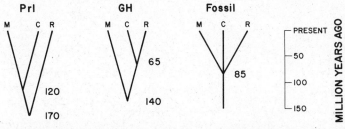

Figure 11. Evolutionary divergence diagrams for men (M), cattle (C), and rats (R), as calculated from a comparison of the amino acid sequences of prolactin (left) and growth hormone (center), assuming a unit evolutionary period of 4.5 (see text). Numbers refer to the millions of years since precursors to the modern species are calculated to have diverged. For comparison, the pattern of divergence determined by the fossil record is shown at right.

changes) and for nucleotide changes resulting in the same amino acid (silent changes) (52, 53). This system is based on the "selectionist" Darwinian theory of molecular evolution, which states that nucleotide replacements are "fixed" in the evolution of genes by positive environmental selection of the altered amino acid sequence (100–102–104). An alternative hypothesis, the "neutral" theory of molecular evolution, argues that most of the nucleotide changes and consequent amino acid substitutions that become fixed in evolution are selectively neutral, thus accounting for the many polymorphisms found among proteins with identical functions (103). Based on this hypothesis, Kimura devised two different ways to compare nucleotide sequences (104, 105). We have applied each of these three elaborate mathematical models to the nucleotide sequences for GH and Prl in the three species. The results shown in Figure 12 are striking: All three procedures give exactly the same patterns determined by the simpler amino acid comparisons.

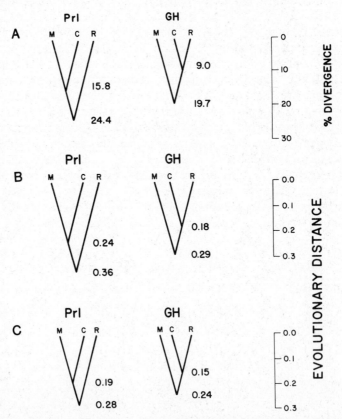

Figure 12. Evolutionary divergence diagrams for men (M), cattle (C), and rats (R) based on nucleotide sequence comparisons. (A) "Percent divergence" calculated according to Perler et al. (52); (B) "evolutionary distance" calculated according to the "three-substitution-type" model of Kimura (104); (C) "evolutionary distance" calculated according to the "two-frequency-class" model of Kimura (105).

2.3   Concerted Evolution

Since the evolution of the GH and Prl genes cannot be described by a simple model, we shall explore how the apparent inconsistencies might be resolved. The evolutionary clock is certainly a useful concept which has been successfully applied to several systems. The difficulty with the various ways of applying this concept is that all of the procedures described above deal with the probability of point mutations occurring and becoming fixed in a gene, and they assume that mutations occur and become fixed at a constant rate in evolutionary time. Although point mutation is a major mechanism of evolution, it is not the only one. DNA may be duplicated, rearranged, deleted, or appended, often in large chunks. When multiple nonallelic genes or pseudogenes exist for a particular peptide, the rate of evolutionary divergence can be slowed and the genes will exhibit the phenomenon of "concerted evolution" (106–109). Concerted evolution is said to occur when two or more genes appear to evolve in concert with each other rather than evolving independently and acquiring divergent sequences. The diagnostic hallmark of concerted evolution is that two different genes within the same genome (e.g., hGH and hCS) that have different functions are more similar to one another than are the genes having the same function in other, related species (e.g., hGH, rGH, and bGH). This phenomenon has been described previously for the families of genes encoding immunoglobulins, ribosomal RNA, and α globin (106–109).

The principal mechanism of concerted evolution appears to be unequal crossover events. Unequal crossovers first lead to polygenic states that subsequently permit the functional suppression of mutant genes while normal ones continue to be expressed. Subsequent unequal crossovers can again replace mutated genomic material with normal material. The net effect is a slowing of the rate at which the functioning gene evolves, because its duplicated neighbors can supply "spare parts" to replace mutant regions. Concerted evolution is favored by gene configurations that favor unequal crossovers, such as multiple nonallelic genes or long, homologous flanking regions or intervening sequences. Thus gene duplications increase the opportunities for concerted evolution, thereby slowing the rate of fixation of point mutations in the parental, wild-type gene, while a homolog of the gene may mutate rapidly without functional constraints. Such a gene may then acquire new properties that can confer selective advantage to the organism.

Human growth hormone and human chorionic somatomammotropin exhibit the hallmark of concerted evolution (107) in that the two peptides are more alike within the human species than is hGH with the growth hormone in various other species. Human GH and hCS have 80% amino acid and 92% nucleotide homology (92), whereas human and rat or bovine GH have 64–67% amino acid and 75–77% nucleotide homologies, respectively (91). The genes for hGH and hCS are closely

linked on chromosome 17 (71), and both genes exist in multiple copies
(N. Eberhardt, unpublished results). Furthermore, the mRNA for hCS
shares several features with the mRNAs for human, bovine, and rat GH:
(i) it has a high G and C content in codon third positions; (ii) it has a
UAG termination codon; (iii) its 3' untranslated region is homologous
with the 3' untranslated regions in the three growth hormone mRNAs;
(iv) it is more homologous with each of the three growth hormone
mRNAs than it is with human prolactin mRNA. These observations suggest that the human chorionic somatomammotropin gene is a duplicated, slightly variant growth hormone gene that has evolved by concerted
evolution.

Concerted evolution may not be so important in the evolution of prolactin genes. The human prolactin gene probably cannot interact with
growth hormone genes, being segregated on chromosome 6 (72), and it
appears to be a single-copy gene (J. Martial, personal communication).
Furthermore, there seems to be only one rat prolactin gene, but this
gene has much larger intervening sequences than do the growth hormone genes (96, 110). It is possible that the prolactin and growth hormone genes are evolving by several different mechanisms, and that the
dominant mechanism may differ between the two hormones and among
various species. These observations imply that the evolutionary analysis of related protein and gene sequences may be less straightforward
than one might initially expect.

2.4 Structure of Chromosomal Genes

In addition to the seven known cDNA structures (57, 91–99), the structures of the chromosomal genes for rat (111) and human (40) GH, rat Prl
(96, 110), and human CS (112; N. L. Eberhardt, unpublished results) are
now known. As discussed previously (Section 1.3), gene structure is
generally organized into three regions, the 5'-flanking region, the sequences that encode the pre-mRNA including the intervening sequences,
and the 3'-flanking region. Within the 5'-flanking regions, the sequences
surrounding the TATAAA box and the CATAAA box are higly homologous among the various GH and Prl genes, but other portions of the
5'-flanking regions show less homology. An additional feature of the
hGH gene is that it contains the region of dyad symmetry discussed
above, which has also been observed in other eukaryotic promoters,
such as human insulin and mouse α globulin (37, 39).

Although the expression of these genes is regulated by other hormones, no specific sequences relating to hormonal regulation have yet
been identified on the 5' ends of the genes. Nevertheless, evidence accumulated from experiments involving transfer of rGH and hGH genes
into mouse L-cells indicates that such regulatory sequences probably
exist on the 5' end of the rat and human GH gene but may lie relatively

far upstream from the promotor sequence. In general, the known homologies are confined to the first 120 nucleotides that immediately precede the genes. As shown in Figure 13, there is considerable homology in this region between the genes for rGH and hGH. By contrast, there is little significant homology between the genes for rGH and rPrl in the 5' flanking region. There is also extensive homology between the genes for hGH and hCS, which extend about 500 base pairs 5' from the CAP sites; as discussed above, this may be related to the close linkage of this family of genes on chromosome 17 and to the recent duplications that have occurred. This homology is particularly noteworthy in light of the fact that these genes are expressed in different tissues and this expression is differentially regulated by hormones. These data may imply that only a few nucleotide differences can have a marked influence on the actions of regulatory factors that direct differential gene expression.

The genes for GH, Prl, and CS are all interrupted by 4 introns (termed A, B, C, and D). The splice points in the rPrl and rGH genes have been preserved despite the fact that the rPrl introns are much larger than those of rGH and the two genes retain only 25% overall amino acid homology (110). The identical pattern of splice junctions is also observed for hGH and hCS (N. L. Eberhardt, unpublished results). The conservation of exon–intron boundaries in individual members of other gene families has been observed previously (53). The preservation of the splice sites in GH, CS, and Prl provides additional evidence that these three genes evolved from a common precursor and suggests that the common precursor possessed similar exon–intron boundaries.

The larger size of the rPrl introns indicates that there is no selective pressure to retain the size of these structures. Moreover, it has been observed that in general the rate of intron divergence is much more rapid than the rate of exon divergence. This suggests that except for exon–intron boundaries, preservation of specific sequences within introns confers little selective advantage to the organism.

Three types of repetitive DNA have been found either flanking or within introns of the growth hormone gene family. Sequences similar to the Alu family of repetitive DNA are found flanking the hGH and hCS genes and are also found within intron D of the rPrl gene. The locations

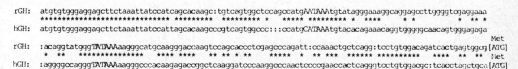

Figure 13. Comparison of the 5'-flanking region of the rat and human growth hormone genes. Gaps have been introduced to maximize the homology. Identical nucleotides are indicated by asterisks. Significant homology is confined to the first 120 nucleotides upstream from the transcription initiation site and the 5' untranslated regions. The complete nucleotide sequence of the rGH gene is shown in Figure 14.

of these Alu family sequences, which contain RNA polymerase III promotors, suggest that these sequences may have been involved in the extensive duplication of the GH/CS locus. This could have occurred by crossover events or by reverse transcription of RNA polymerase III transcripts originating in Alu sequences, as described in Section 1.4 on molecular evolution. Analysis of the human Alu family of dispersed middle-repetitive DNA indicates that the direct terminal repeats flanking the DNA differ in each case, suggesting that these repeats were generated by duplication of chromosomal DNA during an insertional event. Such structures may represent a class of mobile elements (113). Intron B of the rGH gene contains repetitive DNA with a 195 base pair tandem repeat with 96% homology (8 nucleotide substitutions and three insertion–deletions). This structure is followed by a 73 base pair fragment which is 66% homologous to the 5′ portion of the 195 base pair repeat (Figure 14). An homologous structure is found at three other positions in 9 kb of DNA 3′ to the rGH gene. These structures show high homology with transfer RNA genes. Repetitive elements of these types may be involved in the expansion or contraction of intron size, by unequal crossover or by other mechanisms. The middle repetitive DNA sequences within introns may represent sites for genetic recombination resulting in the rearrangements of genes and exons (111). Insertional events within introns may help to explain the more rapid divergence of these structures compared with the coding regions of a large variety of eukaryotic genes.

As described earlier, Gilbert has proposed that exons may represent primitive genetic units encoding different "functional domains" (15). Examination of the structures of the GH/CS/Prl family of genes suggests that the DNA upstream from exon I may be a "regulatory exon." This is suggested by the finding in both rGH (Figure 14) and rPrl that exon I was flanked by direct repeats. In both cases the repeats enclose at least a part of the probable promoter region (TATAAA), the mRNA CAP sites, and the ATG sequence within exon I. The presence of these direct repeats suggests that the regulatory region may have been inserted into these genes by an insertional event similar to that described in

---

Figure 14. Primary structure of the gene encoding rat growth hormone. The 5′-flanking, 3′-untranslated and 3′-flanking regions and introns are designated by nucleotides in lowercase letters. The 195 base pair (bp) tandem repeat structure within intron B is designated by nucleotides in capital letters. The 18 bp direct repeat flanking the tandem repeat structure is enclosed in boxes. The first member of the 195 bp repeat is underlined; the second member is overlined and the partial third repeat is underlined. Nucleotides at the intron–exon boundaries that agree with the consensus sequence are indicated by overlines. The TATAAA sequence is designated by capital letters and the transcription initiation site and polyadenylation sites are indicated by vertical arrows. Data adapted from Barta et al. (111).

```
tcaacaaattaagaggaataagacaatcatgggaaaatacctccttggagaggctctgttgcccctcgtc
 .[-400]                                                  .[-350]
ccagtgaacaaacgatggtaccctgccagagtatcctaccccctggattcaaaaatactctcaaaaggacac
                            .[-300]
attgggtggtctctgtagctgatcttgcgtgaccattgcccataaacctgagcaaaggcggcggtggaa
      .[-250]                                          .[-200]
aggtaagatcagggacgtgaccgcaggagagcagtggggacgacgatgtgtgggaggagcttctaaattatc
                                        .[-150]
catcagcacaagctgtcagtggctccagccatgaataaatgtataggaaaggcaggagccttggggtcga
            .[-100]                         s'y      .[-60]
ggaaaacaggtatgggTATAAAagggcatgcaagggaccaagtccAGCACCCTCGAGCCCAGATTCCAAA
                                  -25              .[1]
CTGCTCAGGTCCTGTGGACAGATCACTGAGTGGCG ATG GCT GCA G gtaagcatgcgcagatccgc
                                Met Ala Ala A
tgggtgtggtttggaccaaagagccttgaagatggatctgaggcttctagtgtgagggcatcccaacttc
    .[100]                                              .[150]
gcccatgttgggaacattctgggaccctatggggattgggagagattggtccttgctcccagcctcctcct
                            -21  .[200]
gtcctcctgtctctctcttttctag AC TCT CAG ACT CCC TGG CTC CTG ACC TTC AGC CTG
                        sp Ser Gln Thr Pro Trp Leu Leu Thr Phe Ser Leu
                        -9 .[250]                        2
Leu Cys Leu Leu Trp Pro Gln Glu Ala Gly Ala Phe Pro Ala Met Pro Leu Ser
CTC TGC CTG CTG TGG CCT CAA GAG GCT GGT GCT TTC CCT GCC ATG CCC TTG TCC
    10 .[300]                                  20
Ser Leu Phe Ala Asn Ala Val Leu Arg Ala Gln His Leu His Gln Leu Ala Ala
AGT CTG TTT GCC AAT GCT GTG CTC CGA GCC CAG CAC CTG CAC CAG CTG GCT GCT
    .[350]    30
Asp Thr Tyr Lys Glu Phe   gtaagttcctcggtgttgggtgcctgactgtggaagcaggaaggggg
GAC ACC TAC AAA GAG TTC
 .[400]                                                  .[450]
cagatcccaccctcgccccgagtccctgccctaggaagtcataggaggaaactatgccgttagatgagca
                            .[500]
gaaacagaatgggtcgtccatAACAGTAATGACAGAGGGCTGGAGAGATGGCTCAGTGGTTAAGAGCAC
                  .[550]
CCGACTGCTCTTCCAAAGGTCCTGAGTTCAATTCCCAGCAACCACATGGTGGCTCACAACCATCTGTAAAG
      .[610]                                  .[650]
AGATCCGATGCCCTCTTCTGGTGTGTCTGAAGACAGCTACAGTGTACTTATATAATAAACAAATAAATCTT
                      .[700]
TAAAAAAAAAAACAAAAACGGGGCTGGAGAGATGGCTCAGCGGTTAAGAGCGCCGACTGCTCTTCCAGAG
    .[750]                                  .[800]
GTCATGAGTTCAATTCCCAGCAACCACATGGTGGCTCACAACCATCTGTAAAGAGATCTGATGCCCTCTTC
                  .[850]
TGGTGTATCTGAAGACAGCTACAGTGTACTTATATATAATAAATAAATAAATCTTTAAAAAAAAACAAAAC
        .[900]
AGGGGCTGGGGATTTAGCTCAGTGGTAGAGCGCTTACCTAGGAAGCGCAAGGCCCTGGGTTCGGTCCCCAG
              .[1000]
CTCCGaaaaaaaagaacccaaaaaaaaaaaaaaaaaaaaccAAAACAAAAACAAAACAGTAATGACAGAGAGgtcac
                  .[1050]
                                39
                              Glu Arg Ala Tyr Ile Pro Glu Gly Gln
aagctggtccctcagtgactaccctcctccag GAG CGT GCC TAC ATT CCC GAG GGA CAG
            .[1110]                    50          .[1150]
Arg Tyr Ser Ile Gln Asn Ala Gln Ala Ala Phe Cys Phe Ser Glu Thr Ile Pro
CGC TAT TCC ATT CAG AAT GCC CAG GCT GCG TTC TGC TTC TCA GAG ACC ATC CCA
    60                                  70  .[1200]
Ala Pro Thr Gly Lys Glu Glu Ala Gln Gln Arg Thr
GCC CCC ACC GGC AAG GAG GAG GCC CAG CAG AGA ACT   gtgagtaggcccaggccttgtc
                                            .[1250]
tgtacagatcctctttcctccccaagcagccctaactgcagtctaggccagggaccagctcttccctgag
                      .[1300]
                                                    Asp
gctgaggtaacttgggagtcccaggcagaggtcactagctaatgcacagccccttttttccctcag GAC
 .[1350]                                          .[1400]
Met Glu Leu Leu Arg Phe Ser Leu Leu Leu Ile Gln Ser Trp Leu Gly Pro Val
ATG GAA TTG CTT CGC TTC TCG CTC CTG CTC ATC CAG TCA TGG CTG GGG CCC GTG
90                                  100  .[1450]
Gln Phe Leu Ser Arg Ile Phe Thr Asn Ser Leu Met Phe Gly Thr Ser Asp Arg
CAG TTT CTC AGC AGG ATC TTT ACC AAC AGC CTG ATG TTT GGT ACC TCG GAC CGC
    110                                  .[1500] 121
Val Tyr Glu Lys Leu Lys Asp Leu Glu Glu Gly Ile Gln Ala Leu Met Gln
GTC TAT GAG AAA CTG AAG GAC CTG GAA GAG GGC ATC CAG GCT CTG ATG CAG   gt
                                        .[1550]
caggatgaccgggggcgctagcctgaggttatactgacctttgcctctgcttggagcctagctgggggggc
            .[1600]
tcactgagctctgtttaccggtcagacccttaaaccttgagaaggcttcctactcactttcccttatgaagc
 .[1650]                      .[1690]
ctctaggcctttctctaggttctggagttgggggaggggcacggctctgagttcttctttcccacaacag
            130 .           .[1750]              140.
Glu Leu Glu Asp Gly Ser Pro Arg Ile Gly Gln Ile Leu Lys Gln Thr Tyr Asp
GAG CTG GAA GAC GGC AGC CCC CGT ATT GGG CAG ATC CTC AAG CAA ACC TAT GAC
                      .[1800] 150                   160
Lys Phe Asp Ala Asn Met Arg Ser Asp Asp Ala Leu Leu Lys Asn Tyr Gly Leu
AAG TTT GAC GCC AAC ATG CGC AGC GAT GAC GCT CTG CTC AAA AAC TAT GGG CTG
                  .[1850]          170
Leu Ser Cys Phe Lys Lys Asp Leu His Lys Ala Glu Thr Tyr Leu Arg Val Met
CTC TCC TGC TTC AAG AAG GAC CTG CAC AAG GCA GAG ACC TAC CTG CGG GTC ATG
    180 .[1900]                              190
Lys Cys Arg Arg Phe Ala Glu Ser Ser Cys Ala Phe AM
AAG TGT CGC CGC TTT GCG GAA AGC AGC TGT GCT TTC TAG gcacacactggtgtctct
    .[1950]                                  .[1990]
gcggcactcccccgttacccccctgtactctggcaactgccacccctacactttgtcctaataaaattaag
 .y3'                                         .[2050]
atgcatcatatcactctgctagacatctttttttttttttaaggcgtccggtttttttttttttagatttatta
                  .[2100]
tttattataag
 .[2150]
```

transposons which result in duplication of the chromosomal DNA at the site of insertion. The presence of such direct repeats is consistent with but does not prove the occurrence of an insertional event. These recombinations or insertions might directly influence the quantitative expression of GH-related genes.

Exon III of the rPrl gene, like exon I discussed above, is flanked by a direct repeat that occurs in introns B and C. This repeat contains 25 nucleotides maintaining 80% homology with one another, followed by an insertion–deletion and 9 perfectly matched nucleotides. This could indicate that exon III, including the intron flanking regions, was inserted into the developing Prl gene.

In the case of the rPrl gene, there is some evidence that the individual exons may represent discrete biological activities. When the amino acids encoded by exon III are removed proteolytically from Prl, the receptor binding activity is reduced 87% compared with the intact protein (114). This would suggest that the sequences in exon III are either directly involved in receptor binding or are required to maintain the structural integrity of the binding site. Exon II contains most of the signal peptide sequences and may also encode sequences of the mature hormone that are responsible for its lactogenic properties. Antigenic sites localized to exon IV and exon V may provide conformational stability or, possibly, mitogenic functions, or both.

From the structural analysis of the GH, CS, and Prl genes discussed above, a hypothetical model for the evolution of this gene family can be constructed as shown in Figure 15. An ancestral gene may have been duplicated into four copies, and this structure evolved into a single gene, thus accounting for the presence of duplicated regions of amino acid homology in GH, CS, and Prl (87–90). These regions of internal homology are located within exons II, IV, and V. A putative intron between the third and fourth copies of the ancestral gene is postulated to have been removed, accounting for the presence of two regions of internal homology within exon V. This basic structure was probably duplicated, with subsequent divergence leading to the genes for the three hormones. Subsequently, the genes appear to have acquired distinct regulatory sequences, which may explain their differential regulation. In other, separate evolutionary events, the gene for growth hormone acquired carbohydrate-regulating properties, which occur in part within exon III.

3 INSULIN AND RELAXIN GENES

Although insulin and relaxin are functionally unrelated, these two polypeptide hormones share common structural features. Both hormones consist of two polypeptide chains (A and B chains) linked by disulfide

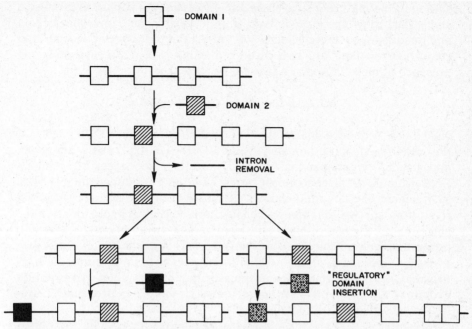

Figure 15. Model of the evolution of the genes encoding growth hormone, prolactin, and chorionic somatomammotropin. The model depicts the fourfold duplication of an ancestral gene (domain 1, open box), accounting for the presence of regions of internal homology in each of these hormones. Subsequently, the information coding for the carbohydrate-regulating properties (domain 2, hatched box) was inserted and the intron between the last two original ancestral gene domains was removed. This entire unit was duplicated (secondary duplication), and the divergence of these genes gave rise to the genes for growth hormone, prolactin, and chorionic somatomammotropin. The insertion of separate regulatory domains (solid and stippled boxes) occurred after the secondary duplication, possibly providing signals required for the unique expression of each of the individual gene products.

bridges and synthesized from a common precursor. The precursors are processed similarly by the proteolytic removal of a connecting peptide that links the A and B chains. Based on these and other structural similarities, it is possible that these two hormones may have evolved from a common precursor (115). Consequently, they are considered together.

3.1   Insulin

The insulin molecule is composed of two different polypeptides (A and B chains) joined by two interchain disulfide bridges. In the precursor polypeptide, the A and B chains are separated by a connecting C peptide that orients them before the formation of the intermolecular disulfide linkages. This precursor (preproinsulin) includes the signal peptide sequence (116–118). The C peptide is removed by peptidase action, resulting in the mature insulin molecule. Most species appear to possess a single insulin polypeptide derived from a single gene. However, in tuna and toadfish and three species of rodent (laboratory rat, mouse, and spiny mouse) there are two distinct insulins (119, 120), suggesting the presence of more than one nonallelic insulin gene.

3.1.1 Structure of Cloned cDNAs

Nucleotide sequence information is available for the cDNA copies of the mRNAs encoding human (121, 122), rat (123–125), anglerfish (126), and hagfish preproinsulins (127). In addition, sequences of genomic DNA isolated from genomic libraries have been obtained for rat (128, 129), human (39, 130), and chicken (52) insulins. These structures are derived from species that span a considerable period of evolutionary time, since the divergence of birds and mammals occurred about 250–300 million years ago and the hagfish diverged from the main line of vertebrate evolution approximately 500–600 million years ago. In addition, the hagfish represents a species that occupies a key branch point in vertebrate evolution. Consequently, studies of these structures is particularly useful for evolutionary comparisons.

A comparison of the structures of the mRNAs for human, rat, chicken, anglerfish, and hagfish is shown in Figure 16. The data indicate that the overall structure of the various insulins has been conserved. Amino acid substitutions have occurred with greater frequency in the signal and C peptide regions. This is particularly apparent in the C peptide region, where the NH_2-terminal sequence has diverged considerably. The lack of sequence conservation in the C peptide suggests that this peptide does not possess independent biological activities. Moreover, the lack of sequence conservation in the C peptide is consistent with its proposed role in converting the bimolecular A and B chain combination to a concentration-independent, first-order reaction (131). For example, the A and B chains may be oriented properly for sulfhydryl oxidation when the C peptide is replaced with nonpeptide linkers (132). Although the sequence of the C peptide appears to serve no functional role, the length of this segment is relatively conserved and in no known instance is it shorter than the 27 amino acid residues found in dog insulin (133).

Figure 16. Comparisons of the complementary DNAs and the mRNAs for human, rat I, rat II, chicken, anglerfish, and hagfish insulins. The complete sequence of the human mRNA is shown and nucleotide and amino acid differences are designated below for each of the other species. The symbol X designates uncertainty in the nucleotide determination. The data are adapted from the mRNA structures for human (121, 122), rat I and rat II (123–125), chicken (52), anglerfish (126), and hagfish (127) insulin. The structure of the chicken insulin mRNA has been deduced from genomic sequence information.

```
Human:     XXXXXXXXXGGACUGGCUCCXXXUGAAGAGAGCCAUCXAGCACAGAUCUGUCCUUCUGCC
Rat I:     AACCCUAAGUGACCAGCCUACAAUCAUAGACCAUCAGGAACGCAGGUCAUDGUUCCAAC
Rat II:    G              G  GG A
Chicken:   AGCCUGCAUGAAUAAAAUAUUCCUUUCCUCUUCAGAAGGCCUCCCCCACUCAUC
Anglerfish: AAACCAACCAGCUCUAAGCGUAUCCACUCCGUCCUCUUCAUCAACUCAUUCAACUCACCUCCUCCUUACUCUUACAGUCUACUCGCUC
Hagfish:   CCAACUUGUCGCACUAGAGGGACGGAGACCAUUAUCCAAAAGCAACCAA
```

```
                              -20                      -10
           Met    AlaLeuTrpMetArgLeuLeuProLeuLeuAlaLeuLeuAlaLeuTrpGlyProAspProAlaAlaAla------
Human:     AUG---GCCCUGUGGAUGCGCCUCCUGCCCCUGCUGGCGGCCUGCCUGGGCCUGUGGGGACCUGACCCAGCCGCAGCC---

                                            Val    Glu Lys      Gln
Rat I:     ---          U               C    C U    AG  CA G U    CAG  U------
                    Ile                           Ile Glu Arg   Gln
Rat II:    ---      C  U               C    CAU    AG  CCG U     CAG  U____
                    Ile Ser                       ValPheSer     GlyThrSerTyr
Chicken:   --- U C  C  AUCA     U U     U    C UUUU CU C    GAA CAG UAU  A____
           Ala       LeuGlnSerPheSer        Val   ValValSerTrp GlySerGln
Anglerfish: GCG U    C C AGUCUU CU UU     UCU A   U G A C U G  A GAU CCAG  U------
                    SerProPhe  AlaAlaValIlePro    ValLeu  LeuSerArgAla   ProSer    AspThr
Hagfish:   --- G    CUCACCAUUC  UGCCGCAGUGAUACCC  UG CU U  CU A UA G CA   C AAGU    AGAUACA
```

```
                   1                10                      20
           PheValAsnGlnHisLeuCysGlySerHisLeuValGluAlaLeuTyrLeuValGlyArgGlyPhePheTyrThrProLysThr
Human:     ---UUUGUGAACCAACACCUGUGCGGCUCACACCUGGUGGAAGCUCUCUACCUAGUGUGCGGGGAACGAGGCUUCUUCUACACACCCAAGACC
               Lys         Pro                                                      Ser
Rat I:     ---  C A G     UU  UCU        G     G  G    U                              U
               Lys                                                                   MetSer
Rat II:    ---  C A G     UU U U U       G     G  U A                                 U U
           AlaAla                                                         Ser    Ala
Chicken:   --GC CC   G    C U   C U      G     G     U A G U                U C    AG
           ValAlaProAla                  Asp                       Asp              Asn
Anglerfish: GCGCGCCC GCG  G    U   U      A C C C U    G C U A CA    U              AC
           ArgThrThrGly       LysAsp     Asn              IleAla    Val             Asp    ThrLysMet
Hagfish:   --CGCACC CGGC U U   AAGCG      C  A U A U  A C C         A UU U A          GAU    A CC AGAUG
```

```
           ArgArgGluAlaGluAspLeuGlnGlnValGlyGlnValGluLeuGlyGlyGlyProGlyAlaGlySerLeuGlnProLeuAlaLeuGluGlySerLeuGln----------LysArg
                           40                     50                          60
Human:     CGCCGGGAGCAGAGGACCUGCAGGUGGGGCAGGUGGAGCUGGGCGGGGGCCCUGGUGCAGGCCGGGCCUGCCCUUGGCCCUGGAGGGGUCCCUGCAG----------AAGCGU
                       Val    Pro      Pro  Leu              Glu      Asp      Thr         ValAlaArg
Rat I:     U U A UG    C A    CCA  AC   U A  G AG C GGAU U A   A        A         UUG  G    ------
                       Val    Pro      Ala  Leu              Asp      Thr         ValAlaArg
Rat II:    C A UG      CA A   CA  UGA U  A    U A GG C UGA U   A A     G  G        U G G     ------      C
                       AspVal  GlnProLeu     SerSerProLeuArg  GluAlaGlyValLeuProPheGln GluGluTyrGluLysVal
Chicken:   A   U UC  C G CC UA  A CAGUCCCUU GU  A CAGGA UG GCCUUC A     GAGGAAUA GA A UC---
           AspValGlnLeuValGlyPheLeuProProLysSerGly AlaAlaAla    AspAsnGluValAlaGluPheAlaPheLysAspArgMetGluMetMetVal
Anglerfish: A AGAC U CA CU CUGGGUUUCC CCCC CAAA UCUGGC   A U A GA GUG  A A AGA GUG A UUUGCCUUCAAGGA A AU GAGAUGAUGGUG        A
           Lys    AspThrGlyAlaLeuAlaAlaAlaPheLeuProLeuAlaTyrArgGluAspAsnGluSerGlnAsnAspAspSerIleGlyIleAsnGluVal LysSer
Hagfish:   AAA C CA C GA CAU  GCU CAUUUUU CCAUU GCCUAU CU AGGA AAC AGUCCCAAGAUG UU  A A GAA AA C AAGUG    A AGC          G
```

```
                   70                          80
           GlyIleValGluGlnCysCysThrSerIleCysSerLeuTyrGlnLeuGluAsnTyrCysAsn
Human:     GGCAUUGUGGAACAAUGCUGUACCAGCAUCUGCUCCCUCUACCAGCUGGAGAACUACUGCAAC
               Asp
Rat I:         U G  C                              A
               Asp
Rat II:    C   U G  C                        U     A
               HisAsnThr
Chicken:   G   U G  CCAU A CG  U                  A A
               HisArgPro      AsnIlePheAsp  Gln
Anglerfish: C   G G  CCAU ACCC  AA A  U G C   C U
               HisLysArg      Ile  Asp
Hagfish:   A C A    CCA AGCG  U  A  GC  A
```

```
Human:  UAGACGCAGCCCGCCAGGCAGCCCCCCACCCCGCCGCCUCCCCCACCCGAGACAGAGAUGGAAUAAAGCCCUUGAACCAGCCGpolyA
Rat I:  CA--------GUCCACCACUCCCC-CCCCACCCCCUCUGCAAAU---------CAAUAAAGCCUUUGAAUGAGCC
Rat II:           C    A UU           U                A       A
Chicken: CCAAGAAGCCAGAACGCGGCCACAGACAUACACUUACUCUAUCGCACCUUCAAAGCAUUUGAAUAAACCUUGUUGGUCUAC
```

```
Anglerfish: UGAACAGUUUCCCUGCCUUCCUUAGCAUCGCUUCAUGUCCCGGCUAACUUUGCCUGAACAUCCCGAAUCCCCCCAACCCGGCAUCGAAGAGUGGCAGCUCUGUCUU
CUCUCUCUCUCUCUCUCUCUCUCUCUCUCAACAAAUGAAACAACGCGCUGUCAAAUGUUGUCUCGAAGAGAGAUUCAAUUAUUUUUUCCUAGAAAAUAAAGUUUUGUGAAUUGAG
```

```
Hagfish: UGAAACGUCCCGGCGCAUCUUUCGCUGGCUUCAUUACUAUUGAAGCGCUUUUAGGAUUAAGAGCAAGUCCUGAAUUGAAAGAAGGAAUCCGGCUGUGUACUCCCAUGCAUCGCAAAUGU
CUUCAAAUUGCUUAAUUGCACACUUCAAAAAUGUGGUCAACUUCUUUCGUUUACCGUUCUUUGCUGCAGUCAGGUCAAUUGAUCACCAACUUAAGCUGAUUGGAUGAUGAUGUUACAUUGUAAUUC
UAAAAUCUUAGUAUACCUAUCUAUGAAAUUUGUCUUCCAAUCCCAAAUCCUAUCCCGCCAAUCCCCCUUACCUCGGCGACCAAUGCUAGGGCAUUGGAUGGAUCCUUUCAUGCAGGAACGUUUUUCUCGGUGAUUCA
GUUUCUAACCGCUGUUCGUUGUUAAUUCGCUCAAUAAAAUUGUUUUUG
```

51

It has been proposed that conservation of overall length may be related
to the efficient segregation of insulin into the cisternae of the rough endoplasmic reticulum (134, 135). Thus the structural analogs of proinsulin,
the insulin-like growth factors I and II, have C peptides 11 residues
long; however, the A chain region of these molecules is extended at the
COOH terminus, resulting in conservation of the length of the molecule
relative to insulin.

An interesting difference in the structure of the teleost insulins is the
presence of a much larger 3' untranslated region. For the hagfish and
anglerfish this region is 530 and 222 nucleotides long, respectively,
whereas in the human, rat I and II, and chicken mRNAs the 3'
untranslated region contains 74, 52, 53, and 80 nucleotides, respectively.
This may indicate that the large 3' untranslated region may be a unique
feature of the more primitive teleost insulin mRNAs (127). Alternatively,
this might suggest that preproinsulin was derived from a larger ancestral protein, as has been suggested for serine proteases (136, 137).

The pairing of basic amino acid residues at the cleavage sites of the
C peptide has been conserved in all proinsulins. This observation suggests that the modified tryptic-like cleavage mechanism for proproteins
may have existed before the appearance of vertebrates. In anglerfish insulin, the carboxy-terminal lysine residue of the B chain is derived from
the basic residue pair linking the B chain to the C peptide. By contrast,
in other vertebrate insulins the single lysine residue at B_{29} is followed
by a neutral or acidic residue at B_{30}, which is followed by a pair of basic residues connecting the B chain to the C peptide. This suggests that
anglerfish proinsulin does not require the action of an enzyme similar to
carboxypeptidase B for final processing to remove the first arginine residue of the C peptide left at the carboxy terminus of the peptide (126).

As shown in Figure 16, the sequences of the prepeptide region of hagfish and anglerfish preproinsulins differ considerably, and the hagfish
prepeptide is two amino acid residues longer than the other preproinsulins. The general molecular features are conserved, including a strongly
hydrophobic central region. The first 17 amino acids of the human and
rat signal peptides are strongly conserved, whereas the corresponding
sequence for the teleost prepeptides have diverged significantly. In human, rat, chicken, and anglerfish insulins the Ala-Leu-Trp sequence near
the initiating methionine and the sequence Leu-Leu-(Ala or Val)-Leu-Leu
have been conserved. Consequently, it has been proposed that these sequences may have a specific function in the vectorial transport process
(134). The Trp in this leader sequence near the amino terminus may not
be essential, since this amino acid is not present in the more primitive
hagfish mRNA. In addition, the exact sequence Leu-Leu-(Ala or Val)-
Leu-Leu is missing. Interestingly, there is a similar sequence of five neutral amino acids in the hagfish mRNA (Leu-Val-Leu-Leu-Leu), which is
displaced three amino residues toward the carboxy terminus of the

prepeptides. It is possible that the function of these residues is to maintain a central hydrophobic core. The prepeptides of all the insulin mRNAs also contain a predicted β turn near the cleavage site (138).

Comparison of the nucleotide sequence of the A and B chains reveals regions that are highly conserved, and some of these regions have been demonstrated to be important for insulin activity. For example, studies of the biological activity, receptor affinities, and amino acid sequences of insulin indicate that a largely invariable region on the surface of the insulin monomer may be the receptor-binding region (102, 139–144). This region, composed of both A-chain residues (A_1Gly, A_5Glu, A_{19}Tyr, and A_{21}Asn) and B-chain residues (B_{24}Phe, B_{25}Phe, B_{26}Tyr, B_{12}Val, and B_{16} Tyr), is perfectly conserved in the human, rat, chicken, anglerfish, and hagfish insulins (Figure 16). In addition, the region of the B chain (B_{24}, B_{25}, B_{26}, and B_{27}) corresponds to the region responsible for the negative cooperativity observed when insulin binds to its cell surface receptor (145). In addition, several residues adjacent to those indicated above have also been perfectly conserved. Nevertheless, comparison with the more primitive hagfish sequence indicates that the overall homology is low. In view of the high percentage of changes in the amino acid sequences and the rapid rate of fixation of silent mutations within the codons (128), the lack of extensive homology is not unexpected.

3.1.2 Structure of Native Genes

As mentioned previously, genomic DNA sequences for the insulin genes from rat (128, 129–135), human (39, 130), and chicken (52) have been analyzed. The overall structures of these genes conform to the general features described in the introduction (Section 1.3).

In humans there appears to be a single gene containing two introns located in the 5′ untranslated region of the insulin mRNA and in the DNA region encoding the C peptide (39). This gene has been localized to the distal end of the short arm of chromosome 11 at Giemsa band p15 by *in situ* hybridization techniques (146) and hybridization of DNA from mouse-human somatic cell hybrids (147).

In the rat, there are two distinct insulin genes differing in intron structure. One gene, rII, contains two introns, one interrupting the connecting C peptide and the other interrupting the segment encoding the 5′ noncoding region of the mRNA. The other gene, rI, contains only the smaller of the two introns. Both genes are functional (148, 149), therefore the presence of the second intron in rII insulin is not needed for insulin expression. The possibility that the small intron plays a regulatory role has not been excluded. The similarity of the two rat genes suggests that they are the result of a recent duplication, it has been estimated that this event occurred about 20–35 million years ago (128). Since the human and chicken insulin genes contain two introns in the same relative position as the rII gene, it is concluded that the rI gene lost an intron either concurrent with or subsequent to the duplication event. These results also suggest that the insulin ancestral gene contained two introns. The two introns in the rII and human insulin genes also differ in size. Intron A contains 119 and 179 base pairs of DNA in rat and human genes, respectively; corresponding sizes of intron B are 499 and 786 base pairs. In addition, except for the exon–intron boundaries, there is no obvious homology in the sequences of the corresponding introns.

The human insulin gene contains a highly polymorphic region located 363 base pairs upstream from the transcription initiation site (150, 151). Sixty-three precent of nondiabetic Caucasians appear to be heterozygous at this site; two major and one minor class of alleles have been identified (150). Within each class there appear to be many different alleles at this locus. Preliminary data indicate that there are racial differences in the frequency of alleles and that the polymorphism is inherited in a Mendelian fashion. The nucleotide sequence of this polymorphic region in the human insulin gene has been determined; it seems to be generated by variation in the number and arrangement of a family of tandemly repeating nucleotides with a structure (151) related to ACAGGGGTGTGGGG.

The function of the polymorphic region is unknown. Since the region exhibits a bimodal distribution of insertion sizes, it is probably not involved in recombinative processes (152) such as proposed for other simple repeating elements in the β-globin genes (153). It might represent an intergenic or spacer DNA (65, 66). Its proximal location to the transcriptional control regions suggests that it might be involved in the regulation of insulin gene expression. Nevertheless, similar regions have not been found in any of the other insulin genes that have been sequenced.

The 15 base pair sequence flanking the tandemly repeated polymorphic region is of interest, since one member of this structure lies within the promoter region. This suggests that it might be involved in the function of the polymorphic region or that it is involved in insulin gene expression. As discussed previously (Section 2.3), the presence of direct repeats flanking the polymorphic region suggests that this region may have been inserted into the insulin gene.

Further analysis of the DNA flanking the human insulin gene indicates that the 5650 base pairs of 5′-flanking DNA and the 11,500 base pairs of 3′-flanking DNA are single copy sequences except for the presence of a single segment of DNA approximately 500 base pairs long located 6000 base pairs from the 3′ end of the gene (113). This segment is composed of a member of the Alu family of dispersed middle repetitive sequences and a less highly repeated homopolymeric segment. The Alu repeat is flanked by 19 base pair direct repeats and also contains a tandemly repeated 83 base pair sequence. Comparison of the sequences flanking the human and rat I insulin genes indicated that the homology between the two genes is restricted to the coding regions and a short segment of about 60 base pairs flanking the proximal 5′ ends of the genes (39). The lack of extensive sequence conservation between the rat and human genes suggests either that the presumptive regulatory sequences are close to the gene or that these regions are less highly conserved and species specific.

The sequence of the Alu family member in the insulin gene is homologous with one of the seven partly characterized Alu family members present in the β-globin gene cluster (154), but the direct repeats flanking the Alu family members in these two genes are different. This probably reflects the concept that the direct repeats are not part of the Alu family member but represent short segments of the chromosomal DNA that are duplicated during the insertion of the Alu sequences. The Alu family member was also found to be identically located in an allelic insulin gene, suggesting that these elements are not highly mobile. The function of these sequences is unknown.

Some members of the Alu family are transcribed (154), and the transcribed RNA appears to be restricted to the nucleus, suggesting the possibility that it is involved in posttranscriptional processing of hnRNA. It has also been proposed that these sequences may be origins of chromosome replication; since there is homology between a 14 base pair segment of the Alu repeat and regions in the vicinity of the origin of replication of papovaviruses (154). Alternatively, such sequences might represent examples of selfish genes that do not possess phenotypes which can be operated upon by natural selection; however, they may be preferred replicators (67, 68). The dispersed middle repetitive sequences in the β globin gene cluster, all of which are probably Alu family members (155), separate the globin genes into three developmentally regulated families (embryonic, fetal and adult). This suggests that the Alu sequences might have a role in the developmental expression of these genes.

The divergence of the chicken, rat, and human insulin gene sequences has been analyzed in detail (52) and extends a similar analysis of the two rat preproinsulin genes (128; Table 2). It is evident that silent changes increase in proportion to the divergence time. As discussed previously (Figure 16), the C-peptide area of the molecule represents a region of rapid accumulation of both replacement and silent substitutions, whereas the A and B chains are constrained (51, 156). Thus, the C peptide serves as an internal standard for testing the neutral hypothesis (51, 103, 156). When the data (Table 2) are plotted as a function of time, the accumulation of replacement changes in the C peptide is linear with time and the rate is approximately five times that for the A and B chains. By contrast, the accumulation of silent changes in the C peptide occurs more rapidly and is not linear with time. There is a possible break in the accumulation rate at about 85 million years; the initial rate

TABLE 2 Percent Corrected Divergence of Insulin Gene Sequences[a]

Preproinsulin	Replacement Sites				Silent Sites				
	A and B Chains	C Peptide	C'Peptide[b]	Not-C	A and B Chains	C Peptide	C'Peptide	Not-C[c]	Small Intron[c]
Rat I/II	1.8	3.2		3.5	32.3	18		23.5	21
Human/rat	5.2	19.2	21	7.5	76	91.4	110.2	64.8	
Human/chicken	8		62.5	13.5	122		139.5	133.3	
Rat/chicken	10.7		49.4	15.2	64		150	141	163

[a] The calculation of these percentages has been described in detail (52).
[b] The C' peptide refers to an alternate alignment of C-peptide sequences (52).
[c] "Not-C" refers to the DNA encoding all regions except the C peptide, i.e., the signal peptide (except for the ATG initiation codon), the A and B chains, and the four basic amino acids which function as cleavage signals.

corresponds to 7×10^{-9} substitutions per nucleotide site per year. A similar situation occurs when the α and β globin genes of human, rat, mouse, and chicken are compared (52). Thus, the rapid accumulation rate of silent mutations appears to saturate at 85–100 million years. These data indicate that the initial rapid accumulation of nucleotide changes is confined to a fraction of the neutral sites. The more rapid accumulation of silent changes in the C peptide is due to the existence of fewer constraints, that is, a higher fraction of neutral sites. These studies suggest that the driving force for fixation of nucleotide changes is selection that operates on a fraction of the replacement changes. In addition, replacement changes but not silent changes may serve as an evolutionary clock. However, this same type of analysis gives inconsistent results in the GH/CS/Prl system (see Section 2.3).

3.2 Relaxin

Relaxin, a polypeptide hormone, is produced by the corpus luteum of pregnancy. It plays a role in mammalian reproductive physiology, where it is involved in the softening and lengthening of the pubic symphysis and the softening of the cervix prior to parturition (157). Amino acid sequence data are available for rat (158), pig (159), and shark (160) relaxins. The structure of relaxin is very similar to insulin; it is composed of two nonidentical polypeptide chains (A and B chains) linked by one intra- and two inter-disulfide bridges. In porcine relaxin, the A and B chains contain 22 and 31 amino acid residues, respectively.

Complimentary DNA to relaxin mRNA has been obtained by means of synthetic oligonucleotide primers that were used to initiate reverse transcription of mRNA derived from pregnant rat and porcine ovaries (161). Primers were used in both cases, since under stringent conditions there was no significant cross-hybridization between the rat relaxin cDNA and porcine cDNA clones, indicating significant divergence of these molecules. In both cases nucleotide sequence information of the entire relaxin precursor has been obtained (Figure 17). Knowledge derived from these studies has greatly extended knowledge of the similarity of the relaxin molecule to insulin.

In the case of rat and porcine relaxins, the C peptide linking the A and B chains is 105 and 104 amino acid residues long, respectively. This sequence information confirmed earlier cell-free translation studies (162) indicating that the relaxin precursor was large (ca. 23,000 daltons) compared with the insulin precursor (11,000 daltons).

A comparison of the structures of rat and pig relaxin mRNAs and their corresponding amino acid sequences is shown in Figure 17. Both preprorelaxins contain signal peptides (22 and 24 amino acids for rat and porcine, respectively) that are rich in hydrophobic amino acids. These peptides share little homology with other signal peptides of se-

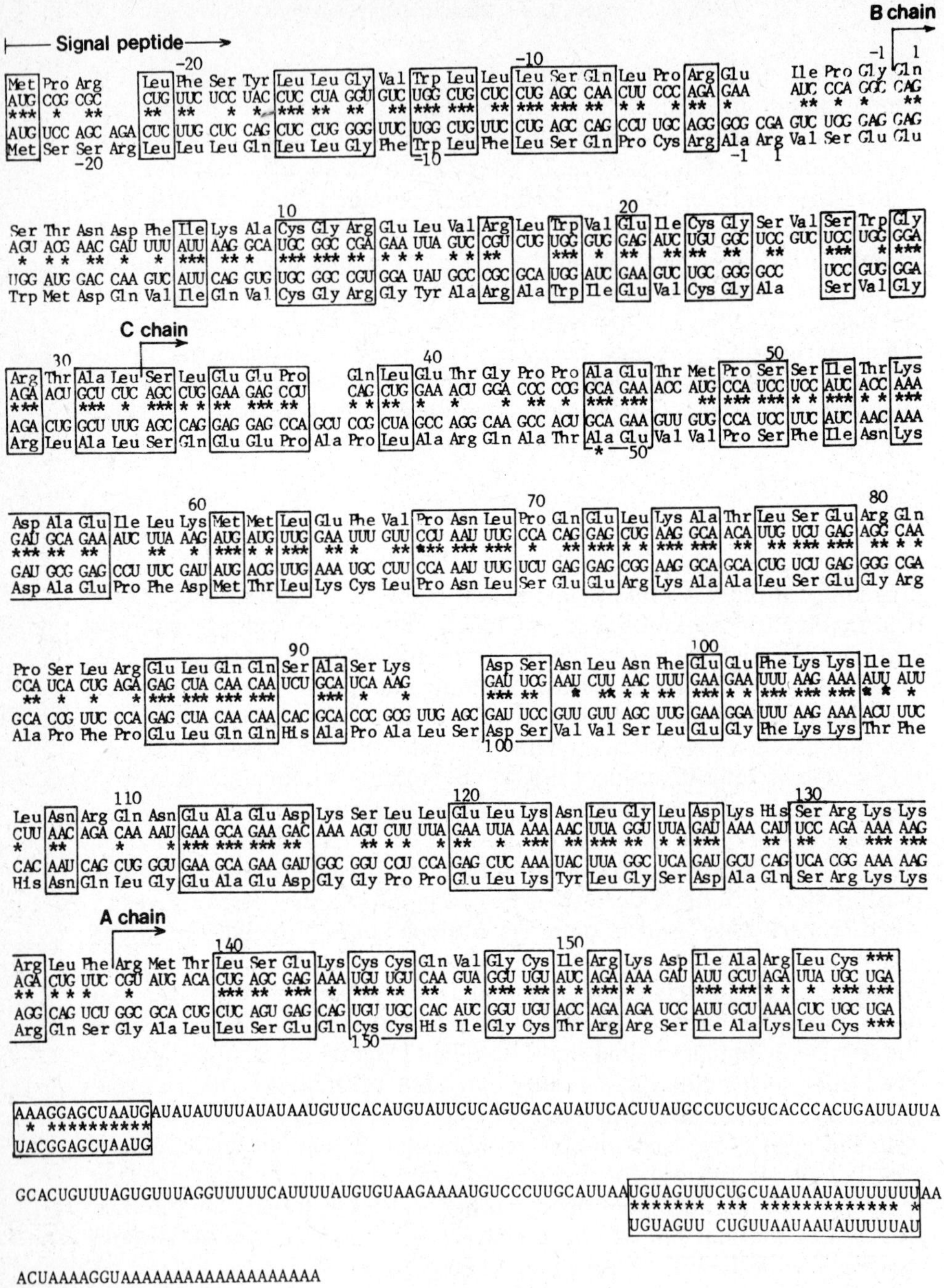
Signal peptide
B chain
-20 -10 -1 1
Met Pro Arg Leu Phe Ser Tyr Leu Leu Gly Val Trp Leu Leu Leu Ser Gln Leu Pro Arg Glu Ile Pro Gly Gln
AUG CCG CGC CUG UUC UCC UAC CUC CUA GGU GUC UGG CUG CUC CUG AGC CAA CUU CCC AGA GAA AUC CCA GGC CAG
*** * ** ** ** * * *** ** ** ** *** *** ** *** *** ** * * * ** * ** * * **
AUG UCC AGC AGA CUC UUG CUC CAG CUC CUG GGG UUC UGG CUG UUC CUG AGC CAG CCU UGC AGG GCG CGA GUC UCG GAG GAG
Met Ser Ser Arg Leu Leu Leu Gln Leu Leu Gly Phe Trp Leu Phe Leu Ser Gln Pro Cys Arg Ala Arg Val Ser Glu Glu
-20 -10 -1 1
10 20
Ser Thr Asn Asp Phe Ile Lys Ala Cys Gly Arg Glu Leu Val Arg Leu Trp Val Glu Ile Cys Gly Ser Val Ser Trp Gly
AGU ACG AAC GAU UUU AUU AAG GCA UGC GGC CGA GAA UUA GUC CGU CUG UGG GUG GAG AUC UGU GGC UCC GUC UCC UGG GGA
* * ** * * *** ** * *** *** ** * * * * * ** *** * ** ** ** ** ** *** * ***
UGG AUG GAC CAA GUC AUU CAG GUG UGC GGC CGU GGA UAU GCC CGC GCA UGG AUC GAA GUC UGC GGG GCC UCC GUG GGA
Trp Met Asp Gln Val Ile Gln Val Cys Gly Arg Gly Tyr Ala Arg Ala Trp Ile Glu Val Cys Gly Ala Ser Val Gly
C chain
30 40 50
Arg Thr Ala Leu Ser Leu Glu Glu Pro Gln Leu Glu Thr Gly Pro Pro Ala Glu Thr Met Pro Ser Ser Ile Thr Lys
AGA ACU GCU CUC AGC CUG GAA GAG CCU CAG CUG GAA ACU GGA CCC CCG GCA GAA ACC AUG CCA UCC UCC AUC ACC AAA
*** *** * *** * * ** *** ** * * ** * * * ** * *** *** ** *** *** * * *** * * ***
AGA CUG GCU UUG AGC CAG GAG GAG CCA GCU CCG CUA GCC AGG CAA GCC ACU GCA GAA GUU GUG CCA UCC UUC AUC AAC AAA
Arg Leu Ala Leu Ser Gln Glu Glu Pro Ala Pro Leu Ala Arg Gln Ala Thr Ala Glu Val Val Pro Ser Phe Ile Asn Lys
50
60 70 80
Asp Ala Glu Ile Leu Lys Met Met Leu Glu Phe Val Pro Asn Leu Pro Gln Glu Leu Lys Ala Thr Leu Ser Glu Arg Gln
GAU GCA GAA AUC UUA AAG AUG AUG UUG GAA UUU GUU CCU AAU UUG CCA CAG GAG CUG AAG GCA ACA UUG UCU GAG AGG CAA
*** ** ** ** * *** ** * *** ** * ** *** *** *** * ** *** * * *** *** ** ** *** *** ** * *
GAU GCG GAG CCU UUC GAU AUG ACG UUG AAA UGC CUU CCA AAU UUG UCU GAG GAG CGG AAG GCA GCA CUG UCU GAG GGG CGA
Asp Ala Glu Pro Phe Asp Met Thr Leu Lys Cys Leu Pro Asn Leu Ser Glu Glu Arg Lys Ala Ala Leu Ser Glu Gly Arg
90 100
Pro Ser Leu Arg Glu Leu Gln Gln Ser Ala Ser Lys Asp Ser Asn Leu Asn Phe Glu Glu Phe Lys Lys Ile Ile
CCA UCA CUG AGA GAG CUA CAA CAA UCU GCA UCA AAG GAU UCG AAU CUU AAC UUU GAA GAA UUU AAG AAA AUU AUU
** * * * *** *** *** *** *** * * *** ** * ** * * * *** * * *** *** *** * * *
GCA CCG UUC CCA GAG CUA CAA CAA CAC GCA CCC GCG UUG AGC GAU UCC GUU GUU AGC UUG GAA GGA UUU AAG AAA ACU UUC
Ala Pro Phe Pro Glu Leu Gln Gln His Ala Pro Ala Leu Ser Asp Ser Val Val Ser Leu Glu Gly Phe Lys Lys Thr Phe
100
110 120 130
Leu Asn Arg Gln Asn Glu Ala Glu Asp Lys Ser Leu Leu Glu Leu Lys Asn Leu Gly Leu Asp Lys His Ser Arg Lys Lys
CUU AAC AGA CAA AAU GAA GCA GAA GAC AAA AGU CUU UUA GAA UUA AAA AAC UUA GGU UUA GAU AAA CAU UCC AGA AAA AAG
* ** * * *** *** *** ** ** * * * ** * *** ** *** ** * * *** ** ** * *** ***
CAC AAU CAG CUG GCU GAA GCA GAA GAU GGC GGU CCU CCA GAG CUC AAA UAC UUA GGC UCA GAU GCU CAG UCA CGG AAA AAG
His Asn Gln Leu Gly Glu Ala Glu Asp Gly Gly Pro Pro Glu Leu Lys Tyr Leu Gly Ser Asp Ala Gln Ser Arg Lys Lys
A chain
140 150
Arg Leu Phe Arg Met Thr Leu Ser Glu Lys Cys Cys Gln Val Gly Cys Ile Arg Lys Asp Ile Ala Arg Leu Cys ***
AGA CUG UUC CGU AUG ACA CUG AGC GAG AAA UGU UGU CAA GUA GGU UGU AUC AGA AAA GAU AUU GCU AGA UUA UGC UGA
** * * * * *** ** *** * *** ** ** * *** *** * * *** * * *** *** * * * *** ***
AGG CAG UCU GGC GCA CUG CUC AGU GAG CAG UGU UGC CAC AUC GGU UGU ACC AGA AGA UCC AUU GCU AAA CUC UGC UGA
Arg Gln Ser Gly Ala Leu Leu Ser Glu Gln Cys Cys His Ile Gly Cys Thr Arg Arg Ser Ile Ala Lys Leu Cys ***
150
AAAGGAGCUAAUGAUAUAUUUUAUAUAAUGUUCACAUGUAUUCUCAGUGACAUAUUCACUUAUGCCUCUGUCACCCACUGAUUAUUA
* **********
UACGGAGCUAAUG
GCACUGUUUAGUGUUUAGGUUUUUCAUUUUAUGUGUAAGAAAAUGUCCCUUGCAUUAAUGUAGUUUCUGCUAAUAAUAUUUUUUUAA
******* *** ************* *
UGUAGUU CUGUUAAUAAUAUUUUUAU
ACUAAAAGGUAAAAAAAAAAAAAAAAAAA

creted hormones except for typically high Leu contents, which can generate some random sequence homologies. In rat relaxin the signal peptide is cleaved at the Ala residue at position −1; in the porcine molecule this cleavage probably occurs between the Gly-Glu residues. In the latter case, concomitant or subsequent cyclization of the N-terminal Glu residue to pyroglutamic acid would generate the blocked N-terminus of the relaxin B chain (163).

The exact processing of the C peptide is unknown since the amino acid sequence of this peptide is lacking. Consequently, the C peptide is referred to as the C region. Cleavage at the carboxyl terminus of the B chain may be at Leu_{32}-Ser_{33}, which is identical in both rat and porcine relaxins. This would require subsequent removal of Leu_{32} to generate the major form of the porcine B chain. Alternatively, cleavage could result at Ala_{31}-Leu_{32}. These cleavages would require a protease with chymotrypsin-like specificity.

At the junction of the C peptide and A chain, the most likely cleavage point would be carboxyl terminal to the four basic residues Arg-Lys-Lys-Arg at positions 131–134 for both rat and porcine relaxins. This cleavage is consistent with the common prohormone processing at basic amino acid clusters. Such cleavage would require removal of the Leu-Phe dipeptide at the amino terminus of the A chain by a dipeptidyl aminopeptidase. Alternatively, an enzyme with chymotrypsin-like activity could cleave at Phe_{136}-Arg_{131}.

Rat and porcine relaxin exhibit little homology in the 3′ untranslated region except for the sequence AAUAAUA, which occurs 17 and 19 bases upstream from the polyadenylation start site for porcine and rat relaxins, respectively. This probable polyadenylation signal is slightly different from the AAUAAA signal found in most other eukaryotic mRNAs (36). There is some homology in the two sequences in the 10 bases following the termination codon and in the 25 bases surrounding the AAUAAUA sequence. This is consistent with other eukaryotic gene families that show a generally higher rate of sequence divergence in the 3′ untranslated regions than in the coding regions.

The number of amino acid replacements between rat and porcine relaxins represents 50.3% of the prorelaxin primary structure and underscores the great divergence of this protein between the two species. Nevertheless, in regions of amino acid homology, nucleotide sequence is retained, since 33.3% of the codon usage is conserved and only 15% of

Figure 17. Comparison of the porcine preprorelaxin mRNA sequences (top) with corresponding rat relaxin sequences (bottom). Homology is indicated by asterisks and the amino acid homologies are designated by the boxed areas. The asterisks beneath Ala denote the putative intron processing site in rat relaxin. The 3′ untranslated region of the rat nucleotide sequence is omitted (except for the boxed region surrounding the AAUAAA sequence), since little homology occurs in this region between the porcine and rat relaxins. Reprinted with permission from Haley et al. (161).

the prorelaxin sequence represents silent mutations. Consequently, the nucleotide sequence homologies for the B, C, and A chains are 63.0, 66.8, and 64.2%, respectively, whereas the amino acid homologies are 41.2, 52, and 54.5%. Despite the extensive divergence in amino acid sequence between rat and porcine relaxins, the relative amounts of hydrophobic, uncharged polar, acidic, and basic amino acids remain very similar. This conservation may be important for maintenance of the structure and biological activity of the molecule.

An interesting feature of the C region of relaxin, which contrasts with the C peptide of insulin, is its unusual length (104–105 amino acids in relaxin versus 27–41 amino acids in insulin) and the finding that it maintains the same relative nucleotide conservation between the rat and pig genes as the A and B chains. In comparing rat and porcine C region homology (Figure 17), two gaps corresponding to three amino acids have been inserted at positions 37 and 93 in order to maximize the homology. The finding of extensive sequence conservation over the entire length of the relaxin C region suggests that this peptide may have another biological function in addition to its possible role in facilitating proper disulfide bond formation between the A and B chains.

4 PRO-OPIOMELANOCORTIN GENES

Pro-opiomelanocortin (POMC) is a protein of about 240 amino acids, which is cleaved to yield ACTH, β-endorphin, melanocyte-stimulating hormone (MSH), β-lipotropin (LPH), and other peptides. The mRNA for POMC encodes the various peptides (164–167). The size and amino acid sequence of POMC vary slightly among species, but in general it follows the structure shown in Figure 18. DNA complementary to mouse (168) and bovine (169) POMC mRNA has been cloned. Fragments of the chromosomal genes for rat (170), human (171), and bovine (172) POMC were cloned subsequently. Recently, Whitfeld et al. (173) determined the structure of the entire human POMC gene.

The processing of POMC varies, depending upon the tissue in which it is expressed. Human POMC is synthesized principally in the anterior pituitary; other mammals including rats, mice, cattle, and sheep synthesize POMC primarily in the intermediate lobe of the pituitary. There is also evidence that POMC is synthesized by the normal human placenta (166, 174) and hypothalamus (166, 175). In the human anterior pituitary, the demonstrable products of POMC are adrenocorticotrophic hormone (ACTH), β-LPH, β-endorphin, and another peptide termed the 16K N-terminal glycopeptide (see below). In the intermediate lobes of rodents and cattle, ACTH is cleaved further to α-MSH and corticotropin-like intermediate lobe peptide (CLIP), and β-LPH is cleaved to β-MSH and β-endorphin. Thus, the single POMC protein may be variously processed to a wide variety of products with different biological activities.

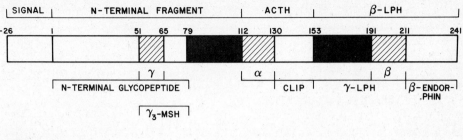

Figure 18. Diagrammatic representation of the structure of human prepro-opiomelanocortin as suggested by amino acid sequencing of various fragments and proved by the gene structure. The numbers refer to amino acid positions, with No. 1 assigned to the first amino acid of POMC following the 26 amino acid signal peptide. The α-, β-, and γ-MSH regions, which characterize the three "constant" regions, are indicated by diagonal lines; the "variable" regions are stippled.

There is a very high degree of homology in POMC throughout three regions for the bovine, rat, and human genes. These are the 16K N-terminal glycopeptide, ACTH, and the β-MSH/β-endorphin region. These "constant" regions are separated by two highly variable regions lying on either side of the ACTH sequence. These structures are shown in Figure 19 with gaps introduced in the amino acid sequences to align regions of obvious homology. The gaps were introduced by the procedure described above (57, 58).

POMC begins with a 26-amino-acid leader peptide rich in hydrophobic amino acids. In rat and man, the only species for which its sequences are known, there are only two amino acid differences. By contrast, the leader peptides of rat and human GH differ in 12 of 26 sites, and those of rat and human Prl differ in 12 of 28 sites.

Following the leader sequence is a long peptide (109 amino acids in humans) that precedes the ACTH sequence. This region is generally termed the "N-terminal fragment" of POMC because of its location at the amino-terminal end and the lack of an identified biological activity. The presence of three pairs of basic amino acids in the human N-terminal fragment suggests it may be proteolytically cleaved. The first and second pairs of basic amino acids bound a dodecapeptide having considerable amino acid homology with the α-MSH region of ACTH and the β-MSH region of β-LPH. This homology has engendered the name γ-MSH for this region (169), but present evidence indicates it is not a significant cleavage product of rat or human POMC (176, 177), hence the term γ-MSH is used only to refer to this structure. When human pituitaries are extracted with acidified acetone, the only peptide derived from this 109 amino acid N-terminal region that is found in significant amounts is a 76 amino acid glycopeptide comprising amino acids 1–76

```
       -26                                                                              -1
b                   Leu       Ser
r
h   Met Pro Arg Ser Cys Cys Ser Arg Ser Gly Ala Leu Leu Leu Ala Leu Leu Leu Gln Ala Ser Met Glu Val Arg Gly


       +1                                                                   18    ┌IVS┐   20
b                                                                                 └─┬─┘
r                                                                                   Ala
h   Trp Cys Lue Glu Ser Ser Gln Cys Gln Asp Leu Thr Thr Glu Ser Asn Leu Leu  } Ala          Arg
                                                                                   Glu Cys Ile Arg Ala Cys Lys
        └───────── S-S ─────────┘                                                       └──── S-S ────┘
    ├────► N-TERMINAL GLYCOPEPTIDE                           40                     CHO
b                                        Val
r   Leu                                  Val
h   Pro Asp Leu Ser Ala Glu Thr Pro Met Phe Pro Gly Asn Gly Asp Glu Gln Pro Leu (Thr) Glu Asn Pro │Arg Lys│ Tyr


                          60                      CHO
b                                               Gly                      Val Gly              Ala
r                                       │Pro                    Ser Ala Gly         Ser Ala
h   Val Met Gly His Phe Arg Trp Asp Arg Phe Gly │Arg Arg (Asn)── Ser Ser Ser Ser Gly Ser Ser Gly Ala Gly Gly
    └──────────────── γ-MSH
            80                                                              Gly           Gly       Asp
b   │Arg      Ala    Glu    Ala Val   ── ── ── ── ── ── ── ── ── ──           Gly                   Asp
r   │    │Ala        Glu Glu Thr          Gly  ── ── ── ── ── ── ── ──                        Gly Arg
h   │Lys Arg│── Glu Asp Val Ser Ala Gly Glu Asp Cys Gly Thr Leu Pro Glu Gly Gly Pro Glu Pro Arg Ser Asp Gly


                        112                      120
b   Glu Thr                        Asp
r   Pro Glu     Ser
h   Ala Lys Pro Gly Pro Arg Glu Gly │Lys Arg│ Ser Tyr Ser Met Glu His Phe Arg Trp Gly Lys Pro Val Gly Lys │Lys
                        ├────► ACTH                      α-MSH

                        140                      CHO
b   Glu Thr                        Val              Gln
r                                  (Asn)
h   Arg│Arg Pro Val Lys Val Tyr Pro Asn Gly Ala Glu Asp Glu Ser Ala Glu Ala Phe Pro Leu Glu Phe │Lys Arg│ Glu
            ├──────► CLIP                                                                    153
                                                                                            ├──►
            160                                              200
b            Glu    Glu Gln Ala Arg           Glu Ala Gln       Glu Ser Ala     Ala Arg Ala Glu Leu Glu
r        Glu Glu Gln Pro Asp Gly  ── ── ──           Glu Ala Gln
h   Leu Thr Gly Gln Arg Leu Arg Glu Gly Asp Gly Pro Asp Gly Pro Ala Asp Asp Gly Ala Gly Ala Gln ── ── ──
    ├────► β-LPH

                                        191                  Ser         Lys
b   Tyr Gly Leu Val Ala Glu Ala Glu Ala Glu                      │Ala          Val
r   ── ── ──           Gln Val     Glu Pro Asp Thr │Lys Lys │ ── Ser ── ── Lys ── Val
h   ── Ala Asp Leu Glu His Ser Leu Leu Val Ala Ala Glu │Lys Lys │Asp Glu Gly Pro Tyr Arg Met Glu His Phe Arg
                                                                                             β-MSH

            211                              220
b
r               Asn                    │Asp Lys │
h   Trp Gly Ser Pro Pro Lys │Asp Lys │ Arg Tyr Gly Gly Phe Met Thr Ser Glu Lys Ser Gln Thr Pro Leu Val Thr Leu
    └──────────           ├────► β-ENDORPHIN

                                        240
b                               His         Gln
r               Val His │            │ Gln
h   Phe Lys Asn Ala Ile Ile Lys Asn Ala Tyr │Lys Lys │ Gly Glu OP
```

of hPOMC (177, 178). In hPOMC, a lysine-arginine pair follows the 76 amino acid region. This Lys-Arg pair may be cleaved in a fashion similar to the Lys-Arg pairs defining the boundaries of ACTH and β-endorphin. The 30 amino acid peptide of the N-terminal fragment that remains following cleavage of this 76 amino glycopeptide has been isolated only in trace amounts (177), suggesting that it is rapidly degraded. This 76 amino acid region is highly homologous among the three species, with significant differences only in its carboxy-terminal end (amino acids 65–76) (Figure 19).

Processing of the N-terminal region of rat POMC may differ in various tissues. Two major products termed 11K γ-MSH and 6K $γ_3$-MSH were found in both the rat anterior and neurointermediate lobes (176). The 11K material appears to represent the intact N-terminal glycopeptide, which is usually termed a 16K peptide, and the 6K or $γ_3$-MSH represents the MSH sequence connected to the 12 conserved amino acids on the carboxy-terminal end of the γ-MSH sequence. This processing scheme requires that both pairs of basic amino acids found in the rat N-terminal glycopeptide are cleaved, whereas two pairs of basic amino acids must remain uncleaved in the human N-terminal fragment in order to generate a 76 amino acid peptide. The N-terminal region has been frequently termed the "16K glycopeptide" because of an apparent molecular weight of 16,000–18,000 daltons on SDS-polyacrylamide gels. However, the rodent N-terminal glycopeptide has two major glycosylation sites having the sequence Asn-X-Ser/Thr, in addition to a third site (179), all of which are glycosylated. Similarly, the N-terminal fragment from human POMC has only one canonical glycosylation site having the sequence Asn-X-Ser, but it also contains at least one other glycosylated residue (Trp 45) and may contain still others (177, 180). As SDS-polyacrylamide gels may overestimate the molecular weight of glycoproteins (181), accurate determination of the molecular weights of the N-terminal peptides will be difficult.

The possible physiological role of such a glycopeptide is still uncertain. A significant body of data suggests that either the human 76 amino acid N-terminal glycopeptide (182) or the $γ_3$-MSH fragment of murine

---

Figure 19. Homologies among bovine, rat, and human POMC. Amino acid sequences were taken from the established gene sequences. Only the complete sequence of human pre-POMC is shown. For the bovine and rat sequences, the amino acids that differ from the human sequence are shown; those that are the same are represented as blanks. Where a sequence lacks an homologous amino acid, the gap is indicated as a dash. The amino acid numbers correspond only to the human sequence. The various known glycosylation sites are encircled and indicated with "CHO." The sequence of rat pre-POMC proximal to the intervening sequence (IVS) is unknown. The pairs of basic amino acids that represent major cleavage sites are enclosed in heavy boxes; other possible cleavage sites are enclosed in light boxes.

(183) or bovine (184) POMC may generally stimulate adrenal steroido-genesis. Other data (177, 178) suggest that this adrenocortical stimulatory effect occurs primarily in the aldosterone pathway.

Following the N-terminal glycopeptide and the first highly variable region is the 39 amino acid ACTH moiety. The structure of ACTH is known for many species and shows a very high degree of homology. Among the few amino acid changes seen among various species, all occur in the carboxy-terminal portion of the molecule. Since only the first 24 of the 39 amino acids are required for full biological activity, it is not surprising to find the known amino acid variation concentrated distal to the first 24 amino acids. Although ACTH has a Lys-Arg pair in its center, this sequence, unlike the other Lys-Arg pairs in human POMC, is not cleaved in the anterior pituitary. This lack of cleavage may be due to the presence of two other adjacent basic amino acids so that the sequence of the region is Lys-Lys-Arg-Arg, but this is purely speculative. However, the intermediate lobe of rodents and cattle does cleave this sequence so that α-MSH and CLIP and not ACTH, are the principal products of this region of POMC in those species.

The β-LPH region that follows the ACTH sequence is composed of three parts. The first is a region that is highly variable among the three species, again raising the question whether this region has any function other than acting as a spacer to permit proper processing, perhaps in a manner somewhat analogous to the C peptide of insulin. Following this spacer region is the highly conserved β-MSH region, which taken together with the preceding variable region is sometimes termed γ-LPH. The variable region of γ-LPH ranges in length from 19 amino acids in the rat to 40 amino acids in cattle, of which only 4 amino acids are homologous among cattle, rats, and humans. By contrast, the conserved portions of βLPH, β-MSH, and the opiate-like peptide β-endorphin are highly homologous, having only 7 of 51 amino acids different among the three species.

Thus the general structure of the POMC molecule is best conceptualized as consisting of five components. Three evolutionarily highly conserved regions, each containing an "MSH" sequence, are separated by two spacer regions. These spacer regions exhibit little homology of length or amino acid sequence among the various species, and, at least in the human anterior pituitary, appear to be degraded as by-products of the processing of POMC.

This model suggests the possibility that the POMC gene arose by two duplications yielding three generally homologous regions (the three conserved sequences), in a manner analogous to the model described above for GH and Prl.

Such a hypothesis would lead one to expect several intervening sequences in the POMC molecule, since it contains several different functional domains. But the genomic arrangement of the rat, bovine, and human POMC genes offers no support for this hypothesis. In all three species, all of the genomic DNA beginning with that encoding amino acid 19 and extending distally through the end of the POMC molecule and to the end of the region encoding the 3'-untranslated portion of the mRNA is contiguous and uninterrupted. The region "upstream" from amino acid 19 is equally surprising. In all three species, the DNA encoding amino acids 18 and 19 is separated by an intervening sequence of DNA about 3000 bases long. The structural arrangement of the hPOMC gene is shown in Figure 20 (173).

In addition to the 3.0 kb intervening sequence between the codons for amino acids 18 and 19, a second intervening sequence of 3.6 kb is found in the transcribed portion of the gene proximal to the first codon encoding the leader peptide. This arrangement is unusual. Many other genes, such as the members of the GH/CS/Prl family, have intervening sequences located shortly after the DNA encoding the 5' untranslated region of the mRNA. As discussed in Section 2.4, these have sometimes been termed "regulatory exons" as these regions contain the mRNA CAP site, the ribosome binding site, the AUG sequence that initiates translation, and possibly other regulatory elements as well. What is unusual about the POMC gene is that the first intervening sequence is found in the midst of this regulatory region. Thus the POMC gene illustrates that the "functional domain" hypothesis may not be applicable in all cases.

It is, of course, possible that the hPOMC gene contained other intervening sequences in the past and has lost them, as in the case of the rat insulin II gene. If such a loss occurred, it was probably mediated by DNA transposition rather than by unequal crossover or reverse transcription and reinsertion into the genome. Unequal crossovers are more likely where genes are duplicated, and reverse transcription and reinsertion favor creation of gene duplications. Present evidence indicates that the human genome contains only one POMC gene, located at the distal end of the short arm of chromosome 2 (173, 185). Cloning of POMC genes from submammalian species may reveal different structures, thus clarifying the evolutionary history of POMC.

5   OTHER POLYPEPTIDE HORMONE GENES

5.1   Somatostatin

Somatostatin regulates the secretion of several peptide hormones. Originally, somatostatin was isolated from the hypothalamus as an inhibitor of pituitary growth hormone release (186). Recently it has been shown to be localized in D cells of the endocrine pancreas (187, 188), where it inhibits the secretion of insulin and glucagon. It is localized also in se-

5'....cccggggagctgctccttgtgctgccgggaaggtcaaagtcccgcgccccaccaggagagctcggcaagTATATAAggacagagaggagcgcgga

*
cc AAGCGGCGGCGAAGGAGGGGAAGAAGAGCCGCCGACCCGAGAGAGGCCCGCCCGAGCCGTCCCCGCCCTCAGAGAGCAGCCTCCCGAGACAG GTAAG

GGCGCAGCGTGGGGGACCCGTGCTCTTTCCCCGGGATCC------------------IntronA -3.6kbp----------------AATGTTGGT
                              SmaI BamHI

TCAAGGTCCTCCTTGGTGAGTGGCCAACATTGTTTTGTCCTTGCAGGGGTCCCACCAATCTTGTTTGCTTCTGCAG AGCCTCAGCCTGCCTGGAAG

pre-peptide   -20   -10
Met Pro Arg Ser Cys Cys Ser Arg Ser Gly Ala Leu Leu Leu Ala Leu Leu Leu Gln Ala Ser Met Glu Val Arg
ATG CCG AGA TCG TGC TGC AGC CGC TCG GGG GCC CTG TTG CTG GCC TTG CTG CTT CAG GCC TCC ATG GAA GTG CGT
                            AvaI

16 K - PEPTIDE
    -1 1   10
Gly Trp Cys Leu Glu Ser Ser Gln Cys Gln Asp Leu Thr Thr Glu Ser Asn Leu Leu
GGC TGG TGC CTA GAG AGC AGC CAG TGT CAG GAC CTC ACC ACG GAA AGC AAC CTG CTG GTACGTGGGCCATGACTGCCATC

TTGGCTAGACATTA----------------IntronB -3kbp-------------ATTCAGTAGACTTTGGTCCTGTTCACAAAAGCTAGGGGTGGCT

AGATGGCTAGACAAACCATGGAATGGGAATGGGAAGTGTGTTGCAGTTGCCAGGCAGAAGCATGAAGGGGATGGGACAAAAGAGGCGGTGGCAAGATCT
                                                                                          BglII

TAGATGCCCACGAGTGCCAAGAAAGCAGGTGGGCAGACCTGCTCTGTAGGGAGGCCTCGACACCTTGACACGCCCGACACTGTGCCCTGTGTCCTCGGC

ACGTGGCCGAGGGCGGCCAGGGCCTAGGCGCAGTGACGGGCGCGCAACCGGGCCGGGTGCGGGGCACGGGCTGCCCTCATGCCCTCGCGTCTTCCCCCAG

          20   30   40
Glu Cys Ile Arg Ala Cys Lys Pro Asp Leu Ser Ala Glu Thr Pro Met Phe Pro Gly Asn Gly Asp Glu Gln Pro
GAG TGC ATC CGG GCC TGC AAG CCC GAC CTC TCG GCC GAG ACT CCC ATG TTC CCG GGA AAT GGC GAC GAG CAG CCT

          50   60
Leu Thr Glu Asn Pro Arg Lys Tyr Val Met Gly His Phe Arg Trp Asp Arg Phe Gly Arg Arg Asn Ser Ser Ser
CTG ACC GAG AAC CCC CGG AAG TAC GTC ATG GGC CAC TTC CGC TGG GAC CGA TTC GGC CGC CGC AAC AGC AGC AGC

          70   80   90
Ser Gly Ser Ser Gly Ala Gly Gln Lys Arg Glu Asp Val Ser Ala Gly Glu Asp Cys Gly Thr Leu Pro Glu Gly
AGC GGC AGC AGC GGC GCA GGG CAG AAG CGC GAG GAC GTC TCA GCG GGC GAA GAC TGC GGC ACG CTG CCT GAG GGC

                                                              110   **ACTH**
Gly Pro Glu Pro Arg Ser Asp Gly Ala Lys Pro Gly Pro Arg Glu Gly Lys Arg Ser Tyr Ser Met Glu His Phe
GGC CCC GAG CCC CGC AGC GAT GGT GCC AAG CCG GGC CCG CGC GAG GGC AAG CGC TCC TAC TCC ATG GAG CAC TTC

          120   130   140
Arg Trp Gly Lys Pro Val Gly Lys Lys Arg Arg Pro Val Lys Val Tyr Pro Asn Gly Ala Glu Asp Glu Ser Ala
CGC TGG GGC AAG CCG GTG GGC AAG AAG CCG CGC CCA GTG AAG GTG TAC CCT AAC GGC GCC GAG GAC GAG TCG GCC

                            ß-LPH   160
Glu Ala Phe Pro Leu Glu Phe Lys Arg Glu Leu Thr Gly Gln Arg Leu Arg Glu Gly Asp Gly Pro Asp Gly Pro
GAG GCC TTC CCC CTA GAG TTC AAG AGG GAG CTG ACT GGC CAG CGA CTC CGG GAG GGA GAT GGC CCC GAC GGC CCT

          170   180   190
Ala Asp Asp Gly Ala Gly Ala Gln Ala Asp Leu Glu His Ser Leu Leu Val Ala Ala Glu Lys Lys Asp Glu Gly
GCC GAT GAC GGC GCA GGG GCC CAG GCC GAC CTG GAG CAC AGC CTG CTG GTG GCG GCC GAG AAG AAG GAC GAG GGC

          200   210   **ß-ep**
Pro Tyr Arg Met Glu His Phe Arg Trp Gly Ser Pro Pro Lys Asp Lys Arg Tyr Gly Gly Phe Met Thr Ser Glu
CCC TAC AGG ATG GAG CAC TTC CGC TGG GGC AGC CCG CCC AAG GAC AAG CGC TAC GGC GGT TTC ATG ACC TCC GAG

          220   230   240
Lys Ser Gln Thr Pro Leu Val Thr Leu Phe Lys Asn Ala Ile Ile Lys Asn Ala Tyr Lys Lys Gly Glu ***
AAG AGC CAG ACG CCC CTG GTG ACG CTG TTC AAA AAC GCC ATC ATC AAG AAC GCC TAC AAG AAG GGC GAG TGA GGG

CACAGCGGGGCCCCAGGGCTAACCTCCCCCAGGAGGTCGACCCCAAAGCCCCTTGCTCTCCCCTGCCCTGCTGCCGCCTCCCAGCCTGGGGGGTCGTGG
                                    SalI

CAGATAATCAGCCTCTTAAAGCCGCCTGTAGTTAGGAAATAAACCTTTCAAATTTCACA tccacctctgactttgaatgtaaactgtgtgaataaa
                                            ↑
                                          poly A

gtaaaaatacgtagccgcaata....3'

66

lected endothelial cells that line the gastrointestinal tract, where it inhibits release of the gastrointestinal hormones, secretin (189), gastrin (190), and cholecystokinin (191). In addition, somatostatin is thought to play a role in neurotransmission, since it has been found in other brain regions (192, 193), spinal cord (194), and sympathetic nerve fibers (195).

Somatostatin contains 14 amino acids and is synthesized as part of a larger precursor molecule of about 120 amino acids, which is processed to yield the mature polypeptide (for a review, see ref. 196). Some of the precursor somatostatin-containing polypeptides retain immunoreactivity with somatostatin antibodies (197–202) and biological activity (203); such a peptide of 28 amino acid residues has been isolated from porcine intestinal tissue (204).

Complementary DNA to the mRNAs for somatostatins have been cloned and characterized by sequence analysis from the anglerfish (205, 206), channel catfish (207), and humans (208). Analysis of the anglerfish somatostatin cDNA predicted a 121 amino acid polypeptide precursor that contained somatostatin at its carboxy terminus. A second cDNA was also isolated that contained a carboxy-terminal somatostatin-like moiety with two amino acid differences, a Tyr in place of Phe_7 and a Gly in place of Thr_{10}. The sequence corresponding to the known somatostatin amino acid sequence was designated somatostatin I and the other somatostatin II. The latter molecule has been chemically synthesized; it inhibits insulin release selectively with no observable effect on glucagon release. Two different forms of channel catfish somatostatin have also been isolated (207, 209, 210). These data indicate that the diverse biological effects of somatostatin may be due to the presence of several related polypeptides. In humans only the sequence coding for somatostatin I has been identified at the present time. This precursor contains both somatostatin 14 and somatostatin 28.

The precursor to somatostatin contains a signal peptide, which is involved in the secretion of the hormone. Comparison of the human sequence with that of anglerfish somatostatin indicates that this region has diverged extensively. Nevertheless, it contains an abundance of neutral amino acids common to signal peptide regions of other secreted proteins. The general organization of the human and anglerfish mRNA precursors is essentially the same. Both contain a signal sequence, a large translated region whose function is unknown, and sequences for somatostatin 28 and somatostatin 14 at the carboxy terminus. Somatostatin 28 contains somatostatin 14 at its carboxy terminus. Generation

---

Figure 20. Structure of the human POMC gene. Nucleotides that are transcribed into pre-mRNA are indicated with capital letters; the 5′ and 3′ flanking DNA is indicated with lower-case letters. The CAP site is indicated with an asterisk. Reproduced with permission from Whitfeld et al. (173).

of the mature forms of the hormone is thought to proceed via posttranslational processing of the prohormone. This is supported by the finding of a basic dipeptide (Arg-Lys) immediately preceding the somatostatin 14 sequence. There is only a single Arg residue preceding the somatostatin 28 sequence. These data suggest that trypsin-like proteases may be involved in the processing of these hormones. Currently, it is not known whether the formation of somatostatin 14 requires the prior formation of somatostatin 28 or whether these two moieties are independently processed.

Comparison of the human and anglerfish mRNAs (208) reveals that the somatostatin 14 sequence is precisely conserved and the somatostatin 28 sequences are 79% homologous. Homology of somatostatin 28 sequences between the two species is greatest near the cleavage sites, suggesting that maintenance of the cleavage sites is important for processing. The conservation of the somatostatin 28 peptide among mammals suggests that this protein may have separate biological functions. Moreover, these two peptides (somatostatin-14 and -28) bind to the somatostatin receptors in various cells with different affinities (211). Nevertheless, the amino terminal sequences of somatostatin 28 in anglerfish and humans are quite divergent. The functional significance of this is currently unknown.

The propeptide that precedes the somatostatin sequences displays conservation of acidic, basic, and hydrophobic and hydrophilic residues. Thus it is possible that the propeptide may have a biological function either to maintain the correct structure of the molecule for proper processing or to serve some separate biological activity.

5.2   Calcitonin and Parathyroid Hormone

5.2.1   Calcitonin

Calcitonin is a peptide of 32 amino acids that has serum calcium-lowering activities. It may also have other actions such as regulating the appetite (212). Calcitonin is produced in the parafollicular cells of the thyroid gland of mammals and in the ultimobranchial glands in lower vertebrates. It is also produced by medullary thyroid carcinomas.

Data from the cell-free translation of calcitonin mRNA suggest that the hormone is synthesized as a larger precursor protein of molecular weight 15,000–17,500 daltons (213, 214). The rat calcitonin cDNA has now been cloned and sequenced (213, 214), and information about the precursor has been obtained. Based on the cDNA sequence and other analyses, it is known that the calcitonin coding sequence arises from an mRNA that codes for a protein of 136 amino acids (214). The precursor protein contains a leader peptide of 25 amino acids that presumably is cleaved as the protein is inserted into the endoplasmic reticulum. The 32 amino acid calcitonin sequence is flanked on its amino terminus by a Lys-Arg basic dipeptide that presumably serves as a site for peptidase action in cleaving calcitonin from the precursor protein. The carboxy-terminal proline is flanked by a glycine followed by three basic amino acids, Lys-Lys-Arg, that also are presumably a site for proteolytic cleavage. The carboxy-terminal proline is amidated, and for this to occur the glycine may be required (as in other systems). Between the spacer sequence and the calcitonin sequence are 59 amino acids (214) that do not have known homology with any other known hormone or other protein. They may reflect a protein with a potential functional role, although there is no evidence for this and it is not known whether this sequence or a portion of it is produced as a distinct peptide.

Calcitonin mRNA has been estimated to contain approximately 1050 nucleotides; the 3' untranslated region of the mRNA contains 600 nucleotides (214, 215). The function of this sequence is not known. A number of larger-molecular-weight RNA species from 6400 to 1200 nucleotides have also been detected, by Northern blot analysis (215).

Older rats have a high incidence of medullary thyroid carcinoma (215). When propagated in tissue culture, these tumors produce calcitonin (215). The production usually decreases with time, but in this case, surprisingly, the content of calcitonin mRNA shows little or no change. Instead, the size distribution of the mature and precursor mRNA forms changes (215). The major mRNA becomes approximately 1250 nucleotides and there is a marked increase in a 3800 nucleotide species (215). The primary translation product of this "pseudocalcitonin" mRNA does not react with antiserum to calcitonin and is about 16,000 daltons (instead of 17,500 daltons) (216). It appears that this mRNA form is generated by different processing of a primary mRNA transcript (216).

Although the complete structure of the calcitonin gene has not yet been elucidated, the gene has been found to contain at least four introns (216). Two of these introns divide the coding region for the peptide that is amino-terminal to calcitonin, a third intron precedes the calcitonin coding sequence, and a fourth precedes a coding sequence downstream from calcitonin. Differential processing of the pre-mRNA generated from this gene results in two different mRNAs. Both mRNAs contain the region that is amino-terminal to calcitonin. However, in the pseudocalcitonin mRNA, the 32 amino acid calcitonin coding sequence is absent and is replaced by a 37 amino acid coding sequence (located downstream from the calcitonin coding sequence in the gene) followed by a Gly-Arg-Arg-Arg-Arg sequence that may be a site for cleavage of the 37 amino acid peptides from a larger precursor. This provides another example of a single gene that has evolved to produce more than one form of mRNA.

5.2.2 Parathyroid Hormone

Parathyroid hormone (PTH) is an 84 amino acid polypeptide involved in calcium homeostasis (217). It is synthesized as a preprohormone; after cleavage of a 25 amino acid signal peptide sequence to yield pro-PTH, a hexapeptide is subsequently removed in the processing to yield PTH. There is information about the structure of cDNAs to human (218) and bovine (219) PTH mRNA; no genomic DNA structural data are yet available. Furthermore, PTH is not known to have sequence homology with other hormones. Despite this limited information, several structural features are noteworthy. Bovine PTH and hPTH do not exhibit a preference for G or C in the third position of codons as do bGH and hGH; only 43% of bPTH codons and 40% of hPTH codons end in G or C. There is significant homology between the amino acids of bPTH and hPTH (72 of 84 amino acids). Furthermore, all 6 amino acids in the hexapeptide "prosequence" and 20 of 25 amino acids of the signal peptide "presequence" are identical. The number of silent nucleotide replacements that have occurred is much less than theoretically expected; this may imply that selective pressure acts to preserve structure at the nucleic acid sequence level as well as at the amino acid sequence level. Major homology also exists in the 5' and 3' untranslated portions of the mRNA. The 5' noncoding portion of the mRNA is relatively shorter (ca. 25 nucleotides); the significance of this is not known. In the 3' noncoding region of the human but not the bovine mRNA exist two AAUAAA structures separated by about 65 nucleotides. These two structures also share homology surrounding the AAUAAA, implying the possibility that partial gene duplication occurred to generate the extra site.

5.3 Glycoprotein Hormones

The glycoprotein hormones include thyroid stimulating hormone (TSH), follicle stimulating hormone (FSH), luteinizing hormone (LH) and chorionic gonadotropin (CG).

All four hormones contain two glycosylated subunits. Th e α subunit (92 amino acids in the case of humans) is common to all of them; the β subunits of CG, LH, FSH, and TSH contain 145, 115, 118, and 112 amino acids, respectively. The β subunits of CG and LH are very similar, differing mostly by the existence of 28–30 extra carboxy-terminal amino acids in CG that are not present in the LH subunit. It is thought that the β subunit confers target tissue specificity for hormone binding and that the α subunit is involved in post-receptor binding and information transfer.

The primary structure of cDNA to mRNA for the α subunit of mouse TSH (220) and hCG (221) and for the β-subunit of hCG (222) has been reported. Cloning of the cDNA for the α and β subunits of mouse TSH was also reported by a different group, but sequence information was not provided (223). This cDNA had a restriction map completely different from the one published by Chin et al. (220), and therefore its identity is in question (220).

The sequence of mouse TSH α subunit (220) displays 93% homology with the bovine (224), 91% homology with the ovine (225), 98% homology with the porcine (226), 82% homology with the equine (227), and 75% homology with the human subunits (221, 228). The amino acids that differ represent conservative substitutions, thereby preserving the hydrophobic or hydrophilic properties of the amino acids. These changes can be explained largely by single base substitutions. There are regions of strict conservation of sequence including positions 31–44, 49–53, 62–67, and 81–85 (218, 229, 230); these may be critical for the hormone's activity. Whereas the homology between the nucleotide sequences for the mouse and human apoprotein and signal peptide sequences is high (85 and 77%, respectively), there is little homology in the 5' and 3' untranslated sequences (220, 221).

The β subunits differ among the glycoprotein hormones; however, they are related as documented by amino acid sequence homology that ranges from 30% between hCG and hFSH to about 80% between hCG and hLH (222); 12 cysteine residues are completely conserved as well as 34–38 amino acids (222). The β subunits of hLH and hCG are similar except for differences in carbohydrate content and a carboxy-terminal extension of about 30 amino acids for hCG not found in hLH. Interestingly, an examination of the nucleotide sequences of hCG suggests that there could have been a mutation at the termination codon for a precursor to the present hCG β subunit, converting it to an amino acid codon that would permit translation read-through into the 3' nontranslated portion until a UAA terminator was reached about 30 codons downstream (222). This termination sequence is located in the AAUAAA structure, thought also to be the signal for polyadenylation. A similar mechanism for the evolution of an abnormal hemoglobin gene (Constant Spring) has also been proposed (222).

There is some homology between the α and β subunits of hCG, which have 16.1% amino acid sequence homology (not including deletions and insertions). Further, 6 of the 12 cysteine residues are conserved (222). The nucleic acid sequence homology is a modest 31%, but this is probably significant; also, certain areas are more homologous, especially in the regions of the cystine residues. In spite of these similarities, there are differences in the base composition; the G + C content of hCG α cDNA is 44.5%, whereas that of hCG β cDNA is 66%. Taken together, these data suggest that the α and β subunit genes are evolutionarily related and probably emerged from a common ancestral gene.

J.C. Fiddes and N.C. Vamvakopoulos (personal communication) have studied the chromosomal genes for the glycoprotein hormones. They find only one α gene, providing further support for the notion that the α subunit is common for the four hormones. As expected, they have found a family of β subunit genes (at least seven) and in some instances have found that these are located closely together on the same chromosome. Some also have homology in their intervening sequences. Two of these linked genes appear to be in opposite orientations. In summary, it appears that a precursor gene was duplicated and that a single α subunit gene and a family of β subunit genes evolved from this duplicated pair.

REFERENCES

1. W. Wickner, *Science* **210**, 861 (1980).
2. V. R. Lingappa and G. Blobel, *Recent Prog. Horm. Res.* **36**, 451 (1980).
3. W. Gilbert and L. Villa-Komaroff, *Sci. Am.* **242**, 74 (1980).
4. J. D. Baxter, *Hosp. Pract.* **15**, 57 (1980).
5. W. L. Miller, *J. Pediatr.* **99**, 1 (1981).
6. B. Lewin, *Gene Expression Vol. 3, Plasmids and Phages*, Vol. 3, Wiley, New York, 1977.
7. D. Nathans and H. O. Smith, *Ann. Rev. Biochem.* **44**, 273 (1975).
8. D. Baltimore, *Nature* **226**, 1209 (1970).
9. H. M. Temin and S. Mizutani, *Nature* **226**, 1211 (1970).
10. A. C. Y. Chang, J. H. Nunberg, R. J. Kaufman, H. A. Erlich, R. T. Schimke, and S. N. Cohen, *Nature* **275**, 617 (1978).
11. F. Bolivar, R. L. Rodriquez, P. J. Greene, M. C. Betlach, H. L. Heyneker, H. W. Boyer, J. H. Crosa, and S. Falkow, *Gene* **2**, 95 (1977).
12. P. Leder, D. Tiemeier, and L. Enquist, *Science* **196**, 175 (1977).
13. F. R. Blattner, B. G. Williams, A. E. Blechl, K. Dennison-Thompson, H. E. Faber, L. A. Furburg, D. J. Grunwald, D. O. Kiefer, D. D. Moore, E. L. Schinn, and O. Smithies, *Science* **196**, 161 (1977).
14. F. G. Grosveld, H.-H. M. Dahl, E. deBoer, and R. A. Flavell, *Gene* **13**, 227 (1981).
15. W. A. Gilbert, *Nature* **271**, 501 (1978).
16. J. Darnell, *Science* **202**, 1257 (1978).
17. F. H. C. Crick, *Science* **204**, 264 (1979).
18. P. A. Sharp, *Cell* **23**, 647 (1981).
19. B. Lewin, *Cell* **22**, 645 (1980).
20. D. H. Hamer and P. Leder, *Cell* **18**, 1299 (1979).
21. V. Murry and R. Holliday, *FEBS Lett.* **106**, 5 (1979).
22. J. Rogers and R. Wall, *Proc. Natl. Acad. Sci. USA* **77**, 1877 (1980).
23. M. R. Lerner, J. A. Boyle, M. S. Mount, L. S. Wolin, and J. A. Steitz, *Nature* **283**, 220 (1980).
24. V. W. Yang, M. R. Lerner, J. A. Steitz, and S. J. Flint, *Proc. Natl. Acad. Sci. USA* **78**, 1371 (1981).
25. V. E. Avvedimento, G. Vogeli, Y. Yamada, J. V. Maizel Jr., I. Pastan, and B. Crommbrugghe, *Cell* **21**, 689 (1980).
26. E. M. DeRobertis, P. Black, and K. Nishikura, *Cell* **23**, 89 (1981).
27. R. P. Perry and D. E. Kelly, *Cell* **1**, 37 (1974).
28. A. J. Shatkin, *Cell* **9**, 635 (1976).
29. C. M. Wei and B. Moss, *Proc. Natl. Acad. Sci. USA* **71**, 3014 (1974).
30. J. K. Rose and H. F. Lodish, *Nature* **262**, 32 (1976).

31. S. Muthukrishnan, M. Morgan, A. K. Bannerjee, and A. J. Shatkin, *Biochemistry* **15**, 5761 (1976).
32. H. F. Lodish and J. K. Rose, *J. Biol. Chem.* **252**, 1181 (1977).
33. J. Shine and L. Delgarno, *Proc. Natl. Acad. Sci. USA* **71**, 1342 (1974).
34. B. Lewin, *Gene Expression Vol. 2, Eukaryotic Genes*, Vol. 3, Wiley, New York, 2nd edition 1980, pp. 675–683.
35. J. A. Steitz and K. Jakes, *Proc. Natl. Acad. Sci. USA* **72**, 4734 (1975).
36. N. J. Proudfoot and G. G. Brownlee, *Nature* **263**, 211 (1976).
36a. Y. Nishioka and P. Leder, *Cell* **18**, 875 (1979).
37. C. Benoist, K. O'Hare, R. Breathnach, and P. Chambon, *Nucleic Acids Res.* **8**, 127 (1980).
38. M. Goldberg, Ph.D. Thesis, Stanford University, 1979.
39. G. I. Bell, R. L. Pictet, W. J. Rutter, B. Cordell, E. Tischer, and H. M. Goodman, *Nature* **284**, 26 (1980).
40. F. M. DeNoto, D. D. Moore, and H. M. Goodman, *Nucleic Acids Res.* **9**, 3719 (1981).
41. D. T. Kurtz, *Nature* **291**, 629 (1981).
42. E. Buetti and H. Diggelmann, *Cell* **23**, 335 (1981).
43. F. Lee, R. Mulligan, P. Berg, and G. Ringold, *Nature* **294**, 228 (1981).
44. M. Karin, N. L. Eberhardt, R. I. Richards, A. Barta, N. Malich, J. Martial, J. D. Baxter, and G. Cathala, submitted.
45. D. M. Robins, I. Paek, P. H. Seeburg, and R. Axel, *Cell*, **29**, 623 (1982).
46. V. M. Ingram, *The Hemoglobins in Genetics and Evolution*, Columbia University Press, New York, 1963.
47. A. Kornberg, *DNA Replication*, W. H. Freeman and Co., San Francisco, 1980, pp. 607–650.
48. E. Zuckerkandl and L. Pauling, in M. Kasha and B. Pullman, Eds., *Horizons in Biochemistry*, Academic Press, New York, 1962, pp. 189–225.
49. E. Zuckerkandl and L. Pauling, in V. Bryson and H. J. Vogel, Eds., *Evolving Genes and Proteins*, Academic Press, New York, 1965, pp. 97–166.
50. M. O. Dayhoff, R. V. Eck, and C. M. Park, in M. O. Dayhoff, Ed., *Atlas of Protein Sequence and Structure*, Vol. 5, National Biomedical Research Foundation, Washington, D. C., 1972, pp. 89–99.
51. A. C. Wilson, S. S. Carlson, and J. T. White, *Ann. Rev. Biochem.* **46**, 573 (1977).
52. F. Perler, A. Efstratiadis, P. Lomedico, W. Gilbert, R. Kolodner, and J. Dodgson, *Cell* **20**, 555 (1980).
53. A. Efstratiadis, J. W. Posakony, T. Maniatis, R. M. Lawn, C. O'Connell, R. A. Spritz, J. K. DeRiel, B. G. Forget, S. M. Weissman, J. L. Slightom, A. E. Blechl, O. Smithies, F. E. Baralle, C. C. Shoulders, and N. J. Proudfoot, *Cell* **21**, 653 (1980).
54. N. E. Cooke, D. Coit, J. Shine, J. D. Baxter, and J. A. Martial, *J. Biol. Chem.* **256**, 4006 (1981).
55. M. O. Dayhoff, R. M. Schwartz, and B. C. Orcutt, in M. O. Dayhoff, Ed., *Atlas of Protein Sequence and Structure*, Vol. 5, Suppl. 3, National Biomedical Research Foundation, Washington, D. C., 1978, pp. 345–352.
56. T. Miyata, S. Miyazawa, and T. Yasunaga, *J. Mol. Evol.* **12**, 219 (1979).
57. W. L. Miller, D. Coit, J. D. Baxter, and J. A. Martial, *DNA* **1**, 37 (1981).
58. W. L. Miller and S. H. Mellon, in K. W. Mc Kerns, Ed., *Regulation of Gene Expression by Hormones*, Plenum Press, New York, 1983, pp. 177-202.
59. A. Deisseroth, A. Nienhuis, P. Turner, R. Valez, W. F. Anderson, J. Lawrence, R. Creagan, and R. Kucherlapati, *Cell* **12**, 205 (1977).
60. A. Deisseroth, A. Nienhuis, J. Lawrence, R. Giles, P. Turner, and F. H. Ruddle, *Proc. Natl. Acad. Sci. USA* **75**, 1456 (1978).
61. F. W. Alt, R. E. Kellems, J. R. Bertino, and R. T. Schimke, *J. Biol. Chem.* **253**, 1357 (1978).
62. R. J. Britten and D. E. Kohne, *Science* **161**, 529 (1968).

63. G. F. Saunders, S. Shirakawa, P. P. Saunders, F. E. Arrighi, and T. C. Hsu, *J. Mol. Biol.* **63**, 323 (1972).

64. C. W. Schmid and P. L. Deininger, *Cell* **6**, 345 (1975).

65. A. S. Perelson and G. I. Bell, *Nature* **265**, 304 (1977).

66. G. P. Smith, *Science* **191**, 528 (1976).

67. W. F. Doolittle and C. Sapienza, *Nature* **284**, 601 (1980).

68. L. E. Orgel and F. H. C. Crick, *Nature* **284**, 604 (1980).

69. C. Baglioni, *Proc. Natl. Acad. Sci. USA* **48**, 1880 (1962).

70. R. W. Jones, J. M. Old, R. J. Trent, J. B. Clegg, and D. J. Weatherall, *Nature* **291**, 39 (1981).

71. D. Owerbach, J. A. Martial, J. D. Baxter, W. J. Rutter, and T. B. Shows, *Science* **209**, 289 (1980).

72. D. Owerbach, W. J. Rutter, N. E. Cooke, J. A. Martial, and T. B. Shows, *Science* **212**, 815 (1981).

73. J. M. Bishop, *New Engl. J. Med.* **303**, 675 (1980).

74. J. M. Bishop, *Cell* **23**, 5 (1981).

75. L. H. Wang, P. Snyder, T. Hanafusa, and H. Hanafusa, *J. Virol.* **35**, 52 (1980).

76. M. P. Calos and J. H. Miller, *Cell* **20**, 579 (1980).

77. P. Jagadeeswaran, B. G. Forget, and S. M. Weissman, *Cell* **26**, 141 (1981).

78. H. F. Acevedo, M. Slifkin, G. R. Pouchet, and M. Pardo, *Cancer* **41**, 1217 (1978).

79. T. Mauro, H. Cohen, S. J. Segal, and S. S. Koide, *Proc. Natl. Acad. Sci. USA* **76**, 6622 (1979).

80. J. Roth, D. LeRoith, J. Shiloah, J. L. Rosenzweig, M. A. Lesniak, and J. Havrankova, *New Engl. J. Med.* **306**, 523 (1982).

81. D. LeRoith, J. Shiloach, J. Roth, and M. A. Lesniak, *Proc. Natl. Acad. Sci. USA* **77**, 6184 (1980).

82. D. LeRoith, J. Shiloach, J. Roth, and M. A. Lesniak, *J. Biol. Chem.* **256**, 6533 (1981).

83. M. Berelowitz, D. LeRoith, and H. von Schenk, *Endocrinology*, in press.

84. D. LeRoith, A. S. Liotta, J. Roth, J. Shiloach, M. E. Lewis, C. B. Pert, and D. T. Krieger, *Proc. Natl. Acad. Sci. USA* **79**, 2086 (1982).

85. Z. Rosenzweig and S. H. Kindler, *FEBS Lett.* **25**, 221 (1972).

86. J. -O. Josefsson and P. Johansson, *Nature* **282**, 78 (1979).

87. K. J. Catt, B. Moffat and H. D. Niall, *Science* **157**, 321 (1967).

88. L. M. Sherwood, *Proc. Natl. Acad. Sci. USA* **58**, 2307 (1967).

89. C. H. Li, J. S. Dixon, T. B. Lo, Y. M. Pankov, and K. D. Schmidt, *Nature* **224**, 695 (1967).

90. H. D. Niall, M. L. Hogan, R. Sayer, I. Y. Rosenblum, and F. C. Greenwood, *Proc. Natl. Acad. Sci. USA* **68**, 866 (1971).

91. W. L. Miller, J. A. Martial, and J. D. Baxter, *J. Biol. Chem.* **255**, 7521 (1980).

92. J. A. Martial, R. A. Hallewell, J. D. Baxter, and H. M. Goodman, *Science* **205**, 602 (1979).

93. W. G. Roskam and F. Rougeon, *Nucleic Acids Res.* **7**, 305 (1979).

94. P. H. Seeburg, J. Shine, J. A. Martial, J. D. Baxter, and H. M. Goodman, *Nature* **270**, 486 (1977).

95. N. L. Sasavage, J. H. Nilson, S. Horowitz, and F. M. Rottman, *J. Biol. Chem.* **257**, 678 (1982).

96. E. J. Gubbins, R. A. Maurer, M. Lagrimini, C. R. Erwin, and J. E. Donelson, *J. Biol. Chem.* **255**, 8655 (1980).

97. N. E. Cooke, D. Coit, R. I. Weiner, J. D. Baxter, and J. A. Martial, *J. Biol. Chem.* **255**, 6502 (1980).

98. J. Shine, P. H. Seeburg, J. Martial, J. D. Baxter, and H. M. Goodman, *Nature* **270**, 494 (1977).

99. H. M. Goodman, F. DeNoto, J. C. Fiddes, R. A. Hallewell, G. S. Page, S. Smith, and E. Tischer, in W. A. Scott, R. Werner, D. R. Joseph, and J. Schultz, Eds., *Mobiliza-*

tion and Reassembly of Genetic Information, Academic Press, New York, 1980, pp. 155–179.

100. B. Clarke, *Science* **168**, 1009 (1970).
101. R. C. Richmond, *Nature* **225**, 1025 (1970).
102. T. I. Blundell and S. P. Wood, *Nature* **257**, 197 (1975).
103. M. Kimura, *Sci. Am.* **241**, 98 (1979).
104. M. Kimura, *J. Mol. Evol.* **16**, 111 (1980).
105. M. Kimura, *Proc. Natl. Acad. Sci. USA* **78**, 454 (1981).
106. L. Hood, J. H. Campbell, and S. C. R. Elgin, *Ann. Rev. Genet.* **9**, 305 (1975).
107. E. A. Zimmer, S. L. Martin, S. M. Beverley, Y. W. Kan, and A. C. Wilson, *Proc. Natl. Acad. Sci. USA* **77**, 2158 (1980).
108. N. Arnheim, M. Krystal, R. Schmickel, G. Wilson, O. Ryder, and E. Zimmer, *Proc. Natl. Acad. Sci. USA* **77**, 7323 (1980).
109. S. A. Liebhaber, M. Goossens, and Y. W. Kan, *Nature* **290**, 26 (1981).
110. N. E. Cooke and J. D. Baxter, *Nature*, **297**, 603 (1982).
111. A. Barta, R. I. Richards, J. D. Baxter, and J. Shine, *Proc. Natl. Acad. Sci. USA* **78**, 4867 (1981).
112. J. C. Fiddes, P. H. Seeburg, F. M. DeNoto, R. A. Hellewell, J. D. Baxter, and H. M. Goodman, *Proc. Natl. Acad. Sci. USA* **76**, 4294 (1979).
113. G. I. Bell, R. Pictet, and W. J. Rutter, *Nucleic Acids Res.* **8**, 4091 (1980).
114. T. -M. Wong, C. H. K. Li, and C. H. Li, *Proc. Natl. Acad. Sci. USA* **78**, 88 (1981).
115. T. L. Blundell and R. E. Humbel, *Nature* **287**, 781 (1980).
116. S. J. Chan, P. Keim, and D. F. Steiner, *Proc. Natl. Acad. Sci. USA* **73**, 1964 (1976).
117. T. P. Lomedico, S. J. Chan, D. F. Steiner, and G. F. Saunders, *J. Biol. Chem.* **252**, 7971 (1977).
118. D. Shields and G. Blobel, *Proc. Natl. Acad. Sci. USA* **74**, 2059 (1977).
119. R. E. Humbel, H. R. Bosshard, and H. Zain, in D. F. Steiner and H. Freinkel, Eds., *Handbook of Physiology*, Sect. 7, Vol. 1, Williams and Wilkins, Baltimore, 1972, pp. 111–132.
120. L. Balant, I. M. Burr, W. Stauffacher, D. P. Cameron, H. F. Buenzi, R. E. Humbel, and A. E. Renold, *Endocrinology* **88**, 517 (1971).
121. G. Bell, W. Swain, R. Pictet, B. Cordell, H. Goodman, and W. J. Rutter, *Nature* **282**, 525 (1979).
122. I. Sures, D. V. Goeddel, A. Gray, and A. Ullrich, *Science* **208**, 57 (1980).
123. A. Ullrich, J. Shine, J. Chirgwin, R. Pictet, E. Tischer, W. J. Rutter, and H. M. Goodman, *Science* **196**, 1313 (1977).
124. L. Villa-Kamaroff, A. Efstradiadis, S. Broome, P. Lomedico, R. Tizard, S. P. Naber, W. L. Chick, and W. L. Gilbert, *Proc. Natl. Acad. Sci. USA* **75**, 3727 (1978).
125. S. J. Chan, B. E. Noyes, K. L. Agarwal, and D. F. Steiner, *Proc. Natl. Acad. Sci. USA* **76**, 5036 (1979).
126. P. M. Hobart, L. Shen, R. Crawford, R. L. Pictet, and W. J. Rutter, *Science* **210**, 1360 (1980).
127. S. J. Chan, S. O. Emdin, S. C. M. Kwok, J. M. Kramer, S. Falkner, and D. F. Steiner, *J. Biol. Chem.* **256**, 7593 (1979).
128. P. Lomedico, N. Rosenthal, A. Efstradiadis, W. Gilbert, R. Kolodner, and R. Tizard, *Cell* **18**, 545 (1979).
129. B. Cordell, G. Bell, E. Tischer, F. M. DeNoto, A. Ullrich, R. Pictet, W. J. Rutter, and H. M. Goodman, *Cell* **18**, 533 (1979).
130. A. Ullrich, T. J. Dull, A. Gray, J. Brosius, and I. Sures, *Science* **209**, 612 (1980).
131. D. F. Steiner, *Diabetes* **27**, Suppl. 1, 145 (1978).
132. A. Wollmer, D. Brandenburg, H. P. Vogt, and W. Schermutzki, *Hoppe-Seyler's Z. Physiol. Chem.* **355**, 1471 (1974).
133. D. F. Steiner, in G. D. Fasam, Ed., *Handbook of Biochemistry and Molecular Biology*, Vol. 3, 3rd ed. CRC Press, Cleveland, 1976, pp. 378–381.

134. D. F. Steiner, P. S. Quinn, S. J. Chan, J. Marsh, and H. S. Tager, *Ann. N.Y. Acad. Sci.* **343**, 1 (1980).

135. C. Patzelt, S. J. Chan, J. Dugrid, G. Hortin, P. Klein, R. L. Heinlikson, and D. F. Steiner, in S. Magnusson, Ed., *Regulatory Proteolytic Enzymes and Their Inhibitors,* Pergamon Press, New York, Vol. 47, 1978, pp. 69–78.

136. C. DeHaen, E. Swanson, and D. C. Teller, *J. Mol. Biol.* **106**, 639 (1976).

137. S. J. Chan, S. C. M. Kwok, and D. F. Steiner, *Diabetes Care* **4**, 4 (1981).

138. P. Y. Chow and G. D. Fasman, *Annu. Rev. Biochem.* **47**, 251 (1978).

139. T. L. Blundell, G. G. Dodson, D. C. Hodgkin, and D. A. Mercola, *Adv. Protein Chem.* **26**, 279 (1972).

140. S. P. Wood, T. L. Blundell, A. Wollmer, N. R. Lazarus, and R. W. J. Neville, *Eur. J. Biochem.* **55**, 531 (1975).

141. R. A. Pullen, J. A. Jenkins, I. J. Tickle, S. P. Wood, and T. L. Blundell, *Mol. Cell. Endocrinol.* **8**, 5 (1975).

142. P. Freychet, D. Brandenburg, and A. Wollmer, *Diabetologia* **10**, 1 (1974).

143. J. Gleinmann and S. Gammeltuft, *Diabetologia* **10**, 105 (1974).

144. R. A. Pullen, D. G. Lindsay, S. P. Wood, I. J. Tickle, T. L. Blundell, A. Wollmer, G. Krail, D. Brandenburg, H. Zahn, J. Gliemann, and S. Gammeltoff, *Nature* **259**, 369 (1976).

145. P. DeMeyts, E. VanObberghen, J. Roth, A. Wollmer, and D. Brandenburg, *Nature* **273**, 504 (1978).

146. M. E. Harper, A. Ullrich, and G. F. Saunders, *Proc. Natl. Acad. Sci. USA* **78**, 4458 (1981).

147. D. Owerbach, G. I. Bell, W. J. Rutter, and T. B. Shows, *Nature* **286**, 82 (1980).

148. L. F. Smith, *Am. J. Med.* **40**, 662 (1966).

149. J. L. Clark and D. F. Steiner, *Proc. Natl. Acad. Sci. USA* **62**, 278 (1969).

150. G. I. Bell, J. H. Karam, and W. J. Rutter, *Proc. Natl. Acad. Sci. USA* **78**, 5759 (1981).

151. G. I. Bell, M. F. Selby, and W. J. Rutter, *Nature* **295**, 31 (1982).

152. G. P. Smith, *Science* **191**, 528 (1975).

153. J. L. Slightom, A. E. Blechl, and O. Smithies, *Cell* **21**, 627 (1980).

154. W. R. Jelinek, T. P. Toomey, L. Leinwand, C. M. Duncan, P. A. Biro, P. V. Choudary, S. M. Weissman, C. M. Rabin, C. M. Houck, P. L. Deininger, and C. W. Schmid, *Proc. Natl. Acad. Sci. USA* **77**, 1398 (1980).

155. E. F. Fritsch, R. M. Lawn, and T. Maniatis, *Cell* **19**, 959 (1980).

156. M. Kimura and T. Ohta, *Proc. Natl. Acad. Sci. USA* **71**, 2848 (1974).

157. F. L. Hisaw, *Proc. Soc. Exp. Biol. Med.* **23**, 661 (1926).

158. M. J. John, J. R. Walsh, B. W. Borgesson, and H. D. Niall, *Endocrinology* **108**, 726 (1981).

159. C. Schwabe, J. K. McDonald, and B. C. Steinetz, *Biochem. Biophys. Res. Comm.* **75**, 503 (1977).

160. C. Schwabe, B. Steinetz, G. Weiss, A. Segaloff, J. K. McDonald, E. O'Byrne, J. Hochman, B. Carrier, and L. Goldsmith, *Recent Prog. Horm. Res.* **34**, 123 (1978).

161. J. Haley, P. Hudson, D. Scanlon, M. John, J. M. Cronk, J. Shine, G. Tregar, and H. Niall, *DNA* **1**, 155 (1982).

162. M. J. Gast, R. Mercado-Simmeer, H. Niall, and I. Boime, *Ann. N.Y. Acad. Sci.* **343**, 148 (1980).

163. R. James, H. Niall, S. Kwock, and G. Bryant-Greenwood, *Nature* **267**, 544 (1977).

164. J. L. Roberts, M. Phillips, P. A. Rosa, and E. Herbert, *Biochemistry* **17**, 3609 (1978).

165. B. A. Eipper and R. E. Mains, *Endocr. Rev.* **1**, 1 (1980).

166. D. T. Krieger, A. S. Liotta, M. J. Brownstein, and E. A. Zimmerman, *Recent Prog. Horm. Res.* **36**, 277 (1980).

167. W. L. Miller, L. K. Johnson, J. D. Baxter, and J. L. Roberts, *Proc. Natl. Acad. Sci. USA* **77**, 5211 (1980).

168. J. L. Roberts, P. H. Seeburg, J. Shine, E. Herbert, J. D. Baxter, and H. M. Goodman, *Proc. Natl. Acad. Sci. USA* **76**, 2153 (1979).

169. S. Nakanishi, A. Inoue, T. Kita, M. Nakamura, A. C. Y. Chang, S. N. Cohen, and S. Numa, *Nature* **278**, 423 (1979).

170. J. Drouin and H. M. Goodman, *Nature* **288**, 610 (1980).

171. A. C. Y. Chang, M. Cochet, and S. N. Cohen, *Proc. Natl. Acad. Sci. USA* **77**, 4890 (1980).

172. S. Nakanishi, Y. Teranishi, M. Noda, M. Notake, Y. Watanabe, H. Kakidani, H. Jingami, and S. Numa, *Nature* **287**, 752 (1980).

173. P. L. Whitfeld, P. H. Seeburg, and J. Shine, *DNA* **1**, 133 (1982).

174. E. Odagiri, B. J. Sherrell, C. D. Mount, W. E. Nicholson, and D. N. Orth, *Proc. Natl. Acad. Sci. USA* **76**, 2027 (1979).

175. A. S. Liotta, D. Gildersleeve, M. J. Brownstein, and D. T. Krieger, *Proc. Natl. Acad. Sci. USA* **76**, 1448 (1979).

176. R. C. Pederson, N. Ling, and A. C. Brownie, *Endocrinology* **110**, 825 (1982).

177. N. G. Seidah, and M. Chretien, *Proc. Natl. Acad. Sci. USA* **78**, 4236 (1981).

178. N. G. Seidah, J. Rochemont, S. Hamelin, M. Lis, and M. Chretien, *J. Biol. Chem.* **256**, 7977 (1981).

179. M. A. Phillips, M. L. Budarf, and E. Herbert, *Biochemistry* **20**, 1666 (1981).

180. W. L. Miller and L. K. Johnson, *J. Clin. Endocrinol. Metab.*, **55**, 441 (1982).

181. J. P. Segrest and R. L. Jackson, *Methods Enzymol.* **288**, 54 (1972).

182. E. A. S. Al-Dujaili, J. Hope, F. E. Estivariz, P. J. Lowry, and C. R. W. Edwards, *Nature* **291**, 156 (1981).

183. R. C. Pedersen and A. C. Brownie, *Proc. Natl. Acad. Sci. USA* **77**, 2239 (1980).

184. R. C. Pedersen and A. C. Brownie, *Science* **208**, 1044 (1980).

185. D. Owerbach, W. J. Rutter, J. L. Roberts, P. L. Whitfeld, J. Shine, P. H. Seeburg, and T. B. Shows, *Somatic Cell Genet.* **7**, 359 (1981).

186. W. Vale, P. Brazeau, G. Grant, A. Nussy, R. Burgus, J. Rivier, N. Ling, and R. G. Guillemin, *C. R. Hebd. Seanc. Acad. Sci. Paris* **275**, 2913 (1972).

187. R. Luft, S. Efendic, T. Hokfelt, O. Johansson, and A. Arimura, *Med. Biol.* **52**, 428 (1974).

188. M. Dubois, *Proc. Natl. Acad. Sci. USA* **72**, 1340 (1975).

189. G. Boden, M. Sivitz, and D. Owen, *Science* **190**, 163 (1975).

190. S. R. Bloom, C. H. Mortimer, M. O. Thorner, G. M. Besser, R. Hall, A. Gomez-Parr, V. M. Roy, R. C. G. Russell, D. H. Coy, A. J. Kastin, and A. V. Schally, *Lancet* **2**, 1106 (1974).

191. S. Konturek, J. Tasler, W. Obtulowicz, D. Coy, and A. Schally, *J. Clin. Invest.* **58**, 1 (1976).

192. W. Vale, C. Rivier, M. Palkovitz, J. Saavedra, and M. Brownstein, *Endocrinology* **94**, 14 (1974).

193. M. Brownstein, A. Arimura, H. Sato, A. Schally, and J. Kizer, *Endocrinolgy* **96**, 1456 (1975).

194. W. Vale, P. Brazeau, C. Rivier, M. Brown, B. Boss, J. Rivier, R. Burgus, N. Ling, and R. G. Guillemin, *Recent Prog. Horm. Res.* **31**, 365 (1975).

195. T. Hokfelt, R. Elde, O. Johansson, R. Luft, G. Nilsson, and A. Arimura, *Neuroscience* **1**, 131 (1976).

196. B. D. Noe, D. J. Fletcher, and G. E. Baver, in S. J. Cooperstein and D. T. Watkins, Eds., *Biochemistry, Physiology, and Pathology of the Islets of Langerhans*, Academic Press, New York, 1981.

197. C. Patzelt, H. S. Trager, R. Carroll, and D. F. Steiner, *Proc. Natl. Acad. Sci. USA* **77**, 2410 (1980).

198. R. H. Goodman, P. K. Lund, J. W. Jacobs, and J. F. Habner, *J. Biol. Chem.* **255**, 6549 (1980).

199. D. Shields, *Proc. Natl. Acad. Sci. USA* **77**, 4074 (1980).
200. M. Lauber, M. Camier, and P. Cohen, *Proc. Natl. Acad. Sci. USA* **76**, 6004 (1979).
201. B. D. Noe, D. J. Fletcher, G. E. Bauer, G. C. Weir, and Y. Patel, *Endocrinology* **102**, 1675 (1978).
202. B. D. Noe, D. Fletcher, and J. Spiess, *Diabetes* **28**, 724 (1979).
203. C. A. Meyers, W. A. Murphy, T. W. Redding, D. H. Coy, and A. V. Schalley, *Proc. Natl. Acad. Sci. USA* **77**, 6171 (1980).
204. L. Pradayrol, H. Jornvall, V. Mutt, and A. Ribet, *FEBS Lett.* **109**, 55 (1980).
205. P. Hobart, R. Crawford, L. Shen, R. Pictet, and W. J. Rutter, *Nature* **288**, 137 (1980).
206. R. H. Goodman, J. W. Jacobs, W. W. Chin, P. K. Lund, P. C. Dee, and J. F. Habner, *Proc. Natl. Acad. Sci. USA* **77**, 5869 (1980).
207. W. L. Taylor, K. J. Collier, R. J. Deschenes, H. L. Weith, and J. E. Dixon, *Proc. Natl. Acad. Sci. USA* **78**, 6694 (1981).
208. L. -P. Shen, R. L. Pictet, and W. J. Rutter, *Proc. Natl. Acad. Sci. USA* **79**, 4575 (1982).
209. H. Oyami, R. A. Bradshaw, O. J. Bates, and A. Permutt, *J. Biol. Chem.* **255**, 2251 (1980).
210. P. C. Andrews and J. E. Dixon, *J. Biol. Chem.* **256**, 8267 (1981).
211. C. B. Srikant and Y. C. Patel, *Nature* **294**, 259 (1981).
212. W. J. Freed, M. J. Perlow, and R. J. Wyatt, *Science* **206**, 850 (1979).
213. S. G. Amara, D. N. David, M. G. Rosenfeld, B. A. Roos, and R. M. Evans, *Proc. Natl. Acad. Sci. USA* **77**, 4444 (1980).
214. J. W. Jacobs, R. H. Goodman, W. W. Chin, P. C. Dee, and J. F. Habner, *Science* **213**, 457 (1981).
215. M. G. Rosenfeld, S. G. Amara, B. A. Roos, E. S. Ong, and R. M. Evans, *Nature* **290**, 63 (1981).
216. S. Amara, V. Jonas, M. G. Rosenfeld, E. S. Ong, and R. M. Evans, *Nature* **298**, 240 (1982).
217. B. Kemper, C. A. Weaver, and D. F. Gordon, in D. V. Cohn, R. V. Talmage, and J. L. Matthews, Eds., *Hormonal Control of Calcium Metabolism*, Excerpta Medica, Amsterdam, 1981, pp. 19–27.
218. G. A. Hendy, H. M. Kronenberg, J. T. Potts, and A. Rich, *Proc. Natl. Acad. Sci. USA* **78**, 7365 (1981).
219. H. M. Kronenberg, B. E. McDevitt, J. A. Majzoub, J. Nathans, P. A. Sharp, J. T. Potts, and A. Rich, *Proc. Natl. Acad. Sci. USA* **76**, 4981 (1979).
220. W. W. Chin, H. Kronenberg, P. C. Dee, F. Maloof, and J. F. Habner, *Proc. Natl. Acad. Sci. USA* **78**, 5329 (1981).
221. J. C. Fiddes and H. M. Goodman, *Nature* **281**, 351 (1979).
222. J. C. Fiddes and H. M. Goodman, *Nature* **286**, 684 (1980).
223. N. C. Vamvakopolous, J. J. Monahan, and I. A. Kourides, *Proc. Natl. Acad. Sci. USA* **77**, 3149 (1980).
224. T.-H. Laio and J. G. Pierce, *J. Biol. Chem.* **246**, 850 (1971).
225. M. R. Sairam, H. Papkoff, and C. H. Li, *Arch. Biochem. Biophys.* **153**, 554 (1972).
226. G. Maghuin-Rogister, Y. Combarnous, and G. Hennen, *Eur. J. Biochem.* **39**, 255 (1973).
227. P. Rathman, Y. Fujiki, T. D. Landefeld, and B. B. Saxena, *J. Biol. Chem.* **253**, 5355 (1978).
228. F. J. Morgan, S. Birken, and R. E. Canfield, *J. Biol. Chem.* **250**, 5247 (1975).
229. M. O. Dayhoff, in *Atlas of Protein Sequence and Structure*, Vol. 5, Suppl. 2, National Biomedical Research Foundation, Washington, D.C., 1975, pp. 116–119.
230. J. G. Pierce, G. A. Bloomfield, and L. C. Givdici, *Biochem. Soc. Trans.* **6**, 57 (1978).

3

Biosynthesis and Processing of Neuropeptides

Y. PENG LOH

HAROLD GAINER

Laboratory of Developmental Neurobiology
National Institute of Child Health and Human Development
National Institutes of Health
Bethesda, Maryland

1 INTRODUCTION

Peptides are molecules in which variable numbers of amino acids are linked together by peptide bonds (-$\overset{\text{O}}{\overset{\|}{\text{C}}}$-NH-), thereby forming unique chemical structures that may have highly specific biological activities. In principle, such chemical bonds could be formed by the catalytic actions of enzymes and, indeed, a number of biologically active peptides are produced in this manner. The most common of these is glutathione (γ-glutamyl-cysteinyl-glycine). This tripeptide is synthesized in living cells by a series of six enzyme-catalyzed reactions (1, 2). Although it is well known that peptide-bond hydrolysis equilibria are thermodynamically unfavorable for synthesis (3), certain specific conditions *in vitro* are capable of shifting this equilibrium towards synthesis (4), even when the enzymes involved are proteinases. The latter conditions involve the addition of organic cosolvents to the reaction mixture in order to restrict the influence of the aqueous environment (4), a condition that is unlikely but conceivable in living tissues. Mechanisms exist in bacteria to synthesize peptide antibiotics by enzymes (5–7), but these mechanisms do not appear to be widely found in other living systems.

In view of the above, it is interesting that most biologically active peptides and proteins are synthesized using mRNA-template and ribosomally-based protein synthesis mechanisms. In the case of secretory peptides the synthesis occurs on ribosomes associated with endoplasmic reticulum (i.e., the rough endoplasmic reticulum). The reasons for the evolutionary preferences for this mechanism of peptide biosynthesis are not entirely clear. It might be due to the relative unreliability of enzymatic peptide-synthesizing mechanisms (7, 8) or to the inherent constraints found in the structural organization of cells, which are necessary to perform its many other functions. One aim of this review is to demonstrate that although the primary structures of peptides are mainly determined by conventional protein synthesis mechanisms, many of their characteristics (and indeed, their very existence) are also determined by various enzymatic mechanisms involved in posttranslational modification processes. Therefore, what peptide or peptides are produced and secreted by a cell (e.g., a neuron) is a function not only of the particular mRNAs expressed in the cell but also of the production and distribution of the specific enzymes involved in the fashioning of the final peptide product. Also of consequence in this regard are the intracellular routing mechanisms, which determine the fates of the newly synthesized peptides (e.g., secretion, degradation, intracellular function).

These considerations are of potential physiological significance for neuropeptides, which are secreted as intercellular messengers. Because of the structure of neurons, the ribosomally directed biosynthesis in the perikaryon occurs at a considerable distance from the secretory site, that is, at the axon terminal. Therefore, local synthesis and recycling mechanisms occurring in the axon terminals for enzymatically synthesized neurotransmitters (e.g., acetylcholine, biogenic amines) cannot be easily applied to neuropeptides. This distinction between neurotransmitter agents that are exclusively synthesized by enzyme mechanisms and the neuropeptides that require ribosomes has been complicated by the observations that both types of molecules are often released from the same nerve endings (9–11) and may even reside in the same secretory vesicles (12). How the synthesis of these diverse molecules can be regulated in a coordinated way in such nerve terminals, when one type must be regulated in the cell soma and the other in the nerve terminals during recycling, remains unclear. It is possible that during periods of intensive impulse activity and secretion the vesicles are depleted of their neuropeptides and the recycled vesicles are refilled only with nonpeptide transmitters (13). The physiological consequences of such events should be profound, and this issue awaits further experimental investigation.

Most of the current information available about peptide biosynthesis is derived from non-neuronal tissues. Much of the data discussed in this review comes from these experimental studies. We have not intended to be exhaustive in our review of this extensive literature but rather to direct the reader's attention to certain peptides of interest to neurobiologists that illustrate some general principles.

2 ROLES OF PRECURSORS

Experimental work over the past 15 years has shown that, in addition to the peptide hormones, a wide variety of other proteins and polypeptides are derived from the posttranslational proteolytic cleavage of larger precursor molecules (14–16). These include such diverse polypeptides as albumin, immunoglobulins, cytochrome c oxidase, catalase, insulin, mellitin, cholera toxin, nerve growth factor, zymogens, and various membrane and viral proteins.

2.1 Intracellularly and Extracellularly Processed Precursors

Steiner and his colleagues (14, 17) have suggested a tentative classification of precursors into those that are proteolytically processed intracellularly and those that are processed extracellularly. The extracellularly processed precursors include the well-known zymogens (15, 18), procollagens (15, 19), the protoxins (e.g., promellitin; 15, 20), and the provitellogenins (15, 21). As can be surmised from the nature of some of these cleaved products, one role of the precursors is to allow the peptide to be synthesized in an inactive form (e.g., the zymogens and protoxins) until release from the cell interior. In other cases (e.g., procollagen), it has been suggested that the proform is soluble and hence can be intracellularly translocated and secreted, whereas the final product (collagen) is relatively insoluble and hence would be best processed near its site of deposition (extracellularly).

2.2 Preproteins and Proproteins

The intracellularly processed precursors are further divided by Steiner's classification (14, 17) into preproteins and proproteins. These are operationally defined by differences in their cleavage kinetics and their intracellular sites of cleavage—the preproteins are rapidly processed in association with the membrane of the rough endoplasmic reticulum, often before the polypeptide is fully translated (i.e., cotranslational cleavage). The proproteins, which include all the polypeptide prohormones, some serum proteins (e.g., proalbumin) but not others (fibrinogen), and viral polyproteins (14–16), are posttranslationally cleaved at sites more distal from the translation site in the RER (e.g., in Golgi and in secretory vesicles) and hence, their proteolytic cleavage occurs more slowly in the cell, in part due to translocation time. The role of the preproteins is to provide a signal sequence at the N-terminal of the polypeptide, which is used to translocate the translated product into the RER cisterna (14–16, 22, 23). Thus, by this mechanism the segregation process for the routing of secretory polypeptides in Palade's general scheme (24) is determined during the translation event itself. The roles of the proproteins are somewhat more diverse. In the case of proinsulin, the C-peptide, which is ultimately cleaved from the prohormone, serves to ensure the correct folding and disulfide formation between the A and B chains of insulin. A similar role has been suggested for the proneurophysins (25). The viral polyproteins (precursors) appear to contain multiple functional groups (e.g, a replicase, various coat proteins, and in some cases, the protease for the cleavage) which are used for the efficient assembly of the complete virion (16). This coordinating function of viral precursors may be analogous to that of some eukaryotic precursors where coordinate synthesis, packaging, and secretion of different specific peptides can be encoded in a single "common precursor" (e.g., ACTH-endorphin, Leu- and Met-enkephalin). A more complete discussion of the potential roles of precursor sequences can be found elsewhere (14, 16, 17).

What is clear from the above is that the precursor represents a general biological mechanism subserving a variety of purposes in living systems. Although it is possible to speculate about the potential roles of each of the individual proproteins, their diversity and our limited knowledge prevent a *general* statement about their functions. The preproteins, on the other hand, appear to constitute a distinct group with respect to function. A newly synthesized protein may be both a pre and proprotein (e.g., preproinsulin); the "pre" simply indicates that there is an N-terminal presequence of amino acids on the nascent protein (see below) that is rapidly cleaved and rarely found on the protein *in situ*.

2.3   Signal Sequences and Intracellular Routing

A significant step in our understanding of how secretory (and membrane) proteins are appropriately compartmentalized in the cell came from the proposal of the "signal hypothesis" (26, 27). Subsequent work based on this hypothesis has established that there is an N-terminal sequence in newly synthesized secretory and membrane proteins composed of between 15 and 30 amino acids rich in hydrophobic residues (i.e., the "signal" sequence) that participates in directing the preprotein through the RER membrane into its cisternae, where the signal sequence is immediately cleaved off the protein by an endopeptidase (see refs. 14–17, 23, 28 for reviews).

The nature of the specific mechanisms involved in the translocations and cleavages of the preproteins are still a matter of debate. Many presequences have been elucidated, and some are illustrated in Table 1. As a rule, the sequences are quite diverse in length and amino acid composition. Their common features are hydrophilic N-terminals, a central hydrophobic region of about 10 residues long (usually from -17 to -7), the latter being at a relatively fixed distance from the cleavage site, which is dominated by amino acids with small neutral side chains (e.g., Ala, Cys, Ser, Thr, and Gly). The absence of any required specific amino acids at the cleavage site (the gap in the sequence in Table 1) suggests that the endopeptidase may recognize molecular configuration signals as opposed to specific amino acids. Several authors have noted that the cleavage sites often contain amino acids (e.g., Ala and Gly) that are likely to form β turns, and that this in combination with the hydrophobic central region of the presequence may provide an adequate signal for endopeptidase action. In addition, this cleavage mechanism appears to be highly conserved in that bacterial cells, *Xenopus* (African clawed frog) oocytes, and microsomal membranes from diverse sources can cleave signal sequences from the preproteins of equally diverse sources.

One of the difficulties in characterizing the endopeptidase has been in developing proper *in vitro* assay procedures. In one case (41), deoxychlolate extracts of dog pancreas rough microsomes (but not smooth microsomes) were shown to contain an enzyme activity that correctly cleaved preprolactin. Using this assay the authors were able to provide evidence that the cleavage enzyme was located within the microsome interior (or associated with the inner membrane) as opposed to its exterior surface. Some evidence exists to indicate that the enzyme

TABLE 1 N-Terminal Sequences of Preproteins[a]

Preprotein	Length	Signal Sequence[b] N-Terminal ← ... −1	Processed Protein +1 +5	Reference
Hormones				
Preproinsulin I (rat)	24	MALWMRFLPLLALLVLWFPKPAQA	FVKQH	29
Prepro-PTH (bovine)	25	MMSAKDMVKVMIVMLAICFLARSDG	KSVKK	30
Pregrowth hormone (bovine)	26	MAADSQTPWLLTFSLLCLLWPQEAGA	LPAMS	31
Prepro-opiomelanocortin (rat)	26	MPRLCSSRSGALLLALLLQASMEVRG	WCLES	32
Preproenkephalin (bovine)	24	MARFLGLCTWLLALGPGLLATVRA	ECSQD	33
Preprovasopressin (bovine)	19	MPDATLPACFLSLLAFTSA	CYFQN	34
Other				
Preproalbumin (rat)	18	MKWVTFLLLFISGSAFSAFS	RGVFR	35
Pre-α_{51}casein (ovine)	15	MKLLILTCLVAVALA	RPKHP	36
Preglycoprotein (VSvirus)	16	MKCLLYLAFLFI[HVN]C	KFXIX	37
Pre-IgG(L chain) (mouse MOPC-41)	22	MDMRAPAQIFGFLLLLFPGTRC	DIQMT	38
Prepromellitin (bee)	21	MKFLVXVALVFMVVYIXYIYA	APEPE	39

[a] The gap in the sequences indicates the point of cleavage between the signal sequence (left) and the beginning of the processed protein (right).
[b] The one-letter notation for amino acids used here (40) is A, Ala; B, Asx; C, Cys; D, Asp; E, Glu; F, Phe; G, Gly; H, His; I, ILe; K, Lys; L, Leu; M, Met; N, Asn; P, Pro; Q, Gln; R, Arg; S, Ser; T, Thr; V, Val; W, Trp; X, undetermined; Y, Tyr; Z, Glx. Asx is Asp or Asn (undistinguished) and Glx is Glu or Gln (undistinguished). The hydrophobic amino acids are F, I, L, M, P, V, W, and Y.

is a metalloprotease (42). Although this enzyme : substrate relationship is conserved in an evolutionary sense, the problem is that it is still dependent on features of the molecule other than the amino acids at the cleavage site. Hence, it is difficult to make easily assayed artificial substrates for *in vitro* assays. A substantial portion of the presequence and processed protein is necessary for the substrate; therefore, radioactively labeled preproteins synthesized *in vitro* have been generally used as substrates (41–43). Given this substrate, tedious assays for correct cleavage (amino terminus, peptide sequence analysis, etc.) are necessary. Even under these circumstances, the natural substrate may be inaccessible to the enzyme because of the artificial microenvironment (e.g., absence of membranes to anchor the hydrophobic region of the presequence) or because of premature folding of the completely translated preprotein used in the assay. Indeed, even in the case of the preprolactin assay (41) discussed above, only 50% of the substrate molecules were able to be cleaved in the assay. This problem in assaying highly specific enzyme activities may be a general one; it is discussed again later in the context of proprotein processing, where the cleavage site does contain specific amino acids as signals.

It becomes apparent from this work on preproteins that fundamental biochemical processes such as translation of proteins and their specific enzymatic cleavages cannot be divorced from the structural organization of the cell. The experience with the signal sequences serves to focus attention on the coupled nature of protein biosynthesis and the intracellular routing (e.g., segregation) processes described by Palade (24).

3 STATE OF THE ART: PRECURSOR IDENTIFICATION

3.1 Experimental Approaches

The initial approach to precursor identification was simply to employ a pulse-chase paradigm using radioactive amino acids and, as in the classical case of proinsulin (44), to demonstrate that a larger labeled form of the peptide (putative precursor) was first synthesized in the tissues and that this subsequently decreased in radioactivity as the labeled peptide increased. In the early phases of this work, identification of the precursors and products were based on the simple physical characteristics (size, charge) of the molecules, on various peptide mapping procedures, and the like. With the subsequent availability of antisera to specific peptides, immunological probes could be used to extend identification procedures to include the demonstration that putative precursors and peptide products contain similar or identical immunoreactivities. A particularly useful approach was to employ the antisera in immunoprecipitation procedures following pulse-chase incubation (for pro-opiocortin, see ref. 45). The labeled immunoprecipitates were then further analyzed to fulfill other criteria of identification (e.g., peptide maps, N-terminus and amino acid composition).

Immunoprecipitation strategies provided the opportunity to enhance the signal-to-noise ratios in *in vitro* translation experiments, in which purified mRNA and heterologous cell-free translation systems (e.g., wheat germ and reticulocyte lysates) were used for precursor synthesis. The newly synthesized proteins were then selectively immunoprecipitated by specific antibodies. This approach was essential in early experiments to identify the preproteins (described earlier) since cleavage of the presequence was too rapid in the *in situ* experiments to detect the preproteins. A wide variety of proproteins have also been detected by this approach (14–17, 46–50). By the addition of dog liver microsome membranes to the cell-free translation systems (41), it is possible to demonstrate several posttranslational processes as well (e.g., signal sequence cleavage, glycosylation).

The most sophisticated approach to precursor identification comes from recent advances in recombinant DNA research. Because of the availability of restriction endonucleases (51) and rapid DNA sequencing techniques (52, 53), it is now possible to clone cDNA from a purified mRNA template, using reverse transcriptase. The cDNA can be easily and rapidly sequenced, and from this nucleotide sequence the amino acid sequence of the precursor can be determined. This approach has been used to elucidate the amino acid sequences of prepro-opiocortin (32), preproenkephalin (33), preprovasopressin (34), preprocalcitonin (54), and others. A possible alternative to isolating purified mRNA by conventional procedures is to chemically synthesize oligodeoxynucleotide probes (55) with which one can "fish out" appropriate mRNAs (56, 57). This requires knowing enough about the amino acid sequence of the peptide in question to be able to synthesize a DNA probe representing a sequence of 4–8 amino acids in the peptide which have unique or low degeneracy codons (58). The mRNA isolated in this manner can then be used, as described above, for molecular cloning and nucleotide sequencing of the cDNA (59). In addition to providing the most complete information about the sequence of the precursor, the recombinant DNA approach has two other virtues. First, it allows for the analysis of potential precursors even in situations where there is no tissue available with an abundant synthesis of the peptide of interest. Pulse-chase experiments, even with effective immunoprecipitation methods, require that enough synthesis be occurring to incorporate labeled amino acids at detectable levels. Similarly, cell-free translation experiments require sufficient mRNA template to be isolated from the tissues to yield enough labeled precursor to be detected by immunoprecipitation. In the recombinant DNA approach, there is amplification of the nucleotide by

cloning so that smaller amounts of mRNA can suffice. The second benefit is that the recombinant DNA approach can provide radioactive
cDNA probes for the precursor's mRNA and therefore provide a tool for
the analysis of gene complexity and expression in tissues.

3.2   Secretory Proproteins

Figures 1 and 2 and Table 2 illustrate the properties of some proproteins
that have been recently elucidated. The proproteins differ widely in
size, ranging from the 86 amino acid proinsulin to the 588 amino acid
proalbumin. Similarly, the size of the secreted product does not correlate with the size of the proprotein. For example, in proalbumin the secreted form accounts for almost 99% of the amino acids in the proform,
whereas in somatostatin this value is less than 14%. The biologically active residues can occur at the N-terminus of the proproteins (e.g., vaso-

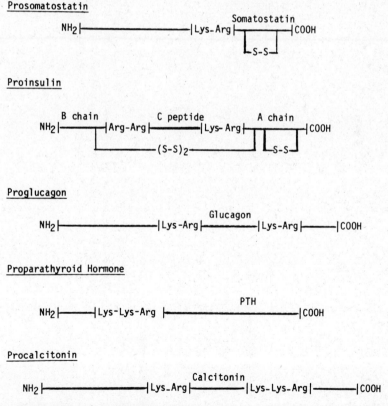

Figure 1.   Diagrammatic representations of the structures of several proproteins, showing
the basic amino acid cleavage sites.

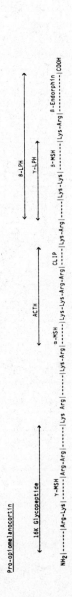
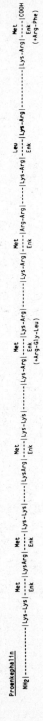

Figure 2. Diagrammatic representations of the structure of pro-opiomelanocortin, provasopressin, and proenkephalin, showing locations of basic amino acids within those molecules that are cleaved (see refs. 32, 33, 34, and 35 for sources).

TABLE 2 Characteristics of Some Secretory Proproteins

Proprotein	No. of Residues in Proprotein	Secreted Products	No. of Residues in Product	Residues at Cleavage Site		Other Processings of Product Before Secretion
				N-terminus	C-terminus	
Proinsulin	86	Insulin	51	—	—	—
		C-peptide		Arg-Arg	Lys-Arg	—
Proalbumin	588	Albumin	582	Arg-Arg	—	—
Prosomatostatin	103	Somatostatin	14	Arg-Lys	—	—
Proglucagon	78	Glucagon	29	Lys-Arg	Lys-Arg	—
Proparathrin	90	Parathyroid hormone	84	Lys-Arg	—	—
Progastrin	110	Gastrin	17	Arg-Arg	Lys-Lys	Amidation
Procalcitonin	118	Calcitonin	32	Lys-Arg	Lys-Lys-Arg	Glycosylation
Pro-opiomelanocortin	243	N-terminal glycopeptide	109	—	Lys-Arg	Glycosylation
(Pro-opiocortin Pro-ACTH/endorphin)		ACTH	39	Lys-Arg	Lys-Arg	Phosphorylation
		β-LPH (bovine)	93	Lys-Arg	—	Acetylation
		α-MSH	13	Lys-Arg	Arg-Arg	Amidation
		CLIP	22	Arg-Arg	Lys-Arg	Glycosylation
		β-Endorphin	31	Lys-Arg	—	Acetylation
Pro-vasopressin	147	Vasopressin	9	Lys-Arg	Lys-Arg	Amidation
(Pro-pressophysin)		Neurophysin	95	Lys-Arg	Arg	
		C-terminal glycopeptide	39	Arg	—	Glycosylation
Proenkephalin	239	Met-Enkephalin₁	5	Lys-Lys	Lys-Arg	—
		Met-Enkephalin₂	5	Lys-Arg	Lys-Lys	—
		Met-Enkephalin₃	5	Lys-Arg	Lys-Lys	—
		Met-Enkephalin₄	7	Lys-Arg	Lys-Arg	—
		Met-Enkephalin₅	5	Lys-Arg	Arg-Arg	—
		Met-Enkephalin₆	7	Lys-Arg	—	—
		Leu-Enkephalin	5	Lys-Arg	Lys-Arg	—

pressin, B chain of insulin), in the middle (e.g., glucagon, calcitonin, ACTH, enkephalin), or at the C-terminus (somatostatin, A chain of insulin, parathyroid hormone, β-endorphin) (Figures 1 and 2). In some cases, the biologically active peptide cleaved from the proprotein can itself serve as a proform for other biological peptides. The best example of this is for pro-opiomelanocortin (Figure 2, Table 2), where adrenocorticotrophic hormone (ACTH) can be converted to α-melanocyte stimulating hormone (α-MSH) and corticotropin-like intermediate lobe peptide (CLIP), the 16K glycopeptide can be converted to γ-MSH, and the β-LPH to γ-LPH (or β-MSH) and β-endorphin.

Unlike the preproteins, the proproteins do appear to have specific amino acids at the proteolytic enzyme cleavage sites. With the exception of one site in provasopressin (which contains a single Arg at the cleavage site between neurophysin and the C-terminal glycopeptide), most of the proproteins have pairs of basic amino acids at the cleavage sites. The most common of these is the Lys-Arg sequence, although Arg-Arg and Lys-Lys can also be found (Figures 1 and 2, Table 2). This structural pattern suggests that the proprotein converting enzymes usually exhibit a specificity for pairs of basic amino acid residues. In earlier work it was shown that immunoreactive secretory peptides could be cleaved from proproteins by pancreatic trypsin, which cleaves at the COOH side of Lys or Arg residues. Hence, it was originally believed that a trypsin-like enzyme was involved in these cleavages *in situ*. However, the *in situ* converting enzyme appears to be more selective than trypsin in that, as a rule, it does not cleave at single basic amino acid residues. Another structural feature in the proproteins which is suggestive is that amidation of the C-terminal amino acids in peptides appears to be signaled by a glycine residue on the N-terminal side of the basic amino acid pair (e.g., in vasopressin by Gly-Lys-Arg, α-MSH by Gly-Lys-Lys-Arg-Arg, and calcitonin by Gly-Lys-Lys-Arg).

Several other posttranslational modifications of the proproteins can occur *in situ*. Some of these (e.g., acetylation of the N-terminal and amidation of the C-terminal) occur after proteolytic cleavage of the peptide from the proprotein. Others, such as glycosylation and possibly phosphorylation, occur on the intact proprotein before cleavage. Proproteins may contain more than one biologically significant product (Figures 1 and 2). Pro-opiomelanocortin may be converted into MSH, ACTH, β-LPH, and β-endorphin. Similarly, provasopressin contains arginine vasopressin (AVP) and its carrier protein, neurophysin. Proenkephalin contains six Met-enkephalin sequences as well as one Leu-enkephalin. Proproteins can thus be "common precursors" and/or multivalent. It is especially apparent for pro-opiomelanocortin and proenkephalin that the nature of the processing enzymes found *in situ* will be important determinants for the types of peptides secreted by any cells that synthesize these proproteins.

3.2.1 Pro-Opiomelanocortin

Excellent reviews of the historical development and significance of this fascinating proprotein (14–16, 45, 60) are available; only a brief commentary is presented here. Although suggestions of precursor forms of ACTH, α-MSH, and β-endorphin were available from various earlier observations on pituitary peptide sequences and heterogeneous immunological forms, the key experiments in support of a biosynthetic precursor for ACTH came from pulse-chase experiments using AtT-20 mouse anterior pituitary tumor cell lines. In these studies, antibodies against ACTH and β-endorphin were used to immunoprecipitate and identify the relevant newly synthesized peptide. Evidence for a high-molecular-weight precursor of ACTH in AtT-20 cells (of around MW 31,000) was obtained using whole cells (45, 61) and cell-free translation of mRNA (62, 63). These experiments also showed that the precursor was a glycoprotein (64, 65). The same procedures were used to demonstrate that the ACTH precursor was also the precursor for β-endorphin (66, 67).

Successful application of recombinant DNA techniques to this proprotein was first performed using mRNA obtained from bovine neurointermediate lobe (32). In addition to providing information about the presequence and the amino acid sequences interposed between the N-terminal glycopeptide, ACTH, and β-LPH, the complete sequence of the N-terminal glycopeptide also revealed within it a third MSH sequence (i.e., γ-MSH). Since this study on bovine intermediate lobe pro-opiomelanocortin, recombinant-DNA techniques have been applied to the AtT-20 cells and to rat, bovine, and human genomic DNA fragments coding for this precursor molecule (see Chapter 26 in this volume).

3.2.2 Proenkephalin

An alternative putative precursor, other than pro-opiomelanocortin, for the opioid peptides Leu- and Met-enkephalin was indicated by the finding that adrenal medulla contains large quantities of these peptides (68, 69) but few pro-opiomelanocortin products. Furthermore, these and related peptides could be derived from higher-molecular-weight proteins extracted from adrenal medulla by the action of trypsin and carboxypeptidase B (70–73). Such studies suggested that there was a unique precursor in adrenal medulla containing multiple copies of Met-enkephalin and at least one Leu-enkephalin.

Pulse-chase analyses and *in vitro* translation experiments using mRNA from adrenal medulla were limited by the relative inability of available antibodies to enkephalin to react well with the putative precursor (74). Furthermore, enkephalin mRNA accounts for less than 0.1% of the total poly(A) RNA in adrenal medulla. In the case of this proprotein, recombinant DNA approaches elucidated the complete structure of bovine proenkephalin (33, 75) before convincing pulse-chase or *in vitro* translation experiments had been done. The preproenkephalin is composed of 263 amino acids and has a calculated molecular weight of 29,786. It contains 4 Met-enkephalins and one copy each of Leu-enkephalin, Met-enkephalin-Arg^6-Phe, and Met-enkephalin-Arg^6-Gly^7-Leu^8. Each of these enkephalin peptides is bounded by basic amino acid pairs (see Figure 2).

Proenkephalin may be glycosylated, since the sequence Asn-Ser-Ser at positions 149–151 is appropriate for asparagine-linked glycosylation mechanisms. Whether such events actually occur *in situ* awaits further experimentation. Since there are two other naturally occurring opioid peptides, dynorphin (Leu-enkephalin-Arg^6-Arg^7-Ile^8-Arg^9-Pro^{10}-Lys^{11}-Leu^{12}-Lys^{13}; ref. 76) and α-neoendorphin (Leu-enkephalin-Arg^6-Lys^7-Arg^8-Pro^9; ref. 77), which cannot be from the pro-opiomelanocortin or proenkephalin sequences, it is anticipated that at least two more proproteins with the Leu-enkephalin sequence may exist (see ref. 197).

3.2.3   Pro-Vasopressin-Neurophysin

A precursor mode of biosynthesis for vasopressin was first hypothesized in 1964 by Sachs and his colleagues (78, 79), who later proposed that the proprotein was a "common precursor" containing both vasopressin and neurophysin (80, 81). This hypothesis was based on the results of extensive pulse-chase experiments (81) that were compelling but which failed to identify the proprotein. Later pulse-chase experiments on the hypothalamo-neurohypophysial system of the rat identified a MW 20,000 protein that appeared to be a precursor of neurophysin (82). Further experiments along these lines using isoelectric focusing, immunoprecipitation, affinity chromatography, and peptide mapping procedures showed that the pro-vasopressin-neurophysin was approximately MW 20,000 had an isoelectric point of 6.1, and was a glycoprotein (83–85). In contrast, pro-oxytocin-neurophysin was smaller (around MW 15,000), had an isoelectric point of 5.4, and was not a glycoprotein (84, 85). These pulse-chase experiments, performed *in vivo* in the rat, suggested that there were a pI 6.1 vasopressin precursor and a pI 5.6 intermediate plus a pI 5.4 oxytocin precursor and a pI 5.1 intermediate (84, 85). Both forms of the vasopressin precursor were absent in homozygous Brattleboro rats with hereditary diabetes insipidus (84). Cyanogen bromide cleavage and peptide mapping experiments indicated that the pro-vasopressin-neurophysin contained AVP at the N-terminus, neurophysin in the middle, and glycopeptide at the C-terminus (85). The oxytocin proprotein contained oxytocin at the N-terminus, followed by neurophysin, and possibly a small peptide at the C-terminus. (See refs. 34 and 202).

Cell-free translation studies using mRNA from hypothalamic tissues confirmed the *in vivo* studies, in that a higher-molecular-weight (around MW 20,000–25,000) form of immunoreactive neurophysin and/or vasopressin was synthesized in the *in vitro* experiments (86–89). Immunological evidence in favor of a common precursor for AVP and neurophysin II was also demonstrated in these *in vitro* studies (90). Furthermore, by including dog liver microsomes in the reticulocyte translation cocktail, it was possible to show that the pro-vasopressin-neurophysin was glycosylated and the oxytocin proprotein was not (89). In the cell-free translation experiments the vasopressin pre-pro-protein has a molecular weight (on SDS gels) of 21,000, is cleaved to the proform of MW 19,000 by microsomes, and is then glycosylated to a form equal to MW 23,000 (88, 89). In agreement with the *in vivo* data, the preprooxytocin is smaller (MW 16,500) and is converted to the proform (MW 15,500) by liver microsomes *in vitro* (88, 89). Tryptic mapping of the vasopressin pre- and proproteins indicated that the vasopressin follows the signal sequence and precedes the neurophysin in the preproprotein (90).

Recently the nucleotide sequence of cloned cDNA encoding the bovine vasopressin-neurophysin II preproprotein was reported (34). The corresponding amino acid sequence contains 166 amino acids, of which 19 appear to belong to the signal sequence. The order of the peptide components in the proprotein is the same as predicted from the *in vivo* (85) and *in vitro* (90) experiments (see Figure 2). From the cDNA sequencing (34) it was possible to determine which amino acids are interposed between the peptide components (Figure 2) and to evaluate the amino acid sequence of the C-terminal glycopeptide. The latter is a 39 amino acid peptide with the glycosylation signal Asn-Ala-Thr in residues 6–8. Curiously, this glycopeptide sequence had been isolated before from the pituitaries of various species (91–93) without the recognition that it was associated with the vasopressin proprotein.

In view of the reports of higher-molecular-weight forms (MW 80,000) of immunoreactive neurophysin and vasopressin (94–97), it is important to note that such forms have not yet been reported in *in vivo* or *in vitro* biosynthesis experiments or in recombinant DNA studies. Until such studies are done, it would be best to be cautious with regard to these putative precursors (96, 97).

4 POSTTRANSLATIONAL MODIFICATIONS OF PROPROTEINS AND PEPTIDES

4.1 Overview

It has become clear in recent years that many proteins undergo further modifications posttranslationally and cotranslationally (for a review, see ref. 15). The most common of these modifications include proteolytic processing, glycosylation, formation of disulfide bonds, and phosphorylation/dephosphorylation (see Table 3). Other modifications such as hydroxylation of prolyl and lysl groups [e.g., procollagen (98)], carboxylation of glutamyl residues [e.g., prothrombin and other blood clotting factors (99)], deamidation of asparaginyl and glutaminyl groups [e.g., aldolase (100, 101)], and carboxyl methylation [e.g., neurophysin, calmodulin (102)] are restricted to a smaller number of proteins.

Posttranslational modifications of proteins are important for synthesis, activation of biological function, subcellular movement, and regulation of degradation (see Table 3). As described in the previous sections, synthesis of neuropeptides and peptide hormones involves posttranslational limited proteolysis of larger precursors (66, 82, 103, 113). In the zymogen systems, activation of function requires the limited proteolysis of an inactive protein precursor (114, 115). For some other proteins, activation and deactivation of their enzymatic function is regulated by reversible phosphorylation and dephosphorylation (116–118) and oxidation-reduction of their SH groups (119). Examples where posttranslational limited proteolysis plays a role in subcellular translocation can be found in the secretory proteins. As described earlier, the "pre" sequence of secretory proteins plays a role in directing the insertion of the growing polypeptide chain into the RER cisternae and is subsequently cleaved within the cisternae (Section 2.3 of this chapter; 29, 121–125). The lysosomal enzyme cathepsin B, a glycoprotein, provides an example of the importance of posttranslational glycosylation as a signal for subcellular movement (i.e., the presence of mannose-6-phosphate). The inhibition of glycosylation of cathepsin B in fibroblasts prevents its routing into lysosomes, resulting in its alternative routing and subsequent secretion from the cells (126). Although the role of posttranslational modification in the regulation of degradation of proteins has not been extensively studied, there is some evidence that modifications such as glycosylation and phosphorylation may stabilize proteins against proteolytic degradation, perhaps through conformation effects (127, 128). For example, nonglycosylated forms of adrenocorticotropin are degraded by blood proteases more rapidly than glycosylated forms (129), and phosphorylation of phosphorylase giving rise to phosphorylase "a" renders this protein more resistant to degradation than the dephosphorylated form "b" (130).

Thus far, proneuropeptides and prohormones have been shown to undergo four types of post- and cotranslational modifications: limited proteolysis, glycosylation, phosphorylation, and disulfide bonding (Table 3). Further studies may reveal other types of posttranslational modifications. After cleavage from the proproteins, the peptides may also undergo further modifications, such as amidation, acetylation (Table 2) and cyclization of the glutamic acid to form pyroglutamate. The cellular organization, enzymology, and significance of these posttranslational modifications are discussed in the following sections.

TABLE 3 Posttranslational Modification of Proteins

Function	Limited Proteolysis	Posttranslational Modifications		
		Phosphorylation/ Dephosphorylation	Glycosylation	Formation of Disulfide Bonds
Synthesis	Proparathormone (103)[a] Progastrin (104) Proglucagon (105) Procalcitonin (106) Proinsulin (105, 107) Pro-opiomelanocortin (66, 108–110) Provassopressin (82) Pro-oxytocin (82) Prosomatostatin (105) Proalbumin (111) Procollagen (112) Promellitin (113)		Pro-opiomelanocortin (122)	Proinsulin (131, 132) Prosomatostatin (133)
Regulation of protein activity	Trypsinogen (114, 115) Pepsinogen (114, 115) Chymotrypsinogen (114, 115) Plasminogen (114, 115)	Phosphorylase kinase (116, 117) Glycogen phosphorylase Tyrosine hydroxylase (116, 118) Phosphofructose kinase (116) Glycogen synthetase (116) Pyruvate kinase (116)		Pineal serotonin N-acetyltransferase (119) Liver glycogen synthetase (120)
Subcellular movement	Preproinsulin (29, 121) Prepro-opiomelanocortin (122) Preproparathormone (123) Preproalbumin (35, 124)		Cathepsin B (126)	
Regulation of degradation		Phosphorylase (13)	ACTH (129)	

[a] Numbers in parentheses are references.

4.2   Cellular Organization of Posttranslational Processing of Proproteins and Peptides

As we reviewed in Section 2.3, neuropeptides and peptide hormones are synthesized as preproproteins (121–124), which are then routed to the RER cisternae where the "pre" sequence is cleaved off (125). Electron microscopic and autoradiographic evidence suggest that after the presequence is removed, the proproteins are transported into the Golgi apparatus (24, 133–135). Depending on the system studied, some proproteins undergo their first cleavage step at the Golgi and the final steps of processing occur after packaging into secretory granules, whereas other proproteins are primarily cleaved after packaging into secretory granules. Examples of both have been found in the nervous system.

Studies of the biosynthesis of the egg-laying hormone in the bag cell neurons of the mollusc *Aplysia* have shown that the MW 29,000 egg-laying peptide precursor undergoes its first cleavage to one 11,300 dalton and two 6000 dalton products, apparently in the RER or Golgi (136–139). Only the two 6000 dalton products (a basic peptide egg-laying hormone and an acidic peptide) appear to be packaged into neurosecretory granules for transport to the nerve terminals for storage and secretion. The 11,300 dalton peptide appears to remain in the perikaryon (136, 137). Further processing of one or both of the 6000 dalton peptides occurred within the secretory granules to < 3000 dalton peptide product or products (138). In another neurosecretory neuron in *Aplysia*, R_{15}, a MW 12,000 neuropeptide precursor synthesized by this neuron appears to be first packaged into secretory granules and then processed intragranularly (139).

Biosynthesis and axonal transport studies on the neuropeptides vasopressin and oxytocin in the rat hypothalamo-neurohypophysial system have also implicated the secretory granule as the intracellular site of processing of the precursors for these peptides (82). In these studies, ^{35}S cysteine was injected into the supraoptic nucleus (containing the cell bodies of the neurons). At various times after injection the ^{35}S labeled proteins present within the axons of these neurons (median eminence) were examined. Provasopressin and pro-oxytocin were found in the axons at the earliest times and these were processed to their respective peptides and neurophysins at later times. This observation indicated that the precursors were processed during axonal transport in a movable compartment, presumably within the secretory granules (82).

The cellular organization of proprotein processing has also been studied in a number of non-neuronal systems. The work of Steiner and his coworkers indicates that processing (limited proteolysis) of proinsulin begins at the Golgi level and continues within the secretory granules (133). Processing of pro-opiomelanocortin within the secretory granule has been observed in the mouse, toad, and rat intermediate lobe and in mouse anterior lobe tumor (AtT-20) cells (134, 140–142). In dissociated cell cultures of rat intermediate lobe and mouse anterior lobe tumor cells, partial processing of pro-opiomelanocortin occurs within the Golgi (134, 142). In the case of proalbumin, proteolytic processing occurred after packaging within vesicles (143, 144). The available experimental evidence from neuronal and non-neuronal systems therefore indicates that the secretory granule (or vesicle) is a major site for proteolytic processing of proproteins, although in some cases limited proteolysis of proteins also may occur in the Golgi. In those cases where limited proteolysis of the proproteins to peptide products occurs intragranularly, it would be expected that further modification of the cleaved peptides before secretion (e.g., amidation, acetylation) would take place within the granules as well.

The mechanisms underlying the packaging of the proproteins and the processing enzymes in the same subcellular processing compartment are poorly understood at the present time. One possibility is that the enzyme and precursors are cosegregated and copackaged. This would suggest that there are "signals" on the precursors and enzymes that would direct them to certain Golgi membrane regions where subsequent formation of the secretory granule occurs. Another idea is the fusion model suggested by the experimental work of Judah and Quinn (144). These authors found that processing of endogenously labeled proalbumin is Ca^{2+} dependent. Reagents that promote membrane fusion greatly increased the rate of processing and those that block fusion (e.g., colchicine) inhibited processing. Hence, they proposed that intragranular conversion of proalbumin requires the fusion of vesicles containing the processing enzymes with the granules containing the proalbumin. A third possible mechanism is the fusion of vesicles containing the processing enzymes with the Golgi, at the budded-off area, just before the complete formation of the secretory granules. All three possibilities provide working hypotheses for future studies on mechanisms.

4.3 Limited Proteolysis

4.3.1 Nature of Proprotein-Converting Enzymes

As indicated in Section 3.2 and Figures 1 and 2, virtually all proproteins have pairs of basic amino acid residues flanking the biologically active peptide sequences to be cleaved (32, 34, 131–133, 145–147). It was therefore proposed that synthesis of peptides from their proproteins involves limited proteolysis, beginning with a cleavage at the paired basic amino acid residues (131). Such a cleavage has often been thought to involve the action of a trypsin-like enzyme. However, since the active peptides do not actually terminate with arginines or lysines, it was further proposed that a second enzyme resembling carboxypeptidase B in action was necessary to subsequently trim these basic residues from the C-terminus. Recent studies have provided evidence for the existence, within secretory granules, of prohormone converting enzymes that are specific for pairs of basic amino acids (148) and carboxypeptidase B-like enzymes that can trim the basic residues from the C-terminus of cleaved peptides.

4.3.2 Experimental Evidence for Trypsin-like Converting Enzymes

Several enzymatic activities that are specific for paired basic amino acid residues of proproteins have been found in different tissues (Table 4). Within the nervous system, an enzyme activity localized in rat and bovine pituitary neural lobe secretory granules that cleaves at the paired basic amino acid residues has been reported (148–150). In these studies, toad pro-opiomelanocortin (pro-opiocortin) was used as a model substrate. The major products formed were a 21K (K=1000) molecular weight molecule with both ACTH and β-endorphin immunoreactivity (ACTH + β-LPH) and a 16K glycopeptide (Figures 3 and 4B), indicating a cleavage at the pair of basic amino acid residues between the N-terminal glycopeptide and ACTH of pro-opiocortin (Figure 2). *In vivo*, this enzyme probably serves to cleave the proproteins containing vasopressin and oxytocin that are found within these granules (82, 84, 85). This converting enzyme activity has a pH optimum of 5.0, and is a thiol protease that is distinct from lysosomal cathepsin B, since it is not inhibited by several cathepsin B inhibitors and is unable to cleave typical cathepsin B substrates. The activity appears to be present in a soluble and membrane-associated form.

Similar pro-opiocortin converting activity has been found in rat intermediate lobe secretory granules (148, 149). This enzyme activity, which was found in both a soluble and a membrane-associated form, catalyzed the cleavage of toad pro-opiocortin to 21K and 13K forms of ACTH, β-LPH, α-MSH, β-endorphin, a β-endorphin-like peptide (β-ELP), and a 16K glycopeptide (16K GP), as shown in Figures 3 and 4A. These *in vitro* generated products are similar to those synthesized within the toad intermediate lobe *in situ* (Figure 5; refs. 109, 151), which suggests that the cleavages occurred at the Lys-Arg pairs of amino acid residues of pro-opiocortin (Figure 2). That the cleavages occurred at these sites is supported by similar experiments in which [³H]-arginine-labeled pro-opiocortin was exposed to the granule converting enzyme. When the cleaved products in this experiment were treated with carboxypeptidase B, free ³H-labeled arginine was released, which suggests that the cleavage occurred at the peptide bond just after the arginine residue of the lysine-arginine pair (Chang and Loh, unpublished data). In addition to the formation of the normal products found in toad intermediate lobe

TABLE 4 Trypsin-like Proprotein-Converting Enzymes in Different Tissues

Source	Substrate	Specificity	Subcellular[a] Localization	pH Optima	Inhibitors	No Inhibition	Reference
Rat pituitary neural lobe	Pro-opiocortin	Lys-Arg	Secretory granules (membrane > sol.)	5.0	PCMB Leupeptin Pepstatin A	DFP Chloroquine EDTA	148, 149
Bovine pituitary neural lobe	Pro-opiocortin	Lys-Arg	Secretory granules	5.0	PCMB Leupeptin Pepstatin A Antipain	DFP Chloroquine EDTA	154, 156
Rat pituitary intermediate lobe	Pro-opiocortin	Lys-Arg	Secretory granules (membrane > soluble)	5.0	PCMB Leupeptin Pepstatin A	DFP Chloroquine EDTA	148, 149
Porcine pituitary	Synthetic hexapeptide Lys-Asp-Lys-Arg-Tyr-Gly	Lys-Arg	Secretory granules (soluble)	8.8		DFP SBTI	152, 153
Anglerfish pancreatic islet cells	Proinsulin Proglucagon, prosomatostatin	{ Arg-Arg Lys-Arg Lys-Arg Lys-Arg	Secretory granules (membrane > soluble)	5.2	PCMB Leupeptin Antipain	DFP Chloroquine EDTA SBTI TPCK TLCK	154–156
Rat pancreas	Proinsulin	Arg-Arg	Secretory granules (membrane and soluble activity)	6.0	DFP TLCK	SBTI BPTI	157–158

(Continued)

TABLE 4 (*Continued*)

Source	Substrate	Specificity	Subcellular[a] Localization	pH Optima	Inhibitors	No Inhibition	Reference
Bovine parathyroid	Proparathormone	Lys-Arg	Particulate fraction of microsomal pellet	7.0–9.0	EDTA Benzamidine Chloroquine	BPTI "Trasylol" TLCK	159, 160
			Widespread in cell particulate fraction		EDTA	BPTI SBTI TLCK	161
Rat liver	Proalbumin	Arg-Arg	Large granules	6.0	Leupeptin TLCK	Pepstatin	143

[a] Secretory granules are lysed and then pelleted by centrifugation. The pellet represents the membrane fraction and the supernatant, the soluble fraction. Enzyme activity is assayed in both the membrane and soluble fraction. Membrane > soluble means more activity was found in the membrane versus the soluble fraction.

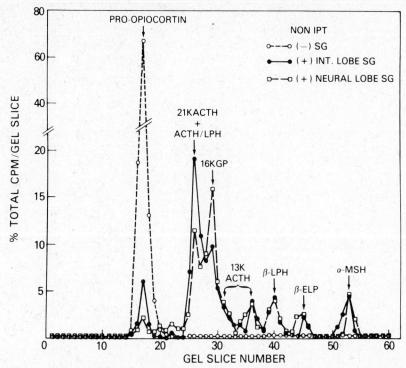

Figure 3. Acid-urea gel profiles of labeled proteins and peptides following a 5 h incubation (pH 5.0, 37°C of [³H] phenylalanine-labeled toad pro-opiocortin in the absence (○ · · · ○) and presence (•———•) of rat intermediate lobe or neural lobe lysed secretory granules (□ · · · □). The products cleaved from pro-opiocortin have been identified immunologically and by size (K = 1000), and the identity of each peak is indicated (see also Figure 4). Note that conversion of the pro-opiocortin to peptide products occurred only in the presence of the secretory granule lysates. Incubation of pro-opiocortin in the presence of neural lobe granule lysate yielded a 16K glycopeptide (16K GP) as the major product; relatively smaller amounts of 16K GP were produced when incubated with the intermediate lobe granule lysate.

in situ, a 21K cleavage product was produced that had the antigenic determinants of both ACTH and β-endorphin. The existence of this product indicates that a proportion (∼30%) of the pro-opiocortin was cleaved between the 16K glycopeptide and ACTH. This cleavage occurs only minimally in the toad intermediate lobe *in situ*. Characterization of the nature of the intermediate lobe pro-opiocortin converting activity shows that it is an acid thiol protease with a pH optimum of 5.0, similar to the neural lobe enzyme (149). However, the converting activities in the two lobes appear to have differential preferences for the various paired basic amino acid cleavage sites on the pro-opiocortin molecules (Figure 3, ref. 149). The neural lobe enzyme primarily cleaves pro-opiocortin at the pair of basic residues between the 16K glycopeptide

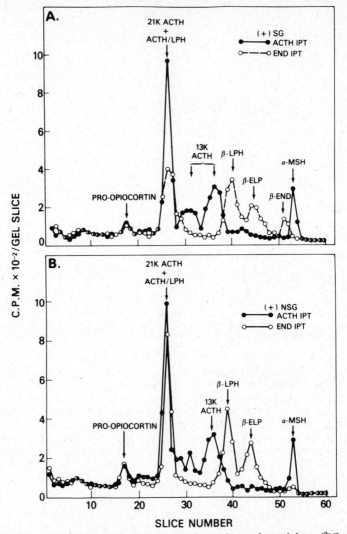

Figure 4. Immunological identification of peptide products cleaved from [³H] phenylala-nine-labeled pro-opiocortin (at pH 5.0, 37°C for 5 h) by lysed rat intermediate lobe (A) or neural lobe (B) secretory granules. The acid-urea gel profiles show labeled peptides immunoprecipitated by anti-ACTH (●———●) and anti β-endorphin (○···○).

and ACTH. [Note the greater amount of 16K glycopeptide (Figure 3) and ACTH/LPH (Figure 4) generated by neural lobe compared with interme-diate lobe enzyme activities.] Whether this difference in conversion of pro-opiocortin by neural lobe and intermediate lobe secretory granule lysates *in vitro* is due to different converting enzymes or to other fac-tors is still under study.

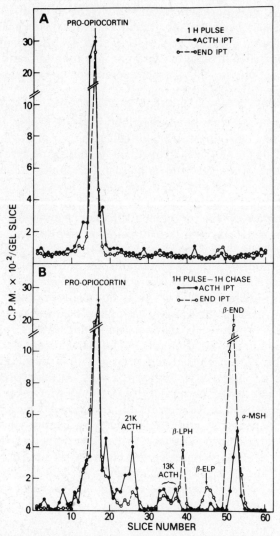

Figure 5. Acid-urea gel profiles of anti-ACTH (●——●) and anti-β-endorphin (○ - - - ○) immunoprecipitated labeled peptides synthesized by toad (*Xenopus leavis*) pituitary intermediate lobe (A) after a 1 h pulse in [^{3}H]phenylalanine, and (B) after a 1 h pulse, followed by a 1 h chase in the presence of dopamine to inhibit release of the newly synthesized peptides. The molecular weight and identity of the peaks are indicated. Note that the common precursor of ACTH and endorphin (pro-opiocortin), synthesized after a 1 h pulse is partly converted (by 1 h chase) to various forms of ACTH, β-LPH, β-endorphin, (β-End), α-MSH, and an endorphinlike peptide (β-ELP). Note similarity of peptide products in Figure 4 using granule converting enzyme activity *in vitro*.

Another enzyme activity that is specific for pairs of amino acids but has properties unlike trypsin has been found in porcine pituitary granules (152, 153). This porcine enzyme activity is quite different in its pH optimum (pH 8.8) from that described for the rat intermediate and rat and bovine neural lobe granules (see Table 4). The assay for this enzyme was carried out using a synthetic hexapeptide, and the relationship of this activity to the pro-opiomelanocortin conversion described above remains to be determined.

A converting enzyme activity for proinsulin, proglucagon, and prosomatostatin has also been described (154–156). This enzyme activity, found within the pancreatic islet cell granules of anglerfish, cleaves at the paired basic amino acid residues of the respective prohormones to form insulin, glucagon, and somatostatin. Inhibitor studies suggest that the activity is due to a thiol protease. The optimum pH of the enzyme activity is 5.2 and appears to be present in the membrane and soluble components of the granules. Whether conversion of the three prohormones of the pancreatic islet cells are due to a single enzyme or three different enzymes remains to be determined. If these are separate activities, the nature of the enzymes appears to be very similar.

Kemmler, Steiner, and coworkers have reported a different enzyme activity in rat pancreatic islet granules that cleaves proinsulin to insulin (157, 158). The converting activity described by these workers suggests that it is a serine protease, distinct from pancreatic trypsin (Table 4), with a pH optimum of 6.0. (See ref. 198 for more recent data).

Two groups have reported the presence of a parathyroid hormone (PTH) converting activity in bovine parathyroid that converts pro-PTH to PTH (159, 160, 161). The activity reported by McGregor et al. (160) is found in the particulate fraction of the microsomal pellet and has a pH optimum of between 7 and 9. The enzyme activity is inhibited by benzamidine and chloroquine and is calcium sensitive. The PTH converting enzyme activity reported by Habener et al. (161) is less well characterized, but it is also calcium sensitive. The nature of the activities described by both groups are very similar. Inhibitor studies suggest that the PTH converting enzyme reported by both groups is not pancreatic trypsin.

Although albumin is not a neuropeptide or peptide hormone, it is worth mentioning that a proalbumin converting activity that has all the characteristics of lysosomal cathepsin B has been found in the large granules of rat liver (143). The enzyme is specific for the Arg-Arg residues of proalbumin, has a pH optimum of 6.0, and is inhibited by leupeptin and TLCK but not pepstatin.

Docherty and Steiner (17) have proposed several criteria for the identification of proprotein converting proteases. Amongst these are: (i) whether the enzyme activity correctly cleaves the prohormone to all known products, (ii) whether the enzyme activity is localized in an appropriate organelle, that is, where conversion occurs *in vitro*, and (iii) whether the pH optimum and stability of the enzyme activity are consistent with the internal pH of the organelle in which the activity is localized. Several studies have considered these criteria. The prohormone converting activities found in the anglerfish pancreatic islet, rat pituitary intermediate lobe, and neural lobe secretory granules fulfill all these criteria. The action of these enzymes is very specific and appears to yield the proper cleavage products from the respective prohormones. These activities are found in secretory granules, consistent with the observations implicating these granules as the site for prohormone processing in these tissues *in vivo* (134, 141, 162). The acidic pH optima and ranges (between pH 5 and 6) of these enzyme activities correlate with the acidic intragranular pHs (between pH 5 and 6) found in virtually all secretory granules studied (163–165). The converting activity found in the neural lobe secretory granules clearly fulfills criteria (ii) and (iii). Although it has been shown that the enzyme activity in neural lobe granules does specifically cleave at the paired basic amino acid residues of pro-opiocortin, the experiments have not yet been reported showing that the proproteins for vasopressin and oxytocin (the relevant substrates) are correctly processed by this enzyme activity.

In our studies on the intermediate and neural lobe, the converting activities were found to cleave the proprotein, pro-opiocortin, but not small synthetic peptides with either single or double basic amino acid residues (150; unpublished data). This might explain why many earlier attempts to study these enzyme activities with small synthetic peptide substrates have proved unsuccessful. It has been suggested that, in addition to the pairs of basic amino acids, the conformation of the substrate may be critical for successful enzyme–substrate interactions to occur (166). Since these prohormone converting activities appear to be clearly different from pancreatic trypsin or lysosomal cathepsin B, it might be more appropriate to refer to them as being due to prohormone converting enzymes rather than trypsin-like enzymes.

4.3.3 Experimental Evidence for Carboxypeptidase B-like Converting Enzymes

The conversion of proproteins to peptides requires, in addition to an enzyme that cleaves at paired basic residues, one that trims the basic amino acids from the C-terminus of the cleaved peptide.

Studies on rat pancreatic islet cells have provided evidence for the existence of a carboxypeptidase B-like (CBP-like) activity in the secretory granules (157, 158). The activity cleaved the basic residues from the C-terminus of the B chain of insulin and the C peptide (split from proinsulin) at pH 7.0. Ethylenediaminetetraacetic acid (EDTA) and orthophenanthroline inhibited the activity; diisopropylphosphofluoridate

(DFP) and thiol reagents were without effect. From the inhibitor study it was suggested that the activity was due to a metalloenzyme, similar to pancreatic carboxypeptidase B (167).

More recently, using ^{125}I-labeled enkephalin-arginine (labeled in the tyrosine residue) or dansyl-Phe-Leu-Arg as a substrate, CPB-like activity was detected in bovine chromaffin granules (168, 170). The bovine chromaffin granule CPB-like activity cleaved enkephalin-arginine to enkephalin, and has a pH optimum of 6.0. The activity was inhibited by antipain and leupeptin as well as by mercurial and copper compounds (PCMPSA,* HgCl$_2$, CuCl$_2$) that inhibit thiol proteases. Potato inhibitor (169), "by-product" analogs of arginine and lysine (GPSA, AMPSA, B$_2$1SA, MGTA),† EDTA and phenanthroline, which inhibit pancreatic carboxypeptidase B activity, also inhibited the chromaffin granule enzyme (Hook et al., unpublished data).

Using the ^{125}I enkephalin in a similar assay, CPB-like activity has also been detected in rat neural, intermediate, and anterior lobe secretory granules and in bovine neural lobe secretory granules (Hook et al., unpublished data). The activities found in the granules of all three lobes of the pituitary have pH optima of about 5.5–6.0 and were inhibited by GPSA, MGTA, B$_2$1SA, and AMPSA. These preliminary studies on the CPB-like activities in pituitary granules from different lobes suggest that they have properties similar to the chromaffin granule CPB activity.

4.3.4   Regulation of Limited Proteolysis (Processing) of Proproteins

Although there appear to be common recognition sites for processing of propeptides, i.e., cleavage at paired basic amino acid sites, it is also apparent that in a number of prohormones—for example, residues 33–35 and 58–60 of proparathyroid hormone and residues 15 and 16 of preglucagon (166)—there are paired basic amino acid residues that are not cleaved. These basic amino acid pairs are probably made inaccessible to the proteolytic enzyme by the conformational constraints in the proprotein molecule. Geisow and Smyth have made extensive theoretical calculations based on the structure of the prohormones and have proposed that pairs of lysine or arginine that are not cleaved are frequently found in the α-helix structure of the protein where the regular pattern of hydrogen bonds can stabilize the polypeptide against proteolytic attack (166). The basic residues that are cleaved are probably located in superficial and aperiodic regions of a globular prohormone. According to this model, the conformation of the prohormone may play a critical role in regulating its limited proteolysis.

---

*PCMPSA, p-chloromercuriphenylsulfonic acid.
†GPSA, guanidinopropylsuccinic acid; APMSA, aminomercaptosuccinic acid; B$_2$1SA, benzylsuccinic acid; MGTA, 2-mercaptomethyl-3-guanidinoethyl thiopropanoic acid.

While the conformation of the prohormone may contribute to the specificity of the processing, it cannot account for the differential processing of the same prohormone by two different tissues, as in the case of pro-opiomelanocortin. In the pituitary anterior lobe this prohormone is processed to ACTH, β-LPH, a 16K glycopeptide, and small amounts of β-endorphin, whereas in the intermediate lobe, the ACTH and β-LPH are further cleaved at paired basic amino acid sites to α-MSH and β-endorphin (140). Such differential processing in the two tissues cannot be accounted for by the conformation of the substrate, but may be due to the existence of different enzymes in the two tissues or the presence of an additional enzyme in the intermediate lobe that can catalyze the further cleavage of ACTH and β-LPH to form α-MSH and β-endorphin, respectively.

4.3.5 Other Proteolytic-Converting Enzymes

Synthesis of some neuropeptides, such as angiotensin I and II and cholecystokinin dodecapeptide (CCK_{12}) and octapeptide (CCK_8), from larger protein precursors requires enzymes that cleave at sites other than pairs of basic amino acids.

The enzymes and substrates involved in angiotensin synthesis are known collectively as the angiotensin-renin system (171–173). The enzyme renin (EC 3.4.99.19) is a neutral protease that cleaves angiotensinogens at Leu-Leu bonds to yield angiotensin I (proangiotensin). The angiotensin converting enzyme (EC 3.4.15.1) then converts angiotensin I (a decapeptide) to angiotensin II (an octapeptide) by splitting a Phe-His bond, resulting in the removal of a His-Leu sequence at the C-terminal. Angiotensin converting enzyme appears to be a rather nonspecific dipeptidylcarboxypeptidase that removes COOH-terminal dipeptides from a variety of substrates, some as small as tripeptides. The angiotensin-renin system has been studied extensively in various tissues, including brain, and reviewed elsewhere (see Chapter 32 in this volume and refs. 171–173).

Studies on the conversion of CCK_{33} have revealed enzymes in brain that cleave the peptide bonds between Arg-Isoleu and Arg-Asp of CCK_{33} to yield CCK_{12} and CCK_8 (174, 175). There appear to be two different enzyme activities, one yielding CCK_{12} and the other CCK_8 as end-products. These enzymes are distinct from trypsin in size and lack of inhibition by SBTI. They will also cleave synthetic dipeptides such as Arg-Val and Arg-Leu and therefore are not hormone (CCK_{33})-specific. Further work is necessary to determine the physiological role of these enzymes in CCK_{12} and CCK_8 biosynthesis.

An enkephalin generating enzyme has been partially purified from rat brain (176). This enzyme is a thiol endopeptidase with chymotryptic-like specificity for peptide bonds following hydrophobic residues Met and Leu. The enzyme is able to cleave a model substrate Leu-Trp-Met-Arg-Phe-Ala and endogenous enkephalin precursors from striatum (176). It has therefore been proposed that such an enzyme may be involved in the cleavage of proenkephalin or its tryptic fragments to yield enkephalin.

A number of other proteinases that may be relevant in proprotein conversion have been found in pituitary and brain. One of these enzymes is a neutral proteinase reported by Graf et al. (177) to be present in porcine anterior pituitary granules. The enzyme cleaves at the Arg of the synthetic substrate Z-Lys-Pro-Arg-pNa and the Arg^{60}-Tyr^{61} bond of β-LPH_{1-91} to release β-LPH_{1-60} (177). Acid-thiol proteinases in pituitary and brain that are able to cleave Bz-Arg-Nap have been reported by Marks et al. (178). However, these enzymes also degrade a number of other protein substrates such as histones, glucagon, the lipotropins, and myelin basic protein. In addition to these proteinases, Cathepsin D-like enzymes have been found in anterior pituitary and brain. These are able to cleave the Leu^{77}-Phe^{78} bond in β-endorphin to form γ-endorphin (177). North et al. (179) have reported the presence in the neural lobe of the rat pituitary of an acidic (pH optimum 4.5) chymotryptic-like enzyme in neurosecretory granules that converts rat neurophysin II to neurophysin III and neurophysin I to neurophysin I'.

4.4 Other Posttranslational Modifications of Neuropeptides

After being cleaved from their precursor, peptides often undergo further posttranslational modifications, usually at the N- and C-termini. Amidation of the C-terminus occurs in α-MSH, thyrotropin releasing hormone (TRH), luteinizing hormone releasing hormone (LHRH), substance P, calcitonin, and CCK (180–185). The most common modifications found at the N-terminus of peptides are acetylation [e.g., α-MSH, β-endorphin (180, 186)] and cyclization of the glutamic acid to form pyroglutamate [e.g., TRH, gastrin, bombesin (181, 187, 188)]. In the case of the chemotactic peptide, N-formylmethionine has been found (189). Other modifications in the internal residues of peptide sequences include sulfation of tyrosine in CCK (185), glycosylation of ACTH (186), and phosphorylation of ACTH (190). In the case of the glycosylation of ACTH, it is likely that the modification took place before cleavage from the proprotein since N-aspargine-linked glycosylations begin in the RER and are completed in the Golgi (191).

The enzyme systems for glycosylation (192), phosphorylation (116), and acetylation (193, 194) of proteins have been studied in various tissues and reviewed elsewhere. However, caution is necessary before accepting these exact enzymes as being involved in the posttranslational modification of neuropeptides. Enzymes catalyzing the neuropeptide modifications should also fulfill the criteria stated by Docherty and Steiner (17). It is likely that "late" modifications such as acetylation and amidation of neuropeptides occur within the secretory granules (see Section 4.2), and therefore one might expect that the enzymes catalyzing these events would reside within this organelle.

Recently, acetylation enzyme activities have been found in highly purified secretory granules from rat neurointermediate lobe (Loh and O'Donohue, unpublished data). Using labeled acetyl coenzyme A as the acetyl group donor and desacetyl α-MSH (ACTH$_{1\text{-}13}$NH$_2$) and β-endorphin$_{1\text{-}31}$ as substrates, α-MSH and acetylated β-endorphin were formed respectively, by the granule lysates. The activities have an operating pH range consistent with an acidic intragranular pH. Further work is necessary to determine if the acetylation activities for α-MSH and β-endorphin are due to the same enzyme. (See ref. 199, 200 for more recent studies.)

Little is known about the enzymes involved in other posttranslational modifications such as sulfation of CCK or the cyclization of the N-terminal glutamic acid residues. C-terminal amidation appears to require an extra glycine between the amino acid in the proprotein that is to be amidated and the pairs of basic amino acids serving as cleavage sites. The mechanisms and enzyme candidates for this reaction are still unknown. (See ref. 201 for more recent studies.)

4.4.1 Functions of Posttranslational Modification of Peptides

Experimental evidence suggests that acetylation of the N-terminus of α-MSH and β-endorphin can greatly alter their biological activities. Deacetylated α-MSH is a much less potent melanotropic hormone (180), and acetylated β-endorphin loses its opiate activity (186). Sulfated CCK has also been found to be more potent than nonsulfated CCK (195). Such modifications can therefore provide a regulatory mechanism for neuropeptide potency.

It has also been reported that peptides that are "blocked" at the C- or N-terminus, or both [e.g., α-MSH (196)], and glycosylated peptides [e.g. ACTH (129)], are more resistant to proteolytic degradation. Thus N- and C-terminal modifications and glycosylation may serve to extend the half-lives and hence the duration of action of the neuropeptides.

5 CONCLUDING REMARKS

Considerable progress has been made in the field of peptide biosynthesis since the discovery of the first prohormone, proinsulin (49), some 15 years ago. Not only have many more prohormones been discovered and sequenced but the concepts of the precursor protein have been shown to be applicable to a wide variety of proteins with diverse functions completely unrelated to hormonal activities. The common theme connecting these diverse precursor proteins is their linkage to the intracellular membrane systems of the cell, through which they are translocated, chemically and physically modified, packaged, and ultimately fused with the plasma membrane (for the purposes of secretion, membrane turnover and modification, uptake of extracellular materials, etc.). The biosynthesis of a precursor protein is therefore intimately associated with the organization of its intracellular membranes, from its initial translation as a preprotein to its final disposition in a secretory granule (or vesicle) being readied for exocytosis. Given this perspective, one might then expect to find that the various processes occurring within these membrane-bounded organelles (e.g., proteolytic activities within secretory vesicles) will be related to but yet different from similar processes occurring extracellularly, or even in the cytosol of the cell itself. For heuristic reasons, we have focused on only one aspect of the microenvironment within these membrane systems (i.e., pH); other factors (ionic concentrations, cofactors, etc.) could also prove to be significant. The prohormone converting enzyme activity found in secretory granules does appear to be of a unique sort, similar to but not identical with lysosomal enzymes.

Much more work is needed to characterize these enzymes and others involved in posttranslational modification. If indeed such enzymes are specific, then recombinant DNA studies currently being directed at the mechanisms of gene expression for specific proproteins should also be directed at the specific expression of the mRNA coding for these enzymes. A complete understanding of how a particular cell type elaborates a specific peptide obviously involves the mechanisms of regulation of both of these types of molecules. We have pointed out that the proteolytic conversion of precursor proteins is not the exclusive property of secretory vesicles (e.g., in some cases the RER and Golgi appear to be involved). Nor do we believe that all peptide secreting cells will be organized in an identical manner. In fact, multiple sites of posttranslational processing events may increase the range of possibilities available to a cell (neuron) in order to regulate specific peptide secretion. Given a common precursor with multifunctional peptides (e.g., the precursor of ACTH and endorphin), cleavage before packaging may allow the separate peptides to be compartmentalized differently in the Golgi so that they can be placed in separate vesicles with different fates (e.g., destined for secretion, degradation, or different posttranslational processing steps). Alternatively, restricting the conversion of a proprotein to the secretory vesicle site would allow for coordinate release of all the functional peptides.

The cell biological organization and specific biochemical character of posttranslational processing in a peptidergic neuron may be as much a determinant of the neuron's properties as is the transcription and translation of gene-encoded messages for specific precursors. Further work in this area will undoubtedly reveal important clues relevant to the mechanisms responsible for the diversity of peptidergic neurons.

REFERENCES

1. A. Meister, *Science* **180**, 33 (1973).
2. A. Meister, *Life Sci.* **15**, 177 (1973).
3. H. Borsook, *Adv. Protein Chem.* **8**, 127 (1953).
4. G. A. Homandberg, J. A. Mattis, and M. Laskowski, *Biochemistry* **17**, 5220 (1978).
5. F. Lipmann, *Science* **173**, 875 (1971).
6. F. Lipmann, W. Gevers, H. Kleinhauf, and R. Roskowski, *Adv. Enzymol.* **35**, 1 (1971).
7. K. Kurahashi, *Ann. Rev. Biochem.* **43**, 445 (1974).
8. S. G. Laland and T. L. Zimmer, *Essays Biochem.* **9**, 31 (1973).
9. T. Hökfelt, O. Johansson, A. Lungdahl, J. Lundberg, and M. Schultzberg, *Nature* **284**, 515 (1980).
10. S. Konishi, A. Tsuno, and M. Otsuka, *Proc. Japan Acad., Ser B*, **55**, 525 (1979).
11. J. M. Lundberg, A. Anggard, P. Emson, J. Fabrenkrug, and T. Hökfelt, *Proc. Natl. Acad. Sci., USA.* **78**, 5255 (1981).
12. G. Pelletier, H. W. M. Steinbusch, and A. A. J. Verhofstad, *Nature* **293**, 71 (1981).
13. J. A. Kessler, J. E. Adler, M. C. Bohn, and I. B. Black, *Science* **214**, 336 (1981).
14. M. Zimmerman, R. A. Mumford, and D. F. Steiner, Eds., *Precursor Processing in the Biosynthesis of Proteins*, Vol. 343, Annals of the New York Academy of Sciences, 1980.
15. R. B. Freedman and H. C. Hawkins, Eds., *The Enzymology of Post-Translational Modification of Proteins*, Vol. 1, Academic Press, New York, 1980.
16. G. Koch and D. Richter, Eds., *Biosynthesis, Modification, and Processing of Cellular and Viral Polyproteins*, Academic Press, New York, 1980.
17. K. Docherty and D. F. Steiner, *Ann. Rev. Physiol.*, **79**, 4613 (1982).
18. B. Kassell and J. Kay, *Science* **180**, 1022 (1973).
19. J. H. Fessler and L. J. Fessler, *Ann. Rev. Biochem.* **47**, 129 (1978).
20. G. Kreil, C. Molloy, R. Kaschnitz, L. Haiaml, and U. Vilas, *Ann. N.Y. Acad. Sci.* **343**, 338 (1980).
21. H. S. Wiley and R. A. Wallace, *J. Biol. Chem.* **256**, 8626 (1981).
22. G. Blobel and B. Dobberstein, *J. Cell Biol.* **67**, 835 (1975).
23. G. Kreil, *Ann. Rev. Biochem.* **50**, 317 (1981).
24. G. Palade, *Science* **189**, 347 (1975).
25. I. M. Chaiken, R. E. Randolf, and H. C. Taylor, *Ann. New York Acad. Sci.* **248**, 442 (1975).
26. G. Blobel and D. D. Sabatini, L. A. Manson, Eds., *Biomembranes*, Vol. 2, Plenum Press, New York, 1971, pp. 193.
27. C. Milstein, G. G. Brownlee, T. M. Harrison, and M. B. Matthews, *Nature New Biol.* **239**, 117 (1972).
28. R. Harwood, in R. B. Freedman and H. C. Hawkins, Eds., *The Enzymology of Post-Translational Modifications of Proteins*, Vol. 1, Academic Press, London, 1980, p. 3.
29. L. Villa-Koraroff, A. Efstratiadia, S. Broome, P. Lomedico, R. Tizard, S. P. Naber, W. L. Chick, and W. Gilbert, *Proc. Natl. Acad. Sci. USA* **75**, 3727 (1978).
30. B. Kemper, J. F. Habener, M. D. Ernst, J. T. Potts, and A. Rich, *Biochemistry* **15**, 15 (1976).
31. P. H. Seeburg, J. Shine, J. A. Martial, J. D. Baxter, and H. M. Goodman, *Nature* **270**, 486 (1977).
32. S. Nakanishi, A. Inone, T. Kita, M. Nakamura, A. C. Y. Chang, S. N. Cohen, and S. Numa, *Nature* **278**, 423 (1979).
33. M. Noda, Y. Furutani, H. Takahashi, M. Toyosato, T. Hirose, S. Inayama, S. Nakanishi, and S. Numa, *Nature* **295**, 202 (1982).
34. H. Land, G. Schütz, H. Schmale, and D. Richter, *Nature* **295**, 299 (1982).

35. H. W. Strauss, C. D. Bennett, A. M. Donohue, J. A. Rodkey, and A. W. Alberts, *J. Biol. Chem.* **252**, 6846 (1977).
36. P. Gaye and J. P. Gautron, *Biochem. Biophys. Res. Comm.* **79**, 903 (1977).
37. V. A. Lingappa, F. N. Katz, H. F. Lodish, and G. Blobel, *J. Biol. Chem.* **253**, 8667 (1978).
38. Y. Burstein and I. Schechter, *Biochemistry* **17**, 2392 (1978).
39. G. Sachanek, G. Kreil, and M. A. Hermodson, *Proc. Natl. Acad. Sci. USA* **75**, 701 (1978).
40. IUPAC-IUB Commission on Biochemical Nomenclature, *J. Biol. Chem.* **243**, 3557 (1968).
41. R. Jackson and G. Blobel, *Proc. Natl. Acad. Sci. USA* **74**, 5598 (1977).
42. C. Zwizinski and W. Wickner, *J. Biol. Chem.* **255**, 7973 (1980).
43. A. W. Strauss, M. Zimmerman, I. Boime, B. Ashe, R. A. Mumford, and A. W. Alberts, *Proc. Natl. Acad. Sci. USA* **76**, 4225 (1979).
44. D. F. Steiner, D. Cunningham, L. Spiegelman, and B. Aten, *Science* **157**, 697 (1967).
45. B. A. Eipper and R. E. Mains, *Endocr. Rev.* **1**, 1 (1980).
46. W. W. Chin, F. Maloof, and J. F. Habener, *J. Biol. Chem.* **256**, 3059 (1981).
47. J. E. Godine, W. W. Chin, and J. F. Habener, *J. Biol. Chem.* **255**, 8780 (1980).
48. J. E. Godine, W. W. Chin, and J. F. Habener, *J. Biol. Chem.* **256**, 2475 (1981).
49. P. K. Lund, R. H. Goodman, J. W. Jacobs, and J. F. Habener, *Diabetes* **29**, 583 (1980).
50. H. Schmale and D. Richter, *Proc. Natl. Acad. Sci. USA* **78**, 766 (1981).
51. D. Nathans and H. W. Smith, *Ann. Rev. Biochem.* **44**, 273 (1975).
52. A. Maxam and W. Gilbert, *Proc. Natl. Acad. Sci. USA* **74**, 560 (1977).
53. F. Sanger, S. Nicklen, and A. R. Coulson, *Proc. Natl. Acad. Sci. USA* **74**, 5463 (1977).
54. J. W. Jacobs, R. H. Goodman, W. W. Chin, P. C. Dee, J. F. Habener, N. H. Bell, and J. T. Potts, *Science* **213**, 457 (1981).
55. K. Agarawal, A. Yamazaki, P. Cashion, and H. Korana, *Angew. Chem. Int. Ed. Eng.* **11**, 451 (1972).
56. B. E. Noyes, M. Mevarech, R. Stein, and K. L. Agarawal, *Proc. Natl. Acad. Sci. USA* **76**, 1770 (1979).
57. P. Hudson, J. Haley, M. Cronk, J. Shine, and H. Niall, *Nature* **291**, 127 (1981).
58. T. H. Jukes, *Science* **213**, 973 (1980).
59. A. K. Sood, D. Pereira, and S. M. Weissman, *Proc. Natl. Acad. Sci. USA* **78**, 616 (1981).
60. D. T. Krieger, A. S. Liotta, M. J. Brownstein, and E. A. Zimmerman, *Recent Prog. Horm. Res.* **36**, 277 (1980).
61. R. E. Mains and B. A. Eipper, *J. Biol. Chem.* **251**, 4115 (1976).
62. R. E. Jones, P. Pulkralsek, and D. Grunberger, *Biophys. Biochem. Res. Commun.* **74**, 1490 (1977).
63. J. L. Roberts and E. Herbert, *Proc. Natl. Acad. Sci. USA* **74**, 4826 (1977).
64. B. A. Eipper and R. E. Mains, *J. Biol. Chem.* **252**, 8821 (1977).
65. B. A. Eipper, R. E. Mains, and R. E. Guenzi, *J. Biol. Chem.* **251**, 4121 (1976).
66. R. E. Mains, B. A. Eipper, and N. Ling, *Proc. Natl. Acad. Sci. USA* **74**, 3014 (1977).
67. J. L. Roberts and E. Herbert, *Proc. Natl. Acad. Sci. USA* **74**, 5300 (1977).
68. M. Schultzberg, T. Hökfelt, J. M. Lundberg, L. Terenius, L. G. Elfvin, and R. Elde, *Acta Physiol. Scand.* **103**, 475 (1978).
69. O. H. Viveros, E. J. Dilberto, E. Hazum, and K.-J. Chang, *Mol. Pharmacol.* **16**, 1101 (1979).
70. A. S. Stern, R. V. Lewis, S. Kimura, J. Rossier, L. D. Gerber, L. Brink, S. Stein, and S. Udenfriend, *Proc. Natl. Acad. Sci. USA* **76**, 6680 (1979).
71. R. V. Lewis, A. S. Stern, S. Kimura, J. Rossier, S. Stein, and S. Udenfriend, *Science* **208**, 1459 (1980).
72. S. Kimura, R. V. Lewis, A. S. Stern, J. Rossier, S. Stein, and S. Udenfriend, *Proc. Natl. Acad. Sci. USA* **77**, 1681 (1980).

73. D. L. Kilpatrick, T. Taniguchi, B. N. Jones, A. S. Stern, J. E. Shively, J. Hullihan, S. Kimura, S. Stein, and S. Udenfriend, *Proc. Natl. Acad. Sci. USA* **78**, 3265 (1981).
74. P. Girard and L. E. Eiden, *Biochem. Biophys. Res. Comm.* **99**, 969 (1980).
75. U. Gubler, P. Seeburg, B. J. Hoffman, L. P. Gage, and S. Udenfriend, *Nature* **295**, 206 (1982).
76. A. Goldstein, S. Tachibana, L. I. Lowry, M. Hunkepiller, and L. Hook, *Proc. Natl. Acad. Sci. USA* **76**, 6666 (1979).
77. K. Kanawaga, H. Matsuo, and M. Igarashi, *Biochem. Biophys. Res. Commun.* **86**, 153 (1979).
78. H. Sachs and Y. Takabatake, *Endocrinology* **75**, 943 (1964).
79. Y. Takabatake and H. Sachs, *Endocrinology* **75**, 1934 (1964).
80. C. P. Fawcett, A. E. Powell, and H. Sachs, *Endocrinology* **83**, 1299 (1968).
81. H. Sachs, P. Fawcett, Y. Takabatake, and R. Portanova, *Recent Prog. Horm. Res.* **25**, 447 (1969).
82. H. Gainer, Y. Sarne, and M. J. Brownstein, *J. Cell Biol.* **73**, 366 (1977).
83. M. J. Brownstein, J. T. Russell, and H. Gainer, *Science* **207**, 373 (1980).
84. J. T. Russell, M. J. Brownstein, and H. Gainer, *Endocrinol.* **107**, 1880 (1980).
85. J. T. Russell, M. J. Brownstein, and H. Gainer, *Neuropeptides* **2**, 59 (1981).
86. L. C. Guidice and I. M. Chaiken, *Proc. Natl. Acad. Sci. USA* **76**, 3800 (1979).
87. C. Lin, P. Joseph-Bravo, T. Sherman, L. Chan, and J. F. McKelvy, *Biochem. Biophys. Res. Comm.* **89**, 943 (1979).
88. H. Schmale, B. Leipold, and D. Richter, *FEBS Letters* **108**, 311 (1979).
89. H. Schmale and D. Richter, *Proc. Natl. Acad. Sci. USA* **78**, 766 (1981).
90. H. Schmale and D. Richter, *Neuropeptides* **2**, 47 (1981).
91. D. A. Holwerda, *Eur. J. Biochem.* **28**, 340 (1972).
92. D. G. Smyth and D. E. Massey, *Biochem. Biophys. Res. Comm.* **87**, 1006 (1979).
93. N. G. Seidah, S. Benjannet, and M. Chretien, *Biochem. Biophys. Res. Comm.* **100**, 901 (1981).
94. M. Lauber, M. Camier, and P. Cohen, *FEBS Lett.* **97**, 343 (1979).
95. M. Camier, M. Lauber, J. Mohring, and P. Cohen, *FEBS Lett.* **108**, 369 (1979).
96. M. Lauber, P. N. Nicholas, H. Boussetta, C. Fahy, P. Beguin, M. Camier, H. Vaudry, and P. Cohen, *Proc. Natl. Acad. Sci. USA* **78**, 6086 (1981).
97. P. Beguin, P. Nicolas, H. Boussetta, C. Fahy, and P. Cohen, *J. Biol. Chem.* **256**, 9289 (1981).
98. K. I. Kivirikko and R. Myllyla, in R. B. Freedman and H. C. Hawkins, Eds., *The Enzymology of Post-Translational Modification of Proteins*, Vol. 1, Academic Press, London, 1980, p. 53.
99. J. W. Suttie, in R. B. Freedman and H. C. Hawkins, Eds., *The Enzymology of Post-Translational Modification of Proteins*, Vol. 1, Academic Press, London, 1980, p. 213.
100. C. F. Midelfort and A. H. Mehler, *Proc. Natl. Acad. Sci. USA* **69**, 1816 (1972).
101. A. B. Robinson, *Proc. Natl. Acad. Sci. USA* **71**, 885 (1974).
102. Y. Kloog and J. Axelrod, *Acta Physiol. Scand. Supp.*, in press (1983).
103. J. T. Potts, H. M. Kronenberg, J. F. Habener, and A. Rich, *Ann. N.Y. Acad. Sci.* **343**, 38 (1980).
104. R. Gregory and H. Tracy, in J. Thompson, Ed., *Gastrointestinal Hormones*, University of Texas Press, Austin, 1975, p. 13.
105. H. S. Tager, C. Patzett, R. K. Assoian, S. J. Chan, J. R. Duguid, and D. F. Steiner, *Ann. N.Y. Acad. Sci.* **343**, 133 (1980).
106. J. W. Jacobs, J. T. Potts, N. H. Bell, and J. F. Habener, *J. Biol. Chem.* **254**, 10600, (1979).
107. D. F. Steiner, J. L. Clark, C. Nolan, A. H. Rubenstein, E. Margoliash, B. Aten, and P. E. Oyer, *Recent Prog. Horm. Res.* **25**, 207 (1969).
108. M. B. Hinman and E. Herbert, *Biochem.* **19**, 5392 (1980).
109. Y. P. Loh, *Proc. Natl. Acad. Sci. USA* **76**, 797 (1979).

110. P. Crine, F. Gossard, N. G. Seidah, L. Blanchette, M. Lis, and M. Chretien, *Proc. Natl. Acad. Sci. USA* **76**, 5085 (1979).

111. J. D. Judah and M. R. Nicholls, *Biochem. J.* **123**, 649 (1971).

112. J. M. Davidson, L. S. G. McEneany, and P. Bernstein, *Biochem.* **14**, 5188 (1975).

113. G. Kreil, G. Suchanek, and I. Kindas-mügge, *Fed. Proc.* **36**, 2081 (1977).

114. H. Neurath and K. A. Walsh, *Proc. Natl. Acad. Sci. USA* **73**, 3825 (1976).

115. J. Kay, in R. B. Freedman and H. C. Hawkins, Eds., *The Enzymology of Post-Translational Modification of Proteins*, Vol. 1, Academic Press, London, 1980, p. 423.

116. P. J. England, in R. B. Freedman and H. C. Hawkins, Eds., *The Enzymology of Post-Translational Modification of Proteins*, Vol. 1, Academic Press, London, 1980, p. 291.

117. H. G. Nimmo and P. Cohen, *Adv. Cyclic Nucleotide Res.* **8**, 145 (1977).

118. T. Yamauchi and M. Fujisawa, *Biochem. Biophys. Res. Comm.* **82**, 514 (1978).

119. S. Binkley, D. Klein, and J. W. Weller, *J. Neurochem.* **26**, 51 (1976).

120. M. J. Ernst and K-H Kim, *J. Biol. Chem.* **248**, 2550 (1973).

121. D. F. Steiner, P. S. Quinn, S. J. Chan, J. Marsh, and H. Tager, *Ann. N.Y. Acad. Sci.* **343**, 1 (1980).

122. E. Herbert, M. Budarf, M. Phillips, P. Rosa, P. Policastro, E. Oates, J. L. Roberts, N. G. Seidah, and M. Chretien, *Ann. N.Y. Acad. Sci.* **343**, 79 (1980).

123. J. F. Habener, B. W. Kemper, A. Rich, and J. T. Potts, *Recent Prog. Horm. Res.* **33**, 249 (1977).

124. A. W. Strauss, M. Zimmerman, R. A. Mumford, and A. W. Alberts, *Ann. N.Y. Acad. Sci.* **343**, 168 (1980).

125. V. R. Lingappa, J. R. Lingappa, and G. Blobel, *Ann. N.Y. Acad. Sci.* **343**, 356 (1980).

126. J. B. Parent, H. C. Bauer, and K. Olden, *Biochem. Biophys. Res. Comm.* **108**, 552 (1982).

127. J. G. Beeley, *Biochem. Biophys. Res. Comm.* **76**, 1051 (1977).

128. D. Small, P. Y. Chou, and G. D. Fasman, *Biochem. Biophys. Res. Comm.* **79**, 341 (1977).

129. Y. P. Loh and H. Gainer, *Mol. Cell. Endocrinol.* **20**, 35 (1980).

130. R. J. Beynon, in R. B. Freedman and H. C. Hawkins. Eds., *The Enzymology of Post-Translational Modification of Proteins*, Vol. 1, Academic Press, London, 1980, p. 363.

131. D. F. Steiner, W. Kemmler, J. L. Clark, P. E. Oyer, and A. H. Rubenstein, in D. F. Steiner and N. Freinkel, Eds., *Handbook of Physiology: Endocrinology, Vol. I*, Williams and Wilkins, Baltimore, Md., 1972, p. 175.

132. R. E. Chance, R. M. Ellis, and W. W. Bromer, *Science* **161**, 165 (1968).

133. C. Patzett, H. S. Tager, R. C. Carroll, and D. F. Steiner, *Proc. Natl. Acad. Sci. USA*, **77**, 2410 (1980).

134. C. C. Glembotski, *J. Biol. Chem.* **256**, 7433 (1981).

135. J. T. Potts, Jr., H. M. Kronenberg, J. F. Habener, and A. Rich, *Ann. N.Y. Acad. Sci.* **343**, 38 (1980).

136. S. Arch, in D. Farner and K. Lederis, Eds., *Proceedings of the 8th International Symposium on Neurosecretion*, Plenum Press, New York, p. 129, 1982.

137. S. Arch, T. Smock, and P. Early, *J. Gen. Physiol.* **68**, 211 (1976).

138. Y. P. Loh, Y. Sarne, M. Daniels, and H. Gainer, *J. Neurochem.* **29**, 135 (1977).

139. H. Gainer, Y. P. Loh, and E. A. Neale, in B. Haber, J. R. Perez-Polo, and J. D. Coulter, Eds., *Proteins in the Nervous System: Structure and Function*, Alan R. Liss, New York, 1982, p. 131.

140. Y. P. Loh and H. Gainer, *Endocrinology* **105**, 474 (1979).

141. Y. P. Loh and H. A. Gritsch, *Eur. J. Cell Biol.* **177** (1981).

142. B. Gumbiner and R. B. Kelly, *Proc. Natl. Acad. Sci. USA*, **78**, 318 (1981).

143. P. S. Quinn and J. D. Judah, *Biochem. J.* **172**, 301 (1978).

144. J. D. Judah and P. S. Quinn, *Nature (London)* **271**, 384 (1978).

145. C. Patzelt, H. S. Tager, R. J. Carroll, and D. F. Steiner, *Nature* **282**, 260 (1979).
146. J. W. Hamilton, H. D. Niall, J. W. Jacobs, H. J. Keutmann, J. T. Potts Jr., and D. V. Cohen, *Proc. Natl. Acad. Sci., USA* **71**, 653 (1974).
147. J. W. Jacobs, R. H. Goldman, W. W. Chin, P. C. Dee, J. F. Habener, N. H. Bell, and J. T. Potts Jr., *Science* **213**, 457 (1981).
148. Y. P. Loh and H. Gainer, *Proc. Natl. Acad. Sci. USA* **79**, 108 (1982).
149. Y. P. Loh and T. L. Chang, *FEBS Lett.* **137**, 57 (1982).
150. T. L. Chang, H. Gainer, J. T. Russell, and Y. P. Loh, *Endocrinology*, **11**, 1607 (1982).
151. Y. P. Loh and B. G. Jenks, *Endocrinology* **109**, 54 (1982).
152. A. F. Bradbury, D. G. Smyth, and C. R. Snell, in E. D. W. Fitzsimmons, Ed., *Polypeptide Hormones: Molecular and Cellular Aspects*, Ciba Foundation Symposium 41, Elsevier/North-Holland, Amsterdam, 1976, p. 61.
153. D. G. Smyth, B. M. Austen, A. F. Bradbury, M. J. Geisow, and C. R. Snell, in J. Hughes, Ed., *Centrally Acting Peptides*, Macmillan, London, 1977, p. 231.
154. D. J. Fletcher, B. D. Noe, G. E. Bayer, and J. P. Quigley, *Diabetes* **29**, 593 (1980).
155. D. J. Fletcher, J. P. Quigley, G. E. Bauer, and B. D. Noe, *J. Cell Biol.* **90**, 312 (1981).
156. B. D. Noe, *J. Biol. Chem.* **256**, 4940 (1981).
157. W. Kemmler, D. F. Steiner, and J. Borg, *J. Biol. Chem.* **248**, 4544 (1973).
158. D. F. Steiner, W. Kemmler, H. S. Tager, H. H. Rubenstein, A. Lernmark, and H. Zühlke, In E. Reich, D. B. Rifkin, and E. Shaw, Eds., *Proteases and Biological Control*, Cold Spring Harbor Laboratory, 1975, p. 531.
159. R. R. MacGregor, L. L. H. Chu, and D. V. Cohn, *J. Biol. Chem.* **251**, 6711 (1976).
160. R. R. MacGregor, J. W. Hamilton, and D. V. Cohn, *J. Biol. Chem.* **253**, 2012 (1978).
161. J. F. Habener, H. T. Chang, and J. T. Potts, Jr., *Biochem.* **16**, 3910 (1977).
162. D. F. Steiner, W. Kemmler, H. S. Tager, and J. D. Peterson, *Fed. Proc.* **33**, 2105 (1974).
163. H. B. Pollard, C. J. Pazoles, C. E. Greutz, and O. Zinder, *Int. Rev. Cytol.* **58**, 159 (1979).
164. A. Scarpa and R. G. Johnson, *J. Biol. Chem.* **251**, 2189 (1976).
165. J. T. Russell and R. W. Hotz, *J. Biol. Chem.* **256**, 5950 (1981).
166. M. J. Geisow and D. G. Smyth, in R. B. Freedman and H. C. Hawkins, Eds., *The Enzymology of Post-Translational Modification of Proteins*, Vol. 1, Academic Press, London, 1980, p. 259.
167. D. V. Marinkovic, J. N. Marinkovic, E. G. Erdos, and C. J. G. Robinson, *Biochem. J.* **163**, 253 (1977).
168. V. Y. H. Hook, L. E. Eiden, and M. J. Brownstein, *Nature* **295**, 341 (1982).
169. C. A. Ryan, G. M. Hass, and R. W. Kuhn, *J. Biol. Chem.* **249**, 5445 (1974).
170. L. D. Fricker and S. H. Snyder, *Proc. Natl. Acad. Sci. USA* **79**, 3886 (1982).
171. M. J. Peach, *Physiol. Reviews* **57**, 313 (1977).
172. E. G. Erdos, *Circ. Res.* **36**, 247 (1975).
173. N. Marks, in H. Gainer, Ed., *Neurobiology of Peptides*, Plenum Press, New York, 1977, p. 221.
174. A. Malesci, E. Straus, and R. S. Yalow, *Proc. Natl. Acad. Sci. USA* **77**, 597 (1980).
175. S. W. Ryder, E. Straus, and R. S. Yalow, *Proc. Natl. Acad. Sci. USA* **77**, 3669 (1980).
176. M. Knight, C. Plotkin, and C. Tamminga, *Peptides*, **3**, 461 (1982).
177. L. Graf and A. Kenessey, in C. H. Li, Ed., *Hormonal Proteins and Peptides*, Vol. 10, Academic Press, New York, 1980, p. 35.
178. N. Marks, A. Suhar, and M. Benuck, in J. B. Martin, S. Reichlin, and K. L. Bick, Eds., *Neurosecretion and Brain Peptides*, Raven Press, New York, 1981, p. 49.
179. W. G. North, H. Valtin, J. F. Morris, and F. T. La Rochelle, *Endocrinology* **101**, 110 (1977).
180. A. Eberle and R. Schwyzer, *Helv. Chim. Acta* **58**, 1528 (1975).
181. R. Burgus, T. F. Dunn, D. Desiderio, and R. Guillemin, *C.R. Acad. Sci. Paris, Ser. D* **269**, 1870 (1969).

182. Y. Baba, H. Matsuo, and A. V. Schally, *Biochem. Biophys. Res. Comm.* **44**, 459 (1971).

183. S. E. Leeman, E. A. Mroz, and R. E. Carraway, in H. Gainer, Ed., *Neurobiology of Peptides*, Plenum Press, New York, 1977, p. 99.

184. J. T. Potts, Jr., H. T. Kentmann, H. D. Niall, and G. W. Tregear, *Vitam. Horm.* **29**, 41 (1971).

185. A. Anastasi, V. Erspamer, and J. M. Cei, *Arch. Biochem. Biophys.* **125**, 57 (1968).

186. D. G. Smyth, S. Zakarian, I. F. W. Deakin, and D. E. Massey, in D. Evered and G. Lawrenson, Eds., *Intermediate Lobe of the Pituitary*, Ciba Symposium No. 81, Pitman Medical, London, 1981, p. 79.

187. G. W. Kenner, and R. C. Sheppard, in S. Anderson, Ed., *Nobel Symposium 16: Frontiers in Gastrointestinal Hormone Research*, Almquist and Wiksell, Stockholm, 1973, p. 137.

188. R. Endean, V. Erspamer, G. Falconieri-Erspamer, G. Improta, P. Melchiorri, L. Negri, and N. Sapranzi, *Brit. J. Pharmacol.* **55**, 213 (1975).

189. H. J. Showell, *J. Exp. Med.* **143**, 1154 (1976).

190. H. P. J. Bennett, C. A. Browne, and S. Solomon, *Proc. Natl. Acad. Sci. USA* **78**, 4713 (1981).

191. U. Czichi, and W. J. Lennarz, *J. Biol. Chem.* **252**, 7901 (1977).

192. C. F. Phelps, in R. B. Freedman and H. C. Hawkins, Eds., *The Enzymology of Post-Translational Modification of Proteins*, Vol. 1, Academic Press, London, 1980, p. 105.

193. T. A. Woodford and J. E. Dixon, *J. Biol. Chem.* **254**, 4993 (1979).

194. K. A. Pease and J. E. Dixon, *Arch. Biochem. Biophys.* **212**, 177 (1981).

195. R. T. Jensen and J. D. Gardner, *Fed. Proc.* **40**, 2486 (1981).

196. T. L. O'Donohue, G. E. Handelmann, T. Chaconas, R. L. Millers, and D. M. Jacobowitz, *Peptides* **2**, 333 (1981).

197. H. Kakidani, Y. Furutani, H. Takahashi, M. Noda, Y. Morimoto, T. Hirose, M. Asai, S. Inayama, S. Nakanishi and S. Numa, *Nature* **298**, 245 (1982).

198. K. Docherty, R. J. Carroll, and D. F. Steiner, *Proc. Natl. Acad. Sci. USA* **79**, 4613.

199. M. Chappell, Y. P. Loh and T. L. O'Donohue, *Peptides* **3**, 405 (1982).

200. C. C. Glembotski, *J. Biol. Chem.* **257**, 10501 (1982).

201. A. F. Bradbury, M. D. A. Finnie and D. G. Smyth, *Nature*, **298**, 686.

202. H. Land, M. Grez, S. Ruppert, H. Schmale, M. Rehbein, D. Richter, and G. Schutz, *Nature*, **302**, 342.

4

Enzymatic Degradation of Brain Peptides

JEFFREY F. McKELVY

Department of Neurobiology and Behavior
State University of New York at Stony Brook
Stony Brook, New York

1 INTRODUCTION

This chapter focuses on the question of how the degradation of nervous system peptides is related to the regulation of their actions as signals in intercellular communication within the nervous system and in neuroendocrine communication. By degradation we mean enzymatically catalyzed peptide bond hydrolysis, mediated by peptidases or proteases, that results in the loss of a defined biological activity of a given peptide without the generation of any new defined biological activity. With this definition we distinguish "inactivation" from "processing": for example, the loss of α-melanocyte stimulating hormone (α-MSH) biological activity due to endopeptidase-catalyzed cleavage of the Pro^{12}-Val^{13}-NH_2 bond (1) vs. the generation of α-MSH from ACTH (2) by peptide bond cleavage. It is clear, however, that this definition will have to account for many new examples of proteolytic "processing," since evidence is already accumulating that products derived from both endopeptidase and exopeptidase catalyzed reactions on "mature" peptides may have new biological activities. For example, the action of pyroglutamyl aminopeptidase on thyrotropin releasing hormone (TRH: pGlu-His-Pro-NH_2) yields His-Pro diketopiperazine, devoid of thyroid stimulating hormone (TSH) releasing activity but able to inhibit prolactin release from the pituitary (3). Similarly, the action of an aminopeptidase on γ-endorphin (β-lipotropic hormone 61–77) removes only N-terminal tyrosine (4), abolishing opiate activity but producing a peptide, des-Tyr-γ-endorphin, with activity in various adaptive behaviors. In fact, with respect to the nervous system, it is possible that peptide "processing" even to the level of free amino acids may be physiologically meaningful in terms of signal generation, since several amino acids have been described as putative neurotransmitters (γ-amino butyric acid, glutamic acid, aspartic acid, proline, glycine). Another point to be made about the definition of degradation given above, is that it should be emphasized that enzyme-catalyzed reactions other than proteolysis can influence the biological activity of a mature peptide, such as N- and O-acylation reactions (5), phosphorylation (6), and possibly sulfation covalent modifications.

In spite of the likelihood that our appreciation of the extent of the proteolytic liberation of information from oligopeptides will increase, it is relevant to consider the inactivation of a given peptide with respect to a given site of peptide action. *A priori*, the most attractive framework for conceptualizing the action of a peptidase at a site of peptide action in the nervous system would seem to be that in which the enzyme was situated at the external surface of the peptide-sensitive cell, and there catalyzed the hydrolysis of peptide released into the synaptic cleft, contributing to primary regulation of excitability changes in that cell. As we will see in the forthcoming discussion, alternative conceptualizations may be adopted. Since brain peptides have been so recently discovered, and since so relatively little is known about their genesis and actions at a molecular level, it is not possible to analyze a large body of data about the enzymatic degradation of a given brain peptide at a defined site of action. Most of the existing information on the enzymatic breakdown of brain peptides derives from four sources: (i) studies on crude preparations of CNS tissue in which bond cleavage sites were not determined and in which no physiological changes were occurring (7), (ii) studies of the enzymatic degradation of a brain peptide in a defined physiological context in which an indirect method of estimation of peptide degradation was used (8); (iii) studies of the kinetic properties of purified peptidases on brain peptides (4), and (iv) studies on the enzymatic degradation of a brain peptide at a specific peptide bond and in a physiological context in which functional demand on the particular peptidergic system was being altered (9, 10). The body of data taken as a whole is weighted toward the first two sources. Encouragingly, more studies are now being carried out at the level of the latter two sources; though few, they are the only studies we will treat in this review.

Before discussing such studies on the enzymatic degradation of brain peptides, some recent information deriving from the study of the degradation of hormonal peptides and of low molecular weight amine neurotransmitters offers a useful perspective. Analysis of actively secreting endocrine glands suggests that intracellular degradation of the hormonal polypeptide may be regulated and may contribute to the control of the amount of hormone secreted. In the parathyroid gland, a fast-acting system extremely sensitive to calcium concentration in the extracellular fluid, a substantial proportion of newly synthesized parathormone (PTH), is degraded, and the rate of PTH degradation decreases when circulating calcium levels drop below a set point (11). The mechanism of this regulation of degradation has not yet been elucidated, but there are several possibilities: (i) The enzyme or enzymes catalyzing the degradation may be regulated directly; evidence exists that cathepsin B cleavage of the Ala^{36}-Leu^{37} bond of PTH (and pro-PTH), followed by exopeptidase-catalyzed hydrolysis of the amino terminal fragment, may be principally responsible for intracellular PTH degradation (12), but there is also evidence for the presence of calcium-sensitive protease activity in the gland (13). (ii) Regulation could occur by fusion of secretory granules with lysosomes, as has been proposed to occur with prolactin in the anterior pituitary (14) and insulin in pancreatic islet β cells (15). Although less well studied from the point of view of intracellular degradation, pancreatic insulin secretion under the influence of glucose stimulation results in a stimulation of insulin-degrading activity by islet tissue (16). These observations suggest a coupling between intracellular peptide hormone degradation and physiological stimulation of peptide hormone biosynthesis and release. Degradation can be stimulated, concomitant with stimulation of the cell to secrete, to promote an ultimate return to prestimulation steady state levels. Alternatively, peptide hormone can be continuously produced at a high level and degraded after production, with degradation being inhibited during stimulation of secretion. Thus, enzymatic degradation of peptide signals could be either increased or decreased in the peptide-secreting cell when functional demand is placed on that cell. A model in which "overproduction" and continuous degradation of peptide occurred, with inhibition of degradation upon stimulation, is an attractive one for peptide-secreting neurons since it would allow for stores of releasable peptide that could be relatively independent of axoplasmic transport and for presynaptic terminal regulation of degradation.

Recent studies of the fate of endocrine peptide hormones at their target cells do not point toward termination of hormone action at the receptor by degradation of the peptide, as originally suggested [17]. Rather, the internalization of hormone–receptor complexes and their interaction with intracellular organelles in the target cell appear to be of great potential significance in the regulation of peptide target cells [18]. In the case of insulin action on the liver, for example, recent evidence [19] suggests that the route of internalization proceeds through Golgi elements, where insulin receptors can be demonstrated, and through various other vesicular structures, including possibly secretory granules, prior to lysosomal degradation of the hormone–receptor complex. Thus, internalized peptide–receptor complexes are implicated in the regulation of protein biosynthesis and processing in target cells. This process should be kept in mind when considering the actions of peptides in the nervous system. Studies dealing with the question of neuropeptide–receptor internalization are needed, and investigation of brain peptide degradation must consider that an observed degrading activity for a given peptide may reflect either pre- or postsynaptically located enzymes responsible for internal degradation, or both. As can be inferred from the above discussion, such degradative enzymes can exhibit membrane association.

Currently available information on the enzymatic degradation of low-molecular-weight amine neurotransmitters suggests that such enzymes contribute to the regulation of the concentration of neurotransmitter in some compartments but probably do not directly regulate the lifetime of a neurotransmitter molecule at its receptor site. Thus, studies on biogenic amine-secreting neurons suggest that diffusion and concentrative uptake are of major importance in terminating transmitter action [20], whereas enzymes such as monoamine oxidase and catechol-*O*-methyl transferase act to scavenge free monoamine, either intra- or extracellularly [21], and are not regulated in concert with synaptic transmission. The importance of enzymatic inactivation of neurotransmitter has been most vigorously proclaimed for acetylcholine at the neuromuscular junction [22]. But there is still considerable controversy over whether the cholinesterase is physiologically most relevant in terms of contributing to the regulation of postsynaptic quantal events or to the concentrative uptake of choline. The decay time of stimulation-induced permeability changes may increase only twofold in the presence of cholinesterase inhibitor (23). The possibilities that diffusion may principally regulate the interaction of acetylcholine molecules with their receptors, and that experiments employing cholinesterase inhibition may reflect presynaptic effects, do not permit firm conclusions about the primacy of enzymatic degradation in regulating the primary events in cholinergic neurotransmission.

To sum up this introduction, current evidence on the interaction of signals with their target cells in the peptide endocrine system and the aminergic nervous system does not support rapid enzymatic inactivation at the receptor site as the major means of control of the action of the signal. The possibility that this may also hold for the peptide nervous system must be entertained in approaching studies of the biophysical actions of peptides and the actions of brain peptidases. This does not mean that peptidase action in the nervous system cannot be of importance to synaptic transmission involving peptides. As noted above, the regulation of peptide degradation in the peptide secreting neuron and in the cell responsive to the peptide might be important determinants of the physiological roles of peptide-secreting neurons. As a final consideration, however, it should be noted that the apparent diversity of use of peptides by the nervous system might involve the use of peptidases as the primary means of cessation of the synaptic action of a peptide.

2 PHYSIOLOGICALLY RELEVANT BRAIN PEPTIDASES

In this section, evidence for a physiological relevance of peptidase activity in the nervous system is reviewed. Two sources of information have been considered: (i) the properties of peptidases purified from nervous tissue, and (ii) the investigation of peptidase activity as being of possible importance in the operation of a defined "peptidergic" neuronal subsystem. The body of data from these two sources is small.

As an introduction to this section, it should be noted that enzymes catalyzing the breakdown of nervous system peptides have been purified from blood (24) and anterior pituitary tissue (25). These enzymes are not considered here.

2.1 Enkephalin-Degrading Enzymes

Currently available evidence suggests that both of the enkephalin pentapeptides, Met⁵-enkephalin (MENK: H-Tyr^1-Gly^2-Gly^3-Phe^4-Met^5-OH) and Leu^5-enkephalin (LENK: H-Tyr^1-Gly^2-Gly^3-Phe^4-Leu^5-OH) can be inactivated—that is, agonist activity at certain opiate receptors can be abolished—at three bond cleavage sites: Tyr -Gly ("enkephalin amino-peptidase"; "aminopeptidase"); Gly^2-Gly^3 ("enkephalinase B"), and Gly^3-Phe^4 ("enkephalinase"; "enkephalinase A"; angiotensin converting enzyme, or ACE). The history of research on the activities catalyzing these cleavages has been comprehensively reviewed by Schwartz et al. (26). This group has also carried out the most extensive studies attempting to implicate enkephalin degrading activity as being of importance in a defined neural subsystem. Using primarily the mouse corpus striatum as a model, they have proposed (26) that at or near opiate receptor sites on striatonigral dopaminergic neurons, "enkephalinase" catalysis may be responsible for acutely terminating the action of enkephalin as a neurotransmitter at this and other CNS synapses involving enkephalins. These conclusions were reached on the basis of the following principle assumptions and lines of experimental evidence: (i) the assumption that enkephalins are likely to have actions at CNS synapses closely similar to those of "classical neurotransmitters" and involving a need for rapid turnoff of the signal either by concentrative uptake or enzymatic breakdown; (ii) the assumption that since no concentrative processes for peptides have been defined in neural tissue, while avid peptidase activity has been observed, peptidase activity could effect the inactivation of synaptically released enkephalins; (iii) the observation that, in mouse striatal membrane preparations, an activity, "enkephalinase," could be observed which cleaved the Gly^3-Phe^4 bond of both MENK (apparent K_m 1.4 μM) and LENK (apparent K_m 27 μM), which was classifiable as a dipeptidyl carboxypeptidase with a specificity favoring enkephalins and which was distinguishable from ACE action on enkephalins by physical separation, kinetic, and regional-distribution criteria; (iv) the observation that the subcellular distribution of "enkephalinase" activity and ^{3}H-(D-Ala^2-Met^5)- enkephalinamide binding activity in rat cerebral cortex was parallel throughout subsynaptosomal fractionation; (v) the observation that pharmacological perturbation of brain opiate receptors, by chronic morphine treatment of mice, resulted in a 20–25% increase in striatal membrane "enkephalinase" activity by four days after implantation of a morphine pellet, whereas neither ACE nor aminopeptidase activity exhibited change; (vi) the observation that a synthetic inhibitor of "enkephalinase," thiorphan (3-mercapto-2-benzylpropanoyl-glycine), a metal-chelating peptide derivative reflecting the apparent metallo-enzyme nature of "enkephalinase," exhibits *in vitro* enkephalinase inhibition at nanomolar concentrations, *in vitro* protection of MENK released by brain slices, while inhibitors of ACE and aminopeptidase do not, and *in vivo* naloxone-sensitive potentiation of the antinociceptive activity of an exogenously administered enkephalin analog.

This is an impressive beginning body of data that suggests "enkephalinase" activity is intimately involved with enkephalin-utilizing neuron systems in the brain. But the central question, whether a highly specific enzyme is situated on the external surface of enkephalin-oceptive neurons and rapidly clears the synaptic cleft of enkephalin molecules liberated during synaptic transmission, is still far from being answered. First, the actions of peptides in the nervous system are not well defined; the notions that enkephalins are ubiquitously fast-acting and rapidly degraded are not well founded on experimental evidence. Given the diversity of effects of enkephalins on neuronal excitability already observed (27), the number of different enkephalin-utilizing systems in the nervous system (28), and the likely chemical heterogeneity of most synapses (29), it is possible enough that even in the brain different actions of enkephalins, with different time courses, may exist to warrant cognizance of this possibility. And the observation that peptides can be rapidly degraded *in vivo* or by various tissue preparations does not necessarily mean that this occurs at synapses. Currently, there are no data available on the quantitative relationship between an excitability change on an enkephalin-sensitive preparation and the kinetics of enkephalinase activity. As in the case of the neuromuscular junction, as discussed above, only this kind of information and not *in vivo* pharmacological data can provide critical evidence about the *primacy* of degradation in the cessation of synaptic events. In fact, with regard to both of the above points, there is evidence from studies on dorsal root ganglion primary cell cultures (30) that (i) enkephalin actions on sensitive (presumably primary sensory) neurons can be of prolonged duration, and (ii) enkephalin molecules are relatively stable in this experimental situation in which intact cells are interacting. This culture system is well established, and it would be of great interest to study it for the possible regulation of enkephalinase activity.

Second, studies on brain peptide hydrolases are truly in their infancy. Few of the enzymes catalyzing the several bond cleavages in the several peptides believed to be acting in neurotransmission in the brain have been purified; the history of enzymology rings with the abjuration not to waste clean thoughts on dirty enzymes. In the case of striatal enkephalinase, for example, attempts were directed toward the kinetic characterization of the activity in a membrane fraction that was still a crude mixture of proteins and enzymes, resulting in an erroneously low estimation of the Michaelis constant for LENK, which led to the inference that a highly selective enzyme was present. Purification and extensive kinetic characterization of this activity are needed to answer several other important questions related to whether enkephalinase selectively cleaves the Gly^3-Phe^4 bonds of enkephalins at synapses. For example, the evidence that the activity is a carboxypeptidase, and not an endopeptidase, is not extensive (26) and is especially lacking for longer peptides, in particular those naturally occurring opiates bearing the enkephalin sequence. It is interesting in this regard that the soluble homogeneous bovine brain aminopeptidase (31), which cleaves LENK with a K_M virtually identical with that of enkephalinase, has been found to act with substantial turnover numbers on α- and γ-endorphins only to yield the des-Tyr derivatives and at a much slower rate on β-endorphin (4). Conformational effects on peptide hydrolase activity are probably of general importance, and the specificity estimates of striatal enkephalinase at residues 4 and 5 of the pentapeptide as assayed by dipeptide inhibition are confounded by this, and do not by this measure appear to be stringent for Phe- (Met, Leu). Thus, it is possible that enkephalinase may be able to act on other known brain peptides, but the significance of any such action would depend on appropriate neuronal connectivity among other things. Finally, the achievement of purification of enkephalinase activity will allow for the ability to identify a discrete molecular form of the enzyme by antibody techniques and thus provide the opportunity for welcome information, such as enzyme biosynthesis and turnover, and cytological disposition.

This subcellular localization of enkephalinase in relation to enkephalin binding, and the ability of thiorphan to protect MENK released from striatal slices, are strong indications that enkephalinase activity could be associated with synaptic release of enkephalins. Further evidence is needed, however, to rule out the possibility that enkephalinase acts presynaptically, especially intracellularly to regulate releasable pentapeptide. In this regard, the above-mentioned studies on endocrine peptide systems suggest that a particulate localization of enzyme can occur owing to the ability of organelles involved in secretion, degradation, and endocytosis to communicate. It would be of interest to look for the appearance of enkephalinase activity in the medium following a striatal slice depolarization-induced enkephalin release experiment, and for the subcellular distribution of enkephalinase activity in control and chronically stimulated (actively releasing) slices. Additional useful information on the role of enkephalinase in slice preparations could be gained by comparing the effects of recently described highly potent inhibitors of aminopeptidase activity (32) side by side with thiorphan, to more accurately assess aminopeptidase and enkephalinase contributions to enkephalin degradation than is possible in a paradigm employing a specific enkephalinase inhibitor and a less specific aminopeptidase inhibitor.

The recent reports that carrier mediated processes for peptide uptake may be observable in neural tissue *in vitro* (33, 34) suggest that it would be profitable to explore this possibility for enkephalins in striatal slices, and, if observable, study its relationship to enkephalinase activity.

In summary, the study of the hydrolysis of enkephalins by "enkephalinase" has provided a compelling avenue of research in pursuit of the mechanisms of regulation of synaptic actions of peptides. It is anticipated that future studies will be most rewarding in this regard.

2.2 LHRH-Degrading Enzymes

The enzymatic degradation in the hypothalamus of luteinizing hormone releasing hormone (LHRH: $pGlu^1$-His^2-Trp^3-Ser^4-Tyr^5-Gly^6-Leu^7-Arg^8-Pro^9-Gly^{10}-NH_2) has been studied in an attempt to implicate peptidase action in neuroendocrine regulation (for a recent comprehensive review, see Advis and Krause, ref. 35). The context within which degradation studies have been carried out has been that of the regulation of gonadotropin secretion, in which the advantages of relatively well defined physiological processes—the integration of peripheral steroid and central neuronal regulatory signals by anatomically defined "final common pathway" hypophysiotropic LHRH secreting neurons—allows for several kinds of correlations to be made between LHRH degradation and physiological change. In spite of these advantages, however, until recently no clearly defined role had emerged for peptidases acting on LHRH at the hypothalamic level. This was most likely due to several factors: (i) the demonstrated existence of activities in hypothalamic extracts that could cleave LHRH at several potential sites ($pGlu^1$-His^2, Tyr^5-Gly^6, Gly^6-Leu^7, Pro^9-Gly^{10}-NH), with no knowledge of the intrahypothalamic distribution or compartmentation of these activities; (ii) the use of inappropriate assays for hypothalamic LHRH degradation, for example, the measurement of (a more convenient) oxytocinase activity based on the belief that such activity and LHRH degrading activities ran parallel, or the use of synthetic arylamidase substrates based on similar assumptions, or the use of LHRH radioimmunoassay in which cross-reactivities with possible LHRH degradation fragments were not assessed; and (iii) the use of nonoptimal conditions in physiological modeling (35). Recently, studies were carried out in our laboratory which attempted to take all of these factors in account (10, 36, 37). The physiological model chosen was that of the positive feedback of ovarian steroids on the hypothalamus in the rat to promote activation of LHRH neurons projecting from the medial preoptic area (POA) to the median eminence (ME) and a subsequent preovulatory surge of luteinizing hormone (LH) by the anterior pituitary gland during the first estrus cycle at puberty. The strategy concerning the measurement of peptidase activity was threefold: (i) To carry out tissue sampling discretely, in individual animals, reflecting the compartmentization of the intrahypothalamic LHRH neuron system; thus, the POA (site of cell bodies of origin of the hypophysiotropic LHRH system) was "punched" from coronal sections and the ME (site of hypophysiotropic LHRH nerve terminals) discretely dissected. (ii) To measure initially total LHRH degradation as initial rates of degradation of exogenous LHRH in crude homogenates of these sites without the addition of exogenous stabilizing agents, such as thiols or chelators, to display enzyme activity as a reflection of the status of the tissue during the estrus cycle. (iii) To carry out a *chemical* analysis of LHRH degradation; here we decided to utilize high performance liquid chromatographic (HPLC) analysis of the loss of LHRH by measurement of the absorbance at 210 nanometers, the isosbestic point of the peptide bond $\pi \rightarrow \pi^*$ transition, combined with quantitation by digital integration. Of particular importance was the need to use rapid HPLC analysis, to process the large number of samples generated for correlations involving initial rate measurement to physiological status and yet unambiguously measure chemically the activity that gave rise to a loss of LHRH. This was achieved by use of an isocratic system based on the triethylammonium phosphate-acetonitrile system described for peptides by Rivier (38), which could separate the LHRH peak from all degradation products with a run time of six minutes per sample (36). The lack of cochromatography of any degradation product with the LHRH peak was assured by initially showing that collection of the latter peak from experimental samples gave amino acid analysis data consistent with only LHRH being present.

As additional aspects of the experimental design, we took advantage of these facts: (i) The sensitivity of detection of LHRH loss enabled us to retain sufficient sample after isocratic measurements were complete to carry out gradient HPLC analysis of degradation products to define specific bond-cleaving activities that might be changing. (ii) An enzyme cleaving LHRH at a specific bond—Pro^9-Gly^{10}-NH_2, postproline cleaving enzyme (39), or proline endopeptidase—had been purified from brain and could be assayed in the remainder of our tissue sample if a sufficiently sensitive rapid assay could be developed. Such an assay would probe for changes in a defined peptidase capable of acting on LHRH. Accordingly, we developed a sensitive fluorometric assay for this activity based on its specificity for the carboxyl side of L-prolyl residues, the hydrolysis of carbobenzoxy-Gly-Pro-methylcoumarineamide to give the fluorophore 7-amino-3-methylcoumarine (40).

On this basis we made the following findings, which suggested that LHRH degradation at a specific bond cleavage site is regulated in the hypothalamus during positive feedback:

1. During the first estrus cycle at puberty, total LHRH degradation in the median eminence was highly correlated with the ME content of LHRH throughout the estrus cycle, except during an interval 3h before the preovulatory surge of LH, when it decreased and was dissociated from the still-rising ME content of LHRH, the latter expected as a prelude to active release of LHRH to the portal vessels.

2. There was no such correlation between LHRH degradation and content in the POA, the site of LHRH cell bodies, and neither was there

any significant change in postproline cleaving enzyme activity during the estrus cycle, suggesting that nonspecific changes were not contributing to the level of activity of LHRH degradation.

3. The same pattern of inhibition of LHRH degradation and dissociation of level of degradation from LHRH content was observed following progesterone administration to estrogen-primed castrated animals.

4. The administration to ovariectomized, steroid-treated rats of diethyldithiocarbamate (DDC), a norepinephrine synthesis inhibitor that can abolish the LH surge due to blockade of its noradrenergic requirement at the hypothalamic level, resulted not only in failure of progesterone administration to elicit an LH surge but in the failure of progesterone administration to effect the transient inhibition of LHRH degradation prior to the LH surge seen in non-DDC-treated animals (37).

5. The analysis of LHRH degradation products in all of these physiological situations revealed that Tyr^5-Gly^6 cleavage accounted for the LHRH degradation observed, probably by a metalloendopeptidase similar to the partially purified pituitary "non-chymotrypsin-like" endopeptidase that cleaves LHRH, described by Bauer and associates (41). Moreover, this activity could be observed in both a soluble and a particulate fraction (42).

These observations suggest that degradation may be regulated in LHRH nerve terminals undergoing active and phasic LHRH release. The mechanism of this regulation could involve either progesterone effects at the transcriptional level to decrease the rate of synthesis of the peptidase (if it turns over rapidly), or the steroid could effect changes in the compartmentation of the enzyme in nerve terminals, resulting in its inability to gain access to LHRH, perhaps by inhibiting lysozome-secretory granule fusion. Analysis of the subcellular distribution of the enzyme in the median eminence during the time course of progesterone effects on peptidase activity would be of great interest in this regard. Further studies require purification and characterization of the activity and the development of specific inhibitors of it.

3   PROPERTIES OF PEPTIDASES PURIFIED FROM BRAIN

In this section we briefly review some features of peptidases purified from brain to homogeneity that are relevant to the possible roles of such enzymes in the nervous system.

3.1   Postproline Cleaving Enzyme (Proline Endopeptidase)

This enzyme has been purified from rat (43), rabbit (44), and bovine brain (L. Hersh, personal communication) and found to be a serine protease of molecular weight 70,000–74,000, which can cleave on the carboxyl side of L-prolyl residues in several brain peptides, such as thyrotropin releasing hormone (TRH), LHRH, substance P, neurotensin, vasopressin, oxytocin, bradykinin and α-melanocyte stimulating hormone (α-MSH) (1, 39, 44, 45). To date, no defined physiological role has been established for it (see above); however, certain features of its action suggest the possibility of a role for the enzyme in brain peptide regulation. Although the range of neuropeptide substrates of the enzyme is large, it exhibits certain structural specificities: for L-prolyl residues; endopeptidase action, for example, it will cleave only the Pro^4-Gln^5 bond in substance P, and not the Pro^2-Lys^3 bond (45) and different affinities for its various neuropeptide substrates. Thus, it acts on substance P with a K_M of 1 μM and a K_{cat}/K_M value approaching that exhibited by acetylcholinesterase and differing from those of other substrates, such as neurotensin and LHRH, by order of magnitude differences (S. Blumberg and J. F. McKelvy, unpublished observations). The recent observations that the products of the action of the enzyme on both substance P and neurotensin have actions on fixed tissue cells: stimulation of phagocytosis by macrophages and of histamine release by mast cells (46), suggest that enzymatic cleavage of these peptides, released in the periphery from primary sensory neurons and innervated vascular elements, could be involved in response to injury and neurogenic inflammation. In addition, the possibility has been proposed that the enzyme could catalyze the production of a synaptically active fragment of substance P (5-11-NH$_2$) and a basic tetrapeptide with growth-promoting properties (45, 34). Recent preliminary immunocytochemical observations, utilizing antibodies to homogeneous rat and bovine enzyme, suggest an unequal but perplexing appearance of the enzyme in neural tissue: (i) In rat brain, reaction product was seen at a low level diffusely throughout brain regions, but with some prominence in neurons in the cerebral cortex and especial prominence in the intermediate lobe of the pituitary (S. Watson, J. Dixon, L. Hersh, and J. F. McKelvy, unpublished observations); the staining pattern in the intermediate lobe is similar to that for monoamine oxidase activity (J. Roberts, personal communication). (ii) In rat hypothalamus, reaction product could be observed most prominently in neurons and glia in the supraoptic nucleus, and in undefined cells in the median eminence, with the preoptic area silent; most strikingly, intense staining could be seen in the organum vasculosum laminae terminalis (OVLT) in DDC-treated animals (J. King, J. P. Advis, J. Dixon, L. Hersh, and J. F. McKelvy, unpublished observations). It must be stressed that these observations are preliminary and that the specificity of the observed staining is uncertain because of a lack of sufficient quantities of purified antigen for displacement controls. It is noteworthy, however, that both antisera gave virtually identical results. Perhaps, however, these observations suggest that the enzyme is involved in the peptide-mediated regulation of transport and exchange phenomena or in the catabolism of peptides at tissue interfaces.

3.2   Enkephalin Aminopeptidase

As mentioned above, on the basis of its greater apparent solubility than "enkephalinase," its lack of adaptive change during chronic morphine addiction, and the lack of protective effect of puromycin on the "depolarization"-induced release of MENK from brain slices (26), aminopeptidase is not regarded as important to "synaptic" enkephalin regulation. However, the possible physiological relevance of this enzyme cannot yet be ruled out for the following reasons: (i) The aminopeptidase can exhibit membrane association depending on the mode of isolation (26), with kinetic properties (K_M, V_{max}) identical to those of the soluble form (L. Hersh and J. F. McKelvy, unpublished observations). For this reason, and since the aminopeptidase is also likely a metalloenzyme, the particulate aminopeptidase activity should also be thoroughly characterized in the above-mentioned types of experiments. (ii) The effects of aminopeptidase inhibition in biological assays should be assessed utilizing recently described aminopeptidase inhibitors of greater potency (32).

3.3   Substance P Endopeptidase

Evidence has recently been presented for a membrane-associated metalloendopeptidase able to cleave substance P at three internal sites: Gln^6-Phe^7, Phe^7-Phe^8 and Phe^8-Gly^9 (47). This enzyme, purified about a thousandfold from a particulate fraction of human diencephalon, exhibited a K_M for substance P of 29 μM and showed a high degree of selectivity for substance P among several other biologically active peptides tested. This interesting and well-characterized enzyme has been proposed by the authors as a candidate for a synaptic peptidase, and further studies on the physiological actions and localization of the enzyme are anticipated.

3.4   Peptidase Specificity

One of the properties most valued for biological processes is that of specificity. In the model for "synaptic peptidases" alluded to above, for example, it is obviously desirable to have an enzyme facing the synaptic cleft and recognizing only a specific bond in a specific peptide, which it could cleave to effect inactivation of the synaptic effects of that peptide. What is the evidence that proteases or peptidases can exhibit such properties? In fact, there is no compelling evidence for the existence of a peptidase exclusive to neural tissue, or represented only in innervated somatic tissues, that could be considered to recognize a particular substrate peptide with such a high degree of residue specificity at the bond cleavage site, or of sequence specificity for the entire substrate, that cleavage of other peptides by the enzyme would seem highly unlikely. This is certainly true for the peptidases purified from brain and described above, but it is also true for the "enkephalinase" activity which, although not purified to homogeneity and characterized as such, has been extensively investigated in other ways. Thus, as alluded to above, existing specificity studies are not adequate to firmly establish the carboxypeptidase nature of this activity, and the activity is distributed in non-neural tissue. Recent studies have also shown that peptides such as substance P and neurotensin, which have internal sequences that could conform to the specificity "rules" deduced so far for enkephalinase, are capable of inhibiting mouse striatal enkephalinase with IC50 values in the micromolar range, that is, at concentrations close to the K_M for the enkephalins (48).

Does this mean that peptidase action cannot exhibit sufficient specificity to be of importance to brain peptide regulation? The answer to this would seem to be no. The important concepts here are that certain peptide bond hydrolases are capable of limited proteolysis and that this is highly conformationally determined. Thus, the proteolysis observed during bacterial sporulation, or even in the blood clotting cascade, is highly limited (49) and therefore specific, but it does not mean that no other substrate proteins could be found which these enzymes could cleave with comparable avidity. Another example of conformationally directed limited proteolysis dealt with in this chapter is the cathepsin B catalyzed hydrolysis of the Ala[36]-Leu[37] bond in parathormone. The enzyme activity was named on the basis of an apparent preference for basic amino acid residues deduced from specificity studies on small peptides. In the conformational context of an 84 (PTH) or 90 (pro-PTH) amino acid protein, a bond involving amino acid side chains of a hydrophobic character comprise the actual site of peptide bond cleavage.

With respect to cleavage of peptides in the nervous system, and considering an extracellular, "synaptic" locus of a peptidase, the specificity properties exhibited for peptidases could confer an even more important role for such enzymes in synaptic regulation by virtue of their ability to cleave more than one peptide signal at a synapse many of which, by widening current perception, will be chemically heterogeneous even with respect to peptide, especially considering the co-liberation of processing-derived precursor fragments for a given peptide.

4   METHODS FOR THE ASSAY OF BRAIN PEPTIDASES

For the investigator wishing to study the possible importance of peptidase action for a brain peptide of interest, there is a growing and already well developed body of analytical methods. In general, investigation of peptidase action is best pursued with knowledge of the bond or bonds undergoing cleavage. Thus, experimental design must include provision for establishing the peptide cleavage pattern in any particular experiment, if that is not directly part of the analysis of degradation. This is especially true in physiological experiments where physiological changes might elicit changes in the activity of only one of several enzymes that might act on a brain peptide. HPLC has proven to be a powerful tool in both enzymological and physiological studies on brain peptide degradation. For example, in the studies on LHRH degradation described above, a rapid chemical assay for peptide substrate disappearance allowed for the analysis of hundreds of samples throughout the estrus cycle at 6–8 min per sample, and it is currently being used for the purification of the Tyr^5-Gly^6 endopeptidase in which it is as rapid as any kind of assay traditionally used in enzyme purification. Given the K_M values exhibited by most of the peptidases shown to act on brain peptides (1–100 μM) and the sensitivity of quantitation by detection at 210_{nm} with digital integration (50 pmoles in the case of LHRH), isocratic HPLC analysis of peptide loss is preferred over radioimmunoassay estimation of peptide loss. The latter technique suffers from lack of knowledge of cross-reactivity of possible degradation products and is more time-consuming. The quantitative aspects referred to above also allow in most cases for routine use of HPLC in combination with amino acid analysis to determine peptidase cleavage sites. If care is taken to desalt fractions collected from gradient HPLC analysis by use of disposable columns packed with HPLC sorbents and conveniently eluted with volatile solvents, amino acid analysis at current high-sensitivity levels is compatible with analytical HPLC fractionation of peptidase digests.

There is an increasing number of synthetic substrates for peptidases with chromogenic or fluorogenic groups that also permit rapid assays for physiological studies and continuous assay for kinetic characterization of peptidases. In physiological or developmental experiments, however, care must be taken to "calibrate" cleavage of the synthetic substrate with that of the native peptide before the latter is used routinely.

For reference, several types of peptidase assay described in the literature are listed in Table 1.

ACKNOWLEDGMENTS

Research was supported with a grant from the National Science Foundation (BNS 7684506) and a Research Career Development Award (AM 00751) from the National Institutes of Health. The skilled typing of Sandra Donaldson is gratefully acknowledged.

TABLE 1 Methods of Assay of Brain Peptidase Activity

Method	Substrate	Enzyme	Reference
Thin-layer chromatography of radiolabeled peptide	Enkephalins	Enkephalinase	9, 26
Tyrosine release coupled to L-amino acid oxidase	Enkephalins	Aminopeptidase	31
Fluorometric detection of β-naphthylamine from Tyr β-naphthylamide	Enkephalins	Aminopeptidase	32
Isocratic HPLC/UV detection of intact LHRH	LHRH	Tyr^5-Gly^6 brain endopeptidase	10, 36
CM-cellulose paper chromatography of [^{3}H]-LHRH	LHRH	Tyr^5-Gly^6 pituitary endopeptidase	41
Isocratic HPLC analysis/UV detection of partial sequences/ amino acid analysis	Substance P	Postproline-cleaving enzyme	45
Fluorometric detection of β-naphthylamine	CbZ-Gly-Pro-β-naphthylamide	Postproline cleaving enzyme	41
Fluorometric detection of aminomethyl-coumarine	CbZ-Gly-Pro-coumarineamide	Postproline cleaving enzyme	40

REFERENCES

1. J. F. McKelvy, submitted.
2. B. A. Eipper and R. E. Mains, *Endocr. Rev.* **1**, 1 (1980).
3. K. Bauer, K. J. Graf, A. Faivre-Bauman, S. Beier, A. Tixier-Vidal, and H. Kleinkauf, *Nature* **274**, 174 (1978).
4. L. B. Hersh, T. E. Smith, and J. F. McKelvy, *Nature* **286**, 160 (1980).
5. D. G. Smyth, D. E. Massey, S. Zackarian, and M. D. Finnie, *Nature* **279**, 252 (1979).
6. B. A. Eipper and R. E. Mains, *J. Biol. Chem.* **257**, 4907 (1982).
7. N. Marks and F. Stern, *Biochem. Biophys. Res. Commun.* **61**, 1458 (1974).
8. H. Kuhl, C. Rosniatowski, and H. D. Taubert, *Endocrinol. Exp.* **13**, 29 (1979).
9. B. Malfroy, J. P. Swerts, A. Guyon, B. P. Roques, and J. C. Schwartz, *Nature* **276**, 523 (1978).
10. J. P. Advis, J. E. Krause, and J. F. McKelvy, *Endocrinology* **110**, 1238 (1982).
11. J. F. Habener, B. Kemper, and J. T. Potts, *Endocrinology* **97**, 431 (1975).
12. R. R. MacGregor, J. W. Hamilton, G. N. Kent, R. E. Shofstall, and D. V. Cohn, *J. Biol. Chem.* **254**, 4428 (1979).
13. J. A. Fischer, S. B. Oldham, G. W. Sizemore, and C. D. Arnaud, *Proc. Natl. Acad. Sci. USA* **69**, 2341 (1972).

14. R. E. Smith and M. G. Farquhar, *J. Cell Biol.* **31**, 319 (1966).
15. B. Chertow, *Endocr. Rev.* **2**, 137 (1981).
16. P. A. Halban and C. B. Wolheim, *J. Biol. Chem.* **255**, 6003 (1980).
17. S. Terris and D. F. Steiner, *J. Biol. Chem.* **250**, 8389 (1975).
18. M. C. Willingham and I. Pastan, *Cell* **21**, 67 (1980).
19. M. N. Khan, B. I. Posner, R. J. Khan, and J. J. Bergeron, *J. Biol. Chem.* **257**, 5969 (1982).
20. J. T. Coyle and S. H. Snyder, *J. Pharmacol. Exp. Ther.* **170**, 221 (1969).
21. J. T. Coyle and S. H. Snyder, *Basic Neurochemistry*, Little Brown, New York, 1981, pp. 205–217.
22. T. Rosenberry, *Biophys. J.* **26**, 263 (1979).
23. D. Colquhoun, W. A. Large, and H. P. Rang, *J. Physiol.* **266**, 361 (1977).
24. W. L. Taylor and J. E. Dixon, *J. Biol. Chem.* **253**, 6934 (1978).
25. H. Knisatschek and K. Bauer, *J. Biol. Chem.* **254**, 10936 (1979).
26. J. C. Schwartz, B. Malfroy, and S. DeLaBaume, *Life Sci.* **29**, 1715 (1981).
27. J. L. Barker, T. G. Smith, and J. H. Neale, *Brain Res.* **154**, 153 (1978).
28. N. C. Brecha and H. J. Karten, Chapter 18 in this volume.
29. T. Hokfelt, O. Johansson, A. Ljungdahl, J. M. Lundberg, and M. Schultzberg, *Nature* **284**, 515 (1980).
30. A. W. Mudge, S. E. Leeman, and G. D. Fischbach, *Proc. Natl. Acad. Sci. USA* **76**, 526 (1979).
31. L. B. Hersh and J. F. McKelvy, *J. Neurochem.* **36**, 171 (1981).
32. G. W. Wagner and J. E. Dixon, *J. Neurochem.* **37**, 709 (1981).
33. M. F. Pacheco, D. J. Woodward, J. F. McKelvy, and W. S. T. Griffin, *Peptides* **2**, 283 (1981).
34. Y. Nakata, Y. Kusaka, H. Yajima, and T. Segawa, *J. Neurochem.* **37**, 1529 (1981).
35. J. P. Advis and J. E. Krause, *Current Methods in Cellular Neurobiology*, vol. 2, Wiley, J. L. Barker and J. F. McKelvy, eds., New York, in press.
36. J. P. Advis, J. E. Krause, and J. F. McKelvy, *Anal. Biochem.*, **125**, 41 (1982).
37. J. P. Advis, J. E. Krause, and J. F. McKelvy, *Endocrinology* **112**, 1147 (1983).
38. J. Rivier, *J. Liq. Chromatogr.* **1**, 343 (1978).
39. L. B. Hersh and J. F. McKelvy, *Brain Res.* **168**, 553 (1979).
40. J. P. Advis, S. Blumberg, J. E. Krause, and J. F. McKelvy, submitted.
41. B. Horsthemke and K. Bauer, *Biochemistry* **19**, 2873 (1980).
42. J. E. Krause, J. P. Advis, and J. F. McKelvy, *Biochem. Biophys. Res. Commun.* **108**, 1475 (1982).
43. J. H. Rupnow, W. L. Taylor, and J. E. Dixon, *Biochemistry* **18**, 1206 (1979).
44. M. Orlowski, E. Wilk, S. Pearce, and S. Wilk, *J. Neurochem.* **33**, 461 (1979).
45. S. Blumberg, V. I. Teichberg, J. L. Charli, L. B. Hersh, and J. F. McKelvy, *Brain Res.* **192**, 477 (1980).
46. Z. Bar-Shavit, R. Goldman, Y. Stabinsky, P. Gottlieb, M. Fridkin, V. I. Teichberg, and S. Blumberg, *Biochem. Biophys. Res. Commun.* **94**, 1445 (1980).
47. C. M. Lee, B. E. B. Sandberg, M. R. Hanley, and L. I. Iversen, *Eur. J. Biochem.* **114**, 315 (1981).
48. R. L. Hudgin, S. E. Charleson, N. Zimmerman, R. Mumford, and P. L. Wood, *Life Sci.* **29**, 2593 (1981).
49. H. Holzer and P. C. Heinrich, *Ann. Rev. Biochem.* **49**, 63 (1980).

5

Principles of Evolution: The Neural Hierarchy Model

R. ACHER

Laboratory of Biological Chemistry
Université d Pierre et Marie Curie
Paris, France

The neo-Darwinian conception assumes that evolutionary changes are determined by random mutations followed by selection. Selective pressure, however, can act at different levels of the biological hierarchy: population, organism, organ, cell, organelle, molecular assembly, free molecule, and it is not clear at all how random modifications in genes (deoxyribonucleic acids) may be filtered to program appropriate changes at various levels.

Directly regulated evolution (somewhat similar to the excommunicated Lamarckism) that means the heredity of acquired characters or the learning of the genome, could have the great merit of explaining both adaptation and speciation. A recording of the organisms experience at the level of the genome is, however, not easy to imagine. The mosaic structural gene found in eukaryotes has introduced a new flexibility in genetic dogma, though, and reverse transcriptase could provide a mechanism for molecular back-information. Study of the regulatory sequences of deoxyribonucleic acids is just beginning and new regulatory mechanisms controlling polymolecular systems will probably be discovered; these sequences could be privileged targets for the retro-information.

Apparently, to become hereditary an adaptative variation must be recorded in a genomic nucleotide sequence; but an adaptative answer to an environmental pressure is primarily physiological and must be reflected in an integrated polymolecular system. The difficulty is in analyzing the adaptative answer in molecular terms: how can a coordinated system send instructions to the genome and how can coordination be maintained at this level? Our concepts of regulatory mechanisms are still rudimentary.

1   HIERARCHIC ASPECTS OF EVOLUTION: THE ASSEMBLY PRINCIPLE

1.1   Hierarchy of Assemblies in Living Matter

Living matter appears to us as a hierarchy of assemblies, each structural unit being itself an assembly. Each assembly has its own internal interactions. Among assemblies, "messenger" elements determine the hierarchic relationships. The variations in the system are in some way interdependent, but how much are the upper levels, such as cells or organisms, submitted to the rules governing the particles? Is the motor of evolution only at the nucleotide level (mutation, recombination) and the direction of evolution at the social level (competition)? What physicochemical law is sexuality masking?

1.1.1 Molecular Assembly: The Neuropeptide

Polypeptides can be regarded as linear assemblies of amino acids. But the amino acid sequence dictates a three-dimensional structure, the conformation; thus the meaning of a given sequence is to build a given shape. Unfortunately, the deduction of conformation from sequence is not yet possible, and the so-called "predictive" theories are in a very early stage. In some cases, X-ray radiocrystallography can give the atomic structure but the conformations may be different in the crystal and in solution. Furthermore the flexibility of the polypeptide chain is hardly revealed by X-ray pictures and this flexibility, which may be amplified by ligands or cofactors, is probably essential to specific interactions with a biological partner.

The size of a polypeptide chain must be determined by its function, but our knowledge of the relationship between conformation and function of molecules is sketchy at best. It can be noted that enzymes are built with one or several polypeptide chains having at least 100 residues, whereas active peptide hormones usually have between 10 and 100 residues and transmitters between 1 and 15 residues. Because of their small size, peptide hormones or transmitters do not have strong tertiary structures so that they are very flexible in solution; for this reason, perhaps, crystals of peptides appropriate for X-ray analysis are usually difficult to obtain and only a few of the largest peptide hormones have been characterized at the three-dimensional level (e.g., insulin and glucagon).

Most of the peptide hormones have been identified immunologically in the brain and therefore qualify as neuropeptides. In fact, all the cells of a given species have the same genome, and for this reason all the proteins theoretically can be expressed in the neuron.

1.1.2 Cellular Assembly: The Neuron

Neurons are the structural units of the brain and the nerves. Like other eukaryotic cells, they comprise a nucleus and a number of organelles with their own specific membranes, so that neurons can be regarded as assemblies of subcellular elements. Some organelles such as mitochondria have their own genome (mtDNA) and may have been derived from a captive prokaryotic cell by a process of endosymbiosis. The same general mechanism of protein biosynthesis (transcription, translation, processing) applies to both nuclear and mitochondrial genomes (for a discussion on the human mtDNA and its peculiar characteristics, see ref. 1). Subcellular assemblies involve sub-subcellular structures such as membranes, microfilaments (actin, etc.), microtubules (tubulin, MAPs*,

*MAP = Microtubule-Associated Proteins.

etc.), neurofilaments, and microtrabecular systems. Molecular assemblies, in particular protein–protein associations, can be analyzed in conformational terms and they depend upon the physicochemical properties of the molecules. In the eukaryotic cell, metabolism cascades are driven not only by the mass action law but also by the channeling created by internal membranes.

The specialization of the neuron includes a distinctive cell shape (cell body with several dentrites and a single axon), an outer membrane for generating nerve impluses, and the synapse, a particular structure for transmitting the impulse to another neuron or to another cell. The transmission involves the secretion of a neurotransmitter from vesicles so that both conductive and secretory functions characterize a neuron.

Although a reticular neuroid tissue complex is found in sponges, the first primitive neurons with elementary synaptic contacts appear in the coelenterates (2). Cytoplasmic secretory granules comparable to those of higher animals and appearing membrane-bounded with diameters of 1000–1700 A can be distinguished, and it seems that at this level of differentiation, the nervous system subserves all the existing endocrine functions (2).

Several peptides, previously identified in mammalian brain and gut, have been recognized immunologically in the nerve net of *Hydra* (3) or in the brain of *Ciona* (4), suggesting that similar precursors exist throughout the animal kingdom (Figure 1). Furthermore the neuronal and non-neuronal peptide-producing cells in vertebrates may arise from the same neuroectodermal cells (5), and differentiated neurons and endocrine cells preserve a common biosynthetic machinery. However, specific biosynthetic amplification and specific processing of neuropeptides leads to particular functions and to specialization among neurons. If the neuron is defined by its chemical products, it would be of interest to observe the ontogenic variations of these latter in order to compare the early neural cells of vertebrates not only to the adult neurons of the most primitive invertebrates but also to their stem cells such as the interstitial cells and even the epithelial cells in *Hydra* (6).

1.1.3 Organ Assembly: The Brain

Because the human brain is an assembly of about 10^{10} neurons, the degree of complexity of organization and internal relationships is probably much higher than that found in an eukaryotic cell. As in any type of assembly, general rules of construction exist despite the huge amount of dispersed data given by paleontology, zoology, anatomy, physiology, embryology, and chemistry. How the genome, regarded today as a sequence of nucleotides, can program such a structure is very difficult to

	VERTEBRATES (mammals)		UROCHORDATES (Ciona)	INVERTEBRATES (Hydra)
HEAD ACTIVATOR	brain	gut		nerve net
SUBSTANCE P	brain	gut	brain	nerve net
NEUROTENSIN	brain	gut	brain	nerve net
SOMATOSTATIN	brain	gut	brain	
CCK / GASTRIN	brain	gut		nerve net
ACTH / MSH	brain		brain	
VASOPRESSIN-LIKE	brain			nerve net
EK / ENDORPHIN	brain	gut	brain	nerve net
BOMBESIN	brain		brain	

Figure 1. Distribution of some neuropeptides in members of the phylum Chordata (vertebrates and urochordates) and the phylum Coelenterata (radially symmetrical invertebrates), which are located at the two ends of the animal scale. Identification of neuropeptides was both immunological and chemical when the tissue source is underlined and only immunological when it is not.

understand, consequently how evolutionary changes have been integrated into the genome seems beyond our understanding. Comparative anatomy and paleontology through endocasts show the progressive increase of the relative size of the brain in the course of evolution. Furthermore, quantitative amplification is associated with an increase in structural and functional complexity (7).

The development of the brain raises many questions dealing with the induction of the neural plate, the localized proliferation of cells in different regions, the migration of these cells from their birthplace to their definitive location, their association to form identifiable parts of the brain, the differentiation of the neurons, and the formation of connections. These mechanisms most likely involve cascades of gene inductions and several types of intercellular messengers. Growth factors may stimulate mitosis, migration factors may direct migration, differentiation factors may determine the neuronal shaping as well as the internal subcellular specific organization, and aggregation factors may trigger the proper associations. These factors may be peptides similar to the nerve growth factor or to the *Hydra* head activator that have been chemically characterized.

In the gigantic assembly that is the brain, apart from the question of the specific cellular differentiation, the architectural settling of the neuron network with its myriad of connections is the main problem. However, the same general rules for cell–cell recognition and association could apply to the building of any organ assembly.

1.2   Evolutionary Barriers

The apparent diversity of living forms masks a great parsimony in their fundamental assembly. As mentioned above, heredity is based on four nucleotides, the structures of which are similar since there are two purine and two pyrimidine bases. On the other hand, the various proteins (perhaps 100–200 billion) that exist result from the combination of only 20 amino acids. Thus the molecular "building blocks" are very limited in number.

Cellular assembly is also fundamentally limited since only two cell types, the prokaryotic and the eukaryotic cells, have been successful. Multicellular eukaryotes are an amplification and diversification of the basic unicellular eukaryotes.

The nervous system and the brain have virtually the same fundamental organization in the entire animal kingdom, though the number of animal species is over a million (8).

Thus, evolution seems rather conservative rather than rich in solutions, at least at certain levels of the hierarchy of the assemblies. Why is the genetic code universal and based on only four molecules? This can be an argument for the unique appearance of life but shows that some "barriers" have existed to the progressive diversification of the living matter. Prokaryotic cells emerged some 3.2–3.5 billion years ago, the first unicellular eukaryotes appeared at least 2.0 billion years later, so that the constitution of the eukaryotic structure with cooperative organelles delimited by internal membranes (intracellular channeling) was the result of a very long labor. Apparently here also there was a barrier to progress that was overcome with difficulty.

Differentiation and coordination between cells in multicellular eukaryotes involved recognition molecules, either fixed in the membranes for cell–cell interactions or free to move among cells for chronologically ordered growth and differentiation. These substances must at least cross or contact two membranes (those of the secretory cell and the target cell) and should have peculiar features. It is rather surprising to observe the same type of peptide processing through the animal realm and to find that peptides can serve as growth factors, differentiation factors, hormones, neurotransmitters or neuromodulators. Apparently the number of keys for the intercellular communications is also very limited.

2 CONSERVATIVE ASPECTS OF MOLECULAR EVOLUTION: THE RECAPITULATION PRINCIPLE

2.1 The Ontogenic Program and Phylogeny

Perhaps because fundamental structures are difficult to evolve, they are in some way preserved during development. Are these early forms found in fetus or larva passages which must be traversed before reaching adulthood or imago forms, or are they just the expression of genomic relics? In the last century, Haeckel proposed the so-called fundamental biogenetic law that could be formulated as "ontogeny recapitulates phylogeny." During development each species passes through different steps that remind one of its evolutionary precursors. For example, the "gills" of the mammalian fetus as well as its two-compartment heart can be regarded as fish features.

At the protein level it is well known that there are changes in mammals between fetus and adult. For instance, the two chains of embryonic hemoglobin, ζ and ξ, are changed into α and γ, respectively, in the fetal hemoglobin, then into α and β in the adult hemoglobin. Are these ontogenic changes related to the phylogenic order of variations? To prove such a hypothesis, it is necessary to compare embryonic or fetal mammalian proteins to fish or amphibian proteins. However, it is known that in amphibians there is also a replacement of the two chains of tadpole hemoglobin by two new chains of frog hemoglobin. It seems that comparison should be made between the early proteins of the two classes since the morphological similarity is mainly found in these forms.

The neurohypophysial hormone vasotocin is found in the adults of all the nonmammalian vertebrates (9). However, this molecule has been detected in fetal sheep or seal at midgestation and it is replaced by vasopressin at birth, apparently an example of molecular recapitulation.

2.2 Schedule and Modulation of Gene Expression

2.2.1 Processing and Cellular Differentiation

Secretory peptides and proteins are produced by cleavages from larger precursor polypeptide chains. Thus, a preproprotein, emerging from the ribosome attached to reticular endoplasmic epithelium by its recognition sequence, is truncated by a specific enzyme to form a proprotein. This proprotein may be truncated again, excised, or divided into fragments by specialized enzymes belonging either to the cathepsin B family (trypsin-like specificity) or to the cathepsin D family (pepsin-like specificity). Each fragment may have its own function so that the initial chain acts as a polyprecursor and may be processed differently at different locations in the body.

In the case of cholecystokinin (CCK), an intestinal hormone responsible for gall bladder contraction and pancreatic secretion, these differences in processing have been clearly demonstrated (see below, Section 3.3.2). The CCK precursor is mainly processed into a 33/39 residue peptide (CCK-33 or CCK-39) in the gut and into an eight-residue fragment (CCK-8) in the brain and myenteric plexus (10).

2.2.2 Processing and Ontogeny

Another interesting observation is the change in peptide processing during development. Corticotropin (39 residues), the adrenocorticoptropic hormone (ACTH), is primarily found in the anterior lobe of the pituitary gland whereas α-melanocyte stimulating hormone (α-MSH), which represents the first 13 residues of corticotropin, is found in the intermediate lobe (11–13). These molecules have both been detected immunologically in the brain. Using the complementary DNA to the mRNA, the sequence of a macromolecular precursor (265 residues) which includes a glycopeptide, corticotropin, and endorphin has been deduced (11–13). Silman and coworkers (14) have found a switch in the processing of this precursor during the development of rhesus monkey (though this has not been confirmed in other laboratories). The fetal pituitary mainly produces α-MSH, whereas the infant or adult gland mainly makes corticotropin. Likewise, the fetal adrenal gland is stimulated by α-MSH but not by corticotropin and this response is reversed in the adult organ. Most important, the metamorphosis of the adrenal at birth is temporally associated with the change in polypeptide processing in the pituitary. Thus, the same precursor may give rise to different products at different stages of development.

2.2.3 Processing and Phylogeny

Concerning the phylogenetic distribution of neuropeptides it is interesting that caerulein, a decapeptide that has been isolated from the skin of an Australian hylid frog, *Hyla caerulea*, has a C-terminal sequence identical with CCK-8 except for the substitution of a methionine residue by threonine (Figure 2). At the N-terminus a pyroglutamyl group is found. This is usually the result of the spontaneous conversion of glutamine after cleavage of an adjacent peptide bond, and it indicates that caerulein is probably a fragment of a larger precursor. The role of caerulein in frog skin is unknown but it is clear that a CCK-like precursor not only exists in the frog but is processed in the same way as the CCK precursor in the sheep brain.

Bombesin, a tetradecapeptide purified from the skin of the frog *Bombina bombina*, is probably also derived from a larger precursor because of its N-terminal pyroglutamyl and its amidated C-terminal end.

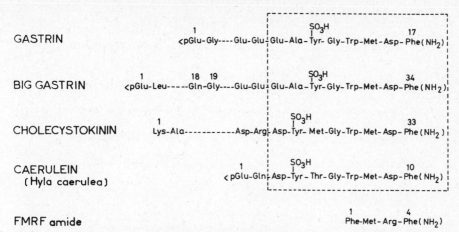

Figure 2. The gastrin–cholecystokinin family. Gastrin (G-17), Big gastrin (G-34), cholecystokinin (CCK-33), and caerulein share a similar C-terminal amidated octapeptide (boxed). Free CCK-8 is found in the brain. The FMRF amide (one-letter symbols for amino acids) was first discovered in molluscan ganglia and later immunologically identified in central nervous system and gut endocrine cells of vertebrates.

In the rat, two populations of bombesin-containing neurons have been detected immunologically. One is found in the brain and intestine and mainly contains a form similar in size to the amphibian peptide, the other is found in the stomach and is larger (10).

Similarly, peptides structurally and pharmacologically related to substance P have been isolated from amphibian skin and from octopod salivary glands (15). The so-called tachykinin peptide family lowers blood pressure and stimulates intestinal smooth muscle. A C-terminal amino acid amide and an N-terminal pyroglutamyl residue are usually found, showing that these peptides are excised from longer precursors (Figure 3).

Structural genes seem, therefore, to have essentially been conserved through the animal kingdom, and their protein products often appear to be processed in the same way by enzymes endowed with similar specificities. Apparently, during development genes are successively turned "on" and "off" and the question is whether present-day mammals have inherited the genes of their ancestors expressed in order of their evolutionary succession. If so, several genes are present for each "adult" protein (multigene family), and mammalian genomes are essentially living archives. On the other hand, in some cases the processing itself may have been subjected to evolution and variations may be observed during the development, the same structural gene remaining turned "on" permanently. Some kind of coevolution should have existed between protein substrate genes and processing enzyme genes.

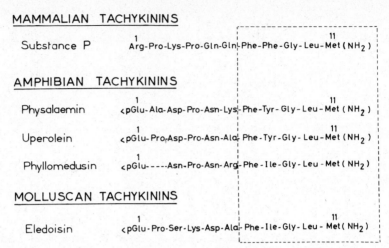

Figure 3. The tachykinin family. The tachykinin peptides are very likely to be excised from longer precursors, as indicated by pGlu (pyrrolidone carboxylic acid) residue at the N-terminal and amide residue at the C-terminal. The pharmacologically active sequence is boxed.

2.3   Co-Recapitulation: Effector and Receptor

Receptors are generally assumed to be intrinsic membrane proteins with a structure permitting both insertion into the lipid bilayer and recognition of the effector (hormone, transmitter, etc.). These proteins are probably built as secretory proteins, synthesized on cytoplasmic ribosomes, and transfered through the rough endoplasmic reticular membrane to reach, after processing and maturation in the Golgi complex, the plasma membrane. Their biosynthetic fate resembles that of the protein hormones except that they are not secreted, and their structural genes have been subjected to similar events in the course of evolution. Because of the specific recognition between the transmitter or the hormone and the receptor, the two conformations (and therefore the two amino acid sequences) are co-adapted and must have co-evolved. It is possible that the receptor gene was turned "off" in one type of cell and turned "on" in another. In this case, there was a change of target cells but the new recipient cells should also have the integrative molecular system to exploit the message.

If a series of hormone genes are successively expressed in development, a series of corresponding receptor genes are probably turned "on" and "off" synchronously. If functional recapitulation is a necessity, it involves co-recapitulations at the molecular level.

3   ADAPTATIVE ASPECTS OF MOLECULAR EVOLUTION: THE RECLAMATION PRINCIPLE

Morphological or molecular adaptation can be regarded as a new integration of preexisting structures. In other words the cell or the molecule can change from one assembly to another. The result is a new function made with ancient material.

3.1   Morphological Reclamation

One bone structure was successively used in the course of evolution, to construct organs of respiration, nutrition, and audition. The bone sustaining the first gill in agnathans, the branchial arch, was first converted into the lower jaw in gnathostomes. In reptiles, this lower jaw was built by several bones, in particular, the dentary and the articular, the latter assuming the articulation with the quadrate. In mammals, the dentary remained the single element of the lower jaw, and the old quadrate-articular joint shifted to a new dentary-squamosal joint; the now unneeded articular and quadrate were taken for the construction of the middle ear as accessory ossicles, the malleus ("hammer") and the incus ("anvil"), respectively (16).

3.2   Molecular Reclamation

Polypeptide material lends itself to shape modification in the same way that bone does in the skeletal system. Variations in the nucleotide sequence of DNA, splicing in mRNA, and processing in proteins can greatly modify the size and the aminoacid sequence of a peptide, that is, the conformation of the final product. However, because several similar proteins have been recognized in lower and higher eukaryotes, it seems that the prototype proteins have in some way resisted evolutionary changes and that preexisting structures have been spared and reemployed in new integrative systems. The initial co-adaptation between two conformations, similar to a key–lock coupling, was probably very difficult to achieve through the two corresponding genes so that this type of acquisition was likely often preserved, particularly the "messenger–receptor" association involving precise molecular recognition. This association could have been inserted in different physiological systems as the articular-quadrate coupling was used either for chewing or for hearing. If so the development of "recent" functions, such as lactation in mammals, may have been expedited by the reclaimation of old proteins.

3.2.1 Molecular Reclamation with a Switch in the Target Cell

Prolactin, the lactogenic hormone of mammals found in adenohypophysis, has a specific receptor present in the secretory (epithelial) cells of the mammary gland. However, several other cells, in particular, those of the corpus luteum, respond to prolactin (17). Furthermore, prolactin, like many other peptide hormones, has been detected in the brain (18). Apparently prolactin is involved in several types of cell–cell signaling.

Prolactin-like proteins existed long before the appearance of lactation since this type of protein is present in virtually all vertebrates. In fish, prolactin is concerned with the regulation of water and electrolyte balance. Purified prolactin of *Tilapia mossambica*, the amino acid composition of which is similar to that of ovine prolactin, exerts a powerful sodium-retaining activity in suitably treated fish (17). However prolactins with mammotropic activity are found only at the level of amphibians and upward (17). The "prolactin"-receptor relationship is probably a very ancient one. By changing the cells expressing the receptor, evolution could use an old message for a new task, the integration depending on the differentiation of the cell. The result is a change from regulation of water homeostasis to control of milk production. This reconversion seems a very clear example of molecular reclaimation.

While prolactin is the lactogenic hormone, oxytocin is the milk-ejecting principle that acts on mammary myoepithelial cells in placental mammals. Oxytocin receptors are also present on uterine smooth muscle cells, another type of target cell with contractile activity (19). The evolutionary precursor of oxytocin found in nonmammalian tetrapods is mesotocin and this peptide is assumed to act on the oviduct. It is rather surprising to note that mesotocin has been preserved in Australian marsupials (20) and in these species likely plays both the milk-ejecting and uterotonic roles given over to oxytocin in eutherians. In metatherians, gestation is very short and the young are almost embryonic in form; lactation, on the other hand, is very long. In macropodids, the milk-ejection response to oxytocin-like peptides has been refined in order to permit simultaneous feeding of both newly born pouch young and young at foot (21). The pre-extant mesotocin has been reclaimed. A mesotocin receptor is expressed by mammary myoepithelial cells the contractile system of which is used for milk-ejection instead of egg laying as was formerly the case. It is striking that the complete hormonal control of lactation has apparently been built with pre-extant messenger molecules.

The change of target cells is also spectacular in the case of vasotocin. This neuropeptide is present in all adult vertebrates except mammals in which it seems to exist in the foetus (22). In fish, vasotocin acts on the gills and the kidneys (23); in amphibians it usually acts on the skin, the urinary bladder and the kidney, except in newts and salamanders in which it has a single site of action, the kidney (24). In reptiles and birds, extrarenal osmotic sites of action no longer exist although vasotocin does act on the oviduct (24). The propensity of vasotocin to adopt different target tissues shows that various cells have the potential for receptor expression and that organisms can make use of coadapted molecular coupling in the course of evolution. The possibility of receptor polymorphism in the same organism with a family of related receptor genes exists, of course, but the ability to switch a specific receptor gene on or off seems an important factor in cellular differentiation.

3.2.2 Molecular Reclamation with a Switch in Processing

A macromolecular precursor can be fragmented into a number of pieces. According to a cell's state of differentiation, the processing of the same precursor may differ, yielding active peptides with different lengths. Cholecystokinin, responsible for gallbladder contraction and pancreatic secretion, has been isolated from hog intestine in two major forms, one having 33 residues (CCK-33) and the other with an N-terminal extension of six residues (CCK-39) (Figure 2; refs. 25, 26). In the brain and myenteric plexus, precursors (27) are converted almost completely (95%) to the C-terminal CCK-8 (10). It may be assumed that CCK-8 found in central and peripheral neurons is a neuromodulator whereas CCK-33 and CCK-39 have hormonal functions in digestion.

4 ADDITIVE ASPECTS OF MOLECULAR EVOLUTION: THE DUPLICATION PRINCIPLE

4.1 Morphological Duplication

Duplication of a structural unit and use of the duplicated unit for more than one task is one of the easiest ways to achieve a polyfunctional system. Eukaryotic multicellular organisms may be regarded as end products of the repetitive duplication and differentiation of a single eukaryotic cell, the egg. Chromatids are duplicated forms of chromosomes and a living species is a permanent duplicative system.

When the two duplicated units remain attached, some kind of symmetry may appear. Organisms are usually symmetric, and the control of symmetric growth is not easy to explain. But the two symmetric elements may act complementarily, and if two hands are efficient to catch prey, eight tentacles may be better, although the millepede is not faster than the snake. Duality or multiplicity suggests a duplicative mechanism, first for reasons of simplicity, but the 10^{10} neurons of the brain arise by repetitive division and differentiation from a limited number of cells in the neural plate.

4.2 Molecular Duplication

Repetitive sequences presenting a high degree of homology have been observed in both proteins and nucleic acids. Although this repetition suggests a duplicative mechanism inside the genes, the mechanism of duplication remains obscure.

On the other hand, several peptide or protein families displaying distinct biological properties present so high a degree of homology in their amino acid sequences that they are thought to share a common evolutionary precursor. Conformational studies based on X-ray crystallography have revealed that two proteins showing 30% or more homology in their sequences have virtually the same general three-dimensional structures. Molecular specialization seems to occur after duplication by particular mutations so that the same prototype may lead to several specialized conformations with specific interactions, that is, to several distinct functions.

4.2.1 Tandem Duplication

One of the clearest examples of tandem duplication is the chains of immunoglobulins, particularly the heavy chain of immunoglobulin G in which four consecutive homologous sequences, and therefore four homologous domains, have been found. The extensive repertoire of immunoglobulins can be accounted for in two ways: multiplicity of germline variable-region genes (V_1 and V_4) and somatic diversification of V genes. In the case of κ chains, which constitute the bulk of the light chains of the mouse, the pattern of variability is extensive and can be explained at least in part by multiple germline genes (28). On the other hand the joining (J) segments of mouse immunoglobulin λ light chain genes, λ_2, λ_3, and a presumptive λ_4, were cloned and their sequences were compared with that of λ_1. All the λJ segments share sequence homology. These sequence data, together with the fact that present day λ genes occur in two clusters, substantiate a probable evolutionary duplication unit, $J_{II}C_{II}J_IC_I$ with II the precursor of λ_3 and λ_2 and I the precursor of λ_1 and λ_4 (29).

Similarly, in the case of human hemoglobin chains, tandem homologous genes, $\zeta_2\zeta_1$, $\alpha_2\alpha_1$, Gγ Aγ, and $\delta\beta$, have been observed with tandem switching during development (30).

Tandem duplication also occurred in neuropeptide precursors. Both α-MSH and its putative precursor, corticotropin, have been detected in the brain and in the pituitary gland. On the other hand, the active melanocyte-stimulating heptapeptide is also contained within the pituitary peptide β-MSH and in the corresponding putative precursor, lipotropin, which also contains the endorphin sequence. A large common precursor which includes a glycopeptide, corticotropin, and lipotropin, termed proopiocortin, has been synthesized using the appropriate mRNA. Finally, the complementary DNA (cDNA) of the mRNA has been made using reverse transcriptase and directly sequenced. In this manner the complete aminoacid sequence of preproopiocortin (265 residues) has been deduced and a third repetition of the melanocyte-stimulating peptide, called γ-MSH, has been found within the decoded N-terminal sequence of the protein (11–13). Peptide fragments containing γ-MSH have now been isolated from the pituitary.

A second example concerns the opioid pentapeptides Leu- and Met-enkephalins. These were first discovered in the brain (31) but have now been identified in many tissues, particularly the adrenal medulla. Two putative precursors, which upon digestion with trypsin yield peptides that bind to opiate receptors, have been purified from adrenal chromaffin granules. One, peptide F, is apparently a Met-enkephalin precursor containing two copies of the peptide, the other, peptide I, contains both Leu- and Met-enkephalin and is presumably a common precursor of the two forms (Figure 4). Recently the nucleotide sequence of a complete cDNA copy of enkephalin precursor mRNA from human phaeochromocytoma has been reported. The corresponding aminoacid sequence shows that the precursor is 267 amino acids long and contains six interspersed Met-enkephalin sequences and one Leu-enkephalin sequence. Five of the seven enkephalins are flanked on both sides by pairs of basic amino acid residues (32, 33). This precursor contains the sequences of peptides F and I previously characterized but not those of the opioid peptides, dynorphin, α-neoendorphin or β-endorphin (Figure 4). The name preproenkephalin A has been suggested for this precursor.

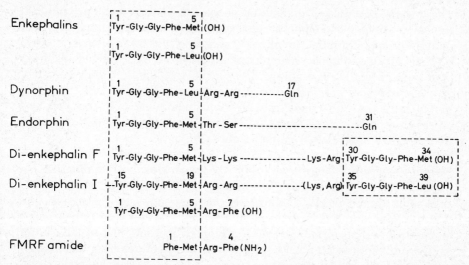

Figure 4. The enkephalin sequences (boxed) exist in at least three distinct polypeptides: dynorphin, endorphin, and a 267-residue precursor that includes peptides F and I and contains six interspeed Met-enkephalins and one Leu-enkephalin.

The primary structure of a precursor protein that contains α-neo-endorphin, dynorphin, and a third Leu-enkephalin sequence with a carboxyl extension, has been deduced from the nucleotide sequence of cloned DNA complementary to the porcine hypothalamic mRNA encoding it (34). The three peptides are each bound by Lys-Arg. This precursor, termed preproenkephalin B or preprodynorphin, therefore comprises three repetitive units of Leu-enkephalin (34).

The three chromosomal genes of preproopiocortin, preproenkephalin A, and preproenkephalin B display a similar structural organization (35–37). A single exon codes for the repetitive units; the absence of introns within the region encoding the multiple units may imply that the repetitive structure has evolved by duplication of primordial DNA segments at adjacent positions.

It has been shown, furthermore, that the intron of the human genome contains at least 400,000 copies of the 300 base-pair *Alu* repeat sequence, the predominant repetitive sequence in the human species (38). Gene amplification, with as many as 200 tandem copies, occurs in peculiar tissues during development (39). Some duplicative mechanisms therefore seem involved in the extension of the gene nucleotide sequence leading to long polypeptide chains with multiple identical amino acid sequences. The repetitive domains may remain bound and give long polyfunctional proteins (e.g., immunoglobulins), or they may be separated by processing enzymes giving structurally related peptides with distinct functions (e.g., proopiocortin).

4.2.2 Separate Duplication

The protein products of duplicated genes are distinct and not bound in the same polypeptide chain as observed for immunoglobulins. Independent mutations can affect duplicated genes so that the evolution of each product is autonomous. When duplication is recent, the two proteins may be very similar in aminoacid sequence and function, and are usually termed "*isoproteins*". But the divergence may increase with the number of mutations and each protein may acquire its own function and therefore receive a specific name. Thus, two structurally-related peptide lineages may arise from a common ancestor gene.

Neurohypophysial Hormones and Neurophysins.   Examination of about 50 species representing the entire vertebrate phylum has revealed that each animal usually makes two neurohypophysial hormones, and that oxytocin and vasopressin appear as the final links of two lineages of molecules—the former probably involved in reproduction, the latter in hydromineral regulation (9, 40). Ten active peptides have been characterized to date. All are nonapeptides with the same molecular pattern, and with substitutions occurring at positions 4 and 8, and very rarely in positions 2 and 3 (Table 1). Because of the similarity between

TABLE 1 Structures of the Neurohypophysial Hormones

Oxytocin-like Peptides

1 2 3 4 5 6 7 8 9

Cys-Tyr-Ile-Gln-Asn-Cys-Pro-Leu-Gly(NH$_2$)
Oxytocin
(prototherian and eutherian mammals)

Cys-Tyr-Ile-Gln-Asn-Cys-Pro-Ile-Gly(NH$_2$)
Mesotocin
(Australian marsupials, birds, reptiles, amphibians, lungfishes)

Cys-Tyr-Ile-Ser-Asn-Cys-Pro-Ile-Gly(NH$_2$)
Isotocin
(bony fishes)

Cys-Tyr-Ile-Ser-Asn-Cys-Pro-Gln-Gly(NH$_2$)
Glumitocin
(cartilaginous fishes: rays)

Cys-Tyr-Ile-Gln-Asn-Cys-Pro-Val-Gly(NH$_2$)
Valitocin
(cartilaginous fishes: sharks)

Cys-Tyr-Ile-Asn-Asn-Cys-Pro-Leu-Gly(NH$_2$)
Aspargtocin
(cartilaginous fishes: sharks)

Vasopressin-like Peptides

1 2 3 4 5 6 7 8 9

Cys-Tyr-Phe-Gln-Asn-Cys-Pro-Arg-Gly (NH$_2$)
Arginine vasopressin
(prototherian, metatherian, and eutherian mammals)

Cys-Tyr-Phe-Gln-Asn-Cys-Pro-Lys-Gly(NH$_2$)
Lysine vasopressin
(eutherians: pig; metatherians: macropodids)

Cys-Phe-Phe-Gln-Asn-Cys-Pro-Arg-Gly (NH$_2$)
Phenypressin
(metatherians: macropodids)

Cys-Tyr-Ile-Gln-Asn-Cys-Pro-Arg-Gly(NH$_2$)
Vasotocin
(nonmammalian vertebrates)

the two hormone lineages and because only a single hormone is found in one of the most primitive vertebrates, the lamprey, it has been assumed that a gene duplication occurred between Cyclostomes (lampreys) and true fishes. After this, the two lines of molecules evolved separately. Thus each vertebrate species usually has an "oxytocin-like" peptide and a "vasopressin-like" peptide. Oxytocin and vasopressin themselves are characteristic of placental mammals whereas mesotocin and vasotocin are found in non-mammalian tetrapods, isotocin and vasotocin in bony fishes, glumitocin and vasotocin in rays, valitocin and aspargtocin, as well as vasotocin, in sharks.

Australian marsupials appear rather peculiar. On one hand the vasopressin-like peptide has been duplicated in *Macropodidae* (kangaroos and wallabies) so that two pressor hormones are found, lysine vasopressin (lysipressin) and phenypressin [Phe^2,Arg^8]-vasopressin. They are present in all the individual glands and are encoded by two distinct genes. In *Phalangeridae* (possum), a single vasopressin, arginine vasopressin is identified. On the other hand the oxytocin-like peptide is not oxytocin as in eutherians but mesotocin as is typically the case in nonmammalian tetrapods. Mesotocin is very likely involved in regulatory lactation of Australian marsupials; it is very surprising to observe that the marsupials use this reptilian hormone. However, the presence of oxytocin in the prototherian echidna might suggest reverse mutation (a leucine–isoleucine interchange in the nonapeptide), and if this is so, the passage from mesotocin to oxytocin or vice versa would represent "neutral" evolution. Fig. 5 depicts the evolution of neurohypophysial hormones in upper tetrapods.

The duality in eutherian hormone structures is also observed for neurophysins. Two types have been characterized in each species: MESL-neurophysins (fully sequenced for ox, sheep, pig, horse, whale, rat and man) and VLDV-neurophysins (sequenced for ox, pig, horse, rat and man) (9, 40, 57). These proteins were named on the basis of the one-letter symbols for aminoacids located in positions 2, 3, 6, and 7, the N-terminal sequence being a specific antigenic site. The two proteins are 93–95 residues long (Figures 6 and 7) and in a given species show about 80% homology. The central sequences (residues 10–75) are nearly identical within and between the families. Variations between families occur in the N-terminal part (residues 1–9) and in the C-terminal part (76–95) within the families (Figure 8).

Neurohypophysial hormones and neurophysins share common precursors. Preliminary research initiated by Sachs (41) revealed in hypothalamus a macromolecular precursor of vasopressin and several indirect data suggested that a neurophysin might be a part of this precursor. Brownstein et al. (42) have shown, by labeling experiments, the presence in rat supraoptic nuclei of two electrophoretically distinct M_r-20,000 proteins supposed to be the precursors of oxytocin and vasopres-

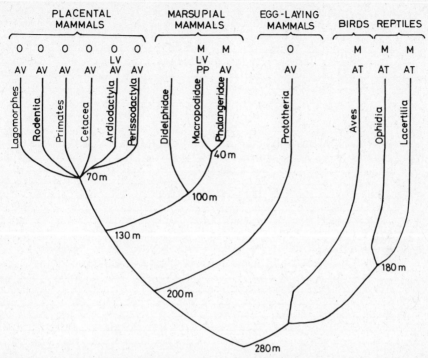

Figure 5. Neurohypophysial hormones and tetrapod evolution according to paleontological data. Letters indicate hormones identified in modern representatives of the groups: O, oxytocin; AV, arginine vasopressin; LV, lysine vasopressin; M, mesotocin; PP, phenypressin; AT, arginine vasotocin. The numbers give the time in millions of years (m) since the divergence.

sin, respectively. The common precursor of vasopressin and a neurophysin, detected by reaction with respective antisera, is split by trypsin into a Mr-10,000 protein reacting only with antineurophysin, and several peptides, one reacting with anti-vasopressin. Several groups of workers (43–45) have confirmed that such precursors can be generated by cell-free translation of mRNA and finally Land et al. (46) have deduced the amino-acid sequence of the vasopressin precursor from the nucleotide sequence of the corresponding cDNA. Three domains can be distinguished in this 147-residue protein : arginine vasopressin, MSEL-neurophysin and a glycopeptide (Figure 9).

Vasopressin or oxytocin-like peptides have been immunologically detected in several invertebrates, including one of the most primitive, *Hydra* (3), and neurophysin-like material has been found associated with hormone-like peptides in two insects (47). The role of these substances in invertebrates is not clear, but it can be assumed that a molecule similar to the vertebrate precursor gives rise to peptides

Bovine 1 2   5   10   15   20   25
Ala-Met-Ser-Asp-Leu-Glu-Leu-Arg-Gln-Cys-Leu-Pro-Cys-Gly-Pro-Gly-Gly-Lys-Gly-Arg-Cys-Phe-Gly-Pro-Ser
Ovine   ——
Porcine ——
Equine ——
Whale   ——
Rat   ——Thr—————————Met——
Human   ——

Bovine   29 30   35 36   40   45   48   50
Ile-Cys-Cys-Gly-Asp-Glu-Leu-Gly-Cys-Phe-Val-Gly-Thr-Ala-Glu-Ala-Leu-Arg-Cys-Gln-Glu-Glu-Asn-Tyr-Leu
Ovine   ——Ile————
Porcine ——
Equine ——
Whale   ————————————————————————————Met——————————————————————————————————
Rat   ————————Ala————————————Leu——————————————————————————————————————
Human   ————————Ala——

Bovine   55   60   65   70 72   75
Pro-Ser-Pro-Cys-Gln-Ser-Gly-Gln-Lys-Pro-Cys-Gly-Ser-Gly-Gly-Arg-Cys-Ala-Ala-Ala-Gly-Ile-Cys-Cys-Asn
Ovine   ——
Porcine ——
Equine ——
Whale   ——
Rat   ——Ser
Human   ————————————————————————Ala————————————————————————Phe————Val——

Bovine   80 81   85   89 90 91 92   94 95
Asp-Glu-Ser-Cys-Val-Thr-Glu-Pro-Glu-Cys-Arg-Glu-Gly-Ile(Val)-Gly-Phe-Pro-Arg-Arg-Val
Ovine   ——————————————————————————————————————Ile——————————
Porcine ————————————————————————————————————Ala-Ser——Leu——————Ala
Equine ————————————————————————————————————Ala——Leu——————Ala
Whale   ————————————————————————————————————Ala-Ser——————Ala
Rat   ——————————————————Ala——————————————Phe-Phe[   ]——Leu-Thr
Human   ————————————————————————————————————Phe-His[   ]——Ala

Figure 6. Amino acid sequences of some mammalian MSEL-neurophysins. Solid lines indicate residues identical with those of the bovine protein.

homologous to neurohypophysial hormones and neurophysins. In lamprey, only a single hormone has been detected to date so that a single protein precursor can be postulated. The duality of neurohypophysial hormones at the level of bony fish suggests a duality of precursors arising by duplication and two evolutionary lines leading to oxytocin and VLDV-neurophysin on one hand and to vasopressin and MSEL-neurophysin on the other (Figure 10).

The Glucagon-Secretin Family. Glucagon is a peptide that produces hyperglycemia that was first isolated from pancreas and subsequently detected in brain. It is a linear peptide consisting of 29 aminoacid residues. Although glucagons from birds or fish show substitutions when compared with mammalian peptides, they all have 29 residues, indicating a constant and precise processing in the vertebrate kingdom.

VLDV · NEUROPHYSINS

	1 2 5 7 9 10 15 20 25
Bovine	Ala·Val·Leu·Asp·Leu·Asp·Val·Arg·Thr·Cys·Leu·Pro·Cys·Gly·Pro·Gly·Gly·Lys·Gly·Arg·Cys·Phe·Gly·Pro·Ser
Porcine	——————————————Lys——————
Equine	—Ala————————Lys———
Rat	—Ala——————Met——Lys———
Human	—Ala·Pro————————Lys——————————————————Asn

	26 29 30 35 40 45 50
Bovine	Ile·Cys·Cys·Gly·Asp·Glu·Leu·Gly·Cys·Phe·Val·Gly·Thr·Ala·Glu·Ala·Leu·Arg·Cys·Gln·Glu·Glu·Asn·Tyr·Leu
Porcine	———————————————————
Equine	———————————————————
Rat	————————Ala———————
Human	————————Ala·Glu———————

	51 55 60 64 65 69 70 72 75
Bovine	Pro·Ser·Pro·Cys·Gln·Ser·Gly·Gln·Cys·Pro·Cys·Gly·Ser·Gly·Gly·Arg·Cys·Ala·Ala·Ala·Gly·Ile·Cys·Cys·Ser
Porcine	———————————Glu————————Asn
Equine	———————————————————
Rat	————————————————Thr———
Human	——————————Ala————————Val·Leu——Leu———

	76 80 81 84 85 86 87 89 90 93
Bovine	Pro·Asp·Gly·Cys·His·Glu·Asp·Pro·Ala·Cys·Asp·Pro·Glu·Ala·Ala·Phe·Ser·Gln
Porcine	——————Arg·Phe————————Thr———
Equine	——————Leu·Ala———Ser——His·Asp———
Rat	——————Arg·Thr—————————Ser———
Human	——————Ala——————Ala———Thr———

Figure 7. Amino acid sequences of some mammalian VLDV-neurophysins. Solid lines indicate residues identical with those of the bovine protein.

Secretin, an intestinal hormone stimulating pancreatic bicarbonate secretion, is a 27-residue linear basic peptide, showing a rather great homology with glucagon (Figure 11); it has been immunologically recognized in the brain of *Ciona* (4). Vasoactive intestinal polypeptide (VIP) has 28 residues and belongs to the same structural family (Figure 11); it has also been immunologically identified in human (18) and *Ciona* (4) brains. Recently a new member of the glucagon-secretin family, the porcine intestinal peptide PHI-27, a peptide (P) having an NH_2-terminal histidine (H), a COOH-terminal isoleucine (I) amide, and 27 residues (Figure 11), has been characterized (48). All these peptides appear structurally related and could be products of genes deriving from a common ancestral gene by duplication and subsequent mutation. They seem processed in the same way although secretin, VIP and PHI are amidated while glucagon is not. The gastric inhibitory peptide (GIP) from duodenal mucosa, the largest gastrointestinal hormone (42 residues) is related. Interestingly, a preproglucagon from angler fish islets has been sequenced through glucagon-specific cDNA. It is 124 residues in length, contains a 29-residue glucagon sequence and a peptide of 34 residues highly homologous to GIP, VIP, and secretin (49). The genes of the glucagon–secretin family seem to be easily duplicated.

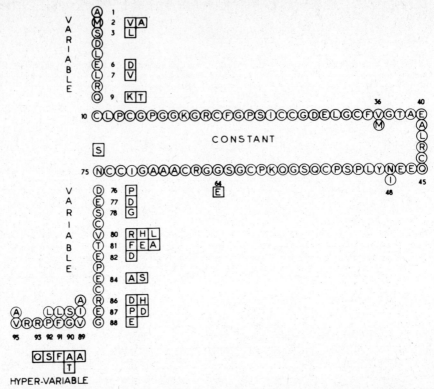

Figure 8. Comparison between MSEL-neurophysin and VLDV-neurophysin families. Bovine MSEL-neurophysin amino acid sequence is indicated by circles and substitutions in other MSEL-neurophysins by adjacent circles. Positions substituted in VLDV-neurophysins are indicated by squares. The N-terminal part (1–9) is variable between the two types of neurophysins, but the C-terminal part (76–95) is also variable within the families. The central region (10–75) is virtually constant.

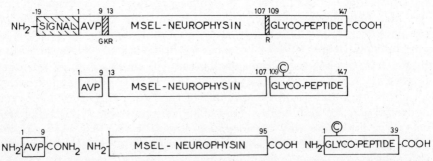

Figure 9. The common precursor of vasopressin (AVP) and MSEL-neurophysin is split into three fragments by two types of enzymatic cleavages, one involving a glycyl-lysyl-arginyl sequence (10–12) and leaving a carboxamid group at the C-terminal end of vasopressin, the other involving a single arginine residue (108) and giving MSEL-neurophysin and a glycopeptide. Redrawn from Land et al. (46).

156

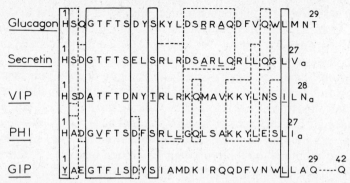

Figure 10. Hypothetic evolution of common neurohypophysial hormone–neurophysin precursors. A duplication between cyclostomes and bony fishes gave two distinct macromolecular precursors; subsequent mutations led to two evolutionary lines, an oxytocin-like/VLDV-neurophysin line and a vasopressin-like/MSEL-neurophysin line. A similar processing in each vertebrate class made the nonapeptide hormones and the corresponding neurophysins.

4.2.3 Duplication and Splicing

Duplication may affect a particular nucleotide sequence in the chromosome which encodes only a part of the final protein. For example an immunoglobulin light chain is encoded by three DNA segments, variable (V), joining (J) and constant (C) that are separated in the germline (24, 25). The light chains are termed according to the constant C-terminal

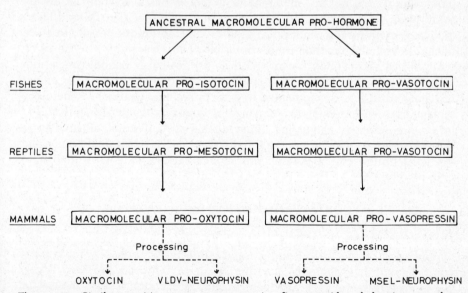

Figure 11. Similar positions or sequences in five peptides belonging to the glucagon/secretion family are boxed (solid lines, virtually in all the peptides; dashed lines, in some peptides). The one-letter symbols for amino acid residues are used.

half (κ or λ). Several homologous genes, supposed to be derived by duplication from a common ancestral variable gene, explain the great diversity of the variable region. The primary transcript (p-mRNA) may be subjected to several types of splicing, each bringing together only one of the variable gene transcript and the unique nucleotide sequence encoding for the constant region; the different type of mature mRNAs would finally be translated into corresponding proteins having the same C-terminal half but different N-terminal moieties.

Joining two distinct sequences to the same nucleotide sequence provides an economical method of peptide diversification. Gastrins and cholecystokinins have the same C-terminal pentapeptide (Figure 3) but very different N-terminal sequences so that they would hardly arise from a common ancestor sequence by duplication and clustered substitutions. Theoretically they could be generated by splicing two different nucleotide sequences to the one coding for the pentapeptide. In fact, calcitonin and a recently discovered calcitonin gene related peptide (CGRP) are made in just this way (50).

5   COORDINATIVE ASPECTS OF MOLECULAR EVOLUTION: THE MESSENGER PRINCIPLE

Because each analytical unit is itself an assembly of subunits, which in turn are themselves assemblies, and so on, between the different levels of the hierarchy precise interrelationships must exist through messenger molecules. If we regard an organ or a physiological system as an assembly of cells, intercellular messengers such as transmitters, hormones, growth factors, migration factors, and differentiation factors are necessary for the functional coordination of this assembly. In the same way, the cell itself may be regarded as an assembly of molecules, and intracellular regulatory mechanisms must be involved in order to adjust the concentrations of molecules and dictate their locations. Regulatory molecules such as allosteric enzymes or coenzymes may be considered internal messenger molecules. Biosynthesis or activation of such messenger molecules must be regulated by some kind of feedback. The chemical nature of the messengers should be determined by their specific binding sites.

5.1   Intercellular Morphogenic Coordination

Among the different kinds of intercellular messengers, some, produced by so-called "target cells," induce and guide the growth of remote partner cells so that contacts are finally made between the two types. Nerve growth factor (118 residues), originally isolated from a mouse tumor (sarcoma-180) but subsequently found to be secreted in trace

amounts by a variety of normal and neoplastic cells, induces the extension of nerve fibers from immature sympathetic neurons. Under normal
conditions, target cells that are innervated by sympathetic neurons
manufacture and secrete small amounts of nerve growth factor. The latter diffuses into the intercellular space and binds to specific membrane
receptors of immature sympathetic neurons. The interaction triggers organization of the growth cone through assembly within the neuron of
filamentous proteins (microtubules, microfilaments, etc.). The growth
cone possesses motile and exploratory microspikes that confer movement and directionality upon the growing axon. Once definitive connections are made with target cells, the contact is consolidated as a
synapse (51).

Other specific growth factors are known, such as epidermal growth
factor (53 residues) and somatomedins (70 residues), but the definition
of growth factors is still vague and may include mitogenic factors and
differentiation factors as well (52, 53).

"Morphogens" such as the *Hydra* head activator are able not only to
induce differentiation in several types of cell (nerve cells, nematocytes)
but also to cause morphological organization [of a mouth, for example,
with a precise number of differentiated tentacles (6)]. This class of coordinating molecules seems to be of fundamental importance though their
mechanism of action remains obscure.

5.2   Intermolecular Cascade Coordination

Apart from intercellular regulators such as hormones or growth factors,
intracellular messengers such as 3'-5'-adenosine monophosphate (cyclic
AMP or cAMP) or calcium govern several critical processes.

The so-called second messenger, cAMP, through cAMP-dependent
protein kinase, stimulates phosphorylation of proteins at serine residues. Phosphorylated proteins serve as effectors or modulators of various cellular reactions or physiological responses (54). The protein
kinase consists of two regulatory and two catalytic subunits and the enzyme is activated when the regulatory subunits bind cAMP, leaving the
catalytic subunits free and active. The cAMP–protein kinase system can
act on different cascades of enzymes, playing a molecular coordination
function.

Calcium ion exerts a profound influence on many biological processes, such as cell motility, muscle contraction, axonal flow, cytoplasmic
streaming, chromosome movement, neurotransmitter release, endocytosis and exocytocis. Calmodulin, an ubiquitous eukaryotic protein with a
Ca^{2+}-dependent conformation, is a primary receptor of calcium and appears to be a multifunctional messenger (55). It seems that a homologous class of Ca^{2+}-binding proteins serves as receptors for Ca^{2+}, just as
protein kinases act as receptors for cAMP or cyclic guanosine

monotriphosphate (cGMP). In mammalian cells, the steady-state concentration of Ca^{2+} in cytosol ranges from 10^{-8} to 10^{-7} M but stimulation of the cell may increase the concentration to 10^{-6} M, a level sufficient to cause the binding to receptor proteins such as calmodulin, triggering a change in protein conformation. The "active" complex in turn combines with the target apoenzyme or effector protein to evoke a biochemical reaction, leading to a physiological response (55).

The primary structure of calmodulin appears to have been conserved throughout the phylogenetic scale since antibodies against rat testis calmodulin cross-react with that from coelenterates. This suggests a precise structure-function relationship. Calmodulin regulates many enzymes such as adenylate cyclase, phosphodiesterase, phosphorylase kinase, myosin light chain kinase, phospholipase A_2, and cellular processes such as membrane phosphorylation, microtubule disassembly, neurotransmitter release, and perhaps postsynaptic and nuclear functions (55).

The multiplicity of actions of cAMP and calcium reveal that coordination among several molecular cascades culminating in physiological events may be performed with a limited number of messengers. Although it is difficult to imagine how this is effected, it is clear that specific binding proteins are involved. Why has cAMP rather than other types of nucleotides been used? Why has Ca^{2+} rather than other ions been selected for this messenger function? How have peculiar proteins with proper binding sites, such as protein kinases and calmodulin-like proteins, been shaped in the course of evolution? Were these cAMP or Ca^{2+} protein complexes originally devoted to simple actions and later used for coordination of multiple functions? All these important questions cannot yet be answered, but we can assume that the messenger molecules were essential to the building of integrated systems.

6 CONCLUSIONS

To explain the hierarchic organization of living matter and the regulatory mechanisms at each level in terms of gene nucleotide sequences, just as a linear program, does not seem reasonable without discovering new biological properties of deoxyribonucleic acids. Apparently DNAs are the molecular vectors of heredity, the units of which are the genes. Genes are usually defined by their phenotypes, but their chemical nature may be more complex than believed. Eukaryotic structural genes encoding for protein sequences are often built with coding regions (exons) separated by noncoding parts (introns) so that the individual phenotype (the protein) is determined by a plurality of dispersed genetic elements. For instance, the gene of proopiocortin (or corticotropin-β-lipotropin) is approximately 7.3 kilobase pairs (kbp) long and has three relatively small exons separated by two large introns (56). Exon 1 (108 bp) at the 5'-end is separated by intron A (4 kbp) from exon 2 (152 bp), itself separated by intron B (2.2 kbp) from exon 3 (838 bp) at the 3' -end. Ninety percent of the gene is noncoding, and the biological significance of the introns remains obscure. A "unit of heredity" could be built by noncontiguous parts of DNA, as an active domain of a protein can be built by several sequences separated on the polypeptide chain. The genetic properties of DNAs are not necessarily linear, and some may not be alphabetical.

If we assume that DNAs are the only hereditary vectors, we must clarify the role of so-called regulatory nucleotide sequences in order to imagine how molecular ontogenesis occurs. The first genes to be expressed could be "integrator" genes coding for molecules, such as morphogens or organogens, that control integrated biosynthetic programs. Mutations in these "integrator" genes could affect a whole program and lead, for example, to the leg of a basset or of a giraffe. Phylogenetic variations should cause irreversible deviations in regulation of programs that have already been integrated. What the features of these variations were and how they were recorded and directed remain essential and unsolved questions.

REFERENCES

1. S. Anderson, A. T. Bankier, B. G. Barrell, M. H. L. De Bruijn, A. R. Coulson, J. Drouin, I. C. Eperon, D. P. Nierlich, B. A. Roe, F. Sanger, P. H. Schreier, A. J. H. Smith, R. Staden, and I. G. Young, *Nature* **290**, 457–465 (1981).
2. B. Scharrer, An evolutionary interpretation of the phenomenon of neurosecretion, Forty-Seventh James Arthur Lecture on the Evolution of Human Brain, The American Museum of Natural History, New York, 1977.
3. C. J. P. Grimmelikhuijzen, K. Dierickx, and G. J. Boer, *Neuroscience* **7**, 3191–3199 (1982).
4. A. G. E. Pearse, *Proc. R. Soc. Lond. Ser. B* **210**, 61–62 (1980).
5. A. G. E. Pearse, The APUD Concept and its Verification by the use of Molecular Markers, in *The Evolution of Hormonal Systems*, Leopoldina-Symposium (in press) (1983).
6. C. J. P. Grimmelikhuijzen and H. C. Schaller, *Trends in Biochem. Sci.* **4**, 265–267 (1979).
7. J. M. Petras and C. R. Noback, Eds. *Ann. N.Y. Acad. Sci.* **167**, 1–513 (1969).
8. Lord Rothschild, *A Classification of Living Animals*, Longmans, London, 1965, pp. 1–134.
9. R. Acher, J. Chauvet, and M. T. Chauvet, Neurohypophysial Hormones and Neurophysins: Structures, Precursors and Evolution, in *Medicinal Chemistry Advances*, F. G. De Las Heras and S. Vega, Eds., Pergamon Press, Oxford, 1981, pp. 473–485.
10. G. J. Dockray and R. A. Gregory, *Proc. R. Soc. Lond. Ser. B* **210**, 151–164 (1980).
11. S. Nakanishi, A. Inoue, T. Kita, M. Nakamura, A. C. Y. Chang, S. N. Cohen, and S. Numa, *Nature* **278**, 423–427 (1979).
12. R. Håkanson, R. Ekman, F. Sundler, and R. Nilsson, *Nature* **283**, 789–792, 1980.

13. S. Benjannet, N. G. Seidah, R. Routhier, and M. Chretien, *Nature* **285**, 415–416 (1980).
14. R. E. Silman, D. Holland, T. Chard, P. J. Lowry, J. Hope, J. S. Robinson, and G. D. Thorburn, *Nature* **276**, 526–528 (1978).
15. V. Erspamer, *Trends in Neurosci.* **4**, 267–269 (1981).
16. A. S. Romer, *Vertebrate Paleontology*, University of Chicago Press, Chicago, 1966.
17. C. S. Nicoll, Physiological Actions of Prolactin, in *Handbook of Physiology*, Sec. 7, Vol. 4, Part 2, E. Knobil and W. H. Sawyer, Eds. American Physiology Society, Washington D.C., 1974, pp. 253–292.
18. M. J. Browstein, *Proc. R. Soc. Lond. Ser. B* **210**, 79–90 (1980).
19. M. S. Soloff, Oxytocin Receptors in the Mammary Gland and Uterus, in *Methods in Receptor Research*, Vol. 9, Part II, M. Blecher, Ed., Marcel Dekker, New York, 1976, pp. 511–531.
20. M. T. Chauvet, D. Hurpet, J. Chauvet, and R. Acher, *FEBS Lett.* **129**, 120–122 (1981).
21. D. W. Lincoln and M. B. Renfree, *Nature* **289**, 504–506 (1981).
22. E. Vizsolyi and A. M. Perks, *Nature* **223**, 1169–1171 (1969).
23. J. Maetz and B. Lahlou, Actions of Neurohypophysial Hormones in Fishes, in *Handbook of Physiology*, Sec. 7, Vol. 4, Part 2. E. Knobil and W. H. Sawyer, Eds. American Physiology Society, Washington D.C., 1974, pp. 521–544.
24. P. J. Bentley, Action of Neurohypophysial peptides in amphibias, reptiles and birds, in Handbook of Physiology, Sec. 7, Vol. 4, Part 2. E. Knobil and W. H. Sawyer, Eds. American Physiology Society, Washington D.C., 1974, pp. 545–563.
25. J. E. Jorpes and V. Mutt, *Handbook of Experimental Pharmacology* **34**, 1–179 (1973).
26. W. Mutt, *Clin. Endocrinol.* **5** Suppl., 175s–183s (1976).
27. J. F. Rehfeld, *Trends in Neurosci.* **3**, 65–67 (1980).
28. O. Valbuena, K. B. Marcu, M. Weigert, and R. P. Perry, *Nature* **276**, 780–784 (1978).
29. B. Blomberg and S. Tonegawa, *Proc. Natl. Acad. Sci. USA* **79**, 530–533 (1982).
30. S. H. Boyer, G. J. Dover, K. D. Smith, and A. Scott, in A. R. Liss, Ed., *Hemoglobins in Development and Differentiation*, New York, pp. 225–241 (1981).
31. J. Hughes, T. W. Smith, H. W. Kosterlitz, L. A. Fothergill, B. A. Morgan, and H. R. Morris, *Nature* **258**, 577–579 (1975).
32. M. Comb, P. H. Seeburg, J. Adelman, L. Eiden, and E. Herbert, *Nature* **295**, 663–666 (1982).
33. U. Gubler, P. H. Seeburg, B. J. Hoffman, L. P. Gage, and S. Udenfriend, *Nature* **295**, 206–208 (1982).
34. H. Kakidani, Y. Furutani, H. Takahashi, M. Noda, Y. Morimoto, T. Hirose, M. Asai, S. Inayama, S. Nakanishi, and S. Numa, *Nature* **298**, 245–249 (1982).
35. M. Noda, Y. Teranishi, H. Takahashi, M. Toyosato, M. Notake, S. Nakanishi, and S. Numa, *Nature* **297**, 431–434 (1982).
36. H. Takahashi, Y. Teranishi, S. Nakanishi, and S. Numa, *FEBS Lett.* **135**, 97–102 (1981).
37. S. Numa, 12th International Congress of Biochemistry (Perth, Western Australia) Abstracts, Plenary Session, PLE 002-1, p. 7.
38. B. Calabretta, D. L. Robberson, H. A. Barrera-Saldana, T. Lambrou, and G. F. Saunders, *Nature* **296**, 219–225 (1982).
39. R. Chisholm *TIBS*, **7** 161–162 (1982).
40. R. Acher, *Trends in Neurosci.* **4**, 226–230 (1981).
41. H. Sachs, P. Fawcett, Y. Takabatake, and R. Portanova, *Recent Prog. Horm. Res.* **25**, 447–492 (1969).
42. M. J. Brownstein, J. T. Russell, and H. Gainer, *Science* **207**, 373–378 (1980).
43. L. C. Giudice and I. M. Chaiken, *Proc. Natl. Acad. Sci. USA* **76**, 3800–3804 (1979).
44. C. Lin, P. Joseph-Bravo, T. Sherman, L. Chan, and J. F. McKelvy, *Biochem. Biophys. Res. Commun.* **89**, 943–950 (1979).
45. H. Schmale, B. Leipold, and D. Richter, *FEBS Lett.* **108**, 311–316 (1979).
46. H. Land, G. Schütz, H. Schmale, and D. Richter, *Nature* **295**, 299–303 (1982).

47. C. Remy, J. Girardie, and M. P. Dubois, *Gen. Comp. Endocrinol.* **37**, 93–100 (1979).
48. K. Tatemoto and V. Mutt, *Proc. Natl. Acad. Sci. USA* **78**, 6603–6607 (1981).
49. J. F. Habener, P. K. Lund, J. W. Jacobs, and P. C. Dee, Polyprotein Precursors of Regulatory Peptides, in *Peptides: Synthesis, Structure, Function*, D. H. Rich and E. Gross, Eds., Pierce Chemical Company, Rockford, 1981, pp. 457–469.
50. M. G. Rosenfeld, C. R. Lin, S. G. Amara, L. Stolarsky, B. A. Roos, E. S. Ong, and R. M. Evans, *Proc. Natl. Acad. Sci. USA* **79**, 1717–21 (1982).
51. R. Levi-Montalcini, *Harvey Lectures*, **60**, 217–259 (1966).
52. D. Gospodarowicz and J. S. Moran, *Ann. Rev. Biochem.* **45**, 531–558 (1976).
53. A. B. Roberts, M. A. Anzano, L. C. Lamb, J. M. Smith, and M. B. Sporn, *Proc. Natl. Acad. Sci. USA* **78**, 5339–5343 (1981).
54. P. Greengard, *Cyclic Nucleotides, Phosphorylated Proteins and Neuronal Function*, Raven, New York, 1978.
55. W. Y. Cheung, *Science* **207**, 19–27 (1980).
56. S. Numa, and S. Nakanishi, *Trends Neurosci.* **6**, 274–277 (1981).
57. M. T. Chauvet, D. Hurpet, J. Chauvet, and R. Acher *Proc. Natl. Acad. Sci. USA* **80**, (1983) in press.

6

Insect Neuropeptides

JAMES W. TRUMAN

Department of Zoology
University of Washington
Seattle, Washington

PAUL H. TAGHERT

Department of Biological Sciences
Stanford University
Stanford, California

1 INTRODUCTION

The roots of the study of insect neuropeptides extend back to the early part of this century, when Kopeć (1) published his classic work on the gypsy moth, *Lymantria dispar*. His experiments indicated that the brain of this insect liberated a blood-borne substance that was essential if metamorphosis was to occur. This was the first demonstration of the phenomenon that later became known as neurosecretion, a concept developed by the Scharrers from their pioneering work on the insect retrocerebral complex and the vertebrate hypothalamic–hypophyseal system (2). In recent years the work on insect neuropeptides has burgeoned. There have been a number of recent reviews (3–5) as well as a book (6) devoted to insect peptides, and the reader is referred to these for more detailed information. Because of space limitations this review is by necessity quite selective. We have chosen to focus on systems in which some information is available on the cellular origins of the peptides and on the regulation of their production or release.

2 ANATOMY OF PEPTIDERGIC SYSTEMS

The central nervous system (CNS) in insects observes the general metameric structure of the body. Each of the three body regions (cephalic, thoracic, and abdominal) contains a portion of the segmented CNS. The basic plan for the insect CNS includes the brain (supraesophageal ganglion), the subesophageal ganglion, and 3 thoracic and 11 abdominal ganglia, although fusion of ganglia to form compound structures is common in all insect orders. The insect CNS contains on the order of 10^5 neurons with the thoracic and abdominal ganglia typically having 500–3000 nerve cells each. The organization of individual ganglia is common to all arthropods: Neuronal somata are situated superficially in one to five cell layers and form a cortex that surrounds the neuropil and fiber tracts.

2.1 Distribution of Peptidergic Neurons

Historically, peptidergic neurons in insects have been studied within the possibly broader category of neurosecretory cells (NSC's). The most important tools used in these earlier studies were histochemical dyes (e.g., chrom alum-hemotoxylin and paraldehyde fuchsin) that selectively stained a subpopulation of CNS neurons. Where examined, such histochemically defined NSC's have almost always shown ultrastructural correlates of neurosecretion such as the abundant presence of dense-core vesicles. The term NSC does not discriminate between peptidergic and aminergic cells.

Rowell (7) reviewed the literature on neurosecretory staining in insects and compiled cell numbers for the purpose of comparison. The insect brain contains 2–5 clearly recognizable groups of NSC's. The most prominent and commonly studied are the median and lateral groups in the protocerebrum (Figure 1A). Cell numbers range 10–100 in the median groups and 2–80 in the lateral groups. The major neurohemal release site for these NSC's is a pituitary-like structure at the base of the brain known as the retrocerebral complex. Its two major components are the corpora cardiaca and corpora allata. Both receive axon terminals from brain and subesophageal ganglion NSC's, and both contain their own intrinsic secretory cells as well. The complex is the source of many hormones that are released into the circulation via a closely positioned aorta.

No more than 10–15% of the cells in the segmental ganglia appear to be neurosecretory (7). In individual ganglia, the cell bodies of these neurons are scattered in various locations (Figure 1B), but in successive ganglia of the chain, homologous NSC's are usually found in similar positions. Each ganglion has its own major neurohemal site, the perivisceral organ, which is the proximal (often swollen) region of the segmentally repeated transverse nerve (8). In addition to storing a large number of peptides, both the perivisceral organs and the retrocerebral complex contain significant amounts of octopamine (9). The neurons that send axons to each perivisceral organ range in number from 15 in some moths (10) to more than 140 in cockroaches (11). Besides their clear endocrine functions, the NSC's in the segmental ganglia subserve a variety of "secretomotor" functions including the innervation of viscera, epidermis, and cardiac musculature (12). In some insect orders, peripheral neurosecretory cells are located along nerves and make either endocrine (13) or secretomotor endings (12).

2.2 Peptidergic Pathways in the Insect CNS

The axonal and dendritic morphologies of some peptide-containing neurons have been described using intracellular dye-injection techniques (10, 14). These studies show common features in the morphologies of an array of known and presumed peptidergic neurons. In the segmental abdominal ganglion of the tobacco hornworm moth, *Manduca sexta*, 20 neurosecretory neurons have been individually identified on biochemical, ultrastructural, or histological grounds. These neurons make up a heterogeneous set of cells but they nevertheless show overlapping dendritic fields whose overall geometry is clearly distinct from other neuron types (15, 16). The fine neurite branches of these cells form a shell around the integrative regions of the neuropil. Most fine branching occurs in three dorsoventral planes: along the two lateral edges and at the midline in between the 2 hemineuropils (Figure 1C). Within these areas, processes of identified peptidergic neurons have been shown to sur-

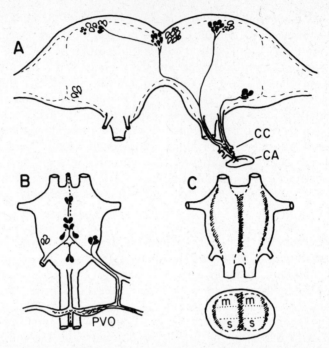

Figure 1. Organization of the main neurosecretory cell groups in the insect CNS. (A) Brain and retrocerebral complex of pupal *Manduca sexta*, showing locations of cell bodies and axon paths that project to the right corpora cardiaca–corpora allata complex (*CC, CA*). Filled cells project to the right complex, open cells to the left (axon paths and the left complex are not shown). (B) Abdominal ganglion of adult *Manduca* showing cells that project to the right perivisceral organ (*PVO*). Filled and open cells are as above, midline cells project to both right and left structures. (C) Dorsal (top) and cross-sectional view (bottom) of an abdominal ganglion showing the distribution of the majority of fine branching of peptidergic neurons (cross-hatched). Margins of the neuropil are shown by the dashed lines. The main projections of motor neurons (*m*) and sensory neurons (*s*) are in the horizontal plane. (A) is based on data from H. F. Nijhout (94).

round fiber tracts and individual axons (17). Processes that connect these three main areas travel superficially along dorsal and ventral surfaces. That such a neurosecretory neuropil may be a general feature of the insect CNS is suggested in the morphological studies of NSC's from other insects (14, 18, 19). Although this neurogeometry suggests specific types of central functions for neurosecretory cells (e.g. paracrine), no direct central effects due to *local* release by insect peptidergic neurons has yet been demonstrated.

3   CHEMISTRY AND PHYSIOLOGY OF INSECT PEPTIDES

A number of peptides having biological activity have been isolated from insect nervous tissue; many are summarized in an extensive table found in ref. 3. Table 1 lists peptides characterized after that review and up-

TABLE 1 Biologically Active Neuropeptides from Insects[a]

Peptide	Action	Molecular Weight (daltons)	Source	Reference
Proctolin	Visceral muscle excitation	648	CNS (*Periplaneta*)	20, 21
Adipokinetic hormone	Lipid mobilization	1,158	Corpora cardiaca (*Locusta*)	22
		≈1,000	Corpora cardiaca (*Schistocerca, Locusta*)	23
Prothoracicotropic hormone	Stimulates ecdysteroid secretion	4,400	Adult heads (*Bombyx*)	24, 25
		25,000	Larval heads (*Manduca*)	26
		18,000, 8,000	Pupal brains (*Manduca*)	27
Diuretic hormone	Stimulates water excretion	<2,000	Thoracic ganglia (*Rhodnius*)	28[b]
Eclosion hormone	Induces ecdysis behaviors	8,500	Brain, corpora cardiaca, ventral ganglia (*Manduca*)	29, 30
Bursicon	Tanning of cuticle	$20-60 \times 10^3$	Brain, ventral ganglia (*Calliphora, Periplaneta, Manduca*)	31, 32
Cardioactive peptides	Accelerates heart rate	1,800, 1,300	Corpora cardiaca (*Periplaneta*)	33
		1,000, 500	Ventral ganglia (*Manduca*)	34
Diapause hormones A and B	Induces egg diapause	(A) 3,300, (B) 2,000	Heads (*Bombyx*)	35
Hyperglycemic hormone	Increases levels of blood sugar	≈1,000	Corpora cardiaca (*Periplaneta*)	33, 36
		≈3,500	Corpora cardiaca (*Manduca*)	37, 38
Cytochromogenic factor	Cytochrome synthesis	1,000	Corpora cardiaca (*Blaberus*)	39, 95
Melanization hormone	Control larval pigmentation	6,400–8,000	Heads (*Bombyx*)	40
Pupariation factors	Puparium tanning	26,000[c]	Blood, CNS (*Sarcophaga*)	41
	Anterior retraction	90,000[c]		
	Puparium immobilization	$(10-30) \times 10^4$	Blood (*Sarcophaga*)	42

[a] See ref. 3 for earlier work.
[b] For various other insects see ref. 28.
[c] Subunit size.

169

dates information on various of the previously known insect peptides. The following account deals with peptides that have received considerable recent attention; they are discussed in the context of specific aspects of peptidergic regulation later in this review.

3.1 Proctolin

The pentapeptide proctolin is one of two insect peptides for which the amino acid sequence has been determined. Proctolin has actions on visceral, cardiac, and skeletal muscles (43) as well as on central neurons (44). It was first studied as one of a number of myotropic substances from the insect CNS that are capable of increasing the spontaneous activity of the cockroach hindgut. Proctolin action conforms to a number of criteria proposed for neurotransmitter function, and this led Brown (45) to propose that proctolin was an excitatory transmitter in the neural control of hindgut motility.

Brown and Starratt (20) outlined their methods for the purification of proctolin. Starting with 125,000 cockroaches they succeeded in isolating 180 μg of a peptide with the sequence Thr-Pro-Leu-Tyr-Arg (21). It was estimated that one cockroach contains about 12 ng of the peptide. More recently, Bishop et al. (46) developed a proctolin radioimmunoassay capable of detecting femtomole quantities of the peptide. They reported detectable levels in all ganglia of the cockroach CNS, the lowest levels being in the brain and the highest in the terminal abdominal ganglion. Total proctolin-like immunoreactivity in the CNS was estimated at 2 ng. Proctolin-like activity is found widely throughout the arthropods; it is reported in six orders of insects (43) as well as crustaceans (47, 48) and the horseshoe crab, *Limulus* (49).

3.2 Adipokinetic Hormone (AKH)

The second sequenced insect peptide is the adipokinetic hormone (AKH) of locusts. This peptide is produced in the locust corpora cardiaca in intrinsic NSC's that are separated off into a discrete "glandular lobe." The peptide is liberated during prolonged flight and stimulates lipid mobilization (50). Material from 3000 locusts was purified to yield a substance that was eventually identified as the blocked decapeptide PCA-Leu-Asn-Phe-The-Pro-Asn-Trp-Gly-Thr-NH$_2$ (22). The structure was subsequently confirmed by synthesis (51). This sequence proved to be very similar to that of the red pigment concentrating hormone isolated earlier from a crustacean: PCA-Leu-Asn-Phe-Ser-Pro-Gly-Trp-NH$_2$ (52). The corpora cardiaca of a locust contains 0.3–0.8 μg of adipokinetic hormone.

Recently, a second small peptide with lipid mobilizing action was isolated from locust corpora cardiaca (23). This peptide has not yet been sequenced but its amino acid composition suggests that its sequence is closer to the crustacean hormone than to the original adipokinetic hormone.

3.3 Prothoracicotropic Hormone (PTTH)

The prothoracicotropic hormone (PTTH), the object of Kopeć's early studies, is released from the brain-retrocerebral complex. It acts on the prothoracic glands, which in turn secrete the ecdysteroids that induce molting. Work on the nature of PTTH has progressed slowly, in large part because of rather cumbersome bioassays that were costly both in terms of time and amounts of hormone consumed. Studies on PTTH have been speeded by the recent development of *in vitro* bioassays that involve measuring by ecdysteroid RIA the amount of steroid secreted by cultured prothoracic glands in response to extracts that contain the PTTH (27).

As indicated in Table 1, considerable disagreement exists concerning the molecular weight of PTTH. Recent reports of hormone purified from adult heads of the commercial silk moth *Bombyx mori* estimate its molecular weight (MW) at 4400 daltons (25), whereas hormone extracted from heads of larval *Manduca sexta* showed a MW of about 25,000 as determined by SDS gel electrophoresis (26). Some resolution to these disparate results is seen in the report that two forms of PTTH have been extracted from pupae of *Manduca sexta* (27). The forms have MW of 18,000 and 8,000, respectively, and appear to be distinct peptides rather than one being a subunit or an aggregate of the other. Both forms act on the prothoracic glands to induce ecdysteroid secretion, but they show different kinetics of activation of the glands. Both are apparently released from the retrocerebral complex but at different times in the insect's life history (27).

The only known function of PTTH is to induce secretion of ecdysteroids from the prothoracic gland or homologous structures of larvae and pupae. Over the past 10 years it has become apparent that a second source of ecdysteroids is the ovaries of adult females (53). In mosquitoes (54) and in locusts (55) there is now good evidence that ecdysteroid secretion by the ovaries is regulated by a peptide hormone from the brain. The mosquito peptide has been partially purified and may turn out to be very similar to the larval PTTH (54).

3.4 Diuretic Hormone

Peptides which promote fluid excretion have been described in a number of insects (see ref. 28 for a review). The most extensive data have been collected for the blood sucking bug, *Rhodnius prolixus*. In this insect diuretic hormone is released from the mesothoracic ganglionic mass within 1 min after initiating blood feeding. It acts on the distal segment of the Malpighian tubules to stimulate the transport of fluids which give rise to the copius amounts of urine that the bug excretes after a blood meal. A simple *in vitro* assay utilizing isolated Malpighian tubules has made possible the measurement of hormone activity in blood, tissue extracts, and even single neurosecretory cells (56).

The *Rhodnius* hormone is rather unstable after it is extracted from tissue. Two forms have been isolated: one greater than 60,000 and the other less than 2000 in molecular weight (28). The large form can be converted to the small form during some of the purification steps (28). Also, only the small form is released from *Rhodnius* ganglia that are bathed in elevated K^+solutions to depolarize neurosecretory endings (57). Consequently, it appears as if the small form is the secreted form of the peptide and the large molecule is a precursor or an aggregate of the smaller.

3.5 Eclosion Hormone

In general, each molt that an insect undergoes is concluded by ecdyses —the shedding of the old cuticle. Studies of adult ecdysis in silkmoths first indicated that a neurosecretory hormone might be involved in this process (58). This hormone, the eclosion hormone, appears at the end of each molt to trigger ecdysis behaviors and to activate behavioral programs that are characteristic of the new stage that the animal attained (59). Besides behavioral actions the hormone also acts to increase the extensibility of the cuticle and to initiate the death of some muscles (59).

Enzyme sensitivity studies indicate that eclosion hormone is a peptide. The activity extracted from retrocerebral complexes of preadult *Manduca sexta* is acidic, with an isoelectric point (pI) of 4.8, and the apparent molecular weight is 8500 daltons (29). Eclosion hormone is found in various regions of the *Manduca* CNS including the brain-retrocerebral complex and the chain of segmental ganglia (30). The peptides produced in these two regions of the nervous system are extremely similar, if not identical (30). Circulating peptide is released from both areas but at different times in the insect's life history (59).

3.6 Bursicon

Ecdysis is usually followed by the expansion and hardening of parts of the new cuticle. Cottrell (60) and Fraenkel and Hsiao (61) first reported that a blood-borne factor induced tanning of the adult cuticle of newly emerged flies. The time of release of this neurohormone, which was later named bursicon, can occur before, during, or just after ecdysis depending on the insect considered. Bursicon has a range of activities in addition to cuticular tanning (see refs. 31, 62 for reviews). These include a transient plasticization of the cuticle prior to tanning, the stimulation of endocuticle deposition, epidermal cell death, and postecdysis diuresis.

The chemical properties of bursicon are consistent with its being a small protein: estimates of its molecular size range from 30,000 to 60,000 (31, 32). It is widely though unequally distributed in the CNS with higher amounts found in the abdominal ganglia and lower amounts in the brain. The sites of bursicon release are typically the segmental perivisceral organs. The hormone lacks specificity when tested between various orders. Since no systematic study of the relative potencies of bursicon from different insect orders has been made, possibly there are differences in the molecules isolated from the various orders.

3.7 Cardioactive Peptides

A number of putative cardioactive factors have been isolated from the insect CNS (33), but until recently their physiological roles have remained unclear. Two newly identified cardioactive peptides, with estimated molecular weights of 1000 and 500, respectively, have been isolated from the perivisceral organs of *Manduca sexta* (34; Tublitz, personal communication). Both peptides increase heart rate when tested on an *in vitro* pharate adult heart bioassay. *In vivo* cardiac recordings indicate a dramatic elevation in heart rate during adult eclosion and wing-spreading behaviors (63). At this time the neurohaemal storage sites show a marked depletion of both cardioactive peptides which is accompanied by their appearance in the blood (34; Tublitz, personal communication). Thus, the two peptides appear to function physiologically to regulate heart rate in this moth.

4 INSECT PEPTIDES THAT ARE IMMUNOLOGICALLY SIMILAR TO VERTEBRATE PEPTIDES

In the mid 1970s Tager et al. (37) reported the presence of glucagon-like and insulin-like immunoreactivity in extracts of the corpora cardiaca from *Manduca sexta*. This report was followed by a number of studies that to this time have shown that antibodies reared against at least nine different vertebrate peptides show cross-reactivity with insect material (Table 2). In a number of cases the immunoreactive material has been localized to specific neurons within the insect CNS.

Of course the demonstration of immunoreactive material does not prove the presence of the peptide against which the antibody was originally directed. In a few cases the immunoreactive substances have been partially characterized and their properties compared with that of the vertebrate peptide (37, 80). The most compelling evidence that insects

TABLE 2   Presence in Insects of Material that Cross-Reacts with Antisera Against Various Vertebrate Peptides

Peptide	Insect	References
Pancreatic polypeptide	*Calliphora, Bombyx* *Eristalis*	64–69
Gastrin/Cholecystokinin	*Calliphora, Manduca, Bombyx*	65, 67, 68
α-Endorphine	*Thaumetopoea, Bombyx, Calliphora*	69–71
Somatostatin	*Locusta*	72
Enkephalin	*Locusta*	73, 74
Vasopressin	*Acheta, Locusta, Clitumnus*	70, 75, 78
Glucagon	*Manduca, Apis*	37, 79
Insulin	*Manduca, Calliphora, Bombyx* *Apis*	37, 76, 77, 79

use peptides that are structurally similar to those of vertebrates comes from the work of Duve and Thorpe on the fly *Calliphora*. This fly has peptides that react with antisera against mammalian insulin and against pancreatic polypeptide (PP). The insulin-like material has been localized by immunocytochemistry to cells in the median neurosecretory cluster of the brain; these cells have axons that project to the corpora cardiaca (77). Lesions in this region of the brain render the flies hyperglycemic, but blood sugar levels in these insects can be reduced by injection of purified brain fractions that contain the immunoreactive material (76). The purified insect peptide also acts on rat epididymal fat cells to stimulate conversion of glucose to lipid, and it displaces labeled porcine insulin that is bound to liver plasma membrane (76). Besides this biological cross-reactivity with mammalian insulin, the insect peptide has a comparable molecular weight and many similarities with the vertebrate hormone in its amino acid composition (71).

The PP-like activity from *Calliphora* is also localized to specific neurons in the fly brain (64). Interestingly, cells reactive to antisera against PP have also been found in the gut of some insects (81). Although the function of the *Calliphora* PP-like peptide is not known, its amino acid composition is almost identical to that seen for the mammalian pancreatic polypeptides (82).

The above examples argue that the insect nervous system may contain peptides that are structurally very similar to those found in vertebrates. Moreover the recent report that high affinity binding sites for opioid peptides occur in the insect CNS (83) suggests that these peptides have biological roles in the insects. Except for the insulin-like material, the function of the immunoreactive peptides in insects is unknown. Presumably in the future the action of some of these peptides will become associated with some of the biological activities listed in Table 1.

The possibility that many of the neuropeptides have ancient associations with the CNS indicates that novel invertebrate peptides should also be examined for their possible presence in the vertebrate CNS. For example, a peptide from coelenterates that has the structure pGlu-Pro-Pro-Gly-Gly-Ser-Lys-Val-Ile-Leu-Phe (84) and that promotes "head regeneration" in *Hydra* has recently been isolated from bovine and human hypothalami as well as rat intestine.

5 IDENTIFICATION OF SPECIFIC PEPTIDERGIC NEURONS

The existence of very sensitive bioassays coupled with the relatively large size and stereotyped location of various neurosecretory cell somata has allowed for the association of particular peptides with specific identified cells. The feasibility of this approach was first demonstrated for the neurons that make diuretic hormone in *Rhodnius* (85). The contents of single cell bodies dissected from thoracic ganglia gave positive assay scores when tested on isolated Malpighian tubules *in vitro*. This technique was then used to follow the changes in the titer of diuretic hormone in the cell body during a complete secretory cycle (86). In *Rhodnius* the time from taking a blood meal by the larva to the subsequent ecdysis of the adult is 21 days. Diuretic hormone is released during the 4 h after the onset of feeding. Hormone activity extractable from perikarya began to decline within 1 h of feeding and continued to fall through the next 5 days. From day 10 through adult ecdysis, a gradual recharging of the cell body was then observed.

In *Manduca*, Agui et al. (87) localized the cells that store PTTH by assaying the contents of single cells on cultured prothoracic glands as described in Section 3.3. By this technique they traced the source of the brain PTTH to one cell located in each of the paired lateral neurosecretory cell groups. The hormone contained in the cell bodies of these paired neurons appears to account for most of the hormone that can be extracted from the whole brain (87).

A similar approach, single cell dissections coupled with bioassays, was used to find the cells that produce bursicon (10). Bursicon appears to be produced primarily by four pairs of cells that are found in each abdominal ganglion. Staining of the cells by intracellular injection of cobalt showed that each of the four cells has a unique dendritic morphology (Figure 2). Although they apparently release the same peptide under the same conditions, each cell nevertheless has its own characteristics that make it unique.

The most rigorous cell identification has been on the proctolin cells of cockroaches. Bioassayable proctolin activity was demonstrated in the contents of a single identifiable cell from a cockroach segmental ganglion. The contents of the cell body were then subjected to a variety

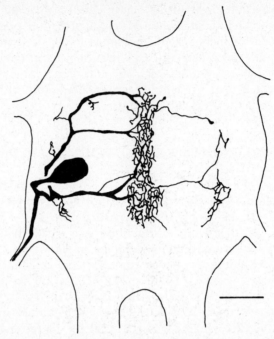

Figure 2. Dorsal view of a bursicon-containing neuron that was injected with cobalt. From the adult stage of *Manduca sexta*. Scale bar, 50µm. From Taghert and Trumen (10).

of HPLC and TLC systems, and biological activity was identical to that of synthetic proctolin (14). More recently, similar biochemical and bioassay data have also shown proctolin activity in an identifiable thoracic ganglion neuron. The cell body and processes of this neuron also specifically and consistently stain with an antibody reared against synthetic proctolin (46; O'Shea and Bishop, personal communication).

6 RELEASE OF MULTIPLE BIOLOGICALLY ACTIVE AGENTS

A number of insect peptides appear to exist in multiple forms. At least two forms have been reported for AKH, PTTH, diapause hormone, and the cardioactive peptides (Table 1). For none of these has it yet been shown that both forms coexist in the same cells. Evidence for co-release has been provided only for the cardioactive peptides; both forms simultaneously appear in the blood and both are released when the perivisceral organs are depolarized by exposure to high-K$^+$ saline (34; Tublitz, personal communication). By contrast, the large and small forms of PTTH are thought to be released independently of each other (27). If there is indeed only one pair of PTTH neurons, as is presently believed, then the cells must actively regulate the ratio of the products they secrete.

Besides the possibility of the existence and release of multiple forms of peptides from the same cell, peptides may also exist with other small molecules such as amines or acetylcholine. In insects there is preliminary evidence that at least one of the proctolin-containing neurons of cockroaches may also contain a biogenic amine (14).

7   REGULATION OF PEPTIDE SYNTHESIS AND RELEASE

At this time little is known about the regulation of neuropeptide synthesis in insects. The precursors for these peptides are as yet unstudied. In the case of the *Rhodnius* diuretic hormone, the secreted form is thought to arise from a 60K molecule (28) but the large form could be an aggregate of the secreted form rather than a true precursor.

Information on peptide synthesis has been largely inferred from accumulations of bioactive material. The studies on the diuretic hormone cells of *Rhodnius* (Section 5) indicate that after peptide release the cell bodies show a continuing reduction in hormone activity that is eventually followed by a recharging of the cell (86). But without a direct measurement of syntheses one cannot tell whether a cell body devoid of activity is synthetically inactive or is transporting hormone as rapidly as the hormone is being made. In the segmental ganglia of larval *Manduca* one sees a depletion of eclosion hormone just prior to ecdysis, followed by peptide accumulation during the intermolt period and then a plateau during the molt until just before the next ecdysis (88). Interestingly, at these same times the brain also accumulates hormone, even though the larval brain does not release the peptide. Thus, in these cells a cycle of synthesis may not be tied to prior release but may be controlled by factors extrinsic to the neurosecretory cell itself.

The regulation of the activity of peptidergic cells has received considerable attention. In many cases the proximate stimulus for peptide secretion is known (e.g., abdomen distension caused by the blood meal in *Rhodnius* is the cause of the release of diuretic hormone). Yet, the circuitry between the receptors and the peptidergic cell is largely unknown. Aminergic pathways have been implicated in the release of some insect peptides (89). The best case has been established for the control of AKH secretion in the locust. The neurons that release this peptide are intrinsic cells in the glandular lobe of the corpora cardiaca. These cells appear to be controlled through axons that enter the corpora cardiaca through the nervus corpus cardiacum II (NCC II), since stimulation of this nerve results in release of AKH.

Orchard and Loughton (90) exploited the above preparation in examining the role of aminergic pathways in peptide secretion. Pretreatment of preparations with reserpine to deplete endogenous amines rendered the stimulation paradigm ineffective. The AKH cells themselves were unaffected by the treatment because direct depolarization of the intrinsic cells with high K$^+$ saline resulted in peptide release. Also α-adrenergic but not β-adrenergic antagonists blocked only neurally stimulated release of AKH; neither prevented high K$^+$ induced release. Previous studies using Falch-Hillarp fluorescence, ultrastructure, and radioenzymatic assays indicated the presence of octopamine containing terminals in the glandular region of the corpora cardiaca. Incubation of locust corpora cardiaca in 10^{-7} M octopamine induced release of AKH and this release was inhibited by the same drugs that blocked release due to nerve stimulation. Thus, it appears likely that AKH secretion is regulated by octopaminergic fibers from the brain.

Circulating hormones comprise another set of chemicals that may regulate the activity of peptidergic neurons. For example, the two centers that release eclosion hormone in *Manduca* are sensitive to circulating levels of ecdysteroids and will not release the peptide until the steroid titer has dropped below a critical level (91). Also, the subsequently released eclosion hormone appears to act back on the release system to shut off further secretion (92).

8   ACTIONS OF PEPTIDES ON THE CNS

In vertebrates, peptides have very marked effects on CNS activity. In the case of the insects, one peptide, the eclosion hormone, is known to have dramatic effects on the CNS. Exposure of the isolated abdominal CNS from the moth *Hyalophora cecropia* to the peptide releases a long stereotyped program of spontaneous motor activity. The pattern of motor activity faithfully mimics that seen from *in situ* recordings during normal ecdysis behavior. Besides these transient actions, the peptide permanently activates a number of behavioral pathways. In one simple reflex circuit that has been analysed in detail, the action of the peptide appears to result in the turning-on of a previously nonfunctional synapse in the pathway (see 93 for a review).

Other peptides also appear to have actions on the insect CNS. One of the most intriguing is a recent report that an identified set of octopaminergic neurons in the ventral ganglia is sensitive to proctolin (44).

9   FUTURE DIRECTIONS

Insects provide convenient material for the study of peptidergic neurons. In a number of instances it has been possible to associate a given peptide with a specific identified cell. Thus, one has the prospect of studying various aspects of the regulation of peptide synthesis, production of multiple forms, co-release, and so on in the context of identified cells.

One hinderance to this goal is the limited knowledge that is currently available on the structure of bioactive peptides in insects. Increased knowledge of the amino acid sequences of these molecules will provide answers as to possible homologies between various invertebrate peptides as well as between those of insects and vertebrates. Antibodies against specific insect peptides are badly needed. Not only will these provide for new immunohistochemical and RIA techniques but also they can be used as probes to detect biologically inactive precursor peptides and thus open up the area of processing of insect peptides.

The availability of these tools in the coming years coupled with a continued emphasis on study of identified neurons should greatly expand our understanding of the regulation of peptidergic systems.

ACKNOWLEDGMENTS

We thank Dr. Lynn M. Riddiford and Mr. Nathan J. Tublitz for a critical reading of the manuscript. We are grateful to Mick O'Shea, Cindy Bishop, and Nathan Tublitz for allowing us to cite their unpublished results.

REFERENCES

1. S. Kopeć, *Biol. Bull.* (*Woods Hole*) **42**, 323 (1922).
2. E. Scharrer and B. Scharrer, *Neuroendocrinology*, Columbia University Press, New York, 1963, p. 289.
3. N. Frontali and H. Gainer, in H. Gainer, Ed., *Peptides in Neurobiology*, Plenum Press, New York, 1977, p. 259.
4. L. W. Haynes, *Progr. Neurobiol.* **15**, 205 (1980).
5. J. V. Stone and W. Mordue, *Insect Biochem.* **10**, 229 (1980).
6. T. A. Miller, Ed., *Neurohormonal Techniques in Insects*, Springer-Verlag, New York, 1980, p. 282.
7. C. H. F. Rowell, *Adv. Insect Physiol.* **12**, 63 (1976).
8. M. Raabe, N. Baudry, J. P. Grillot, and A. Provansal, in F. Knowles and L. Vollrath, Eds., *Neurosecretion: The Final Common Pathway*, Springer-Verlag, Berlin, 1974, p. 60.
9. P. D. Evans, *J. Neurochem.* **30**, 1009 (1978).
10. P. H. Taghert and J. W. Truman, *J. Exp. Biol.*, **98**, 385 (1982).
11. Z. I. Ali and R. Pipa, *Gen. Comp. Endocrinol.* **396** (1978).
12. T. A. Miller, in P. N. R. Usherwood, Ed., *Insect Muscle*, Academic Press, New York, 1975, p. 545.
13. L. H. Finlayson and M. P. Osborne, *J. Insect. Physiol.* **14**, 1793 (1968).
14. M. O'Shea and M. Adams, *Science* **213**, 567 (1981).
15. P. H. Taghert and J. W. Truman, *Soc. Neurosci. Abstr.* **6**, 373 (1980).
16. P. H. Taghert, in D. Farner and K. Lederis, Eds., *Neurosecretion: Molecules, Cells, and Systems*, Plenum Press, New York, 1981, p. 456.
17. C. Remy and J. Girardie, *Gen. Comp. Endocrinol.* **40**, 27 (1980).
18. C. M. Buys and D. Gibbs, *Cell Tissue Res.* **215**, 505 (1981).
19. M. Eckert, H. Agricola, and H. Penzer, *Cell Tissue Res.* **217**, 633 (1981).
20. B. E. Brown and A. N. Starratt, *J. Insect Physiol.* **21**, 1879 (1975).

21. A. N. Starratt and B. E. Brown, *Life Sci.* **17**, 1253 (1975).
22. J. V. Stone, W. Mordue, K. E. Batley, and H. R. Morris, *Nature* (*London*) **263**, 207 (1976).
23. J. Carlsen, W. S. Herman, M. Christensen, and L. Josefsson, *Insect Biochem.* **9**, 497 (1979).
24. H. Nagasawa, A. Isogai, A. Suzuki, S. Tamura, and H. Ishizaki, *Dev. Growth Differ.* **21**, 29 (1979).
25. H. Ishizaki and A. Suzuki, in T. A. Miller, Ed., *Neurohormonal Techniques in Insects,* Springer-Verlag, New York, 1980, p. 244.
26. T. G. Kingan, *Life Sci.* **28**, 2585 (1981).
27. W. E. Bollenbacher and L. I. Gilbert, in D. S. Farner and K. Lederis, Eds., *Neurosecretion: Molecules, Cells, and Systems,* Plenum Press, New York, 1981, p. 361.
28. R. J. Aston and L. Hughes, in T. A. Miller, Ed., *Neurohormonal Techniques in Insects,* Springer-Verlag, New York, 1980, p. 91.
29. S. E. Reynolds and J. W. Truman, in T. A. Miller, Ed., *Neurohormonal Techniques in Insects,* Springer-Verlag, New York, 1980, p. 196.
30. P. H. Taghert, J. W. Truman, and S. E. Reynolds, *J. Exp. Biol.* **88**, 339 (1980).
31. I. M. Seligman, in T. A. Miller, Ed., *Neurohormonal Techniques in Insects,* Springer-Verlag, New York, 1980, p. 137.
32. P. H. Taghert and J. W. Truman, *J. Exp. Biol.,* **98**, 373 (1982).
33. M. E. Traina, M. Bellino, L. Serpietri, A. Massa, and N. Frontali, *J. Insect Physiol.* **22**, 323 (1976).
34. N. J. Tublitz and J. W. Truman, *Soc. Neurosci. Abstr.* **7**, 256 (1981).
35. I. Kubota, M. Isobe, T. Goto, and K. Hasegawa, *Z. Naturforsch.* **31**, 132 (1976).
36. J. Jones, *Physiologically Active Factors in the Corpora Cardiaca of Insects.* Ph.D. Theses, University of London, 1978 (as cited in ref. 5).
37. H. S. Tager, J. Markese, K. J. Kramer, R. D. Speirs, and C. N. Childs, *Biochem. J.* **156**, 515 (1976).
38. R. Ziegler, in F. Sehnal, A. Zabza, J. J. Menn, B. Cymborowski, Eds., *Regulation of Insect Development and Behavior,* Wroclaw Technical University Press, Wroclaw, Poland, 1981, p. 17.
39. T. K. Hayes and L. L. Keeley, *Gen. Comp. Endocrinol.* **45**, 115 (1981).
40. S. Matsumoto, A. Isogai, A. Suzuki, N. Ogura, and H. Sonobe, *Insect Biochem.* **11**, 725 (1981).
41. P. Sivasubramanian, S. Friedman, and G. Fraenkel, *Biol. Bull., Marine Biol. Lab., Woods Hole* **147**, 163 (1974).
42. J. Zdarek, R. Rohlf, J. Blechl, and G. Fraenkel, *J. Exp. Biol.* **93**, 51 (1981).
43. A. N. Starratt and R. W. Steele, in T. A. Miller, Ed., *Neurohormonal Techniques in Insects,* Springer-Verlag, New York, 1980, p. 1.
44. R. J. Walker, V. A. James, C. J. Roberts, and G. A. Kerkut, in D. B. Satelle, L. M. Hall, and J. G. Hildebrand, Eds., *Receptors for Neurotransmitters Hormones and Pheromones in Insects,* Elsevier/North Holland, Amsterdam, 1980, p. 41.
45. B. E. Brown, *Life Sci.* **17**, 1241 (1975).
46. C. A. Bishop, M. O'Shea, and R. J. Miller, *Proc. Nat. Acad. Sci. USA* **78**, 5899 (1981).
47. R. E. Sullivan, *J. Exp. Zool.* **210**, 543 (1979).
48. T. L. Schwartz, G. Lee, and E. A. Kravitz, *Soc. Neurosci. Abstr.* **7**, 253 (1981).
49. W. Watson, K. Neill, and E. Tillinghast, *Soc. Neurosci. Abstr.* **7**, 254, (1981).
50. J. V. Stone and W. Mordue, in T. A. Miller, Ed., *Neurohormonal Techniques In Insects,* Springer-Verlag, New York, 1980, p. 31.
51. C. E. Broomfield and P. M. Hardy, *Tetrahedron Lett.* **25**, 2201 (1977).
52. P. Fernlund, *Biochem. Biophys. Acta* **371**, 304 (1974).
53. H. H. Hagedorn, J. D. O'Connor, M. S. Fuchs, B. Sage, D. A. Schlaeger, and M. K. Bohm, *Proc. Natl. Acad. Sci. USA* **72**, 3255 (1975).
54. H. H. Hagedorn, J. P. Shapiro, and K. Hanaoka, *Nature (London)* **282**, 92 (1979).
55. J. A. Hoffman, M. Lagueux, C. Hetro, M. Charlet, and F. Gottzene, in J. A. Hoffmann,

Ed., *Progress in Ecdysone Research*, Elsevier/North Holland, Amsterdam, 1980, p. 431.

56. S. H. P. Maddrell, in T. A. Miller, Ed., *Neurohormonal Techniques in Insects*, Springer-Verlag, New York, 1980, p. 81.
57. R. J. Aston, *Insect Biochem.* **9**, 163, (1979).
58. J. W. Truman and L. M. Riddiford, *Science* **167**, 1624 (1970).
59. J. W. Truman, in M. Locke and D. S. Smith, Eds., *Insect Biology in the Future*, Academic Press, New York, 1980, p. 385.
60. C. B. Cottrell, *J. Exp. Biol.* **39**, 418 (1962).
61. G. Fraenkel and C. Hsiao, *Science* **138**, 27 (1962).
62. S. E. Reynolds, in H. Laufer and R. G. H. Downer, Eds., *Insect Endocrinology*, Liss, New York, in press.
63. L. T. Wasserthal, *Experientia* **32**, 577 (1976).
64. H. Duve and A. Thorpe, *Cell Tissue Res.* **210**, 101 (1980).
65. R. Yui, T. Fujita, and S. Ito, *Biomed. Res.* **1**, 42 (1980).
66. M. El-Salhy, R. Abou-El-Ela, S. Falkner, L. Grimelius, and E. Wilander, *Reg. Peptides* **1**, 187 (1980).
67. H. Duve and A. Thorpe, *Gen. Comp. Endocrinol.* **43**, 381 (1981).
68. K. J. Kramer, R. D. Spiers, and C. N. Childs, *Gen. Comp. Endocrinol.* **32**, 423 (1977).
69. C. Remy, J. Girardie, and M. P. Dubois, *C. R. Acad. Sci., (Paris), Ser. D* **286**, 651 (1978).
70. C. Remy, J. Girardie, and M. P. Dubois, *Gen. Comp. Endocrinol.* **37**, 93 (1979).
71. H. Duve and A. Thorpe, in *Proceedings of the 9th International Symposium on Comparative Endocrinology*, Hong Kong University Press, Hong Kong, in press.
72. J. Doerr-Schott, L. Joly, and M. P. Dubois, *C. R. Acad. Sci., (Paris), Ser. D* **286**, 93 (1978).
73. C. Gros, M. Lafon-Cazal, and F. Dray, *C. R. Acad. Sci. (Paris), Ser. D* **287**, 647 (1978).
74. C. Remy and M. P. Dubois, *Cell Tissue Res.* **218**, 271 (1981).
75. C. Strambi, G. Roygan-Rapuzzi, A. Cupo, N. Martin, and A. Strambi, *C. R. Acad. Sci. (Paris), Ser. D* **288**, 131 (1979).
76. H. Duve, A. Thorpe, and N. R. Lazarus, *Biochem. J.* **184**, 221 (1979).
77. H. Duve and A. Thorpe, *Cell Tissue Res.* **200**, 187 (1979).
78. C. Remy, J. Girardie, and M. P. Dubois, *C. R. Acad. Sci. (Paris), Ser. D* **285**, 1495 (1977).
79. V. Maier, G. Witznick, R. Keller, and E. F. Pfeiffer, *Acta Endocrinol.* **87**, 69 (1978).
80. J. Proux and G. Rougan-Rapuzzi, *Gen. Comp. Endocrinol.* **42**, 378 (1980).
81. T. Iwanaga, T. Fujita, J. Nishiitsutsuji-Uwo, and Y. Endo, *Biomed. Res.* **2**, 202 (1981).
82. H. Duve, A. Thorpe, N. R. Lazarus, and P. J. Lowry, *Biochem. J.* **201**, 429 (1982).
83. G. B. Stefano and B. Scharrer, *Brain Res.* **225**, 107 (1981).
84. H. Bodenmuller and H. C. Schaller, *Nature (London)* **293**, 579 (1981).
85. S. H. P. Maddrell, *Amer. Zool.* **16**, (1976).
86. A. Berlind and S. H. P. Maddrell, *Brain Res.* **166**, 459 (1979).
87. N. Agui, N. A. Granger, L. I. Gilbert, and W. E. Bollenbacher, *Proc. Nat. Acad. Sci. USA* **76**, 5694 (1979).
88. J. W. Truman, P. H. Taghert, P. F. Copenhaver, N. J. Tublitz, and L. M. Schwartz, *Nature (London)* **291**, 70 (1981).
89. M. Gersch, *J. Insect Physiol.* **18**, 2425 (1972).
90. I. Orchard and B. G. Loughton, *J. Neurobiol.* **12**, 143 (1981).
91. J. W. Truman, *Am. Zool.* **21**, 665 (1981).
92. J. W. Truman, in P. J. Gaillard and H. H. Baer, Eds., *Comparative Endocrinology*, Elsevier/North Holland, Amsterdam, 1978, p. 123.
93. J. W. Truman and R. B. Levine, in J. Barker and J. McKelvy, Eds., *Current Methods in Cellular Neurobiology*, Wiley, New York, in press.
94. H. F. Nijhout, *Int. J. Insect Morphol. Embryol.* **4**, 529 (1975).
95. L. L. Keeley, personal communication.

7

Peptidergic Neurons and Neuroactive Peptides in Molluscs: From Behavior to Genes

FELIX STRUMWASSER

Division of Biology
California Institute of Technology
Pasadena, California

Original research has been supported by grants from the NIH (NS 07071, NS 13896, NS 15183).

1 INTRODUCTION

1.1 Why Study Molluscs?

The reader of this chapter might wonder why someone might want to study peptidergic systems in molluscs. Will the studies of molluscan systems offer insights into vertebrate peptidergic systems? Part of the answer is that certain molluscs provide major advantages for understanding the physiology and biochemistry of peptidergic systems. They have a relatively simple system in that the number of interacting subsystems appears to be fewer compared with the higher vertebrates. Certain molluscan systems are more readily accessible for physiology and biochemistry because of the ganglionic organization of the nervous system, with each ganglion more or less specialized for a major function such as visceral regulation vs. control of locomotion. Often (but not always) the peptidergic systems include a homogeneous "large" population of neurons or single large identifiable neurons, which simplifies biochemical interpretation. The *in vitro* maintenance of molluscan ganglia for periods of a day or more does not usually require special conditions such as nutrient media or oxygenation, and often one can reversibly cool the preparation to slow the process of interest without cellular damage.

As to the relevance for mammalian systems of what we learn from molluscan peptidergic systems, the most powerful argument is to examine what we presently know about the evolution of peptidergic systems, in particular with respect to the control of reproduction.

1.2 Conservation of Peptidergic Neurons and Their Principles of Operation in Evolution of the Nervous System

1.2.1 Phylogenetic Spectrum of Peptides

The synthesis, storage, and release of peptides by specialized neurons with wide-ranging target effects is a principle that is probably conserved from the earliest nervous systems. In addition, the mediation by cyclic nucleotides of many peptide actions on target cells also appears to date to have no phylogenetic distinctions. In echinoderms, the factor extracted from the radial nerves that causes egg-shedding is a peptide [1]. In opisthobranch [2–4] and pulmonate gastropod molluscs [5], the egg-shedding factor is generated in the central nervous system (CNS). Egg-laying hormone (ELH), a peptide of known structure [6], is synthesized in $\sim$800 bag cell neurons of the abdominal ganglion of the opisthobranch mollusc *Aplysia*, a marine gastropod. In mammals, ovulation is mediated by a hypothalamic neuropeptide, luteinizing hormone releasing hormone (LHRH), and an endocrine polypeptide, luteinizing hormone (LH), synthesized in the anterior pituitary gland. In *Aplysia*, two peptides purified from the atrial gland of the reproductive tract are potent activators of bag cell discharge (7). The fact that reproductive control is mediated by peptides in such diverse phyla suggests evolutionary conservation.

The presence of enkephalin-immunoreactive substances in leech neurons (8) and lobster photoreceptors (9), β-endorphin-like neurons in earthworms (10), substance P-immunoreactive axons in the optic neuropiles of the lobster eyestalk (9), and the presence of other vertebrate peptides in a gastropod mollusc, the fresh-water snail *Lymnaea* (11), suggest interesting relationships between certain vertebrate and invertebrate neuropeptides that will be more fully understood in the future. It will certainly be essential to chemically isolate the immunoreactive substances in these cases to establish their identities. In one case so far, somatostatin-like material in the CNS, gut, and hemolymph of a pond snail appears to have multiple forms, most of which are not chemically identical to mammalian somatostatin (12). However, in the coelenterate *Hydra*, the morphogenetic head activator is an undecapeptide with a primary structure that is similar to a new peptide enriched in the hypothalamus of mammals including humans (13). Recently, a molluscan cardioactive neuropeptide, FMRF (Phe-Met-Arg-Phe-NH$_2$) has been localized, by RIA and immunocytochemistry, in the brain of several vertebrate species (14).

Thus, well-known vertebrate peptides are now being found in invertebrate systems and vice versa. While chemical identities remain to be established in most of these cases, one can no longer maintain that there is little or no relationship between vertebrate and invertebrate peptidergic systems. It is more likely than ever that what we find out about invertebrate peptidergic systems will shed light on vertebrate systems, and of course physiological and biochemical knowledge will flow in both directions. For a recent phylogenetic review of peptidergic systems the interested reader can consult Haynes (15).

1.2.2   Cyclic Nucleotide-Mediated Peptide Actions

A similar view that evolution was conservative with regard to the mechanisms of peptide action on cells emerges from the following examples. It is widely thought that peptide actions are mediated by cyclic nucleotides acting as intracellular messengers, and this concept appears to operate across diverse phyla. The cyclic nucleotides, in particular 3', 5'-cyclic adenosine monophosphate (cyclic AMP or cAMP), are in turn thought to regulate protein phosphorylation by activating cyclic nucleotide-dependent substrate-specific protein kinases (16, 17). In insects, growth of the larva and eventual metamorphosis is associated with periodic shedding (ecdysis) of the old cuticle at molting. Eclosion hormone

(EH), a neuropeptide produced in the brain and ventral nerve cord, is secreted near the end of each molt (larval or adult) and is responsible for the behaviors associated with ecdysis. Truman and Levine (18) review the evidence that cyclic GMP mediates the response of target neurons located in the ventral nerve cord of the moth *Hyalophora cecropia*. They also describe their studies of a three-neuron pathway that operates the abdominal-segment gin traps, which can crush potential intruders. The gin-trap reflex is "turned on" by EH at pupal ecdysis in the moth *Manduca sexta*, and cyclic 3′, 5′-guanosine monophosphate (cyclic GMP or cGMP) by itself can mimic this response.

The peptidergic bag cell neurons of *Aplysia* release the peptide ELH during a long-lasting (30 min) electrical discharge initiated by stimulation of an afferent pathway for a few seconds (19). This long-lasting electrical discharge, termed afterdischarge, is correlated with a rise of cAMP and can be initiated by the application of appropriate cAMP analogs without any electrical stimulation (20). We have shown that during afterdischarge two proteins termed BC-1 and BC-2 (BC is for bag cell) increase their state of phosphorylation at different times (21). Thus in arthropods and molluscs, cyclic nucleotides play an important role in mediating the targets of peptide actions as well as modulating membrane ion channels, as is thought to be the case for vertebrates.

2   A MODEL MOLLUSCAN PEPTIDERGIC SYSTEM REGULATING REPRODUCTION

2.1   The Bag Cells of *Aplysia*: Overview of the System

The bag cell neurons of the opisthobranch mollusc *Aplysia* are a remarkable and model neuroendocrine system. The properties of this system are summarized in Table 1. These neurons synthesize, and release on stimulation, several peptides, one of which, ELH, is directly involved in the reproductive process of egg-laying. Egg-laying in *Aplysia* normally results after mating although isolated animals can also spontaneously lay eggs. The main function of the bag cell neurons, part of the abdominal ganglion, is no less than to propagate the species—an important function entrusted to this population of some 800 peptidergic neurons. Some of the advantages in studying this neuroendocrine system are evident from the following features. These 800 neurons are distributed symmetrically in two identifiable clusters at the base of the pleurovisceral connectives which link the abdominal ganglion and pleural ganglia in the head region. The peptide that induces egg-laying, ELH, has been purified and sequenced so that the primary structure of this neuropeptide, molecular weight (MW) 4400, is now known. ELH has profound behavioral effects and there is direct evidence for actions on the central nervous system as well as on the ovotestis.

TABLE 1   Properties of the Bag Cell Neuroendocrine System

$\sim$800 "Homogeneous" neurons with neurohaemal specialization synthesize and release peptides.

Extensive electrical coupling allows synchronization.

Brief synaptic input causes $\sim$30′ afterdischarge.

Prolonged refractoriness (hours) follows afterdischarge.

Afterdischarge can be initiated by atrial gland peptides or cyclic AMP analogs.

Afterdischarge can be suppressed by serotonin and enhanced by dopamine.

During afterdischarge four peptides are released.

One of these peptides, ELH, causes egg-laying.

ELH releases eggs from ovotestis.

ELH inhibits feeding in hungry *Aplysia*.

ELH inhibits locomotion.

ELH activates buccal, pedal, and abdominal ganglia neurons.

Studied *in vitro* in the intact abdominal ganglion, the bag cell neurons are normally electrically silent cells—they show no spontaneous activity. During and after a brief synaptic stimulation, lasting a few seconds, these cells generate action potentials in synchrony and continue to do so for about 30 min. Afterdischarge is the normal mode by which ELH is released into the circulation. Presumably, mating triggers afterdischarge in the bag cells of an intact hermaphroditic *Aplysia* performing as a female. There is evidence that the atrial gland, a part of the reproductive tract, contains peptides, two of which have been purified, that initiate afterdischarge of bag cells. After a single afterdischarge the bag cells become refractory in that another lengthy afterdischarge is not normally possible until several hours have elapsed. The long nature of the afterdischarge and recovery processes may in themselves be useful models for long-lasting processes in the nervous system and may even have significance for "abnormal" neuronal discharges, such as epilepsy. We show in this chapter that cyclic AMP and cyclic AMP-dependent protein phosphorylation are intimately involved in the afterdischarge mechanism. Interestingly, afterdischarge can also be modulated. We see later in this chapter that serotonin, an indoleamine, is a powerful inhibitor of afterdischarge.

The bag cell neurons can be maintained *in vitro*, as a primary culture of disconnected cells, and this provides a distinct advantage for electrophysiological studies. Such neurons maintain electrical excitability, regenerate their neurites, and produce functional synaptic connections with one another. Antibodies have been raised to ELH and by indirect immunofluorescence the bag cells, in primary culture, have been shown to stain for ELH.

This section deals in part with the current status of this model neuroendocrine system, some questions that have been answered, and questions that remain to be answered. Within this single molluscan system, we are beginning to unravel the physiological inputs, the long-term cellular response to these inputs, and the resultant hormonal effects on both neuronal and non-neuronal targets.

2.2   Morphology of Bag Cells and Neurohemal Specialization

The morphology of the bag cell neurons was first described by Coggeshall (22) and Frazier et al. (23), based on light and electron microscopic studies. It was concluded that they were neurosecretory cells because of the presence of numerous, $\sim$200 nanometer (nm) granules, each with a 100 nm electron-dense core, in the cytoplasm and somewhat modified, crenulated, less osmophilic granules in the axoplasm. In addition, it was found that the processes ended in the vascularized connective tissue sheath without apparent functional contact with other axons or cells in the sheath. These authors concluded, correctly, that such bag cell processes constituted part of a neurohemal organ (see below). Coggeshall (22) also reported, in a survey of five abdominal ganglia, that the numbers of bag cells (and other abdominal ganglion neurons) increased by about 40% between 5 g and 200–375 g animals. The latter two animals were reported to contain 961 and 787 bag cells, respectively.

Present evidence suggests that the bag cells are a homogeneous population with respect to hormone production. Antibodies raised against ELH coupled to thyroglobulin have been prepared in rabbits. After removing antibodies directed against thyroglobulin, through affinity chromatography, the antibodies to ELH bind all bag cell neurons in the cluster as judged by the peroxidase-antiperoxidase (PAP) immunohistochemical method (Figure 1; 24). These results are consistent with earlier studies suggesting that all bag cells in a cluster share common electrophysiological and morphological properties (25, 23).

The earliest drawings of bag cells in the literature depicted these neurons as monopolar (e.g., Figure 3A in ref. 23), but with the passage of time more processes appeared in the literature. The processes of bag cells have been traced, in the pleurovisceral connectives by electron microscopy, no further than the midpoint of the connectives, between the abdominal and pleural ganglia in *Aplysia californica* (23). Recently, lucifer yellow fills of individual bag cells in the intact cluster have indicated that these cells range from monopolar to heteropolar with typically three or four processes emanating from each soma (26). These processes extend into the connective tissue sheath over both the abdominal ganglion proper and the pleurovisceral connectives. Thus it is likely that the extent of the neurohemal organ of the bag cells is distributed more widely than was first thought (23). The finding that extracts of the abdominal ganglion (without bag cell clusters) induce egg-laying is consistent with this view (3).

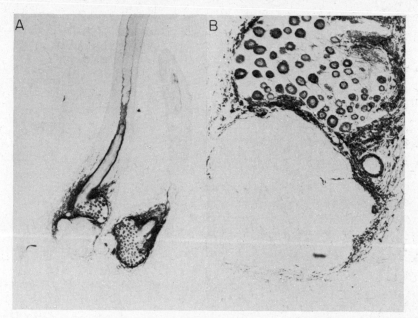

Figure 1. Cryostat sections of the abdominal ganglion of *A. californica* immunostained with ELH antiserum by the peroxidase-antiperoxidase method. (A) Transverse section shows symmetrical bag cell clusters; immunoreactive processes ramify into the connective tissue sheath of the ganglion and the pleurovisceral connective (PVC). A dense cuff of processes lines the PVC nerve, extending anteriorly for up to 2 cm. Scale bar, 500 μm in both frames. (B) At higher magnification, it can be seen that all somata within the bag cell cluster show perikaryal immunoreactivity; nuclei remain unstained. Note lack of staining between bag cell somata, a zone occupied by glial cells. Other neurons of the abdominal ganglion are not immunoreactive. From Strumwasser et al. (56).

The bag cells in primary culture are also generally heteropolar, with as many as six individual neurites emanating from the soma (16, 26). Figure 2 illustrates the heteropolar nature of three apparently connected bag cells in primary culture. In the complexity of their processes, these cells are indistinguishable from cultures of mammalian neurons reported in the literature (28) and are unusual among invertebrate neurons, which are conventionally considered mono- or bipolar neurons.

The availability of an antibody to ELH has helped to clarify the exact distribution of the neurohemal organ by immunohistochemistry, as is evident in Figure 1 (24). Immunohistochemical studies using the PAP technique show a dense cuff of ELH-containing processes wrapped around the posterior 2 cm of the nerve trunk within the pleurovisceral connective (PVC) nerves (Figure 1; 24). Earlier studies by Coggeshall (22) had suggested that this cuff of processes was from the bag cells based on the $\sim$200 nm dense core granules contained within them.

It is generally accepted that the bag cell processes in the connective tissue are part of the neurohemal areas, for there are sinus spaces in the connective tissue. But the functional significance of the dense cuff

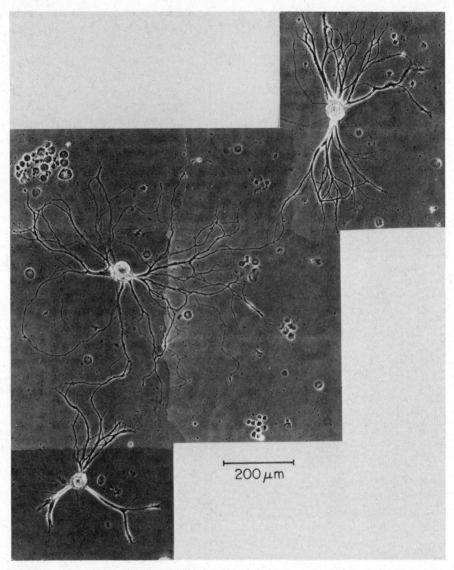

Figure 2. Three bag cell neurons fully developed and interconnected at 20 days in primary culture. The heteropolar condition, the occurrence of three or more major neurites, is typical for cultured bag cell neurons. Phase contrast. From Strumwasser et al. (63).

of ELH-containing fibers wrapped around the posterior portion of the PVC nerve trunk remains obscure at the moment. There are at least three possibilities, not mutually exclusive: the bag cell cuff is a zone that allows electrical coupling between the distal neurites of widely separated bag cells; the cuff is a specialized zone of secretion that allows mutual influence between bag cells and/or between bag cells and other axons in the nerve trunk; the cuff is a functional zone for afferent input from axons descending in the nerve trunk from the head ganglia.

2.3   Primary Structure of Egg-Laying Hormone (ELH)

The first evidence for the peptide nature of ELH was obtained by Toevs (29) as part of her thesis research in this laboratory. She found that the factor causing egg-laying was inactivated by either trypsin or pronase (4). She determined an apparent molecular weight of about 6000 for this factor by gel filtration on Sephadex G50 (29). Arch and colleagues (30) confirmed the apparent molecular weight by gel filtration on Bio-Rad P10 and determined its isoelectric point as ∽9.3. The basic nature of ELH has played an important role in its purification. A two-step purification procedure consisting of cation exchange chromatography (Sephadex SP C25) followed by gel filtration (Bio-Rad P6) provides a homogeneous bio-active product with pI 9.2, enriched by 100-fold and with a 36% recovery. Hunkapiller and Hood (31) have described a microsequencer capable of sequencing about 200 pmole of cytochrome c (12,400 MW). Utilizing their microsequencer, the primary amino acid sequence of ELH has been determined (6) as:

10

NH_2-Ile-Ser-Ile-Asn-Gln-Asp-Leu-Lys-Ala-Ile-Thr-Asp-Met-Leu-Leu-Thr-

20   30

Glu-Gln-Ile-Arg-Glu-Arg-Gln-Arg-Tyr-Leu-Ala-Asp-Leu-Arg-Gln-Arg-

Leu-Leu-Glu-Lys-OH

ELH contains 36 amino acids with a calculated molecular weight of 4385. Seven amino acids are not represented in ELH, all of which excepting histidine, possess either non-polar or neutral polar side chains. One of the interesting regions of the ELH molecule spans amino acids

20

20–25 where there is an alternating Arg-Glu-Arg-Gln-Arg sequence terminating in Tyr. This is the most polar portion of the molecule (i.e., it has the greatest charge density), with a net positive charge, which could be the region which binds to receptive sites on targets. The fact that trypsin inactivates ELH is compatible with this working hypothesis because trypsin is specific for arginine and lysine peptides (and esters) and should produce seven peptide fragments, three of them in the postulated critical region.

There is no homology between the ELH molecule and other well known vertebrate neuropeptides such as vasopressin, oxytocin, Substance P, LHRH, TRH, somatostatin, neurotensin or a molluscan cardioexcitatory tetrapeptide isolated from the ganglia of clams (32). However, a small portion of ELH, residues 24–26, is identical with the first three amino acids of the insect neuropeptide Proctolin, a pentapeptide isolated from the cockroach hindgut (33). Proctolin (Peninsula) injected into *Aplysia* does not induce egg-laying even in amounts as high as 200 nanomoles.

2.4   Afterdischarge and Peptide Release

Kupfermann and Kandel (25, 34) first described the normal property in bag cells of afterdischarge in response to brief stimulation of either pleurovisceral nerves in the excised abdominal ganglion. Bag cells are normally silent but during electrical stimulation of the anterior pleurovisceral connective they begin to produce action potentials that are synchronous in all the cells of the cluster. At the termination of a few seconds of electrical stimulation, the bag cells continue to discharge synchronous action potentials for an average time of 30 min at 14°C (20). A surprising result was that synaptic activation of afterdischarge could occur in the isolated bag cell neurites (20), a preparation consisting of the PVC severed from the bag cell somata at the junction between the connective and the cluster. Whatever the mechanism of this afterdischarge, which will be discussed later, it is clear that the cell bodies themselves are not essential for the process. Afterdischarge in isolated neurites may reflect the emergence, in evolution, of a safety factor to ensure release of large amounts of ELH to sustain egg-laying and propagation of the species.

During a single afterdischarge in an isolated bag cell cluster, prelabeled simultaneously with two radioactive amino acids, at least four peptides are released, compared with the preceding control period as shown in Figure 3A (19). Two of these released peptides have been identified by their isoelectric point (pI) and apparent molecular weight (19). Egg-laying hormone was shown by Arch and colleagues (30) to be quite basic (pI of $\sim$9.2). Released (and bioactive) ELH appears in the included volume of a gel filtration column (Bio-Rad P6) with an average K_{av} of 0.2; when this radioactive peak (fraction 36 in Figure 3) is run on IEF gels, over 90% of the counts in the gel run at pI 9.2 along with marker ELH. The second identified peptide released during afterdischarge is quite acidic (pI 4.8, see Figure 4 in ref. 19) and its apparent molecular weight is about 6000 daltons. This peptide was first described by Gainer and Wollberg (35) as existing in homogenates of bag cell clusters and had been speculated by them to be the egg-laying hormone. This is clearly not the case because Arch et al. (30) have shown that this acidic peptide does not induce egg-laying whereas the basic peptide does.

At least two other factors of lower apparent molecular weight are released from bag cells during afterdischarge (the fourth and fifth peaks in Figure 3B, counting the void as the first peak). These factors are presumably peptides because they incorporate arginine and leucine, but they are otherwise not well characterized. The biological functions of

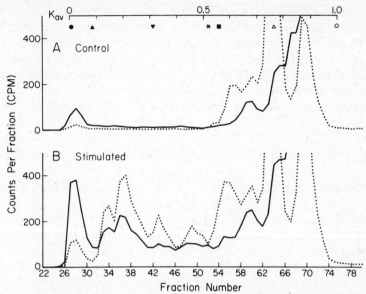

Figure 3. P-6 fractionation of consecutive 1 h perfusates from a single bag cell cluster. The profile in (A) is from the control hour and in (B) from the second hour where the cluster was stimulated briefly and produced an afterdischarge for more than 25 min. The cluster was labeled with ^{3}H-Arg and ^{14}C-Leu. The profiles for both ^{3}H(——) and ^{14}C(...) are shown. The ELH region, K_{av} = 0.2, shows a 15-fold to 100-fold increase in released counts in B. The ^{14}C counts in the leucine region or the ^{3}H counts in the ^{3}H$_2$O region are not changed. The markers, not run concurrently are ▪ blue dextran 2000,MW = 2 million; bovine pancreatic trypsin inhibitor (Kunitz), MW = 6,500; ▲ cytochrome c, MW = 12,384;* glucagon, MW = 3485; ▼ α-bungarotoxin, MW = 7904; ▪ bacitracin, MW = 1411; △ leucine; ○ ^{3}H$_2$O. For both ^{3}H and ^{14}C, 59% of the applied radioactivity was recovered in the collected fractions of the control period, and 42 46%, respectively, in the stimulation period. From Stuart et al. (19).

these presumed peptides and the acidic peptide are not known; however, they do not induce egg-laying. They could be "discard" peptides, part of the molecular makeup of the neurosecretory granule, but in the absence of much information they could just as well be modulatory or even trophic factors acting on the nervous, endocrine, or reproductive system.

The role of Ca^{2+} in secretion of ELH has only been investigated with regard to high potassium-stimulated release of presumed ELH from either the intact abdominal ganglion or isolated bag cell clusters. Arch (36) showed that 107 mM K$^+$ released radiolabeled material from a prelabeled isolated bag cell cluster. This material migrated on an SDS-polyacrylamide gel with an apparent molecular weight of <10,000 daltons. Such high potassium-stimulated release of this material was not apparent in a medium containing 1.0 mM Ca^{2+} and 77 mM Mg^{2+}. Loh et al. (37) have reported the Ca^{2+}-dependent release of MW 12,000, 6,000, and <3,000 peptides with high potassium stimulation of isolated bag cell clusters. While high potassium is a convenient method for depolarizing bag cell neurons, it also depolarizes glia and connective tissue cells in the intact bag cell cluster preparations. The selective activation of an afterdischarge in an isolated bag cell cluster, while more physiological and specific in studying peptide release, could still initiate release from glial cells for it is known that neural activity causes a depolarization of adjacent glia, mediated by K^+ released from active neurons (38).

2.5   Behavioral and Electrophysiological Consequences of ELH

It was Kupfermann (2) who discovered that an extract of bag cells caused egg-laying. In his report, based on five animals, he assayed for the presence of an egg mass some hours after injection of crude extract but did not mention the profound repertoire of behavioral changes that are now known to occur and the latency for egg-laying. Cessation of locomotion, onset of head weaving movements and inhibition of feeding all occur as part of egg-laying behavior. At 14°C, the latency between injection of ELH-containing extracts and onset of egg-laying is 72 ± 2.5 (SEM, $n = 52$) min (3). During this interval a number of behavioral phenomena occur. Within 20 min of injection, locomoting animals become relatively quiescent. ELH-injected animals, during this period, come to rest on the wall or at a corner of the aquarium. Within the period 40 min after injection until appearance of the egg string, lateral head weaving movements appear. Such movements continue during extrusion of the egg strand and serve to package it, once attached to the substrate, into a compact assembly. A typical egg-laying resonse at 14°C, yields about 2.3 ± 0.3 (SEM, $n = 32$) gm of eggs (13). We now know that 2.5 nmoles of pure ELH will consistently induce egg-laying in *Aplysia* at 20°C (6).

The egg string, a translucent gelatinous tube, is assembled in the albumen gland, part of the reproductive tract. Single eggs, released from the gonad most likely in direct response to ELH (39), collect in the little hermaphroditic duct. There, presumably by ciliary sweeping and/or peristalsis, they are passed into the albumen gland. In this gland the strand is secreted and serves to package and protect the eggs which are located within highly regular compartments or capsules. Either ELH and/or some of the other peptides, released during bag cell afterdischarge, serve to directly or indirectly trigger ciliary sweeping and/or peristalsis in the reproductive tract along with secretion of the egg strand by the albumen gland.

Besides cessation of locomotion, extrusion of the egg string, and egg-winding behavior, animals show an inhibition of feeding, which commences before the egg strand actually appears (40). Two paired groups of 24-h starved *Aplysia*, maintained at 20°C, were injected with ELH-containing extracts (experimentals) or extracts of head ganglia (controls). When 1 g of algae (*Plocamium coccinium*) was presented as food 10 min after injection, both groups ate but the ELH-injected group stopped feeding at 17 $\pm$ 4 (SD, $n = 7$) min, leaving 60% of their food, whereas the control group finished all their food by 22 $\pm$ 8 minutes (SD, $n = 7$) without interruption. Eggs were laid at 29 min (at 20°C) in the ELH-injected group. In two additional paired groups of starved animals, when food was presented at 20 min after injection, none of the five ELH-injected animals fed while all five controls did.

One would expect that if ELH was mediating inhibition of feeding there would be direct effects of ELH on the nervous system, especially at sites directly concerned with feeding such as the buccal ganglion. In fact, purified ELH activates at least four neurons in the isolated buccal ganglion, one pair having been identified by intacellular recording (40). The identified neuron pair, one in each buccal ganglion, lie between identified neurons B3 and B4 according to Gardner's (41) map of the buccal ganglion, and each sends an axon into the ipsilateral buccal nerve (b.n. 3). The B4 neuron is classified as a command cell for protracting and opening the radula halves of the buccal mass (42). The b.n. 3 neuron is normally silent in unstimulated preparations except for activity synchronized with the end of the spontaneous intermittent bursts of impulses, presumably the expression of the feeding motor program that occurs in a number of different gastropod buccal ganglia preparations (43–47). After pure ELH is added to the dish (or is released by activating an afterdischarge in bag cells neurally disconnected from the head ganglia) the b.n. 3 neuron becomes active for hours until the dish is flushed free of ELH (40).

During activation by ELH, the b.n. 3 neuron produces a relatively regular pacemaker discharge with maximal rates approaching 90 spikes/min. The time course of activation indicates that the b.n. 3 neuron reaches half-maximal response by 8 minutes after addition of ELH to isolated but otherwise intact buccal ganglion preparations. The response to ELH is likely to be a direct effect on the b.n. 3 neuron because it occurs in a high Mg^{2+}, low Ca^{2+} solution which blocks the synaptic activity in the buccal ganglion. A dose/response curve remains to be generated but 200 nM ELH (about 1.5 nmoles) produces a moderately strong response. This compares favorably with the quantity of ELH that consistently induces egg-laying.

The relationship between activation of the b.n. 3 neuron by ELH and inhibition of feeding has not been directly investigated but there is reasonable suggestive evidence for a connection. In the first place the neuron is half maximally activated at 8 minutes (*in vitro*) and reaches its peak activity at the same time that intact starved *Aplysia* stop feeding (at 17 min) when offered food at 10 min. Secondly, the intracellular recordings indicate a short duration action potential, and a constant latency and one to one relationship between the soma spike and the b.n. 3 nerve spike. The neuron is then likely to directly innervate muscle or peripheral nerve terminals innervating muscle. This nerve includes motoneurons that excite the accessory radula closer muscle (42, 43). It will not, therefore, be surprising if the net action of the b.n. 3 neuron is to allow retraction and closing of the radula but that remains to be directly demonstrated. This possibility is also in agreement with the fact that the b.n. 3 neuron fires at the end of a "feeding" burst.

Mayeri and colleagues (48, 49) have described specific excitatory and inhibitory effects of bag cell activation on a number of neurons in the intact abdominal ganglion. These experiments, per se, do not allow a conclusion as to which of the several bag cell peptides mediate these effects. Recent evidence, using purified ELH, indicates that some of these effects, the inhibition of the left upper quadrant bursters (L2,3,4,6), are not mediated by ELH (50) but that the excitatory effects on R 15 (51) and cells of the LB and LC cluster (50) are. The abdominal ganglion itself does not appear to be required for the act of egg-laying other than as a source of ELH. *Aplysia* in which the abdominal ganglion has been surgically removed still respond to ELH with behavioral egg-laying (52). However, there may still be subtle, even if not primary, effects that the abdominal ganglion contributes to behavioral egg-laying. These effects remain to be clarified.

2.6 Electrical Coupling and the Mechanisms of Synchronous Discharge

The synchronous activity and afterdischarge property of bag cells were recognized as important attributes of this neuroendocrine system by the earliest investigators (25) but direct evidence for mechanisms remained to be worked out. Kupfermann and Kandel (25) tested for electrical coupling between pairs of impaled bag cells as a means of synchrony, but they could not find any coupling in *A. californica* and concluded that this was probably accounted for by electrical coupling at a site remote from the somata. Blankenship and Haskins (53) were able to find evidence for electrical coupling in *A. dactylomela*, as measured between somata, but the coupling was quite weak. They reported mean nonrectifying coupling ratios (post : pre) of $\sim$0.008 between 84 pairs of bag cells and concluded that the site of coupling was likely to be remote but within the first 3 mm of the PVC's. The coupling was insensitive to solutions with high Mg^{2+} (136.4 mM) and low Ca^{2+} (2mM). The fact that we can obtain a synchronous afterdischarge in the isolated (asomatic) neurites of the posterior PVC's (20) is certainly consistent with one of the coupling sites being remote in *A. californica*.

Primary cell cultures of bag cells have helped establish that bag cells in *A. californica* are electrically coupled to one another (26). In cell culture, bag cells connect with each other after neurite outgrowth (see Figure 2), and when closely adjacent cell pairs are tested we always find strong bidirectional coupling (e.g., ratio 0.8). An induced action potential in either cell of a pair generates a delayed action potential in the other cell. Thus it seems likely that the formation of electrical (vs. chemical) synapses in cell culture reflects the normal development of bag cells in the intact cluster.

The morphological basis of electrical coupling between bag cells has been investigated in the intact bag cell cluster by freeze-fracture studies (26). These studies have revealed numerous gap junctions (made up of 9–11 nm particles) between bag cell processes within the cluster and in the connective tissue of the pleurovisceral connectives. The numbers of particles or size of the gap junction were always greater within the cluster than in the connective. Therefore, it seems likely that the extensive synchrony among bag cells in the intact cluster during afterdischarge is mediated by gap junction coupling between processes within the cluster as well as within the pleurovisceral connectives.

The synchronization of bag cells can be best assessed by simultaneous extracellular and intracellular recordings (54). The extracellular recordings on a bag cell cluster, or proximal PVC nerve, record population spikes. Intracellularly recorded bag cell spikes discharge in a one-to-one relationship with these population spikes. The studies of Dudek and Blankenship (54) have clearly shown that at the start of an afterdischarge bag cell spikes are initiated in the distal neurites in the PVC nerve and propagate toward the cell bodies in the cluster.

2.7 Afterdischarge: Questions about Synaptic Input

It was demonstrated a decade ago that a fundamental property of the bag cell system is the property of afterdischarge (25). Brief stimulation of the anterior end of the PVC nerve produces a long-lasting depolarization and repetitive discharge which considerably outlasts the stimulus. In 19 preparations the afterdischarge averaged 30 min ($\pm$ 4.3, SEM) at 14°C (20). Bag cell action potentials and afterdischarge can also be triggered by stimulation of the pleurocerebral connective nerve (20) or of the caudodorsal region of the cerebral ganglion (Kaczmarek, Chiu, and Strumwasser, unpublished).

A fundamental question concerns the mechanism of activation of the bag cells when either the anterior end of the PVC nerve or those regions in the head ganglia are stimulated. It is likely that in this type of activation synapses are involved between descending axons from the head ganglia and bag cell processes. The best evidence for synapses is indirect at the moment. ELH immunohistochemistry indicates that the bag cell processes do not continue anteriorly for more than 2 cm from the posterior end of the PVC nerve while the full length of the PVC in adult animals ranges between 7 and 10 cm. The location of these synapses is likely to be in the PVC nerve itself because the isolated nerve is capable of afterdischarge when stimulated form the anterior end (20). However, it remains unclear whether these synapses on bag cell processes in the posterior PVC are chemical or electrical or both. High magnesium, low calcium experiments to block chemical synaptic transmission are difficult to interpret because the action potentials in the bag cells appear to have a large calcium component, as shown by experiments in the intact cluster (55) as well as their sensitivity to tetrodotoxin in primary culture (56).

2.8   Cyclic AMP Involvement in Afterdischarge

We had originally considered the possibility that afterdischarge might be due to a positive feedback of released ELH on the bag cells. Perhaps ELH released in the first few seconds of electrical stimulation excites bag cells, which release more ELH, and so on. When the supply of releasable ELH is exhausted or the membrane receptors to ELH are desensitized, then afterdischarge would stop. We were unable to find any evidence for this working hypothesis. Removing and replacing the bathing solution with fresh solution during afterdischarge did not shorten the afterdischarge but rather tended to lengthen it. Furthermore, recent attempts to measure ELH release by an enzyme-linked immunosorbent assay during afterdischarge indicates that there is little release during the first few minutes of afterdischarge (Chiu, Jennings, and Strumwasser, unpublished).

Insight into the mechanisms of the long-lasting afterdischarge came from investigations on the nature of the relative refractoriness to producing a second afterdischarge soon after the first. Typically, stimulation following a long-lasting afterdischarge produces either no afterdischarge or, with more intense stimulation, a much shorter afterdischarge of lower firing rate. A second normal long-lasting afterdischarge can only be produced after several hours of recovery. We were able to overcome this refractoriness, however, by the use of any one of a number of phosphodiesterase inhibitors (theophylline, caffeine, isobutyl methylxanthine, or papaverine) applied at the end of the first afterdischarge (20). If the phosphodiesterase inhibitor is applied within 1–2 min of the end of afterdischarge, the afterdischarge is reinitiated without further electrical stimulation and lasts on the average approximately seven times longer than the partial second afterdischarge due to electrical stimulation (20). However, these phosphodiesterase inhibitors were never able to initiate afterdischarge by themselves in an unstimulated preparation.

Although these phosphodiesterase inhibitors, particularly the methylxanthines, may have mixed cellular effects, the fact that they extended afterdischarge suggested that cyclic nucleotides might be important in mediating this phenomenon. Measurements of cyclic AMP concentration by radioimmunoassay during afterdischarge indicated that by 1 min, the earliest time point measurable, it had already doubled; by 2 min it had reached a maximum increase of threefold above baseline; and by 5–6 min it was near the resting level (20).

The cyclic AMP increase in bag cells during afterdischarge could be a correlative phenomenon. Perhaps a number of metabolic events are set into motion by membrane activity, for example, increased glucose utilization and glycogenolysis and the cAMP increase is related to control of these secondary events. On the other hand, the cAMP increase might be more intimately related to a modulation of membrane channels, which causes the generation of afterdischarge. These working hypotheses are not mutually exclusive. The cAMP increase in bag cells could be causal to afterdischarge and at the same time setting metabolic processes into motion as preparation for expected metabolic demands on the system.

Evidence that the cAMP elevation is causal to the afterdischarge comes from the finding that any one of four cAMP analogs can initiate discharge in bag cells in the absence of any electrical stimulation. These analogs include 8-benzylthio (8-BT) or 8-methylthio cAMP (20), orthonitrobenzyl cAMP ester (Nerbonne, Kaczmarek, and Strumwasser, unpublished), and a disubstituted analog N^6-n-butyl-8-(benzylthio-cAMP (Strumwasser, unpublished) obtained from Dr. J. P. Miller (57). The characteristics of cAMP-initiated discharge are quite similar to the electrically initiated afterdischarge in bag cells. In afterdischarge, the frequency of action potentials rises and peaks at $\sim$2.5-6 hz at about 1 min into afterdischarge, falling slowly over minutes to $\sim$0.5 hz, which is maintained for the rest of the afterdischarge (Figure 4, 58). The duration of action potentials also increases during afterdischarge but follows a somewhat different time course, reaching its maximum at about 2 min (Figure 4).

2.9 Protein Phosphorylation During Afterdischarge

A decade ago Siggins, Bloom, and colleagues provided the first neurophysiological evidence for the importance of cAMP-mediated hyperpolarization in the Purkinje neurons of the mammalian cerebellum in response to norepinephrine (59, 60). Since then progress on the mechanisms by which cyclic nucleotides control electrical excitability has been slow. The principal drawbacks to investigations of these phenomena in vertebrates are that complicated interactions occur among neuron types, that the individual neurons are too small for a comprehensive electrophysiological analysis, and that samples of brain tissue for biochemical analysis are often heterogeneous. The study of the bag cells and other invertebrate preparations frees the investigator from most of

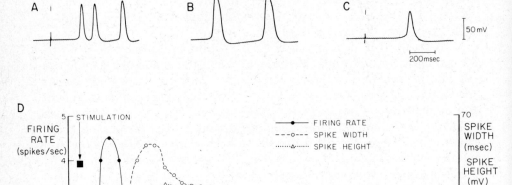

Figure 4. (A, B, and C) Intracellularly recorded bag cell action potentials. Trace (A) shows spikes evoked by extracellular stimulation (20 V, 2.5 msec) of a pleuroabdominal connective nerve at the onset of a bag cell afterdischarge. Trace (B) shows the shape of the enhanced action potentials 10 min. after the onset of afterdischarge. Trace (C) shows an action potential evoked after the end of afterdischarge. (D) A plot of the firing rate, spike width, and spike height at the onset of a bag cell afterdischarge triggered by extracellular stimulation (20 V, 2.5 msec, 1 Hz, 10 secs) of a pleuroabdominal connective nerve in a normal seawater medium. From Kaczmarek et al. (58).

these limitations and promises to disclose basic cellular mechanisms that underly long-lasting changes in neural excitability.

Since 1968 it has been known that there are cAMP-dependent protein kinases. The first was discovered in rabbit skeletal muscle (17); subsequently, Kuo and Greengard (61) discovered that such cAMP-dependent protein kinases are widespread among the organs and tissues of the mammal, including the nervous system. These cAMP-dependent protein kinases also occur in the tissues of the nine phyla examined so far (61). Greengard (16) has postulated that the mechanism of action of the cyclic nucleotides as second messengers is indeed mediated by cAMP-dependent protein kinases, the specificity of a cellular response being determined by which substrate phosphoproteins are present within the cell.

One of the possible ways in which protein phosphorylation might initiate afterdischarge in bag cells is by directly modifying the properties of a membrane ion channel. The catalytic subunit of cAMP-dependent protein kinase from beef heart has been found to phosphorylate proteins from the nervous system of *Aplysia* (21, 62), indicating that the mammalian enzyme recognizes presumably foreign proteins. We have used this feature to back-phosphorylate or postlabel with [γ^{32}P]-ATP the bag cell proteins extracted at various times into afterdischarge (21). If enhanced phosphorylation occurs during afterdischarge then the postlabel paradigm should result in reduced phosphorylation measured *in vitro* because phosphorylation sites are already occupied due to the activation of cyclic AMP-dependent protein kinases during afterdischarge. Using the postlabel technique on crude homogenates of the bag cell organ, we find that a bag-cell-specific protein (BC-2, $\sim$21,000 daltons) on SDS polyacrylamide gels shows a 73% ($\pm$ 9%, $n = 4$) reduction in *in vitro* phosphorylation at 20 min but no change at 2 min into afterdischarge when compared with unstimulated ganglia (Figure 5).

We were able to confirm this change in the phosphorylation of the BC-2 protein by using the more classical prelabeling paradigm. Intact abdominal ganglia were incubated in inorganic ^{32}PO$_4$ for $\sim$24 h in order to maximize the intracellular pools of labeled ATP. At 2 and 20 min into afterdischarge, the bag cell organs were homogenized in 10% trichloroacetic acid and the pellet was extracted with acetone-ethanol to remove lipids and treated with ribonuclease A to digest RNA. The pattern of labeled phosphoproteins on SDS polyacrylamide gels showed that the BC-2 phosphoprotein was increased by 92% ($\pm$ 23%) at 20 min but not at 2 min into afterdischarge (Table 2). With use of the prelabel paradigm there was an early increase (82%) in the labeling of another phosphoprotein (BC-1, $\sim$33,000 daltons) at 2 min, and this increase was sustained at a lower level even at 20 min into afterdischarge (Table 2). More recently, with the use of the postlabeling technique, this protein has also been demonstrated to change with afterdischarge (DeRiemer, Greengard, and Kaczmarek, unpublished).

In summary, using two different paradigms, the BC-2 protein, a bag-cell-specific protein, shows an enhanced phosphorylation at 20 min but not 2 min into afterdischarge. On the other hand, the BC-1 protein, which is not specific to bag cells, shows an early enhancement of phosphorylation during afterdischarge. Our present evidence indicates that this elevation in phosphorylation is still sustained at a moderately lower level 20 min into afterdischarge. We have also determined that both of these proteins are specific substrates for cAMP-directed phosphoryla-

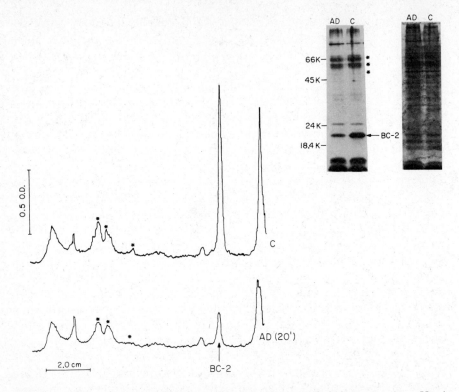

Figure 5. Afterdischarge-dependent phosphorylatin: postlabeled preparation. Hemi-ganglion preparation where the left bag-cell cluster was electrically stimulated to afterdis-charge, then dissected at 20 min. into the afterdischarge and "back-phosphorylated" with protein kinase. The densitometer traces illustrate the change in phosphorylation of protein BC-2 with afterdischarge (AD) compared with the control (C) from the undischarged clus-ter. The inset photograph shows the autoradiogram (left two tracks) from which the densi-tometer traces were made and the corresponding Coomassie blue protein stained gel (right two tracks). The three reference phosphoprotein bands used in quantitating the changes in BC-2 (9) are denoted by an asterisk (*). From Jennings et al. (21).

tion. Preliminary evidence indicates that the phosphorylation state of at least one other protein ($\approx$50,000 daltons) is also enhanced with afterdis-charge but that this is due to a calcium-calmodulin-dependent kinase presumably activated by calcium ion entry into the cells during afterdis-charge (DeRiemer, Greengard, and Kaczmarek, unpublished).

2.10   The Action of Cyclic AMP Analogs and Intracellularly Injected Protein Kinase on Isolated Bag Cells

The results described so far allow us to conclude that cyclic AMP ana-logs can initiate a discharge with characteristics similar to the electri-cally initiated afterdischarge in the intact bag cell clusters. Furthermore, two substrate proteins for cAMP-dependent protein kinase in the bag

TABLE 2   Phosphorylation Changes of Phosphoproteins Prelabeled for 22–24 Hours with Inorganic ^{32}P During Afterdischarge

Protein (mw)	% Phosphorylation Change[a]			
	2 min		20 min	
BC-2	$-19 \pm 28\%$	(5)	$+92 \pm 23\%$[b]	(4)
BC-1	$+82 \pm 14\%$[c]	(8)	$+69 \pm 43\%$[d]	(4)
45K	$-11 \pm 12\%$	(8)	$-9 \pm 32\%$	(4)

[a] Data are plotted as percentage change ($\pm$ SEM) in the area under the peak on a densitometer scan relative to a 28,000 dalton reference peak observed not to change with afterdischarge. The number of separate experiments is shown in parentheses. The BC-1 and BC-2 phosphoproteins were observed to undergo significant increases in phosphorylation during afterdischarge. The 45,000 dalton phosphoprotein is included as a representative phosphoprotein that did not undergo a change in phosphorylation during afterdischarge. Statistical significance was calculated using a one-tailed paired t-test.
[b] $P < 0.02$
[c] $P < 0.005$
[d] $P < 0.05$

cells increase their phosphorylation during electrically initiated afterdischarge with apparently different time courses. For the study of the electrical consequences of these biochemical changes, isolated bag cells have distinct advantages over the cells in the intact cluster. In the intact cluster the cells are electrically coupled, making the study of membrane channels by voltage clamping difficult. Moreover, results from intracellular injection of agents could be difficult to interpret. We found it possible to dissociate the bag cells with neutral protease and to establish viable primary cultures of these cells (27). When initially seeded, these cells have few processes due to the shearing forces during trituration. They quickly regenerate their neurites, however, and also form electrical connections with other bag cells (26, 63). One can then select isolated cells in the dish with simple or complex neuritic patterns for electrophysiological studies.

We found that totally isolated bag cells are normally electrically quiescent but are induced to discharge action potentials with either 8-BT cyclic AMP (64) or N^6-n-butyl-8-(benzylthio)-cyclic AMP (Strumwasser, unpublished). This discharge due to 8-BT-cyclic AMP is preceded by an average 68% increase in membrane input resistance (64); a similar result has recently been obtained for the disubstituted cyclic AMP analog. An actual afterdischarge can be produced in the presence of these agents in isolated bag cells immediately after direct spikes are elicited, as shown in Figure 6. It appears likely that some aspect of the action potential itself facilitates the production of further action potentials in the presence of the cyclic AMP analog. The action potentials in the isolated bag cells in primary culture are mainly calcium-mediated since for the

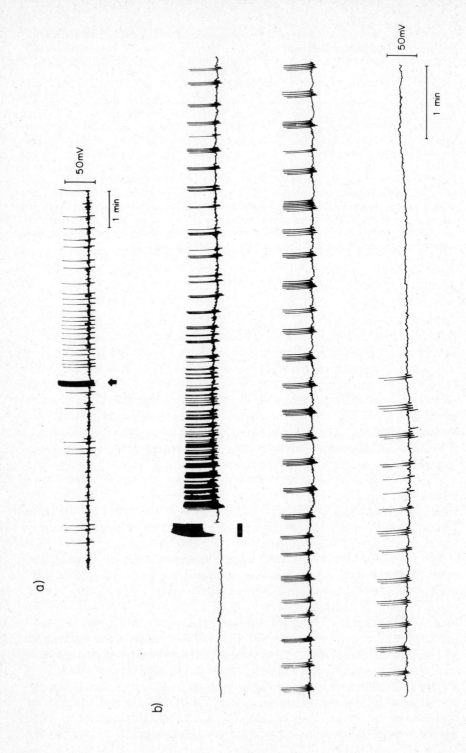

majority of cells tetrodotoxin does not block the spikes but cobaltous ions do (56). The role of calcium influx in the further long-lasting excitability increase following a burst of directly elicited spikes remains to be worked out.

If protein phosphorylation induced by cAMP can indeed modify membrane excitability then a most compelling test could be made by inducing protein phosphorylation through intracellular injection of the catalytic subunit of cAMP-dependent protein kinase (PKC) into an isolated bag cell, thus bypassing the cAMP step. We injected PKC purified from beef heart into isolated bag cells (62). As mentioned above, calcium spikes are predominant in isolated bag cells in cell culture. The rate of rise and amplitude of the calcium spikes were enhanced after PKC injection by 73 and 35% respectively, in 11 of 16 cells injected. These enhanced amplitude spikes were not blocked by tetrodotoxin (50 μM) but were partly or totally blocked by $CoCl_2$ (12 mM). In 24 bag cells used for control intracellular injections, only one showed an increase (7.5%) in spike height. These control experiments included injections with heat-inactivated PKC or the various carrier solutions (62).

In order to obtain insight into the enhanced calcium spikes of bag cells after intracellular injection of PKC, we measured membrane input resistance by determining the steady-state electrotonic potential to constant-current hyperpolarizing pulses. In the nine cells in which membrane input resistance was measured before and after PKC injection, with enhanced spikes, five showed a mean increase of 65%, and the overall increase in the nine cells averaged 32%. Thus the enhancement of calcium spikes by PKC was associated with an increased membrane resistance, as is also the case for the extracellular application of cAMP analogs.

We have done voltage-clamp experiments on isolated bag cells to gain more insight into the nature of the membrane-resistance increase obtained with either extracellularly applied 8-BT-cAMP or intracellularly applied PKC (65). We find that 8-BT-cAMP causes a significant reduction in the net steady state outward current and thereby induces a region of negative slope resistance in the steady state I-V relations (Figure 7). However, 8-BT-cAMP, does not affect the peak inward currents, which are abolished by Co^{2+} or Ni^{2+}. We therefore believe that one ac-

Figure 6. (A) An intracellular record from a bag cell neuron in cell culture after repetitive discharge had been induced by 8-BT-cAMP. At the time marked by the arrow, a series of 10 depolarizing current pulses (250 msec, 0.25 nA, 0.83 pulses/sec) was applied to the cell. Following the pulses, an increase in the frequency of discharge was observed. (B) Afterdischarge in a bag cell neuron in cell culture. After addition of 8-BT-cAMP (0.5 mM) to the extracellular medium, a hyperpolarizing current (0.06 nA) was applied to the cell to prevent the onset of a repetitive discharge. For the duration indicated by the bar, this bias current was released, resulting in repetitive firing by the cell. After reapplication of the bias current, a prolonged afterdischarge was generated. From Kaczmarek and Strumwasser (64).

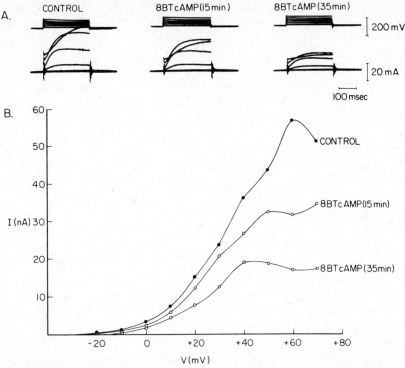

Figure 7. The outward currents observed during depolarizing current pulses (250 msec) are diminished by 8-BT-cAMP (0.5 m*M*). (B) shows I-V relations at the end of a 250 msec pulse before and after 8-BT-cAMP. This represents the most profound diminution observed in 16 experiments. We have also investigated the effects of 8-BT-cAMP on outward currents in the presence of calcium channel blockers (5–10 m*M* Ni^{2+2+} or 20m*M* Co^{2+}). Under these conditions we have seen no effect of 8-BT-cAMP on outward currents. From Kaczmarek and Strumwasser, unpublished (see ref. 65).

tion of this cyclic AMP analog is to suppress a potassium current, the identity of which remains to be clearly established. We have suggested that phosphorylation of the proteins controlling the membrane channel could modulate the voltage-dependent behavior of either or both potassium and calcium channels (56). Analysis of single-channel currents by the patch-clamp gigaseal technique (66, 67) in isolated bag cells in culture might reveal whether the open time is decreased for certain potassium channels and perhaps increased for calcium channels with the cAMP analogs or PKC injection.

2.11   Intracellular Modulation of Membrane Channels

The concept that there exists a class of actions in excitable membranes where an intracellular control can modulate a membrane channel is not entirely new. To account for bursting activity and its slow modulation in the *Aplysia* neuron, R 15, there had been postulated an intracellularly synthesized "depolarizing substance," perhaps a peptide, with actions on the inner surface of the membrane (68, 69). There is no direct evidence for this hypothesis at the moment but the striking effects of protein-synthesis or RNA-synthesis inhibitors or X rays on the circadian rhythm of impulse rate in the isolated eye of *Aplysia* (70–73) are compatible with such a concept.

Intracellular calcium is another important internal control that modulates membrane activity. It was first shown in the R15 neuron that there is a calcium-activated potassium channel (74, 75), and such channels appear to be fairly common in a variety of cell types (76, 77). There is good evidence that the postburst hyperpolarization that partly accounts for the silent interval between bursts in R15 is due to a calcium-activated potassium conductance (78).

The evidence that protein phosphorylation is another important intracellular modulator of membrane channels, a concept originating with Greengard (16), is becoming very compelling for two systems in *Aplysia* in addition to the bag cell neurons described here. These include the serotonergic-induced inhibition of bursting in R15 (79) and the serotonergic-induced enhancement or sensitization at the synapse of the siphon sensory neuron and gill motor neuron (80). It is likely that there are yet other intracellular controls waiting to be discovered, and molluscan as well as other model neurons will have distinct advantages for such research.

2.12 Transmitter Modulation of Afterdischarge

One may question whether afterdischarge can be stopped once it is in progress because it has the appearance, in spite of its long-lasting nature, of a triggered all-or-none reaction. Such a suppressing mechanism at the source of the neurohormone ELH would be advantageous in evolution because otherwise after a maximum release the multiple targets of ELH action would have to be individually deactivated in order to stop egg-laying. Arousing stimuli, such as the presence or actual contact with a predator or sudden change in the marine environment that made it nonadaptive for egg-laying, can be imagined as appropriate stimuli for prematurely terminating afterdischarge and hence aborting an egg-laying episode.

It is interesting that serotonin suppresses bag cell afterdischarge (20) because serotonin has been shown to enhance monosynaptic transmission in the sensory neuron-gill or siphon motor neuron pathway (81), a process equated with sensitization. The dose dependency and pharmacology of suppression of bag cell afterdischarge is illustrated in Figure 8 (82). Reliable suppression of afterdischarge is achieved at low concentrations of serotonin ($0.5 \times 10^{-6} M$) and the suppressing action of sero-

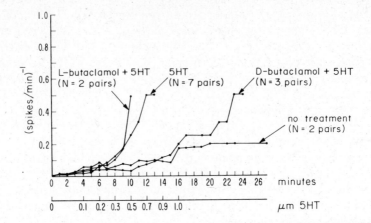

Figure 8. Serotonergic inhibition of bag cell afterdischarge. Abdominal ganglia were preincubated for 30 min at 14°C in a recording chamber containing either filtered seawater alone or filtered seawater containing 10^{-5} M(D) or (L) butaclamol. Afterdischarge was initiated by electrical stimulation to the right pleurovisceral connective. Afterdischarge was recorded by suction electrodes placed on the right and left bag cell clusters. At 4 min into the afterdischarge (and 2 min intervals thereafter) 100–200 μL aliquots of a stock serotonin solution were applied extracellularly to a final concentration as illustrated. D-Butaclamol (but not its inactive isomer L-butaclamol) was an effective antagonist of the serotonergic inhibition of bag cell afterdischarge (p < 0.01). From Jennings et al. (82).

tonin can be partially reversed by D-butaclamol (10^{-5} M), a presumed serotonergic receptor blocker (83, 84). The fact that serotonin acts to suppress afterdischarge at such low concentrations and rather rapidly (within 1 min in an intact bag cell cluster) suggests that the effect is quite physiological and probably of great adaptive value.

Arousing or sensitizing stimuli enhance monosynaptic transmission in the gill and siphon withdrawal pathway but would be expected to suppress afterdischarge and hence ELH release in the bag cell neuroendocrine system. Presumably serotonin will be found to have suppressing effects in other systems in *Aplysia* where arousal dictates turning these systems off for behaviorally adaptive reasons.

Sensitization of the gill or siphon withdrawal motor neurons is currently thought to be a presynaptic process whereby serotonergic terminals innervate the synaptic terminals of the sensory neurons from gill or siphon. Klein and Kandel (85) have shown that serotonin prolongs the duration of the calcium spike in such sensory neurons when they are in Na^{+}-free artificial seawater combined with the K^{+}-channel blocker tetraethylammonium (TEA). Klein and Kandel (85) have also shown that intracellular injection of cAMP also prolongs the duration of TEA-treated sensory neurons in normal seawater. These observations have led Kandel (86) to suggest that mediation of sensitization of synaptic actions by serotonin involves a cAMP-dependent protein phosphorylation that enhances Ca^{2+}-channels. We have observed a reduction of spike width and amplitude in BCs in the intact cluster treated with serotonin up to 5×10^{-5} M. The mechanism of the powerful serotonin suppression of afterdischarge in bag cells may involve a conductance increase to K^+ and/or Cl^- ions. What remains puzzling is that serotonin causes a significant increase in cAMP in the intact bag cell cluster (20).

In the mammalian hypothalamus, dopamine plays an important role in modulation of anterior and intermediate lobe pituitary function. In *Aplysia*, dopamine has excitatory effects on bag cell afterdischarge. Prolactin secretion is thought to be under tonic inhibitory control by dopamine released into the hypophysial portal system (87, 88). Prolactin cells actually generate action potentials; in favorable preparations with large prolactin cells that can be maintained in primary culture, such as those of the alewife fish (*Alosa pseudoharenngus*), dopamine will slow (10^{-8} M) or arrest (10^{-6} M) spontaneous discharge (89). Recent evidence indicates that there may be two types of dopamine receptors on prolactin cells in rats because a rather low concentration of dopamine (10^{-12} M) actually stimulates release of prolactin, and when the inhibitory receptors are blocked by haloperidol, apomorphine acts as an agonist for the excitatory receptors (90).

In *Aplysia*, application of 10^{-4} M dopamine during BC afterdischarge produces an excitatory effect on spike frequency and population spike amplitude; however, dopamine cannot initiate afterdischarge (20). When an electrically initiated afterdischarge is completed, a profound refractoriness occurs in that the duration of subsequent electrically initiated afterdischarge is at best $\sim$20% of normal (20). Dopamine can overcome this refractoriness; when added within 1–2 min after the end of a normal afterdischarge, the afterdischarge is extended. Similar disruptions of refractoriness, as evidenced by prolongations of afterdischarge, occur with a number of phosphodiesterase inhibitors (theophylline, caffeine, isobutylmethylxanthine, and papaverine). In summary, both dopamine and serotonin modulate afterdischarge in opposite ways but the behavioral situations in which each of these two transmitter systems predominates remain to be worked out.

2.13 Peptide Initiation of Afterdischarge

Afterdischarge in bag cells causes the release of ELH as well as at least three other peptides whose functions are not presently known (19). In the intact *Aplysia* it is not known how afterdischarge in bag cells is initiated. The normal dominant stimulus for egg-laying in *Aplysia* is presumably mating. Hence one possibility is that the act of natural mating triggers the bag cells into afterdischarge. The most elegant proof of this working hypothesis would have to come from the use of implanted electrodes around the PVC nerve to record afterdischarge in an *Aplysia* acting as a female during mating. This should be technically feasible but remains to be accomplished.

If mating is a dominant stimulus for egg-laying in *Aplysia*, one can inquire whether purely neural or hormonal pathways (or some combination of both) mediate this behaviorally fixed action pattern, the ethologist's term for a triggered but complex behavioral program.

There is excellent evidence that at least two potent chemical factors endogenous to the atrial gland, a specialized part of the reproductive tract, are capable of initiating afterdischarge in bag cells. These two factors have been purified and the amino acid sequences are known (7). In Table 3 we summarize some of the characteristics of the atrial gland peptides (Peptides A and B) and compare them with those of ELH. In Figure 9 we compare the structures of ELH and the two atrial gland peptides. Although peptide B has an isoelectric point that coincides with that of ELH (pI 9.1), its amino acid sequence is quite different. Both peptides A and B initiate egg-laying in intact *Aplysia* as well as afterdischarge in *in vitro* experiments with either the intact bag cell cluster or the isolated PVC nerve (7).

Based on these results, we have postulated that peptides A and B might be released from the atrial gland during copulation to act on the bag cell trigger neurons (in the head ganglia) and/or more directly on the bag cells (63) (Figure 10). In order to test this hypothesis further, we have investigated the effects of purified peptide B on egg-laying in *Aplysia* with the abdominal ganglion and full length PVC nerves removed (Strumwasser, Yeakley, Mailheau, unpublished). We demonstrated previously that *Aplysia* without abdominal ganglia can feed, survive for months, produce a normal free-running circadian locomotor rhythm, and respond normally to ELH by egg-laying (52, 91).

Peptide B (40–80 μg) did not induce egg-laying in *Aplysia* without an abdominal ganglion and PVC nerves ($n = 3/3$), although these same animals all responded to ELH with egg-laying when tested within a few hours after the peptide B injection (Strumwasser, Yeakley, and Mailheau, unpublished). Furthermore, each batch of Peptide B was shown to be bioactive by inducing egg-laying in intact controls. We conclude from these experiments that peptide B requires the presence of the bag cells in order to induce egg-laying and most likely has no direct action on the gonad, that is, the egg-releasing function, unlike ELH.

TABLE 3   Characteristics of Atrial Gland Peptides

	Extracted From	Amino-Acid Residues	Molecular weight	pI[a]
ELH	Bag cell neurons	36	4385	9.1
Peptide A	Atrial gland	34	3924	8.0
Peptide B[b]	Atrial gland	34	4032	9.1

[a] Isoelectric point.

[b] Peptide B is identical to A in all but four amino-acid positions.

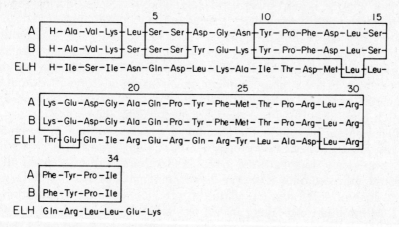

Figure 9. Comparison of amino acid sequences of egg-laying hormone (ELH), extracted from bag cells, and peptides A and B, extracted from the atrial gland of the reproductive tract. Boxes identify homologous amino acid sequences.

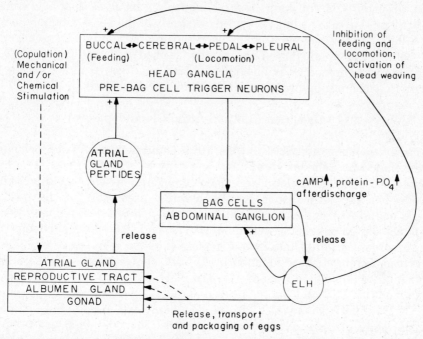

Figure 10. Summary of the neuroendocrine bag cell system. Although there is good evidence for ELH being a hormone, we only suggest, since experiments are lacking, that the atrial gland peptides are likely to be hormones. From Strumwasser et al. (63).

211

Whether peptide B (and other atrial peptides) is released during copulation remains to be determined. It is known that atrial gland factors other than peptides A and B can cause egg-laying, for example, fraction I obtained from Bio-Gel A-0.5 m chromatography (7) and other fractions as described by Arch et al. (92). Since we have recently determined that crude extract of atrial gland will cause egg-laying in *Aplysia* without an abdominal ganglion, it seems likely that one factor will be found in Fraction I and that this factor has direct effects on the gonad.

Since peptide B requires the abdominal ganglion to induce egg-laying, one can inquire whether serotonin can effectively antagonize its actions —we previously demonstrated a profound suppression of ongoing afterdischarge by serotonin (20). We have demonstrated in intact *Aplysia* that a dose of serotonin, calculated to produce a final concentration of $10-5\ M$ inhibited egg-laying in 8/8 animals whether primed with peptide B ($n = 4$) or crude atrial gland homogenate (82). Since ELH still produces egg-laying in the presence of serotonin, it is unlikely that there is a significant direct action of serotonin on egg release from the gonads. These results clearly reinforce the hypothesis that the site of action of peptide B for induction of egg-laying involves the bag cells directly or through the bag cell trigger neurons in the head ganglia.

A third atrial gland peptide has been recently purified and sequenced by Schlesinger et al. (93). This peptide, termed egg-releasing peptide, has extensive homology with both ELH and peptides A and B and appears to cause egg-laying in the absence of the abdominal ganglion.

2.14   Genes for ELH and Atrial Gland Peptides

Recently the genes for ELH and the atrial gland peptides A and B have been cloned by Scheller et. al. (94). The gene for the putative ELH precursor codes for 358 amino acids whose molecular weight would be 41.8 kilodaltons (kd). The genes for the putative precursors of the atrial gland peptides A and B code for 181 and 122 amino acids, respectively, with calculated molecular weights of 20.6 kd and 13.8 kd, respectively.

The organization of these three genes, which code for three peptides involved in reproductive function in *Aplysia*, shows interesting features and inter-relationships (Figure 11). The ELH gene codes for one complete copy of ELH and the acidic peptide and a partial copy of peptide B. The peptide A gene codes for one complete copy of peptide A and a partial copy of ELH and the acidic peptide. The peptide B gene only codes for one complete copy of peptide B and the first six amino acid residues of ELH. Thus these three genes are related even though their products are synthesized in distinctly different tissues and systems.

Another important feature of the three genes is the presence of numerous putative cleavage sites for endopeptidases. Independent of the putative signal sequence cleavage sites, there are nine putative cleav-

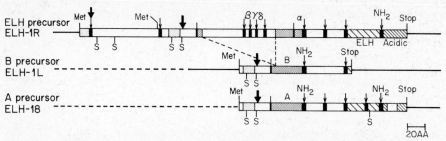

Figure 11. Diagram of the organization of the three peptide genes, involved in reproduction in *Aplysia*. The putative signal sequences are indicated by ☐, peptides A and B by ▨, ELH by ◣ and the acidic peptide by ▧. Redrawn from Scheller et al. (94).

age sites for the ELH gene, five for the peptide A gene and two for the peptide B gene. There is limited information at present as to how many peptide fragments are actually released under physiological conditions from either bag cells or the atrial gland. There is good evidence that during a single bag cell cluster afterdischarge, ELH, the acidic peptide and at least two other smaller peptides are released (19 and Figure 3). While the putative cleavage sites for the three peptide genes may suggest processing steps, such possibilities will have to be checked by actual experiments which are already in progress (95, 96).

REFERENCES

1. H. Kanatani and H. Shirai, *Dev. Growth Differ.* **13**, 53–64 (1971).
2. I. Kupfermann, *Nature* **216**, 814–815 (1967).
3. F. Strumwasser, J. W. Jacklet and R. B. Alvarez, *Comp. Biochem. Physiol.* **29**, 197–206 (1969).
4. L. A. Toevs and R. W. Brackenbury, *Comp. Biochem. Physiol.* **29**, 207–216 (1969).
5. W. P. M. Geraerts and S. Bohlken, *Gen. Comp. Endocrin.* **28**, 350–357 (1976).
6. A. Y. Chiu, M. W. Hunkapiller, E. Heller, D. K. Stuart, L. E. Hood, and F. Strumwasser, *Proc. Natl. Acad. Sci. USA* **76**, 6656–6660 (1979).
7. E. Heller, L. K. Kaczmarek, M. W. Hunkapiller, L. E. Hood, and F. Strumwasser, *Proc. Natl. Acad. Sci. USA* **77**, 2328–2332 (1980).
8. B. Zipser, *Nature* **283**, 857–858 (1980).
9. J. R. Maneillas, J. F. McGinty, A. I. Selverston, H. Karten, and F. E. Bloom, *Nature* **293**, 576–578 (1981).
10. J. Alumets, R. Haranson, F. Sundler, and J. Thorell, *Nature* **279**, 805–806 (1979).
11. H. H. Boer, L. P. C. Schot, E. W. Roubos, A. Ter Maat, J. C. Lodder, D. Reichett, and D. F. Swaab, *Cell Tissue Res.* **202**, 231–240 (1979).
12. Y. Grimm-Jorgensen, *Gen. Comp. Endocrinol.*, in press (1982).
13. H. Bodenmüller and H. C. Schaller, *Nature* **293**, 579–580 (1981).
14. G. J. Dockray, C. Vaillant, and R. G. Williams, *Nature* **293**, 656–657 (1981).
15. L. W. Haynes, *Prog. Neurobiol.* **15**, 205–245 (1980).
16. P. Greengard, Raven Press, New York, 1978, p. 124.
17. D. A. Walsh, J. P. Perkins, and E. G. Krebs, *J. Biol. Chem.* **243**, 3763–3765 (1968).
18. J. W. Truman and R. B. Levine, *Fed. Proc.* **41**, (1982).
19. D. K. Stuart, A. Y. Chiu, and F. Strumwasser, *J. Neurophysiol.* **43**, 488–498 (1980).

20. L. K. Kaczmarek, K. Jennings, and F. Strumwasser, *Proc. Natl. Acad. Sci. USA* **75**, 5200–5204 (1978).
21. K. R. Jennings, L. K. Kaczmarek, R. M. Hewick, W. J. Dreyer, and F. Strumwasser, *J. Neurosci.* **2**, 158–168 (1982).
22. R. E. Coggeshall, *J. Neurophysiol.* **30**, 1263–1287 (1967).
23. W. T. Frazier, E. R. Kandel, I. Kupfermann, R. Waziri, and R. E. Coggeshall, *J. Neurophysiol.* **30**, 1288–1351 (1967).
24. A. Y. Chiu and F. Strumwasser, *J. Neurosci.* **1**, 812–826 (1981).
25. I. Kupfermann and E. R. Kandel, *J. Neurophysiol.* **33**, 865–876 (1970).
26. L. K. Kaczmarek, M. Finbow, J.-P. Revel, and F. Strumwasser, *J. Neurobiol.* **10**, 535–550 (1979).
27. F. Strumwasser, L. K. Kaczmarek, and D. Viele, *Soc. Neurosci. Abstr.* **4**, 207 (1978).
28. P. G. Nelson, in S. Fedoroff and L. Hertz, Eds., *Cell, Tissue, and Organ Cultures in Neurobiology*, Academic Press, pp. 347–368 (1977).
29. L. A. Toevs, Ph.D. Dissertation, California Institute of Technology, 1970.
30. S. Arch, P. Earley, and T. Smock, in *Aplysia californica, J. Gen Physiol.* **68**, 197–210 (1976).
31. M. Hunkapiller and L. E. Hood, *Biochemistry* **17**, 2124–2133 (1978).
32. D. A. Price and M. J. Greenberg, *Science* **197**, 670–671 (1977).
33. B. E. Brown, *Life Sci.* **17**, 1241–1252 (1975).
34. I. Kupfermann, E. Kandel, and R. Coggeshall, *The Physiologist* **9**, 223 (1966).
35. H. Gainer and Z. Wollberg, *J. Neurobiol.* **5**, 243–262 (1974).
36. S. Arch, *J. Gen. Physiol.* **60**, 102–119 (1972).
37. Y. P. Loh, Y. Sarne, and H. Gainer, *J. Comp. Physiol.* **100**, 283–285 (1975).
38. S. W. Kuffler, *Proc R. Soc. Lond.* (Biol.) **168**, 1–21 (1966).
39. F. E. Dudek and S. S. Tobe, *Gen. Comp. Endocrinol.* **36**, 618–627 (1978).
40. D. K. Stuart and F. Strumwasser, in *Aplysia californica, J. Neurophysiol.* **43**, 499–519 (1980).
41. D. Gardner, *Science* **173**, 550–553 (1971).
42. K. R. Weiss, J. L. Cohen, and I. Kupfermann, *J. Neurophysiol.* **41**, 181–203 (1978).
43. J. L. Cohen, K. R. Weiss, and I. Kupfermann, *J. Neurophysiol.* **41**, 157–180 (1978).
44. W. J. Davis, M. V. S. Siegler, and G. J. Mpitsos, *J. Neurophysiol.* **36**, 258–274 (1973).
45. S. B. Kater, *Amer. Zool.* **14**, 1017–1036 (1974).
46. S. B. Kater and C. H. F. Rowell, *J. Neurophysiol.* **36**, 142–155 (1973).
47. M. V. S. Siegler, G. J. Mpitsos, and W. J. Davis, *J. Neurophysiol.* **37**, 1173–1196 (1974).
48. E. Mayeri, P. Brownell, W. D. Branton, and S. B. Simon, *J. Neurophysiol.* **42**, 1165–1184 (1979).
49. E. Mayeri, P. Brownell, and W. D. Branton, *J. Neurophysiol.* **42**, 1185–1197 (1979).
50. B. S. Rothman, P. Brownell, and E. Mayeri, *Soc. Neurosci. Abstr.* **5**, 260 (1979).
51. W. D. Branton, S. Arch, T. Smock, and E. Mayeri, *Proc. Natl. Acad. Sci. USA* **75**, 5732–5736 (1978).
52. F. Strumwasser, F. R. Schlechte, and S. Bower, *Fed. Proc.* **31**, 405 (1972).
53. J. E. Blankenship and J. T. Haskins, *J. Neurophysiol.* **42**, 347–355 (1979).
54. F. E. Dudek and J. E. Blankenship, *Science* **192**, 1009–1010 (1976).
55. J. Acosta-Urqidi and F. E. Dudek, *Soc. Neurosci. Abstr.* **5**, 239 (1979).
56. F. Strumwasser, L. K. Kaczmarek, K. R. Jennings, and A. Y. Chiu, in D. S. Farmer and K. Lederis, Eds., *Neurosecretion: Molecules, Cells, Systems*, Plenum Press, 1981, pp. 251–270.
57. J. P. Miller, K. H. Boswell, R. B. Meyer Jr., L. F. Christensen, and R. K. Robins, *J. Med. Chem.* **23**, 242–251 (1980).
58. L. K. Kaczmarek, K. R. Jennings, and F. Strumwasser, *Brain Res.*, in press (1982).
59. G. R. Siggins, A. P. Oliver, B. J. Hoffer, and F. E. Bloom, *Science* **171**, 192–194 (1971).
60. G. R. Siggins, E. F. Battenberg, B. J. Hoffer, F. E. Bloom, and A. L. Steiner, *Science* **179**, 585–588 (1973).

61. J. F. Kuo and P. Greengard, *Proc. Natl. Acad. Sci. USA* **64**, 1349–1355 (1969).
62. L. K. Kaczmarek, K. R. Jennings, F. Strumwasser, A. C. Nairn, U. Walter, F. D. Wilson, and P. Greengard, *Proc. Natl. Acad. Sci. USA* **77**, 7487–7491 (1980).
63. F. Strumwasser, L. K. Kaczmarek, A. Y. Chiu, E. Heller, K. Jennings, and D. Viele, in F. Bloom, Ed., *Peptides: Integrators of Cell and Tissue Functions*, Raven Press, 1980, pp. 197–218.
64. L. K. Kaczmarek and F. Strumwasser, *J. Neurosci.* **1**, 626–634 (1981).
65. L. K. Kaczmarek and F. Strumwasser, *Soc. Neurosci. Abstr.* **7**, 932 (1981).
66. E. Meher and B. Sakmann, *Nature* **260**, 799–802 (1976).
67. F. J. Sigworth and E. Neher, *Nature* **287**, 447–449 (1980).
68. F. Strumwasser, in J. Aschoff, Ed., *Circadian Clocks*, North-Holland, Amsterdam, 1965, pp. 442–462.
69. F. Strumwasser, in G. C. Quarton, T. Melnechuk, and F. O. Schmitt, Eds., *The Neurosciences: An Intensive Study Program*, Rockefeller University Press, New York, 1967, pp. 516–528.
70. J. W. Jacklet, *J. Exp. Biol.* **85**, 33–42 (1980).
71. B. S. Rothman and F. Strumwasser, *J. Gen. Physiol.* **68**, 359–384 (1976).
72. B. S. Rothman and F. Strumwasser, *Fed. Proc.* **36**, 2050–2055 (1977).
73. J. C. Woolum and F. Strumwasser, *Proc. Natl. Acad. Sci. USA* **77**, 5542–5546 (1980).
74. R. W. Meech, *Comp. Biochem. Physiol.* **42**, 493–499 (1972).
75. R. W. Meech and F. Strumwasser, *Fed. Proc.* **29**, 834 (1970).
76. A. Marty, *Nature* **291**, 497–500 (1981).
77. B. S. Pallotta, K. L. Magleby, and J. N. Barrett, *Nature* **293**, 471–474 (1981).
78. A. L. F. Gorman and M. V. Thomas, *J. Physiol.* **275**, 357–376 (1978).
79. I. B. Levitan and W. B. Adams, *Adv. Cyclic Nucleotide Res.* **14**, 647–653 (1981).
80. V. F. Castellucci, E. R. Kandel, J. H. Schwartz, F Wilson, A. C. Nairn, and P. Greengard, *Proc. Natl. Acad. Sci. USA* **77**, 7492–7496 (1980).
81. M. V. Brunelli, V. Castellucci, and E. R. Kandel, *Science* **194**, 1178–1181 (1976).
82. K. R. Jennings, J. J. Host, L. K. Kaczmarek, and F. Strumwasser, *J. Neurobiol.* **12**, 579–590 (1981).
83. S. J. Enna, J. P. Bennett Jr., D. R. Burt, I. Creese, and S. H. Snyder, *Nature* **263**, 338–341 (1976).
84. A. H. Drummond, F. Bucher, and I. B. Levitan, *Nature* **272**, 368–370 (1978).
85. M. Klein and E. R. Kandel, *Proc. Natl. Acad. Sci. USA* **75**, 3512–3516 (1978).
86. E. R. Kandel, *Soc. Neurosci. Monogr.*, 1978 p. 90.
87. R. M. Macleod, in L. Martini and W. F. Ganong, Eds., *Frontiers in Neuroendocrinology*, Vol. 4, Raven Press, New York, 1976, pp. 169–194.
88. G. A. Gudelsky and J. C. Porter, *Endocrinology* **104**, 583–587 (1979).
89. P. S. Taraskevich and W. W. Douglas, *Proc. Natl. Acad. Sci. USA* **74**, 4064–4067 (1977).
90. C. Denef, D. Manet, and R. Dewals, *Nature* **285**, 243–246 (1980).
91. F. Strumwasser, *The Physiol.* **16**, 9–42 (1973).
92. S. Arch, T. Smock, R. Gurvis, and C. McCarthy, *J. Comp. Physiol.* **128**, 67–70 (1978).
93. D. H. Schlesinger, S. P. Babirak, and J. E. Blankenship, in D. H. Schlesinger, Ed., *Symposium on Neurohypophyseal Peptide Hormones and Other Biologically Active Peptides*, Elsevier/North-Holland, Amsterdam, in press.
94. R. H. Scheller, J. F. Jackson, L. B. McAllister, B. S. Rothman, E. Mayeri and R. Axel, *Cell* **32**, 7–22 (1983).
95. R. W. Berry, *Biochemistry* **20**, 6200–6205 (1981).
96. R. W. Berry, M. J. Trump and J. T. Baylen, *Biochemistry* **20**, 6206–6211 (1981).

8

Crustacean Neuropeptides

DAVID A. PRICE
C. V. Whitney Laboratory
St. Augustine, Florida

1 PHYLOGENETIC RELATIONS

All the invertebrate groups considered in this book are included in only
one of the two major lines of animal evolution, the protostomes. The
other line, the deuterostomes, culminates in the vertebrates. Thus, one
can expect the invertebrate groups discussed here to have more similarities to each other than to the vertebrates. Actually, the three invertebrate groups discussed, crustaceans, insects, and molluscs, represent
only a very small part of the taxonomic diversity present in the animal
kingdom. Though the insects and crustacea are given separate chapters,
this is more a reflection of the popularity of these groups as experimental animals than of their distinctiveness of form and function. There is
some tendency to elevate the crustaceans and insects to the rank of distinct phlya (1), but the two groups are very similar and the important
question is whether or not they should be given equal status in the arthropod phylum or lumped together in one subphylum, the mandibu-
lates. In any event, there are many close similarities between insect
and crustacean neuropeptides and endocrine systems, and it is certainly
advantageous to think of them as variants of a single theme. In contrast, the molluscs, and their peptides, are distinct from the arthropods.
Finally, much of the work on invertebrates has been done on only a
very small selection of species. In particular, most crustacean studies
were of one order, the Decapoda, so throughout this chapter the term
crustacean usually carries the more restricted sense of decapod crustacean.

The endocrine physiology of the decapods has been studied for
years, so that a number of references can be consulted for historical
perspective and general background on the physiology and anatomy (2–
4). More current information about the neuropeptides themselves has
also been summarized (5, 6). Here, I briefly review the endocrine structures found in these animals, describe the major homeostatic systems
for which endocrine regulation is known, and discuss the chemistry and
physiology of those neuropeptides which have been well characterized.

2 ENDOCRINE STRUCTURES

Crustaceans have three known non-neural endocrine glands: the Y-organ, the ovary, and the androgenic gland (2–4). The Y-organ serves the
same function as, and is probably homologous to, the prothoracic
(ecdysial or molting) gland of insects (see J. W. Truman and P. H.
Taghert, Chapter 6 in this volume): it secretes ecdysteroids involved in
the initiation of molt. The ovary secretes hormones involved in the development and maintenance of secondary female sex characteristics.
The androgenic gland, usually located adjacent to the vas deferens, is

responsible for the development of male sexual characteristics, including the development of the gonad as a testes.

Three neurohemal organs (neurohormone storage and release areas) are also known: the sinus gland, the postcommissural organs, and the pericardial organs. The sinus gland is located in the eyestalks of those species with stalked eyes; thus, it is very amenable to experimental extirpation by removal of the entire eyestalk. Eyestalk ablation actually removes part of the source of hormone in addition to the release site. One group of neuronal cell bodies that supply axons to the sinus gland is located right in the eyestalk: this is the medulla terminalis ganglionic X-organ (MTGXO), often called simply the X-organ. The sinus gland X-organ complex, or either part alone, can be removed leaving the rest of the eye intact, but this is technically more difficult. The pericardial organs and the postcommissural organs are located deep within the body of the animal and are supplied extensively by neurosecretory cells in the central nervous system (CNS), making them very difficult to study by simple ablation. Consequently, the eyestalk hormones have been associated with many more physiological processes than either the pericardial organs or the postcommissural organs.

3 HOMEOSTATIC SYSTEMS

3.1 Ecdysis (Molting)

Like all arthropods, crustaceans are covered with a hard exoskeleton. Molting, the periodic shedding and replacement of this exoskeleton, is one of the most characteristic features of arthropod physiology. One tends to think of molting as an intermittent phenomenon, but except for some species that undergo a terminal molt and never molt again, the process is more or less continuous for the lifetime of the animal, with recovery from one molt followed by preparation for the next. The actual act of molting, ecdysis, is initiated by ecdysteriod hormones secreted by the Y-organs. Once the first external signs of impending molt appear, molting will go to completion even if the Y-organs are removed. The Y-organs are under inhibitory neuroendocrine control by the X-organ-sinus gland complex, so that eyestalk ablation usually leads to accelerated molt cycles. Most of the tissue growth of the animal takes place between molts, but there is often a dramatic size increase at the molt caused by uptake of water. Eyestalk ablation often leads to an abnormally large uptake of water at the molt; but this effect seems to be independent of the molt inhibiting hormone.

Significant changes in mineral metabolism occur at the molt as minerals are removed from the old exoskeleton and deposited in various tissue stores, and there are also changes in carbohydrate and possibly protein metabolism at the molt. It is not known if these changes are under independent hormonal control. Though the most obvious reason for molting is to accommodate increases in tissue mass, molting is not only associated with size increase but also serves other functions, such as appearance or loss of secondary sexual characteristics, metamorphosis, and the regeneration of lost appendages (7). Loss of appendages does accelerate the molt cycle, but it is not known how.

3.2 Reproduction

The eyestalks contain a gonad inhibiting hormone. Eyestalk ablation often leads to increased gonadal (particularly ovarian) growth. To a certain extent there seems to be an antagonism between somatic and reproductive growth. Depending on time of year, age of the animal, and other factors, eyestalk removal leads either to gonadal growth or accelerated molt cycles, but in most species, not both (8). In males the androgenic gland, rather than the testes, is responsible for the development of secondary sexual characteristics and is probably the target of the gonad inhibiting hormone (9). The possibility that the gonad inhibiting hormone is also the molt inhibiting hormone has been discussed (8).

3.3 Metabolism and Activity

Factors from the eyestalk are thought to have a general inhibitory or depressing action on metabolism. Destalked animals exhibit a higher oxygen consumption; this effect can be at least partially reversed by injection of eyestalk extracts. A factor isolated from various crustacean eyestalks, neurodepressing hormone, has been shown to reduce spontaneous neural activity (10, 11).

A hyperglycemic hormone is also present in the eyestalks (12). Destalked animals do not always show reduced blood glucose levels, but they do lose the ability to elevate their blood sugar in response to environmental stimuli.

The secretions of the pericardial organ seem to work in opposition to those of the eyestalk so far as activity is concerned. These organs release both peptide and nonpeptide materials (amines) into the blood returning from the gills to the heart, from which they can be rapidly distributed throughout the animal. Both the peptides and amines have excitatory actions on the heart and seem to be positive modulators of neuromuscular transmission. There is now evidence that one peptide is very similar to, if not identical with, proctolin (see Section 4.4).

3.4 Color Change and Light Adaptation

Crustaceans have pigment cells, or chromatophores, located in the hypodermis and also in the deeper-lying tissues of the body. The pigment granules in the chromatophores can be of various colors, and the cells

are often named for the pigment they contain: erythrophores, melano-
phores, leucophores, and so on. The number and distribution of different
colored chromatophores varies with species from as few as two colors
evenly distributed to four or more arranged in complex patterns.

Chromatophores show rapid changes in the distribution of their pigment granules. Various environmental factors affect the degree of dispersion of the pigments, and there is also an underlying circadian
rhythm of dispersion in many species. Pigment movement is not neurally mediated. The changes in dispersion are in part hormonally controlled and in part a direct response of the chromatophores to
environmental factors such as light and temperature. The relative contributions of the hormonal and environmental factors to the degree of
dispersion found in normal animals is poorly understood for the chromatophores, but somewhat better known for the pigments of the eye.

In the compound eye of crustacea three pigments can be distinguished. The proximal pigment is the primary screening pigment of excess light; it is contained in the retinal cells and migrates almost
exclusively in response to illumination of the eye and not to hormonal
levels. The distal pigment is controlled almost exclusively by hormones.
The third pigment is the reflecting pigment; it responds to both illumination and hormones. The reflecting pigment is white, like the pigment of
the leucophores, and it is interesting that the leucophores, too, are relatively insensitive to pigment effector hormones and are more directly
sensitive to light than the other chromatophores.

There has been much discussion in the past about the number of distinct hormones affecting the pigment cells (13). Confusion was created
by many factors, but it now appears, at least in shrimp, that there are
only two hormones: one causing dispersion of the chromatophores and
light adaptation of the eye, and the other causing concentration of the
chromotophores and possibly dark adaptation of the eye. There may be
species variation in these hormones and their receptors, but the evidence is not at all clear. This question is discussed further in Section
4.2 on the pigment dispersing hormone.

4 NEUROPEPTIDES

4.1 Pigment Concentrating Hormone (PCH)

In a series of very elegant studies, Fernlund and Josefsson (14–16) purified the red pigment concentrating hormone of a prawn and determined
its sequence (Table 1). Since this peptide is found at very low concentrations in the prawn eyestalk (about 5 pmole/animal), a considerable
degree (about 10^6 fold) of purification was required and still only small
amounts were available for sequencing. The first sequence determination depended partially on mass spectroscopy, but later chemical se-

TABLE 1 Some Arthropod Neuropeptides

Peptide Name	Species	MW (daltons)	Structure (or Composition)	Reference
Pigment concentrating hormone (PCH)	*Pandalus borealis*	950	Glp-Leu-Asn-Phe-Ser-Pro-Gly-Trp-NH$_2$	15
Adipokinetic hormone (AKH)	*Locusta migratoria*	1150	Glp-Leu-Asn-Phe-Thr-Pro-Asn-Trp-Gly-Thr-NH$_2$	18
Locust factor II	*Schistocerca americana gregaria*	1000	Glx$_1$Leu$_1$Asx$_1$Phe$_1$Thr$_1$Ser$_1$Gly$_1$Gly$_1$Trp$_1$ (NH$_3$)$_1$[a]	20
Neurodepressing hormone	*Procambarus bouvieri*	1000	Glx or Asx Val Thr Pro Gly Ala Ser (NH$_3$)[a] with Leu/Ile	11
Pigment dispersing hormone (PDH)	*Pandalus borealis*	2000	Asn-Ser-Gly-Met-Ile-Asn-Ser-Ile-Leu-Gly-Ile-Pro-Arg-Val-Met-Thr-Glu-Ala-NH$_2$	23
Hyperglycemic hormone	*Carcinus maenus*	6700	Asx$_9$ Thr$_2$ Ser$_4$ Glx$_5$ Pro, Gly, Ala$_4$ Cys$_4$ Val$_4$ Met$_3$ Ile, Leu$_5$ Tyr$_4$ Phe$_2$ Trp, His, Lys$_2$ Arg$_4$	27
Proctolin	*Periplaneta americana*	650	Arg-Tyr-Leu-Pro-Thr	36

[a] Glx is either Glp (pyroglutamic acid) or Gln; Asx is Asn; and the carboxyl terminal is amidated to account for the electrophoretic immobility of these peptides.

222

quencing of the entire molecule was also done. The sequence was borne out by synthesis which, of course, is always the ultimate test. This peptide should be renamed pigment concentrating hormone (PCH) since synthetic samples of this peptide are active on chromatophores other than the erythrophores. In shrimp, leucophore (*Palaemon*) (17) and melanophore (*Cragon*) (18) pigments are also concentrated by this peptide.

No immunoassay has yet been reported for the pigment concentrating hormone. This is probably because the hormone has the very unusual property (for a peptide) of having no ionizable groups. Thus, it is immobile during electrophoresis at any pH and cannot be easily conjugated to a carrier protein for the production of antibodies. A further deterrent is that the peptide, lacking histidine and tyrosine, cannot be iodinated, and though its Tyr[4] analog is active and can be iodinated, iodination has led to a complete loss of biological activity (19).

Pigment concentrating hormone is homologous to the adipokinetic hormone (AKH) of locusts (see Chapter 6), which also lacks ionizable groups. It is interesting that AKH has a glycyl residue in the position corresponding to the terminal amide of PCH (see Table 1). It has been suggested that a C-terminal glycine is the signal for the cellular amidifying system (20). Thus, a single base-change of a Thr codon (ACA) to an Arg codon (AGA) in the AKH gene might have led to processing changes giving rise to an octapeptide amide instead of a decapeptide amide. A second electrophoretically immobile peptide has been isolated from locusts (21); judged by its amino acid composition (see Table 1), it seems to have structural affinities with both peptides.

Physiological studies with synthetic PCH and AKH have shown that PCH has adipokinetic activity in locusts and AKH has pigment-concentrating activity in shrimp (18). Both hormones also have hyperglycemic activity, but their potencies vary independently with species. For example, in crabs, AKH has hyperglycemic activity but not PCH, whereas in cockroaches both peptides have hyperglycemic activity but PCH is the more potent (18). Extracts of cockroach corpora cardiaca have adipokinetic activity in locusts and hyperglycemic activity in the roaches themselves (22). These activities reside in two distinct electrophoretically immobile peptides, neither identical with AKH.

To further complicate matters, the neurodepressing hormone of crayfish is another electrophoretically immobile peptide, similar in size to AKH and PCH (about 1000 daltons). However, it does not appear to have any aromatic residues or an N-terminal pyroglutamyl residue, though the N-terminal is blocked (11). An amino acid composition has been reported, but since it was not quantitative, it must be considered very tentative (see Table 1). The neurodepressing hormone is found at only very low levels in the eyestalks of crayfish (5 pmole/animal), similar to the levels of PCH in prawns (5 pmole/animal) but much less than the levels of other characterized eyestalk neuropeptides.

All of the electrophoretically immobile peptides of arthropods should be considered as homologs. Though many neuropeptides have blocked terminals, only those above completely lack ionizable side chains. Insects probably have two distinct but related peptides of this group while the number in crustacea is still uncertain, but may be only one. The peptides in this family clearly have a variety of actions and their physiological roles are, in several species, still very much undetermined.

4.2 Pigment Dispersing Hormone (PDH)

The light adapting hormone from *Pandulus borealis* was purified and sequenced by Fernlund (23, 24). This peptide is larger than the PCH and is present in much greater (about 30-fold) quantity than PCH; however, as if to make up for this, it is much less stable. It contains two methionyl residues; but the appearance of multiple peaks of activity suggests that some oxidation can be tolerated without complete loss of activity. This instability makes it hard to determine if there are distinct physiological forms of this peptide, but this is unlikely, at least in *Pandulus*, because all of the peaks separated have the same spectrum of activities. No immunoassay has been described for the pigment dispersing hormone. Fernlund used migration of the distal retinal pigment to the light adapted position as his bioassay, but as soon as synthetic peptide became available, it was shown to disperse pigment in the chromatophores also (25). Pigment-dispersing activity can be extracted from the nervous system of the horseshoe crab (26), but it is not known how similar this substance is to the crustacean peptide. Keller (27) found no significant differences in the electrophoretic mobilities of pigment dispersing hormones from several species, so there probably is not very much variation within the crustacea (or at least the decapods).

The lack of radioimmunoassays for both pigment effector hormones has greatly hindered progress in crustacean neuropeptides. Hormones are still measured by bioassays which respond in as yet uncharacterized ways to mixtures of the two pigment effector hormones. It is not known whether chromatophores respond to the ratio of concentrating-to-dispersing activity or if one is dominant above a certain threshold or even if the various chromatophores respond to the same parameter. Crabs seem to be less responsive to PCH, but is this due to a very high titer of PDH or some difference in the receptor. These questions and many more could be answered if an assay were developed to quantitate the levels of the two hormones in mixtures—they are unanswerable without such an assay.

4.3 Hyperglycemic Hormone

The hyperglycemic activity of eyestalk extracts is still enigmatic. The hyperglycemic activity in crustacean eyestalk extracts resides in peptides of fairly large size (6000–7000), which have considerable species specificity (12, 27). In particular, the peptides from crabs seem to be active only in crabs while those in crayfish and lobsters are only active within this group. Yet the adipokinetic hormone of locusts is hyperglycemic in crabs at concentrations comparable to those of the native hormone, whereas the pigment concentrating hormone of prawns, with a very similar structure, has no such effect (18). Thus there is marked specificity on the one hand and marked nonspecificity on the other. Perhaps these hyperglycemic effects are pharmacological rather than physiological; it has already been mentioned that eyestalk ablation often has no effect on blood glucose levels (Section 3.3) but does block the hyperglycemic response to stress.

Recently Keller and Wunderer (28) purified the hyperglycemic hormone from isolated sinus glands rather than whole eyestalks. Since the sinus gland consists almost entirely of neurosecretory axon terminals, it would be expected to be a purer source of hormone than the whole eyestalks, and it is. The hyperglycemic hormone is the major peptide in aqueous extracts of the sinus gland and accounts for 10–20% of the water-soluble protein.

The extremely high concentration of the hyperglycemic hormone in sinus gland is, at first, disturbing; particularly, considering the number of hormonal activities the eyestalk is reputed to contain. Of course, one peptide might have several hormonal activities. The possibility raised by Jaros and Keller (29), that the hyperglycemic hormone might be the molt inhibiting hormone, deserves serious consideration. The molt inhibiting hormone is synthesized in the medulla terminalis ganglionic X-organ (MTGXO) as determined by extirpation experiments (discussed in ref. 2) and this organ appears to be chiefly devoted to synthesis of the hyperglycemic hormone (by immunocytochemistry). Furthermore, it seems to be the same group of large neurons that stain for the hyperglycemic hormone that also show marked change in secretory activity correlated with the molt cycle (2, 30).

This hypothesis is exciting because the techniques needed to test it are in hand. Jaros (28) has used extracts of sinus gland to raise antibodies in rabbits. Not unexpectedly the antisera obtained gave positive staining of terminals in the sinus gland and cell bodies in the X-organ. Perhaps less expected, is the abolition of specific staining by preincubation with purified hyperglycemic hormone. It was also possible to develop a radioimmunoassay using iodinated hyperglycemic hormone (31). With these two techniques it should be possible to determine if the hyperglycemic hormone is also a molt inhibiting hormone.

4.4 Proctolin

Proctolin (see Chapter 6) is a pentapeptide first isolated from the hindgut of cockroaches. A peptide having the biological activity of proctolin on several assay systems and very similar, if not identical, mobility on several chromatographic and electrophoretic systems was found in the pericardial organs of a crab (*Cardisoma carnifer*) (32). Immunoreactive proctolin is found throughout the lobster nervous system, but the bulk is in the pericardial organs and associated structures, and the specific activity (per mg protein) in the pericardial organs is 400 times that in the brain (33). These results, taken together, are good evidence for the presence of proctolin or a close homolog in the crustacean nervous system.

Proctolin has many actions on crustacean muscle and nerve. It has an excitatory action on crustacean heart, activity long associated with the pericardial organ peptides, and it appears to be mediated through the cardiac ganglion rather than by a direct action on the muscle (34). Proctolin acts directly on certain muscles to increase the force of neurally invoked contractions or even to initiate contractions. In the opener muscle of the dactyl of the walking leg of the lobster (*Homarus*), such effects occur without any measurable change in membrane potential or resistance. Furthermore, such effects occur at very low peptide concentrations (threshold is $10^{-10}\,M$ for effects on the opener muscle), below the levels measured in lobster hemolymph by radioimmunoassay ($4 \times 10^{-10}\,M$), so that these effects appear to be physiological.

There are some interesting parallels between proctolin and the molluscan neuropeptide FMRFamide (36). Both peptides are cardioexcitatory, both are small (500 daltons) and basic; both seem to be released into the blood, and both have excitatory actions on many different, but not all, muscles in the animals. They are clearly not homologous peptides, but they do seem to perform analogous functions.

5 SUMMARY

Three distinct, well-characterized peptides are found in the crustacean sinus gland. One, the hyperglycemic hormone, is synthesized primarily, if not exclusively, in the medulla terminalis ganglionic X-organ and is the major peptide in the sinus gland. Another, the pigment dispersing hormone, is also found in other parts of the central nervous system and is probably released from the postcommissural organs as well as the sinus gland. Very little is known about the synthesis and distribution of the third peptide, the pigment concentrating hormone.

Each of these peptides may have several hormonal activities. The pigment dispersing hormone is also the light adapting hormone of the distal retinal pigment; the hyperglycemic hormone may be the molt inhibiting hormone (Section 4.3), and the pigment concentrating hormone may be the neurodepressing hormone (Section 4.1). It remains to be seen if other hormonal activities attributed to the sinus gland reside in these three peptides.

One peptide of known structure, proctolin, has been detected in the crustacean pericardial organ, and others may be present; several hormonal activities have been ascribed to the pericardial organs. Little is known about the peptides of the postcommissural organs except that pigment-dispersing activity is present.

There is no endocrine organ equivalent to the pituitary in the crustacea. All of the known peptide hormones are secreted directly by neurons. Of the non-neural glands described, the Y-organs secrete steroids and the chemical nature of the androgenic gland hormone and the ovarian hormone are unknown. Since the neuroendocrine organs must take the place of the pituitary, they should contain high levels of peptide, more comparable to those of the pituitary than to those of the hypothalamus. The very high levels of egg-laying hormone in the bag cells of *Aplysia* (see F. Strumwasser, Chapter 7 in this volume) are similar to the high levels of hyperglycemic hormone in sinus gland, suggesting that this may be the general protosome arrangement.

REFERENCES

1. S. M. Manton, *The Arthropoda: Habits, Functional Morphology, and Evolution*, Clarendon Press, Oxford, 1977.
2. D. B. Carlisle and F. Knowles, *Endocrine Control in Crustaceans*, Cambridge University Press, Cambridge, 1959.
3. A. P. M. Lockwood, *Aspects of the Physiology of Crustacea*, W. H. Freeman, San Francisco, 1967.
4. A. S. Tombes, *An Introduction to Invertebrate Endocrinology*, Academic Press, New York, 1970.
5. N. Frontali and H. Gainer, in H. Gainer, Ed., *Peptides in Neurobiology*, Plenum Press, New York, 1977, pp. 259–294.
6. L. W. Haynes, *Prog. Neurobiol.*, **15**, 205 (1980).
7. D. E. Bliss, S. M. E. Wang, and E. A. Martinez, *Am. Zool.* **6**, 197 (1966).
8. K. G. Adiyodi and R. G. Adiyodi, *Biol. Rev.* **45**, 121 (1970).
9. T. Subramoniam, *J. Sci. Ind. Res.* **40**, 396 (1981).
10. H. Arechiga, A. Huberman, and E. Naylor, *Proc. R. Soc. Lond., B.* **187**, 299 (1974).
11. A. Huberman, H. Arechiga, A. Cimet, J. De La Rossa, and C. Aramburo, *Eur. J. Biochem.* **99**, 203 (1979).
12. L. H. Kleinholz and R. Keller, *Gen. Comp. Endocrinol.* **21**, 554 (1973).
13. L. H. Kleinholz, *Am. Zool.* **16**, 151 (1976).
14. P. Fernlund and L. Josefsson, *Biochim. Biophys. Acta* **158**, 262 (1968).
15. P. Fernlund and L. Josefsson, *Science* **177**, 173 (1972).
16. P. Fernlund, *Biochim. Biophys. Acta* **371**, 304 (1974).
17. L. Josefsson, *Gen. Comp. Endocrinol.* **25**, 199 (1975).
18. W. Mordue and J. V. Stone, *Gen. Comp. Endocrinol.* **33**, 103 (1977).
19. M. Christensen, J. Carlsen, and L. Josefsson, *Hoppe-Seyler's Z. Physiol. Chem.* **360**, 1051 (1979).
20. G. Suchanek and G. Kreil, *Proc. Natl. Acad. Sci.* **74**, 975 (1977).
21. J. Carlsen, W. S. Herman, M. Christensen, and L. Josefsson, *Insect Biochem.* **9**, 497 (1979).
22. D. A. Holwerda, E. Weeda, and J. M. Van Doorn, *Insect Biochem.* **7**, 477 (1977).
23. P. Fernlund, *Biochim. Biophys. Acta* **237**, 519 (1971).
24. P. Fernlund, *Biochim. Biophys. Acta* **439**, 17 (1976).
25. L. H. Kleinholz, *Nature* **258**, 256 (1975).

26. P. D. Pezalla, R. M. Dores, and W. S. Herman, *Biol. Bull. (Woods Hole),* **154,** 148 (1978).
27. R. Keller, *J. Comp. Physiol.* **122,** 359 (1977).
28. R. Keller and G. Wunderer, *Gen. Comp. Endocrinol.* **34,** 328 (1978).
29. P. P. Jaros, *Histochemistry* **63,** 303 (1979).
30. P. P. Jaros and R. Keller, *Cell Tissue Res.* **204,** 379 (1979).
31. P. P. Jaros and R. Keller, *Experientia* **35,** 1252 (1979).
32. R. E. Sullivan, *J. Exp. Zool.* **210,** 543 (1979).
33. T. L. Schwarz, G. Lee, and E. A. Kravitz, *Neurosci. Abstr.* **7,** 253 (1981).
34. M. W. Miller and R. E. Sullivan, *J. Neurobiol.* **12,** 629 (1981).
35. T. L. Schwarz, R. M. Harris Warrick, S. Glusman, E. A. Kravitz, *J. Neurobiol.* **11,** 623 (1980).
36. M. J. Greenberg, in B. Lofts, Ed., *Proceedings of the 9th International Symposium on Comparative Endocrinology,* Hong Kong University Press, in press (1983).
37. A. N. Starratt and B. W. Brown, *Life Sciences* **17,** 1253 (1975).

9

Mechanisms Governing Peptidergic Phenotypic Expression and Development

J. A. KESSLER

I. B. BLACK

*Division of Developmental Neurology
Cornell University Medical College
New York, New York*

1 INTRODUCTION

The study of neuronal ontogeny has elucidated mechanisms governing neurotransmitter phenotypic expression and has helped define the phenomenon of neuronal plasticity. Recent work has indicated that neuronal function, capability, and even phenotype may be altered by changes in the extracellular and extraembryonic milieu (1–9). Moreover, neuronal mutability is not restricted to the conventional developmental period but extends into adult life: appropriate evironmental stimuli alter transmitter phenotypic expression in mature as well as immature neurons (10, 11). Indeed, emerging evidence suggests that continuing neuronal change is the rule, not the exception, and that transmitter mutability may be central to neuronal function.

The potential scope of plasticity has been vastly expanded by the discovery that peptides may function as neurotransmitters, and that peptides and "conventional" transmitters, such as norepinephrine, may coexist in the same neuron (12, 13). Since there are now close to 30 identified putative peptide transmitters, the potential field for neuronal flexibility and variability is immense. However, the study of peptide neurotransmitter development is just beginning, and knowledge of the molecular mechanisms governing peptidergic ontogeny is limited. Consequently, it may be helpful to review principles of development derived from studies of conventional transmitters before focusing on peptidergic ontogeny and regulation.

The study of peripheral sympathetic and sensory ganglia has been particularly useful in defining mechanisms governing neuronal ontogeny, since these structures provide readily accessible and easily manipulated systems, allowing a variety of experimental perturbations. Moreover, autonomic neurons use a number of well-characterized transmitters, including norepinephrine and acetylcholine, and extremely sensitive techniques are available to measure noradrenergic and cholinergic gene products. This has permitted detailed examination of the development of individual characters which, in aggregate, constitute the noradrenergic and cholinergic phenotypes.

This introductory section examines autonomic and sensory development in sequence, from embryonic neural crest formation to postnatal ganglion regulation, to illustrate the variety of influences affecting transmitter phenotypic expression (for a more detailed review, see ref. 14). In particular, the events governing expression of noradrenergic and cholinergic traits are examined to provide the background for considering peptidergic development in autonomic and sensory neurons. We then discuss the development of peptides in peripheral sensory ganglia and proceed to outline ontogeny and regulation in the sympathetic superior cervical ganglion. These sections, in turn, provide the background for considering regulation in different neuronal populations and for analyzing the role of specific environmental stimuli, such as calcium, in peptide regulation. Finally, comparisons are made between processes regulating different peptide transmitters, to begin defining general rules that may govern peptide development throughout the nervous system.

2 NEURAL CREST MIGRATION AND INITIAL PHENOTYPIC EXPRESSION

Peripheral autonomic and sensory neurons arise from the neural crest, a transient embryonic structure which develops from the neural plate, neural folds, and neural tube (15–17). From a dorsal, midline position adjacent to the neural tube, crest cells migrate throughout the embryo, giving rise not only to neurons, but also to chromatophores, nonneuronal cells of the peripheral nervous system, chromaffin cells, calcitonin-producing cells, and mesenchymal derivatives of the cephalic region (18). What processes lead to the emergence of multiple cell lines from this common progenitor? Recent studies suggest that the embryonic microenvironment encountered during migration, and at the definitive site, are crucial in determining cell fate (for review see ref. 19). In particular, increasing evidence suggests that cellular interactions are pivotal in determining neuronal phenotype.

In the chick embryo, the appearance of catecholamine histofluorescence in presumptive sympathoblasts is influenced by interactions with somitic mesenchyme, and therefore may require ventral crest migration (20). Moreover, ventral neural tube ablation reduces the quantity of nervous tissue formed, suggesting that critical interactions occur between neural tube, somitic mesenchyme, and neurons. These observations are supported by studies in culture showing that crest must be contiguous with somite for catecholaminergic expression, and that ventral neural tube may act across a Millipore filter to induce appropriate changes in somite (21). The crucial role of the embryonic environment is further illustrated by a series of studies in avian species involving transplantation of neural crest tissue. Normally the neural crest in the trunk region gives rise to catecholaminergic sympathetic ganglion and adrenomedullary cells, whereas the "vagal" region (somites 1–7) gives rise to cholinergic enteric ganglion cells. However, if trunk (sympathoadrenal) crest is grafted to the vagal region, cells colonize the gut to form cholinergic enteric populations. Conversely, cephalic trunk transplanted to the trunk region gives rise to catecholaminergic adrenomedullary chromaffin tissue (22). These studies suggest that preferential migratory pathways are located at precise levels of the crest in the embryo, and that the expression of a given phenotype may be regulated by the environment of the migratory pathway or the definitive site or both.

In contrast with these observations, other studies suggest that environmental cues may not be necessary for crest cells to express transmitter phenotypes. Crest neuroblasts in culture can express noradrenergic traits in the absence of the normal embryonic microenvironment (23). Moreover, cells derived from a single clone in the same cell culture initially express catecholamine fluorescence or melanin (23), suggesting that interaction with somite, neural tube, or other crest cells may not be an absolute requirement for differentiation. Consequently, at least some noradrenergic traits can be expressed in artificial environments of undefined composition. Thus the crest neuroblast is neither wholly predetermined regarding initial transmitter expression nor a true blank slate simply reflecting environmental signals.

3   MUTABILITY OF NEURONAL PHENOTYPE

Does the early expression of neurotransmitter characters during embryogenesis represent irrevocable commitment to that phenotype? Recent work suggests that under certain conditions, neurotransmitter phenotypic development may be mutable. For example, a population of cells in the embryonic gut transiently expresses noradrenergic characters including the biosynthetic enzymes tyrosine hydroxylase and dopamine-β-hydroxylase and catecholamine itself. These traits disappear during the ensuing days, although the cells themselves apparently persist (24–26). The ultimate transmitter fate of this population is unknown, but it is clear that noradrenergic characters may be expressed and subsequently lost. Similar observations have been made in the sympathetic innervation of rat eccrine sweat glands, in which noradrenergic fibers apparently convert to cholinergic nerves (27). Thus the early expression of neurotransmitter phenotypic characters does not necessarily represent an irrevocable commitment to that transmitter.

The foregoing *in vivo* studies are complemented by extensive *in vitro* experiments indicating that noradrenergic sympathetic neurons may acquire cholinergic characteristics under appropriate conditions. Neonatal rat sympathetic neurons grown in dissociated cell culture develop catecholaminergic properties, as indicated by morphological and biochemical criteria (3, 28). Under appropriate conditions, the cultured neurons continue to develop catecholaminergic properties, qualitatively paralleling ontogeny *in vivo*. In particular, norepinephrine synthesis increases when cells are grown in the presence of depolarizing stimuli (9). Conversely, growth under certain conditions reverses early catecholaminergic development, and cholinergic differentiation occurs instead. Sympathetic neurons grown in the presence of certain types of non-neuronal cells synthesize and store acetylcholine and form functional cholinergic synapses with appropriate cholinergic morphologic junctions (3, 7, 29, 30). The non-neuronal cells apparently produce a factor that enhances cholinergic expression without altering overall neuronal survival and growth (4, 6). Moreover, cholinergic–noradrenergic "dual function" cells have been identified in culture (31), indicating that these choices are not mutually exclusive. Consequently, there is apparently no cellular mechanism that *a priori* prevents simultaneous expression of more than one transmitter phenotype.

4 POSTNATAL DEVELOPMENT AND REGULATION

Since the foregoing studies employed neonatal ganglia, it is clear that phenotypic expression remains mutable long after neuroblast migration has terminated in the embryo. In fact, such plasticity apparently extends into adult life (32). Once the adult phenotype is expressed qualitatively, environmental cues regulate the developmental increase of phenotypic characters in the maturing neuron, ultimately resulting in adult levels. During postnatal development, tyrosine hydroxylase activity increases sixfold to eightfold in the sympathetic superior cervical ganglion. Transection of the presynaptic nerve innervating the ganglion (33, 34), or ablation of the target organs (35), prevents the normal accumulation of enzyme in sympathetic neurons. Consequently, both anterograde and retrograde transsynaptic factors regulate the ontogeny of postnatal autonomic neurons.

In the adult neuron, phenotypic characters are expressed within precise, quantitative limits, resulting in stable baseline values for any single trait. The maintenance of normal transmitter character levels during maturity is an active process, dependent on continued exposure to extracellular factors. For example, denervation of an adult sympathetic ganglion (36) or ablation of the target organs (37) results in reduced tyrosine hydroxylase and dopamine-β-hydroxylase activities. Although the factors governing phenotypic expression during development and maturity are often identical, neuronal responses may differ temporally and quantitatively. During the development, the presence of appropriate factors, such as transsynaptic stimulation or nerve growth factor, assures normal sympathetic maturation and leads to long-term increases in the concentrations of phenotypic gene products. In contrast, increased transsynaptic stimulation in the adult results in a well-circumscribed, transient increase in the concentration of characters such as tyrosine hydroxylase and dopamine-β-hydroxylase (33).

5 PEPTIDE ONTOGENY

With this background, it may be helpful to enunciate several broad questions to approach the problem of peptidergic ontogeny as well as the related issues of neuronal plasticity and specificity. What mechanisms regulate peptide development? Does a set of common mechanisms operate in diverse neuronal populations, or are these mechanisms fundamentally population-specific? On this basis, is it biologically and experimentally useful to classify peptidergic neurons by transmitter phenotype? Do similar mechanisms govern peptide ontogeny and function during maturity? Do the well-defined mechanisms which influence development of conventional transmitter phenotypic characters similarly regulate peptide ontogeny?

To begin addressing the foregoing issues, this chapter examines the development of substance P and somatostatin. These peptides are chosen as prototypes because recent work has begun to elucidate mechanisms underlying their development. Moreover, current studies are defining the relationship of mechanisms regulating substance P and somatostatin development to those regulating conventional transmitter ontogeny. Finally, substance P and somatostatin are of particular interest because their physiological function in certain loci is best characterized: increasing evidence suggests that these peptides are primary sensory transmitters, possibly mediating pain perception (39–48). Both peptides, for example, are present in high concentrations in some perikarya of the dorsal root ganglion and in projections to the substantia gelatinosa of the spinal cord (39–44), providing relatively simple models of ontogeny (49–51). Nevertheless, since substance P and somatostatin are also heterogeneously distributed throughout the central and peripheral nervous systems, regulatory mechanisms may be characterized and compared in neurons that differ embryologically, anatomically and functionally.

6   INITIAL APPEARANCE OF SUBSTANCE P AND SOMATOSTATIN IN SENSORY NEURONS

To define the normal developmental profiles of substance P and somatostatin in the dorsal root ganglion, the sixth cervical (C_6) ganglia from rats of different ages have been examined (49–51; Figure 1). Here substance P and somatostatin are initially detectable by radioimmunoassay on day 16 of gestation (E16). A variety of studies employing both immunohistochemical and radioimmunoassay techniques, obtain similar results in the brain and periphery (52–58). In contrast, catecholamines are detectable as early as E10.5 (59), suggesting that the regulation of initial peptidergic expression may differ from initial catecholaminergic expression. It is not yet clear whether the relatively late expression of peptidergic traits results from delayed transcriptional or translational events or whether it is a posttranslational phenomenon. For example, it is entirely possible that nonimmunoreactive (and hence undetectable) precursor molecules are expressed much earlier in gestation.

After initial appearance on E16, the developmental profiles for substance P and somatostatin in the dorsal root ganglion are similar,

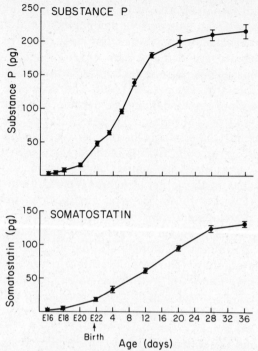

Figure 1. Development of substance P (SP) and somatostatin (SS) in dorsal root ganglia. The C_6 DRG was removed from animals at different ages and examined for SP and SS content. Each point represents eight animals. SP and SS are expressed as mean pg per ganglion ($\pm$ SEM).

suggesting that their respective populations develop contemporaneously and that critical regulatory events may occur simultaneously for the two peptides. However, recent work in culture suggests that not all processes regulating SP and SS are identical. When sensory neurons from embryonic chick dorsal root ganglia are grown together with ganglionic nonneuronal cells, neuronal content of SS is increased without any change in SP (60). Consequently, the influences of nonneuronal cells on SP and SS apparently differ. The effects of the nonneuronal cells on SS are mediated by a diffusable factor which alters peptide levels without affecting overall neuronal survival (60). The role of this factor in the normal development of sensory neurons is not yet clear.

7   DEVELOPMENTAL REGULATION BY TARGETS AND NERVE GROWTH FACTOR

To define the factors regulating development of DRG peptides *in vivo*, the role of target organs in SP and SS development has been defined (49–51). Previous studies had demonstrated that normal morphologic maturation of sensory ganglia is dependent upon the integrity of the peripheral field of innervation; limb amputation in the embryo prevents normal growth of the innervating DRG (55, 56). To begin to characterize the relationship between ganglion SP development and its field of innervation, unilateral forelimb amputation has been performed in neonates. Limb amputation prevented the normal development of ipsilateral ganglion SP, whereas contralateral ganglion SP and that in sham-operated rats develops normally (Figure 2; ref. 49). The failure of SP to increase normally may reflect direct damage to peripheral nerve fibers as well as loss of the field of innervation. To help differentiate between these alternatives, similar experiments have been performed in embryos, in which peripheral nerve outgrowth is much less extensive. The effects of amputation are quantitatively similar in neonates and embryos (50), suggesting that loss of the target structure represents the critical perturbation. It is noteworthy that even after amputation, however, impaired but significant development does occur, suggesting that targets are not the sole determinants of dorsal root ganglion maturation.

What factor or factors mediate the apparent limb–ipsilateral dorsal root ganglion interaction? The trophic protein nerve growth factor was examined initially, since it is well documented that it alters dorsal root ganglion morphologic development in the *embryo* (57, 61). However, the role of nerve growth factor in *postnatal* ganglion maturation has been unclear. Neonatal sensory ganglia reportedly lack nerve growth factor receptors (62) and do not respond *morphologically* to nerve growth factor either *in vivo* or in culture (62–64). In fact, however, more recent studies indicate that NGF administration elicits a twofold increase of C_6 DRG substance P (Figure 2; 49) and somatostatin (51). Consequently, postnatal sensory ganglia do respond to the protein.

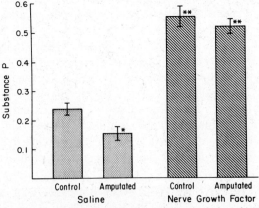

Figure 2. Effects of combined amputation and nerve growth factor (NGF) treatment. Unilateral forelimb amputation was performed in neonates. Animals were then injected subcutaneously with 100 μL of either NGF (10 μg) in saline or saline daily for 9 days. The C_6 ganglia on both the amputated side and the contralateral control side were examined for content of substance P, expressed as mean pg per ganglion (± SEM). (*) Differs from saline control at $P < 0.01$; (**) differs from saline control at $P < 0.001$. Reprinted with permission from Kessler and Black (49).

To determine whether nerve growth factor can prevent the effects of amputation on substance P development, rats have been treated with the factor after surgery (Figure 2; 49). In summary, nerve growth factor prevents the effects of amputation on substance P development, suggesting that nerve growth factor may substitute for limb factors that are necessary for substance P development. This raises the possibility that cells in the limb elaborate a nerve growth factor-like molecule that regulates peptidergic development in the dorsal root ganglion.

Recent experiments lend support to this possibility. Treatment of neonates with anti-nerve growth factor antiserum prevents normal development of substance P in the dorsal root ganglion (65). Consequently, endogenous nerve growth factor is apparently *required* for normal postnatal development of substance P. Moreover, the recent demonstration that NGF is transported in a retrograde fashion from limb to innervating dorsal root ganglion (66) suggests a plausible mode of action. But *in situ* elaboration of nerve growth factor by cells of the target limb has yet to be demonstrated; a number of additional experiments are required to define the factors that mediate the limb–dorsal root ganglion interaction.

Regardless of ultimate mediating mechanisms, the regulation of substance P development by the target limb is entirely consistent with target regulation of development of other transmitter phenotypes. For example, it is well-documented that the field of innervation governs noradrenergic (52, 67, 68) and cholinergic (69–71) maturation. Consequently, this mode of regulation is certainly not transmitter-specific and may occur throughout the nervous system. It should be noted, parenthetically, that target regulation is independent of nerve impulse direction, governing the afferent dorsal root ganglia as well as the efferent superior cervical ganglia.

The lack of transmitter specificity of target regulation is paralleled by the actions of nerve growth factor. This single molecular species influences development of neurons using a variety of transmitters, including catecholamines and acetylcholine (1, 57, 72) as well as somatostatin and substance P. In turn, this suggests that NGF does not elicit expression of a single, specific transmitter but rather stimulates development of the transmitter (or transmitters) normally expressed by receptive neurons. In summary, the foregoing mechanisms that regulate substance P and somatostatin development in the dorsal root ganglion appear to be generalized, not peptide-specific, and govern development of a variety of transmitters.

8   SUBSTANCE P IN SYMPATHETIC GANGLIA

The foregoing studies indicate that peptidergic ontogeny in sensory neurons is regulated by mechanisms that influence development of a variety of other transmitter phenotypes. On the other hand, to define processes that *specifically* foster peptidergic expression and development in neurons that also express conventional transmitters, other systems must be examined. A particularly convenient model is the superior cervical ganglion, in which noradrenergic and cholinergic development have been studied extensively (52).

Traditional teaching maintains that sympathetic neurons use only norepinephrine or acetylcholine as neurotransmitters, and that nerves innervating ganglia are cholinergic (73). However, the recent demonstration of substance P in ganglion nerve fibers (74, 75) suggests that the biochemical organization of the sympathetic nervous system is more complicated. Moreover, substance P appears to subserve a physiologic role in sympathetic ganglia, since the peptide is released from ganglia by a high potassium stimulus in a calcium-dependent manner, and since application of substance P to sympathetic neurons elicits membrane depolarization and neuronal discharge (76, 77). These observations raise interesting questions regarding the relationship between catecholamine and peptidergic expression in autonomic ganglia. Recent experiments have focused on a number of specific issues. Are classical sympathetic catecholamine neurons capable of expressing peptide phenotypic characters? What molecular mechanisms foster peptidergic expression? Do these processes influence catecholamine expression and metabolism? Can we begin to formulate general rules that govern peptidergic development in different classes of neurons?

9 TRANSSYNAPTIC REGULATION OF SUBSTANCE P *IN VIVO*

It has long been recognized that transsynaptic factors regulate the activity and amount of catecholamine biosynthetic enzymes in both developing and adult sympathetic ganglia (78–80). For example, decentralization (denervation) of the superior cervical ganglion in adults decreases ganglion content of tyrosine hydroxylase (TOH) (36, 79), the rate-limiting enzyme in catecholamine biosynthesis (80), while increased transsynaptic impulse-flow biochemically induces TOH (81). In neonates, transsynaptic factors regulate the normal developmental increase in TOH (52).

To determine whether transsynaptic factors also regulate substance P, ganglia were unilaterally decentralized in adult rats, with the contralateral (intact) ganglia and ganglia of sham-operated animals serving as controls. Decentralization, which decreases catecholamine phenotypic characters, increased ganglion substance P after 12 days (82), suggesting that preganglionic nerves normally suppress substance P. In contrast, postganglionic axotomy produced no change in substance P, suggesting that retrograde factors are less important (82).

To determine whether the influences of preganglionic nerves are mediated by ganglionic transmission, rats were treated with chlorisond-amine, a specific ganglionic-blocking agent. The drug prevents postsyn-aptic depolarization by competing with acetylcholine for postsynaptic nicotinic receptor sites (83). Treatment significantly increased ganglion substance P, reproducing the effects of surgical decentralization. These observations suggest that presynaptic fibers normally decrease ganglion peptide through the mediation of transsynaptic acetylcholine and post-synaptic depolarization (82).

To assess whether increased presynaptic nerve impulse activity de-creases substance P, rats were treated with phenoxybenzamine, an α-receptor blocking agent which reflexly increases sympathetic nervous system activity (84). Treatment significantly decreased substance P, suggesting that ganglion substance P, content is inversely related to im-pulse activity (82). However, administration of reserpine or phentol-amine, two drugs that also stimulate sympathetic impulse activity, had variable effects. It is possible that the effects of phenoxybenzamine on substance P resulted from an action of the drug unrelated to nerve im-pulse activity.

These observations suggest that impulse activity has opposite effects on ganglion peptidergic and catecholaminergic characters. Surgical de-centralization, or pharmacologic blockade of transmission, decreases amine enzyme activities (36, 79) but increases ganglion substance P. Conversely, pharmacologic stimulation of sympathetic activity increases amine biosynthetic enzymes and catecholamine synthesis (81) but de-creases substance P. Transsynaptic impulse activity, mediated by ace-tylcholine release, may regulate the quantitative relationship between ganglion noradrenergic and peptidergic characters.

Interpretation of the foregoing studies requires anatomic localization of substance P in the adult superior cervical ganglion. Immuno-histochemical studies of the superior cervical ganglion *in vivo* by Hökfelt et al. (74, 75) demonstrated substance P-containing nerve fibers but no substance P immunoreactive perikarya. However, the putative peptide transmitters are generally more difficult to demonstrate in cell bodies than in nerve fibers (10). Other indirect evidence has suggested that substance P in the superior cervical ganglion might be localized to sensory fibers innervating the ganglion (85). Nevertheless, the results of the foregoing decentralization and axotomy experiments, as well as oth-er studies (86), exclude the possibility that substance P is derived pri-marily from fibers entering the superior cervical ganglion via afferent or efferent connections. Nevertheless, to more definitively localize gangli-on substance P, neonates were treated with 6-hydroxydopamine, which selectively destroys noradrenergic neurons in sympathetic ganglia. One month after treatment the superior cervical ganglion was assayed for substance P and for TOH, a specific marker for postsynaptic noradren-

ergic neurons (78). Treatment significantly decreased both substance P
and TOH, to 44 and 14%, respectively, strongly suggesting that substance P is localized to intraganglionic, noradrenergic neurons (82). Subsequent studies *in vitro* (87, *vide infra*) have confirmed the localization
of substance P to principal sympathetic neurons in the superior cervical
ganglion. Although substance P in the superior cervical ganglion is primarily localized to ganglion neurons, the distribution of the peptide may
not be the same in every sympathetic ganglion. For example, mesenteric
ganglia, which have significantly higher substance P levels than the superior cervical ganglion, appear to have at least some substance P–containing fibers arising from extrinsic sources (77).

In summary, the foregoing studies suggest that in the adult superior
cervical ganglion presynaptic nerves decrease substance P in postsynaptic sympathetic neurons through the transsynaptic release of acetylcholine and postsynaptic nicotinic stimulation. Transsynaptic factors
similarly regulate substance P levels in neonates; decentralization of the
superior cervical ganglion in neonates increases substance P 36 h postoperatively (Figure 3; ref. 87). This regulatory process appears to occur
throughout life. Transsynaptic depression of ganglion substance P could
result from: (i) decreased synthesis or mobilization of the peptide from
precursor molecules; (ii) increased catabolism; (iii) increased release of
substance P. Although the precise processes mediating transsynaptic
regulation of substance P have not yet been established, recent studies
performed *in vitro* have begun to define a number of molecular regulatory mechanisms.

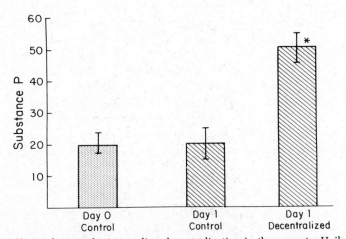

Figure 3. Effects of sympathetic ganglion decentralization in the neonate. Unilateral surgical denervation of the superior cervical ganglion was performed on the day of birth. The
denervated and contralateral control ganglia were examined 36 h later for substance P
content, expressed as mean pg per ganglion ($\pm$ SEM). (*) Differs from control at $P < 0.001$.
Reprinted with permission from Kessler et al. (87).

10   REGULATION OF SUBSTANCE P *IN VITRO*

Explanted neonatal ganglia have provided a model system for delineating the cellular processes that regulate substance P metabolism. Neonatal ganglia may be maintained in medium without added NGF, since the trophic protein does not substantially alter *short-term* observations *in vitro* (88). In fact, substance P content increases dramatically in cultured ganglia (Figure 4; ref. 87); by 12 h, substance P increases more than fivefold, by 24 h more than twentyfold, and by 48 h more than fiftyfold.

To determine whether protein, RNA, or DNA synthesis is required for this striking increase in substance P, ganglia have been cultured for 12 h in the presence of appropriate inhibitors (87). Cycloheximide completely prevents the increase in substance P, suggesting that protein synthesis is necessary for the rise. By contrast, arabinosylcytosine, an inhibitor of DNA synthesis, has no significant effect, and actinomycin D and camptothecin, inhibitors of RNA synthesis, partially inhibit the elevation in substance P. Therefore, ongoing protein synthesis and to a lesser extent RNA synthesis are required for the rise in ganglion substance P *in vitro*.

To correlate regulatory mechanisms *in vivo* and *in vitro*, the effects of membrane depolarization have been examined in culture, since nerve

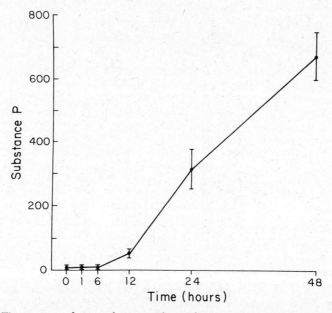

Figure 4.   Time course of sympathetic ganglion substance P accumulation in culture. The SCG was explanted for varying times and examined for SP content, expressed as mean pg per ganglion (± SEM). Reprinted with permission from Kessler et al. (87).

impulse activity decreases ganglion substance P *in vivo*. Veratridine, which increases membrane sodium flux by binding to sodium channels (89), abolishes the rise in substance P (87; Figure 5). Tetrodotoxin, which specifically antagonizes the sodium ion effects of veratridine (90, 91), blocks the effects of veratridine on substance P (Figure 5), suggesting that the inhibitory effects of veratridine are related to increased sodium influx. Potassium-induced membrane depolarization similarly prevents the rise of substance P in the explants (92), suggesting that membrane depolarization rather than sodium influx *per se* may mediate the effects of veratridine. Viewed in aggregate, the foregoing observations *in vivo* and in culture suggest that transsynaptic impulses, mediated by postsynaptic sodium influx and membrane depolarization, decrease substance P in the superior cervical ganglion. Future experiments, employing dissociates as well as explants, may help to precisely localize the site of action of the aforementioned pharmacologic agents.

Although the studies of adult ganglia after 6-hydroxydopamine treatment suggest that substance P is localized within sympathetic perikarya (see above; 82), previous immunohistochemical studies had failed to visualize substance P-containing cell bodies (74, 75). However, the dramatic increase of SP in cultured ganglia afforded a unique opportunity to localize substance P immunohistochemically. Examination of ganglia after 48 hours in culture demonstrated striking substance P-like immu-

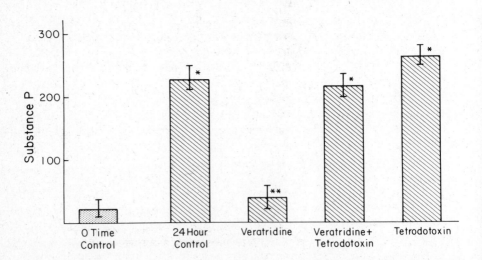

Figure 5. Effects of membrane depolarization on sympathetic ganglion substance P. The SCG was cultured in the presence of veratridine ($2 \times 10^{-4} M$), tetrodotoxin ($10^{-7} M$), or both. After 24 h, ganglia were examined for substance P content, expressed as mean pg per ganglion ($\pm$ SEM). (*) Differs from 0 time control at $P < 0.001$; (**) differs from 24 h control at $P < 0.001$. Reprinted with permission from Kessler et al. (87).

nofluorescence in the principal (postsynaptic) neuron perikarya (87). Substance P-like immunofluorescence is also observed in varicose fibers coursing within the ganglion and in boutons apposed to substance P-containing perikarya.

These observations suggest that the apparent putative transmitter of a neuron, as defined immunohistochemically, may depend on the functional state of the neuron. Thus external stimuli, such as transsynaptic impulse flow, may alter the apparent phenotype, and negative immunohistochemical data may simply reflect unfavorable environmental and physiologic conditions. Consequently, neurotransmitter expression and metabolism may represent a dynamic, changing process that reflects the physiologic state of the neuron.

To determine whether the foregoing regulatory processes represent generalized mechanisms governing metabolism of different peptides in a variety of neuronal types, two separate but related questions have been examined: (i) Is substance P similarly regulated in anatomically, functionally, and embryologically different neuronal populations? (ii) Are other putative peptide transmitters subject to the same regulatory processes?

11 REGULATION OF SUBSTANCE P IN DIFFERENT NEURONAL POPULATIONS

To approach the first question, substance P regulation in sensory neurons of the nodose ganglion, dorsal root ganglion, and trigeminal ganglion were examined *in vivo* and *in vitro*. In the nodose ganglion the peptide is localized to a population of sensory neurons (93) derived from the epibranchial placode (94). By contrast, dorsal root ganglion neurons, like sympathetics, are neural crest derivatives (95), while the trigeminal ganglion contains neural crest as well as epibranchial derivatives (94, 95). Consequently, these ganglia contain a variety of peptidergic populations, allowing comparison with peptidergic sympathetic neurons.

To compare the maturation of substance P in sympathetic and sensory neurons *in vivo*, the normal developmental profiles of the peptide in the superior cervical, nodose, trigeminal, and dorsal root ganglion have been defined (92). Substance P increases approximately fourfold in each of the three sensory ganglia (nodose, trigeminal, and dorsal root) during the first five weeks of life (92). In the nodose ganglion, the peptide rises from 65 pg/ganglion at birth to 250 pg, while in the dorsal root ganglion it rises from 56 to 210 pg/ganglion. The larger trigeminal ganglion contains considerably more peptide, increasing from 200 pg at birth to 750 pg/ganglion at 5 weeks. By contrast, substance P in the sympathetic superior cervical ganglion increases only twofold over the same period to

40 pg/ganglion. Thus the ontogeny of substance P varies to some extent in different neuronal populations.

To determine whether sodium flux is important in the regulation of substance P in different populations of neurons, the effects of veratridine *in vitro* have been examined in the nodose ganglion as well as in the superior cervical ganglion. The placodal-derived nodose ganglion was chosen for comparison because it differs embryologically, functionally, and anatomically from the superior cervical ganglion derived from neural crest. In culture, substance P increases twelvefold in the latter and threefold in the former over 24 hours (92). In each instance the elevation is prevented by veratridine, and tetrodotoxin blocks the veratridine effect (92). Consequently, sodium influx and membrane depolarzation appear to decrease substance P in both sympathetic and nodose ganglion sensory neurons, suggesting that this mechanism may represent a general process, governing substance P levels in diverse neuronal populations. It is not yet clear whether this effect is due to increased neuronal release of substance P, decreased synthesis or mobilization from precursor molecules, increased catabolism, or a combination of these processes. However, preliminary studies have detected insufficient release of substance P into the culture medium to account for the effects of veratridine (92), suggesting that depletion due to increased release is not the sole mechanism.

12   ROLE OF CALCIUM IN SUBSTANCE P REGULATION

Extracellular factors may influence neurotransmitter metabolism by altering membrane ionic permeability and thus the internal ionic composition of the neuron. For example, the foregoing experiments suggested that veratridine-induced changes in sodium flux decrease peptidergic characters in sympathetic and sensory neurons. Sympathetic and sensory neurons also have membrane calcium "channels," and it is well recognized that Ca^{2+} regulates a variety of cellular functions (96), including noradrenergic and cholinergic traits in sympathetic ganglia (97). To examine the effects of decreasing extracellular calcium and consequently calcium flux, ganglia have been cultured in calcium-free medium in the presence of EGTA, a chelator of polyvalent cations. EGTA blocks the increase of substance P in the superior cervical and nodose ganglia, suggesting that extracellular calcium is necessary for the rise in culture (92). Moreover, the increase in substance P is prevented by culture in the presence of ions that decrease transmembrane calcium flux (96), including manganese, cobalt, zinc, and lanthanum, but not magnesium (92). In contrast, strontium, which may substitute for calcium in many cellular processes (96), and calcium itself did not block the increase (92). Finally, phenytoin, which also inhibits calcium flux (98), also blocked the rise in substance P, supporting the contention that calcium flux is required (92).

13 REGULATION OF OTHER PEPTIDES: SOMATOSTATIN

To determine whether similar regulatory mechanisms govern the expression and metabolism of other peptide transmitters, somatostatin has been examined in the superior cervical ganglion *in vitro* (92). Like substance P, somatostatin increases dramatically in culture, rising sixfold in 24 h, and the rise is blocked by veratridine. Moreover, tetrodotoxin prevents the effects of veratridine on somatostatin, suggesting that sodium influx and depolarization decrease somatostatin as well as substance P in the superior cervical ganglion. Finally, culture of the superior cervical ganglion in calcium-free medium in the presence of EGTA inhibits the rise in ganglion somatostatin, reproducing effects on substance P and suggesting that calcium flux is necessary for elevation of both peptides (92).

Despite small differences among the ganglia examined, the most striking aspect of these studies is the remarkable similarity in the regulation of both substance P and somatostatin in diverse populations of neurons. Peptidergic neurons, under the influences of sodium and calcium fluxes, as well as other environmental stimuli, can rapidly and profoundly alter transmitter metabolism. Therefore there may be a group of regulatory mechanisms governing peptide transmitter metabolism throughout the nervous system. More generally, these studies support the concept that the expression of neurotransmitter phenotypes is a dynamic, changing process that reflects the physiologic state of a neuron.

REFERENCES

1. L. L. Y. Chun and P. H. Patterson, *J. Cell Biol.* **75**, 694 (1977).
2. L. L. Y. Chun and P. H. Patterson, *J. Cell Biol.* **75**, 705 (1977).
3. M. Johnson, D. Ross, M. Meyers, R. Reese, R. Bunge, E. Wakshull, and H. Burton, *Nature (London)* **262**, 308 (1976).
4. P. H. Patterson, *Ann. Rev. Neurosci.* **1**, 1 (1978).
5. R. Rees and R. P. Bunge, *J. Comp. Neurol.* **157**, 1 (1974).
6. P. H. Patterson and L. L. Y. Chun, *Dev. Biol.* **56**, 263 (1977).
7. P. H. Patterson and L. L. Y. Chun, *Dev. Biol.* **60**, 473 (1977).
8. S. S. Varon and R. P. Bunge, *Ann. Rev. Neurosci.* **1**, 327 (1978).
9. P. A. Walicke, R. B. Campenot, and P. H. Patterson, *Proc. Natl. Acad. Sci. USA* **74**, 5567 (1977).
10. I. A. Hendry, L. L. Iversen, and I. B. Black, *J. Neurochem.* **20**, 1683 (1973).
11. H. Thoenen, R. A. Mueller, and J. Axelrod, *J. Pharmacol. Exp. Ther.* **169**, 249 (1969).
12. T. Hökfelt, O. Johansson, A. Ljungduhl, J. Lundberg, and M. Schultzberg, *Nature (London)* **284**, 515 (1980).

13. S. H. Snyder, *Science* **209**, 976 (1980).
14. I. B. Black, *Science* **215**, 1198 (1982).
15. S. R. Detwiler, *Am. J. Anat.* **61**, 63 (1937).
16. J. Pick, *J. Comp. Neurol.* **120**, 409 (1963).
17. V. Tennyson, *J. Comp. Neurol.* **124**, 267 (1965).
18. A. J. Coulombre, M. C. Johnston, and J. A. Weston, *Dev. Biol.* **36**, f15 (1974).
19. N. M. LeDouarin, *Nature* **286**, 663 (1980).
20. A. L. Cohen, *J. Exp. Zool.* **179**, 167 (1972).
21. S. L. Norr, *Dev. Biol.* **34**, 16 (1973).
22. N. M. LeDouarin, D. Renaud, M. A. Teillet, and G. H. LeDouarin, *Proc. Natl. Acad. Sci. USA* **72**, 728 (1975).
23. M. Sieber-Blum and A. L. Cohen, *J. Cell Biol.* **79**, 31A (1978).
24. P. Cochard, M. Goldstein, and I. B. Black, *Proc. Natl. Acad. Sci. USA* **75**, 2986 (1978).
25. G. Teitelman, H. Baker, T. H. Joh, and D. J. Reis, *Proc. Natl. Acad. Sci. USA* **76**, 509 (1979).
26. G. M. Jonakait, J. Wolf, P. Cochard, M. Goldstein, and I. B. Black, *Proc. Natl. Acad. Sci. USA* **76**, 4683 (1979).
27. S. C. Landis and D. Keefe, *Soc. Neurosci. Abstr.* **6**, 379 (1980).
28. R. E. Mains and P. H. Patterson, *J. Cell Biol.* **59**, 329 (1973).
29. P. H. Patterson and L. L. Y. Chun, *Proc. Natl. Acad. Sci. USA* **71**, 3607 (1974).
30. P. H. O'Lague, D. D. Potter, and E. J. Furshpan, *Dev. Biol.* **67**, 384 (1978).
31. E. J. Furshpan, P. R. MacLeish, P. M. O'Lague, and D. D. Potter, *Proc. Natl. Acad. Sci. USA* **73**, 4225 (1976).
32. E. Wakshull, M. I. Johnson, and H. Burton, *J. Cell Biol.* **79**, 121 (1978).
33. I. B. Black, I. A. Hendry, and L. L. Iversen, *Brain Res.* **34**, 229 (1971).
34. I. B. Black, I. A. Hendry, and L. L. Iversen, *J. Neurochem.* **19**, 1367 (1972).
35. M. D. Dibner and I. B. Black, *Brain Res.* **103**, 93 (1976).
36. I. A. Hendry, L. L. Iversen, and I. B. Black, *J. Neurochem.* **20**, 1683 (1973).
37. I. A. Hendry and H. Thoenen, *J. Neurochem.* **22**, 999 (1974).
38. P. B. Molinoff, S. Brimijoin, R. Weinshilboum, and J. Axelrod, *Proc. Natl. Acad. Sci. USA* **66**, 453 (1970).
39. B. Pernow, *Acta Physiol. Scand.* **105**, Suppl. 29, 1 (1953).
40. T. Takahashi and M. Otsuka, *Brain Res.* **87**, 1 (1977).
41. T. Hökfelt, R. Elde, O. Johansson, R. Luft, G. Nilsson, and A. Arimura, *Neuroscience* **1**, 131 (1976).
42. V. Seybold and R. Elde, *J. Histochem. Cytochem.* **28**, 367 (1980).
43. T. Hokfelt, J. Kellerth, G. Nilsson, and B. Pernow, *Brain Res.* **100**, 235 (1975).
44. T. Hokfelt, J. Kellerth, G. Nilsson, and B. Pernow, *Science* **190**, 889 (1975).
45. S. Konishi and M. Otsuka, *Nature (London)* **252**, 734 (1974).
46. M. Otsuka and S. Konishi, *Cold Spring Harbor Symp. Quant. Biol.* **40**, 135 (1976).
47. M. Randic and V. Miletic, *Brain Res.* **152**, 196 (1978).
48. J. L. Henry, *Brain Res.* **114**, 436 (1976).
49. J. A. Kessler and I. B. Black, *Proc. Natl. Acad. Sci. USA* **77**, 644 (1980).
50. J. A. Kessler and I. B. Black, *Brain Res.* **208**, 135 (1981).
51. J. A. Kessler and I. B. Black, *Proc. Natl. Acad. Sci. USA* **78**, 4644 (1981).
52. I. B. Black, *Ann. Rev. Neurosci.* **1**, 183 (1978).
53. P. H. Patterson, *Ann. Rev. Neurosci.* **1**, 1 (1978).
54. S. S. Varon and R. P. Bunge, *Ann. Rev. Neurosci.* **1**, 327 (1978).
55. V. Hamburger, *J. Exp. Zool.* **68**, 449 (1934).
56. M. L. Shorey, *J. Exp. Zool.* **7**, 25 (1909).
57. R. Levi-Montalcini and P. U. Angeletti, *Physiol. Rev.* **48**, 534 (1968).
58. R. F. T. Gilbert and P. L. Emson, *Brain Res.* **171**, 166 (1979).
59. P. Cochard, M. Goldstein, and I. B. Black, *Proc. Natl. Acad. Sci. USA* **75**, 2488 (1978).

60. A. W. Mudge, *Nature* **292**, 764 (1981).
61. L. A. Greene and E. M. Shooter, *Ann. Rev. Neurosci.* **3**, 353 (1980).
62. K. Herrup and E. Shooter, *J. Cell Biol.* **67**, 118 (1975).
63. P. Burnham, C. Raiburn, and S. Varon, *Proc. Natl. Acad. Sci. USA* **69**, 3556 (1972).
64. S. Varon, L. Raiborn, and E. Tysku, *Brain Res.* **54**, 51 (1973).
65. U. Otten, M. Goedert, N. Mayer, and F. Lembeck, *Nature* **287**, 158 (1980).
66. J. Brunso-Bechtold and V. Hamburger, *Proc. Natl. Acad. Sci. USA* **76**, 1494 (1979).
67. M. Dibner and I. B. Black, *Brain Res.* **103**, 93 (1975).
68. M. Dibner, C. Mytilineou, and I. B. Black, *Brain Res.* **123**, 301 (1977).
69. V. Hamburger, *Am. J. Anat.* **102**, 365 (1958).
70. M. C. Prestige, *J. Embryol. Exp. Morphol.* **18**, 359 (1967).
71. L. Landmesser and G. Pilar, *J. Physiol. (London)* **241**, 715 (1974).
72. J. A. Kessler and I. B. Black, *Brain Res.* **184**, 157 (1980).
73. S. E. Mayer, in A. C. Gilman, L. A. Goodman, and A. Gilman, Eds., *Pharmacologic Basis of Therapeutics*, Macmillan, New York, 1980, p. 56.
74. T. Hokfelt, L.-G. Elfvin, M. Schultzberg, M. Goldstein, and G. Nilsson, *Brain Res.* **132**, 29 (1977).
75. T. Hokfelt, L.-G. Elfvin, M. Schultzberg, M. Goldstein, and R. Luft, *Proc. Natl. Acad. Sci. USA* **74**, 3587 (1977).
76. N. J. Dun and A. G. Karczmar, *Neuropharmacology* **18**, 215 (1979).
77. S. Konishi, A. Tsunoo, and M. Otsuka, *Proc. Jpn. Acad., Ser B.* **55**, 525 (1979).
78. I. B. Black, I. A. Hendry, and L. L. Iversen, *Brain Res.* **34**, 229 (1971).
79. J. A. Kessler and I. B. Black, *Brain Res.* **171**, 415 (1979).
80. M. Levitt, S. Spector, A. Sjoerdsma, and S. Udenfriend, *J. Pharmacol. Exp. Ther.* **148**, 1 (1960).
81. H. Thoenen, R. A. Mueller, and J. Axelrod. *J. Pharmacol. Exp. Ther.* **169**, 249 (1969).
82. J. A. Kessler and I. B. Black, *Brain Res.*, in press.
83. K. Crimson, A. Tarazi, and J. Frazer, *Circulation* **11**, 733 (1955).
84. A. S. Dontas and M. Nickerson, *J. Pharmacol. Exp. Ther.* **120**, 147 (1954).
85. R. Gamse, A. Wax, R. E. Zigmond, and S. E. Leeman, *Neuroscience* **6**, 437 (1981).
86. S. E. Robinson, J. P. Schwartz, and E. Costa, *Brain Res.* **182**, 11 (1980).
87. J. A. Kessler, J. E. Adler, M. C. Bohn, and I. B. Black, *Science* **214**, 335 (1981).
88. M. D. Coughlin, D. M. Boyer, and I. B. Black, *Proc. Natl. Acad. Sci. USA* **74**, 3438 (1977).
89. W. Ulbricht, *Ergeb. Physiol. Biol. Chem. Exp. Pharmacol.* **61**18, (1964).
90. M. H. Evans, *Int. Rev. Neurobiol.* **15**, 83 (1973).
91. W. A. Catterall and M. Nirenberg, *Proc. Natl. Acad. Sci. USA* **70**, 3579 (1979).
92. J. A. Kessler, J. E. Adler, and I. B. Black, in preparation.
93. D. M. Katz and H. J. Karten, *J. Comp. Neurol.* **193**, 549 (1980).
94. E. vanCampenhout, *Bull. Acad. R. Med. Belg.* **2**, 169 (1937).
95. J. A. Weston, *Adv. Morph.* **8**, 41 (1970).
96. S. Hagiwara and L. Byerly, *Ann. Rev. Neurosci.* **4**, 69 (1981).
97. P. Walicke and P. Patterson, *J. Neuroscience* **1**, (1981).
98. R. Sohn and J. Ferrendelli, *J. Pharmacol. Exp. Ther.* **185**, 272 (1973).

PART
2

Role of Peptides in Major Homeostatic Systems

10

Feeding Behavior

BRUCE S. SCHNEIDER
JEFFREY M. FRIEDMAN
JULES HIRSCH
Rockefeller University
New York, New York

Supported in part by grants from NIH AM 30583 and the Irma T. Hirschl Trust.

1 INTRODUCTION

In this discussion of recent investigations into the function of brain peptides in the control of feeding behavior, we have thought it helpful and appropriate to provide an overview of theory and methodology, followed by an account of current research on brain peptides that have been sufficiently investigated to serve as concrete examples of experimental approaches to the problem. (Space limitations have precluded an exhaustive review of the published experiments on every brain peptide.)

2 THE CONTROL OF FEEDING BEHAVIOR

The assimilation, storage, and disposition of nutrient energy constitute a complex homeostatic system central to the survival of both prokaryotic and eukaryotic organisms. In vertebrates, and especially among land-dwelling mammalian species, the ability to store large quantities of energy-dense fuel in the form of adipose tissue triglyceride permits survival during prolonged periods of food deprivation. In order to maintain such fuel stores without sustaining continual alterations in the size and shape of the organism, some balance between energy intake and expenditure must be achieved. A detailed description of current research in the regulation of feeding behavior is well beyond the scope of this chapter, but it is worth emphasizing that ingestive behavior in mammals is not a random, haphazard series of events but instead comprises two interacting sets of regulated behavioral and metabolic phenomena, a short-term system and a long-term system. The short-term system regulates periods of feeding, or meal patterns, throughout the day. Investigation of animal and human feeding behavior has demonstrated that meals are highly structured events, with very typical meal sizes, intermeal intervals, and satiety-associated behaviors. It is likely that these short-term feeding parameters are individually regulated and can be individually affected by various pharmacological and nutritional manipulations. In addition, it appears highly probable, although not definitively proved, that the mammalian fuel reserve stored within adipocytes as neutral triglyceride is also subject to long-term regulation, by modulations in both food intake and basal energy consumption.

   The regulation of feeding behavior can be best perceived as an integrated homeostatic system comprising a series of complex interacting circuits. Food is ingested and, in an unknown fashion, the amount of nutrient consumed is rapidly quantified and transduced into neural or humoral signals that are ultimately processed by the CNS, terminating a meal. There is certainly evidence to suggest that short-term, preabsorptive satiety signals originate in the gastrointestinal (GI) tract during a meal and cause rapid cessation of feeding (1). The amount of stored adipose tissue triglyceride may also be monitored over longer periods of time, and it is thought by many investigators that the current global nutritional status of the animal is continually assessed and compared against an ideal reference, or "set point," for body weight. Corrections in an upward or downward direction are effected by changes in food intake (modulation of the short-term system) or energy expenditure whenever there are deviations from the ideal. Although one cannot prove the existence of a set point, support for this concept is derived from numerous observations that demonstrate the ability of animals and humans to maintain fairly stable body weights over long periods of time when fed *ad libitum* and to restore normal body weights following periods of over- or undernutrition. If such "set points" do indeed exist, we have little information about their physical, chemical, or neuroanatomical composition. Furthermore, it would be wrong to think of set points as fixed for the life of the organism. For example, the adipose tissue triglyceride stores of laboratory rats are maintained at a stable level if physical activity, temperature, and the quality (palatability) of the diet remain constant (2). Feeding behavior and body weight change drastically in several species during periods of migration or hibernation (3). Animals that have sustained lesions to the ventromedial hypothalamus generally demonstrate an initial phase of hyperphagia and rapid weight gain which persist until a new plateau in body weight is achieved and then maintained (4, 5). Lateral hypothalamic lesions yield directly opposite results, with hypophagia, weight loss, and the maintenance of a lower body weight plateau (6). Thus, if such set points for long-term control of body weight do exist, they are capable of changing in response to a variety of internal or external perturbations, further adding to the complexity of the conceptual framework in which the mechanisms of weight regulation are studied.

Whatever the nature of such short-term or long-term homeostasis, the existence of a regulated system or set of systems necessitates some mechanism of information exchange among multiple loci, including adipose tissue, the gastrointestinal tract, and the central nervous system. In hypothetical terms, this homeostatic system could be regulated at any of three levels: the afferent loop (with signals originating from the gastrointestinal tract, adipose tissue, liver); the integrative center within the central nervous system; and the efferent loop, comprising the neurophysiological events that initiate or constitute a behavioral or metabolic change relevant to nutrition.

It has been suggested that several brain–gut peptides function at each limb of this system. In considering these compounds it is important to avoid the assumption that a CNS peptide functions in a manner parallel to that of its gastrointestinal homolog. Corresponding brain and gut peptides may demonstrate independent biosynthetic regulatory mechanisms (including posttranslational modifications), widely diver-

gent patterns of *in vivo* release in response to stimuli, dissimilar characteristics of receptor binding and postreceptor action on relevant target
cells, and different patterns of ontogenetic development. In dissecting
the relationships between the two tissues, it is also important to determine whether the peptide in question is transported into or out of the
CNS. Specifically, it is possible that a given peptide may act peripherally as a satiety signal yet serve an unrelated function with the CNS. We
will thus discuss the role of brain–gut peptides in terms of peripheral
action (afferent loop), as distinct from possible actions within the CNS
(integrative and effector loops).

3 PEPTIDE SIGNALS FROM THE PERIPHERY: THE AFFERENT LOOP

Over the past 15 years a number of gastrointestinal and pancreatic peptide hormones—such as insulin, cholecystokinin, bombesin, glucagon,
somatostatin, and pancreatic polypeptide—have been thought to function as short-term satiety signals or as modulators of feeding behavior.
Many of these peptides are secreted from portions of the gastrointestinal tract in response to specific ingested substrates (carbohydrates,
amino acids, or fatty acids) and may convey nutritional information to
receptors in the periphery or in the CNS in addition to their established
roles in the assimilation of nutrients. Many metabolites—such as glucose, glycerol, free fatty acids, ketone bodies, and certain amino acids—
may also play a role in modulating feeding behavior (7–9).

Experiments designed to demonstrate the involvement of a given gut
peptide in the production of satiety have proceeded in the following
manner: A well-characterized peptide is administered systemically and
food intake is measured in the experimental animal. If feeding is found
to be suppressed by the peptide, and if stereotypic behavior patterns
normally associated with meal termination in that species are found,
then that peptide is believed to be acting in a physiologically relevant
manner. It is also important to demonstrate that this effect is behaviorally specific, that is, the animal should not stop eating because of an
aversive effect of the peptide, drinking should not be impaired, and the
cessation of eating should not be secondary to the production of competing behaviors. Following the demonstration that a given dose of hormone is capable of causing meal termination or diminished food intake,
and that the above criteria are also satisfied, questions predictably
arise over the interpretation of the results: Are the given doses in the
physiological or pharmacological range? Are we observing a true physiological event or simply a phenomenon caused by a compound administered in a dose, at a site, and with timing that are never normally
encountered? Reliable radioimmunoassays (or other assays) capable of

detecting endogenous plasma levels of these hormones can help clarify these issues.

Experiments of this sort have been undertaken almost exclusively with presently characterized compounds. It is not unlikely that other, as yet unidentified, substances found within the gastrointestinal tract are even more potent controllers of feeding behavior than are any known compounds. Indeed, there may exist substances whose only function is to carry information regarding the long-term or short-term nutritional status of the organism.

4 BRAIN PEPTIDES: INTEGRATIVE SIGNALS WITHIN THE CNS

All the foregoing considerations relevant to peripheral satiety signals apply to the search for endogenous peptides and other compounds mediating satiety within the central nervous system, except that in the latter case the problems encountered are far more complex.

Speculation that brain peptides modulate feeding behavior was stimulated partly by neuropharmacological experiments and, to some extent, by awareness of amino acid homologies between some CNS peptides and those peripheral hormones suspected of mediating meal termination. However, as discussed above, it is important to consider the physiology of a CNS peptide separately from that of its peripheral hormone homolog. Furthermore, a particular brain peptide is almost always concentrated in several discrete, and even unrelated, anatomical loci within the CNS, and consideration should always be given to the possibility, indeed the likelihood, that a peptide may function differently at each of its locations within the brain. It is certain that elucidation of the function of brain peptides in feeding behavior will await further, meticulous neurophysiological investigation and greater understanding of brain function in general. Given the limitations in our current understanding of brain peptides, how can we begin to evaluate their possible function in the control of feeding behavior? Toward this end we have proposed criteria for establishing a physiological role for a given brain peptide in the control of feeding behavior.

4.1 Ideal Criteria

As an ideal, it would be most convincing if an established, well-defined neurophysiological action of a peptide at a specific anatomical locus could be correlated with an observed response or change in an animal's feeding behavior or nutritional status. The data would be most cogent if the locus examined were one known to be involved in the regulation of food intake or energy metabolism. Depending on the technology available, experimentally induced or normally occurring perturbations in nutritional status might be shown to effect variations in the function of the peptide system (afferent or integrative loop); conversely, primary interference with the function of the peptide would produce changes in feeding behavior or nutritional status.

4.2 Criteria Given Constraints of Current Methodology

Given that our current understanding of brain peptide physiology precludes satisfying the above ideal criteria, we will survey the major methodological avenues of brain peptide research currently available to investigators of feeding behavior. Positive experimental results using any or all of the systems described below offer suggestive, but still incomplete, interpretations and conclusions.

4.2.1 Microinjection and Infusion of an Exogenous Peptide into Areas of the CNS

Introduction of a peptide into the CNS allows the investigator to alter drastically its local concentrations in the ventricular fluid or in stereotaxically selected areas of the brain itself. Animals can be carefully prepared with implanted cannulae and allowed to recover from the operation until they resume normal patterns of feeding behavior. Graded doses of (preferably synthetically pure) peptides are injected or infused and the response variable consists of a change in feeding that is, hopefully, behaviorally specific. In addition, behaviors normally associated with satiety—such as resting or grooming, in rats—should be shown to occur with the cessation of food intake. The changes in feeding behavior resulting from the introduction of the peptide into the CNS may be transitory, but it is possible to monitor the responses on a minute-to-minute basis by means of automated computer-linked meal-pattern recording devices (10). This methodology can provide important information about stereo-specificity for agonist and antagonists, peptide structure-activity relationships, and regional anatomic specificity of response. The interaction of peptides with endogenous monoaminergic systems related to feeding behavior can also be studied using microinjection and "push–pull" methodology (11). It must be remembered, however, that experiments of this nature are essentially pharmacological: frequently effects are produced with doses that exceed the total brain quantity of the endogenous peptide under investigation; it is doubtful that one can ever reproduce a truly physiological event, in terms of timing and achievement of local concentrations of peptide, with such techniques. However, when these methods are supplemented by the use of specific blocking agents, or when specific antibody alone produces the reciprocal alteration of a behavior, the data become more than suggestive.

4.2.2 Measurements of Endogenous Tissue Concentrations of the Peptide in Specific Brain Regions

The methodologies routinely employed in endocrine physiology have been successfully applied to the measurement and characterization of peptides present in extracts of brain tissue. Peptide concentrations can be quantified by bioassay, radioreceptor assay, or radioimmunoassay, each method detecting potentially different activities in the tissue extract. As is true of hormone assay in peripheral blood and secreting glands, radioimmunoassay has proven to be the most sensitive, convenient, and reproducible method. Several laboratories have demonstrated that the techniques of regional brain dissection, followed by tissue extraction and radioimmunoassay of the extracts are capable of yielding highly reproducible concentrations of immunoreactive peptides within groups of experimental animals. The technique has thus been employed to compare endogenous regional brain concentrations of peptides in groups of animals under differing nutritional or behavioral conditions. The demonstration of altered local concentrations of a brain peptide in association with nutritional changes can implicate that peptide in the regulation of feeding behavior.

Several considerations relevant to the use of radioimmunoassay in the investigation of this problem are worth emphasizing: (i) Radioimmunoassay is a competitive protein binding assay which compares the immunochemical potency of an unknown with that of a standard. It is not a bioassay. (ii) Depending on the extraction procedure, a given brain extract may demonstrate considerable molecular size heterogeneity of immunoreactivity, that is, molecules of varying size may each contain the immunoreactive peptide sequence recognized by the antibody, representing high molecular weight precursor proteins, partially processed peptides, or even smaller peptide fragments produced artifactually during the extraction process. Without complementary protein separation techniques, such as gel filtration or electrophoresis, a simple determination of total immunoreactivity may be uninterpretable. (iii) Available tissue sampling techniques permit single, static determinations of peptide concentration, rather than yielding dynamic measurements of synthetic, degradative, and release rates. If these rates change in parallel, the measured concentration of the total peptide pool may remain unchanged in the face of nutritionally-induced alterations in peptide turnover. This is especially true of situations in which there is a quantitatively small, physiologically labile compartment and a large storage pool. The situation might then be analogous to attempting to study the dynamics of pituitary growth hormone secretion by measuring concentrations of hormone in the pituitary gland rather than in the peripheral blood. (iv) Choice of denominator in the concentration function (mg wet weight, mg protein, μg DNA, etc.) can also influence the interpretation of experimental results, particularly in studies of animal models of abnormal nutrition in which the brain compositions (and even total brain weight) of experimental animals differ from those of controls. This is especially true of some of the commonly studied genetic models of obesity (e.g., the ob/ob mouse or the Zucker fatty rat, fa/fa) and also of rodent models of pre- or perinatal undernutrition (12–16). In any of these, a unit weight of brain taken from an experimental animal may differ from that taken from a control animal in number of neurons, number of glial cells, amount of myelin, and other parameters.

Sensitive radioimmunoassays may also be used to measure changes in the concentrations of brain peptides in CSF or cerebroventricular fluid; if changes in concentration reflect nutritionally related changes in release rates of peptide from neurons, it is conceivable that physiologically important information about normal function can be obtained. One should ascertain whether CSF immunoreactivity arises from brain or from the peripheral circulation.

4.2.3 Immunohistochemical Staining

More refined peptide localization in single neurons, fiber tracts, and neuronal cell clusters is achieved with immunohistochemical staining. Unfortunately, present staining techniques are only semiquantitative and could be expected to detect only major perturbations in intracellular peptide concentration in association with nutritional abnormalities.

4.2.4 Identification and Characterization of Peptide Receptor

Presumably, the first step in brain peptide action involves binding of the peptide to a specific receptor complex on the surface of target cells, as is true of peptide hormone action in the periphery. Specific receptors have already been described for a number of brain peptides, and in one case (brain CCK), Scatchard analysis has revealed changes in receptor number in association with altered nutrition (17). Elucidation of the relationship between receptor occupancy and biologic action will greatly enhance our understanding of the significance of local alterations in receptor binding kinetics in association with nutritional changes. Further, development of a brain peptide receptor pharmacology, with the identification of cross-reacting peptidal and non-peptidal compounds, offers the exciting possibility of altering such abnormal nutritional conditions as obesity by pharmacotherapy.

4.2.5 Blocking Experiments

In principle, blocking the local action of a given brain peptide, and only that peptide, should reveal aspects of its function. In the case of brain peptides methodological problems have hampered this approach.

Since the biosynthesis of peptides in the brain proceeds via mechanisms common to virtually all proteins, specific inhibition of the transcription or translation of the m-RNA coding for a given peptide has not been possible. Similarly, agents which block the axonal transport, synaptic vesicular packaging, and release of a specific CNS peptide exclusively are not yet available. It is possible that specific converting enzymes which post-translationally cleave the small, active peptides from their high molecular weight precursors are vulnerable to inhibition. Development of specific receptor blocking agents (analogous to naloxone) for other endogenous brain peptides will also help elucidate function. Inhibition of the action of endogenous peptides in the extracellular compartment by injection of specific antibody has been feasible under certain circumstances. The use of monoclonal antibodies (or FAB fragments thereof) to brain peptides and to brain peptide receptors may be useful in future experiments of this type.

Almost all research in this field has employed one or more of the above methodologies. In the following section we describe the ways in which these experimental approaches have been used to evaluate the role of specific brain–gut peptides in the control of feeding behavior.

5 CHOLECYSTOKININ

As a candidate for an endogenous satiety signal, probably no brain–gut peptide has received as much research attention as cholecystokinin (CCK). Consideration that CCK of intestinal origin might function as a satiety signal was stimulated by the work of Smith, Gibbs, and their coworkers on the appetite-suppressing effects of peripherally administered CCK. The investigators reasoned that hormones of the upper gastrointestinal tract were likely candidates for inducers of meal termination because they are released, during feeding, by a variety of intraluminal substrates. Maximum concentrations of these hormones in portal and peripheral blood should be achieved when meal termination is generally observed. Prior to this, Maclagen (18) had demonstrated a suppressive effect of food intake in rabbits by administration of an extract of small intestine; and Schally et al. (19) reported that parenteral administration of an enterogastrone preparation derived from hog duodenum was capable of inhibiting food intake in mice. In 1973, Gibbs, Smith, and their coworkers began to report their studies of the satiety-inducing effects of parenterally administered gut hormones in both intact and sham-feeding rats (i.e., rats with open gastric fistulas). They found that CCK, either in the form of its C-terminal octapeptide or as a 20% pure extract, was capable of inhibiting food intake in the rat in a dose-related manner. Desulfation of the tyrosine residue markedly diminished the potency of CCK, and gastrin, secretin, and GIP showed no effect on satiety over a wide dose range. The satiety-inducing effect of CCK was not accompanied by signs of toxicity, by competing behaviors, or by inhibition of water intake. Cessation of eating was quickly followed by typical postprandial behavior patterns of grooming and resting (20–23). Suppression of food intake by parenterally administered CCK has also been reported in monkeys, pigs, sheep, chickens, rabbits, lean and obese rats and mice, and lean and obese humans (see refs. 24, 25 for recent reviews). In most reports, satiety-inducing effects have not been accompanied by overt evidence of toxicity, although there has been some controversy over this (26, 27).

The nature and general reproducibility of the effects of exogenously administered CCK strongly suggest that injections of this peptide are capable of triggering mechanisms involved in short-term satiety. The demonstration that total and gastric vagotomies block the satiety effect of peripherally administered CCK-8 (in rats, but not rabbits) supports the idea (28–30) that parenterally administered CCK acts at a site outside the CNS. It has been hypothesized that this particular action of CCK is mediated by an effect on gastric or upper intestinal smooth muscle, with information reaching the brain via vagal afferent fibers that innervate that field. Alternatively the CCK may activate CCK receptors in the vagus itself (29, 31).

Whether endogenous CCK of intestinal origin functions physiologically as a humoral satiety signal is still not known. There remains a critical need to fill gaps in our knowledge of the dynamics of CCK release during feeding: the timing of hormone release, the magnitude of plasma concentrations achieved, and the characterization of molecular forms of circulating hormone. Further advances in the development of radioimmunoassay systems for plasma CCK will provide much of this information and will allow us to know whether the minimum doses of exogenous CCK required to inhibit food intake produce plasma concentrations of hormone that fall within physiological range.

Reports that high concentrations of CCK, chiefly in the form of its C-terminal octapeptide, occur in the brains of vertebrates (32–38) appeared just after the initial observations of Gibbs and Smith and stimulated speculation that brain CCK might be involved in the neuromodulation of satiety. In the past seven years numerous neuropharmacological studies have appeared describing the behavioral and metabolic effects of administration of CCK directly into the brains of rats, sheep, and pigs. The results have varied with species tested, experimental-behavioral par-

adigm employed, neuroanatomical site of injection, and mode of introduction of exogenous peptide (bolus injection vs. continuous infusion).

Stern et al. (39) reported that lateral cerebroventricular injections of
caerulein (a decapeptide that has C-terminal 7-amino acid homology
with CCK) suppressed feeding in food-deprived rats, at doses (100
ng/kg) that failed to suppress food intake when injected intraperitoneally. Injections of the peptide directly into the ventromedial hypothalamus
(VMH) suppressed short-term food intake, whereas injections into the
lateral hypothalamus (LH) were ineffective. Studying the effects of a purified CCK preparation on operant feeding responses in the food-deprived rat, Maddison (40) demonstrated that intracranial (lateral
ventricular) injections of as little as 0.05 IDU were capable of suppressing food-rewarded lever pressing, following a 60 min latency period.
The dose required for minimal suppressive effect was less than 5% of
that required to diminish operant responses when administered intraperitoneally. As in other published studies, injections of CCK had no effect on water intake. Consistent results have also been reported in
sheep, in which continuous intracerebroventricular infusions of pico-
molar doses of CCK-8 have been shown to suppress feeding (41, 42).
With an operant feeding paradigm in pigs deprived of food for 17-h,
CCK-8 injected into the lateral cerebral ventricles induced a dose-dependent reduction in feeding but not in drinking (43).

Other studies of the effects of intracranial injections of CCK-8 (or
caerulein) have failed to discern any inhibition of food intake either in
food-deprived or in freely feeding rats (41, 44, 45), even when doses as
high as 4 μg of peptide were employed. Using computer-linked 24-h
monitoring devices, which allow continuous recording of food intake in
freely-feeding rats, our laboratory group has been unable to detect alterations in either meal size or intermeal interval in rats given up to 2 μg
of CCK-8 either into the lateral cerebral ventricles or directly into the
hypothalamus. In the same rats, lower doses of intracranial bombesin
(see below) were effective in suppressing spontaneous feeding (44). In
their study of the suppressive effects of CCK-8 on stress-induced eating
in the rat (46), Nemeroff et al. reported that CCK-8 was effective at
doses of 250 ng if administered intraperitoneally, but that doses of 3 μg
were required to achieve an effect if administered centrally. Thus, it has
been difficult to replicate earlier reports of the pharmacological effects
of intracranially injected CCK in rats. It should be emphasized that the
doses employed in most of these experiments have been equal to if not
greater than the total amount of endogenous CCK found in rat brain. On
the other hand, it is also possible that the putative cellular CCK receptors for mediating satiety in rat brain are relatively unresponsive to or
cannot be reached by the administered CCK preparations.

The mode of action of brain CCK may be quite complex and demonstrable, at least in rats, only within specific feeding paradigms such as

stress- or drug-induced feeding. For example, neuropharmacological studies in rats (47, 48) have demonstrated that CCK, either administered peripherally or microinjected into specific hypothalamic areas, suppressed norepinephrine-induced feeding (that is, feeding induced by injection of norepinephrine into the hypothalamus). It is likely that norepinephrine is a key hypothalamic neurotransmitter involved in the control of feeding behavior, and feeding may be enhanced or reduced depending on the hypothalamic site of release of this monoamine. CCK may interact physiologically with this catecholaminergic feeding system in a complex, site-specific manner.

Stress-induced eating in rats, which may involve dopaminergic systems and possibly endogenous opiates (49–51), can also be suppressed by intracranially administered CCK. This suppressive effect is accompanied by peripheral hyperglycemia and is blocked by prior adrenalectomy (52).

What is known of the relationship of endogenous brain CCK to feeding behavior? There is little doubt that the CCK immunoreactivity, which has been well characterized in vertebrate central nervous systems, is endogenous. Brain tissue is capable of biosynthesis of CCK, and brain receptors for CCK have been identified (53–56). Using cell fractionation techniques combined with radioimmunoassay, a significant proportion of total brain CCK immunoreactivity can be shown to sediment with a synaptosome fraction. In addition, CCK can be released from brain tissue *in vitro* under appropriate stimuli (57–59), suggesting that brain CCK may function in neurotransmission, in the modulation of neurotransmission, or in other modalities of cell-to-cell communication. Studies employing regional brain dissection and radioimmunoassay have yielded generally consistent results across laboratories and have shown that in all species studied, the major proportion of brain CCK is found in the cerebral cortex, with concentrations of roughly 0.5 nmole of peptide per g of tissue. Somewhat lower levels are found in other brain areas, including the olfactory bulbs, hypothalamus, hippocampus, and upper brainstem (32, 37, 16, 60, 61). Immunohistochemical staining studies in rat brain have generally yielded parallel results (38, 62).

Although CCK is present in nerve cell bodies and fibers lying in or near anatomical areas associated with olfaction and with the control of feeding behavior, it is found at highest level in the cerebral cortex and is widely distributed among several other brain regions. Thus, the results of these neuroanatomical mapping studies do not support the conclusion that the major function of the mass of brain CCK is to control ingestive behavior. Ontogenetic studies carried out in our laboratory have shown that the appearance of CCK immunoreactivity in the brain of a particular vertebrate follows a precise time course, one that is quite distinct from that of intestinal CCK. The developmental patterns of brain CCK are closely linked to structural aspects of brain histogenesis and are not specifically associated with the attainment of behavioral milestones or the manifestations of adult patterns of feeding behavior (16, 63).

To test whether endogenous stores of brain CCK are affected by nutritional alterations, we have measured the levels of CCK in major neuroanatomical regions in a variety of altered nutritional states, including: neonatally malnourished rats; fasted adult rats; and rodents made obese as a result of diet, genetic mutation, and brain lesioning. In no instance was any measurable parameter of brain CCK (tissue concentration, regional anatomic distribution, and molecular heterogeneity) found to differ from that of controls (16). These results are in agreement with those reported from other laboratories studying brain CCK concentrations in ob/ob mice, Zucker rats, and short-term food deprivation (64–67) but contrast sharply with the reports from one laboratory of lower levels of cerebral cortical CCK in ob/ob mice and mice subjected to 2–4 days of food deprivation (68, 69). The reason for these discrepancies is not known.

Thus, from all the information this methodology has yielded about brain CCK—its neuroanatomy, ontogenetic development, and regional concentrations in relation to nutritional status—it has been difficult to implicate endogenous brain CCK in the control of appetitive behavior. However, the limitations inherent in studies of tissue peptide concentrations, described above, preclude definitive conclusions about specific function.

There is some indication that aspects of brain CCK receptor function may change in association with nutritional alterations. Saito et al. (54) have demonstrated saturable, reversible binding of ^{125}I-labeled Bolton-Hunter CCK-33 to a membrane fraction of rat brain. Using this methodology, this group (17) has demonstrated increased binding (increased receptor number; unchanged affinity) in hypothalamus and olfactory bulb of mice following a 42-h fast, with no significant changes in binding to cerebral cortical tissue. This group has also reported increases in CCK receptor number in cerebral cortical tissue of ob/ob mice compared with lean littermates, but no changes in binding to brain receptors derived from hypothalamus, olfactory bulb, or other brain areas in these same animals. Brain tissue derived from the obese db/db mouse showed no changes in CCK receptors. Pancreatic receptors were unaltered in the ob/ob mouse (70).

These investigators have suggested that perturbations in normal feeding behavior involve changes in binding of brain CCK to hypothalamic receptors whereas one type of genetically induced obesity (the ob/ob mouse) may be associated with abnormal cerebral cortical CCK function, as manifest by increased receptor number. In similar experiments, Hays et al. reported increases in CCK binding to cerebral cortical, but not hypothalamic, membranes in both ob/ob mice and Zucker fatty rats when compared with lean littermates. However, this group of researchers did not observe alterations in CCK binding to hypothalamic or cerebral cortical membranes of rats fasted for 96-h (71, 72).

These results are provocative but must be treated with some caution because desulfated CCK-8, CCK-4, and gastrin are capable of binding to the receptor (although with somewhat diminished potencies) and these compounds are devoid of satiety-inducing effects at almost any dose.

It should also be noted that db/db and ob/ob mice and Zucker fatty rats are hyperphagic, obese, and manifest numerous peripheral metabolic abnormalities. If changes in feeding behavior are associated with alterations in hypothalamic CCK receptors, it is not clear why changes in hypothalamic binding are not manifest in these obese models. Furthermore, in genetically obese animals with associated derangements in brain morphology (such as the ob/ob mouse), the considerations described above (and relating to radioimmunoassay data expression) apply also to quantifying receptor number per weight of tissue or tissue protein. These studies represent an important avenue of research, and further characterization of brain CCK receptors and postreceptor biologic events will be required.

In separate experiments, attempts have been made in sheep and rats to block the action of endogenous brain CCK with anti-CCK antibody. Injections of anti-CCK antibody into the lateral cerebral ventricles of sheep appear to inhibit normal postprandial satiety and stimulate food intake. Since the effects of antibody infusion were apparent 30 min after injection, it is most probable that the enhanced food intake was due to binding of endogenous CCK within the CSF, for it is unlikely that the antibody could penetrate into the substance of the brain within that time period. This experiment suggests a role for CSF-borne CCK in postprandial satiety. Similar experiments carried out in rats, using the same antisera, failed to demonstrate any effect on food intake (73).

Conclusion

Despite often conflicting results and obvious interspecies variation in responses, the many pharmacologic experiments that demonstrate a suppressive effect of exogenous CCK on food intake, particularly experiments demonstrating interactions of exogenous CCK with monoaminergic feeding circuits, provide valuable probes into possible modes of action of brain CCK. However, it must be emphasized that such experiments do not prove that appetite regulation constitutes part of the normal function of this brain peptide. The nutritionally associated alterations in brain CCK receptor number and the effects of anti-CCK antibody on feeding in sheep suggest that endogenous brain CCK is involved in feeding behavior, but it is difficult to integrate these results into a cohesive framework. A more comprehensive understanding of the physiology of brain CCK is needed before its function in the control of feeding behavior can be established.

6 BOMBESIN

It has also been suggested that bombesin, a 14-amino-acid peptide originally isolated from frog skin (74), functions in the control of mammalian feeding behavior. Bombesin-like immunoreactivity has been identified in many mammalian tissues including gastric fundus, gastric antrum, small and large intestine, fetal lung, and brain (75–80). The complete amino acid sequence of mammalian bombesin is unknown, but there appear to be at least two molecular forms present in the stomach. Functional activity, including appetite-suppressive effects, appears to reside in the same nine-amino-acid carboxy-terminal sequence found in the frog skin peptide, and mammalian "bombesins" are thought to include gastrin-releasing peptide and other uncharacterized family members (81).

The gastrointestinal localization of bombesin and its diverse pharmacologic effects on gastrointestinal function—including gastrin release, CCK release, gall bladder contraction (82–84), pancreatic secretion, and augmented intestinal motility—have led to extensive investigation into this peptide's role as a peripheral satiety signal.

Gibbs and Fauser (85) first demonstrated that parenteral administration of synthetic bombesin reduced feeding behavior by inducing meal termination in freely feeding rats. Martin and Gibbs (86) further showed that bombesin at intraperitoneal doses of 1–10 microgram/kg suppressed food intake in sham-feeding animals. Morley and Levine (87) have demonstrated that bombesin also inhibits tail-pinch-induced feeding. The effect of peripheral bombesin on feeding behavior occurs at a fivefold lower potency than that of CCK but is associated with grooming and resting behavior and is unaccompanied by impaired water intake. The satiety-inducing effects of bombesin are not abolished by truncal or gastric vagotomy, indicating that this action is independent of CCK release. When CCK and bombesin are given conjointly their effects are additive, further suggesting separate mechanisms of action for the two hormones (88). The anatomic loci or mechanisms involved in the satiety-inducing effects of parenteral bombesin are unknown. The peptide could act directly on the CNS, via a neural pathway outside the vagus, or secondarily by permuting gastrointestinal function. There are also conflicting reports as to whether the appetite-suppressive effect of bombesin is secondary to taste aversion (89, 90). It is still a subject of some debate whether these effects of peripheral bombesin are physiological or pharmacological. No one has clearly demonstrated a rise in plasma bombesin with normal feeding but this may reflect technical difficulties with the radioimmunoassays that are

currently available. Until elevated endogenous plasma bombesin is correlated with satiety, the physiological relevance of these data will remain in question.

Bombesin and bombesin receptors are also found in the central nervous system at highest concentrations in the hypothalamus (75, 76, 78–
80, 91, 92). Bombesin is found in synaptosomes and is released in Ca^{2+}-
dependent fashion, suggesting a neurotransmitter function.

Intraventricular administration of bombesin has been shown to reduce feeding in rats, sheep, and pigs, to inhibit stress-induced feeding,
and to cause alterations in peripheral glucose, insulin, and catecholamine metabolism (44, 87, 88, 93–97). In contrast with experiments with
CCK, virtually all laboratories consistently report decreases in food intake with intraventricular administration of bombesin. Unlike CCK or
peripherally administered bombesin, intraventricular dosages of
bombesin also decrease water intake and generally do not produce behaviors characteristic of satiety. This has suggested to several authors
that peripheral bombesin does not act exclusively by gaining access to
the CSF. Intrahypothalamic injection of bombesin is associated with satiety, appropriate postprandial behavior, and normal water intake,
suggesting that bombesin may act at this locus to regulate meal termination (98).

A recent publication (99) has reported that endogenous CNS
bombesin levels change with the nutritional state of the animal; however, interpretation of these findings is difficult, since bombesin levels
changed divergently in different neuroanatomical sites in association
with various nutritional manipulations.

Conclusion

Several reports demonstrate that exogenous bombesin can suppress
feeding, but the physiological relevance of these observations awaits
further experimentation. Bombesin does not appear to control feeding in
a specific fashion when administered into the cerebral ventricles, but it
may function in the hypothalamus to regulate food intake.

7 INSULIN

It has been suggested that the fluctuating plasma concentrations of insulin serve as input signals in control mechanisms that modulate both
short-term feeding behavior and the regulation of adipose tissue triglyceride stores over long periods of time.

Havrankova et al. have reported the presence of high concentrations
of insulin relative to plasma concentrations in rodent brain (100, 101),
although another group has failed to replicate this finding (102–104). It is

therefore still not clear whether the reported brain insulin immunoreactivity represents locally synthesized peptide or that which arises from the peripheral circulation. The observations that whole brain insulin concentrations are ten times higher than normal plasma levels and that concentrations of brain insulin are unchanged despite drastic alterations in peripheral plasma insulin levels have led Havrankova and coworkers to suggest that brain insulin is synthesized within the CNS (100, 101, 105). The half-life of brain insulin is unknown, however, and its appearance in the brain may represent a stable pool of exogenous peptide that turns over very slowly. To our knowledge, no laboratory has described proinsulin or C-peptide in brain, although these compounds might also arise from extra-CNS sources so that their presence would still not provide unequivocal evidence for endogenous brain insulin synthesis. To resolve this issue definitively, demonstration of biosynthesis of insulin by brain tissue will be required. The relationship between brain and plasma insulin thus remains obscure. Brain insulin receptors have also been reported (101, 106) and appear to be similar to insulin receptors found outside the CNS, but the neuroanatomical distribution of insulin receptor concentrations does not parallel that of brain insulin itself.

While the source or function of brain insulin remains unelucidated, several investigators have proposed that the central nervous system may be capable of detecting physiological changes in circulating plasma insulin concentrations. If this proves correct, then it is conceivable that circulating insulin may carry information to the brain regarding the nutritional status of the organism. Of particular significance in the case of insulin, such information may relate both to meal-taking (short-term signaling) and to the global status of adipose tissue triglyceride stores, for not only is pancreatic insulin release acutely responsive to stimulation by substrates during meals, it is also well-established that both basal and peak levels of circulating insulin vary directly with increasing adiposity in mammals. In fact, hyperinsulinemia is a constant finding in virtually all forms of human and animal obesity. Noting this relationship between the size of adipose tissue triglyceride stores and circulating insulin levels, Woods and Porte (107, 108) proposed that although plasma insulin concentrations are labile, if ambient levels are unusually high (as in obesity and overfeeding) the insulin may slowly enter the cerebrospinal fluid, causing a steady elevation of CSF insulin concentrations. Such an elevation may then be "read" by relevant centers in the brain as an integral of insulin secretion over long periods of time. Insulin has been detected in the CSF of experimental animals following intravenous injections of large, supraphysiological doses (109). Endogenous CSF insulin immunoreactivity has also been reported in dogs (109, 110). The CSF insulin concentrations reported in dogs appeared to reflect plasma insulin levels (110). In addition, elevated levels of endogenous insulin have been reported in the CSF of obese patients (111). However, using an antiserum capable of detecting 1–2 pg of human insulin per mL, we have been unable to detect any immunoreactive insulin in spinal fluid specimens derived from numerous obese patients in whom plasma insulin levels were elevated at the time of sampling (unpublished observations). Exogenous human insulin was found to be fully recoverable from CSF. It is conceivable that spinal fluid contains proinsulin or fragments of MW 6000 insulin that react poorly with our antibody, or that the discrepancy is due to sampling site (lumbar in humans vs. cisternal in dogs). Further investigation of the relationship between plasma insulin and spinal fluid insulin will require more complete physicochemical characterization to verify the nature of the reported insulin immunoreactivity in CSF.

There is evidence that blood-borne insulin can reach selected sites within the brain. Using *in vivo* radioautographic methods, van Houten et al. (112–114) have demonstrated specific binding of intravenously administered ^{125}I-insulin to the endothelium of microvessels distributed throughout the brain and to neurons confined to circumventricular organs where there is no effective blood-brain barrier. For example, binding of ^{125}I-insulin to nerve terminals and axons has been demonstrated in the median eminence and arcuate nucleus (115). It is also known that locally applied insulin can alter hypothalamic electrical activity, affect peripheral glucose metabolism, and interfere with norepinephrine turnover (114, 116–118). In addition, centrally administered insulin can suppress feeding in rats and baboons (119, 120). Thus, there is a growing body of experimental evidence indicating that insulin can enter selected sites in the brain, bind to receptors, and activate neurochemical mechanisms central to the control of metabolism and feeding behavior. That ambient, fluctuating levels of plasma insulin actually serve as a physiological short-term or long-term feedback signal to the brain has been difficult to prove, largely because it is difficult to alter endogenous circulating insulin concentrations without producing profound metabolic changes associated with the actions of insulin. This is particularly true of short-term studies in which altered insulin levels are accompanied by changes in carbohydrate, amino acid, and fat metabolism. The methodological problem also exists in long-term nutritional studies in which food intake, adipocyte size, total body fat, body weight, and ambient insulin levels usually co-vary. To approach this problem, we have employed several rodent models in which adipose tissue morphology has been artificially altered (by surgical and other means) so that adipose cell size, total body fat, and food intake can be experimentally dissociated (121). In some models, chronic food intake was dissociated from ambient plasma insulin levels—that is, animals in one paradigm were found to consume equal quantities of food despite great differences in endogenous insulin levels whereas in another model, experimental and control animals consumed different amounts of food while insulin levels remained identical. Thus, at least in these experiments, plasma insulin concentrations are not a major determinant of long-term food intake. In all experimental models, plasma insulin levels correlated directly with fat cell size, suggesting that nutritional information regarding adipose cell size is carried by this hormone.

Conclusion

Insulin and its receptors have been reported in brain, but the origin of the CNS insulin remains unresolved. The concentrations of brain insulin and its receptors are reported to be unchanged despite drastic alterations in nutritional status and in concentrations of plasma insulin and its peripheral target cell membrane receptors. There is evidence that plasma-borne insulin can enter specific sites in brain and initiate or modulate neurochemical pathways involved in metabolism and feeding behavior. The intriguing possibility thus remains that plasma insulin constitutes at least part of the afferent component of long- or short-term nutritional control systems.

The origin of reported CNS insulin immunoreactivity must be clarified before insulin can be established as an endogenous brain peptide involved in the central integration of feeding behavior.

8 ENDOGENOUS OPIATES

Several studies have suggested that the endogenous opiates may stimulate food intake (122). These peptides do not fit neatly into the paradigm presented earlier in this chapter in which a peripheral hormone, the release of which is in part directed by the levels of intestinal or plasma nutrient, signals to the central nervous system the nutritional status of the organism. The situation in this case is complicated by the diverse number of peptides in both the periphery and central nervous system with opiate-like activity. Each of the peptides that needs to be considered in any discussion of opioid effects on feeding—Met-enkephalin, Leu-enkephalin, beta-endorphin, and dynorphin—has its own characteristic anatomical distribution both in the periphery and the central nervous system, and furthermore has distinct receptor populations with which it probably acts under physiologic conditions. However, at high concentrations (pharmacologic doses) a given opioid peptide can interact with other opiate receptors, albeit at lower affinity (123–128).

Early consideration that the opiate receptor system might have some relationship to feeding behavior arose in large part from clinical observations of nutritional status in narcotic addicts, observations which antedated the discovery of the endogenous opiates. Narcotic addicts have been noted to lose weight while addicted, and to regain the lost weight when either entering steady-state methadone maintenance or abstaining from narcotic use. It has never been adequately resolved whether these weight fluctuations reflect the socioeconomic or medical status of the addicted individuals or signify some underlying pharmacologic property of the narcotic. These observations and earlier studies demonstrating that narcotics can alter feeding behavior in animals have led to inquiry into the possible role of the endogenous opiates in the control of food intake (129).

Margules et al. (130) have reported elevated plasma and pituitary endorphin levels in genetically obese rodents and have shown that the hyperphagia characteristic of this syndrome is reduced after administration of the narcotic antagonist naloxone. They have postulated on this basis that circulating beta-endorphin acts at some peripheral locus to augment food intake. The precise nature of this proposed system is unclear and primarily speculative. More recent work by Rossier et al. (131) demonstrates that the development of the obesity of the ob/ob syndrome precedes the elevation of endorphin, suggesting that circulating endorphin is not pathogenic in this system. Furthermore, these animals manifest numerous endocrine abnormalities, including elevated ACTH and corticosterone levels. Since ACTH and beta-endorphin are derived from the same 31K precursor molecule, it is possible that the increased beta-endorphin levels seen in this syndrome reflect a more general hypothalamic–pituitary defect. In a longitudinal hormonal profile of the ob/ob mouse, Garthwaite et al. (132) found only partial temporal correlation between the development of the obesity syndrome and the manifestation of the pro-opiocortin-related hormonal abnormalities. Furthermore, Wallace et al. (133) showed that feeding behavior was not different among groups of rats with high and normal endogenous plasma beta-endorphin levels, nor were those animals with high endorphin levels abnormally sensitive to naloxone.

Peripheral naloxone administration can diminish feeding in ob/ob mice, Zucker fatty rats, and other experimental animal models of hyperphagia, including stress-induced eating (130, 134–141), although there has been controversy about the last effect (142, 139). However, this does not necessarily imply that the reduction in food intake is due to blockade at the peripheral site of action of circulating beta-endorphin, for naloxone at the doses administered will block not only circulating beta-endorphin but any of the endogenous opiates at either peripheral or central receptor sites. Furthermore, in interpreting studies of the effects of a narcotic agonist or antagonist on feeding behavior, it is important to question which system or systems are being perturbed; whether the drug is acting peripherally or centrally; whether the observed effect is behaviorally specific (i.e., the alteration in food intake is not secondary to mood changes); and, with repeated administration of exogenous

opiates, whether the animal's response reflects, in part, narcotic abstinence.

Although the biosynthetic pathway of pituitary beta-endorphin is
well understood and much is known about its patterns of release into
plasma, its biological function remains unelucidated. It is probably premature to ascribe any specific role to circulating beta-endorphin in the
control of feeding behavior until more is known of its physiology. The
effects of endorphin and the enkephalins on gastrointestinal functions
make it possible that these peptides can alter feeding patterns by direct
actions on the gastrointestinal tract (143, 144).

It is intriguing to speculate that opiate-like peptides in foodstuffs, so-
called exorphins (145), might affect appetite although no studies examining the effects of these peptides on feeding behavior have been
published.

The evidence that endogenous opiates found within the central nervous system play a role in the control of feeding behavior is somewhat
more compelling. Experiments demonstrating a relationship between
central opioid peptides and feeding can be generally assigned to one of
four categories: (i) administration of opioid peptides and exogenous opiates directly into discrete regions of the central nervous system, (ii) observation of the effects on feeding after peripheral administration of
narcotics presumed to act centrally, (iii) observation of the effects on
feeding of administration of narcotic antagonists, (iv) measurement of
endogenous opioid peptide levels in brain in various nutritional states.

Beta-endorphin has been shown to stimulate food intake in satiated
rats when injected intraventricularly or into the ventromedial hypothalamus (146–148, 150). Since intracerebral injections of a variety of compounds generally reduce feeding, this finding is of particular interest.
Further studies, using dynorphin, have confirmed these observations
(149). Since the hypothalamus is intimately involved in regulation of
feeding it is attractive to speculate that beta-endorphin, which is present in high levels in the hypothalamus, augments feeding behavior directly or by interacting with brain monoamines. Nevertheless, the
neurophysiological basis for these observation remains unelucidated.
The results must also be considered with some caution because the effective dose of endorphin administered, 1.5 μgm, exceeds the total
amount of beta-endorphin in the hypothalamus by a factor of 1000.

Numerous studies have demonstrated that peripherally and centrally
administered narcotics can increase feeding behavior in animals (122,
152–154). Although it is generally accepted that the classic behavioral
effects of narcotics are mediated directly within the CNS, it is unclear
which CNS (or possibly extra-CNS) loci are involved in narcotic-in-
duced feeding or which opiate receptors at those loci are stimulated. In
fact, at the doses administered, any of the known opiate receptors (mu,
sigma, kappa, or any heretofore undefined receptor) could be activated.

The lack of specificity of these agents limits their utility in dissecting the underlying neurophysiological mechanisms involved in their stimulation of feeding.

It is somewhat satisfying that naloxone can inhibit feeding behavior in the same experimental settings in which narcotics stimulate feeding (151, 152). Naloxone administered directly into the lateral ventricle of the rat suppresses feeding behavior, at doses that are ineffective when given peripherally (153). These observations, coupled with the assumption that naloxone is devoid of narcotic agonist or other intrinsic activities, have suggested to many investigators that endogenous central opiate activity exerts a positive effect on feeding that is blocked by naloxone. It needs to be mentioned however, that naloxone has been shown to have agonist activity in some systems (154, 155), and until the complete biological effects of this compound are clearly established it cannot be assumed that all effects of naloxone are due exclusively to endogenous opiate blockade. The same ambiguity of opiate receptor specificity encountered in narcotic experiments also applies to naloxone, since at the doses generally employed receptor specificity is nonexistent.

In a separate approach to this problem, central beta-endorphin has been measured in various nutritional states. Gambert et al. (156) showed that fasting in rats is associated with a decrease in the levels of hypothalamic beta-endorphin. Gibson et al. (157) reported higher total brain endorphin levels in the Zucker fatty rat, although no differences in hypothalamic endorphin levels were detected. Similarly, Margules et al. (130) found unchanged hypothalamic endorphin concentrations in ob/ob mice, compared with those of their lean littermates. It is difficult at present to integrate these results into a consistent model of endorphin action within the CNS. Specific inquiries into the effects of altered nutrition on opiate receptor number and affinity or post-receptor activities have not been published.

Conclusion

There is growing evidence that endogenous opiates may act within the CNS, possibly at the hypothalamic level, to stimulate food intake. The opiate receptors, post-receptor events and cellular loci which mediate this behavioral action remain to be established.

9   THYROTROPIN RELEASING HORMONE AND RELATED PEPTIDES

Although highest concentrations of TRH in mammalian brain are found within the hypothalamus, this tripeptide is widely distributed through other brain regions, including cerebral cortex, thalamus, brainstem, spinal cord, and cerebellum. The presence of receptors for TRH in brain, its synaptosomal localization and appropriate release from tissue *in vitro*, and demonstration of its biosynthesis by brain tissue all indicate that TRH is an endogenous brain peptide involved in neurotransmission or in the modulation of the action of monoamine neurotransmitters. TRH is also found in several extra -CNS sites, including the pancreas, gastrointestinal tract, placenta, and male reproductive organs. TRH is also phylogenetically very old and ubiquitous: it is present in frog skin, lamprey, amphioxus, snail ganglia, and even in some plants. Clearly, the hypophysiotropic effect of TRH on TSH secretion constitutes only one of a multiplicity of functions performed by this tripeptide.

Administration of TRH into the CNS results in a number pharmacologic and behavioral effects (158–160), one of which is a reduction of food and water intake. Vijayan and McCann found that injections of 0.6 nmole of TRH into the third ventricle of rats diminished food intake while doses of 0.3 nmole diminished water intake. No other behavioral effects or signs of toxicity were observed following intracranial injection of TRH (161). In these experiments somatostatin also diminished food intake, although at higher doses. The precise neuroanatomical locus or pharmacological mode of action of TRH on food intake has not been elucidated. TRH can antagonize effects of opioid peptides, and it is possible that the suppression of feeding is effected by interference with the endogenous opiate system (162). Peripherally administered TRH has also been shown to inhibit food intake (163, 164).

When TRH is metabolized in brain by pyroglutamyl peptidase and the reaction product undergoes spontaneous cyclization, histidyl-proline-diketopipe razine (cyclo-His-Pro) is formed (165, 166). This compound, detected in brain tissue by radioimmunoassay (167), also inhibits food intake when given intraventricularly (168). Using a radioimmunoassay for cyclo-His-Pro, Mori et al. have demonstrated increased hypothalamic levels of this peptide during 24 h of fasting in rats, without concomitant changes in cyclo-His-Pro concentrations in other parts of the brain. TRH levels also did not change during these experiments. Strikingly, the hypothalamic cyclo-His-Pro levels returned to control levels 1 h after refeeding (169). These experiments demonstrate that hypothalamic cyclo-His-Pro is acutely sensitive to alterations in nutritional status, and together with the pharmacological data suggest that endogenous cyclo-His-Pro may function in the hypothalamic integration of appetite regulation.

Trygstad and associates reported the existence of a tripeptide similar to TRH, with the sequence pyro-Glu-His-Gly-OH, in the urine of patients with anorexia nervosa (170, 171). A synthetic preparation of this tripeptide had a profound and prolonged anorectic effect when injected subcutaneously in mice. The anatomical source of this peptide was not established. In a later study, Nance et al. (172) tested this tripeptide and found it had no effect on either food intake or body weight in rats and mice, even in doses higher than those employed by the Trygstad group. Thus, the anorectic effect of this peptide has yet to be confirmed.

10 CONCLUSION

Pharmacological studies have provided evidence that a number of brain peptides can alter feeding behavior, either directly or by interacting with local monoaminergic or possibly other peptidergic systems. All the peptides discussed above have been shown to act on the brain either to suppress or enhance feeding, although in some studies the results have been inconsistent or have depended on the experimental paradigm. Investigations of some brain peptides have also yielded positive results using other experimental modalities designed to demonstrate endogenous action (radioimmunoassay of tissue peptide concentrations, radioreceptor assay, blocking experiments using antibody or nonpeptidal antagonist). In no study has the investigation of any known peptide yielded consistently positive results across all available research modalities.

It is likely that further research will disclose other peptides in brain and gut that are even more potent regulators of feeding. Improved bioassays for such putative substances may help in their identification. Clinical experiments of nature, provided by such pathological conditions as anorexia nervosa or tumor-induced cachexia, may also provide clues if the pathophysiology of these syndromes involves excess or ectopic production of anorexigenic compounds.

REFERENCES

1. P. R. McHugh, T. H. Moran, and G. N. Barton, *Science* **190**, 167–169 (1975).
2. N. Mrovsovsky and T. L. Powley, *Behav. Biol.* **20**, 205–223 (1977).
3. N. Mrovsovsky, *Hibernation and the Hypothalamus*, Appleton Century Crofts, New York, 1971.
4. J. R. Brobeck, *Physiol. Rev.* **23**, 541–559 (1946).
5. B. G. Hoebel and P. Teitelbaum, *J. Comp. Physiol. Psychol.* **61**, 189–193 (1966).
6. R. L. Powley and R. E. Keesey, *J. Comp. Physiol. Psychol.* **70**, 25–36 (1970).
7. L. D. Lytle, in R. J. Wurtman and J. J. Wurtman, Eds., *Nutrition and the Brain*, Vol. 2, Raven Press, New York, 1977, pp. 1–145.
8. R. J. Wurtman, F. Hefti, and E. Melamed, *Pharmacol. Rev.* **43**,4 315–335 (1980).
9. R. J. Wurtman, *Sci. Am.* **246**(4), 50–59 (1982).
10. A. J. Strohmayer, G. Silverman, and J. A. Grinker, *Physiol. Behav.* **24**, 789–791 (1980).
11. R. D. Myers, in R. D. Myers, Ed., *Methods in Psychobiology*, Vol. I, Academic Press, London, 1971, pp. 247–280.
12. P. H. W. Van der Kroon and G. J. A. Speijers, *Metab. Clin. Exp.* **28**, 1–3 (1979).
13. W. J. Shoemaker and F. E. Bloom, in R. J. Wurtman and J. J. Wurtman, Eds., *Nutrition and Brain*, Vol. 2, Raven Press, New York, 1977, pp. 147–192.

14. M. Winick and A. Noble, *J. Nutr.* **89**, 300–306 (1966).
15. I. Fish and M. Winick, *Exp. Neurol.* **25**, 534–540 (1969).
16. B. S. Schneider, J. Monahan, and J. Hirsch, *J. Clin. Invest.* **64**, 1346–1348 (1979).
17. A. Saito, J. A. Williams, and I. D. Goldfine, *Nature* **289**, 599–600 (1981).
18. N. F. Maclagan, *J. Physiol. (London)* **90**, 385–394 (1937).
19. A. V. Schally, T. W. Redding, H. W. Lucien, and J. Meyer, *Science* **157**, 210–211 (1967).
20. J. Gibbs, R. C. Young, and G. P. Smith, *J. Comp. Physiol. Psychol.* **84**(3) 488–495 (1973).
21. J. Gibbs, R. C. Young, and G. P. Smith, *Nature* **245**, 323–325 (1973).
22. J. Antin, J. Gibbs, J. Holt, R. C. Young, and G. P. Smith, *J. Comp. Physiol. Psychol.* **89**, 784–790 (1975).
23. D. N. Lorenz, G. Kreiselsheimer, and G. P. Smith, *Physiol. Behav.* **23**, 1065–1072 (1979).
24. G. P. Smith, in R. F. Beers Jr. and E. G. Bassett, Eds., *Polypeptide Hormones*, Raven Press, New York, 1980, pp. 413–420.
25. G. P. Smith, J. Gibbs, C. Jerome, F. X. Pi-Sunyer, H. R. Kissileff, and J. Thornton, Peptides **2**, Suppl. 2, 57–59 (1981).
26. J. A. Deutsch and W. T. Hardy, *Nature* **266**, 196 (1977).
27. J. Gibbs and G. P. Smith, *Nature* **266**, 196 (1977).
28. D. N. Lorenz and S. A. Goldman, *Soc. Neurosci. Abstr.* **4**, 178 (1978).
29. G. P. Smith, C. Jerome, B. J. Cushin, R. Eterno, and K. J. Simansky, *Science* **213**, 1036–1037 (1981).
30. T. R. Houpt, S. M. Anika, and N. C. Wolff, *Am. J. Physiol.* **235**(1), R23–R28 (1978).
31. M. A. Zarbin, J. K. Wamsley, R. B. Innis, and M. J. Kuhar, *Life Sci.* **29**, 697–705 (1981).
32. J. J. Vanderhaeghen, J. C. Signeau, and W. Gepts, *Nature (London)* **257**, 604–605 (1975).
33. G. J. Dockray, *Nature (London)* **264**, 568–570 (1976).
34. J. E. Muller, E. Straus, and R. S. Yalow, *Proc. Natl. Acad. Sci. USA* **74**, 3035–3037 (1977).
35. G. J. Dockray, R. A. Gregory, J. B. Hutchinson, J. I. Harris, and M. J. Runswick, *Nature* **274**, 711–713 (1978).
36. E. Straus and R. S. Yalow, *Proc. Natl. Acad. Sci. USA* **75**, 486–489 (1978).
37. J. F. Rehfeld, *J. Biol. Chem.* **253**, 4022–2030 (1978).
38. R. B. Innis, F. M. A. Correa, G. R. Uhl, B. Schneider, and S. H. Snyder, *Proc. Natl. Acad. Sci.* **76**, 521–525 (1979).
39. J. J. Stern, C. A. Cudillo, and J. Kruper, *J. Comp. Physiol. Psychol.* **90**(5), 484–490 (1976).
40. S. Maddison, *Physiol. Behav.* **19**, 819–824 (1977).
41. M. A. Della-Fera and C. A. Baile, *Science* **206**, 471–473 (1979).
42. M. A. Della-Fera and C. A. Baile, *Physiol. Behav.* **26**, 979–983 (1981).
43. R. F. Parrott and B. A. Baldwin, *Physiol. Behav.* **26** 419–422 (1981).
44. J. A. Grinker, B. S. Schneider, G. Ball, A. Cohen, A. Strohmayer, and J. Hirsch, *Fed. Proc.* **39**, 1234A (1980).
45. C. Jerome, P. Kulkosky, V. Simansky, and G. P. Smith, *Society for Neuroscience, Abst.* 275.1 (1981).
46. C. B. Nemeroff, A. J. Osbahr III, G. Bissette, G. Jahnke, M. A. Lipton, and A. J. Prange Jr., *Science* **200**, 793–794 (1978).
47. M. L. McCaleb and R. D. Myers, *Peptides* **1**, 47–49 (19)/(1980).
48. R. D. Myers and M. L. McCaleb, *Neuroscience* **6**(4), 645–655 (1981).
49. S. M. Antelman, H. Szechtman, P. Chin, and A. E. Fisher, *Brain Res.* **99**, 319–337 (1975).
50. M. T. Lowy, R. P. Maickel, and G. K. W. Yim, *Life Sci.* **26**, 2113–2118 (1980).

51. J. E. Morley and A. S. Levine, *Science* **209**, 1259–1261 (1980).
52. A. S. Levine and J. E. Morley, *Regul. Peptides*, **2**, 353–357 (1981).
53. N. R. Goltermann, J. F. Rehfeld, and H. Roigaard-Petersen, *J. Biol. Chem.* **255**, 6181–6185 (1980).
54. A. Saito, H. Sankaran, I. D. Goldfine, and J. A. Williams, *Science* **208**, 1155–1156 (1980).
55. R. B. Innis and S. H. Snyder *Proc. Natl. Acad. Sci. USA* **77**, 6917–6921 (1980).
56. S. E. Hays, M. C. Beinfeld, R. T. Jensen, F. K. Goodwin, and S. M. Paul, *Neuropeptides* **1**, 53–62 (1980).
57. M. Pinget, E. Straus, and R. S. Yalow, *Proc. Natl. Acad. Sci. USA* **75**, 6324–6326 (1978).
58. M. Pinget, E. Straus, and R. S. Yalow, *Life Sci.* **25**, 339–342 (1979).
59. P. C. Emson, C. M. Lee, and J. F. Rehfeld, *Life Sci.* **26**, 2157–2162 (1980).
60. L. I. Larsson and J. F. Rehfeld, *Brain Res.* **165**, 201–218 (1979).
61. M. C. Beinfeld, D. K. Meyer, R. L. Eskay, R. T. Jensen, and M. J. Brownstein, *Brain Res.* **212**, 51–57 (1981).
62. J. J. Vanderhaegen, F. Lotstra, J. DeMey, and C. Filles, *Proc. Natl. Acad. Sci. USA* **77**, 1190–1194 (1980).
63. S. A. Goldman and B. Schneider, *Society for Neuroscience, Abst. 32.1*, (1981).
64. J. Hansky and P. Ho, *Austral. J. Exp. Biol. Med. Sci.* **57**, 575 (1979).
65. P. Ho and J. Hansky, *Gastroenterology* **76**, 1155 (1979).
66. J. Oku, Z. Glick, Y. Shimomura, S. Inoue, G. A. Bray, and J. Walsh, *Clin. Res.* **28**, 25A (1980).
67. J. A. Finkelstein, A. W. Steggles, F. W. Lotstra, and J. J. Vanderhaegen, *Peptides* **2**, 19–21 (1981).
68. E. Straus and R. S. Yalow, *Science* **203**, 68–69 (1979).
69. E. Straus and R. S. Yalow, *Life Sci.* **26**, 969–970 (1980).
70. A. Saito, J. A. Williams, and I. D. Goldfine, *Endocrinology* **109**(3), 984–986 (1981).
71. S. E. Hays and S. M. Paul, *Eur. J. Pharmacol.* **70**, 591–592 (1981).
72. S. E. Hays, F. K. Goodwin, and S. M. Paul, *Peptides* **2**, Suppl. 1, 21–26 (1981).
73. M. A. Della-Fera, C. Baile, B. S. Schneider, and J. A. Grinker, *Science* **212**, 687–689 (1981).
74. A. Anastasi, V. Erspamer, and M. Bucci, *Experientia* **27**, 166–167 (1971).
75. J. H. Walsh, H. C. Wong, and G. J. Dockray, *Fed. Proc.* **38**, 2315–2319 (1979).
76. M. Brown, R. Allen, J. Villarreal, J. Rivier, and W. Vale, *Life Sci.* **23**, 2721–2728 (1978).
77. J. Wharton, J. M. Polak, S. R. Bloom, M. A. Ghatei, E. Solcia, M. R. Brown, and A. G. E. Pearse, *Nature* **273**, 769–770 (1978).
78. T. W. Moody, T. B. Nguyen, T. L. O'Donohue, and C. B. Pert, *Life Sci.* **26**, 1707–1712 (1980).
79. J. A. Villarreal and M. R. Brown, *Life Sci.* **23**, 2729–2734 (1978).
80. T. W. Moody, J. L. O'Donohue, and D. M. Jacobowitz, *Peptides* **2**, 75–79 (1981).
81. M. Brown, W. Marki, and J. Rivier, *Life Sci.* **27**, 125–128 (1980).
82. V. Erspamer and P. Melchiarri, in J. C. Thompson, Ed., *Gastrointestinal Hormones*, University of Texas, Austin, 1975, pp. 575–589.
83. V. Erspamer, G. Improta, P. Melchiorri, and N. Sopranzi, *Br. J. Pharmacol.* **52**, 227–232 (1974).
84. G. Bertaccini, V. Erspamer, P. Melchiorri, and N. Sopranzi, *Br. J. Pharmacol.* **52**, 219–225 (1974).
85. J. Gibbs and D. J. Fauser, *Nature* **282**, 208–210 (1979).
86. C. F. Martin and J. Gibbs, *Peptides* **1**, 131–134 (1980).
87. J. E. Morley and A. S. Levine, *Pharmacol. Biochem. Behav.* **14**, 149–151 (1980).
88. J. Gibbs, P. J. Kulkosky, and G. P. Smith, *Peptides* **2**, 179–183 (1981).

89. J. A. Deutsch and S. L. Parsons, *Behav. Neural Biol.* **31**, 110–113 (1981).
90. P. J. Kulkosky, L. Gray, J. Gibbs, and G. P. Smith, *Peptides* **2**, 61–64 (1981).
91. T. W. Moody, C. B. Pert, J. Rivier, and M. R. Brown, *Proc. Natl. Acad. Sci. USA* **75** (11), 5372–5376 (1978).
92. A. Pert, T. W. Moody, C. B., Pert, L. A. Dewald, and J. Rivier, *Brain Res.* **193**, 209–220 (1980).
93. C. A. Baile and M. A. Della-Fera, *Behav. Pharmacol. Physiol.* **40**(3) Abst. no. 421, 1981.
94. R. F. Parrott and B. A. Baldwin, *Physiol. Behav.* **28**, 521–524 (1982).
95. M. Brown, Y. Tache, and D. Fisher, *Endocrinology* **105**(3), 660–665 (1979).
96. M. Brown, *Diabetologia* **20**, 299–304 (1981).
97. P. J. Kulkosky, J. Gibbs, and G. P. Smith, *Physiol. Behav.* **28**(3), 505–512 (1982).
98. J. A. Stuckey and J. Gibbs, *Soc. Neurosci. Abstr.* 275.4 (1981).
99. C. Soveny and J. Hansky, *Regulatory Peptides* **3**, 325–331 (1982).
100. J. Havrankova, D. Schmechel, J. Roth, and M. Brownstein, *Proc. Natl. Acad. Sci. USA*, **75**, 5737–5741 (1978).
101. J. Havrankova, M. Brownstein, and J. Roth, *Diabetologia* **20**, 268–273 (1981).
102. J. Eng and R. S. Yalow, *Proc. Natl. Acad. Sci. USA* **78**(7), 4576–4578 (1981).
103. J. Eng and R. S. Yalow, *Diabetes* **29**, 105–109 (1980).
104. J. Eng and R. S. Yalow, *Proc. Natl. Acad. Sci. USA* **79**, 2683–2685 (1982).
105. J. Havrankova, J. Roth, and M. Brownstein, *J. Clin. Invest.* **64**, 636–642 (1979).
106. J. Havrankova, J. Roth, and M. Brownstein, *Nature* **272**, 827–829 (1978).
107. S. C. Woods and D. Porte Jr., in D. Novin, G. A. Bray, and W. Wyrwichka, Eds., *Hunger: Basic Mechanisms and Clinical Implications*, Raven Press, New York, 1976, pp. 273–280.
108. D. Porte Jr. and S. C. Woods, *Diabetologia* **20**, 274–280 (1981).
109. R. U. Margolis and N. Altszuler, *Nature* **215**, 1375–1376 (1967).
110. A. C. Woods and D. Porte Jr., *Am. J. Physiol.* **233**, E331–334 (1977).
111. O. E. Owen, G. A. Reichard Jr., G. Boden, and C. R. Shuman, *Metabolism* **23**, 7–14 (1974).
112. M. van Houten and B. I. Posner, *Nature* **282**, 623–625 (1979).
113. M. van Houten, B. I. Posner, B. M. Kopriwa, and J. R. Brawer, *Endocrinology* **105**, 666–673 (1979).
114. M. van Houten and B. I. Posner, *Diabetologia* **20**, 255–267 (1981).
115. M. van Houten, B. I. Posner, B. M. Kopriwa, and J. R. Brawer, *Science* **207**, 1081–1083 (1980).
116. Y. Oomura, in D. Novin, W. Wyrwicka, and G. Bray, Eds., *Hunger: Basic Mechanisms and Clinical Implications*, Raven Press, New York, 1976, pp. 145–157.
117. L. H. Storlien, W. P. Bellingham, and G. M. Martin, *Brain Res.* **96**, 156–160 (1975).
118. M. L. McCaleb, R. D. Myers, G. Singer, and G. Willis, *Am. J. Physiol.* **236**, R312–321 (1979).
119. J. S. Hatfield, W. J. Millard, and C. J. V. Smith, *Pharmacol. Biochem. Behav.* **2**, 223–226 (1974).
120. S. C. Woods, E. C. Lotter, L. D. McKay, and D. Porte Jr., *Nature* **282**, 503–505 (1979).
121. B. S. Schneider, I. M. Faust, R. Hemmes, and J. Hirsch, *Am. J. Physiol.* **240** (*Endocrinol. Metab.* **3**), E358–E362 (1981).
122. D. J. Sanger, *Appetite: J. Intake Res.* **2**, 193–208 (1981).
123. C. Kwen-Jen, B. R. Cooper, E. Hazum, and P. Cuatrecasas, *Mol. Pharmacol.* **16**, 91–104 (1979).
124. Chang, K.-J. and P. Cuatrecasas, *J. Biol. Chem.* **25**, 2610–2618 (1979).
125. G. W. Pasternak, *Proc. Natl. Acad. Sci. USA* **77**, 3691–3694 (1980).
126. P. Law, H. Loh, and C. H. Li, *Proc. Natl. Acad. Sci. USA* **76**, 5455–5459 (1979).

127. J. Rossier, T. M. Vargo, S. Minick, N. Ling, F. E. Bloom, and R. Guillemin, *Proc. Natl. Acad. Sci. USA* **74**, 5162–5165 (1977).

128. C. Gramsch, V. Hollt, P. Mehraein, A. Pasi, and A. Herz, *Brain Res.* **171**, 261–270 (1979).

129. R. Kumar, E. Mitchell, and I. P. Stolerman, *Br. J. Pharmacol.* **42**, 473–484 (1971).

130. D. L. Margules, B. Moisset, M. J. Lewis, H. Shibuya, and C. B. Pert, *Science* **202**, 988–991 (1978).

131. J. Rossier, J. Rogers, T. Shibasaki, R. Guillemin, and F. E. Bloom, *Proc. Natl. Acad. Sci. USA* **76**, 2077–2080 (1979).

132. T. L. Garthwaite, D. R. Martinson, L. F. Tseng, T. C. Hagen, and L. A. Menahan, *Endocrinology* **107**(3), 671–676 (1980).

133. M. Wallace, C. D. Fraser, J. A. Clements, and J. W. Funder, *Endocrinology* **108**(1), 189–192 (1981).

134. D. R. Brown and S. G. Holtzman, *Pharmacol. Biochem. Behav.* **11**, 567–573 (1979).

135. S. G. Holtzman, *J. Pharmacol. Exp. Ther.* **189**, 51–60 (1974).

136. S. G. Holtzman, *Life Sci.* **24**, 219–226 (1979).

137. S. J. Cooper, *Psychopharmacol.* **71**, 1–6 (1980).

138. R. Schulz, M. Wuster, and A. Herz, *Eur. J. Pharmacol.* **63**, 313–319 (1980).

139. N. L. Ostrowski and N. Rowland, *Pharmacol. Biochem. Behav.* **14**, 549–599 (1981).

140. J. M. Stapleton, M. D. Lind, V. J. Merriman, and L. D. Reid, *Life Sci.* **24**, 2421–2426 (1979).

141. J. E. Morley and A. S. Levine, *Science* **209**, 1259–1260 (1980).

142. S. M. Antelman, N. Rowland, J. E. Morley, and A. S. Levine, *Science* **214**, 1149–1150 (1981).

143. F. P. Nijkamp and J. M. Van Ree, *Br. J. Pharmacol.* **68**, 599–606 (1980).

144. J. Stanislaw, J. T. Konturek, M. Cieszkowski, E. Mikos, D. H. Coy, and A. V. Schally, *Gastroenterology* **78**:294–300 (1980).

145. C. Zioudrou, R. A. Streaty, and W. A. Klee, *J. Biol. Chem.* **254**(7), 2446–2449 (1979).

146. L. Grandison and A. Guidotti, *Neuropharmacology* **16I**, 533–536 (1977).

147. S. F. Leibowitz and L. Hor, *Soc. Neurosci. Abstr.* **6**, 318 (1980).

148. L. D. McKay, N. J. Kenney, N. K. Edens, R. H. Williams, and S. C. Woods, *Life Sci.* **29**, 1429–1434 (1981).

149. J. E. Morley and A. S. Levine, *Life Sci.* **29**, 1901–1903 (1981).

150. D. J. Sanger and P. S. McCarthy, *Psychopharmacology* **74**, 217–220 (1981).

151. J. E. Jalowiec, J. Panksepp, A. J. Zolovick, N. Najam, and B. H. Herman, *Pharmacol. Biochem. Behav.* **15**, 477–484 (1981).

152. F. S. Tepperman, M. Hirst, and C. W. Gowdey, *Life Sci.* **28**, 2459–2467 (1981).

153. J. F. Jones and J. A. Richter, *Life Sci.* **18**, 2055–2064 (1981).

154. J. Sawynok, C. Pinsky, and F. S. LaBella, *Life Sci.* **25**, 1621–1632 (1979).

155. E. Jean-Baptiste and M. A. Rizack, *Life Sci.* **27**, 135–141 (1980).

156. S. R. Gambert, T. L. Garthwaite, C. H. Pontzer, and T. C. Hagen, *Science* **210**, 1271–1272 (1980).

157. M. J. Gibson, A. S. Liotta, and D. T. Krieger, *Neuropeptides* **1**, 349–362 (1981).

158. I. M. D. Jackson, *N. Engl. J. Med.* **306**(3), 145–155 (1982).

159. J. E. Morley, *Life Sci.* **25**, 1539–1550 (1979).

160. M. Brown, *Diabetologia* **20**, 299–304 (1981).

161. E. Vijayan and S. M. McCann, *Endocrinology* **100**, 1727–1730 (1977).

162. J. E. Morley, *Life Sci.* **27**, 355–368 (1980).

163. R. A. Vogel, B. R. Cooper, T. S. Barlow, A. J. Prange, R. A. Mueller, and G. R. Breese, *J. Pharmacol. Exp. Ther.* **208g**, 161–168 (1979).

164. J. E. Morley and A. S. Levine, *Life Sci.* **27**, 269–274 (1980).

165. C. Prasad and A. Peterkofsky, *J. Biol. Chem.* **251**, 3229–3334 (1976).

166. T. Matsui, C. Prasad, and A. Peterkofsky, *J. Biol. Chem.* **254**, 2439–2455 (1979).

167. M. Mori, C. Prasad, and J. F. Wilber, *Endocrinology* **108**(5), 1995–1997 (1981).

168. J. E. Morley, A. S. Levine, and C. Prasad, *Brain Res.* **210**, 475–478 (1981).

169. M. Mori, J. Pegues, C. Prasad, and J. F. Wilber, *Endocrinology* **110** Suppl., 527 (1982).

170. O. Trygstad, I. Foss, P. D. Edminson, J. H. Johansen, and K. L. Reichelt, *Acta Endocrinol.* **89**, 196–208 (1978).

171. K. L. Reichelt, I. Foss, O. Trygstad, P. D. Edminson, J. H. Johansen, and J. B. Boler, *Neuroscience* **3**, 1207–1211 (1978).

172. D. M. Nance, D. H. Coy, and A. J. Kastin, *Pharmacol. Biochem. Behav.* **11**, 733–735 (1979).

11

Glucoregulation

LAWRENCE A. FROHMAN

Division of Endocrinology and Metabolism
Department of Internal Medicine
University of Cincinnati College of Medicine
Cincinnati, Ohio

1 INTRODUCTION

The role of the central nervous system (CNS) in the regulation of blood glucose and in metabolic homeostasis has been recognized for more than 100 years, ever since the classic experiments of Bernard (1) in which puncture (picûre) of the floor of the fourth ventricle was shown to produce transient glycosuria. Studies during the early part of the present century by Cannon, Britton, Zunz and LaBarre, Gellhorn, and many others provided evidence for the participation of both sympathetic and parasympathetic components of the autonomic nervous system, the adrenals, the endocrine pancreas, and the liver (for detailed reviews, see refs. 2–5). Because of the limited techniques available for studying the CNS components of this highly complex integrative system, much of the effort up to the past 10–15 years was focused on the characterization of the peripheral or extraneural components, and their relative contributions to overall blood glucose regulation has been fairly well defined. Recently, with the availability of stereotaxic, microiontophoretic, and single-unit recording techniques, and with the major advances in monoamine and peptide chemistry and pharmacology, the characterization of the CNS role has also become possible.

The CNS utilizes two mechanisms for communicating with peripheral effector organs: (i) direct neurotransmission involving aminergic or peptidergic neurotransmitters that serve as chemical messengers between nerve terminals and the peripheral cells they innervate; and (ii) neurohormonal means involving the release of amines or peptides from nerve terminals into a regional or systemic circulation with uptake and binding to specific membrane receptors on target cells. Within the past decade the distinction between these processes has become somewhat blurred with respect to the definition of neurotransmitters, neurohormones, and hormones.

This chapter provides an overview of the role of the CNS in glucoregulation including the autonomic nervous system and the hypothalamic-pituitar y axis components, an assessment of the aminergic and peptidergic neurotransmitters participating in the process, and an overall hypothesis of the integrative role of neuropeptides in glucoregulation. The emphasis of the chapter is on the processes involved in short-term regulation rather than on food intake and caloric homeostasis (for which the reader is referred to Chapter 10).

2 ROLE OF THE AUTONOMIC NERVOUS SYSTEM

2.1 Neuroanatomical Basis for Glucoregulation

The belief, held for many years, that individual functions of the CNS could be localized to specific brain nuclei has required modification with the appreciation that an integrative process exists with multiple components contributing to overall neurometabolic control. The hypo-thalamus has been recognized as the critical locus for metabolic inte-gration within the CNS. Both the ventromedial and ventrolateral hypothalamic areas participate in glucoregulation by virtue of the pres-ence, in those loci, of glucose sensitive neurons the electrical activity of which is modified by increases or decreases or both in ambient glucose concentration. The specific connections of the glucoreceptor neurons themselves remain to be fully clarified, though the termination of the pathways involved are generally known.

The most important pathways responsible for glucoregulation involve the autonomic nervous system. The ventral hypothalamus is an impor-tant component of this system and has been divided functionally into two zones: a medial area connected with the sympathetic nervous sys-tem and a more lateral portion connected with the parasympathetic ner-vous system. Within the ventromedial hypothalamus, most attention has been given to the ventromedial hypothalamic nucleus (VMH). Glucose-sensitive neurons in the VMH respond to hypoglycemia by activating the sympathetic nervous system through pathways that travel caudally and laterally from the hypothalamus through the midbrain and pons, in-teract with neurons residing in the floor of the fourth ventricle (site of Bernard's stimulation), and continue through the medulla by polysynap-tic pathways to the intermediolateral column of the spinal cord and the splanchnic nerves. The fibers connect directly with the adrenal medulla and, after reaching the celiac ganglia, with hepatocytes, multiple cell types in the pancreatic islets, and hormone-secreting cells in the gastro-intestinal tract. Some of the neurons in the ventrolateral hypothalamic area (VLH) travel through the dorsal motor nucleus of the vagus and from there to the gastrointestinal tract, the pancreatic islets, and the liv-er. Sympathetic and parasympathetic nerve fibers become integrated in terminal nerve branches, and fibers of both systems frequently enter the organs in association with their blood supply.

The functions of these two systems appear to be in most instances reciprocally related with respect to glucoregulation, though the re-sponses of individual pancreatic hormones are not entirely specific. Studies providing current knowledge of the role of the CNS in glucoregulation have consisted largely of two types: single-unit record-ing studies of individual neurons in response to changes in the local or systemic glucose environment, and measurement of peripheral tissue re-sponses to altered neural activity induced by (i) direct electrical stimu-lation or lesions at various locations within the neuraxis, (ii) chemical stimulation or inhibition using neurotransmitters or antagonists, or (iii) altering substrate or hormonal levels either systemically or locally with-in the CNS.

It has become clear that the neurometabolic response to a single sig-nal is not all-inclusive. Activation of one component of the system such as direct neural stimulation of hepatic glycogenolysis may be unassociated with effects on the endocrine pancreas or the adrenal medulla. Consequently, it has not been possible to differentiate those neurons which activate the liver from those which stimulate the pancreatic A or B cells, and differentiation of primary (hepatic) vs. secondary (pancreatic or adrenal medullary) effects on blood glucose regulation has not always been possible. However, the pattern described below (shown in Figure 1) is generally accepted as the most important physiological control mechanism.

2.2   Effects on the Liver

The most immediate effects of neural control on blood glucose relate to the liver (6). The VMH and VLH act in a reciprocal manner on this organ to provide nearly instantaneous effects on glucoregulation. Stimulation of the VMH causes a rapid rise in hepatic glucose output and a marked reduction in liver glycogen content. Stimulation of the VLH, in contrast, leads to hepatic glycogenesis, though changes in blood glucose and liver glycogen content are difficult to detect. The expected changes

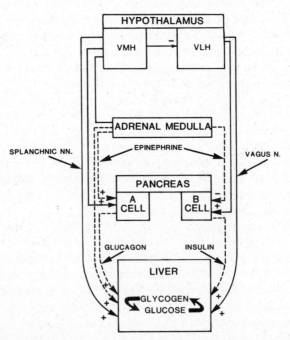

Figure 1.   Integrating actions of the hypothalamus and the autonomic nervous system on the endocrine pancreas, adrenal medulla, and liver serve to regulate blood glucose levels. Neural pathways are indicated by solid lines, hormonal pathways by dashed lines. Reprinted from L. A. Frohman (5).

in hepatic enzymes involved in these processes have also been shown: VMH stimulation produces a rise in phosphorylase A (the active form of phosphorylase, which promotes glycogenolysis) and in glucose-6-phosphatase, but no change in glycogen synthetase I (the active form of synthetase which stimulates glycogenesis). VLH stimulation increases synthetase I activity without affecting phosphorylase A activity. The responses to hypothalamic stimulation can be reproduced by sympathetic or vagus nerve stimulation and can be demonstrated in the absence of the pancreas and the adrenals, indicating that the effects occur directly at the liver. Furthermore, the responses induced by neural stimulation occur much more rapidly than do those produced by administration of glucose or insulin. The VMH and VLH also regulate hepatic gluconeogenesis in a reciprocal manner. Electrical stimulation of the VMH increases the activity of phosphoenolpyruvate carboxykinase, a key gluconeogenic enzyme, and suppresses pyruvatekinase, a glycolytic enzyme. Although several hours are required for changes in enzyme levels to become apparent, chemical stimulation with intracerebroventricular 2-deoxyglucose, which causes central glucocytopenia, enhances gluconeogenesis within 30 min as determined by measurement of alanine conversion to glucose.

The question of whether these stimulatory effects originate with neurons whose perikarya reside within the VMH or with nerve fibers traversing this locus has been resolved by using chemical stimulation which has, in addition, provided some evidence for the monaminergic coding of the responses. Microinjections of norepinephrine in the VMH increase phosphorylase A levels in liver and mimic the changes observed after electrical stimulation. The concentrations required, approximately 5×10^{-10} M, are well within the physiologic range of this neurotransmitter. The effects are blocked by beta- but not by alpha-adrenergic antagonists. Microinjections of acetylcholine, in similar concentrations, into the VLH increase hepatic synthetase I activity, an effect which can be blocked by muscarinic blockers such as atropine. Systemic injection of N-methylatropine, a cholinergic blocker that does not penetrate the blood brain barrier, also inhibits the stimulatory effects of acetylcholine, demonstrating that both central and peripheral components of the pathway are under cholinergic control. It has also recently been recognized that nerve terminals in the liver contain peptidergic as well as aminergic neurotransmitters, and both are most likely involved in these processes.

2.3 Effects on the Endocrine Pancreas

Neural stimulation of insulin secretion is mediated by both parasympathetic and sympathetic fibers that traverse the vagus nerve and celiac ganglia respectively (4). The fibers enter the pancreas as a mixed pancreatic nerve together with the vascular supply of the organ. Nerve terminals can be identified within the islets in juxtaposition to A, B, and D cells in association with cell borders and in relationship to gap junctions. Stimulation of the vagus increases and vagotomy decreases insulin secretion, indicating the existence of a tonic effect of the CNS on insulin release. The responses are acetylcholine-mediated and can be inhibited by atropine, indicating a muscarinic effect. Sympathetic nerve fibers inhibit insulin secretion through alpha-adrenergic receptors on the B cell. These may be activated by direct neural stimulation of sympathetic fibers and also by epinephrine and norepinephrine. Direct neural stimulation constitutes an important regulatory mechanism in all species examined, though circulating catecholamines appear to be more important in rats than in dogs or humans. Beta-adrenergic receptors are also present on the B cells and enhance insulin secretion. The beta$_2$ rather than the beta$_1$ receptor appears to be involved. The role of beta receptors in insulin secretion appears less important than that of alpha receptors, and almost every physiological or pathological condition associated with sympathetic nervous system activation results in predominance of the alpha-receptor-mediated inhibitory effect. The CNS locus responsible for the sympathetic effects is located within the VMH. Stimulation of this locus inhibits insulin secretion even during hyperglycemia. The pathways from the hypothalamus are, in general, similar to those utilized by other components of the sympathetic nervous system. Both epinephrine and norepinephrine, when injected into the VMH, are capable of inducing this inhibitory effect. Destruction of the VMH results in increased insulin secretion in response to hyperglycemia, indicating a tonic effect of this locus under normal physiological circumstances. The VLH has for many years been implicated in the stimulation of insulin secretion, though only recently (7) has it been demonstrated that chemical stimulation of this locus by epinephrine results in a selective increase in insulin secretion. It is of interest that at very low concentrations epinephrine also exhibits a direct stimulatory effect on the beta cell.

The control of glucagon secretion by the autonomic nervous system is in many ways reciprocal to that of insulin, though some differences exist. At peripheral sites both norepinephrine and acetylcholine stimulate glucagon release. Norepinephrine stimulation is predominately beta$_2$-adrenergic, though alpha-adrenergic receptors also appear to be stimulatory. The contribution of catecholamines secreted by the adrenal medulla is less important than for insulin secretion in lower species and in humans is of relatively minor significance. Centrally, the VMH is the stimulatory locus for glucagon secretion. At present it is not known whether there are discrete neurons responsible for the hepatic and pancreatic effects or whether individual neurons activate both pathways. Epinephrine, and to a lesser extent, norepinephrine injected into the VMH stimulate glucagon secretion. Local injections of acetylcholine in the VMH stimulate glucagon release and this effect is mediated through nicotinic receptors present in high concentrations in the hypothalamus. Neither electrical nor chemical stimulation of the VLH influences glucagon secretion, though activation of glucoreceptor neurons in this locus do appear in some species to stimulate glucagon release through parasympathetic pathways.

Somatostatin secretion by the D cells of the pancreas is stimulated by both beta-adrenergic and cholinergic receptors, thus exhibiting similarities to the control of glucagon secretion (8, 9). Gamma aminobutyric acid receptors are present on D cells which mediate inhibitory effects on somatostatin secretion. Although the effect of hypothalamic stimulation on somatostatin secretion is not known, pancreatic somatostatin content and release in response to nutrient stimulation are increased following VMH destruction (10).

3 NEUROPEPTIDE EFFECTS ON GLUCOREGULATION

3.1 Anatomical Considerations

A large number of peptides are common to the brain, gastrointestinal tract, and pancreas. Some of these peptides, originally identified in the CNS, have been labeled as brain peptides whereas others, identified primarily in peripheral sites, have subsequently been demonstrated to be present in brain. They constitute the messengers of what has been termed by Pearse (11) the "diffuse neuroendocrine system" (Table 1).

TABLE 1 Peripheral (Systemic) and Central Effects of Specific Neuropeptides on Blood Glucose, Insulin, and Glucagon Levels[a]

Peptide	Glucose	Insulin	Glucagon
Somatostatin			
Peripheral	↑ or ↓	↓	↓
Central	— (↓)	—	—
Neurotensin			
Peripheral	↓	↓ (↑)	↑
Central	—	—	—
Substance P			
Peripheral	↑	↓ (↑)	↑
Central	—	—	—
Bombesin			
Peripheral	↑	↓	↑
Central	↑	↓	↑
Endorphins			
Peripheral	↑	↑ (↓)	↑ (↓)
Central	↑		
β-Lipotropin (Peripheral)	—	↑	
TRH			
Peripheral	↑ (—)	↑ (—)	↑ (—)
Central	↑	↑	↑

[a] ↑ Increase; ↓ decrease; — No change.

Many of these peptides have been implicated in the control of nutrient homeostasis and glucoregulation primarily as the result of experiments involving their systemic administration or their addition to *in vitro* systems in which specific hormone or metabolic responses have been measured. In this manner, more attention has been given to their hormonal than to their neurotransmitter effects, and the locus of their action has of necessity been restricted to peripheral (i.e., extra-CNS) sites. Antiserum to individual neuropeptides has been administered systemically and effects of circulating neuropeptide deficiencies demonstrated. However, this technique is incapable of distinguishing between endocrine and paracrine effects. Inasmuch as individual neuropeptidergic transmitters are present in multiple areas involved in glucoregulation (CNS, pancreatic islets, and GI tract), it is tempting to propose that their functions at each site are integrated with one another and that they form an overall system analogous to the monoamine neurotransmitters that participate in the autonomic nervous system functions described above.

On the basis of accumulating evidence, it is now fairly certain that CNS neuropeptidergic transmitters must exert their effects on glucoregulation primarily as neurotransmitters and by paracrine rather than hormonal actions. For example, somatostatin of CNS origin has been shown to be released into the hypothalamic-pituitary portal circulation (12). However, somatostatin in the peripheral circulation appears to originate from the GI tract and the pancreas (13). Thus, effects of CNS somatostatin on peripheral target organs and on glucoregulation, if present, must be mediated by changes in neurotransmission within the CNS rather than by neurosecretion. The same conclusions, though based on less extensive data, can be made for other brain peptides. The extent to which individual neuropeptides are utilized to modulate specific homeostatic systems, however, is still uncertain; the question is addressed in the next section.

3.2   Effects of Individual Neuropeptides

3.2.1   Somatostatin

The tetradecapeptide somatostatin was initially isolated from the hypothalamus and identified on the basis of its growth hormone release-inhibiting capabilities (14). Its distribution was soon found to be quite widespread, including many areas of the central nervous system and, in addition, selected non-neural tissues. High concentrations are present in the stomach and pancreas, providing the potential for effects on glucoregulation (see refs. 8 and 9 for detailed reviews). In the stomach, somatostatin is located in D cells, which are closely related to gastrin-producing G cells. In the pancreatic islets somatostatin has been identified in the peripherally located D cells which are in closer proximity to glucagon-containing A cells than to insulin-containing B cells. Exogenously administered somatostatin exerts an inhibitory effect on many hormones involved in glucose homeostasis, including insulin, glucagon, pancreatic polypeptide, gastrin, gastric inhibitory peptide, and secretin. In addition, there is a reduction in splanchnic blood flow, decreased gastrointestinal motility, and decreased glucose absorption from the gut. Somatostatin administration decreases hepatic glucose output, though the majority of studies suggest that this effect is secondary to its inhibition of pancreatic hormone secretion. A direct effect of somatostatin on the liver *in vitro* has been reported (15, 16) though these effects have not been confirmed *in vivo* (17).

The most profound effects of somatostatin are on the inhibition of glucagon and insulin secretion, which can be observed in the presence of virtually all stimuli. The inhibitory effect is believed due to interference with a cAMP-related process, possibly by inhibition of adenylate cyclase (18) or to impairment of calcium transport (19). It was suggested that somatostatin effects are influenced by alpha-adrenergic receptors (20) but this has not been confirmed by other workers (21, 22).

Considerable evidence also exists for a role of endogenous pancreatic somatostatin in the inhibition of insulin and glucagon secretion. Administration of antisomatostatin serum *in vivo* results in increases in insulin levels (23), and exposure of isolated islets *in vitro* to antisomatostatin serum increases both insulin and glucagon release (24). Thus, a paracrine effect of somatostatin on insulin and glucagon secretion is very likely (25). A schematic diagram of the interrelationships of the three islet hormones affecting glucose metabolism is shown in Figure 2. Measurements of somatostatin secretion into the portal circulation, taken as an index of its paracrine activity, have raised questions concerning the physiological importance of these effects. For example, nutrient stimuli such as glucose, which stimulates insulin release, and amino acids, which stimulate insulin and glucagon release, also enhance somatostatin secretion (26). Furthermore, VMH destruction results in heightened responses not only of insulin and glucagon but also of somatostatin to the above stimuli (10). The postulated paracrine action of somatostatin predicts that enhancement of its secretion would result in a suppression of insulin and glucagon release, and the above examples are therefore inconsistent with this hypothesis.

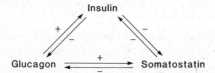

Figure 2. Interrelated effects of insulin, glucagon, and somatostatin in pancreatic islets.

In contrast, somatostatin secretion in response to nutrient stimuli is increased in diabetes and restored to normal by insulin administration. The enhanced secretion consequently appears to be secondary to insulin deficiency rather than to a primary hormonal disturbance.

Pancreatic somatostatin content is also increased in animals with experimental and genetic diabetes and in humans with insulin-dependent diabetes (27–29). A close examination of the temporal relationships of pancreatic somatostatin to the disturbances in carbohydrate metabolism supports the concept that changes in pancreatic somatostatin represent a response to rather than a cause of hypoinsulinemia (30).

Excessive production of somatostatin in humans, associated with somatostatin-producing tumors of the pancreas (31), is associated with mild carbohydrate intolerance and relative hypoinsulinemia. These effects, however, are mediated by circulating somatostatin released from the tumor and do not help to clarify the putative paracrine effects of the peptide. In infants with nesidioblastosis, a disorder characterized by B cell hyperplasia, the presence of clusters of B cells throughout the exocrine pancreas, and severe hypoglycemia, the number of somatostatin-containing D cells in the islets are reduced (32). It is unclear, however, whether this observation has any pathological significance or whether it represents an effect secondary to excessive insulin production.

There is preliminary evidence to suggest that somatostatin acting within the CNS may also exhibit an effect on glucoregulation. Administration of somatostatin into the cisterna magna has no effect on plasma glucose levels under basal conditions. However, when administered in association with beta-endorphin or bombesin, the hyperglycemia produced by each of these agents (see below) is abolished (33, 34). Similar and even more potent effects can be demonstrated with an octapeptide derivative of somatostatin (33), which also exhibits the growth hormone-, insulin-, and glucagon-inhibiting effects of somatostatin. This analog has been shown to inhibit the plasma epinephrine response to insulin hypoglycemia and to 2-deoxyglucose and the epinephrine and norepinephrine responses to central administration of carbachol and bombesin (35); it has not been possible to demonstrate these effects with native somatostatin, raising the possibility that the effect is mediated by a CNS receptor unrelated to somatostatin. Alternatively, the analog could have greater penetrability than does somatostatin from the cerebrospinal fluid to the specific CNS locus involved.

The possibility of related but distinct somatostatin receptors in various brain regions is supported by the recent reports of other forms of somatostatin within the CNS and gastrointestinal tract (somatostatin-28 and somatostatin-25) that contain somatostatin-14 at the C-terminal end of the molecule. Somatostatin-28 exhibits a different relative potency than does somatostatin-14 with respect to inhibition of insulin and glucagon secretion (36). Although some controversy still exists, somatostatin-28 seems considerably more potent than somatostatin-14 on insulin compared with glucagon secretion. When administered centrally, somatostatin-28 is also more potent than somatostatin-14 in inhibiting bombesin-induced hyperglycemia.

If the central actions of somatostatin on glucoregulation are indeed physiological, it might be expected that alterations in glucose availability within the CNS would influence endogenous somatostatin content or release. Several groups have now reported an absence of alterations in hypothalamic somatostatin content in experimental and genetic diabetes (27, 37, 38). However, somatostatin release by the hypothalamus is stimulated by central glucopenia produced by decreased ambient glucose concentrations, by 2-deoxyglucose, 3-O-methylglucose, and cytochalasin B, and suppressed by elevations in glucose concentrations (39). Somatostatin release from the cerebral cortex is not affected in a similar manner. These findings may serve to explain the decreases in growth hormone levels in the rat in response to hypoglycemia (40), but they do not explain the elevations in growth hormone seen in humans under similar circumstances.

3.2.2 Neurotensin

Neurotensin is a tridecapeptide first identified in bovine hypothalamus (41) and subsequently in the gastrointestinal tract. Systemic injections of neurotensin produce a transient hyperglycemic effect (42), a decrease in hepatic glycogen and an increase in phosphorylase activity (43). These effects are not observed *in vitro* (43, 44) indicating that the effects are mediated by a hormonal or neural mechanism. Increases in glucagon and an inhibition of insulin release have been reported (45, 46) in the rat. Whereas the increase in glucagon release very likely represents a direct effect of neurotensin on the A cells, the inhibition of insulin secretion is mediated through the stimulation of epinephrine from the adrenal medulla since this effect is abolished by adrenal demedulation. Many of the effects of systemic neurotensin are reproduced by histamine administration and can be blocked by pretreatment with H_1-histamine, and to a lesser extent, H_2-histamine receptor antagonists. Thus the well-recognized histamine-releasing effects of neurotensin may mediate its action on pancreatic hormone secretion. Administration of neurotensin into the pancreatoduodenal artery stimulates both glucagon and insulin release in dogs (47) and can be blocked by propranolol, suggesting participation of the beta-adrenergic receptor. The effects of neurotensin in vitro vary with experimental conditions. In the presence of basal glucose concentrations neurotensin stimulates the release of insulin, glucagon, and somatostatin whereas in the presence of stimulatory concentrations of glucose or arginine, the effects of neurotensin are inhibitory (48).

Two lines of evidence argue against a possible role of circulating neurotensin as a mediator of central nervous glucoregulation. First, administration of antineurotensin serum in a quantity sufficient to inhibit the hyperglycemic response to neurotensin does not impair the hyperglycemic response to central administration of 2-deoxyglucose, a potent stimulator of sympathetic nervous system–mediated hyperglycemia (44). Second, systemic infusion of neurotensin in quantities sufficient to simlate circulating neurotensin-like immunoreactivity levels in plasma observed after a mixed meal (49) are without effect on plasma glucose, insulin, or glucagon concentrations.

The possibility exists, however, that neurotensin may exhibit paracrine effects on the other islet hormones. Although attempts to identify neurotensin in pancreatic islets using immunohistochemical techniques have thus far been unsuccessful, the peptide has been identified immunologically and is increased in both experimental (50) and genetic (51) diabetes. As with somatostatin, however, it appears that the changes in neurotensin are secondary rather than primary.

There has been no evidence to suggest that neurotensin within the CNS participates in glucoregulation. In contrast to the effects of peripherally administered neurotensin, injection of this peptide into the CNS is without effect on plasma glucose, insulin, or glucagon levels (45).

3.2.3 Substance P

Substance P is an undecapeptide with widespread distribution in the CNS, where high concentrations are found in the hypothalamus and in the dorsal roots. It is also present in nerve plexuses and in endocrine cells of the intestinal tract, particularly the duodenum. Systemic administration of substance P results in a hyperglycemic response associated with hyperglucagonemia and a suppression of insulin secretion, similar to that seen after neurotensin administration (46). In contrast to neurotensin, however, histamine receptor blockade does not inhibit the elevations in glucagon and glucose levels after substance P administration (52). Intrapancreatic infusion of substance P in the dog increases both portal insulin and glucose concentrations (47). An increase in pancreatic blood flow is also observed and may account for part of the hormonal rises. The hormone-releasing effects of substance P are not blocked by baclofen, a gamma-aminobutyric acid analog that suppresses the depolarizing effects of the peptide on spinal reflexes. Thus, the effects of substance P on the islets are unlikely to be mediated by enhanced autonomic nervous system ganglionic synaptic transmission. As with the majority of studies on neurotensin, the quantity of substance P required to demonstrate the hyperglycemic and hyperglucagonemic responses are in the microgram range, suggesting that this neuropeptide is unlikely to exert physiological effects on carbohydrate metabolism as a hormone. The possibility that substance P may function as a neurotransmitter in components of the autonomic nervous system involved in glucoregulation, however, cannot be excluded from these results. To date, there is no evidence that substance P within the CNS exerts any role on glucoregulation or carbohydrate metabolism.

3.2.4 Bombesin

Bombesin is a tetradecapeptide isolated from the skin of the frog. Its mammalian counterpart appears to be a 27-amino-acid peptide, present in both gastrointestinal tract and hypothalamus which exhibits extensive homology in the C-terminal decapeptide region (53, 54). The systemic administration of bombesin produces a hyperglycemic response. However, when administered intracisternally, the peptide exhibits approximately 10,000 times greater potency (55). Mammalian bombesin also exhibits hyperglycemic activity after central administration but appears to be only 10–20% as active as the tetradecapeptide (56). The bombesin effects are blocked by adrenalectomy but not by hypophysectomy, implying a role for the adrenal medulla. The response is mediated by epinephrine release which occurs within 5 min of the central administration of bombesin. Evidence of selectivity of the catecholamine response is provided by the absence of changes in dopamine or norepinephrine release after bombesin administration (57). The stimulatory effects of bombesin can be inhibited by a somatostatin analog but not by somatostatin itself (see Section 3.2.1). The specific site at which bombesin acts to produce its hyperglycemic effect remains to be determined.

3.2.5 Endorphins and Enkephalins

The hyperglycemic effect of morphine has been recognized for many years. With the discovery of the endorphin-enkephalin family of peptides, a number of different effects on glucoregulation and hormones involved in this process have been described. In the perfused dog pancreas, beta-endorphin stimulates glucagon and insulin secretion and concomitantly inhibits somatostatin release (58). In high concentrations met-enkephalin also stimulates insulin and glucagon release in the same model (59). The effects of both peptides are reversible by naloxone. When islets are exposed to beta-endorphin *in vitro*, insulin and glucagon release are inhibited (60). The large concentrations of peptide required for the demonstration of these effects, however, leaves their physiologic significance uncertain.

Beta-lipotropin (beta-LPH) stimulates insulin secretion in rabbits by a non-endorphin mediated mechanism (61) inasmuch as the effect is not blocked by naloxone. Its effects may be related to the heptapeptide sequence shared with ACTH (see Chapter 2) since the N-terminal portion of ACTH exhibits potent insulin-releasing activity (62).

Administration of beta-endorphin intracisternally produces hyperglycemia in the rat. On a molar basis, the effect of beta-endorphin is less than that of bombesin (33). The effects of beta-endorphin are blocked by naloxone and by adrenal denervation, indicating a stimulation of sympathetic outflow (34). Intracerebral hemicholinium and somatostatin also block the hyperglycemic effect indicating the presence of multisynaptic pathway. Beta-endorphin inhibits dopamine turnover but concomitant administration of apomorphine, a dopamine agonist, does not inhibit the hyperglycemic response, indicating an absence of dopamine mediation. Enkephalin (and morphine) have reciprocal effects on glucoregulatory neurons in the hypothalamus (63). Glucoreceptor neurons in the VMH are excited by enkephalin whereas glucosensitive neurons in the VLH are inhibited by the peptide. Thus, the VMH may serve as a locus which mediates the hyperglycemic response to endorphins.

3.2.6   Thyrotropin Releasing Hormone

Thyrotropin hormone (TRH) is widely distributed throughout the CNS. In addition, it is present in the gastrointestinal tract and pancreas with highest concentrations in the pancreas (64). Systemic administration of TRH to fasted rabbits results in increased glucose, insulin, and glucagon levels, and the effect is dose related. The hyperglycemia is not due to the increases in glucagon and insulin secretion since it occurs in fed animals where the hormonal responses cannot be demonstrated (65). Only minimal increases in insulin and glucose are observed during the first 10 min after TRH injection, suggesting that the effects are not directly on the pancreatic islets. Furthermore, TRH does not exhibit a direct stimulatory effect on glucagon or insulin release in the isolated rat pancreas (66). In all other species tested, including humans, systemic administration of TRH is unassociated with changes in glucose, insulin, or glucagon.

When administered directly into the CNS of rats, TRH exhibits effects similar to those of several other peptides already described (67). A moderate hyperglycemia and a significant stimulation of glucagon release occurs, as does an increase in plasma epinephrine and norepinephrine. The rises in both insulin and glucose are not observed in adrenalectomized animals, confirming the mediating role of catecholamine secretion. In contrast to the effects of bombesin, TRH stimulation of catecholamine secretion is not inhibited by analogs of somatostatin. As with several of the other peptides, the dose of TRH required is quite large and the physiological significance of its effect remains uncertain.

3.2.7   Other Structurally Identified Neuropeptides

Several additional peptides common to the brain and to either the gastrointestinal tract or pancreas have effects on glucoregulation directly
or indirectly; most prominent are vasoactive intestinal polypeptide
(VIP), secretin, insulin, and glucagon. The effects of the first two peptides are predominately on the secretion of insulin and glucagon by hormonal mechanisms subsequent to their release from the gastrointestinal
tract. The effects of the latter two are, of course, central to the entire
process of glucoregulation and a discussion of their effects is beyond
the scope of this chapter.

Administration of insulin into the cerebrospinal fluid has been reported to decrease pancreatic insulin secretion (68) suggesting the presence
of a locus within the CNS sensitive to insulin. Neurons in the ventral
hypothalamus have been reported to exhibit electrophysiologic changes
in response to insulin (69) and evidence for insulin uptake and localization in the ventral hypothalamus has also recently been reported (70).
Insulin has been reported to be present in many areas in the brain (71).
The role of brain insulin in glucoregulation is uncertain since the levels
are unaltered by physiological and pathological states in which marked
changes in pancreatic insulin occur, that is, fasting and experimental diabetes.

3.3   Effects of Other Neural Factors

In addition to the structurally identified and characterized brain peptides already described, several peptides of hypothalamic origin have
been reported to effect the secretion of insulin and glucagon and to alter blood glucose levels. These studies have utilized in vivo and/or in
vitro models in which crude or partially purified extracts of hypothalamic tissue have served as stimuli for evaluating hormone release from
pancreatic islets. Three peptides have received the most attention.

3.3.1   Hypothalamic Insulin-Releasing Peptide

A perfusate of mouse lateral hypothalamus has been reported to stimulate insulin release by isolated islets *in vitro* (72) and similar results
have been obtained with an extract of rat lateral hypothalamus (73).
The insulin-releasing activity could be demonstrated in rat plasma but
disappeared following bilateral destruction of the VLH. These same
workers, using an extract of bovine hypothalamus purified by Sephadex
G-25 gel filtration and paper electrophoresis, demonstrated insulin-releasing effects in isolated islets and *in vivo* in the rat (74). At present it
is uncertain whether the biological activity observed in plasma is related to that in the hypothalamic extracts.

3.3.2   Insulin Release-Inhibiting Peptide

A factor present in rat VMH and released into incubation medium has been reported to inhibit the secretion of insulin in isolated islets and *in vivo* (75, 76). The factor is distinct from other hypothalamic peptides known to have direct effects on insulin release such as somatostatin, neurotensin, and substance P. The insulin release-inhibiting activity is destroyed by chymotrypsin, trypsin, carboxypeptidase, and pepsin treatment and appears to be only minimally retarded on Sephadex G-25 gel filtration (77). The physiological significance of this peptide is, of course, unknown. The possibility of direct neurosecretion into the bloodstream, while possible, would appear unlikely in view of the accumulating evidence from studies with other neuropeptides. By analogy, the peptide might also be present in the islets and thus be capable of exhibiting a paracrine effect.

3.3.3   Glucagon-Releasing Peptide

A glucagon-releasing factor has been identified in rat VMH (75) and is distinguishable from neurotensin and substance P by several criteria. Treatment with carboxypeptidase and pepsin destroys its biological activity, but trypsin is ineffective and chymotrypsin enhances its activity (77). The glucagon-releasing peptide is retarded in its elution from Sephadex G-25 and in this manner can be separated from the insulin release-inhibiting peptide described above.

4   SUMMARY

The regulation of blood glucose is a complex process involving the integration of the CNS with both hormonal and neural mechanisms. Although neuropeptide participation in the process is only partly understood at present, several conclusions are evident.

First, neuropeptides are present in various portions of the autonomic nervous system from the central components in the hypothalamus to the peripheral vertebral ganglia and the adrenal medulla. Their mediation of neural impulses involved with glucoregulation is unquestionable, though their interaction with monoaminergic neurotransmitters requires further study.

Second, many of these peptides are present in the gastrointestinal tract and the endocrine pancreas as well as in the CNS. The results of an increasing number of studies involving the systemic administration of the various peptides and the measurement of their endogenous circulating levels indicate that their effects are produced not by a classical hormonal mechanism, secretion into the bloodstream, but by a direct cell-to-cell (paracrine) action or by a neurotransmitter action in the pancreas, adrenal medulla, and liver.

Third, a pattern is beginning to emerge in which specific neuropeptides may exert an integrative role in a specific homeostatic system at different anatomical locations. The involvement of somatostatin in glucose absorption by the gastrointestinal tract, in pancreatic hormone secretion, and in hepatic glucose production, and the stimulation of somatostatin secretion from the hypothalamus by glucopenia, is just one example. Whether these actions are interrelated through a CNS control mechanism or whether they represent evolutionary developments from a single neuropeptide-mediated process in a more primitive species remains to be elucidated. In either case, a fuller understanding of the role of neuropeptides in glucoregulation can be expected in the future and should provide new insights into certain disorders of carbohydrate metabolism.

REFERENCES

1. C. Bernard, *C. R. Soc. Biol. (Paris)* **1**, 60 (1849).
2. S. Woods and D. Porte Jr., *Physiol. Rev.* **54**, 596 (1974).
3. L. A. Frohman, in P. J. Morgane and J. Panksepp, Eds., *Handbook of the Hypothalamus*, Vol. 2, Marcel Dekker, New York, 1980, p. 519.
4. R. E. Miller, *Endocr. Rev.* **2**, 471 (1981).
5. L. A. Frohman, in S. Bleicher and B. Brodoff, Eds., *Diabetes Mellitus and Obesity*, Williams and Wilkins, Baltimore, 1982, p. 200.
6. T. Shimazu, *Diabetologia* **20**, 343 (1981).
7. T. Shimazu and K. Ishikawa, *Endocrinology* **108**, 605 (1981).
8. J. E. Gerich, in K. Fotherby and S. B. Pal, Eds., *Hormones in Normal and Abnormal Tissues*, Vol. 2, Walter de Gruyter, Berlin, 1981, p. 475.
9. M. Berelowitz, in S. Bleicher and B. Brodoff, Eds., *Diabetes Mellitus and Obesity*, Williams and Wilkins, Baltimore, 1982, p. 89.
10. Y. Goto, R. G. Carpenter, M. Berelowitz, and L. A. Frohman, *Metabolism* **29**, 986 (1980).
11. A. G. E. Pearse, *Med. Biol.* **55**, 115 (1977).
12. K. Chihara, A. Arimura, and A. V. Schally, *Endocrinology* **104**, 1656 (1979).
13. V. Schusdziarra, E. Zyznar, D. Rouiller, V. Harris, and R. H. Unger, *Endocrinology* **107**, 1572 (1980).
14. P. Brazeau, W. Vale, R. Burgus, N. Ling, M. Butcher, J. Rivier, and R. Guillemin, *Science* **179**, 77 (1973).
15. J. R. Oliver and S. R. Wagle, *Biochem. Biophys. Res. Commun.* **62**, 772 (1974).
16. H. Sacks, K. Waligora, J. Matthes, and B. Pimstone, *Endocrinology* **101**, 1751 (1977).
17. E. W. Chideckel, J. Palmer, D. J. Koerker, J. Ensinck, M. B. Davidson, and C. J. Goodner, *J. Clin. Invest.* **55**, 754 (1975).
18. P. Borgeat, F. Labrie, J. Drouin, A. Belanger, H. Immer, K. Sestanj, V. Nelson, M. Gotz, A. V. Schally, D. H. Coy, and E. J. Coy, *Biochem. Biophys. Res. Commun.* **56**, 1052 (1974).
19. J. R. Oliver, *Endocrinology* **99**, 910 (1976).
20. P. H. Smith, S. C. Woods, and D. Porte Jr., *Endocrinology* **98**, 1073 (1976).
21. S. Efendic and R. Luft, *Acta Endocrinol.* **78**, 516 (1975).

22. J. K. Schmitt, M. Lorenzi, J. E. Gerich, M. V. Bohannon, J. H. Karam, and P. H. Forsham, *J. Clin. Endocrinol. Metab.* **48**, 880 (1979).
23. V. Schusdziarra, E. Zyznar, E. Rouiller, G. Boden, J. C. Brown, A. Arimura, and R. H. Unger, *Science* **207**, 530 (1980).
24. M. Itoh, L. Mandarino, and J. E. Gerich, *Diabetes* **29**, 693 (1980).
25. L. Orci and R. H. Unger, *Lancet* **2**, 1243 (1975).
26. E. Ipp, R. E. Dobbs, A. Arimura, W. Vale, V. Harris, and R. H. Unger, *J. Clin. Invest.* **60**, 760 (1977).
27. H. Makino, A. Kanatsuka, Y. Matsushima, M. Yamamoto, A. Kumagai, and N. Yanihara, *Endocrinol. Jpn.* **24**, 295 (1977).
28. Y. C. Patel, L. Orci, A. Bankier, and D. P. Cameron, *Endocrinology* **99**, 1415 (1976).
29. L. Orci, D. Baetens, C. Rufener, M. Amherdt, M. Ravazzola, P. Studer, F. Malaisse-Lagae, and R. H. Unger, *Proc. Natl. Acad. Sci. USA* **73**, 1338 (1976).
30. M. Berelowitz, D. L. Coleman, and L. A. Frohman, *Diabetes* **29**, 717 (1980).
31. G. J. Krejs, L. Orci, J. M. Conlon, M. Ravazzola, G. R. Davis, P. Raskin, S. M. Collins, D. M. McCarthy, D. Baetens, A. Rubenstein, T. A. M. Aldor, and R. H. Unger, *New Engl. J. Med.* **301**, 285 (1979).
32. A. E. Bishop, J. M. Polak, P. Garin Chesa, C. M. Timson, M. G. Bryant, and S. R. Bloom, *Diabetes* **30**, 122 (1981).
33. M. Brown, J. Rivier, and W. Vale, *Endocrinology* **104**, 1709 (1979).
34. G. R. Van Loon and N. M. Appel, *Brain Res.* **204**, 236 (1981).
35. D. A. Fisher and M. R. Brown, *Endocrinology* **107**, 714 (1980).
36. M. Brown, J. Rivier, and W. Vale, *Endocrinology* **108**, 2391 (1980).
37. Y. C. Patel, D. P. Cameron, A. Bankier, F. Malaisse-Lagae, M. Ravazzola, P. Studer, and L. Orci, *Endocrinology* **103**, 917 (1978).
38. B. Petersson, R. Elde, S. Efendic, T. Hokfelt, O. Johansson, R. Luft, E. Cerasi, and C. Hellerstrom, *Diabetologica* **13**, 463 (1977).
39. M. Berelowitz, D. Dudlak, and L. A. Frohman, *J. Clin. Invest.*, **69**, 1293 (1982).
40. D. S. Schalch and S. Reichlin, in A. Pecile, and E. E. Muller, Eds., *Growth Hormone*, Excerpta Med., Amsterdam, 1968, p. 211.
41. R. E. Carraway and S. E. Leeman, *J. Biol. Chem.* **248**, 6854 (1973).
42. R. E. Carraway, L. M. Demers, and S. E. Leeman, *Fed. Proc.* **32**, 1 (1973).
43. R. E. Carraway, L. M. Demers, and S. E. Leeman, *Endocrinology* **99**, 1452 (1976).
44. K. Nagai and L. A. Frohman, *Diabetes* **27**, 577 (1978).
45. K. Nagai and L. A. Frohman, *Life Sci.* **19**, 273 (1976).
46. M. Brown and W. Vale, *Endocrinology* **98**, 819 (1976).
47. A. Kaneto, T. Kaneko, H. Kajinuma, and K. Kosaka, *Endocrinology* **102**, 393 (1978).
48. J. Dolais-Kitabgi, P. Kitabgi, P. Brazeau, and P. Freychet, *Endocrinology* **105**, 256 (1979).
49. A. M. Blackburn, D. R. Fletcher, T. E. Adrian, and S. R. Bloom, *J. Clin. Endocrinol. Metab.* **51**, 1257 (1980).
50. M. H. Fernstrom, M. A. Z. Mirski, R. E. Carraway, and S. E. Leeman, *Metabolism* **30**, 853 (1981).
51. M. Berelowitz, C. Nakawatase, and L. A. Frohman, *Diabetes* **29**, 55A (1980).
52. M. Brown, J. Villarreal, and W. Vale, *Metabolism* **25**, 1459 (1976).
53. J. M. Polak, R. Hobbs, S. R. Bloom, E. Solcia, and A. G. E. Pearse, *Lancet* **2**, 1109 (1976).
54. J. Villarreal and M. Brown, *Life Sci.* **23**, 2729 (1978).
55. M. Brown, J. Rivier, and W. W. Vale, *Life Sci.* **21**, 1729 (1977).
56. M. Brown, W. Marki, and J. Rivier, *Life Sci.* **27**, 125 (1980).
57. M. Brown, Y. Tache, and D. Fisher, *Endocrinology* **105**, 660 (1979).
58. E. Ipp, R. Dobbs, and R. H. Unger, *Nature* **276**, 190 (1978).
59. E. Ipp, J. M. Dhorajiwala, A. R. Moossa, and A. H. Rubenstein, *Clin. Res.* **28**, 396A (1980).

60. R. A. Kanter, J. W. Ensinck, and W. Y. Fujimoto, *Diabetes* **29**, 84 (1980).
61. P. Schwandt, W. O. Richter, P. Kerscher, and P. Bottermann, *Life Sci.* **29**, 345 (1981).
62. H. E. Lebovitz, S. Genuth, and K. Pooler, *Endocrinology* **79**, 635 (1966).
63. T. Ono, Y. Oomura, H. Nishino, K. Sasaki, K. Muramoto, and I. Yano, *Brain Res.* **185**, 208 (1980).
64. E. Martino, A. Lernmark, H. Seo, D. F. Steiner, and S. Retetoff, *Proc. Natl. Acad. Sci. USA* **75**, 4265 (1978).
65. J. Knudtzon, *Horm. Metab. Res.* **13**, 371 (1981).
66. J. E. Morley, S. R. Levin, M. Pehlevanian, R. Adachi, A. E. Pekary, and J. M. Hershman, *Endocrinology* **104**, 137 (1979).
67. M. Brown *Life Sci.* **28**, 1789 (1981).
68. S. C. Woods and D. Porte, J., *Diabetes* **24**, 905 (1975).
69. Y. Oomura, T. Ono, H. Ooyama, and M. J. Wayner, *Nature* **222**, 282 (1969).
70. M. van Houten, B. I. Posner, B. M. Kopriwa, and J. R. Brawer, *Endocrinology* **105**, 666 (1979).
71. J. Havrankova, D. Schmechel, J. Roth, and M. Brownstein, *Proc. Natl. Acad. Sci. USA* **75**, 5737 (1978).
72. L.-A. Idahl and J. M. Martin, *J. Endocrinol.* **51**, 601 (1971).
73. J. M. Martin, C. C. Mok, J. Penfold, N. J. Howard, and D. Crowne, *J. Endocrinol.* **58**, 681 (1973).
74. R. B. Lockhart-Ewart, C. Mok, and J. M. Martin, *Diabetes* **25**, 96 (1976).
75. J. H. Moltz, C. P. Fawcett, S. M. McCann, R. E. Dobbs, and R. H. Unger, *Endocrinol. Res. Commun* **2**, 537 (1975).
76. J. H. Moltz, R. E. Dobbs, S. M. McCann, and C. P. Fawcett, *Endocrinology* **101**, 196 (1977).
77. J. H. Moltz, R. E. Dobbs, S. M. McCann, and C. P. Fawcett, *Endocrinology* **105**, 1262 (1979).

12

Thermoregulation

MARVIN R. BROWN

Peptide Biology Laboratory
The Salk Institute
La Jolla, California

1 INTRODUCTION

Regulation of body temperature in mammals ranges from strict endo-
thermic homeothermy to various types of regulated hypothermia and
hyperthermia. The absolute temperature at which an animal regulates
its internal environment results in an optimal set of conditions that no
doubt contributes to its survival. Regulated hypothermia, such as torpor
or hibernation, probably subserves an animal's efforts to maintain caloric homeostasis and adapt to periods of absolute or relative nutrient deprivation. Deviation of body temperature above euthermy in mammals
is generally termed fever; how fever benefits animal survival during
various infectious disease states is at present under debate (1).

Elevation, reduction, or maintainance of normal body temperature involves controlled coordination of heat production and heat loss. Cellular metabolism produces heat that is stored or liberated to maintain
body temperature within the boundaries required by the animal. Heat
production is increased or decreased in accordance with these thermal
requirements. The transfer of heat, that is, heat loss, is enhanced or retarded in animals by three main mechanisms: First, the delivery of heat
to the areas of heat transfer (e.g. skin) is influenced by alterations of
blood flow to those areas. Second, the thermal conductance of heat-ex-
change areas is modulated by processes such as piloerection or sweating. The third mechanism is behavioral in that an animal may seek
alternative thermal environments that either increase or decrease net
heat transfer from the organism to the environment.

The central nervous system (CNS) controls heat production and heat
loss mechanisms. Areas of the CNS that control thermoregulation receive inputs from peripheral afferent receptor systems along with direct
input from their local environment as influenced by local blood flow
and temperature. Presumably these inputs are compared with a CNS
thermoregulatory set point, and if discrepancies exist between the set
point and body temperature, appropriate measures to change body temperature are initiated. Changes in body temperature are achieved by altering heat production or heat loss by a variety of neural efferent
mechanisms. The afferent and efferent systems subserving thermoregulation are multiple and therefore a large number of intercellular regulatory substances might influence this process. Several chemical
transmitters are proposed to be putative regulators of body temperature.
For instance, it is suggested that neurotransmitters such as serotonin
and norepinephrine play important roles within the CNS to increase or
decrease body temperature respectively (2, 3). However, no substance is
unequivocally demonstrated to be involved in these processes.

Peptides are reported to act within the CNS to influence various parameters of body temperature regulation such as body temperature, heat
production and heat loss mechanisms in normal mammals, fever, and

hibernation. Few studies pursue in-depth analysis of the mechanisms whereby peptides influence body temperature regulation. Most studies assess the effects of peptides on body temperature alone without defining what changes occur in heat production, heat loss, or behavioral thermoregulatory mechanisms. This review covers studies examining the CNS effects of thyrotropin releasing factor (TRF), peptides related to somatostatin, vasopressin, opiate-like peptides, bombesin, neurotensin, and corticotropin releasing factor (CRF) on the aspects of animal thermoregulation mentioned above. These peptides are chosen for discussion because of their unique actions or completeness of studies regarding the mechanisms of action that underlie their influences on thermoregulation. Many other peptides have been proposed as having an influence on thermoregulation and some may have roles equivalent to or more important than those cited above.

2 THYROTROPIN RELEASING FACTOR

Thyrotropin releasing factor (TRF) placed into brains of rats or rabbits produces a variety of actions of potential importance to regulation of body temperature. Metcalf [4] and subsequently other investigators [5, 6] report that TRF (0.5–10 μg) placed into the lateral ventricles of rabbits or rats causes a dose-dependent rise of core temperature. TRF produces a larger rise of body temperature when given at high ambient temperatures than when given at low ambient temperatures [7]. These observations are interpreted to indicate that TRF stimulates heat production. Given into the lateral ventricle, TRF reverses hypothermia induced by bombesin, neurotensin, β-endorphin, barbiturates, and ethanol [6, 8–10]. Other effects of TRF administration that appear to be coordinated with its actions to increase body temperature are increased motor activity [11], decreased spreading of saliva with forepaws [12], and increased TSH secretion [13]. Contrary to the above studies, in the cat TRH (10–20 ng) causes a reduction of core temperature, an effect presumed to be secondary to tachypnea [14].

The mechanism whereby TRF increases body temperature may depend on endogenous prostaglandins because TRF-induced hyperthermia is prevented by indomethacin and salicylates [15]. CNS administration of TRF also results in increased plasma levels of epinephrine and norepinephrine [16]. The sites of action of TRF for producing hyperthermia are in the hypothalamus and medial preoptic area [6, 17]. TRF placed into the nucleus accumbens also produces a long-lasting hyperthermia [17].

Evidence to support a physiological role of TRF in the regulation of body temperature is provided by the observations that TRF injected into the hippocampus reverses hibernation [18] and that passive immu-

nization against endogenous TRF by lateral ventricular administration
of anti-TRF sera results in a decrease of core body temperature in rats
(19). As with many other peptides that are putative regulators of body
temperature, TRF is anatomically distributed in brain regions such as
the anterior hypothalamic preoptic region and other areas known to be
involved in thermoregulation (20–22).

The ability of TRF to increase motor activity, enhance sympathetic
nervous system activity, affect behavioral thermoregulation, increase
body temperature, and increase pituitary TSH secretion indicates that
this peptide may initiate a series of coordinated effects that may be of
physiological significance to animals exposed to cold thermal environments.

3   OPIOID PEPTIDES

Before the identification of the opiate-like peptides β-endorphin and the
enkephalins, morphine sulfate was recognized to influence regulation of
body temperature in several species (23, 24). Morphine, like β-endor-
phin, either increases or decreases body temperature depending on the
thermal environment, dose, and state of confinement of the animal (23).
Both morphine (25–27) and β-endorphin (20, 29) given at low doses produce predominantly hyperthermic effects; high doses of these substances produce hypothermia, especially at low ambient temperatures
(26–28, 30). β-Endorphin (2.5–3.0 μg) given icv to rats not only increases
body temperature but also increases salivation (27). These observations
do not support the idea of a coordinated action of β-endorphin to increase body temperature since salivation is a thermoregulatory response to reduce body temperature. By the definition of substances that
affect thermoregulation as outlined by Clark (23), β-endorphin fits into
the category of substances interfering with thermoregulatory efferent
mechanisms rather than altering set point or afferent mechanisms. The
hypothermic effects of β-endorphin (12, 28, 31) are antagonized by naloxone whereas the hyperthermic effects of this peptide are not. Naloxone does not reverse the hypothermic actions of both Met-enkephalin
and Leu-enkephalin (32, 33). These observations suggest that the
enkephalins and endorphins may be working through separate receptors
of the opiate type.

Several lines of evidence suggest that endogenous opiate-like peptides may be involved in the regulation of body temperature. First,
stress-induced hyperthermia is blocked by administration of naloxone
(34). Second, animals exposed to cold or hot environments reduce or increase their body temperatures, respectively, following administration
of naloxone (35, 36). These results suggest that endogenous opiates may
be involved in adaptation to both extremes of thermal environment and

that antagonism of β-endorphinergic transmission by administration of naloxone results in a disorder of thermoregulation. The third line of evidence suggesting that opiate peptides are involved in animal thermoregulation arises from the observation that naloxone awakens animals from hibernation (37). As noted above, TRF also wakens animals from hibernation (18). These findings are of considerable interest since TRF antagonizes opiate-induced hypothermia (8, 12). Whether endogenous opiates are involved in initiating the hibernating state, and whether TRF is involved in reversing this hibernation state, are interesting hypotheses worthy of further investigation.

4 BOMBESIN

Bombesin (1–100 ng) and its mammalian counterpart gastrin-releasing peptide, when administered into the cisterna magnum, lateral ventricle, or specific anterior hypothalamic preoptic sites, produce a decrease of body temperature in animals exposed to low thermal environments, no change of body temperature in animals at thermoneutrality, and an increase of body temperature in animals placed at high thermal environments (38–40). Bombesin-induced hypothermia is reversed by TRF, prostaglandins, and peptides related to somatostatin, and is partially reversed by naloxone (6, 41). Initial studies suggested that bombesin might produce poikilothermia in animals, indicating a complete abolishment of thermoregulatory mechanisms by this peptide (40). Subsequent experiments using calorimetric methods showed that bombesin disrupts the central nervous system component of temperature regulation, that is, it inhibits regulatory heat production (42, 43).

Some investigators suggest that bombesin alters the thermoregulatory set point as evidenced by a behavioral thermoregulatory response to this peptide that parallels its action to inhibit heat production (44). Bombesin's effects on behavioral thermoregulation were demonstrated by placing animals in a thermoneutral environment and allowing bar-pressing to escape radiant heat. While control-injected animals did not bar-press and had elevated rectal temperatures, animals receiving bombesin exhibited increased bar-pressing and no changes in body temperature. These results are consistent with a behavioral attempt to reduce body temperature.

To determine if other putative brain neurotransmitters might be involved in mediating bombesin's effects, antagonists of dopamine and acetylcholine were tested for their ability to inhibit bombesin-induced hypothermia. Haloperidol and atropine prevented hypothermia produced by dopamine or apomorphine and carbachol, respectively, whereas neither haloperidol nor atropine prevented bombesin-induced hypothermia (8). As mentioned above, both TRF and peptides related to somatostatin completely reversed bombesin-induced hypothermia. Whether the mechanisms of bombesin-induced hypothermia involve alterations of endogenous TRF or somatostatin remains to be determined.

Bombesin placed into the lateral ventricle completely prevents cold-induced TSH secretion by inhibiting the secretion or delivery of TRF to the anterior pituitary gland (8). This conclusion is supported by the observation that bombesin does not interfere with TRF-induced TSH secretion either *in vitro* or *in vivo*.

To determine the mechanism of bombesin-induced hypothermia, studies were carried out to analyze the effects of this peptide on heat production and heat loss mechanisms. Although bombesin produces poikilothermic-like effects on body temperature, changes in both oxygen consumption and heat production differ from those observed in true poikilotherms. Animals given bombesin icv and placed in an open circuit calorimeter did not display any significant increase in skin temperature but did show a dramatic reduction of oxygen consumption and developed hypothermia when exposed to low ambient temperatures (42, 43) (Figure 1). In contrast, animals at thermoneutral temperatures did not exhibit any reduction of oxygen consumption following administration of bombesin. Taken together, these results suggest that bombesin does not reduce heat production below the level of minimum heat production, but rather interferes with regulatory heat production. Regulatory heat production, as defined by Girardier (45), is the CNS-dependent heat production necessary to maintain thermal homeostasis in animals exposed to environments below their lower critical temperature.

As with TRF, bombesin appears to produce several coordinant effects that might lead to reduction of body temperature, such as decreased heat production, inhibition of TSH secretion, and behavioral maneuvers that result in reduction of body temperature. To date there is little evidence to support a physiological role of bombesin in the regulation of body temperature, although its potent effects (1–100 ng) on thermoregulation as well as its effects on neuroregulation of metabolism suggest that this peptide may be an important regulator of body temperature and metabolism.

5 NEUROTENSIN

Nemeroff and his associates were the first to demonstrate neurotensin's effects on thermoregulation. Neurotensin lowers body temperature in the mouse, rat, gerbil, guinea pig, hamster, and monkey (8, 46, 47). In contrast with bombesin's effects on temperature regulation, neurotensin does not elevate rectal temperature in animals placed in a warm environment (48).

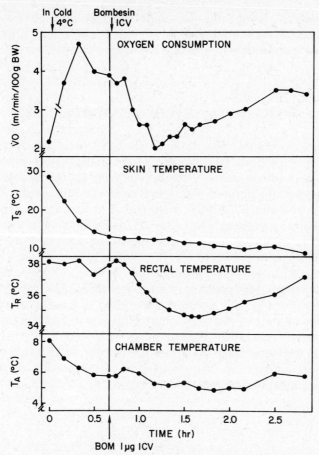

Figure 1. Effects of bombesin placed into the lateral cerebral ventricle (icv) on rat oxygen consumption, tail skin temperature, and rectal temperature. Animals were placed in a cold calorimetry box and a half-hour later given an icv injection of bombesin. Ambient temperature is indicated in the lower panel.

The sites of action of neurotensin to influence temperature regulation are medial preoptic area, anterior hypothalamus, periaqueductal gray, dorsal hypothalamus, and medial hypothalamus (49). Neurotensin placed into the anterior pituitary also lowers rectal temperature, suggesting the possibility that this peptide is transported retrogradely from the pituitary to the hypothalamus (50). Taube et al. (51) have reported that neurotensin placed into the anterior hypothalamic preoptic region of the rat produces hyperthermia.

Neurotensin-induced hypothermia is enhanced by depletion of brain dopamine and suppressed by administration of dopamine agonists (52). Antagonists of norepinephrine, serotonin, acetylcholine, and opiates do not alter neurotensin-induced hypothermia (52).

A physiological role of neurotensin in the regulation of body temperature is supported by the observation that administration of neurotensin antibodies into the lateral ventricle elevates rectal temperature in rats (53).

6 SOMATOSTATIN AND RELATED PEPTIDES

Somatostatin-14 (SS-14) was initially demonstrated by Cohn (54) to cause reduction of body temperature. Other investigators reported that SS-14 had little effect on body temperature (8, 41, 55). Shortened analogs of somatostatin (termed oligosomatostatins), such as desAA[1,2,4,5,12,13] [D-Trp[8]]-somatostatin (ODT8-SS) were found to produce significant elevations of body temperature (41). One of the difficulties in testing SS-14 for its effects on body temperature regulation results from the very close proximity of the LD_{50} to the ED_{50} when placed in the brain. The oligosomatostatins, however, produce very profound hyperthermia with amounts of peptide far less than their toxic doses. The explanation for these observations is still unclear. The initial discovery of the potent hyperthermic actions of the oligosomatostatins suggested the possibility that other somatostatin-like ligands might exist within the central nervous system and that their hyperthermic actions were being mimicked by the oligosomatostatins. The endogenous somatostatin in question is probably somatostatin-28 (SS-28) (41; Figure 2). SS-28 shares complete

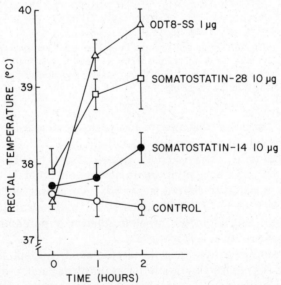

Figure 2. Effects of somatostatin-14, somatostatin-28, and desAA[1,2,4,5,12,13][D-Trp[8]]-somatostatin (ODT8-SS) on rectal temperatures of rats. Peptides were given into the lateral cerebral ventricle of animals in 22°C environment.

C-terminal homology with SS-14 but is extended at the N-terminus by 14 residues. SS-28 is not only an apparently brain-selective somatostatin, it also shows selective actions on the endocrine pancreas to inhibit the secretion of insulin far more potently than that of glucagon (56).

The somatostatin ODT8-SS potently prevents hypothermia induced by bombesin, neurotensin, carbachol, and dopamine (8). However, β-endorphin-induced hypothermia is not antagonized by this oligosomatostatin. These observations may relate to the sites of action of these various substances to influence temperature regulation. In contrast to the inhibition of TRF-induced hyperthermia by indomethacin and salicylates, somatostatin-induced hyperthermia is not influenced by prostaglandin synthesis inhibition (41). ODT8-SS is approximately 10 times more potent than PGE to produce hyperthermia (41).

To determine the mechanisms by which peptides related to somatostatin influence temperature regulation, calorimetry experiments were carried out. Icv administration of ODT8-SS to animals placed at thermoneutrality produced a dramatic rise in oxygen consumption (42, 43). The rise in oxygen consumption of saline-injected animals placed at 4°C did not exceed that of ODT8-SS treated animals placed at thermoneutrality. That is, the rise in oxygen consumption produced by cold exposure alone was equal to the rise in oxygen consumption exhibited by animals receiving ODT8-SS in the absence of cold. Whether these results indicate that somatostatin or a somatostatin pathway is involved in generating the increased heat production observed following cold exposure requires further investigation. Animals given bombesin plus ODT8-SS demonstrated normal oxygen consumption responses to cold exposure. These results suggest that ODT8-SS antagonizes bombesin-induced hypothermia by preventing bombesin's inhibitory effects on heat production.

The best evidence for a possible physiological role of somatostatin or somatostatin-related peptides in regulating body temperature derives from studies done in the ob/ob mouse (41). Homozygous ob/ob mice exposed to cold experience drastic hypothermia and die if not removed from the cold and rewarmed. Administration of ODT8-SS to these animals completely prevents cold-induced hypothermia (Figure 3). Since these animals have decreased levels of somatostatin-like activity in their brains (Vale and Brown, unpublished data), the possibility exists that their failure to thermoregulate results from a defect in a CNS somatostatinergic pathway involved in thermoregulation.

7 VASOPRESSIN

Over the past several years, Kasting, Veale, and Cooper have performed an impressive series of studies which implicates vasopressin as both an endogenous antipyretic and a possible contributing factor in

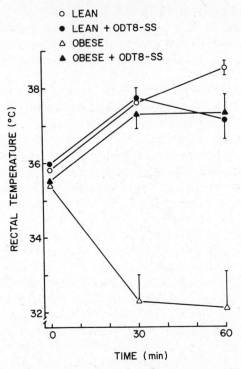

Figure 3. DesAA[1,2,4,5,12,13][D-Trp[8]]-somatostatin (ODT8-SS) prevention of hypothermia in the ob/ob mouse. Peptide was given intracisternally before placement of animals at 4°C.

the etiology of febrile convulsions. The observations that pregnant ewes do not exhibit febrile reponses around the time of parturition and that newborn lambs likewise do not exhibit febrile responses led to question whether an endogenous antipyretic substance might protect these animals against fever (57, 58). Previously, vasopressin was demonstrated to be elevated in the plasma of pregnant ewes around the time of parturition (59) and also was shown to affect animal thermoregulation (60). Furthermore, vasopressin secretion was stimulated by heating the anterior hypothalamic preoptic area, the brain region where prostaglandins as well as antipyretics act to influence animal thermoregulation (61). Recent studies (62, 63) demonstrated that placement of arginine vasopressin into the septal region, 2 to 3 mm anterior to the anterior commisure, prevents pyrogen-induced fever in sheep. Consistent with these data, a specific antivasopressin serum perfused into the same septal area enhanced the fever response to pyrogen administration (62). Similar effects were noted with administration of vasopressin antagonists into this brain region. Other studies, using push-pull cannulae perfusion methods, documented the release of vasopressin into the septal area following induction of fever (64).

Kasting et al. (65) observed that vasopressin, when placed into the brains of rats, produces monoclonic, monotonic convulsions. The possibility that vasopressin is an endogenous antipyretic released during fever that may be responsible for the initiation of febrile seizures in newborns is an attractive hypothesis.

8 CORTICOTROPIN RELEASING FACTOR (CRF)

The recently isolated and characterized 41-amino-acid peptide corticotropin releasing factor (CRF) stimulates the secretion of ACTH and β-endorphin both *in vitro* and *in vivo* (66, 67). In addition to these hypophysiotropic activities, this peptide, when placed into the brain, increases animal activity, stimulates the sympathetic nervous system resulting in increased plasma levels of epinephrine and norepinephrine, increases plasma levels of vasopressin, and produces a profound increase in metabolic rate (68–70) (Figure 4). In some animals, slight increases of core body temperature occur following CRF administration. However, it appears that the increased metabolic rate of these animals is related to their increased physical activity and that any extra heat produced is liberated. CRF is an example of a peptide that acts in the brain to profoundly alter pathways capable of modifying body temperature, but no rise in body temperature occurs following its administration because other components of thermoregulatory activity remain intact. It

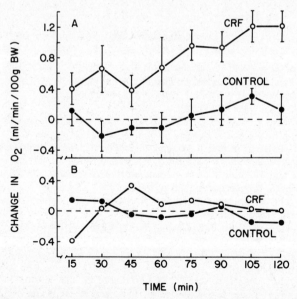

Figure 4. Effects of CRF given into the lateral cerebral ventricle (A) or intravenously (B) on oxygen consumption of rats. Animals were at an ambient temperature of 22°C.

is tempting to speculate that the release of vasopressin following CRF administration might prevent development of hyperthermia.

9   CONCLUSIONS

It is apparent that a variety of peptides act within the CNS to influence various aspects of thermoregulation. No peptide has been demonstrated to be involved unequivocally in the physiological regulation of body temperature. Future studies should be directed towards determining if endogenously released peptides participate in thermoregulatory events. Specific peptide antagonists and methods to assess peptide turnover need development to pursue this goal. In-depth analyses of the mechanisms by which each peptide could influence thermoregulatory neural set point, and analyses of afferent and efferent mechanisms should be carried out.

ACKNOWLEDGMENTS

This research has been supported in part by NIH grants NS-14263 and AM-26741 and in part by The Clayton Foundation for Research, California Division. Dr. Brown is a Clayton Foundation Investigator. Thanks to Dr. L. Fisher for helpful discussions and to S. McCall for manuscript preparation.

REFERENCES

1. D. Rodbard, *New Engl. J. Med.* **305**, 808 (1981).
2. W. Feldberg and R. D. Meyers, *J. Physiol.* **173**, 226 (1964).
3. W. Feldberg and R. D. Meyers, *J. Physiol.* **175**, 464 (1964).
4. G. Metcalf, *Nature* **252**, 310 (1974).
5. M. A. Carino, J. R. Smith, B. G. Weick, and A. Horita, *Life Sci.* **19**, 1687 (1976).
6. M. Brown, J. Rivier, and W. Vale, *Life Sci.* **20**, 1681 (1977).
7. G. Metcalf, P. Dettmar, and T. Watson, in *Thermoregulatory Mechanisms and Their Therapeutic Implications*, S. Karger, Basel, 1980, p. 175.
8. M. Brown and W. Vale, in *Thermoregulatory Mechanisms and Their Therapeutic Implications*, S. Karger, Basel, 1980, p. 186.
9. A. J. Prange, G. R. Breese, J. M. Cott, B. R. Martin, B. R. Cooper, I. C. Wilson, and N. P. Plotnikoff, *Life Sci.* **14**, 447 (1974).
10. G. R. Breese, J. M. Cott, B. R. Cooper, A. J. Prange, and M. A. Lipton, *Life Sci.* **14**, 1053 (1974).
11. D. Segal and A. Mandell, *The Thyroid Axis Drugs and Behavior*, Raven Press, New York, 1974, p. 129.
12. J. Holaday, L. Tseng, H. Loh, and C. H. Li, *Life Sci.* **22**, 1537 (1978).
13. R. Burgus, T. F. Dunn, D. Desiderio, W. Vale, and R. Guillemin, *Acad. Sci. (Paris)* **269**, 226 (1969).

14. R. D. Meyers, G. Metcalf, and J. C. Rice, *Brain Res.* **126**, 105 (1977).
15. M. L. Cohn, M. Cohn, and D. Taube, in *Thermoregulatory Mechanisms and Their Therapeutic Implications*, S. Karger, Basel, 1980, p. 198.
16. M. Brown, *Life Sci.* **28**, 1789 (1981).
17. G. Boschi and R. Rips, *Neurosci. Lett.* **23**, 93 (1981).
18. T. L. Stanton, A. L. Beckman, and A. Winokur, in *Thermoregulatory Mechanisms and Their Therapeutic Implications*, S. Karger, Basel, 1980, p. 195.
19. C. Prasad, J. J. Jacobs, and J. F. Wilber, *Brain Res.* **193**, 580 (1980).
20. A. Winokur and R. D. Utiger, *Science* **185**, 265 (1974).
21. M. Brownstein, M. Palkovits, J. Saavedra, R. Bassiri, and R. Utiger, *Science* **185**, 267 (1974).
22. I. Jackson and S. Reichlin, *Endocrinology* **95**, 854 (1974).
23. W. Clark, *Pharm. Biochem. Behav.* **10**, 609 (1979).
24. T. Burks and G. Rosenfeld, in *Body Temperature*, Marcel Dekker, Inc., New York, 1979, p. 531.
25. B. Cox, M. Ary, W. Chesarek, and P. Lomax, *Eur. J. Pharmacol.* **36**, 33 (1976).
26. J. B. Herrman, *J. Pharmacol. Exp. Ther.* **76**, 309 (1942).
27. H. W. Holaday, H. Loh, and C. H. Li, *Life Sci.* **22**, 1525 (1978).
28. A. S. Bloom and L. Tseng, *Peptides* **2**, 293 (1981).
29. J. Huidobro and E. L. Way, *J. Pharmacol. Exp. Ther.* **211**, 50 (1979).
30. V. Lotti, P. Lomax, and R. George, *J. Pharmacol. Exp. Ther.* **150**, 135 (1965).
31. F. Bloom, D. Segal, N. Ling, and R. Guillemin, *Science* **194**, 630 (1976).
32. S. Ferri, R. Arrigo-Reina, A. Santagostino, F. M. Scoto, and C. Spadaro, *Psychopharmacology* **58**, 277 (1978).
33. W. Clark, *Proc. Soc. Exp. Biol. Med.* **154**, 540 (1977).
34. J. Blasig, V. Hollt, U. Baverle, and A. Herz, *Life Sci.* **23**, 2525 (1978).
35. J. W. Holaday, E. Wei, H. Loh, and C. H. Li, *Proc. Natl. Acad. Sci. USA* **75**, 2923 (1978).
36. J. A. Thornhill, K. E. Cooper, and W. L. Veale, *J. Pharm. Pharmacol.* **32**, 427 (1980).
37. D. L. Margules, B. Goldman, and A. Finck, *Brain Res. Bull.* **4**, 721 (1979).
38. M. Brown, J. Rivier, and W. Vale, *Science* **196**, 998 (1977).
39. Q. Pittman, Y. Tache, and M. Brown, *Life Sci.* **26**, 725 (1980).
40. Y. Tache, Q. Pittman, and M. Brown, *Brain Res.* **188**, 525 (1980).
41. M. Brown, N. Ling, and J. Rivier, *Brain Res.* **214**, 127 (1981).
42. M. Brown, *Fed. Proc.* **40**, 2765 (1981).
43. M. Brown, *Brain Res.*, 242, 243 (1982).
44. D. Avery, M. F. Hawkins, and B. A. Wunder, *Neuropharmacology* **20**, 23 (1981).
45. L. Girardier, *Experientia* **33**, 1121 (1977).
46. G. Bissette, C. B. Nemeroff, P. T. Loosen, A. J. Prange, and M. A. Lipton, *Nature* **262**, 607 (1976).
47. B. V. Clineschmidt, and J. C. McGuffin, *Eur. J. Pharmacol.* **46**, 395 (1977).
48. G. A. Mason, C. B. Nemeroff, D. Luttingen, O. L. Hatley, and A. J. Prange, *Regulatory Peptides* **1**, 53 (1980).
49. G. E. Martin, C. B. Bacino, and N. L. Papp, *Peptides* **1**, 333 (1981).
50. D. M. Dorsa, E. R. DeKloct, E. Mezey, and D. DeWied, *Endocrinology* **104**, 1663 (1969).
51. D. Taube, M. Cohn, and M. L. Cohn, *Fed. Proc.* **39**, 1070 (1980).
52. C. B. Nemeroff, G. Bissette, P. J. Manberg, A. J. Osbahr, G. R. Breese, and A. J. Prange, *Brain Res.* **195**, 69 (1980).
53. M. M. Wallace, R. J. Bodnar, D. Badillo-Martinez, G. Nilaver, and E. A. Zimmerman, *Soc. Neurosci. Abstr. (1981).*
54. M. L. Cohn, *Molecular Anesthesia*, Raven Press, New York, 1975, p. 485.
55. C. B. Nemeroff, A. J. Osbahr, P. Manberg, G. N. Ervin, and A. J. Prange, *Proc. Natl. Acad. Sci. USA* **76**, 5368 (1979).

56. M. Brown, J. Rivier, and W. Vale, *Endocrinology* **108**, 2391 (1981).
57. N. Kasting, W. L. Veale, and K. E. Cooper, *Nature* **271**, 245 (1978).
58. N. Kasting, W. L. Veale, and K. E. Cooper, in *Current Studies of Hypothalamic Function, 1978*, Part II: *Metabolism and Behavior*, S. Karger, Basel, 1978, p. 63.
59. D. P. Alexander, R. A. Bashore, H. G. Britton, and M. A. Forsling, *Biologia Neonat.* **25**, 242 (1974).
60. A. Okuno, M. Yamamoto, and S. Itoh, *Jap. J. Physiol.* **15**, 378 (1965).
61. E. Szczepanska-Sadowska, *Am. J. Physiol.* **226**, 155 (1974).
62. K. E. Cooper, N. W. Kasting, K. Lederis, and W. L. Veale, *J. Physiol.* **295**, 33 (1979).
63. N. W. Kasting, K. E. Cooper, and W. L. Veale, *Experientia* **35**, 208 (197).
64. W. L. Veale, N. W. Kasting, and K. E. Cooper, *Fed. Proc.* **40**, 2750 (1981).
65. N. Kasting, W. L. Veale, K. E. Cooper, and K. Lederis, *Brain Res.* **213**, 322 (1981).
66. W. Vale, J. Spiess, C. Rivier, and J. Rivier, *Science* **213**, 1394 (1981).
67. J. Spiess, J. Rivier, C. Rivier, and W. Vale, *Proc. Natl. Acad. Sci. USA* **78**, 6517, 1981.
68. M. R. Brown, L. A. Fisher, J. Rivier, J. Spiess, C. Rivier, and W. Vale, *Life Sci.* **30**, 207 (1982).
69. L. A. Fisher, J. Rivier, C. Rivier, J. Spiess, W. Vale, and M. R. Brown, *Endocrinology* **110**, 2222 (1982).
70. M. R. Brown, L. A. Fisher, J. Spiess, C. Rivier, J. Rivier, and W. Vale, *Endocrinology*, **111**, 928 (1982).

13

Nociception

THOMAS M. JESSELL

Department of Neurobiology
Harvard Medical School
Boston, Massachusetts

Attempts to resolve the mechanisms underlying the processing and integration of sensory information that is eventually perceived as pain have, until recently, relied almost exclusively on anatomical and physiological techniques (for reviews see refs. 1–3). In particular, the failure to detect any of the classical neurotransmitters within primary sensory neurons has meant that the chemical circuits involved in sensory transmission have been difficult or impossible to analyze. The advent of immunocytochemical techniques for the localization of neuropeptides within mammalian neurons (4) has now revealed the presence of neuropeptides in a significant proportion of neurons located in sensory ganglia, central sensory relay nuclei, and descending pathways that regulate incoming sensory information. The presence of identified peptides thus provides a series of reliable markers for functionally distinct classes of somatosensory neurons and also provides the first information on possible mechanisms of chemical transmission in nociceptive pathways. This chapter reviews current information on the localization and organization of peptide neurons in nociceptive pathways and discusses the preliminary information that is available on the function of individual peptides.

1 PEPTIDES IN PRIMARY SENSORY NEURONS

It has been known for some time that a close correlation exists between the peripheral receptive properties, somatic size, and central terminal arborization of spinal sensory neurons. Small diameter nociceptive neurons that give rise to unmyelinated or thinly myelinated central axons terminate almost exclusively within laminae I and II of the dorsal horn of the spinal cord. Although there is some uncertainty surrounding the precise organization of central terminals, the majority of unmyelinated afferent fibers appear to terminate within lamina II (the substantia gelatinosa) while thinly myelinated A delta fibers project to lamina I (the marginal layer) with occasional axons dropping deeper into lamina V (5, 6). Virtually all other classes of cutaneous afferent fibers give rise to central terminal arbors located within and ventral to lamina III, with little or no incursion across the lamina II–III border (3). In most species, high threshold mechanoreceptive and some thermoreceptive afferents terminate within lamina I (6), and indirect evidence suggests that chemosensitive sensory neurons contribute terminals to the central region of lamina II (7). This reasonably precise mapping of functional classes of primary sensory afferents makes it possible to draw tentative conclusions about the distribution of neuropeptide-containing sensory terminals in the dorsal horn.

About one-third of small diameter sensory neurons have so far been shown to contain neuropeptides (Table 1, Figure 1). Substance P is pres-

TABLE 1 Identified Neuropeptides in Central and Peripheral Neurons that Originate in, or Project to, the Dorsal Horn of the Spinal Cord

Peptide	Cellular Origin	Dorsal Horn Termination	Reference
I. Primary Sensory Neurons			
Substance P	∾20% of small-diameter dorsal ganglion neurons	Lamina I Lamina II Lamina V	8
Somatostatin	∾5–10% of small-diameter dorsal root ganglion-neurons	Lamina I Lamina II	8
Cholecystokinin-like	Small-diameter dorsal root ganglion neurons (some may also contain substance P)	Lamina I Lamina II	8
Vasoactive intestinal polypeptide	Scattered small cells in sensory ganglion	Lamina I	8
Angiotensin	Some sensory neurons	Lamina II	11
Dynorphin	Unidentified cells in dorsal root ganglia	Present in dorsal horn	13
Met-Tyr-Lys	Unidentified cells in dorsal root ganglia	Not known	102
II. Dorsal Horn Interneurons			
Enkephalins	Laminae I–III	Laminae I–III Lamina V	47 48
Substance P	Laminae I–III	Lamina I–II Lamina V	50 47
Somatostatin	Lamina IIi	Lamina I–II	47
Neurotensin	Lamina II	Lamina I–II	47 74
Avian pancreatic polypeptide	Laminae I, III	Laminae I, II	47
Gastrin-releasing peptide/bombesin	Laminae I–II	Lamina I, II	79
III. Supraspinal Neurons			
Substance P	Midline brainstem nuclei	Lamina I, II?	93
Thryotopin releasing hormone	Brainstem nuclei	Little, if any	93
Enkephalin	Brainstem nuclei	Not known	96 98
Cholecystokinin-like	Brainstem	Lamina I, II?	99
Oxytocin/vasopressin	Paraventricular nucleus	Lamina I	100
Angiotensin II	Paraventricular nucleus	Lamina I	11

ent within 10–20% of all sensory ganglion neurons, somatostatin is present within a separate population of about 5–10% of cells, and vasoactive intestinal polypeptide (VIP) can be found in a few scattered neurons within sensory ganglia (8). A peptide related to but not identical with cholecystokinin (CCK) (9) is also present within sensory ganglion cells, but recent studies (Hökfelt, personal communication) have shown that

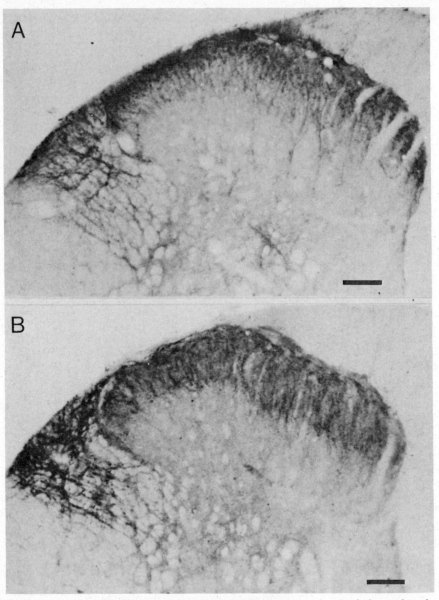

Figure 1. Immunocytochemical localization of substance P and enkephalin within the dorsal horn of rat spinal cord. A Substance P immunoreactivity in the central terminals of primary sensory neurons in laminae I and II of the dorsal horn of rat spinal cord. Immunoreactive fibers in the dorso-lateral funiculus originate from descending brainstem neurons, some of which also contain serotonin. Scale= 100 um. B Leucine-enkephalin immunoreactivity in the terminals of interneurons within laminae I and II of the dorsal horn. The similarity in terminal distribution of substance P and leucine-enkephalin neurons is evident. Scale= 100 um.

many of the CCK-like immunoreactive cells also contain substance P. As might be expected then, the central terminal fields of substance P and CCK containing sensory neurons are strikingly similar and are confined predominantly to lamina I and lamina IIo. Somatostatin neurons of sensory origin project more ventrally into lamina IIi and VIP immunoreactive terminals are located predominantly within lamina I (10). Some sensory neurons that project to lamina II of the dorsal horn may also contain an angiotensin-like peptide (11).

A number of other peptides have been reported to be present within spinal sensory ganglia although detailed information on cellular localization is lacking. Biochemical studies have shown that a number of small di- and tripeptides extracted from sheep sensory ganglia have depressant effects on dorsal horn neurons (12). The opioid peptide dynorphin has also been reported to be present within sensory ganglia although immunocytochemical evidence has not yet been presented (13).

Identified peptide containing neurons account for approximately 25% of all sensory neurons, thus the transmitter or peptide content of over half the small, presumably, nociceptive neurons is still unknown (see Table 1). However, a marker does exist for these neurons. An isoenzyme of acid phosphatase is present in a subpopulation of small-diameter sensory neurons that project to the central region of lamina II. These acid phosphatase-containing sensory neurons have recently been shown to exhibit little or no overlap with sensory neurons that contain substance P and somatostatin, and therefore by implication the CCK-like peptide (14), and thus probably delineate the majority of the remaining small nociceptive neurons. The function of this enzyme is at present unknown although its probable location in secretory granules suggests that it may have a role in chemical transmission at afferent synapses.

Of the peptides localized in sensory ganglia, the role of substance P has been studied in greatest detail. In the central terminals of sensory neurons in laminae I and II of the dorsal horn, substance P immunoreactivity is associated with large, dense core vesicles and probably also with the external membrane of small clear vesicles (15). The presence in sensory terminals of small clear vesicles that are not normally associated with sites of peptide storage is suggestive of the presence of another compound or compounds that may be released together with peptides from these terminals. Some of the physiological evidence on postsynaptic actions of substance P released from sensory terminals (discussed below) is also consistent with this possibility.

The release of substance P from sensory terminals in the dorsal horn has been demonstrated both *in vivo* and *in vitro* (16–18). Experiments in which release of substance P into the spinal subarachnoid space has been measured after intrathecal cannulation of the cat spinal cord have shown that substance P release can be evoked selectively by recruitment of peripheral sensory fibers that have conduction velocities in the A delta and C fibers range (18; Figure 2).

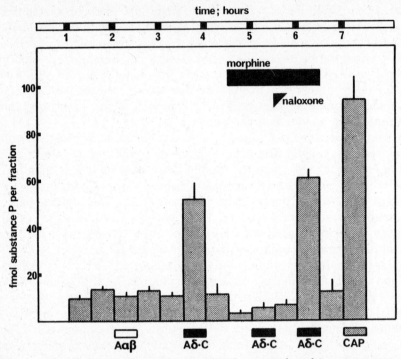

Figure 2. Release of substance P from superfused cat spinal cord in response to sciatic nerve stimulation and capsaicin (CAP). The sciatic nerve was stimulated bilaterally with rectangular pulses (3–4 V, 0.05 msec, 50 Hz for activation of AA and AB fibers and 40-50 V, 0.05 msec, 50 Hz for recruitment of A delta and C fibers). Perfusion samples (3 mL) were collected into glacial acetic acid, frozen, and lyophilized. Samples were reconstituted in 1.0 mL of assay buffer and neutralized, and aliquots of each fraction were used to determine the content of substance P by radioimmunoassay. Each value is the mean ± SEM of four separate experiments. From Yaksh et al. (32).

Although it is clear that the generalized activation of nociceptive afferents leads to the release of substance P from central sensory terminals, it has been more difficult to equate the postsynaptic actions of substance P with the response of dorsal horn neurons to noxious peripheral stimuli. There is also some debate at present whether the actions of substance P in the dorsal horn are confined to neurons that receive a nociceptive input (19) or extend to neurons with low-threshold afferent inputs. There seems no particular reason to expect that the actions of substance P in the dorsal horn need be confined to nociceptive neurons. In fact the excitatory action of substance P on motoneurons (16) and on neurons in the cuneate nucleus (20) illustrates that neurons with other classes of sensory input are responsive to substance P.

In vivo, the iontophoretic application of substance P produces a slow and prolonged activation of dorsal horn neurons that is in many cases slower in onset than the response of the same neuron to peripheral noxious stimuli. However, very little is known at present about the basic characteristics of synaptic transmission between nociceptive primary afferents and dorsal horn neurons. Until more information is available, interpretation of the actions of substance P and other peptides within primary sensory neurons will remain difficult.

Some clues to the possible role of substance P in nociceptive pathways in the dorsal horn can be derived from the recent studies performed by (21) in the guinea pig inferior mesenteric ganglion. Some substance P-containing primary sensory neurons with central terminals in the superficial dorsal horn send peripheral processes through the sympathetic chain, many of which form classical axo-somatic synapses with principal sympathetic neurons in the inferior mesenteric ganglion (22–24). By stimulating the dorsal roots it is possible to elicit a slow depolarization of postganglionic neurons, the time course and characteristics of which can be mimicked by substance P (21). The noncholinergic depolarization has an onset of about 500 msec and disappears after depletion of substance P from terminals within the ganglion by pretreatment with capsaicin. If substance P has a similar time course of action on dorsal horn neurons receiving input from the central projections of the same sensory neurons, one of the functions of substance P could be to sensitize dorsal horn neurons to the actions of a more rapidly acting sensory transmitter released from the same or nearby sensory afferents.

The functional role of other peptides in nociceptive sensory neurons is even more uncertain. Somatostatin has been reported to inhibit nociceptive dorsal horn neurons (25, 26), whereas CCK and VIP have excitatory actions (27, 28).

Capsaicin, the active principal of the capsicum species, has been used for many years to modify the function of nociceptive primary sensory neurons (29, 30). More recently the compound has been extensively studied as a possible chemical probe for investigating peptide-containing sensory afferents. In adult animals administration of capsaicin leads to a series of behavioral responses that probably reflects the activation of nociceptive afferents (31) and results in the release of substance P from the central terminals of nociceptive afferents (17, 32). More prolonged application results in the depletion of substance P from primary sensory neurons and their terminals in the dorsal horn (33). The depletion of substance P is reversible, and ultrastructural studies have shown that systemic administration of capsaicin in adult animals does not lead to overt degeneration of the sensory neuron. The changes in sensory perception associated with capsaicin administration in adult animals have been difficult to define. Intrathecal application of capsaicin has been reported to lead to a loss in response to thermal noxious stimuli (31, 34, 35) although it is not possible at present to correlate sensory deficit with the depletion of specific neuropeptides. In guinea pigs, systemic administration of capsaicin to adult animals does, however, seem to be effective in depleting substance P and lowering responsiveness to thermal stimuli (36).

Capsaicin administration in neonatal animals leads initially to the release of substance P (37), followed soon after by the onset of degeneration of the majority of small-diameter sensory neurons that give rise to unmyelinated afferent fibers (38–40) although higher doses of capsaicin leads to some loss of thinly myelinated afferents (40). The destruction of sensory neurons induced by neonatal capsaicin administration is irreversible and, not surprisingly, is accompanied by a loss of substance P, the CCK-like peptide, somatostatin, VIP, and acid phosphatase from primary sensory neurons (10). The sensory deficit elicited by neonatal capsaicin administration is less dramatic than might be expected, with only small changes in thermal or mechanical response threshold detectable in adult animals treated neonatally with capsaicin (41–43). The depletion of one population of sensory neurons in early postnatal life may allow a functional reorganization of remaining sensory neurons (44) that serves to minimalize the functional deficit initially induced by capsaicin.

Although the general correlation between peptide depletion and sensory deficit induced by capsaicin supports the concept that peptides play a role in sensory transmission at nociceptive afferent synapses, it is possible to dissociate, at least partially, the changes in peptide content, sensory impairment, and electrophysiological response (45). These observations have been interpreted by Wall and colleagues as indicating alternative roles for peptides containing unmyelinated afferents, perhaps in the organization of receptive fields of somatosensory cells (44). While precedents clearly exist for long term actions of peptides and peptide hormones the evidence that peptides act as transmitters in the autonomic nervous system is now quite convincing (46, 21) and it seems unnecessary at present to abandon the idea of similar actions in the central nervous system.

2   LOCAL PEPTIDE CIRCUITS MODIFYING NOCICEPTIVE INPUT TO THE DORSAL HORN

In addition to the high density of peptide-containing nociceptive afferents in the dorsal horn there are at least six classes of peptide-containing neurons that originate within the dorsal horn itself (see Table 1). Enkephalin-immunoreactive neurons have been described throughout laminae I–III with highest density in lamina IIo (47, 48). Whether all enkephalin immunoreactive cells in the dorsal horn are exclusively involved in segmental circuitry is still unclear. A population of lamina I neurons are known to contribute axons to the spinothalamic tract, terminating within various thalamic subnuclei (1). However, the low densi-

ty of enkephalin terminals in these thalamic regions and the lack of
accumulation of enkephalin immunoreactivity caudal to spinal transections suggests that the majority of enkephalin neurons within laminae I
correspond to segmental or short-ranging neurons that have been characterized physiologically (49).

Enkephalin-containing terminals within laminae I and II are in a stra-
tegic position to regulate incoming nociceptive information. Hökfelt et
al. (50) first emphasized the close overlap in distribution of enkephalin
and substance P immunoreactive terminals within the dorsal horn and
proposed that a functional interaction between enkephalin interneurons
and the terminals of substance P nociceptive afferents might underly
the direct spinal analgesic actions of opiates and opioid peptides described by Yaksh and Rudy (51). The suppression of substance P release by opioid peptides *in vitro* (52, 53) and *in vivo* (32) has provided
more direct physiological evidence that substance P-containing sensory
afferents may be under phasic or tonic regulation by opioid peptide systems. *In vivo*, the release of substance P elicited by high-threshold activation of primary sensory neurons can be abolished by intrathecal
administration of opiates at concentrations that produce behaviorally
defined analgesia (32; Figure 2).

These studies, however, do not define the precise anatomical relationship between opioid and substance P neurons. Biochemical and anatomical studies have shown that one population of primary sensory
neurons expresses opiate receptors on cell bodies in the primate dorsal
root ganglion (54, 55). Some of these receptors are transported along the
dorsal roots (56, 57) to afferent terminals in the dorsal horn (58). Dorsal
rhizotomy removes approximately 40–50% of dorsal horn opiate receptors (59, 33, 60) suggesting that at least two populations of opiate receptors exist in the dorsal horn, those on afferent terminals and those that
persist after deafferentation and are presumably located on postsynaptic neural elements. Sensory neurons grown in dissociated cell culture
synthesize substance P (61–63) and express opiate receptors on their somatic membrane (61, 64). Application of opiates to chick sensory neurons at concentrations that suppress substance P release reduces the
duration of the action potential recorded from the sensory neuron cell
soma (53), probably by decreasing inward calcium current (65). These
experiments demonstrate the existence of functional opiate receptors on
cultured primary sensory neurons. Moreover, if similar ionic mechanisms operate at the central terminals of sensory neurons, the decrease
in intracellular calcium might be expected to depress transmitter release.

It is not clear at present whether opiate receptors expressed on the
cell bodies of sensory neurons in adult animals are functional. The application of opiates to isolated adult dorsal root ganglia has so far
failed to reveal the same decrease in action potential duration found in

embryonic neurons in culture (66). However, since only a small proportion of sensory cells (8% in primates, according to ref. 55) express opiate receptors, such effects might be difficult to detect in an intact preparation.

The anatomical substrate for the opiate-mediated suppression of afferent transmitter release in the superficial dorsal horn is not immediately apparent. In extensive ultrastructural studies in the macaque, Ralston and Ralston (67) commented on the infrequency of axo-axonic contacts between dorsal horn neurons and primary afferent terminals in lamina I and II. Similarly, ultra-structural immunocytochemical studies in a number of species have revealed very few enkephalin immunoreactive terminals in contact with identifiable primary afferents (68, 69, 48).

Two possibilities then exist; enkephalin released from interneurons in the dorsal horn could act exclusively on dorsal horn neurons with little interaction with the population of opiate receptors located on primary afferent terminals. Alternatively, the absence of axo-axonic synapses may still permit a physiological interaction between neuronally released enkephalin and primary afferent neurons. Evidence for a physiological action of opioids on C-fiber terminals in the dorsal horn has been provided recently by Fitzgerald and Woolf (70). Two other lines of evidence are also consistent with the latter scheme. Yaksh and Elde (18) have shown that sufficient enkephalin can be released from the dorsal horn in response to peripheral nerve stimulation to enable detection of the peptide in intrathecal superfusates, suggesting that the local concentration of enkephalin in the vicinity of nearby nerve terminals may be quite high. Moreover, Konishi et al. (21) and Jiang et al. (71) have shown that sensory collaterals in the guinea pig inferior mesenteric ganglion are subject to presynaptic modulation by endogenous opioids with no morphological evidence at present for axo-axonic contacts. Furthermore, Jan et al. (72) have shown that the synaptic action of the peptide LHRH in bullfrog paravertebral ganglia is not dependent on direct contact between the peptide-containing presynaptic terminal and the postsynaptic sympathetic neuron.

Although further studies on the relationship between peptide elements in the dorsal horn are clearly required, it is possible that peptides released from terminals within the dorsal horn act in a manner more analogous to local hormones with cellular specificity introduced by the density and location of peptide receptors. The presence in primary afferent fibers of substance P-containing storage vesicles at sites not obviously associated with synaptic specialization provides some indirect anatomical support for this suggestion.

Neurotensin-immunoreactive cell bodies are found along the border of laminae II and III and contribute axons to laminae I and IIi with occasional dendrites entering lamina III (73, 47, 74). The distribution of neurotensin terminal bands in the superficial dorsal horn corresponds quite closely to the pattern of neurotensin receptors in the dorsal horn determined with autoradiographic techniques (60). Very little is known of the functional role of neurotensin-containing interneurons in the dorsal horn. Some reports have indicated that intrathecal application of neurotensin leads to thermal analgesia, (75) although iontophoretic application of neurotensin onto dorsal horn neurons leads to only a modest increase in the firing rate of dorsal horn neurons (27).

In addition to the dense plexus of substance P, somatostatin, and CCK-like terminals arising from neurons in the spinal ganglia, separate populations of dorsal horn neurons contain similar or identical peptides. Somatostatin cells are distributed throughout laminae I–III although little is known of the terminal distribution of these neurons (47). A separate population of cells expresses avian pancreatic polypeptide-like immunoreactivity (47) although the equivalent peptide in mammalian species is likely to be structurally different, with a lower molecular weight (76). Although it is clear that the CCK-like peptide found in sensory ganglia is not authentic CCK octapeptide, immunoassay measurements have shown that CCK-8 is in fact present in quite high concentrations in the dorsal horn although undetectable in the sensory ganglia (9). Capsaicin treatment or dorsal rhizotomy effectively dissociates these two related peptides. After chemical or surgical deafferentiation, CCK-like immunoreaction product observed immunocytochemically disappears while immunoassayable levels of the octapeptide remain unchanged in the dorsal horn (9). All immunocytochemical studies using anti-CCK antisera are therefore probably measuring an as yet unidentified peptide. CCK-8 itself is a potent excitant of dorsal horn neurons (77).

Numerous dorsal horn neurons within laminae I–III contain substance P. Substance P-immunoreactive neurons in lamina III are frequently surrounded by a network of substance P-immunoreactive fibers that may be primary afferent in origin (47). Some of these neurons possess dorsally oriented dendritic arbors and may correspond to the arboreal neurons defined by Gobel (78). Recent studies have also demonstrated the existence of gastrin-releasing-peptide immunoreactivity within dorsal horn neurons (79), some of which may also contain substance P.

Peptide-containing neurons that originate in the dorsal horn appear to contribute primarily to the local and segmental regulation of afferent input. Neurons in laminae I and V that project rostrally via the spinothalamic tract seem to lack any of the known neuropeptides. Moreover, with the exception of the opioids, almost nothing is known of the integrative actions of neuropeptides on dorsal horn neurons. Opioid peptides and possibly neurotensin have been shown to produce analgesia when applied intrathecally. Since neurotensin excites dorsal horn neurons it is possible that the neurotensin may elicit analgesia by activation of local inhibitory neurons within the dorsal horn.

3   ORGANIZATION OF PEPTIDE NEURONS CONTRIBUTING TO THE DESCENDING CONTROL OF AFFERENT SYNAPSES

The observation that electrical stimulation of the periaqueductal gray (PAG) and nucleus raphe magnus (NRM) elicits a strong inhibition of dorsal horn neurons and results in analgesia has prompted a number of studies on the connectivity between midline brainstem nuclei and the dorsal horn. Orthograde and retrograde tracing techniques have shown that a high proportion of cells originating in the nucleus raphe magnus and adjacent nucleus reticularis paragigantocellularis (NRPG) contribute axons to the superficial dorsal horn via a descending projection along the dorsolateral funiculus (56). The inhibitory influence of neurons originating in the NRM and NRPG is most pronounced in dorsal horn laminae that receive A-delta and C-fiber afferent input (80). Other medullary sites that are functionally involved in the regulation of dorsal horn neurons do not project directly to the dorsal horn but exert their actions via neurons in the NRM. In particular, the PAG sends a large direct projection to the ventromedial medulla (81), and electrical stimulation of the PAG has been shown to excite medullospinal neurons (82). The NRM and NRPG therefore appear to be the principal brainstem sites involved in the regulation of sensory input to the dorsal horn.

Early histofluorescence studies had shown the presence of serotonin neurons within the NRM and NRPG and a dense serotonin terminal network in the dorsal horn (83). More recent immunocytochemical studies employing lesions and selective serotonin neurotoxins have confirmed the existence of a major descending serotonin input to both the dorsal and ventral horn (84, 85). Within the dorsal horn, serotonin fibers are found in high density within laminae I and II_o. The inner region of lamina II appears almost devoid of serotonin terminals although scattered fibers are present deeper within the dorsal horn. Ultrastructural studies have shown that serotonin terminals make direct contact with dorsal horn neurons (86). In the dorsal horn virtually all serotonin terminals labeled by serotonin uptake are associated with synaptic specializations (86) in contrast with the observations of Descarries et al. (87) in the cerebral cortex. Much of the descending brainstem control of afferent input to the dorsal horn is therefore likely to be exerted on dorsal horn neurons. However, Lamotte and de Lanerole (88) have recently reported that some serotonin terminals, identified by ultrastructural immunocytochemical techniques, may also make axo-axonic contacts with the terminals of afferent fibers in the superficial dorsal horn. Furthermore, the release of substance P from sensory neurons grown in dissociated culture can be inhibited by serotonin, and the duration of the somatic action potential of the same cells is depressed by serotonin (61, 89). It is possible, therefore, that serotonin may exert both pre- and postsynaptic actions at afferent synapses in the dorsal horn.

Substance P cell groups in the medulla oblongata were originally observed by Ljungdahl et al. (90) and reported to correspond very closely
with the location of known serotonin cell groups. Direct double-labeling
studies have now confirmed that a significant proportion of serotonin
neurons with midline brainstem nuclei contain substance P (91, 92) and
thyrotropin releasing hormone (TRH) (93). By sequential staining of serial cryostat sections, Johansson et al. (93) have further demonstrated
that single brainstem neurons can contain serotonin, substance P, and
TRH.

Many of these neurons project to the spinal cord. Ablation of serotonin nuclei in the brainstem or administration of serotonin neurotoxins
results in a dramatic loss of substance P and TRH from the ventral horn
in addition to the complete disappearance of serotonin itself (85). A
smaller but significant depletion of substance P also occurs from the
dorsal horn. TRH fibers are absent from the normal dorsal horn,
suggesting that brainstem neurons containing both peptides are destined
for the ventral horn. There has so far been no direct demonstration of
the corelease of serotonin and substance P from nerve terminals within
the dorsal horn, although the presence of both transmitter candidates
within single storage vesicles (94) suggests that corelease is likely. The
functional role of substance P within descending brainstem fibers is
unclear at present. Serotonin released from the terminals of the same
population of neurons has pronounced inhibitory action on neurons receiving nociceptive afferent input (95), but there is some evidence that
neurons receiving low-threshold inputs may be excited. Intrathecal application of serotonin agonists results in a selective and specific analgesia. The actions of descending fibers on afferent transmission are
unlikely to be mediated at the spinal level by opioid neurons since naloxone does not block the actions of serotonin on neuronal firing rate or
thermal threshold (see ref. 56). The presence of the predominant substance P-containing primary afferent input to the dorsal horn is likely to
make interpretation of the role of substance P in these descending projections extremely difficult.

Other immunocytochemical studies have reported the presence of a
group of neurons in the NRPG of the brainstem that exhibits
enkephalin-like immunoreactivity (4). Retrograde labeling of these neurons after injection of fluorescent dye or lectin into the spinal cord has
demonstrated the spinal termination of some of these neurons (96, 97).
In addition, Basbaum et al. (98) have reported that some serotonin neurons in the brainstem may also contain enkephalin. Hökfelt (99) has
also observed that some substance P-containing descending neurons
also contain a CCK-like peptide. The identification of additional peptides within brainstem neurons that project to the dorsal horn is almost
certain. All the peptides currently identified in brainstem neurons are
also found within sensory or intrinsic dorsal horn cells, making any

separation of peptide function in different classes of neurons extremely difficult.

The dorsal horn also receives descending peptide input from supraspinal sites other than the brainstem. Retrograde fluorescence studies have shown that at least 25% of neurons in the paraventricular nucleus of the hypothalamus project to the dorsal horn (100). Double labeling studies have shown that some of these neurons contain oxytocin and vasopressin, and a smaller proportion contain enkephalin and angiotensin (11). Oxytocin and vasopressin neurons terminate within lamina I and lamina IIo, although no reports on the sensitivity of dorsal horn neurons to these peptides has been reported.

4   CONCLUSIONS

The studies outlined in this chapter reflect recent advances in the chemical identification of subclasses of neurons that are likely to contribute to the initial processing and regulation of nociceptive afferent input to the dorsal horn of the spinal cord. In very few instances, however, has there been convincing evidence for the transmitter status of any of the peptides that delineate these classes of neurons. The best case at present can be made in support of a role for substance P as a sensory transmitter released by certain classes of small-diameter afferent neurons. However, the postsynaptic actions of substance P on dorsal horn neurons are not entirely consistent with the responses of the same neurons to stimulation of the peripheral receptive field. Enkephalin and related opioid peptides have profound inhibitory effects on sensory and dorsal horn neurons that may underlie the analgesic actions of these compounds (Figure 3). Little is known of the functions of numerous other peptides present in the dorsal horn. The design of drugs that selectively interfere with peptide receptors (101) may provide one of the most promising future approaches for assessing the function of individual peptide circuits within the dorsal horn.

REFERENCES

1.   W. D. Willis and R. E. Coggeshall, Plenum Press, New York, 1978.
2.   F. Cevero and A. Iggo, *Brain* **103**, 717–772 (1980).
3.   A. G. Brown, *Organization in the Spinal Cord*, Springer-Verlag, Berlin, 1981.
4.   T. Hökfelt, O. Johansson, A. Ljungdahl, J. M. Lundberg, and M. Schultzberg, *Nature (London)* **284**, 515–521 (1980).
5.   M. Rethelyi, *J. Comp. Neurol.* **172**, 511–528 (1977).
6.   A. R. Light and E. R. Perl, *J. Comp. Neurol.* **186**, 133–150 (1979).
7.   G. Jancso and E. Kiraly, *J. Comp. Neurol.* **190**, 781–792 (1980).

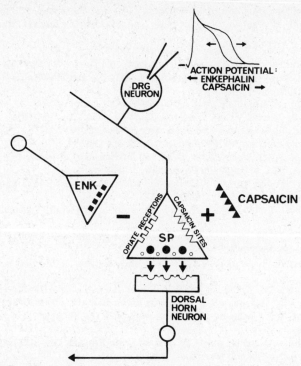

Figure 3. Schematic representation of the possible interactions of opiates and capsaicin with substance P containing primary sensory neurons in the dorsal horn of the spinal cord. For details see text. DRG, dorsal root ganglion; ENK, enkephalin.

8.   T. Hökfelt, *Neurosci. Res. Prog. Bull.* **17**, 425–443 (1979).
9.   M. Schultzberg, G. J. Dockray, and R. G. Williams, *Brain Res.* **235**, 198–204 (1982).
10. G. Jancso, T. Hökfelt, J. M. Lundberg, E. Kiraly, N. Halasz, G. Nilsson, L. Terenius, J. Rehfeld, H. Steinbusch, A. Verhofstad, R. Elde, S. Said, and M. Brown, *J. Neurocytol.* **10**, 963–980 (1981).
11. K. Fuxe, D. Ganten, K. Andersen, L. Calza, L. F. Agnati, R. E. Lang, K. Poulson, T. Hökfelt, and P. Bernardi, *Exp. Brain Res.* **4**, Suppl., 208–232 (1982).
12. S. D. Logan, C. J. Lote, J. H. Wolstencroft, J. P. Gent, J. E. Fox, D. Hudson, and M. Szelke, *Neuroscience* **5**, 1437–1443 (1980).
13. L. J. Botticelli, B. M. Cox, and A. Goldstein, *Proc. Natl. Acad. Sci. USA* **78**, 7783–7786 (1981).
14. J. I. Nagy and S. P. Hunt, *Neuroscience* **7**, 89–97 (1982).
15. R. P. Barber, J. E. Vaughn, J. R. Slemmon, P. M. Salvaterra, E. Roberts, and S.E. Leeman, *J. Comp. Neurol.* **184**, 331–351 (1979).
16. M. Otsuka and S. Konishi, *Cold Spring Habror Symp. Quant. Biol.* **40**, 135–143 (1976).
     M. Otsuka and S. Konishi, *Nature* **264**, 83–84 (1976).
17. R. Gamse, A. Molnar, and F. Lembeck, *Life Sci.* **25**, 629–636 (1979).
18. T. L. Yaksh and R. Elde, *Eur. J. Pharmacol.* **63**, 359–362 (1980).
19. Henry, 1976, Brain Res. **114**, 439–451 (1976).

20. K. Krnjevic and M. E. Morris, (1974) *Can. J. Physiol. Pharmacol.* **52**, 736–744 (1974).
21. S. Konishi, A. Tsunoo, N. Yanaihara, and M. Otsuka, *Biomed. Res.* **1**, 528–536 (1980).
22. L. G. Elfvin and C. J. Dalsgaard, *Brain Res.* **128**, 149–153 (1977).
23. M. R. Matthews and A. C. Cuello, *Proc. Natl. Acad. Sci. USA* **79**, 1668–1672 (1982).
24. C. -J. Dalsgaard, T. Hökfelt, L.-G. Elfvin, L. Skirboll, and P. Emson, *Neuroscience* **7**, 647–654 (1982).
25. M. Randic and V. Miletic, *Brain Res.* **152**, 196–202 (1978).
26. Jeftinija, S., Miletic, V. and Randic M. *Brain Res.* **213**, 231–236 (1981).
27. V. Miletic and M. Randic, *Brain Res.* **169**, 600–604 (1979).
28. Miletic and Randic, 1982, *Pharmacologist* **22**, 204 (1980).
29. N. Jancso, (1968) *Proceedings of the 3rd International Congress of Pharmacology* (Sao Paulo) Vol. 9, Pergamon Press, Oxford, 1968, pp. 33–55.
30. J. I. Nagy, in L. L. Iversen, S. D. Iversen, and S. H. Synder, Eds., *Handbook of Psychopharmacology*, in press (1982).
31. T. L. Yaksh, D. H. Farb, S. E. Leeman, and T. M. Jessell, *Science* **206**, 481–483 (1979).
32. T. L. Yaksh, T. M. Jessell, R. Gamse, A. W. Mudge, and S. E. Leeman, *Nature (London)* **286**, 155–157 (1980).
33. T. M. Jessell, A. Tsunoo, I. Kanazawa, and M. Otsuka, *Brain Res.* **168**, 247–260 (1979).
34. N. N. Palermo, H. K. Brown, and D. L. Smith, *Brain Res.* **208**, 506–510 (1981).
35. J. I. Nagy, P. C. Emson, and L. L. Iversen, *Brain Res.* **211**, 497–502 (1981).
36. S. H. Buck, P. P. Deshmukh, H. I. Yamamura, and T. F. Burks, *Neuroscience* **6**, 2217–2222 (1981).
37. E. Theriault, M. Otsuka, and T. M. Jessell, *Brain Res.* **170**, 209–213 (1979).
38. J. W. Scadding, *J. Anat.* **131**, 471–487 (1980).
39. S. N. Lawson and S. M. Nickels, *J. Physiol.* **303**, 12p (1980).
40. J. I. Nagy, S. P. Hunt, L. L. Iversen, and P. C. Emson, *Neuroscience* **6**, 1923–1934 (1981).
41. P. Holzer, I. Jurna, R. Gamse, and F. Lembeck, *Eur. J. Pharmacol.* **58**, 511–514 (1979).
42. J. I. Nagy, S. R. Vincent, W. A. Staines, H. C. Fibiger, T. D. Reisine, and H. I. Yamamura, *Brain Res.* **186**, 435–444 (1980).
43. A. C. Hayes and M. B. Tyers, *Brain Res.* **189**, 561–564 (1980).
44. P. D. Wall, M. Fitzgerald, J. C. Nussbaumer, H. Van der Loos, and M. Devor, *Nature* **295**, 691–693 (1982).
45. P. D. Wall, in R. Porter and M. O'Connor, Eds., *Substance P in the Nervous System*, Ciba Symposium 91, Pitman Press, in press (1982).
46. Y. N. Jan, L. Y. Jan, and S. W. Kuffler, *Proc. Natl. Acad. Sci. USA* **76**, 1501–1505 (1979).
47. S. P. Hunt, J. S. Kelly, P. C. Emson, J. R. Kimmel, R. J. Miller, and J. Y. Wu, *Neuroscience* **6**, 1883–1898 (1981).
48. E. J. Glazer and A. I. Basbaum, *J. Comp. Neurol.* **196**, 377–389 (1981).
49. F. Cevero, A. Iggo, and V. Molony, *Exp. Brain Res.* **35**, 135–149 (1979).
50. T. Hökfelt, A. Ljungdahl, L. Terenius, R. Elde, and G. Nilsson, *Proc. Natl. Acad. Sci. USA*, **74**, 3081–3085 (1977).
51. T. L. Yaksh and T. A. Rudy, *Science* **192**, 1357–1358 (1976).
52. T. M. Jessell and L. L. Iversen, *Nature (London)* **268**, 549–551 (1977).
53. A. W. Mudge, S. E. Leeman, and G. D. Fischbach, *Proc. Natl. Acad. Sci. USA* **76**, 526–630 (1979).
     K. Murase, V. Nedeljkov, and M. Randic, *Brain Res.* **234**, 170–176 (1982).
54. J. M. Hiller, E. J. Simon, S. M. Crain, and E. R. Peterson, *Brain Res.* **145**, 396–400 (1978).
55. M. Ninkovic, S. P. Hunt, and J. W. R. Gleave, *Brain Res.*, in press (1982).

56. H. L. Fields and A. I. Basbaum, *Annu. Rev. Physiol.* **40**, 193–221 (1978).
H. L., Fields, P. C. Emson, B. K. Leigh, R. F. T. Gilbert, and L. L. Iversen, *Nature* **284**, 351–353 (1980).
57. W. S. Young, J. K. Wamsley, M. A. Zarbin, and M. J. Kuhar, *Science* **210**, 76–78 (1980).
58. S. F. Atweh and M. J. Kuhar, *Brain Res.* **124**, 53–67 (1977).
59. C. LaMotte, C. B. Pert, and S. B. Snyder, *Brain Res.* **112**, 407–412 (1976).
60. M. Ninkovic, S. P. Hunt, J. Gleave, S. D. Iversen, and L. L. Iversen, *Pain*, Suppl. 1, 134 (1981).
61. A. W. Mudge, Studies on Peptides in Cultured Sensory Neurons, Ph.D. Thesis, Harvard University, 1979.
62. T. M. Jessell and M. Yamamoto, in G. R. Fink and L. J. Whalley, Eds., *Neuropeptides; Basic and Clinical Aspects*, Churchill, in press (1982).
63. E. A. Neale, E. Matthew, E. A. Zimmerman, and P. G. Nelson, *J. Neurosci.* **2**, 169–177 (1982).
64. M. A. Werz and R. L. Macdonald, submitted.
65. G. D. Fischbach, K. Dunlap, A. W. Mudge, and S. E. Leeman, in J. B. Martin, S. Reichlin, and K. L. Bick, Eds., *Advances in Biochemical Psychopharmacology*, Vol. 28, Raven Press, New York, 1981, pp. 175–188.
66. J. T. Williams and W. Zieglgansberger, *Neurosci. Lett.* **21**, 211–215 (1981).
67. H. J. Ralston and D. D. Ralston, *J. Comp. Neurol.* **184**, 643–684 (1979).
68. S. P. Hunt, J. S. Kelly, and P. C. Emson, *Neuroscience* **5**, 1871–1890 (1980).
69. N. Aronin, M. Di Figlia, A. S. Liotta, and J. B. Martin, *J. Neurosci.* **1**, 561–577 (1981).
70. M. Fitzgerald and C. J. Woolf, *Neurosci. Lett.* **29**, 67–72 (1982).
71. Z. G. Jiang, M. A. Simmons, and N. J. Dun, *Brain Res.* **235**, 185–191 (1982).
72. L. Y. Jan, Y. N. Jan, and M. S. Brownfield, *Nature* **288**, 380–382 (1980).
73. G. R. Uhl, R. R. Goodman, and S. H. Snyder, *Brain Res.* **167**, 77–91 (1979).
74. V. S. Seybold and R. P. Elde, *J. Comp. Neurol.* **205**, 89–100 (1982).
75. T. L. Yaksh, in Annals of the New York Academy of Sciences, in press (1982).
76. K. Tatemoto, M. Carlquist, and V. Mutt, *Nature* **296**, 659–660 (1982).
77. Randic et al., 1979, V. Miletic and Randic, M. *Brain Res.* **169**, 600–609 (1979).
78. S. Gobel, in J. J. Bonica, Ed., *Advances in Pain Research and Therapy*, Vol. 3, Raven Press, N.Y., 1979, pp. 175–195.
79. K. Fuxe, V. Locatelli, T. McDonald, T. Hökfelt, L. F. Agnati, N. Yonaihara, and V. Mutt, *Neuroscience* **7**, Suppl. 1, S74 (1982).
80. W. D. Willis, L. H. Haber, and R. F. Martin, *J. Neurophysiol.* **40**, 968–981 (1977).
81. I. E. Abols and A. I. Basbaum, *J. Comp. Neurol.* **201**, 285–297 (1981).
82. S. L. Pomeroy and M. M. Behbehani, *Brain Res.* **176**, 143–147 (1979).
83. A. Dahlstrom and K. Fuxe, *Acta Physiol. Scand.* **64**, Suppl. 247, 5–36 (1965).
84. H. W. M. Steinbusch, A. A. J. Verhofstad, and H. W. J. Joosten, *Neuroscience* **3**, 811–820 (1978).
85. R. F. T. Gilbert, P. C. Emson, S. P. Hunt, G. W. Bennett, C. W. Marsden, B. E. B. Sandberg, H. W. M. Steinbusch, and A. A. J. Verhofstad, *Neuroscience* **7**, 69–87 (1982).
E. J. Glazer and A. I. Basbaum, *Soc. Neurosci. Abstr.* **6**, 523 (1980).
86. M. A. Ruda and S. Gobel, *Brain Res.* **184**, 57–83 (1980).
87. L. Descarries, A. Beaudet, and Watkins, *Brain Res.* **100**, 563–588 (1975).
88. C. LaMotte and N. de Lanerole, *Pain*, Suppl. 1, 19 (1981).
89. K. Dunlap and G. D. Fischbach, *Nature (London)* **276**, 837–839 (1978).
90. A. Ljungdahl, T. Hökfelt, and G. Nilsson, *Neuroscience* **3**, 861–943 (1978).
91. T. Hökfelt, A. Ljungdahl, L. Terenius, R. Elde, and G. Nilsson, *Neuroscience* **3**, 517–538 (1978).
92. V. Chan-Palay, G. Jonsson, and S. L. Palay, *Proc. Natl. Acad. Sci. USA* **75**, 1582–1586 (1978).

93. O. Johansson, T. Hökfelt, B. Pernow, S. L. Jeffcoate, N. White, H. M. W. Steinbusch, A. A. J. Verhofstad, P. C. Emson, and E. Spindel, *Neuroscience* **6**, 1857–1881 (1981).

94. G. Pelletier, H. W. M. Steinbusch, and A. A. J. Verhofstadt, *Nature* **293**, 71–72 (1981).

95. G. Belcher, G. Ryall, and R. Schaffner, *Brain Res.* **151**, 307–332 (1978).

96. T. Hökfelt, L. Terenius, H. G. J. M. Kuypers, and O. Dann, *Neurosci. Lett.* **14**, 55–60 (1979).

97. R. M. Bowker, H. W. M. Steinbusch, and J. D. Coulter, *Brain Res.* **211**, 412–417 (1981).

98. A. I. Basbaum, E. Glazer, H. Steinbusch, and A. Verhofstad, *Soc. Neurosci. Abstr.* **6**, 540 (1980).

99. T. Hökfelt, (1982) in R. Porter and M. O'Connor, Eds., *Substance P in the Nervous System*, Ciba Symposium 91, Pittman Medical, 1982, in press.

100. P. E. Sawchenko and L. W. Swanson, *J. Comp. Neurol.* **205**, 260–272 (1982).

101. S. Leander, R. Hakanson, S. Rosell, K. Folkers, F. Sundler, and K. Tornqvist, *Nature* **294**, 467–469 (19—).

102. S. D. Logan, C. J. Lote, J. H. Wolstencroft, J. P. Gent, J. E. Fox, D. Hudson, and M. Szelke, *Neuroscience* **5**, 1437–1443 (1980).

14

Salt and Water Regulation

IAN A. REID

Department of Physiology
University of California
San Francisco, California

1 INTRODUCTION

Several brain peptides influence the intake and excretion of salt and water. Some of the peptides play major roles in salt and water regulation, some play a lesser modulatory role, and others play no physiological role at all. Brain peptides influence salt and water regulation via actions on the brain, kidney, and adrenal cortex.

2 BRAIN AND PITUITARY

A number of peptides influence the intake and excretion of sodium and water through actions on the brain and pituitary. Angiotensin II exerts the most extensive actions, but other peptides, including the opioid peptides, can also produce significant effects.

2.1 Angiotensin II

2.1.1 Relation to the Central Nervous System

Angiotensin II, the physiologically active component of the renin-angiotensin system, acts on the brain and pituitary to produce an impressive number of cardiovascular, endocrine, and behavioral effects. Before these central actions of angiotensin II are discussed, it is appropriate to consider the question whether the actions are normally produced by a brain renin-angiotensin system or whether they are mediated by way of circulating angiotensin II formed by the renal renin-angiotensin system.

The question whether or not there is a brain renin-angiotensin system is discussed in detail in Chapter 32 by W. F. Ganong. However, although the components required for the formation of angiotensin II are present in the brain and pituitary, there is still no convincing evidence that they interact *in vivo* to form angiotensin II (1). The question whether angiotensin II can be considered a brain peptide remains to be resolved.

On the other hand, there is little doubt that circulating angiotensin II formed by the renal renin-angiotensin system can elicit most, and probably all, of the central actions of angiotensin II (2). The effects of circulating angiotensin II are mediated via the circumventricular organs, unique areas of the brain that lack a blood-brain barrier and are therefore accessible to peptides such as angiotensin II, which do not normally cross the blood-brain barrier. Angiotensin II binding sites, presumed to be angiotensin receptors, are present in several circumventricular organs including the area postrema, subfornical organ, organum vasculosum of the lamina terminalis (OVLT), and median eminence (3). As discussed by Ganong, current evidence indicates that angiotensin II can act on the circumventricular organs from the blood side or from the cerebrospinal fluid side, and thus the effects of centrally administered angiotensin II and circulating angiotensin II may be mediated via the same receptors. On this basis, the brain renin-angiotensin system, if it exists, would seem to be redundant.

2.1.2 Central Actions of Angiotensin II

Blood Pressure. Elevations in arterial pressure have been observed following injection of angiotensin II into the vertebral and carotid arteries, the cerebral ventricles, and specific brain regions of several species including the rat and dog (2, 4). These pressor responses result from actions of angiotensin II on the central nervous system rather than from leakage or recirculation of the peptide, since they can be elicited by doses of angiotensin II that are ineffective when administered intravenously. The pressor responses to infusions of angiotensin II into the blood supply to the brain are rapid in onset and offset whereas the responses to intraventricular angiotensin II are slow to develop and are quite prolonged. This latter characteristic probably reflects the slow rate at which angiotensin II is removed from the ventricular system.

The receptors that mediate the pressor response to infusion of angiotensin II into the vertebral arteries are located in the area postrema, a circumventricular organ located in the medulla oblongata (4). Direct application of angiotensin II to the area postrema increases blood pressure; ablation of the structure abolishes the pressor response to intravertebral angiotensin II and reduces the blood pressure response to intravenous angiotensin II. The pressor responses to intraventricular and intracarotid infusions of angiotensin II are not mediated via the area postrema. The receptors that mediate these responses appear to be located in two other circumventricular organs, the subfornical organ and the OVLT, but the relative importance of these two structures remains to be determined.

The pressor responses to centrally administered angiotensin II may result from one or a combination of the following: an elevation in total peripheral resistance resulting from increased sympathetic discharge; an increase in cardiac output secondary to withdrawal of vagal tone to the heart; an increase in vasopressin secretion (see below). The relative importance of these three changes varies with the route of administration and the animal species being studied.

Water Intake and Excretion. One of the most recently discovered actions of angiotensin II is stimulation of drinking. The peptide stimulates drinking when it is administered systemically or directly into the central nervous system of a wide variety of animal species (5). Furthermore, water intake is increased in a number of situations in which renin secretion and hence circulating angiotensin II levels are increased; in at least some of these situations, the increase in water intake can be reduced by angiotensin II antagonists or by converting enzyme inhibitors (5). Drinking responses can be elicited by elevations in plasma angiotensin II concentration within the range generally considered to be physiological (2). Nevertheless, at the present time it appears unlikely that the renin-angiotensin system plays an important role in the physiological control of water intake.

Considerable effort has been directed toward locating the central receptors that mediate the dipsogenic action of angiotensin II. Most attention has been focused on two circumventricular organs, the subfornical organ and the OVLT (2). Evidence exists that angiotensin II can stimulate drinking by actions at either of these sites, but their relative importance is still disputed. It has been proposed that the subfornical organ contains receptors for circulating angiotensin II and that the OVLT mediates drinking responses to centrally administered or circulating angiotensin II, but definitive evidence is not yet available (6).

In addition to stimulating water intake, angiotensin II can promote water reabsorption in the kidney by increasing the secretion of vasopressin. Angiotensin II has been reported to increase vasopressin secretion in several animal species when injected intravenously into the carotid arteries or directly into the cerebral ventricles (2). The most impressive responses are produced when angiotensin II is administered via the ventricular route; the responses to intravenous angiotensin II are much smaller, and some investigators have not observed increases in vasopressin secretion when angiotensin II is administered via this route (2). This difference probably reflects the fact that angiotensin II is distributed into a much smaller volume and degraded at a slower rate when administered intraventricularly than when injected intravenously.

The site at which angiotensin II acts to increase vasopressin secretion has not been definitely established. Possible sites include the subfornical organ, supraoptic nucleus, and posterior pituitary (2).

Sodium Intake and Excretion.   Angiotensin II has been reported to increase sodium appetite in rats and sheep (7, 8). This effect differs from the dipsogenic response to angiotensin II in that it is slow to develop (6–12 h). The increased sodium appetite may not result from a direct central action of angiotensin but could be secondary to sodium loss, since it is known that centrally administered angiotensin II increases urinary sodium excretion (see below). Such an explanation is consistent with the long latency of the increase in sodium appetite.

The doses of angiotensin II required to induce a salt appetite are very high and it is therefore unlikely that the renin-angiotensin system plays a physiological role in the control of sodium intake. Furthermore, intraventricular injections of drugs that block the formation or actions of angiotensin II fail to modify the increased sodium appetite that accompanies sodium deficiency (8).

Intraventricular injection of angiotensin II causes a natriuresis in rats, dogs, and goats (9, 10). This may be due in part to increased blood pressure and glomerular filtration rate, although it is possible to elicit a natriuresis with doses of angiotensin II that do not change blood pressure, renal blood flow, or glomerular filtration rate (10). The natriuretic effect of angiotensin can be dissociated from changes in plasma aldosterone concentration (10); in any case the response is too rapid to be accounted for on the basis of a decrease in aldosterone secretion. The natriuretic effect might result from a decrease in plasma angiotensin II concentration since intraventricular angiotensin II inhibits renin secretion (see below) and angiotensin II acts on the kidney to promote sodium reabsorption. Or the natriuresis might be mediated via vasopressin, since this peptide is released by angiotensin II and at least under some conditions can increase urinary sodium excretion (see below). Finally, the natriuretic effect of centrally administered angiotensin II might result from a decrease in renal sympathetic neural activity (10). Further research is required to distinguish among these possibilities.

ACTH Secretion. There have been reports that angiotensin II increases ACTH secretion when administered into the cerebral ventricles, carotid arteries, or directly into the anterior pituitary gland (2, 11). In dogs, angiotensin II increases ACTH secretion when infused intravenously (12), but in humans it has been reported that intravenous angiotensin II actually suppresses ACTH secretion (13). The site at which angiotensin II acts to increase ACTH secretion is not known. Evidence has been presented for actions at the median eminence and the anterior pituitary (2, 11). It is also possible that angiotensin II increases ACTH secretion indirectly by increasing vasopressin release, since it is known that vasopressin is a corticotropin releasing factor. Evidence in favor of this possibility includes the recent observation that the ACTH response to intraventricular angiotensin II is reduced in vasopressin-deficient Brattleboro rats (14).

Renin Secretion. Angiotensin II inhibits renin secretion when injected into the cerebral ventricles or into the carotid and vertebral arteries (2, 15). The suppression of renin secretion by intraventricular angiotensin II is accompanied by an increase in plasma vasopressin concentration and is inhibited by hypophysectomy, indicating that it is mediated via vasopressin (15). Moreover, intraventricular angiotensin II fails to inhibit renin secretion in Brattleboro rats (14). On the other hand, intracarotid or intravertebral infusions of angiotensin II can suppress renin secretion without increasing plasma vasopressin levels (2). This suppression may result from increased blood pressure or from decreased renal sympathetic neural activity.

2.2 Opioid Peptides

Various opioid peptides including the enkephalins and β-endorphin
have been reported to cause an antidiuresis; this effect can be inhibited
by naloxone (16–18). The antidiuretic effect of these opioids results, at
least in part, from stimulation of vasopressin secretion since it is accompanied by an increase in plasma vasopressin concentration (16) and
a decrease in urinary vasopressin excretion (17). The stimulation of vasopressin by opioids apparently does not result from a direct action on
the posterior pituitary, since β-endorphin fails to increase vasopressin
release when added to isolated rat neural lobes *in vitro* (16). Paradoxically, enkephalins and β-endorphins have been reported to antagonize
the stimulatory effects of angiotensin II on drinking and vasopressin release (19).

A limited amount of information suggests that endogenous opioid
peptides play a role in the regulation of water balance. For example, it
has been reported that naloxone inhibits water-deprivation-induced and
angiotensin II-induced drinking (20, 21). Naloxone does not alter resting
vasopressin secretion (20) but does antagonize the vasopressin secretory responses to osmotic and nonosmotic stimuli (22).

3 KIDNEY

Several peptides are known to exert their effects on the kidney to modify excretion and reabsorption of water and of electrolytes.

3.1 Vasopressin

Vasopressin, which is synthesized and released by neurons of the hypothalamus, reaches the kidney via the systemic circulation to exert effects on renal tubules.

3.1.1 Water Excretion

Vasopressin regulates water reabsorption by the distal tubule and collecting duct and thus plays a key role in osmoregulation of the body fluids. This subject is dealt with in standard textbooks and need not be
discussed here. In addition to its effects on water excretion, vasopressin
inhibits the secretion of renin and under some conditions increases the
excretion of sodium. These actions are discussed next.

3.1.2 Sodium Excretion

Vasopressin causes a natriuresis when it is administered during a water
diuresis in humans and animals (23). This effect is not secondary to inhibition of renin secretion and diminished aldosterone secretion because it persists when mineralocorticoids are administered and it is not

prevented by adrenalectomy. The natriuresis does not result from increased blood volume, blood pressure, or glomerular filtration rate since it occurs when hemorrhage is used as a stimulus to vasopressin secretion (24). Furthermore, a similar natriuretic effect can be produced by analogs of vasopressin that lack vasoconstrictor activity (25). The site at which vasopressin acts to decrease sodium reabsorption has not been identified. Evidence for actions in the proximal tubule and loop of Henle has been presented (23) but further research is needed to distinguish between these two possibilities.

3.1.3 Renin Secretion

Administration of vasopressin in humans and several animal species suppresses the secretion of renin (26, 27). Vasopressin also attenuates the renin secretory responses to various stimuli including sodium deficiency, diuretics, isoproterenol, and ureteral occlusion. The mechanism of the inhibitory effect of vasopressin on renin secretion is not completely understood. It does not appear to involve vasoconstriction since analogs of vasopressin that lack vasoconstrictor activity also suppress renin secretion (25, 27). Shade and associates (28) reported that vasopressin inhibits renin secretion when infused intrarenally in dogs with a single nonfiltering kidney. Since renal blood flow and arterial pressure were unchanged, these investigators suggested that vasopressin acts directly on the juxtaglomerular apparatus.

The concentration of vasopressin required to inhibit renin secretion has been established and is within the range observed during water deprivation and nonhypotensive hemorrhage (29). It is therefore likely that the peptide does play a role in the regulation of renin secretion. Consistent with this conclusion is the finding that plasma renin activity is suppressed in patients with the syndrome of inappropriate secretion of vasopressin and elevated in rats with hereditary diabetes insipidus (26, 27).

3.2 Adrenocorticotropic Hormone (ACTH)

The major action of ACTH is regulation of adrenocortical secretion, but there have also been reports that the hormone can alter the secretion of renin. In rats, ACTH causes a prompt but transient increase in plasma renin activity in association with an increase in corticosterone secretion (30). Such an effect might be expected because corticosteroids can increase plasma renin activity by increasing plasma angiotensinogen concentration (26). This is not the mechanism of the ACTH-induced increase in plasma renin activity, however, since the increase is not prevented by adrenalectomy and can actually be inhibited by treatment with glucocorticoids (30). An action of ACTH on the renin-secreting cells has been suggested, but there is no direct evidence for this.

The effects of ACTH on renin secretion in humans and dogs is less clear cut. ACTH has been reported to increase plasma renin activity in human subjects (31), but in other studies an increase in plasma renin activity was only seen if the subjects were sodium-depleted (32). Acute administration of ACTH does not increase plasma renin activity in dogs (26). In both humans and dogs, chronic treatment with ACTH actually causes suppression of plasma renin activity. This effect is thought to be secondary to expansion of extracellular fluid volume (26).

3.3   Vasoactive Intestinal Peptide

Vasoactive intestinal peptide (VIP) produces a transient increase in renin secretion when infused intravenously or intrarenally in dogs (33). With a high dose of VIP, the increase in renin secretion is accompanied by falls in blood pressure and plasma potassium concentration, but with a lower dose VIP increases renin secretion without changing blood pressure or plasma potassium concentration. VIP causes renal vasodilatation and tends to increase sodium excretion; these changes would be expected to decrease, rather than increase, the secretion of renin (27). The stimulation of renin secretion by VIP results, at least in part, from an action on the kidney since it can be elicited by intrarenal infusion of a low dose of VIP that is ineffective when injected intravenously (33). Furthermore, VIP increases the rate of renin release when added to isolated glomeruli *in vitro* (34). Beyond this, the mechanism of the stimulatory effect of VIP is not known. An action on the juxtaglomerular cells, possibly involving cyclic AMP generation, has been proposed (33) but direct evidence for this is not yet available. The physiological significance of this recently discovered action of VIP remains to be determined.

3.4   Somatostatin

3.4.1   Water Excretion

Somatostatin increases urine flow when administered intravenously or intrarenally in dogs (35, 36) (Figure 1). This increase is not accompanied by changes in blood pressure, renal plasma flow, glomerular filtration rate, electrolyte excretion, or osmolar clearance but is associated with an increase in free water clearance and a decrease in urinary osmolality (35, 36). These changes could result from a decrease in vasopressin secretion or an inhibition of the action of vasopressin on the distal tubule and collecting duct. The latter possibility is the most likely since the diuretic effects of intrarenal somatostatin occurs primarily in the infused kidney and there is little or no effect in the contralateral kidney

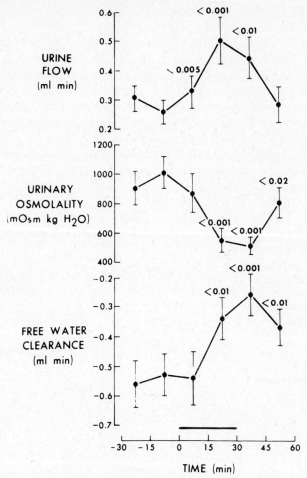

Figure 1. Effect of somatostatin on urine flow, urinary osmolality, and free water clearance in anesthetized dogs. Somatostatin was infused intrarenally at 2.0–3.3 μg/kg/min from 0 to 30 min. From Reid and Rose (35).

(35). Moreover, somatostatin increases free water clearance when it is infused in animals receiving a vasopressin infusion (36).

The mechanism of this antagonistic effect of somatostatin is not known. It may involve a reduction of cyclic AMP formation in the kidney, since the action of vasopressin on water reabsorption is mediated by cyclic AMP, and somatostatin is known to decrease cyclic AMP concentration in other tissues. However, the diuresis is not associated with changes in urinary cyclic AMP excretion (35). Moreover, the effects of parathyroid hormone on calcium and phosphate excretion, which are mediated via the formation of cyclic AMP, are not altered by somatostatin (36). Thus, the details of the interaction between somatostatin and vasopressin remain to be elucidated.

3.4.2 Renin Secretion

Somatostatin has been reported to attenuate the rise in plasma renin activity produced by furosemide in normal subjects (37) and to decrease plasma renin levels in subjects in which basal renin secretion has been increased by the administration of furosemide (38). Somatostatin also attenuates the rise in plasma renin activity produced by β-adrenoceptor stimulation with orciprenaline (39). Somatostatin does not decrease basal plasma renin activity in normal subjects or in patients with low renin or normal renin hypertension (40). However, it does decrease renin secretion in patients with high renin hypertension (40) (Figure 2).

The mechanism of the inhibitory effect of somatostatin on renin secretion is unknown. The finding that somatostatin reduces the renin secretory response to orciprenaline suggests an action on the β-adrenoceptor controlling renin secretion. However, it has been reported that

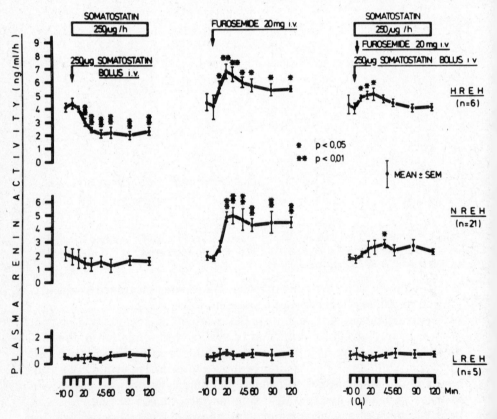

Figure 2. Effect of somatostatin, furosemide, and somatostatin-plus-furosemide on plasma renin activity in patients with high renin (HREH), normal renin (NREH), and low renin (LREH) essential hypertension. From Rosenthal et al. (40). Reprinted by permission of the American Heart Association, Inc.

the renin response to furosemide is not blocked by propranolol (41) and it is unlikely that the attenuation of this response by somatostatin involves β-adrenoceptors.

4 ADRENAL CORTEX

4.1 ACTH and Angiotensin II

One of the major regulators of sodium and water excretion is aldosterone, a steroid hormone secreted by the zona glomerulosa of the adrenal cortex. The secretion of aldosterone is, in turn, controlled by two peptide hormones, angiotensin II and ACTH. Angiotensin II is the major regulator of aldosterone secretion, acting both as an acute stimulus and as a tropic hormone that maintains the responsiveness of the zona glomerulosa (42). ACTH also exerts important effects on aldosterone secretion; indeed, the zona glomerulosa appears to be as sensitive to ACTH as the zona fasciculata and zona reticularis. The effects of angiotensin II and ACTH on aldosterone secretion are mediated by separate populations of specific receptors on the plasma membrane of the target cells. Both peptides act early in the aldosterone biosynthetic pathway, increasing the conversion of cholesterol to pregnenolone. Despite these similarities, the intracellular messengers for the two peptides are different; the response to ACTH is mediated via cyclic AMP, and the response to angiotensin II is thought to be mediated via calcium. Further details of the effects of angiotensin II and ACTH on aldosterone secretion can be found elsewhere (42).

During recent years, it has become apparent that other peptides can influence the secretion of aldosterone. These include β-lipotropin, reported to stimulate aldosterone secretion, and somatostatin and luteinizing hormone releasing hormone (LHRH), which modulate the effect of angiotensin II on aldosterone secretion. These peptides are considered next.

4.2 β-Lipotropin

Recently Matsuoka and associates (43) studied the effects of β-lipotropin (β-LPH) on aldosterone production by dispersed adrenal capsular cells. They found that β-LPH produced dose-related increases in aldosterone production; this effect was observed with β-LPH concentrations as low as 10^{-9} M (Figure 3). The maximum aldosterone response obtained with β-LPH was similar to that obtained with ACTH and was greater than that obtained with angiotensin II. At high concentrations (greater than 10^{-7} M) β-LPH also increased corticosterone production. Met-enkephalin and α- and β-endorphin did not stimulate aldosterone production.

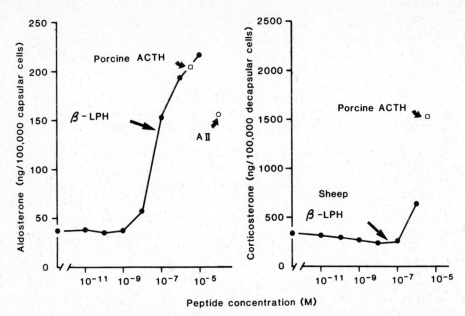

Figure 3. Effect of β-lipotropin (β-LPH), ACTH, and angiotensin II (A II) on aldosterone and corticosterone production by dispersed rat adrenal cells. From Matsuoka et al. (43). Copyright © 1980 by the American Association for the Advancement of Science.

The mechanism by which β-LPH stimulates aldosterone production was not established. However, β-LPH increased aldosterone production without increasing the levels of adenosine 5'-monophosphate (cyclic AMP or cAMP) in the adrenal cells; the aldosterone response to β-LPH thus differs from the response to ACTH which is associated with increased cAMP formation. Matsuoka et al. (43) suggested that β-LPH may be one of the non-ACTH pituitary factors that appear to play a role in the control of aldosterone secretion in situations such as sodium deficiency. Further investigation of this interesting possibility is required.

4.3 Somatostatin

Aguilera and associates (44) recently reported that somatostatin inhibits the angiotensin II-stimulated increase in aldosterone production by dispersed rat adrenal glomerulosa cells. The maximum aldosterone response was reduced 43% by 10^{-9} M somatostatin and completely abolished by 10^{-6} M somatostatin (Figure 4). In marked contrast, the aldosterone responses to other stimuli, including potassium and ACTH, were unaffected by somatostatin.

Aguilera et al. further demonstrated that the inhibition of the angiotensin II-stimulated increase in aldosterone production by somatostatin could not be explained by an interaction between somatostatin and an-

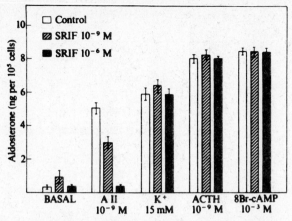

Figure 4. Effect of somatostatin (SRIF) on basal and stimulated aldosterone production in dispersed rat adrenal glomerulosa cells. From Aguilera et al. (44). Reprinted by permission from Nature. Copyright © 1981 Macmillan Journals Limited.

giotensin II receptors. They were able to demonstrate, however, that specific high affinity receptors for somatostatin are present in the zona glomerulosa and suggested that, through actions on these receptors, somatostatin may modulate the second messenger system that mediates the action of angiotensin II on aldosterone biosynthesis. Furthermore, they showed that somatostatin is present in a high concentration in the zona glomerulosa, where it can act as a local modulator of the action of the renin-angiotensin system on aldosterone production (44).

4.4 Luteinizing Hormone Releasing Hormone

Capponi and Catt (45) observed that luteinizing hormone releasing hormone (LHRH), another hypothalamic peptide, inhibits binding of ^{125}I-angiotensin II to dispersed canine adrenal glomerulosa cells. Binding was also inhibited by the analog des-pGlu[1]-LHRH. The inhibition of angiotensin binding by LHRH was thought to result from the fact that the carboxyl terminal sequences of LHRH and angiotensin II are quite similar (Figure 5).

   Although LHRH and des-pGlu[1]-LHRH competed effectively with angiotensin II for binding to adrenal receptors, only the analog displayed aldosterone-stimulating activity, behaving as a weak partial agonist. On the other hand, LHRH behaved as a weak antagonist of the stimulation of aldosterone by angiotensin II.

5 CONCLUDING REMARKS

A variety of brain peptides influence the intake or excretion, or both, of sodium and water. Some of these peptides, for example vasopressin,

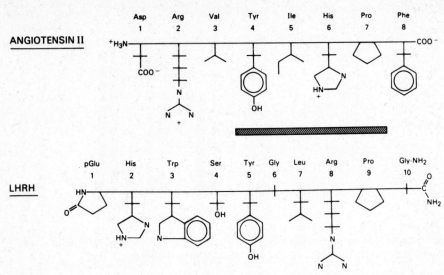

Figure 5. Structural similarities between angiotensin II and LHRH. From Capponi and Catt (45).

ACTH, and angiotensin II, play major roles in salt and water regulation. Other peptides, including somatostatin, VIP, and the opioids, may also exert important effects although somatostatin and the opioids may function primarily as modulators of the action of other hormones; the physiological significance of the actions of these and other brain peptides on salt and water regulation remains to be precisely defined.

REFERENCES

1. I. A. Reid, *Fed. Proc.* **38**, 2255 (1979).
2. I. A. Reid, V. L. Brooks, C. D. Rudolph, and L. C. Keil, *Am. J. Physiol.,* **243**, R82 (1982).
3. M. van Houten, E. L. Schiffrin, J. F. E. Mann, B. I. Posner, and R. Boucher, *Brain Res.* **186**, 480 (1980).
4. C. M. Ferrario, P. L. Gildenberg, and J. W. McCubbin, *Circ. Res.* **30**, 257 (1972).
5. W. B. Severs and J. Summy-Long, *Life Sci.* **17**, 1513 (1975).
6. M. I. Phillips, S. K. Landas, M. K. Raizada, and J. F. Stamler, *Science* **214**, 1376 (1981).
7. J. T. Fitzsimons, *Rev. Physiol. Biochem. Pharmacol.* **87**, 117 (1980).
8. J. P. Coghlan, P. J. Considine, D. A. Denton, D. T. W. Fei, L. G. Leksell, M. J. McKinley, A. F. Muller, E. Tarjan, and R. S. Weisinger, *Science* **214**, 195 (1981).
9. B. Andersson, *Ann. Rev. Physiol.* **39**, 185 (1977).
10. V. L. Brooks and R. L. Malvin, *Proc. Soc. Exp. Biol. Med.,* **169**, 532 (1982).
11. J. W. Maran and F. E. Yates, *Am. J. Physiol.* **233**, E273 (1977).
12. D. J. Ramsay, L. C. Keil, M. C. Sharpe, and J. Shinsako, *Am. J. Physiol.* **234**, R66 (1978).
13. R. Fraser, P. A. Mason, J. C. Buckingham, R. D. Gordon, J. J. Morton, M. G. Nicholls, P. F. Semple, and M. Tree, *J. Steroid Biochem.* **11**, 1039 (1979).

14. W. F. Ganong, J. Shinsako, I. A. Reid, L. C. Keil, D. L. Hoffman, and E. A. Zimmerman, *Ann. N.Y. Acad. Sci.,* **394**, 619 (1982).

15. S. A. Malayan, L. C. Keil, D. J. Ramsay, and I. A. Reid, *Endocrinology* **104**, 672 (1979).

16. R. E. Weitzman, D. A. Fisher, S. Minick, N. Ling, and R. Guillemin, *Endocrinology* **101**, 1643 (1977).

17. G. W. Bisset, H. S. Chowdrey, and W. Feldberg, *Br. J. Pharmacol.* **62**, 370 (1978).

18. J. P. Huidobro-Toro, F. Huidobro, and R. Croxatto, *Life Sci.* **24**, 697 (1979).

19. J. Y. Summy-Long, L. C. Keil, K. Deen, and W. B. Severs, *J. Pharmacol. Exp. Ther.* **217**, 630 (1981).

20. J. Y. Summy-Long, L. C. Keil, K. Deen, L. Rosella, and W. B. Severs, *J. Pharmacol. Exp. Ther.* **217**, 619 (1981).

21. R. P. Maickel, M. C. Braude, and J. E. Zobik, *Neuropharmacology* **16**, 863 (1977).

22. S. Ishikawa and R. Schrier, *Clin. Res.* **30**, 78A (1982).

23. I. A. Reid and W. F. Ganong, in S. M. McCann, Ed., *Physiology, Series One, Vol. 5: Endocrine Physiology,* M.T.P. International Review of Science, Butterworths, 1974, p. 205.

24. M. H. Humphreys, R. M. Friedler, and L. E. Earley, *Am. J. Physiol.* **219**, 658 (1970).

25. S. A. Malayan and I. A. Reid, *Life Sci.* **31**, 2757 (1982).

26. I. A. Reid, B. J. Morris, and W. F. Ganong, *Ann. Rev. Physiol.* **40**, 377 (1978).

27. T. K. Keeton and W. B. Campbell, *Pharmacol. Rev.* **32**, 81 (1980).

28. R. E. Shade, J. O. Davis, J. A. Johnson, R. W. Gotshall, and W. S. Spielman, *Am. J. Physiol.* **224**, 926 (1973).

29. S. A. Malayan, D. J. Ramsay, L. C. Keil, and I. A. Reid, *Endocrinology* **107**, 1988 (1980).

30. J. H. Hauger-Klevene, H. Brown, and N. Fleischer, *Proc. Soc. Exp. Biol. Med.* **131**, 539 (1969).

31. L. Bozovic, S. Efendic, and U. Rosenquist, *Acta Endocrinol.* **138**, 123 (1969).

32. D. C. Kem, C. Gomez-Sanchez, N. J. Kramer, O. B. Holland, and J. R. Higgins, *J. Clin. Endocrinol. Metab.* **40**, 116 (1975).

33. J. P. Porter, I. A. Reid, S. I. Said, and W. F. Ganong, *Am. J. Physiol.,* **234**, F306 (1982).

34. J. P. Porter, S. I. Said, and W. F. Ganong, *Fed. Proc.,* **41**, 1232 (1982).

35. I. A. Reid and J. C. Rose, *Endocrinology* **100**, 782 (1977).

36. N. Brautbar, B. S. Levine, J. W. Coburn, and C. R. Kleeman, *Am. J. Physiol.* **237**, E428 (1979).

37. J. Rosenthal, S. Raptis, F. Escobar-Jimenez, and E. F. Pfeiffer, *Lancet* I, 772 (1976).

38. A. Gomez-Pan, M. H. Snow, D. A. Piercy, V. Robson, R. Wilkinson, R. Hall, and D. C. Evered, *J. Clin. Endocrinol. Metab.* **43**, 240 (1976).

39. J. Rosenthal, F. Escobar-Jimenez, and S. Raptis, *Clin. Endocrinol.* **6**, 455 (1977).

40. J. Rosenthal, S. Raptis, C. Zoupas, and F. Escobar-Jimenez, *Circ. Res.* **43**, Suppl. 1, I-69 (1978).

41. W. F. Ganong, in T. A. Assaykeen, Ed., *Control of Renin Secretion,* Plenum Press, New York, 1972, p. 17.

42. I. A. Reid and W. F. Ganong, in J. Genest, E. Koiw, and O. Kuchel, Eds., *Hypertension,* McGraw-Hill, New York, 1977, p. 265.

43. H. Matsuoka, P. J. Mulrow, and C. H. Li, *Science* **209**, 307 (1980).

44. G. Aguilera, J. P. Harwood, and K. J. Catt, *Nature* **292**, 262 (1981).

45. A. M. Capponi and K. J. Catt, *J. Biol. Chem.* **254**, 5120 (1979).

15

Peptides and Psychiatry

STANLEY J. WATSON

Mental Health Research Institute
and
Department of Psychiatry
University of Michigan
Ann Arbor, Michigan

A. ARIAV ALBALA

Clinical Psychobiology Program
Department of Psychiatry
University of Michigan
Ann Arbor, Michigan

PHILIP BERGER

Department of Psychiatry
Stanford University
Palo Alto, California

HUDA AKIL

Mental Health Research Institute
University of Michigan
Ann Arbor, Michigan

This work was supported in part by NIMH Grant ROd1MH36168 and NIDA Grant DA02265 (to S. J. W. and H. A.), by NIMH Grant MH30854 (to P. B.), and by the Medical Research Service of the Veterans Administration.

The purpose of this chapter is twofold: first, to describe key studies designed to investigate the interface between psychiatry and neuropeptides, and second, to focus on methodological perspectives and logical difficulties encountered in such endeavors. The attempts to link fundamental aspects of neuropeptide biology with various categories of psychiatric illness have taken many routes, including measurement of basal levels of peptides in blood and cerebrospinal fluid (CSF), examination of the regulation of peptide systems as indicated by challenge tests, study of the effects of administration of the peptides (or analogs with agonist or antagonist effects) into peripheral tissues or into brain, and removal of the substance (s) by hemodialysis.

Two aspects of the neuropeptide–psychiatry interface are considered, the hypothalamo-pituitary-thyroid axis (HPT) and the opioid peptide systems in pituitary and hypothalamus. No attempt is made to review all aspects of these two areas nor to discuss experiments on functions of sex hormones, other releasing factors, antidiuretic hormone (arginine vasopressin), or oxytocin. The discussion is restricted to the functions of the central nervous system, pituitary, thyroid, and adrenal in relation to these two aspects.

Recent studies have allowed the generalization of a broad set of principles applicable to neuropeptide-producing cells. The β-endorphin/adrenocorticotropic hormone (ACTH) system serves as an important model for examination of the complexities and perspectives necessary for the successful study of peptide systems. This information base may facilitate and sharpen the study of peptides under pathological circumstances.

The two peptide–psychiatry interfaces chosen for review (HPT axis and opioid peptides) represent different aspects of the biology of regulatory systems. For example, the HPT axis studies are clinically more mature. The logic of these studies is to evaluate the effect of the hypothalamic releasing factor, thyrotropin releasing hormone (TRH), on its pituitary target, the thyrotrope, which produces thyroid stimulating hormone (TSH), as a possible indicator of the state of the limbic system in psychiatric illness. In contrast, the studies of the opioid peptides are clinically less mature, have been much broader in scope, are more diffuse, and are confounded by known effects of opioid peptides in several regulatory systems.

1 THYROTROPIN RELEASING HORMONE IN PSYCHIATRY

Thyrotropin releasing hormone (TRH) has been studied for its possible application as a diagnostic, therapeutic, and prognostic tool in several psychiatric conditions.

Early reports (1–3) suggested that TRH might be of benefit in unipolar depressed women, in whom it was initially found to have rapid but short-lived antidepressant effects. Numerous replications of these studies have been attempted, largely with unsuccessful results. Therapeutic trials for other mental disorders have been equally disappointing (4).

1.1 Diagnostic and Prognostic Applications of TRH

Much more promising are the findings regarding the diagnostic and prognostic value of TRH in certain psychiatric disorders. The diagnostic use of TRH in psychiatry was a natural and logical outgrowth of the study of the regulation of neuroendocrine systems applied to the analysis of mood disorders. The basis of this strategy can be summarized as follows. The limbic system and the hypothalamus are the postulated sites of primary pathology in the affective disorders. Among the many functions influenced by the limbic system, regulation of neuroendocrine function is one of the clearest. Thus, study of this function in psychiatrically disturbed patients may provide indirect knowledge of the integrity of the limbic-hypothalamic system. The use of the dexamethasone suppression test for the diagnosis of endogenous depression is another example of the application of such a neuroendocrine strategy (5).

TRH, a hypothalamic releasing hormone, induces the release of both TSH and prolactin (PRL) from the anterior pituitary. It may also stimulate growth hormone (GH) release in certain conditions, including depression and anorexia nervosa. These neuroendocrine effects of TRH have been studied in a large number of psychiatric patients with a variety of disorders. The findings have resulted in an improved understanding of affective disorders.

1.2   Distribution of Thyrotropin-Releasing Hormone

TRH was the first of the hypothalamic hormones to be identified and synthesized (6, 7). The compound is a tripeptide pyroglutamyl-histidyl-proline-amide. Although the highest concentration of TRH is found in the hypothalamus, it is widely distributed in the extrahypothalamic brain. In fact, about 80% of total brain TRH is found in extra-hypothalamic areas, including the CSF and retina (8). TRH is also present in peripheral blood, in urine, and in the pancreas, gastrointestinal tract, placenta, amniotic fluid, adrenals, and skin (9, 10). Although neurochemical data are still inconclusive, it appears that TRH increases both central noradrenergic and central serotonergic activity (4) and interacts both with endogenous and exogenous opiates (10). It appears that the synthesis or release of TRH, or both, is influenced by catecholaminergic systems (9).

2   THE TRH TEST

The TRH test used in psychiatric studies is identical with the one devised by endocrinologists for the study of the HPT axis. The test is usually conducted in midmorning after an overnight fast, when plasma TSH fluctuations are minimal. TRH is administered intravenously over a 30-sec period after one or two baseline blood samples have been obtained. Subsequent samples are secured at 15, 30, 60, and 90 min after TRH administration. In most studies, TRH doses of either 200 or 500 μg are used. Side effects to TRH administration are in most cases mild and include slight transient hypertension, flushing, sweating, nausea, and a sensation of urinary urgency. TSH (or PRL and GH) concentrations are determined by radioimmunoassay, and a maximal TSH response is obtained by subtracting baseline TSH values from the maximum TSH increment occurring after TRH administration.

2.1   The TRH Test: Endocrinology

The most widely studied effect of TRH is its role in inducing TSH secretion from the pituitary. A dose as low as 15 μg of TRH administered intravenously to a human subject can trigger a TSH response. Changes in TSH concentrations can be detected as early as 5 min and the maximal response occurs at about 30 min after stimulation. Women appear to have greater responses than men, probably due to effects of estrogen on the pituitary. The response declines in men with increasing age and is severely blunted during the seventh and eighth decade of life (11). The responsivity of the pituitary to TRH stimulation is partially regulated by a negative feedback mechanism determined by the concentration of circulating thyroid hormones. The stimulatory effects of TRH on TSH release can be blocked by pretreatment with such hormones (12). A variety of factors can influence the TRH-induced TSH response. Endocrinopathies like hyper-or hypothyroidism and Cushing's disease, and drugs like lithium, aspirin, corticosteroids, phenytonin and morphine may alter the response.

The dose response curve of TRH-induced PRL secretion appears to be parallel to that of the TSH response with peaks also occurring at around 30 minutes after stimulation. Female PRL responses are nearly twice as high as those observed among males of the same age groups (13). In normal individuals there is no response in GH after TRH administration.

2.2   The TRH Test in Depression

Many investigators have now replicated and extended early observations (1, 3) that a certain proportion of depressed patients have blunted TSH responses to TRH. A review of these studies reveals that about 25 to 30 percent of euthyroid depressed patients have blunted responses to TRH after a dose of 200 μg or 500 μg TRH (14–38). A cutoff point of a Δ max TSH of 5 μIU/mL has been the most-used criterion to differentiate between a blunted and a normal response. Gold and collaborators (39), using a cutoff point of 7 μIU/mL to distinguish blunted from normal responses (thereby allowing more subjects to fall into the abnormal category and making the criterion less restrictive and thus increasing the sensitivity of the test), were able to identify correctly 31 out of 41 unipolar depressed patients with major depressive disorder, for a sensitivity of 76%. They reported only one blunted response among twelve patients with bipolar major depressive disorder and none among patients with minor depressive disorder, schizophrenia, or schizoaffective disorder. Although the performance of the test was impressive when used to distinguish *major* from *minor* depressive disorder, it is unclear how useful it would be in differentiating *endogenous* from *nonendogenous* major depressive disorder. The main difficulty in interpreting such studies of depression is that individual investigators use different nosological systems to diagnose their patients. In particular, several studies made no distinctions between two important categories of depression, namely major depressive disorder with melancholia (endogenous depression) and primary major depressive disorder. The former is a more restrictive diagnostic category that shows a particular symptom picture associated with good response to somatic therapy. It includes features like pathological guilt, early morning awakening, weight loss, and diurnal variation of symptoms, all of which suggest a more autonomous or "biological" condition. The validity of this specific category derives not only from analysis of clinical assessments (40) but also from neuroendocrine studies (41). The concept of primary major depressive disorder encompasses melancholic depressions as well as any other reasonably pure depressive syndromes. Therefore, in studies in which this distinction is not made, it is difficult to determine whether blunted responses are typical of melancholic depression only, or of the entire group of primary major depressive disorders.

In some studies, depressed patients have been divided into unipolar (no manic episodes in the past) and bipolar (positive history of past manic episodes) depression; Δ max TSH responses were reported to be no different in the two groups (20, 28, 29). However, there is a disagreement over this finding. Gold et al. (34, 39) have reported substantially different responses between unipolar and bipolar patients, the former showing blunted responses to TRH and the latter showing basically the same responses as normal individuals (see above). The potential use of the TRH test in differentiating unipolar and bipolar major depressive disorders would be an important device, lending further support to the contention that unipolar and bipolar depressive disorders are different clinical and pathophysiological entities. This finding, however, awaits further replication.

2.3 The TRH Test in Mania

Only a few studies have been published on the TSH response to TRH in mania, possibly reflecting the inherent difficulty of conducting catheter studies on acutely manic patients. All studies report basically similar results, namely that the TSH response to TRH is blunted among patients with mania (25, 33, 38, 42, 43). One study (21) showed a normal TSH response among a group of nine manic patients. Some of these patients, however, had received lithium shortly before the study and therefore might have had somewhat exaggerated responses on this basis only. With this exception, all other studies agree that Δ max TSH is reduced in mania as it is in depression. This appears to be a paradoxical finding in view of the usual approach of conceptualizing depression and mania as opposite conditions.

2.4 The TRH Test in Other Psychiatric Disorders

There is one study reporting abnormal TSH responses to TRH in patients with chronic alcoholism (31). The authors found that 6 of 12 patients during acute withdrawal from alcohol and 3 of 7 patients immediately following acute withdrawal from alcohol had blunted responses to TRH. They suggested that these findings provide a biological link between alcoholism and affective disorders. Blunted TSH responses also have been shown in heroin addicts but not among ex-addicts (44).

Patients with anorexia nervosa have been shown to have basically normal TSH responses to TRH when the weight-loss factor per se is disregarded (38, 45–48).

The TSH response to TRH in schizophrenia has been demonstrated to be normal in several studies (20, 31, 38, 49). This is a recurring and important finding that lends validity to the observation that abnormal TSH responses are not the result of nonspecific stress associated with severe mental illness, but in fact reflect a basic abnormality characteristic only of the specific clinical conditions of depression and mania.

In conclusion, it can be stated that the TSH response to TRH is abnormally blunted in a substantial number of depressive patients. The sensitivity of the test may be acceptable for differentiating major from minor depressive disorder, unipolar subtype, but when the more restrictive category of endogenous depression is applied, as is usually the case in clinical practice, the diagnostic utility of the TRH test is very limited. Whether different responses occur between unipolar and bipolar patients still remains to be resolved. Bipolar patients during manic episodes have abnormally blunted responses whereas schizophrenic patients do not differ from normals. This difference may find important application in clinical practice, where the differential diagnosis between acute schizophrenia and acute manic episode is not always simple. Finally, abnormal responses are found in some patients during acute ingestion of alcohol and immediately after withdrawal. The number of patients, however, is small, and further studies are needed.

The abnormal TSH responses observed in patients with major depressive disorder are particularly interesting in view of another deviant neuroendocrine response that has repeatedly been found among patients with endogenous depression: an abnormal cortisol escape following dexamethasone suppression (41). Following the rationale of the neuroendocrine strategy described earlier in this chapter, the dexamethasone suppression test (DST) and the TRH test appear to reflect a disturbed function of the limbic-hypothalamic-pituitary-adrenal axis and the limbic-HPA axis, respectively. Since both tests presumably reflect similar limbic system dysfunctions, it is of importance to see whether the same patients share both neuroendocrine abnormalities. Extein et al. (50) performed TRH tests and DSTs on 50 patients with major depressive disorder, primary unipolar subtype. They found that both tests were abnormal in 30% of the patients. In 34% of the patients, only the TRH test was abnormal, and in 20% of the patients, only the DST was abnormal. Sixteen percent of the patients had normal responses to both TRH stimulation and dexamethasone suppression. They suggested that both tests were complementary as biological markers for unipolar depression. In fact, both tests in combination correctly identified 84% of the patients, compared with 50% with the DST alone or 64% with the TRH test alone.

These findings suggest that there are at least two neuroendocrine abnormalities in patients who are clinically indistinguishable. It is not known whether these abnormalities represent separate neurotransmitter pathologies or different susceptibilities of the HPA axis and HPT axis to common changes in neurotransmitter function. Both catecholamine and indoleamine systems are known to be involved in the regulation of both neuroendocrine axes, but to date no specific neurotransmitter or neuropeptide abnormality has been found to be linked with either disorder.

2.5   The Prognostic Value of the TRH Test in Depression

Following up the observation that abnormal TSH responses to TRH are present in a number of patients during episodes of depression, it is logical to determine whether normalization of the neuroendocrine disturbance accompanies clinical recovery. This has been documented, for example, with the DST test (51). Several studies have reported the results of repeated TRH tests after clinical recovery (15, 18, 19, 23, 28, 32). These studies show that in spite of evident clinical recovery, not all patients show a normalized TSH response to TRH. This suggests that in some patients antidepressant treatment can have a symptomatic effect without altering the underlying neuroendocrine disturbance. It has been shown with the DST (51) that failure to normalize the cortisol response to dexamethasone has ominous prognostic implications; such patients are much more likely to have earlier relapses compared with patients who have experienced both clinical recovery and a normalization of cortisol suppressive patterns. Kirkegaard (35) has reported that in the case of the TRH test, altered TSH responses to TRH after clinical recovery predict early relapses. In 66 "clinically cured" patients in whom antidepressant therapy was withdrawn after clinical recovery and who were followed for at least six months or until relapse, they found that $\Delta\Delta$ max TSH values (Δ max TSH response on discharge $-$ Δ max TSH response on admission) clearly differentiated patients with a good prognosis from those with a poor prognosis. According to the report, a hypothetical patient who had a Δ max TSH of 4 mIUI/mL (a blunted response) on admission and a Δ max TSH of 5 μIU/mL after clinical recovery has a high probability of relapse, since the $\Delta\Delta$ max TSH is only 1 μIU/mL. The risk for early relapse in this patient would be much less if the TRH test performed after clinical recovery had shown a Δ max TSH of, for example, 11 μIU/mL. Kirkegaard's study (35) showed that the limit of 2.0 μIU/mL predicted "cure" in 27 out of 29 patients and relapse in 33 of 37 patients. The majority of patients who showed little improvement in neuroendocrine disturbance following treatment relapsed within four months. In contrast, most of the patients wih Δ max

TSHs above 2 μIU/mL had a good outcome during the first six months after antidepressant treatment was discontinued. These findings appear to be in agreement with those recorded for the DST. However, no prognostic study using the two tests simultaneously on the same patients has been reported.

2.6 Prolactin and Growth Hormone Responses to TRH

As mentioned earlier, TRH normally elicits PRL secretion from the pituitary. The results among depressive patients are inconclusive since normal (26, 27), blunted (23, 52), increased (19), and variable (37) responses of PRL to TRH have been reported among patients with different categories of depression. Kirkegaard et al. (36) studied PRL responses in endogenous depression and found them to be of no diagnostic value. The report by Mendlewicz et al. (52) is of particular interest since the diagnostic category is well defined (bipolar) and patients were controlled for their menopausal status. They reported significantly blunted PRL responses to TRH in the patients compared with controls. This finding has additional relevance in light of the report by Maeda et al. (53) that four manic patients had signficantly increased PRL responses to TRH when compared with controls. Since the PRL response is regulated in part by both serotonergic and noradrenergic mechanisms, the opposite responses found in manic and depressed patients lend some support to the monoamine hypothesis of affective disorders (54).

In summary, the results of the PRL response do not appear to be as clear-cut as those obtained with TSH responses to TRH, and further studies are required. The possible prognostic value of PRL responses to TRH among endogenous depressive patients was studied by Kirkegaard et al. (36) and was found to fall short of that observed for TSH responses to TRH.

Although it is generally accepted that under normal conditions growth hormone (GH) is not released after TRH administration (55, 56), the GH response to TRH has been studied in patients with affective disorder. Maeda et al. (19) reported an increased GH response in patients with "mental depression." They repeated these tests following clinical recovery and found that the GH response was absent. Gold et al. (34, 39) demonstrated the presence of GH secretion following TRH in patients with major depressive disorder, both unipolar and bipolar, but not in patients with minor depression. In this study a response was also observed in patients with anorexia nervosa, opiate addiction, and schizoaffective illness. The authors suggested that GH responses to TRH may be of value in differentiating major depressive disorder from minor depressive disorder, but they found it an unreliable test for unipolar depression. Kirkegaard et al. (36) found the GH response to TRH to be of no diagnostic value in patients with endogenous depression and of only limited predictive value, certainly lower than that of abnormal TSH responses. In general, GH responses seem to be very sensitive to nonspecific stress (57), and therefore the interpretation of these responses is difficult.

2.7 Possible Mechanisms

The impaired TSH response to TRH discussed earlier awaits explanation. Since circulating levels of thyroid hormones play a significant role in the responsivity of the pituitary to TRH stimulation, a possible effect of thyroid hormones accounting for the blunted response in depressive patients has been examined. During depression, serum concentrations of T4 have been reported to be elevated, normal, or reduced (35). Furthermore some studies agree that serum T4 tends to decrease when the depressive symptoms improve (18, 22, 58). However, Kirkegaard and Faber (59) showed that decreases of free T4 and free T3 indices occur among patients recovered from depression regardless of whether the blunted TSH response to TRH normalizes or not. The minor changes in CSF levels of T4 observed in patients treated with electroconvulsive therapy (ECT) (30) were also found to be similar in patients with or without changes on Δ max TSH following treatment.

The hypercortisolemia observed in patients with endogenous depression could explain the blunted TSH response to TRH. It is known that glucocorticoid administration to normal subjects can diminish the TSH response to TRH (60–62). In fact, two studies found an inverse relationship between serum cortisol and Δ max TSH among depressed patients (24, 31). However, studies including larger number of patients (30, 34) found no relationship between serum cortisol and TSH responses to TRH. Furthermore, the fact that Extein et al. (50) found no specific association between these two abnormalities supports the contention that blunted TSH responses to TRH are not an artifact of hypothalamic-pituitary-adrenal overactivity.

Possible disturbances in TRH secretion could explain the abnormal TSH responses reported. Kirkegaard et al. (63) found considerably higher concentrations of CSF TRH in patients with endogenous depression compared with controls. But these levels remained elevated after treatment with ECT, both in patients with normalized Δ max TSH and in those whose response remained unaltered in spite of clinical recovery. The Kirkegaard group concluded that CSF levels of TRH could not explain the abnormal Δ max TSH responses observed in endogenous depression. Furthermore, the fact that 80% of brain TRH is located in extrahypothalamic tissue makes it unlikely that CSF TRH alone serves as a reliable indicator of hypothalamic TRH turnover.

Again, the data in support of a specific hypothesis for the nature of TSH blunting in depression are unclear. If it is true that an excess of TRH is released into the pituitary portal system in depression, then one might observe TRH receptor down regulation as reflected in blunted TSH release after exogenous TRH.

Future studies should be directed towards trying to define further the clinical population with the abnormal neuroendocrine responses to TRH and towards exploring the neurotransmitter and receptor mechanisms underlying it. This will most surely lead to a better understanding of the pathology of affective disorders.

3 ENDORPHINS IN PSYCHIATRY

3.1 Basic Science Summary of β-Endorphin Systems

The opioid peptide studies described below reflect the problems of a substance in search of its physiology (or pathophysiology). The general thrust of these studies has been to examine the role of the endorphin systems in treatment paradigms or to search for abnormalities in endorphins as "markers" for the illnesses in question. The nature of this chapter does not allow space for a review of the fundamental complexities of the several opioid systems in nervous tissue. A review of some issues critical to clinical studies as presented elsewhere (64) can be summarized:

1. There are many peptides in nervous tissue with opioid activity. The list includes β-endorphin, methionine(Met)-enkephalin, leucine(Leu)-enkephalin, dynorphin, α-neo-endorphin, and several enkephalin variants.

2. There are at least three main biosynthetic pathways for the opioid peptides. Beta-endorphin is cosynthesized with ACTH (or α-MSH), β-lipotropin, and γ-MSH from the pro-opiomelanocortin (POMC) precursor. Met- and Leu-enkephalin and Met-enkephalin-Arg[6]-Phe[7] and Met-enkephalin-Arg[6]-Gly[7]-Leu[8] are produced from a 260+ amino acid precursor in adrenal (and most likely in brain) (65–67a). No other identifiable peptides are cosynthesized by proenkephalin; however, several nonenkephalin conserved pieces of that precursor are candidates for biologically active peptides. The primary structure of the dynorphin precursor (which also contains β-neo-endorphin and a third Leu-enkephalin sequence) has just been elucidated (67b).

3. Colocalization of several active peptides in the same cell is the rule for opioid peptides. Beta-endorphin is costored with ACTH, α-MSH, and γ-MSH. The two enkephalins occur together plus the -COOH

extended-Arg^6-Phe^7 and -Arg^6-Gly^7-Leu^8 enkephalins and the nonenkephalin peptides from the same precursor. Finally, dynorphin and α-neo-endorphin can be found together with arginine vasopressin (AVP) in the hypothalamus (68). Colocalization of active peptides suggests corelease and a complex biology of the substances in question. In some cases the several substances coreleased by one neuron are found to synergize or at least to have additive effects with each other (69).

4. There are a variety of opioid receptor subtypes. Some show highest affinity for the enkephalins (delta receptors), some for dynorphin (kappa receptors), and some for β-endorphin (mu and delta receptors). Although this is a substantial oversimplification, the complexity of opioid receptors pales when one considers the receptors for other peptides related to opioid peptide activity. For example, is there an ACTH or α-MSH receptor related to the synaptic activity of these two peptides? How are these receptors related to that of β-endorphin in the same synapse? How about dynorphin and AVP? Are they coreleased in brain to act transsynaptically on their own receptors? Do these combinations of peptides act in concert? How does the postsynaptic receptor complex integrate the several peptide messages it receives? The biology of cotransmitter neurons and endocrine cells is very complex and demands new methods for investigation and new theoretical perspectives.

5. In addition to the issues mentioned above, the question remains whether there are multiple sites of effect by the same peptide system. For example, β-endorphin can be found in four nervous tissue loci. Two in brain (one in hypothalamus and one in brain stem) and two in pituitary (the anterior lobe and intermediate lobe). Thus the same substance (and related peptides), produced by the same biosynthetic route seems to be capable of two functions, that of neurotransmitter or hormone. The enkephalins are similarly distributed in neurons (brain) and endocrine cells (adrenal). Dynorphin also has both neuronal and endocrine distributions, being located both in the hypothalamic magnocellular nuclei that project to the posterior pituitary and in other pathways that terminate in the brain stem. Further, there are many other tissue sites where these peptides play an important role—pancreas, autonomic nervous system, gut, and so on.

These types of observations on the opioid peptide systems can be repeated for a variety of other peptide systems throughout nervous tissue. Many of these observations are now seen as reflecting important principles of organization for peptide-secreting cells.

The basic science complexities outlined above make clinical studies in psychiatry very difficult to design and interpret. For example, systemic administration of a general opiate antagonist (naloxone) might well influence certain psychiatric symptoms, yet the investigator has no way of knowing which peptide or in which of several locations the drug is acting.

3.2 Opioid Peptides in Psychiatric Studies: Evidence Suggesting an Endorphin Deficiency in Schizophrenia

Several types of evidence support the hypothesis that schizophrenia reflects a deficiency of endorphins. Positive reports of the effects of exogenous opiates on schizophrenic symptoms have appeared in the psychiatric literature for the past century; however, none of these reports is based on appropriate study designs (70).

A synthetic analog of Met-enkephalin, FK33824, has been reported to decrease psychotic symptoms in schizophrenic subjects. In an uncontrolled pilot study by Nedopil and Ruther (71), nine patients received 0.5 mg and 1 mg FK33824 for 2 days. The group reported a significant decline in symptoms, lasting from one to seven days. In another single-blind study Jorgensson et al. (72) reported that FK33824 reduced the hallucinations of nine chronic psychotic patients.

Des-tyrosine-gamma-endorphin (DTgE) (β-LPH62-77), another endorphin-like peptide, is undergoing investigation in several settings. This peptide is structurally related to endorphins but is lacking in opiate activity. Burback and De Wied (73) have detected DTgE in rat pituitary, rat brain, and human spinal fluid. They also reported that the incubation of β-endorphin with homogenates of rat forebrain produced DTgE. This suggests that DTgE is an endogenously formed compound derived from β-endorphin. Verhoeven et al. (74) reported a decrease in schizophrenic symptoms in a single-blind study of six patients and in a double-blind study of eight patients after the administration of DTgE. But Emrich et al. (75) have found that DTgE reduced schizophrenic symptomatology in only a subgroup of the patients studied. Of 10 schizophrenic patients in another study (75), only two acute schizophrenics improved on DTgE.

Another endorphin-like peptide without opiate activity (des-enkephalin-gamma-endorphin, DEgE) has been studied in schizophrenia by Verhoeven et al. (77). They report that DEgE is as potent as DTgE in acute hebephrenic schizophrenic patients. These results are promising, but the complexity of the biology of these peptides points to the need for further investigations to determine their practical antipsychotic efficacy.

The rigidity induced by intraventricular injections of β-endorphin in rats has been compared with the catalepsy produced in these animals by neuroleptics (91). Not all investigators agree with this conclusion (79). Yet this finding suggests that β-endorphin is an endogenous neuroleptic and that schizophrenic symptoms might reflect an endorphin deficiency (79). In the single-blind study of Kline and Lehmann (80), three of four schizophrenic subjects were reported to experience symptom reductions from 15 intravenous doses of 1.5 to 9 mg of β-endorphin.

Three groups of investigators have performed double-blind studies using β-endorphin in schizophrenic subjects. Our group found a statistically significant improvement in eight schizophrenic subjects over five days following a single 20 mg intravenous injection of β-endorphin (81). Two other groups found no decline in schizophrenic symptoms on the day of the intravenous injection of β-endorphin (82, 83). In fact, as described in the following section, one of these two groups (82) reported a transient worsening of schizophrenic symptoms following β-endorphin injections. Thus, further investigations are needed to determine whether or not β-endorphin has any antipsychotic activity.

3.3   Evidence Suggesting an Endorphin Excess in Schizophrenia

In contrast to those studies suggesting an endorphin deficiency in schizophrenia, several studies indicate an increase in the activity of endorphin systems in schizophrenia. In the double-blind crossover study by Gerner et al. (82) mentioned above, the symptoms of six of eight schizophrenic subjects worsened after β-endorphin treatment when compared with placebo trials. The symptoms of one schizophrenic subject worsened after placebo injection. The investigators hypothesized that an increase in CNS dopamine activity, due to the β-endorphin administration, might account for the worsening of the schizophrenic condition.

Wahlstrom et al. (84) and Terenius et al. (85) report that endorphin fractions other than β-endorphin and enkephalins appear to be elevated in the CSF of unmedicated schizophrenic patients. When these patients were given neuroleptics, the increased concentrations decreased to normal levels. There are also reports of elevated CSF levels of β-endorphin in some schizophrenic patients. One study reported that normal subjects had values of 72 fmol/mL, whereas neurological controls had values of 92 fmol/mL (86). In contrast, chronic schizophrenic patients had values of 35 fmol/mL and acute schizophrenic patients had values of 760 fmol/mL.

If verified in control studies, the reported improvement in schizophrenic symptoms following hemodialysis would be further evidence for an excess of endorphins in schizophrenia. Wagemaker and Cade (87) and Palmour et al. (88) have attempted to relieve schizophrenic symptoms by the removal of leucine[5]-β-endorphin (Leu[5]-β-endorphin). Unfortunately, their hemodialysis trial was not double-blind and there has been no confirmation that Leu[5]-β-endorphin-like immunoreactivity is elevated in schizophrenic subjects when compared with control subjects (90).

Finally, a lessening of symptoms in schizophrenic patients has been reported in four double-blind studies following intravenous administration of the opiate antagonist naloxone hydrochloride. One study reported a reduction in unusual thought content of schizophrenic patients (92); two of the studies, including our own, reported a decrease in schizophrenic hallucinations following naloxone administration (93–95); and a further study reported a general reduction of psychotic symptoms (96). Although not all investigators have been able to replicate our findings, a recent World Health Organization collaborative study involving more than 30 schizophrenic patients given high doses of naloxone (97) reported decreased auditory hallucinations.

3.4 Endorphins in Affective Illness (Mania)

Terenius et al. (85) extracted and measured in the CSF of patients with affective disorders two endorphin substances (labeled fraction I and II) that are neither β-endorphin nor the enkephalins. Using a radioreceptor assay, the group found fraction I to be elevated in three or four manic subjects. Interestingly, these patients had increased levels of the fraction II opioid during normal mood states. Judd and coworkers (98) studied the effects of the short-lived opiate antagonist naloxone in mania. Four of eight manic patients reported a reduction of symptoms such as irritability, tension, anger, and hostility following the administration of 20 mg of naloxone. In another study, using generally lower doses of naloxone, other investigators found no change in the symptomatology of patients with affective disorders (99). Finally, in the recent collaborative investigation of the World Health Organization a larger number of manic patients showed no change in symptoms following high doses of naloxone (97).

Janowsky et al. (100) observed a recurrence of depressive symptomatology in patients with a history of depression following the infusion of the cholinesterase inhibitor physostigmine. Antimanic properties of physostigmine were also reported (101, 102). In an investigation with normal volunteers the physostigmine-induced mood changes (particularly the depressive components) were correlated with elevated plasma β-endorphin levels. These changes included an increase in reports of depression, hostility, and confusion and a decrease in arousal and mania. This study implies a cholinergic link to β-endorphin and supports the suggestion that an increase in endorphin activity may be a cause of depressive symptoms.

3.5 Endorphins in Affective Illness (Depression)

Several studies indicate an endorphin deficiency in patients with affective disorders. In a study by Angst et al. (103), three of the six depressed patients switched into hypomania after a 10 mg intravenous injection of β-endorphin. This mood swing could be due to an injection of β-endorphin in depressed patients with endogenously low endorphin levels, although other factors such as the stress of the experimental situation or patient expectation may be involved. Kline et al. (104) reported improvement in a variety of psychotic symptoms in depressed patients following intravenous administration of 1–9 mg of β-endorphin. These trials were not double-blind, and a relatively low dose of β-endorphin was given. In one preliminary investigation, β-endorphin was also found to be moderately and transiently effective in reducing the symptoms of depression (105).

In a double-blind, placebo-controlled crossover study by Gerner et al. (82), nine depressed patients manifested significant improvement 2–4 h after β-endorphin administration when compared with placebo trials. A second group of investigators (83) also reported a short-term decline in depressive symptoms in a smaller group of depressed patients who received β-endorphin intravenously in a double-blind design. Taken together these findings support the hypothesis that depressed patients have a deficit in endorphin activity. In an attempt to integrate the schizophrenia and affective disease results, Gerner and associates suggested that an increase in CNS dopamine activity, possibly induced by β-endorphin administration, might account for the antidepressant effects as well as the exacerbation of the schizophrenic symptoms observed in their study (82). More recently this group has reported a transient reduction in depressive symptoms in some patients each time β-endorphin was administered (105). In further support for the opioid deficit hypothesis is a study by Emrich et al. (107) demonstrating the efficacy of buprinorphin in depression.

Apparently unrelated to the direct study of "peptides" in psychiatry are the many excellent studies linking cortisol regulatory problems with affective disease (cf. 41). The gist of this well-established finding is that endogenously depressed patients escape early from the cortisol suppression after dexamethasone. Interestingly, this "adrenal" finding has only very recently been extended upward to pituitary (much less brain) in the form of plasma ACTH or β-endorphin measurements. It is clear that dexamethasone can suppress human ACTH and β-endorphin release and that endogenously depressed patients with abnormal dexamethasone suppressibility also escape with β-endorphin and ACTH, (108–110).

From the logical point of view it is surprising that there has been so little effort to extend this clinical–endocrine correlation into the CNS. Clearly this will be a rich peptide–psychiatry interface in years to come.

4   FINAL IMPRESSIONS

There appears to be the potential for a rich interface between the actions of peptides and a better understanding of psychopathology. As can be seen from the two areas presented above, both the clinical and basic sciences associated with these studies are in need of further sharpening and clarification. There is a basis for these types of studies but one requiring heavy interdependence between the levels of discourse—between the laboratory and the clinical research center.

REFERENCES

1. A. J. Prange, I. C. Wilson, P. P. Lara, L. B. Alltop, and G. R. Breese, *Lancet* **2**, 999 (1972).
2. A. J. Prange and I. C. Wilson, *Psychopharmacologia* **26**, 82 (1972).
3. A. J. Kastin, R. H. Ehrensing, D. S. Schalch, and M. S. Anderson, *Lancet* **2**, 742 (1972).
4. A. J. Prange, C. B. Nemeroff, M. A. Lipton, G. R. Breese, and I. C. Wilson, in L. L. Iverson, S. D. Iversen, and S. H. Snyder, Eds., *Handbook of Psychopharmacology*, Vol. 13, Plenum Publishing, New York, 1978, p. 1.
5. B. J. Carroll, G. C. Curtis, and J. Mendels, *Arch. Gen. Psychiat.* **33**, 1039 (1976).
6. R. Guillemin, *Science* **202**, 390 (1978).
7. A. V. Schally, *Science* **202**, 18 (1978).
8. I. Jackson and S. Reichlin, *Endocrinology* **95**, 854 (1974).
9. J. B. Martin, S. Reichlin, and G. N. Brown, *Clinical Neuroendocrinology*, F. A. Davis, Philadelphia, 1977.
10. J. E. Morley, *Life Sci.* **25**, 1539 (1979).
11. P. J. Snyder and R. D. Utiger, *J. Clin. Endocrinol.* **34**, 380 (1972).
12. P. J. Snyder and R. D. Utiger, *J. Clin. Invest.* **51**, 2077 (1972).
13. L. S. Jacobs, P. J. Snyder, R. D. Utiger, and W. H. Daughaday, *J. Clin. Endocrinol. Metab.* **36**, 1069 (1973).
14. S. Takahashi, H. Kondo, M. Yoshimura, and Y. Ochi, *Folia Psychiatr. Neurol. Jpn.* **27**, 305 (1973).
15. A. Coppen, S. Montgomery, M. Peet, J. Bailey, V. Marks, and P. Woods, *Lancet* **2**, 433 (1974).
16. S. Takahashi, H. Kondo, M. Yoshimura, and Y. Ochi, *Folia Psychiatr. Neurol. Jpn.* **28**, 335 (1974).
17. C. Kirkegaard, N. Norlem, U. Birk Lauridsen, N. Bjorum, and C. Christiansen, *Arch. Gen. Psychiatry* **32**, 1115 (1975).
18. C. Kirkegaard, N. Norlem, U. Birk Lauridsen, and N. Bjorum, *Acta Psychiatr. Scand.* **52**, 170 (1975).
19. K. Maeda, Y. Kato, S. Ohgo, K. Chihara, Y. Yoshimoto, N. Yamaguchi, C. Kuromaru, and H. Imura, *J. Clin. Endocrinol. Metab.* **40**, 501 (1975).
20. P. T. Loosen, A. J. Prange, I. C. Wilson, P. P. Lara, and C. Pettus, *Psychoneuroendocrinology* **2**, 137 (1977).
21. P. W. Gold, F. K. Goodwin, T. Wehr, and R. Rebar, *Am. J. Psychiatry* **134**, 1028 (1977).
22. C. Kirkegaard, N. Bjorum, D. Cohn, J. Faber, U. Birk Lauridsen, and J. Nerup, *Psychoneuroendocrinology* **2**, 131 (1977).
23. F. Gregoire, H. Brauman, R. De Buck, and J. Corvilain, *Psychoneuroendocrinology* **2**, 303 (1977).
24. P. T. Loosen, A. J. Prange, and I. C. Wilson, *Am. J. Psychiatry* **135**, 244 (1978).
25. C. Kirkegaard, N. Bjorum, D. Cohn, and U. Birk Lauridsen, *Arch. Gen. Psychiatry* **35**, 1017 (1978).
26. F. Brambilla, E. Smeraldi, E. Sacchetti, F. Negri, D. Cocchi, and E. E. Muller, *Arch. Gen. Psychiatry* **35**, 1231 (1978).
27. R. Naeije, J. Golstein, D. Zegers De Deyl, P. Linkowski, J. Mendlewicz, G. Copinschi, M. Badawi, R. Leclercq, M. L'Hermite, and L. Vanhaelst, *Clin. Endocrinol.* **9**, 49 (1978).

28. J. Mendlewicz, P. Linkowski, and H. Brauman, *Lancet* **2**, 1079 (1979).
29. J. D. Amsterdam, A. Winokur, J. Mendels, and P. Snyder, *Lancet* **2**, 904 (1979).
30. C. Kirkegaard and B. J. Carroll, *Psychiatr. Res.* **3**, 253 (1980).
31. P. T. Loosen and A. J. Prange, *Psychoneuroendocrinology* **5**, 63 (1980).
32. G. M. Asnis, R. S. Nathan, U. Halbreich, F. S. Halpern, and E. J. Sachar, *Lancet* **1**, 424 (1980).
33. I. Extein, A. L. C. Pottash, M. S. Gold, J. Cadet, D. R. Sweeney, R. K. Davies, and D. M. Martin, *Psychiatr. Res.* **2**, 199 (1980).
34. M. S. Gold, A. L. C. Pottash, N. Ryan, D. R. Sweeney, and D. M. Martin, *Psychoneuroendocrinology* **5**, 147 (1980).
35. C. Kirkegaard, *Psychoneuroendocrinology* **6**(3), 189 (1981).
36. C. Kirkegaard, P. C. Eskildssen, and N. Bjorum, *Psychoneuroendocrinology* **6**(3), 253 (1981).
37. A. Winokur, J. Amsterdam, S. Caroff, P. J. Snyder, and D. Brunswick, *Am. J. Psychiatry* **139**(1), 39 (1982).
38. Y. Papakostas, M. Fink, J. Lee, P. Irwin, and L. Johnson, *Psychiatry Res.* **4**, 55 (1981).
39. M. S. Gold, A. L. C. Pottash, I. Extein, D. M. Martin, E. Howard, E. A. Mueller, and D. R. Sweeney, *Psychoneuroendocrinology* **6**(2), 159 (1981).
40. R. L. Spitzer, J. Endicott, and E. Robbins, *Research Diagnostic Criteria (RDC): Biometrics Research* , New York State Psychiatric Institute, New York (1977).
41. B. J. Carroll, M. Feinberg, J. F. Greden, J. S. Tarika, A. A. Albala, R. F. Haskett, N. McI. James, Z. Kronfol, N. Lohr, M. Steiner, J. P. DeVigne, and E. Young, *Arch. Gen. Psychiatry* **33**, 1051 (1981).
42. S. Takahashi, H. Kondo, M. Yoshimura, and Y. Ochi, *Folia Psychiatr. Neurol. Jpn.* **29**, 231 (1975).
43. I. Extein, A. L. C. Pottash, M. S. Gold, and R. W. Cowdry, *Arch. Gen. Psychiatry* **39**, 77 (1982).
44. V. Chan, C. Wang, and R. T. T. Yeung, *Clin. Endocrinol.* **10**, 557 (1979).
45. R. Moshang, J. S. Parks, L. Baker, V. Vaidya, R. D. Utiger, A. M. Bongiovanni, and P. J. Snyder, *J. Clin. Endocrinol. Metab.* **40**, 470 (1975).
46. M. S. Croxson and H. K. Ibbertson, *J. Clin. Endocrinol. Metab.* **44**, 167 (1977).
47. R. D. G. Leslie, A. J. Isaacs, J. Gomez, P. R. Raggatt, and R. Bayliss, *Br. Med. J.* **2**, 526 (1978).
48. A. Wakeling, V. F. A. De Souza, M. B. R. Gore, M. Sabur, D. Kingstone, and A. M. B. Boss, *Psychol. Med.* **9**, 265 (1979).
49. A. J. Prange, P. T. Loosen, I. C. Wilson, H. Y. Meltzer, and V. S. Fang, *Arch. Gen. Psychiatry* **36**, 907 (1979).
50. I. Extein, A. L. C. Pottash, and M. S. Gold, *Psychiatry Res.* **4**, 49 (1981).
51. J. F. Greden, A. A. Albala, R. F. Haskett, N. McI. James, L. Goodman, M. Steiner, and B. J. Carroll, *Biol. Psychiatr.* **15**, 449 (1980).
52. J. Mendlewicz, P. Linkowski, and H. Brauman, *New Engl. J. Med.* **302**(19), 1091 (1980).
53. K. Maeda, K. Tanimoto, N. Yamaguchi, Y. Iwasaki, K. Chihari, and K. Fujita, *New Engl. J. Med.* **301**, 1400 (1979).
54. J. J. Schildkraut, *Am. J. Psychiatry* **122**, 509 (1965).
55. M. S. Anderson, C. Y. Bowers, A. J. Kastin, D. S. Schalch, A. V. Schally, P. J. Snyder, R. D. Utiger, J. F. Wilber, and A. J. Wise, *New Engl. J. Med.* **285**, 1279 (1971).
56. B. J. Ormston, J. R. Kilborn, R. Garry, J. Amos, and R. Hall, *Br. Med. J.* **2**, 199 (1971).
57. M. Feinberg, B. J. Carroll, and J. F. Greden, *Soc. Biol. Psychiatry Sci. Proc.* Abstract No. 6, 38 (1980).
58. P. Bech, C. Kirkegaard, E. Bock, M. Johannesen, and O. J. Rafaelson, *Neuropsychobiology* **4**, 99 (1978).
59. C. Kirkegaard and J. Faber, *Acta Endocrinol.* **96**, 199 (1981).

60. G. Faglia, C. Gerrari, P. Beck-Peccoz, A. Spada, P. Travaglini, and R. Ambrosi, *Horm. Metab. Res.* **5**, 289 (1973).

61. M. Otsuki, M. Dakoda, and S. Baba, *J. Clin. Endocrinol. Metab.* **36**, 95 (1973).

62. R. N. Re, I. A. Kourides, E. C. Ridgway, B. D. Weintraub, and F. Maloof, *J. Clin. Endocrinol. Metab.* **43**, 338 (1976).

63. C. Kirkegaard, J. Faber, L. Hummer, and P. Rogowski, *Psychoneuroendocrinology* **4**, 227 (1979).

64. H. Akil and S. J. Watson, in L. L. Iverson, S. D. Iverson, and S. H. Snyder, Eds., *Handbook of Psychopharmacology*, Vol. 17, Plenum Publishing, New York, 1982.

65. M. Noda, Y. Furutani, H. Takahashi, M. Toyosato, T. Hirose, S. Inayama, S. Nakanishi, and S. Numa, *Nature* **295**, 202 (1982).

66. M. Comb, P. H. Seeburg, J. Adelman, L. Eiden, and E. Herbert, *Nature*, in press (1982).

67. (a) U. Gubler, P. Seeburg, B. J. Hoffman, L. P. Gage, and S. Udenfriend, *Nature* 296 (1982). (b) H. Kakidani, Y. Furutani, H. Takahashi, M. Noda, Y. Morimoto, T. Hirose, M. Asai, A. Inayama, S. Nakanishi, and S. Numa, *Nature* **298**, 245 (1982).

68. S. J. Watson, C. W. Richard III, and J. D. Barchas, *Science* **200**, 1180 (1978).

69. J. M. Walker, H. Akil, and S. J. Watson, *Science* **210**, 1247 (1980).

70. P. A. Berger, *Neurosci. Res. Program Bull.* **16**, 585 (1978).

71. W. Nedopil and E. Ruther, *Pharmakopsychiatr. Neuropsychopharmakol.* **12**, 277 (1979).

72. A. Jorgensson, R. Fog, and B. Veilis, *Lancet* **1**, 935 (1979).

73. P. Burbach and D. De Wied, *Enzymes and Neurotransmitters in Mental Disease*, Wiley, New York, 1980, p. 103.

74. W. M. Verhoeven, H. M. van Praag, J. M. van Ree, and D. de Wied, *Arch. Gen. Psychiatry* **36**, 294 (1979).

75. H. M. Emrich, M. Zaudig, W. Kissling, G. Dirlich, D. B. Zerssen, and A. Herz, *Pharmakopsychiatr. Neuropsychopharmakol.* **13**, 290 (1980).

76. J. Metz, D. A. Busch, and H. Meltzer, *Life Sci.* **28**, 2003 (1981).

77. W. M. A. Verhoeven, J. M. van Ree, D. De Wied, and M. Van Praagitt: *Arch. Gen. Psychiatry* **38**, 1182 (1981).

78. D. S. Segal, R. G. Brown, A. Arnsten, and D. C. Derrington, *Characteristics and Function of Opioids*, Elsevier/North Holland, Amsterdam, 1978, p. 413.

79. L. F. Tseng, H. H. Loh, and C. H. Li, *Int. J. Peptide Protein Res.* **12**, 173 (1978).

80. N. S. Kline and H. Lehmann, *Endorphins in Mental Health Research*, Macmillan, New York, 1979, p. 500.

81. P. A. Berger, S. J. Watson, H. Akil, G. R. Elliott, R. Rubin, A. Pfefferbaum, K. L. Davis, J. D. Barchas, and C. H. Li, *Arch. Gen. Psychiatry* **37**, 635 (1980).

82. R. H. Gerner, D. H. Catlin, D. A. Gorelick, K. K. Hui, and C. H. Li, *Arch. Gen. Psychiatry* **37**, 642 (1980).

83. D. Pickar, G. C. Davis, C. Schulz, I. Extein, R. Wagner, D. Naber, P. W. Bold, D. P. van Kammen, F. K. Goodwin, R. J. Wyatt, C. H. Li, and W. E. Bunney Jr., *Am. J. Psychiatry* **138**(2), 160 (1981).

84. A. Wahlstrom, L. Johansson, and L. Terenius, *Opiates and Endogenous Opioid Peptides*, Elsevier/North Holland, Amsterdam, 1976, p. 49.

85. L. Terenius, A. Wahlstrom, L. Linstrom, and E. Widerlov, *Neurosci. Lett.* **3**, 157 (1976).

86. W. Domschke, A. Dickschas, and P. Mitznegg, *Lancet* **1**, 1024 (1979).

87. H. Wagemaker and R. Cade, *Am. J. Psychiatry* **134**, 684 (1977).

88. R. Palmour, F. Ervin, H. Wagemaker, and R. Cade, *Endorphins in Mental Health Research*, Macmillan, New York, 1979, p. 581.

89. R. V. Lewis, L. D. Gerber, S. Stein, R. L. Stephen, B. I. Grosser, S. F. Velick, and S. Udenfriend, *Arch. Gen. Psychiatry* **36**, 237 (1979).

90. M. Ross, P. A. Berger, and A. Goldstein, *Science* **200**, 974 (1979).

91. F. E. Bloom, D. Segal, N. Ling, and R. Guillemin, *Science* **194**, 630 (1976).

92. G. C. Davis, W. E. Bunney Jr., M. S. Buchsbaum, E. G. De Fraites, W. Duncan, J. C. Gillin, D. P. van Kammen, J. Kleinman, D. L. Murphy, R. M. Post, V. Reus, and R. J. Wyatt, *Endorphins in Mental Health Research*, Macmillan, New York, 1979, p. 393.

93. S. J. Watson, P. A. Berger, H. Akil, M. J. Mills, and J. D. Barchas, *Science* **201**, 73 (1978).

94. H. M. Emrich, C. Cording, and S. Piree, *Pharmakopsychiatr. Neuropsychopharmakol.* **10**, 265 (1977).

95. P. A. Berger, S. J. Watson, H. Akil, and J. D. Barchas, *Am. J. Psychiatry* **138**(7), 913 (1981).

96. H. Lehman, N. P. Vasavan Nair, and N. S. Kline, *Am. J. Psychiatry* **136**, 762 (1979).

97. D. Pickar, W. E. Bunney Jr., *Proceedings of the 3rd World Conference on Biological Psychiatry*, Elsevier/North Holland, Amsterdam, in press.

98. L. L. Judd, D. S. Janowsky, D. S. Segal, and L. Y. Huey, *Characteristics and Function of Opioids*, Elsevier/North Holland, 1978, p. 173.

99. G. C. Davis, W. E. Bunney Jr., E. G. De Fraites, and I. Extein, paper presented at the Annual Meeting of the American College of Neuropsychopharmacology, Maui, Hawaii, 1978.

100. D. S. Janowsky, M. K. Khaled, and J. M. Davis, *Psychosom. Med.* **36**, 248 (1974).

101. D. S. Janowsky, K. El-Yousef, J. M. Davis, and H. I. Sekerke, *Arch. Gen. Psychiatry* **28**, 542 (1973).

102. K. Davis, P. A. Berger, L. E. Hollister, and E. G. De Fraites, *Arch. Gen. Psychiatry* **35**, 119 (1978).

103. J. Angst, V. Autenrieth, F. Brem, M. Koukkou, H. Meyer, H. Stassen, and U. Storek, *Endorphins in Mental Health Research*, Macmillan, New York, 1979, p. 518.

104. N. S. Kline, C. H. Li, H. E. Lehmann, A. Lajtha, E. Laski, and T. Cooper, *Arch. Gen. Psychiatry* **34**, 1111 (1977).

105. D. H. Catlin, D. Gorelick, R. H. Gerner, K. K. Gui, and C. H. Li, in *Advances in Psychopharmacology: Neural Peptides and Neuronal Communication*, Vol. 22, E. Costa and M. Trabucchi, eds. Raven Press, New York, 1980, pp. 465–472.

106. D. H. Catlin, R. H. Gerner, and D. A. Gorelick, *Proceedings of the 3rd World Conference on Biological Psychiatry*, Elsevier/North Holland, Amsterdam, 1981, in press.

107. H. M. Emrich, P. Vogt, and A. Herz, *Biological Psychiatry*, Elsevier/North Holland, Amsterdam, 1981, p. 380.

108. V. I. Reus, M. S. Joseph, and M. F. Dallman, *New Engl. J. Med.* **306**, 238 (1982).

109. V. S. Fang, B. J. Tricou, A. Robertson, and H. Y. Meltzer, *Life Sci.* **29**, 931 (1981).

110. J. D. Matthews, H. Akil, H. Greden, and S. J. Watson, paper presented at the Society of Biological Psychiatry Annual Meeting, Toronto, Canada, May 1982, Proceedings abstract no. 51

16

Memory, Learning, and Adaptive Behaviors

GEORGE KOOB

FLOYD E. BLOOM

A. V. Davis Center for Behavioral Neurobiology
The Salk Institute
La Jolla, California

1 INTRODUCTION

In this chapter, we deal with the problem of studying how naturally occurring peptides of the endocrine and central nervous system participate in the behavioral phenomena generally termed memory and learning. Our focus here is the effects of endorphins, vasopressin, and corticotropin releasing factor (CRF) on memory, learning, and adaptive behaviors exclusively, as other chapters in this volume consider other families of peptides. This area of research is often viewed quite skeptically, especially by scientists in nonbehavioral fields, because the phenomena to be measured are "behavioral" and because the actual cellular and molecular mechanisms underlying the formation, storage, and retrieval of any operational information in any nervous system remain to be determined. The allure of peptides for studies of memory and learning, especially the two peptide families covered here in depth —endorphins and vasopressin/oxytocin—largely reflects the changing fashions in studies of neurotransmitters. Peptide "regulators" of behavioral phenomena have succeeded to the center of the experimental stage once occupied by protein synthesis inhibitors, cholinergic drugs, and more recently the drugs affecting central and peripheral catecholamine neurotransmission. The never-ending stream of new candidate mediators of complex behavioral events points up the fickle nature of such research: When it proves difficult to explain how behaviors are changed after an endogenous transmitter system is activated or suppressed, or when actions are only found with nonphysiological doses of an endogenous substance injected into unnatural body compartments, then the easy course is to go to the newest "transmitter of the month" and see what it will do to behaving rats or men.

Our recent efforts to understand what actually is happening when we inject minute doses of peptides subcutaneously and observe that some animal behaviors are altered for many hours have lead us to certain interpretative biases, which we wish to acknowledge in advance. We reiterate the inescapable fact that we are sure they *do* affect behavior, and we are pretty sure we don't know *why*. However, our working hypotheses and reflective reviews of the growing literature (see also refs. 1, 2) lead us to the position that the behavioral effects of peptides are an outward expression of specific cellular signals most likely initiated at some visceral receptive relay of the central nervous system. If these effects are in any way relevant to the generally common behavioral effects of endorphins, vasopressin, and other hypothalamo-pituitary peptides, then we infer that the action reflects on a global scale their individual cellular responsibilities for homeostatic regulation of the organism.

One final introductory note deserving explicit recognition is an overview of the strategies and interpretations for investigating how these, or any other peptides, could participate in memory and learning. There is the "top down" approach, generally applied by administering the peptides or their synthetic agonists and antagonists and looking at what happens to animals in spontaneous behaviors or more subtle operant, exploratory, or consummatory behaviors. Although this leads to phenomena, it generally fails to reveal mechanisms or necessary structures for the expression of the response. The opposite approach is from "bottom up"—developing bodies of evidence at the molecular mechanism level for those cells likely to release and respond to peptides, and then devising test paradigms that would reflect on the functional status of these cellular systems. The general practical route of progress has tended to be an eclectic one, moving both from top down and from bottom up simultaneously, and we, therefore, have selected those studies in which such multidisciplinary data bases can be assembled most heuristically.

2 ENDORPHINS

2.1 Opioid Receptor Agonists

The majority of studies in the area of endorphins have employed the strategy of analyzing behaviors after peripheral or central injections of the opiates or the selective antagonist naloxone and inferring from these changes the possible behavioral actions of the endogenous peptide systems. These strategies require the assumption that the natural agonists and synthetic antagonists both act directly and specifically at the same opioid receptors. However, in the case of endorphins, many studies have already suggested that different populations of opiate receptors may exist with different affinities for agonists and antagonists. Martin and colleagues (3, 4) have identified three such receptors, mu, sigma, and kappa. The mu receptor is considered the classical opiate receptor in that morphine-like drugs appear to interact with it; in contrast, dynorphin, a C-terminally extended Leu-enkephalin (5, 6), and certain benzomorphan compounds such as ketocyclazocine appear to act at the kappa receptor (7). Others (8) have identified a fourth receptor, called delta and differentiated from the mu receptor by the enhanced potency of the prototype agonist, D-Ala^2, D-Leu^5, enkephalin, over morphine. Examination of the pharmacological responses of two different *in vitro* physiological preparations provided evidence that there are indeed heterogeneous receptor populations. In the guinea pig ileum, for example, the endorphin peptides appear to interact mainly with the mu receptor, while in the mouse vas deferens, enkephalins probably act more through the putative delta receptor (8). The guinea pig ileum also appears to have more kappa receptors than the mouse *vas deferens*.

In addition, recent findings have called into question the definition of opioid activity by the criterion of naloxone antagonism. Very high concentrations of naloxone also antagonize GABA (9), and naloxone nonreversibility now characterizes at least three classes of well-characterized endorphin or enkephalin action: (i) the behavioral effects of peripheral or central endorphins as observed by Kovacs and De Wied (10) and confirmed by us (see 11) and others (12, 13); (ii) the actions of dynorphin (14, 15) and other sigma or kappa agonists (16, 17) on central or peripheral receptors; and the sites at which beta-endorphin binds to (18) and influences the function of T lymphocytes (19).

2.2 Learning and Memory Actions of Opiates and Endorphins

2.2.1 Opiate Alkaloids and Naloxone

Opiate actions on pain perception have been known for centuries and suggest the primary basis by which opiates can also influence the learning or retention of pain-motivated tasks (20–24). For example, even in studies where the opioid is administered after the presentation of the unconditioned stimulus, its action could conceivably prolong or shorten the motivational state of fear produced by the unconditioned stimulus (25). In early work, morphine disrupted learning and performance of conditioned avoidance responses when injected before testing (20–22, 26) or after the training session (22). The disruption of this avoidance behavior is presumably related to the ability of morphine to reduce the alarm response associated with a conditioned situation motivated by fear or anxiety. Although analgesic doses do produce such effects (20, 26), subanalgesic doses also disrupt acquisition of conditioned avoidance responding (22). Furthermore, withdrawal from morphine improves avoidance responding (22), suggesting that the suppression of the alarm or fear response by morphine may be independent of its analgesic effects.

Consistent with this view are results of studies involving posttraining (consolidation) injections of morphine. Mice injected with morphine or heroin immediately after daily conditioning sessions in a water maze show a naloxone-antagonizable retrograde amnesia for a discriminative avoidance test (23). However, morphine had no effect when injected 2 h after training. Similarly, morphine also produces significant retrograde amnesia in an inhibitory avoidance test with rats (27, 28). When injected intracerebroventricularly immediately after the training (shock) trial a dose of 3.0 ng morphine disrupted retention. In contrast it facilitated retention at a dose of 40 ng (27). Similar results were reported by Stein and Belluzzi (29) at similarly high doses. Interestingly, naloxone increases the latency (time) to reenter the shock compartment in an inhibitory avoidance task (i.e., the opposite results) and facilitates retention of the behavioral response in an active avoidance task (27, 30). These results are consistent with either an increase in the motivational value of the aversive stimulus or a facilitation of associative learning or both. Curiously, little or no work has been reported on the effects of opiates or naloxone on acquisition or retention of appetitively motivated tasks.

Recent work with intracerebral injections of opiates and opiate antagonists has suggested that a specific central endorphinergic neural system may be involved in these opiate effects. Posttraining injections of the opiate agonist levorphanol into the amygdala of rats produced a time-dependent and dose-dependent decrease in the latency of time to reenter the shock compartment in an inhibitory avoidance test (24). These effects appeared to be stereospecific, as dextrophan had no effect. In addition, posttraining administration of naloxone into the amygdala significantly increased the latency to reenter the shock compartment and the combination of levorphanol, and naloxone produced no effect.

Although these results collectively argue for an action of the opiates on the neural processes responsible for the formation of associations, or memory, other explanations cannot be entirely ruled out. For example, as discussed by Gallagher and Kapp (24), it is possible that opiate administration attenuates the "emotional state" associated with aversive situations, particularly the establishment of fear, which presumably outlasts the actual duration of the shock in an inhibitory avoidance task. A theoretical model for this latter explanation of the effects of postconditioning challenge has been proposed (31) and may explain why so many different drugs appear to interfere with the formation of the memory substrate.

2.2.2 Endorphins and Endorphin Analogs: Aversively Motivated Learning

The effects of opiate-like peptides on aversive conditioning are not nearly as clear as those of opiate alkaloids and naloxone. In fact, to a large extent, the results appear to be exactly opposite. In a series of experiments by Rigter and colleagues, endorphins were found to attenuate amnesia in rats after systemic injection (32, 33). Here, beta-endorphin at a low dose (10 μg/rat) injected subcutaneously 1 h before the retention test reversed the disruption of a one-trial inhibitory avoidance task caused by posttraining exposure to carbon dioxide. Like previous results with $ACTH_{4-9}$ (see 34), beta-endorphin only acted when injected 1 h pretest and not when injected 1 h preacquisition. However, extraordinarily low doses of Met- and Leu-enkephalin (0.0003 μg to 30.0 μg/rat, subcutaneously) produced results identical with beta-endorphin when injected 1 h before either the acquisition or the retention test. This attenuation of CO_2-induced amnesia by enkephalins was not reversible by naloxone (32). Although these results are consistent with an interpretation of an antiamnesia action for endorphins (i.e., the opposite of results discussed above with opiates), broader hypotheses regarding changes in arousal, fear motivation, or response to stress were not explored.

Similar results and a similarly difficult interpretation can be found in recent studies by De Wied and his colleagues (34–36). Here peripheral injections of Met-enkephalin, beta-endorphin, and alpha-endorphin (β-LPH$_{61-76}$) all delayed the extinction of a pole jump avoidance task at doses of less than 3.0 μg/rat when injected peripherally and at doses less than 0.1 μg/rat when injected intraventricularly (37). Naltrexone, a long-lasting naloxone, produced the opposite effect, facilitating extinction of the pole jump avoidance task but failing to block the delay in extinction produced by ACTH$_{4-9}$ and alpha-endorphin. These results also appear to be in direct contrast with the memory-enhancing effects of naloxone in the previously cited studies.

Even more curious, gamma-endorphin (β-LPH$_{61-77}$) facilitated the extinction of pole jump avoidance (34, 36). This facilitation of extinction and the fact that Des-Tyr-β-endorphin appeared to have "cataleptogenic" properties similar to haloperidol (36) prompted De Wied to speculate that Des-Tyr-β-endorphin could be an endogenous neuroleptic (10, 34, 35). The differential effects of alpha- and gamma-endorphin on extinction of pole jump avoidance after peripheral injection have been replicated (11), but to date no one aside from the De Wied group has observed cataleptogenic action of Des-Tyr-β-endorphin (38, 39; A. Pert, personal communication).

In contrast with what might be expected from these studies of endorphins given either pretraining or pretest, 40–400 μg/kg Met[5]-enkephalin and Leu[5]-enkephalin, and 4.0 μg/kg D-Ala[2] D-Leu[5]-enkephalin (DADLE) produced morphine-like effects and actually impaired acquisition of an active avoidance task when injected intraperitoneally immediately before a series of eight trials, but it produced no effect when injected 15 min before the training (40). These effects appear therefore to be more opiate-like and thus contrast with other peptide findings listed above and with Rigter's own previous work. Nevertheless, these results reiterate the importance of the time course of training and testing protocols in determining the mechanism of action of peripherally injected endorphins. Indeed it may be that limited penetration into the brain over a short period of time can produce these opiate-like effects.

Several other studies have also attempted to examine the effects of endorphins on retention of inhibitory avoidance, and in general the results appear to be consistent with the findings using carbon-dioxide-induced amnesia and the extinction of active avoidance. Treatment with alpha endorphin 1 h posttraining or preretention, significantly increases latency to re-enter an aversive test chamber, whereas under the same

conditions Des-Tyr-γ-endorphin decreases the latency (36). Similar results were observed in our laboratory, where we have observed that 1 h
preretention treatment with alpha endorphin increased the latency for
reentry whereas gamma endorphin had the opposite effect of decreasing
reentry latency (41).

2.2.3 Endorphin and Endorphin Analogs and Appetitively Motivated Learning

One of the first reports of endorphin learning effects, and the only study
using appetitively motivated learning, indicated that Met⁵-enkephalin
and [D-Ala²]-Met⁵-enkephalin-NH₄ facilitated performance of hungry rats
in a complex 12-choice maze (42), at a dose of 80.0 μg/kg i.p., 15 min
before the test. Interestingly, a Met-enkephalin analog with virtually no
opiate activity [D-Phe²]-Met⁵-enkephalin, also facilitated maze performance, whereas morphine produced the opposite results. This opposite
effect of endorphin peptides and morphine is thus consistent with most
observations on aversive conditioning described above.

We have taken the view that it is essential to extend behavioral observations with peptides to appetitively motivated tasks in order to test
the generality of the conclusions. If the actions of the endorphins were
similar for both the aversive and appetitive tasks, then a primary learning or memory substrate might be proposed as a mechanism of action.
Alternatively, if the effects of the peptides are task-specific, other mechanisms of action such as motivational variables may be more important.

In our laboratory, we examined peptides for ability to alter the extinction of learning motivated by positive reward in order to compare
these effects directly with results obtained with negative reward tasks
[34–37, 43 (De Wied and associates); 11, 41]. In a continuously rein-
forced lever-press task for food reward, alpha-endorphin (30 ng/kg, s.c.)
delayed extinction and gamma-endorphin (30 ng/kg, s.c.) again slightly
facilitated extinction (1, 11). The rats had been trained for 10 days (42),
and on the eleventh day a series of extinction tests were performed every 2 h. As with the active avoidance task, saline or peptide were injected s.c. immediately after the first extinction trial. The peptide-
treated rats were significantly different from control injected rats only
at the first 2 h extinction trial.

A potentially more interesting result, but also one more difficult to
understand, was obtained in a comparable test using water as a reward. Here, rats deprived of water for 23 h/day were trained for 7 days
(one trial per day) to run down an angular alley to lick a water tube for
30 sec. On the eighth day a series of extinction trials were conducted
every 2 h and saline or a peptide was injected (10.0 μg/rat s.c.) after the
first extinction trial. Surprisingly, both alpha- and gamma-endorphin

delayed the extinction of a runway task for water (11). The rats receiving alpha- and gamma-endorphin continued to run to the dry tube even at the fourth extinction trial. In a replication of this water task experiment with gamma-endorphin (11), naloxone (5 mg/kg) not only failed to block the delay in extinction but, in fact, produced similar delays of extinction. The naloxone plus gamma-endorphin group actually ran to the dry tube faster than the gamma-endorphin plus saline group. In both series of water reward experiments, peptide actions on extinction were detectable for 4–6 h after injection.

Thus, in shock motivated tests, alpha-endorphin delays extinction and gamma-endorphin facilitates extinction. Similarly, opposite effects of smaller magnitude were observed in the extinction of a lever press response for food. However, in a water motivated test *both* alpha- and gamma-endorphin delayed extinction. This effect was not blocked by naloxone and, in fact, naloxone appeared to produce results similar to the endorphins. This effect of naloxone would be consistent with the effects observed with naloxone in aversively motivated tasks (see 28).

In summary, opiate alkaloids appear to impair general performance of aversively motivated learning even when injected posttrial in memory tests, whereas naloxone appears to improve performance in similar situations. In dramatic contrast however, exogenously administered opioid peptides, endorphins and enkephalins, appear to reverse amnesia or delay extinction of aversively motivated learned tasks; gamma-endorphin generally produces effects opposite to other endorphins or enkephalins on extinction of either active or passive avoidance. However, when enkephalin analogs are injected immediately before the test session (40) rather than 1 h or more before the test (11, 32, 33, 36, 37), the peptides impair performance like the opiate alkaloids.

With appetitively motivated behavior, the general tendency, seen in a smaller number of studies, is also for endorphins to improve performance or prolong extinction. The results showing differences in the effects of gamma-endorphin on food-motivated vs. water-motivated learning emphasize the need for further studies examining specific motivational states as independent variables. The prolonged effects of peptides on these tasks after subcutaneous injections are difficult to reconcile with the rapid disappearance of endorphins (41) or beta-endorphin from the blood (44). Taken at face value, the behavioral effects of the endorphins appear not to require persistence of the peptide in the blood. Determining the actual active compound, and the site and mechanism by which these peptides produce such delayed effects, is thus of major importance for future work.

The seemingly divergent behavioral results between opiate alkaloids and endorphins are difficult to integrate into a single hypothesis explaining the functional significance of natural endorphins. The role of central endorphins in the relief of pain and in producing behavioral activation is relatively clear, particularly since these effects appear to be naloxone-reversible and since they can be attributed to specific pathways of the central nervous system (45–47). Furthermore, all the endorphin analogs appear to act in the same qualitative direction after *central* injection, yielding analgesia or hyperactivity with varying potencies, and where tested have effects similar to morphine on avoidance learning (29). However, after systemic injection the endorphins can produce effects opposite to that of morphine that in many cases are not naloxone reversible. Whether these effects depend on penetration into the central nervous system is unknown. Also unknown is the relationship between the secondary peripheral physiological effects of endorphins and their subsequent behavioral action following peripheral injection. Similar questions arise in our discussion of the body of evidence accumulated on the behavioral effects of vasopressin-related peptides.

3 VASOPRESSIN

3.1 Classical Endocrinological Actions

Vasopressin, synthesized in the hypothalamo-hypophysial system and released from the posterior pituitary, has the primary physiological action of conserving water, primarily by making the distal renal tubules more permeable to water (for a review, see Sawyer, 48). The usual physiological stimulus for the release of the hormone is dehydration, or plasma hyperosmolarity, and it is generally accepted that osmoreceptors in the region of the brain with the highest concentrations of vasopressin immunoreactivity mediate this response. The other major physiological stimulus for the release of vasopressin is the reduction of the effective plasma volume. A deficiency in vasopressin results in a diuresis of dilute urine, a condition known as diabetes insipidus, and lesions placed anywhere along the hypothalamic neurohypophysial system is associated with permanent diabetes insipidus.

Another important nonrenal action of antidiuretic hormone is its pressor effect (48). This vasopressor effect is mediated directly as vasoconstriction on the smooth muscles of the vascular system (104, 105) and may be physiologically significant during hypovolemic or hypotensive crises (106). This effect also seems to require doses of vasopressin considerably higher than for maximal antidiuresis (49). In other nonrenal actions, vasopressin may function as a releaser of corticotropin (50, 51) in the maintenance of learned avoidance behaviors and in cognitive processing in general (52).

3.2   Learning and Memory Actions of Vasopressin

3.2.1   Effects of Vasopressin on Aversively Motivated Behavior

In early classical work by De Wied and associates, hypophysectomized rats were found to be deficient in a number of behavioral situations, especially the acquisition and extinction of aversively motivated tasks (53), and these deficiencies were reversible by administration of a crude pituitary extract, Pitressin. In later work, arginine vasopressin (AVP) in microgram amounts injected subcutaneously (54) also reversed these deficits.

Further studies then showed that subcutaneous and intracerebroventricular vasopressin delays extinction in active or passive avoidance tasks in normal rats (55–57) and an antivasopressin immune serum injected intracerebroventricularly inhibits retention in the passive avoidance test (58, 59). Arginine vasopressin was reported by the same investigators to enhance retention of the passive (inhibitory) avoidance response when injected subcutaneously either just after the training test (shock) or just before the retention test, but it was not effective at times in between (see 60). This result was interpreted to mean that AVP enhances both consolidation and retrieval of "memory." Finally, rats of the Brattleboro strain expressing a congenital diabetes insipidus, with inability to synthesize vasopressin, were deficient on this passive (inhibitory) avoidance test (52, 54).

Although attempts to replicate these effects of AVP in other laboratories have met with mixed success (61–63), we have reproduced and extended some of the findings of De Wied and associates on active avoidance: both subcutaneous and intracerebroventricular injection of vasopression delayed the extinction of an active avoidance response (64). A pressor antagonist analog of arginine vasopressin, 1-deaminopenicillamine, 2-(o-methyl)tyrosine AVP, [dPTyr (Me)AVP] that prevented the pressor response to subcutaneous AVP (65) also abolished the ability of subcutaneously injected AVP to prolong extinction of active avoidance (66). This dual blockade action of the AVP analog indicates either that signals from peripheral visceral sources may play an important role in the subsequent behavioral changes or that the molecular receptors at which AVP elicits its pressor effect are structurally similar to those leading to its behavioral action.

The hypothesis that vasopressin produces its behavioral effects independently of its classical endocrinological effects has been tested by De Wied and associates. For example, desglycinamide lysine vasopressin, a vasopressin analog that is thought to be practically devoid of classical endocrine activity, has been reported to reverse the behavioral deficits associated with diabetes insipidus (52, 58), to prolong the extinction of pole jump active avoidance (67), and to counteract puromycin and CO_2-induced amnesia (68, 69).

If these effects of desglycinamide vasopressin can be replicated and the lack of peripheral AVP-like actions confirmed, the "nonendocrine" (presumably CNS) effects on behavior would be supported. In contrast, however, recent work in our laboratory has provided evidence that AVP can also produce potent effects on overt behaviors when tested acutely at doses similar to those used in the "memory" experiments. These effects on overt behavior broaden the physiological consequences of AVP actions and highlight the dynamic range of ongoing effects during the memory testing. For example, AVP decreases locomotor activity in a dose-dependent manner (70) and disrupts high rate lever-press responding on a random interval schedule for food reward (71). This latter effect is also reversed by the pressor antagonist dPTyr (Me)AVP and suggests that these doses of AVP are themselves behaviorally disruptive, possibly aversive. This aversive action could reflect the profound hypertensive effects of these doses or other visceral signs associated with altered hemodynamics through the viscera. Consistent with this hypothesis are other observations from our laboratory showing that AVP, in the same dose range, can produce conditioned taste and place aversions (70). In all of the conditions examined to date, desglycinamide AVP has had no action at all. These disruptive and aversive effects of AVP make more important the nature of the task used to determine "memory-enhancing" properties, given that virtually all the data regarding a role for vasopressin in learning come from studies employing aversively motivated tasks. Obviously this limits the nature of the *behavioral* conclusions that can be drawn from such data, and if vasopressin does have "memory" enhancing properties, this effect should also be demonstrable using positively motivated tasks. We next examine such reported effects.

3.2.2   Vasopressin and Appetitively Motivated Learning

Two reports in the literature do, in fact, show some prolongation of extinction of appetitive learning with vasopressin. Rats trained to discriminate sides of a T-maze using a sex reward showed facilitated retention with desglycinamide-lysine vasopressin (60), and rats receiving vasopressin during acquisition training in a black-white discrimination T-maze task showed delayed extinction, but only on the side using the black discriminative stimulus (72). In addition, preliminary experiments in our laboratory (70) have shown that posttraining administration of vasopressin can facilitate subsequent test performance in a one-trial water-finding task initially described by Major and White (73). Curiously enough, however, LiCl—in doses known to be sufficient to produce conditioned taste and place aversion—produces similar effects. Resolution of the relative contribution of these aversive effects of AVP to the "memory" enhancement observed in learning situations will require more effort directed at appetitively motivated tasks where the unconditioned stimulus is not itself aversive. Moreover, the relative contribution of endogenously released AVP, with its accompanying physiological changes, is still unknown, and those effects could also affect behavior. Other untested hypotheses include a direct behavioral role for the AVP- or oxytocin-containing hypothalamic projections to limbic structures such as the septal area, hippocampus, and brain stem regions (locus coeruleus, parabrachial nuclei, and nucleus tractus solitarius) (74).

3.2.3   Site of Action for Vasopressin

Consistent with a hypothesis involving a central nervous system site of action for vasopressin is a series of studies implicating the limbic system in the mechanism of action of vasopressin (52, 59). For example, intracerebral injections of vasopressin into limbic areas prolonged the extinction of active avoidance as seen with peripheral injections (59); and lesions of the dorsal hippocampus attenuated the effects of vasopressin on avoidance behavior (52, 76).

Furthermore, other studies have implicated a specific neurochemical substrate in the limbic system, the dorsal noradrenergic system, in the effects of vasopressin on avoidance behavior (77–82). Initial observations showed that vasopressin injected peripherally and intraventricularly increased apparent turnover of catecholamines in these limbic areas (77–79). More recent work has shown that blockade by central noradrenaline synthesis also blocked the facilitatory action of vasopressin on passive avoidance behavior (79) and on the delayed extinction of active avoidance behavior (80). More specific involvement of a noradrenergic substrate was shown in a complementary study where 6-hydroxydopamine lesions of the dorsal noradrenergic bundle also blocked the facilitation of passive avoidance behavior produced by vasopressin when injected immediately after the learning trial (82, 83).

Further analysis of this hypothesis has revealed a complicated putative relationship between the dorsal noradrenergic system, the dorsal raphe nucleus, and the locus coeruleus, the cell bodies of origin of the dorsal noradrenergic bundle. Vasopressin facilitates avoidance behavior when injected in picogram amounts (25–50 pg) into the dentate gyrus, dorsal septum, and dorsal raphe, all terminal regions of locus coeruleus neurons; but this effect does not occur when AVP is injected into the locus coeruleus itself (82, 83). Moreover, both 6-hydroxydopamine and the serotonin neurotoxin, 5,6 dihydroxytryptamine, when injected into the region of the dorsal raphe nucleus reportedly will prevent the standard facilitation of passive avoidance behavior normally observed by these scientists with AVP (83). A more detailed analysis of this hypothesis can be found in Kovacs et al. (83).

These results provide reasonably compelling evidence that centrally administered vasopressin can also produce behavioral effects on aversively motivated tasks that mimic the effects of peripheral injections. In addition, although somewhat complicated in its interactions, there appears to be an important role for the dorsal noradrenergic system in these AVP effects in the central nervous system.

In contrast with these effects, our recent results showing that a vasopressin-pressor antagonist can also reverse the facilitation of aversively motivated behavior caused by peripheral vasopressin raised the issue of intervening physiological responses as causal in vasopressin behavioral action. Whether similar physiological signals can accompany or precede direct central nervous system action of vasopressin needs to be determined. Indeed, central nervous system injection of vasopressin can produce a pressor response (84). Interestingly, others have concluded that the altered catecholamine metabolism in the brainstem induced by intraventricularly injected vasopressin is due to its action on blood pressure regulation (77, 85).

3.2.4 Clinical Studies

Recent clinical observations have demonstrated that lysine vasopressin, the natural vasopressin of swine, can improve performance in tests involving attention, concentration, and memory in double blind studies involving aged subjects. Others have also reported improvements in retrograde and anterograde amnesia with lysine vasopressin (75, 86). In two recent double-blind studies, a synthetic analog of vasopressin, 1-desamino-D-arginine-8 vasopressin (DDAVP) produced consistent improvements in tests designed to measure long-term memory in patients suffering from affective illness; DDAVP also produced improvements in serial learning, prompted free recall, and prompted recall of semantically related words in both cognitively impaired and unimpaired adults (87, 88). But in animal studies, the substitution of D-Arg for L-Arg markedly decreases the potency to alter extinction of pole jump avoidance behavior (67). Whether this reflects species differences in response to vasopressin or a difference in the nature of the behavioral tests remains to be determined.

In summary, vasopressin and vasopressin analogs clearly alter the maintenance of learned behavior, but as with opioid peptides, these effects appear largely in situations involving motivation by aversive events. Furthermore, when tested on spontaneous behaviors, doses of AVP that alter active or passive extinction rates are found to be directly aversive. Intriguingly, stressful aversive situations can themselves lead to a release of vasopressin and endorphins from the pituitary.

Equally intriguing is the possibility of a link between some primary peripheral hormonal actions of vasopressin and subsequent secondary behavioral actions. Peripheral antecedent events have not yet been
identified in the case of the pituitary-derived endorphins. But recent
studies with a synthetic corticotropin releasing factor (89) known to be
capable of releasing pituitary corticotropin and endorphin may provide
a key link in this schemata of the brain-pituitary role in adaptive behavior. For this reason we shall now discuss some preliminary
nonlearning/memory behavioral effects of corticotropin releasing factor.

4 CORTICOTROPIN RELEASING FACTOR (CRF)

4.1 Classical Endocrinological Actions

After nearly 30 years of intense effort, a corticotropin releasing factor
(CRF) with high potency and intrinsic activity for *in vitro* and *in vivo*
stimulation of ACTH and β-endorphin has been characterized and synthesized by Vale and his associates (89). This 41-residue peptide stimulates the secretion of corticotropin-like and beta-endorphin-like
immunoactivities by cultured anterior pituitary cells (89), and peripherally injected CRF can produce significant elevations of plasma ACTH
(90).

In addition, CRF appears to act centrally to activate the sympathetic
nervous system. Brown et al. (91) administered CRF intracerebroventricularly to rats and found that it produced prolonged elevation of plasma
epinephrine, norepinephrine, and glucose. In addition, they observed an
increase in motor activity and oxygen consumption. These investigators
noted that the physiological changes produced by CRF are similar to effects observed in animals in response to stress.

4.2 The Stress Response

The general concepts of stress theory have undergone little modification
and refinement over the past 40 years. Most investigators would still
generally define "stress" as the response of the pituitary-adrenocortical
system to a wide variety of physical and psychological stimuli. These
stimuli are conveyed via humoral or neural pathways to the anterior pituitary, which responds with secretion of ACTH. The secretion of
ACTH is in turn controlled primarily by one or more corticotropin releasing factors secreted by cells in the hypothalamus (89). ACTH stimulates the adrenal cortex to secrete glucocorticoids that have widespread
effects on metabolism, such as gluconeogenesis, hyperinsulinemia, lysis
of lymphoid tissue, increased gastric secretion, and reduced inflamma-

tory and antibody responses. The glucocorticoids decrease ACTH production by a negative feedback on the hypothalamus and pituitary. These physiological changes in response to increased hypothalamo-pituitary action are also paralleled by alterations in behavior. For example, some authors have argued that ACTH can act as an anxiogenic (92) and that corticosteroids can act as anxiolytic agents in rats (93).

Efforts to identify the antecedent physiological mechanisms of the hypothalamo-pituitary "stress responses" have commonly defined two categories of stress: systemic and neurogenic. Systemic stress is defined as a stress that activates ACTH release by a direct hormonal action on the pituitary, presumably via the median eminence, whereas neurogenic stress is a stress that activates ACTH release by an indirect action on the pituitary via neural connections. This distinction is based on the observation that complete or partial hypothalamic deafferentation or localized hypothalamic lesions can abolish or reduce the adrenocortical response to photic, acoustic, olfactory, and peripheral nerve stimulation, whereas such lesions do not alter the adrenocortical response to systemic stresses such as ether stress or injection of epinephrine (94, 99). Indeed, it is through these central nervous system pathways to the hypothalamus that presumably the adrenocortical response is triggered by psychological factors and may also be the basis for the autonomic arousal associated with anxiety. But there is one alternative means by which behavioral or physiological responses to stress or anxiety might be mediated by hypothalamic-pituitary system in an organism, that is, via direct neurotropic action of CRF in the central nervous system itself. Thus, just as pathways project from the limbic areas to the hypothalamus to activate the pituitary–adrenal axis via CRF, so might CRF feed back to these same areas to mediate appropriate behavioral responses to stress.

These observations of extrahypothalamic control of the corticosteroid response, and preliminary histological evidence suggesting that terminals containing immunoreactive CRF are located in pontine and diencephalic brain regions (100), suggest possible reciprocal connections between CRF and extrahypothalamic structures. This hypothesized relationship makes even more compelling the possibility that CRF mediates some behavioral responses to stress.

4.3 Behavioral Actions of CRF

Indeed, recent work in our laboratories has demonstrated that CRF injected intracerebroventricularly in rats produces a dose-dependent locomotor activation in rats that could not be reproduced by peripheral injection. Besides increases in normal locomotion and sniffing, the rats injected with CRF (dose range 0.015–1.5 nmol) exhibit some unique behavior that appears to reflect a general behavioral activation, such as a bizarre elevated-hindlimb walking and rhythmic forward-and-backward walking (101).

Although other peptides such as the endorphins and ACTH have been shown to produce increases in spontaneous behavioral activity, the nature of the CRF response differs substantially from the responses observed with these other peptides (102, 103). CRF does not produce the initial depressant phase followed by bursts of locomotor activity that characterizes i.c.v. injections of opioid peptides (103), nor does CRF produce the "stretching-yawning syndrome" observed after intraventricular injection of ACTH (102). In contrast, the activation by CRF at the lower doses appeared to be an exaggeration of the normal activation produced by introduction of the animal into a familiar environment.

Rats were also tested in a novel open field following i.c.v. injection of similar doses of CRF 0.0015–0.15 nmol; they showed responses that were consistent with an increased emotionally or increased sensitivity to the stressful aspects of the situation. Here the rats showed *decreases* in locomotion and rearing. Typically a rat injected with 0.15 nmol of CRF and placed 60 min later in the open field moved hesitantly to the outer squares and then either circled the open field remaining nose to the floor or remained in one of the corners grooming or hesitantly moving forward or backward. In contrast, saline-injected animals rapidly circled the open field, rearing and exploring, and eventually made forays into the inner squares of the center of the open field. (101).

These preliminary results suggest that CRF acts centrally to produce a dose-dependent behavioral activation in a familiar environment where control rats rapidly habituate and go to sleep. In contrast, in a novel, more stressful environment rats show behavior consistent with an increase in the stress of the situation. These results are consistent with the hypothesis that CRF in the brain may play a behavioral role consonant with its hypothesized function in the classical endocrine response to stress.

Of future interest will be to determine whether this activation can facilitate learning and, if so, under what conditions. Equally intriguing will be the pursuit of interactions among circulating steroids, endorphins, and vasopressin, and the physiological and behavioral actions of CRF.

5 CONCLUSIONS

At the outset of this examination of the behavioral effects of endorphins, opiate alkaloids, vasopressin, and corticotropin releasing factor, we stipulated that although we were certain these substances could significantly regulate learned or spontaneous behaviors, we also had no firm idea how they did so. Having reached this point in our coverage, it is quite likely the persistent reader will be ready to accept this unsatisfying conclusion. Although the determination of how peptides given peripherally or centrally can affect behavior remains a complex problem, it is at the very least now possible to begin to make a list of testable alternatives. A first step in doing so requires that we reiterate the view that there is no basic understanding of what happens in molecular or cellular terms when we say "learning has taken place" or "memory is being tested."

As a result of this lack of understanding of the mechanisms of this fundamental behavioral phenomenon, it becomes almost impossible to exclude the possibility that these peptides do represent some sort of "memory" or "learning" peptide, either in their native form (i.e., as released by the lobes of the pituitary or the neurons terminating in the median eminence) or in a processed form devoid of detectable endocrine actions. Those who feel that the existing data support such a conclusion on the basis of the effects of exogenously administered peptides have the problem of demonstrating that such actions can also be attributed to the naturally formed peptides in the concentration ranges that can be found during normal physiological variations. Thus, one awaits with interest determinations of the amounts of vasopressin or endorphin normally found within rat or human cerebrospinal fluid and the degree to which the normal ranges of these peptides are altered by injections of what sound like vanishingly small amounts of exogenous peptides.

Given that the plasma ranges of these peptides are known for the conditions of stress or dehydration that provoke their physiologic secretion, it seems clear from available data that the doses given subcutaneously are probably orders of magnitude above the physiologically attained ceilings. Thus, at least in these cases of peripherally injected peptides, one would appear to be dealing with pharmacological actions on behavior, and the site of that series of actions remains unclear. Our view, based heavily on the ability to antagonize the behavioral actions of AVP by a peptide analog able to prevent the early blood pressure effects of behaviorally active doses of AVP, is that nonphysiological visceral signals, such as an inappropriate epoch of hypertension, can in and of itself produce an aversive arousal (as indicated by the homology between the effects on spontaneous behaviors of AVP and LiCl). Until such nonspecific arousing type effects can be eliminated from the repertoire of actions of peptides that influence behavior, we feel that it is unnecessary to postulate peptides acting as memory hormones. Future work may profitably concentrate on the means by which the neuroendocrine and visceral regulatory axes of the brain monitor the results of executive commands to secrete pituitary and peripheral hormones for maintenance of the internal mileu, and may profitably examine whether even "nonendocrine" metabolites of active peptides are able to function as feedback signals.

REFERENCES

1. G. F. Koob, M. LeMoal, and F. E. Bloom, in J. L. Martinez et al., Eds., *Endogenous Peptides and Learning and Memory Processes*, Academic Press, New York, 1981, pp. 249.
2. G. F. Koob and F. E. Bloom, *Annu. Rev. Physiol.* **44**, 571 (1982).
3. W. R. Martin, C. G. Eades, J. A. Thompson, R. E. Huppler, and P. E. Gilbert, *J. Pharmacol. Exp. Ther.* **197**, 517 (1976).
4. P. E. Gilbert and W. R. Martin, *J. Pharmacol. Exp. Ther.* **198**, 66 (1963).
5. A. Goldstein, S. Tachibana, L. I. Lowney, M. Hunkapiller, and L. Hood, *Proc. Natl. Acad. Sci. USA* **76**, 6666 (1979).
6. A. Goldstein, W. Fischli, L. I. Lowney, M. Hunkapiller, and L. Hood, *Proc. Natl. Acad. Sci. USA* **78**, 7219 (1981).
7. C. Chavkin, I. F. James, and A. Goldstein, *Science* **215**, 413 (1982).
8. J. A. H. Lord, A. A. Waterfield, J. Hughes, and H. W. Kosterlitz, *Nature* **267**, 495 (1977).
9. R. Dingledine, L. L. Iversen, and E. Breuker, *Eur. J. Pharmacol.* **47**, 19 (1978).
10. G. L. Kovacs and D. De Wied, in J. L. Martinez et al., Eds., *Endogenous Peptides and Learning and Memory Processes*, Academic Press, New York, 1981, pp. 231–248.
11. M. LeMoal, G. F. Koob, and F. E. Bloom, *Life Sci.* **24**, 1631 (1979).
12. I. Izquierdo, M. L. Perry, and R. D. Dias, in J. L. Martinez et al., Eds., *Endogenous Peptides and Learning and Memory Processes*, Academic Press, New York, 1981, pp. 269–290.
13. F. E. Bloom and D. S. Segal, in J. H. Wood, Ed., *Neurobiology of the Cerebrospinal Fluid*, Plenum Press, New York, 1980, pp. 651–664.
14. R. S. Zukin and S. R. Zukin, *Life Sci.* **26**, 2681 (1981).
15. C. Chavkin and A. Goldstein, *Nature* **293**, 591 (1981).
16. B. L. Wolozin and G. W. Pasternak, *Proc. Natl. Acad. Sci. USA* **78**, 6181 (1981).
17. R. Schulz, M. Wuster, and A. Herz, *Pharmacol. Biochem. Behav.* **14**, 75 (1981).
18. E. Hazum, K. -J. Chang, and P. Cuatrecasas, *Science* **205**, 1033 (1978).
19. S. Gilman, J. Schwartz, R. Milner, J. Feldman, and F. Bloom, *Proc. Natl. Acad. Sci. USA*, in press (1982).
20. L. Cook and E. Weidley, *N.Y. Acad. Sci.* **66**, 740 (1957).
21. E. F. Domino, A. J. Karoly, and F. L. Walker, *J. Pharmacol. Exp. Ther.* **41**, 92 (1963).
22. U. Banerjee, *Psychopharmacology* **22**, 133 (1956).
23. C. Castellano, *Psychopharmacologia (Berlin)* **42**, 235 (1975).
24. M. Gallagher and B. S. Kapp, *Life Sci.* **23**, 1973 (1978).
25. K. J. Chang and Cuatrecasas, *J. Biol. Chem.* **254**, 2610 (1979).
26. T. Verhave, J. E. Owen, and E. B. Robbins, *J. Pharmacol. Exp. Ther.* **125**, 248 (1959).
27. R. A. Jensen, J. L. Martinez, R. B. Messing, V. Speihler, B. J. Vasquez, B. Soumireu-Mourat, K. C. Liang, and J. L. McGaugh, *Soc. Neurosci. Abstr.* **4**, 260 (1978).
28. R. B. Messing, R. A. Jensen, J. L. Martinez Jr., V. R. Spiehler, B. J. Vasquez, B. Soumireu-Mourat, D. C. Liang, and J. L. McGaugh, *Behav. Neural Biol.* **27**, 266 (1979).
29. L. Stein and J. D. Belluzzi, in M. Trabucchi, Ed., *Advances in Biochemical Psychopharmacology*, Vol. 18, Raven Press, New York, 1978.
30. R. B. Messing, R. Jensen, B. J. Vasquez, J. L. Martinez, V. R. Spiehler, and J. L. McGaugh, in J. L. Martinez et al., Eds., *Endogenous Peptides and Learning and Memory Processes*, Academic Press, New York, 1981, pp. 431–444.
31. A. A. Spevak and M. D. Suboski, *Psychol. Bull.* **72**, 66 (1969).
32. H. Rigter, H. Greven, and H. Van Riezen, *Neuropharmacology* **16**, 545 (1977).
33. H. Rigter, *Science* **200**, 83 (1978).

34. D. De Wied, J. M. Van Ree, and H. M. Greven, *Life Sci.* **26**, 1575 (1980).
35. D. De Wied, B. Bohus, J. M. Van Ree, G. L. Kovacs, and H. M. Greven, *Lancet* **1**, 1046 (1978).
36. D. De Wied, G. L. Kovacs, B. Bohus, J. M. Van Ree, and H. M. Greven, *Eur. J. Pharmacol.* **49**, 427 (1978b).
37. D. De Wied, B. Bohus, J. M. Van Ree, and I. Urban, *J. Pharmacol. Exp. Ther.* **204**, 570 (1978c).
38. S. B. Weinberger, A. Arnstein, and D. C. Segal, *Life Sci.* **24**, 1637 (1979).
39. M. LeMoal, O. Gaffori, J. Rossier, N. Ling, G. F. Koob, and F. E. Bloom, *Soc. Neurosci. Abstr.* **6**, 319 (1980).
40. H. Rigter, T. J. Hannan, R. B. Messing, J. L. Martinez, Jr., B. J. Vasquez, R. A. Jensen, J. Veliquette, and J. L. McGaugh, *Life Sci.* **26**, 337 (1980).
41. S. J. Mason and S. D. Iversen, *J. Comp. Physiol. Psychol.* **91**, 165 (1977).
42. A. J. Kastin, E. L. Scollan, M. G. King, A. V. Schally, and D. H. Coy, *Pharmacol. Biochem. Behav.* **5**, 691 (1976).
43. D. De Wied, *Life Sci.* **20**, 195 (1977).
44. R. A. Houghten, R. W. Swann, and C. H. Li, *Proc. Natl. Acad. Sci. USA* **77**, 4588 (1980).
45. H. Takagi, M. Satoh, A. Akaike, T. Shibata, H. Yasima, and H. Ogawa, *Eur. J. Pharmacol.* **49**, 113 (1978).
46. A. E. Kelley, L. Stinus, and S. D. Iversen, *Behav. Brain Res.* **1**, 3 (1980).
47. L. Stinus, G. F. Koob, N. Ling, F. E. Bloom, and M. Le Moal, *Proc. Natl. Acad. Sci. USA* **77**, 2323 (1980).
48. W. J. Sawyer, *Endocrinology* **75**, 981 (1964).
49. M. B. Strauss, *Body Water in Man: The Acquisition and Maintenance of the Body Fluids*, Little Brown, Boston, 1957, p. 286.
50. A. F. Pearlmutter, E. Rapino, and M. Saffran, *Neuroendocrinology* **15**, 106 (1974).
51. G. E. Gillies and P. J. Lowry, *Nature* **278**, 463 (1979).
52. T. J. B. Van Wimersma Greidanus, B. Bohus, and D. De Wied, *Prog. Brain Res.* **42**, 135 (1975).
53. D. De Wied, *Int. J. Neuropharmacol.* **4**, 157 (1965).
54. B. Bohus, T. J. B. Van Wimersma Greidanus, and D. De Wied, *Physiol. Behav.* **14**, 609 (1975).
55. D. De Wied, *Nature* **232**, 58 (1971).
56. R. Ader and D. De Wied, *Psychonomic Sci.* **29**, 46 (1972).
57. D. De Wied, *Life Sci.* **46**, 27 (1976).
58. T. B. Van Wimersma Greidanus, J. Dogterom, and D. De Wied, *Life Sci.* **16**, 637 (1975).
59. T. B. Van Wimersma Greidanus and D. De wied, *Behav. Biol.* **18**, 325 (1976).
60. B. Bohus, *Horm. Behav.* **8**, 52 (1977).
61. J. F. Celestian, R. J. Carey, and M. Miller, *Physiol. Behav.* **15**, 707 (1975).
62. W. H. Bailey and J. M. Weiss, *Brain Res.* **162**, 174 (1979).
63. G. Hostetter, S. L. Jubb, and G. P. Kozlowski, *Neuroendocrinol.* **30**, 174 (1980).
64. G. F. Koob, M. Le Moal, O. Gaffori, M. Manning, W. H. Sawyer, J. Rivier, and F. E. Bloom, *Regul. Peptides* **2**, 153 (1981).
65. K. Bankoski, M. Manning, J. Haldar, and W. H. Sawyer, *J. Med. Chem.* **21**, 850 (1978).
66. M. Le Moal, G. F. Koob, L. Y. Koda, F. E. Bloom, M. Manning, W. H. Sawyer, and J. Rivier, *Nature* **291**, 491 (1981).
67. R. Walter, J. M. Van Ree, and D. De Wied, *Proc. Natl. Acad. Sci. USA* **75**, 2493 (1978).
68. S. Lande, T. B. Flexner, and L. L. Flexner, *Proc. Natl. Acad. Sci. USA* **69**, 558 (1972).
69. H. Rigter, H. Van Riezen, and D. De Wied, *Physiol. Behav.* **13**, 381 (1974).

70. A. Ettenberg, D. Van der Kooy, G. F. Koob, M. Le Moal, and F. E. Bloom, *Behav. Brain Res.*, in press.

71. J. Wenger, G. F. Koob, and F. E. Bloom, *Regul. Peptides*, in press.

72. G. Hostetter, S. L. Jubb, and G. P. Kozlowski, *Life Sci.* **21**, 1323 (1977).

73. R. Major and N. White, *Physiol. Behav.* **20**, 723 (1978).

74. L. Swanson and G. J. Mogenson, *Brain Res. Rev.* **3**, 11 (1981).

75. J. J. Legros, D. Gilot, X. Seron, A. Claessens, J. M. Moeglen, A. Audibert, and P. Berchier, *Lancet* **1**, 41 (1978).

76. T. B. Van Wimersma Greidanus and D. De Wied, *Pharmacol. Biochem. Behav.* **5**, 29 (1976).

77. M. Tanaka, E. R. De Kloet, D. De Wied, and D. H. G. Versteeg, *Life Sci.* **20**, 1799 (1977).

78. M. Tanaka, D. H. G. Versteeg, and D. De Wied, *Neurosci. Lett.* **4**, 321 (1977).

79. G. L. Kovacs, L. Vecsei, G. Szabo, and G. Telegdy, *Neurosci. Lett.* **5**, 337 (1977).

80. G. Telegdy and G. L. Kovacs, in M. A. B. Brazier, Ed., *Brain Mechanisms in Memory and Learning: From Single Neuron to Man*, IBRO Monograph Series, Vol. 4, Raven Press, New York, 1979.

81. G. L. Kovacs, B. Bohus, and D. H. G. Versteeg, *Brain Res.* **172**, 73 (1979).

82. G. L. Kovacs, B. Bohus, D. H. G. Versteeg, E. R. Kloet, and D. De Wied, *Brain Res.* **175**, 303 (1979).

83. G. L. Kovacs, B. Bohus, and D. H. G. Versteeg, *Neurosci.* **4**, 1529 (1979).

84. H. Matsuguchi, F. M. Sharabi, F. J. Gordon, A. K. Johnson, and P. G. Schmid, *Neuropharmacol.* **21**, 687 (1982).

85. J. M. Van Ree, B. Bohus, D. H. G. Versteeg, and D. De Wied, *Biochem. Pharmacol.* **28**, 1793 (1978).

86. J. C. Oliveros, M. K. Jandali, R. R. Timsit-Berthier, A. Benghezal, A. Audibert, and J. H. Moeglen, *Lancet* **1**, 42 (1978).

87. P. W. Gold, H. Weingartner, J. C. Ballenger, F. K. Goodwin, and R. M. Post, *Lancet* **2**, 992 (1979).

88. H. Weingartner, P. Gold, J. C. Ballenger, S. A. Smallberg, R. Summers, D. R. Rubinow, R. M. Post, and F. K. Goodwin, *Science* **211**, 601 (1981).

89. W. Vale, J. Spiess, C. Rivier, and J. Rivier, *Science* **213**, 1394 (1981).

90. C. Rivier, J. Rivier, J. Speiss, and W. Vale, *Endocrinology* **110**, 272 (1982).

91. M. Brown, L. Fisher, J. Rivier, J. Spiess, C. Rivier, and W. Vale, *Life Sci.* **30**, 207 (1982).

92. S. File, *Brain Res.* **171**, 157 (1979).

93. S. File, S. Vellucci, and S. Wendland, *J. Pharm. Pharmacol.* **31**, 300 (1979).

94. N. Conforti and S. Feldman, *Neuroendocrinology* **22**, 1 (1976).

95. S. Feldman, N. Conforti, and I. Chowers, *Neuroendocrinology* **10**, 316 (1972).

96. S. Feldman and N. Conforti, *J. Endocrinol.* **69**, 165 (1976).

97. S. Feldman and N. Conforti, *Neuroendocrinology* **24**, 162 (1977).

98. S. Feldman and N. Conforti, *Neuroendocrinology* **30**, 52 (1980).

99. S. Feldman and N. Conforti, *Neuroscience* **5**, 1323 (1980).

100. F. E. Bloom, E. Battenberg, J. Rivier, and W. Vale, *Regul. Peptides* **4**, 43 (1982).

101. S. Sutton, G. F. Koob, M. LeMoal, J. Rivier, and W. Vale, *Nature* **297**, 331 (1982).

102. A. J. Dunn, E. J. Green, and R. L. Isaacson, *Science* **203**, 281 (1979).

103. D. S. Segal, R. Browne, F. E. Bloom, N. Ling, and R. Guillemin, *Science* **198**, 411 (1977).

104. B. M. Altura, *Am. J. Physiol.* **212**, 1447 (1967).

105. E. Monos, R. B. Cox, and L. H. Peterson, *Am. J. Physiol.* **234**, H167 (1978).

106. M. Rocha, E. Silva, Jr., and M. Rosenberg, *J. Physiol.* **202**, 535 (1969).

17

Reproduction: The Central Nervous System Role of Luteinizing Hormone Releasing Hormone

BRENDA D. SHIVERS

RICHARD E. HARLAN

DONALD W. PFAFF

The Rockefeller University
New York, New York

1   INTRODUCTION

Two principal challenges confront all organisms: preservation of self
and preservation of kind. Multicellular organisms that employ sexual reproduction as a means of preserving kind must assess many factors before accepting the costs of reproducing. Two major systems, the neural
and endocrine, are responsible first for assessing whether the reproductive risks are to be accepted and then for integrating a broad range of
physiological and behavioral responses. There are at least three reasons
that the integration of the reproductive effort in the vertebrate is hierar-
chically organized, with the upper level (or levels) of organization located in the central nervous system: (i) All existing experimental evidence
suggests that to achieve the sophisticated degree of regulation evident
in and necessary for reproduction, a hierarchical organization is required. (ii) Much of the incoming environmental information utilizes
sensory (neural) pathways, which converge in the central nervous system. (iii) Rapid responsiveness is often required, and the shorter time
constants that characterize nerve cells permit these cells to alter their
signals faster than endocrine cells. Within this hierarchy of controls, luteinizing hormone releasing hormone (LHRH) constitutes a signaling
system recognized to play important roles in the central regulation of
reproduction in vertebrates. In this chapter we review the information
currently available on this neuropeptide.

2   WHICH COMPONENTS OF REPRODUCTION ARE LHRH-
PRODUCING CELLS ORGANIZED TO SUBSERVE?

2.1   Pituitary Secretion

It has been known since the 1930s that the central nervous system plays
an integral role in the maintenance of reproduction (1–3). Harris (4) postulated that this action of the brain is mediated through the release of
substances that act on the pituitary, and McCann (5) first demonstrated
the existence of a hypothalamic substance that stimulates pituitary release of luteinizing hormone (LH). The amino acid sequence of this dec-

apeptide was determined in the early 1970s (6–8). This peptide has been demonstrated to stimulate release of both LH and follicle stimulating hormone (FSH) in all species examined. However, the existence of a possible FSH-releasing hormone remains controversial (9). Regardless of this controversy, it is clear that a major function of LHRH is to stimulate the release of pituitary gonadotrophins, which then maintain testicular function in males and stimulate ovarian folliculogenesis and ovulation in females.

2.2   Female Sexual Behavior

LHRH may also be involved in the species-specific behaviors necessary for reproduction to occur. Systemic injection of LHRH into ovariectomized, estrogen-treated rats facilitates lordotic responsiveness (10, 11), an easily quantifiable index of sexual receptivity (12). Since this effect is not dependent on the presence of the pituitary (11), a direct action of the peptide on the central nervous system is indicated. Neural sites at which LHRH was reported to facilitate lordotic responsiveness include the preoptic area and ventromedial hypothalamus but not the cerebral cortex or lateral hypothalamus (13). Additional studies have indicated that a neural site at which LHRH is particularly effective in facilitating lordotic responsiveness is the midbrain, especially in the central gray (14, 15). That LHRH may play a physiological role in the midbrain central gray is supported by the dramatic and prolonged lordosis-inhibitory effect of antiserum to LHRH when infused into the dorsal midbrain (15). Moreover, the presence of a descending LHRH fiber system around the ventral-lateral walls of the cerebral aqueduct (16, 17) provides a morphological basis for such a behavioral effect. Our immunocytochemical evidence suggesting increased release of LHRH in the midbrain central gray in estrogen-treated rats (see Section 5.2.2) is consistent with a physiological role for LHRH in facilitating lordotic responsiveness. Lesion, stimulation, and electrophysiological studies also implicate the midbrain central gray as an important site where estrogen-sensitive hypothalamic neurons may modify the neuronal circuitry for lordosis (18–22).

It is unlikely that the decapeptide LHRH is the only neuroactive substance that facilitates estrogen-induced alterations in the functional activity of the neural circuitry producing lordosis. Estrogen action limited to the ventromedial hypothalamus is sufficient to prime neural substrates for a lordosis-facilitating action of progesterone (23, 24). However, very few LHRH cell bodies can be found in or around the ventromedial nucleus (Figure 1D), where estrogen has its prime effect on lordosis. Moreover, LHRH cannot *substitute* for estrogen but rather acts only when estrogen has been administered previously (10, 11). Finally, the number of LHRH fibers in the midbrain central gray is small;

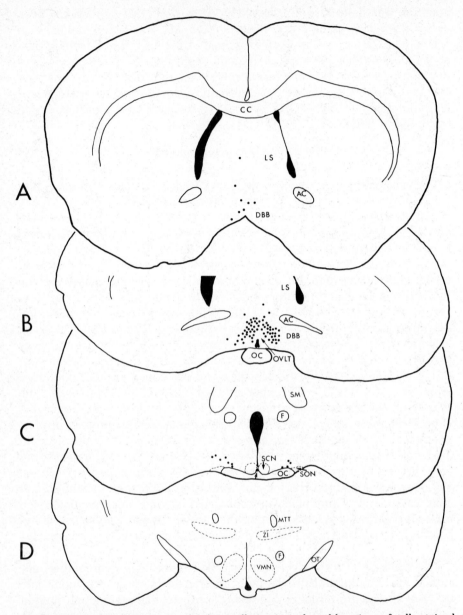

Figure 1. Drawings of four coronal sections illustrating selected locations of cells stained with antiserum to LHRH in an intact male rat. Each section represents 90 μm of tissue. Each dot represents one LHRH cell. Abbreviations: AC, anterior commissure; CC, corpus callosum; DBB, diagonal bands of Broca; F, fornix; LS, lateral septum; MIT, mamillothalamic tract; OC, optic chiasm; OT, optic tract; OVLT, organum vasculosum lamina terminalis; SCN, suprachiasmatic nucleus; SM, stria medullaris; SON, supraoptic nucleus; VMN, ventromedial nucleus; ZI, zona incerta. From Shivers, Harlan, Morrell and Pfaff, manuscript in preparation.

usually fewer than 15 separate LHRH axon fragments can be visualized in a coronal section through the midbrain central gray. Relatively small quantities of LHRH in the midbrain central gray have also been demonstrated by radioimmunoassay (25).

LHRH analogs that have an agonistic or antagonistic action on the pituitary do not always have similar effects on lordotic responsiveness (26; Sakuma and Pfaff, manuscript in preparation). This may be due to differences among target sites in receptor requirements and/or degradative controls.

The concept of a particular neural system having a role in a specific function can be strengthened if evidence is accumulated to indicate that the neural system and the function have been conserved phylogenetically. For instance, the basic pattern of estrogen-concentrating cells in the brain has been well conserved in vertebrate evolution (27). Thus, LHRH has been reported to facilitate sexual receptivity in doves (28), lizards (29), and frogs (30), in addition to rats. The LHRH molecule extracted from rat hypothalami behaves similarly in radioimmunoassay and chromatography procedures to that extracted from frogs but slightly differently from that extracted from birds and reptiles (31). Thus, it is possible that administration of native LHRH in birds and reptiles would facilitate sexual receptivity to a greater degree than does synthetic LHRH.

2.3 Male Sexual Behavior

A role of LHRH in male sexual performance has also been suggested. Moss et al. (32) reported that LHRH given to gonadally intact male rats decreased the latency to intromission and ejaculation, whereas LHRH given to castrated males receiving subthreshold doses of testosterone decreased the latency to ejaculation. However, such a behavior-enhancing effect of subcutaneous administration of LHRH in male rats has been difficult to replicate (33). Although specific neural sites for an action of LHRH on masculine sexual performance have not been identified, administration of LHRH into the lateral ventricle has been reported to facilitate mounting behavior in a paradigm designed to measure sexual arousal in intact male rats (34). A facilitatory effect of LHRH on species-specific masculine reproductive behaviors has been difficult to document in ring doves (35), chimpanzees (36), and normal human males (37).

2.4 Non-Neural LHRH and Reproduction

Recent evidence for the production or presence of LHRH in non-neural organs suggests that the peptide may be involved in additional, as yet unidentified, aspects of reproduction. For instance, LHRH has been reported present in milk from humans, cows, and rats (38), in the placenta of humans, where it apparently is synthesized (39), and in the testis of rats (40).

3 WHICH CENTRALLY LOCATED CELLS GENERATE AN LHRH SIGNAL?

Cells that produce LHRH have been immunocytochemically localized and studied in the brains of numerous vertebrate classes including fish, amphibia, birds, and mammals (for reviews, see refs. 41–43). In general, LHRH-producing cell bodies are localized in olfactory, septal, diagonal bands of Broca, preoptic, and hypothalamic areas. The relative distribution of LHRH cell bodies in each of these anatomical areas varies with each species, though the physiological significance, if any, of these differences among species is unknown. In the baboon (44), golden hamster (45), and rat (17, 46) the relative distributions of LHRH cell bodies have been reported in detail.

In coronally sectioned rat brains, the greatest percentage of LHRH cell bodies is localized at the level of the organum vasculosum lamina terminalis (OVLT), a structure that also represents a major terminal field for LHRH fibers (Figures 1 and 2). This brain level corresponds to the junction of the diagonal bands of Broca and the preoptic area (Figure 1B). A population of LHRH cell bodies is also consistently localized immediately dorsal to the supraoptic nuclei (Figure 1C). Occasionally, LHRH cell bodies are localized in the medial basal hypothalamic area, ventral or lateral to the ventromedial nucleus (Figure 1D), and in or near the arcuate nucleus. However, given the importance of LHRH in the central integration of reproduction, it seems unlikely that the number of LHRH cell bodies routinely visualized by ourselves (Figure 2) and others (45, 47) is sufficient to maintain this function. Recent estimates of

---

Figure 2. Mean ($\pm$ SE) number of LHRH cell bodies per slide (90 μm tissue examined out of every 270 μm) in four different groups of rats, projected below a parasagittal section of the hypothalamus and basal forebrain. Except for one group of male rats, all rats were gonadectomized and sacrificed one week later. Estrogen replacement in gonadectomized females consisted of subcutaneous implantation of a 5 mm Silastic capsule containing crystalline estradiol, inserted immediately after surgery. Numbers below identification of group indicate mean ($\pm$ SE) total number of LHRH cell bodies counted, and thus represent approximately one-third of the estimated total numbers, which were: 507 $\pm$ 52 (intact male); 130 $\pm$ 58 (GDX male); 146 $\pm$ 41 (GDX, E2-treated female); and, 82 $\pm$ 30 (GDX female) LHRH cell bodies per rat brain. Abbreviations as in Figure 1., with these additions: AHA, anterior hypothalamic area; AR, arcuate nucleus; DMN, dorsomedial nucleus; E2, estradiol; GDX, gonadectomized; MB, mamillary body; MS, medial septum; POA, preoptic area. From Shivers et al. (17).

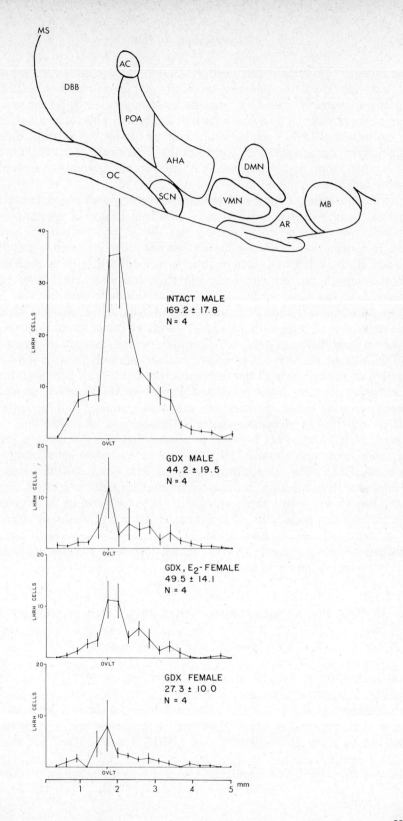

the number of oxytocin and vasopressin cell bodies indicate a presence of 5000–10,000 cell bodies per rat brain (48). Reasons that LHRH cell numbers currently visualized may be underestimated by at least an order of magnitude include the possibilities that (i) physiochemical differences in somal LHRH render it unrecognizable by the antisera directed against the decapeptide, (ii) membranes of granules containing LHRH limit penetration of antisera, and (iii) insufficient amounts of immunoreactive LHRH accumulate in the cell body.

Although Dale's hypothesis is currently being challenged (more than one neuroactive substance has been localized in and is presumably released from single neurons; see, e.g., ref. 49), it appears that the cellular LHRH distribution in the rat brain does not closely resemble the distribution of any other neuroactive substance localized to date. Recently, a short report appeared that both acetylcholine and LHRH may be released from the same neuron in the frog sympathetic ganglia (50).

In addition to anatomical and electrophysiological studies showing the existence of cells in the diagonal bands of Broca, preoptic area, and anterior hypothalamic area, which project to the median eminence (51–53), results of these kinds of experimental manipulations of the LHRH system uniformly support the distribution of LHRH cell bodies in the rat that we and others have described. For example, electrical or electrochemical stimulation directed at areas containing high densities of LHRH cell bodies increases markedly the release of LHRH into portal blood (54, 55) and of LH from rat pituitaries (56, 57). Conversely, lesions of regions containing many LHRH cell bodies decrease substantially the release of LH from rat pituitaries (58, 59) and decrease the amount of immunoreactive staining in the median eminence of the guinea pig (60). And, finally, knife cuts that sever LHRH fiber projections to the median eminence from their cells of origin in anterior hypothalamic areas, or from more rostrally located areas, produce large decreases in both the amount of immunoreactive LHRH in the median eminence (61) and of LH in the systemic circulation (62).

4   HOW IS THE LHRH SIGNAL GENERATED AND TRANSMITTED?

4.1   Properties of LHRH Neurons

Although little is known about the mechanisms of LHRH synthesis, packaging, transport, release, and degradation, the evidence to date can be summarized and compared with knowledge of other peptidergic systems. It is highly likely that synthesis of LHRH occurs by a ribosomal mechanism. It is also possible that LHRH is synthesized by cleavage from a large-molecular-weight species, as is the family of peptides cleaved from pro-opiomelanocortin, and the neurosecretory products of the magnocellular system along with their neurophysins. Little direct proof of such a prohormone for LHRH has accumulated, but Millar et al. (63) have reported that extracts of sheep hypothalami passed through Sephadex G-25 exhibited peaks of immunoreactivity in a molecular-weight range higher than that of the decapeptide LHRH. Digestion of the material in these peaks by trypsin yielded LHRH, suggesting that the higher-molecular-weight substances were precursors to LHRH. Higher-molecular-weight substances with LHRH bioactivity but not immunoreactivity were reported by Gillies and Lowry (64) in chromatographed extracts of the stalk median eminence of rats. However, characterization of these fractions has been limited.

Very little is known about the packaging and transport of LHRH in neurons. It is likely that packaging occurs in the Golgi apparatus, as is thought to be the case of posterior pituitary peptides (65), and that the resulting granules containing LHRH are transported along the axon. Ultrastructural studies have demonstrated the presence of LHRH in neurosecretory granules, in both the median eminence (66, 67) and in cell bodies (68). And cell fractionation studies of the hypothalamus have revealed LHRH in structures that behave similarly to synaptic vesicles (69). Consistent with the proposed mechanisms of transport of LHRH are findings that intraventricular administration of colchicine, which blocks fast axoplasmic transport (70), increased the immunocytochemical stainability of LHRH cells in castrated male rats (71), and that administration of colchicine to hypothalamic fragments incubated *in vitro* decreased the release of LHRH into the medium (72).

Mechanisms for release of LHRH from nerve terminals in the median eminence have been studied in more detail. LHRH release from mediobasal hypothalamic fragments can be evoked by elevated K^+, by veratridine, or by direct electrical stimulation (72–74). This enhanced release is dependent on external Ca^{2+} concentration (72–74), and the effect of calcium is mediated through voltage-dependent calcium channels (73). Electrically stimulated or K^+-stimulated release is not blocked by tetrodotoxin (TTX) (72–74). A requirement for metabolic energy in K^+-stimulated release was demonstrated by an inhibitory effect of ouabain, cyanide, and iodoacetic acid (72).

Release of LH from the pituitaries of several species appears to be episodic, with an interpeak interval of 20–60 min (75, 76). This pattern presumably is induced by a similar episodic release of LHRH, as has been inferred from studies on pituitary response to LHRH (77) and has been demonstrated by direct measurements (78–80). Steroid hormones may modulate the frequency and/or the amplitude of LHRH pulses released from the median eminence (81, 82). The release mechanisms for LHRH are apparently geared toward episodic release, since periodic bursts of electrical stimulation of the mediobasal hypothalamus *in vivo* are more effective in eliciting LH release than is continuous stimulation

(83) and since pulses of cyclic AMP added to incubating hypothalamic fragments are more effective in eliciting LHRH release than is continuous administration (84). The mechanisms underlying such responsiveness to periodic rather than continuous stimulation have not been identified.

Finally, a requirement for electrical activity (action potentials) on the part of LHRH neurons for release of the peptide has not been established. Although it has been known for many years that some anesthetics will block the neural activity necessary to produce an LHRH surge of sufficient magnitude to release an ovulatory LH surge (85), this does not necessarily imply that the electrical activity of LHRH neurons was blocked by the anesthetic. Direct proof that LHRH neurons generate action potentials and that these action potentials are required for release would be difficult to obtain. However, a comparison with the magnocellular system, where physiologically identified oxytocin and vasopressin neurons have been demonstrated to generate action potentials related to release of peptides (86), suggest that similar properties may be surmised for LHRH neurons.

4.2   Comparison with Another Estrogen-Sensitive Neural System of Reproductive Importance

We have begun a series of experiments analyzing the properties of another hormone-sensitive hypothalamic system: those neurons in the mediobasal hypothalamus that receive information concerning circulating estrogen levels and transduce this information into neural signals that ultimately alter lordotic responsiveness. A requirement for estrogen in lordotic responsiveness has been known for many years (87). Major neural targets for estradiol in inducing and maintaining lordotic responsiveness are cells in and around the ventromedial nuclei (VMN) of the hypothalamus (23, 24). Lesions of this area severely disrupt lordotic responsiveness (88), and electrical stimulation of cells in this area facilitates lordotic responsiveness in rats treated with a low dose of estrogen (89). Projections from cells in this area to the dorsal midbrain, especially the central gray, are particularly important for lordosis (22, 90), and some of the VMN neurons that project to the midbrain also concentrate estrogen (91). Estrogenic action on these neurons may be dependent on protein synthesis (92, 93), a finding that is consistent with, but does not prove, a possible peptidergic nature of these cells.

We have found that infusion of colchicine near these VMN cells disrupts estrogenic induction and the maintenance of lordotic responsiveness (94), suggesting that axoplasmic transport within or away from the hypothalamus is necessary for lordosis. In addition, we have found that action potentials generated by hypothalamic neurons are apparently also necessary for estrogenic maintenance of lordotic responsiveness (95). Infusion of TTX into the hypothalamus of estrogen-treated rats disrupts lordotic responsiveness, with a very interesting time course. The first significant decline in lordotic responsiveness occurs 40 min after infusion, and the nadir is reached 2–4 h after infusion of TTX. Recovery of lordotic responsiveness to pre-infusion levels was complete 12–24 h after infusion. In electrophysiological experiments, we found that complete suppression of multiunit electrical activity occurs within 5 min after infusion of TTX and lasts for at least several hours. The difference between disruption of electrical activity (occurring within 5 min after infusion) and disruption of lordotic responsiveness (occurring with a maximum effect at 2–4 h after infusion) is striking. A favorite interpretation is that the neurosecretory products (perhaps peptides) released by these neurons in association with action potentials have a duration of action at least on the order of minutes. It is interesting to compare this duration with that of LHRH on pituitary cells and on principal cells of the frog sympathetic ganglia (see Section 7.2.2), which is also on the order of minutes.

5 WHAT SIGNALS FROM OTHER CELLS AFFECT LHRH-PRODUCING CELLS?

5.1 Neural Signals

Results of numerous studies show that neural inputs from various sensory modalities such as light (96), olfaction (97), or cervical stimulation (98), as well as neural input from a circadian timekeeping system (99, 100), converge at some point or points on the LHRH system of the rat to alter the release of this peptide into portal blood supplying the pituitary. For example, bilateral lesions of the suprachiasmatic nucleus (SCN), as well as horizontal knife cuts above the SCN, block LH release or ovulation or both in the female rat (101, 102). The paucity of LHRH fibers in and around the SCN (unpublished observations) suggests that blockade of ovulation produced by these lesions or knife cuts is not due to severing LHRH fibers projecting to the median eminence. Rather, the lesion data may be interpreted as destroying a circadian timekeeper (103, 104); the knife cut data may also be interpreted as destroying SCN efferents that supply temporal information to LHRH cells. One candidate for these efferents is the vasopressinergic fibers that project dorsally from the SCN (105).

The identities of the neuroactive substances that mediate sensory and timekeeping input onto LHRH cells are unknown, though the effects of many putative neurotransmitters and neuromodulators on LHRH or LH release have been evaluated (for reviews, see refs. 106, 107). Since advances in cytochemistry now permit the cellular localization of many of these substances or the enzymes that synthesize them, combinations of cytochemical methodologies both at the light microscopic and the ultrastructural level will increasingly permit a more precise appreciation of the structural relations between neuroactive substances and the LHRH system. Early examples of the application of these methods showed that biogenic amines and LHRH share some, though not substantial, overlap of fibers in the median eminence (108–111). Colocalization studies at the light level show that biogenic-amine fibers appear closely juxtaposed to LHRH cell bodies (112, 113).

5.2 Endocrine Signals

The effects of various alterations in the endocrine system on the LHRH system are well documented (for a review, see ref. 114), though how this occurs is largely unknown. Accordingly, we have examined the influence of gonadal hormones on the immunocytochemical localization of LHRH. Since many variables besides physiological state may affect the immunocytochemical localization of LHRH—including choice of primary antibody, fixative, and sectioning procedure—we first optimized the procedures (115) and then maintained them strictly to ensure that any alterations measured in the immunocytochemical localization of LHRH were hormonally induced (17). This peptide was examined in the brains of intact and gonadectomized male rats as well as gonadectomized female rats and gonadectomized estradiol-replaced female rats. We determined the effect of gonadal hormones on LHRH cell number, cell distribution, optical density of staining in individual LHRH cells, and on the amount of staining in LHRH fibers in three terminal fields (17).

5.2.1 Effects of Gonadectomy in Male Rats

Intact male rats have 3.9 times more LHRH cell bodies than gonadectomized males (Figure 2). Gonadectomy significantly decreases the number of LHRH cell bodies in the diagonal bands of Broca, preoptic area, and anterior hypothalamic area, but not in the mediobasal hypothalamus (Table 1). Gonadectomy also produces a significant decrease in the optical density of the stain in LHRH cell bodies (Figure 3A,B), presum-

TABLE 1 Mean $\pm$ SE Number of LHRH Cell Bodies in Different Treatment Groups across 4 Anatomical Locations (from ref. 17, reprinted by permission of S. Karger AG, Basel)[a]

Group		MS + DBB	POA	AHA	BH
Intact male	$\bar{x}$	87.8 + 12.7	41.8 + 7.1	28.8 + 5.1	8.8 + 2.3
	%	52.5	25.0	17.2	5.2
Gdx male	$\bar{x}$	19.0 + 8.7[b]	9.5 + 6.5[b]	9.8 + 2.0[b]	5.2 + 2.6
	%	43.7	21.8	22.4	12.1
Gdx, E2-female	$\bar{x}$	22.5 + 5.9[b]	13.2 + 5.5[b]	10.5 + 4.1	2.2 + 1.3
	%	46.4	27.3	21.6	4.6
Gdx female	$\bar{x}$	17.0 + 9.0[b]	3.5 + 0.6[b]	5.0 + 1.6[b]	1.2 + 0.5[b]
	%	63.6	13.1	18.7	4.7

[a] Abbreviations: AHA, anterior hypothalmic area; BH, basal hypothalmus; DBB, diagonal bands of Broca; E2, estradiol; gdx, gonadectomized; MS, medial septum; POA, preoptic area.
[b] Significantly lower than intact male (Mann–Whitney U test).

ably reflecting a decrease in the content of LHRH. Taken together, the results strongly suggest that gonadectomy in the male rat decreases substantially the somal accumulation of immunoreactive LHRH. Results of a morphometric analysis do not reveal any influence of gonadectomy on the percentage of area covered by LHRH fibers in the OVLT but reveal that the percentage of area having LHRH fibers in the middle and caudal aspects of the median eminence decreases following castration (17). In the third LHRH terminal field examined in this study, individual LHRH fibers appearing in each section were counted in the midbrain central gray. Results show that gonadectomy significantly decreases the number of fibers that appear to penetrate into gray matter (Figure 4A). The overall effect of gonadectomy of male rats is summarized in Figure 5. Gonadectomy (i) decreases the number and staining intensity of LHRH cell bodies, (ii) has no effect on LHRH fibers in the OVLT, (iii) decreases the amount of stain in the median eminence, and (iv) decreases the number of stained fibers in the midbrain central gray. The decreased amount of LHRH staining in the median eminence is interpreted to reflect an increased amount of LHRH released into the portal blood, as has been measured by others (55). The decreased number of stained LHRH fibers in the midbrain central gray suggests increased release of the peptide in this structure. Finally, the decreased number and optical density of LHRH cell bodies following gonadectomy provides indirect evidence that maintenance of sustained high levels of LHRH release in gonadectomized males must require more LHRH to be synthesized or less degraded or both; subsequently, LHRH must be transported out of the cell body at a higher rate than that seen in intact male rats.

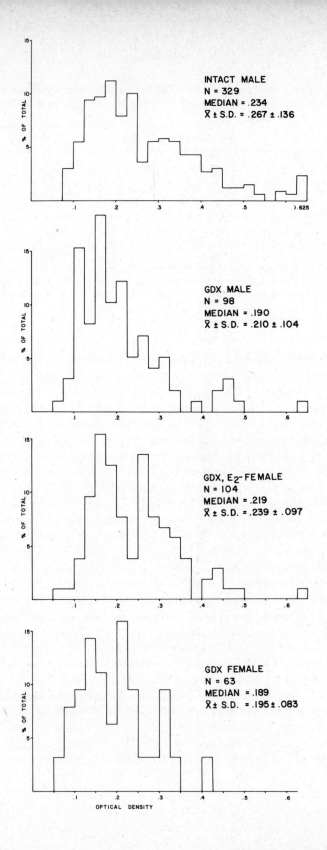

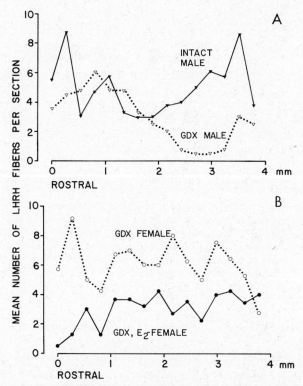

Figure 4. Mean number of LHRH fibers per section from 15 rostral-caudal levels of the midbrain central gray in (A) males and (B) females. Each point represents the mean of four rats. Gonadectomized males and significantly fewer LHRH fibers than intact males; estradiol treatment of gonadectomized females significantly decreased the number of LHRH fibers (Friedman ANOVA in each case). From Shivers et al. (17). Reprinted by permission of S. Karger AG, Basel.

Figure 3. Histograms of optical density of LHRH cell bodies for four experimental groups of rats, normalized to percent of total cell bodies measured. For each group, N = total number of cell bodies measured. The distributions of optical densities of stain in LHRH cell bodies were significantly different between the intact and gonadectomized males, and between the gonadectomized females and gonadectomized estradiol-replaced females (Mann-Whitney U tests and Komolgorov-Smirnov tests). From Shivers et al. (17). Reprinted by permission of S. Karger AG, Basel.

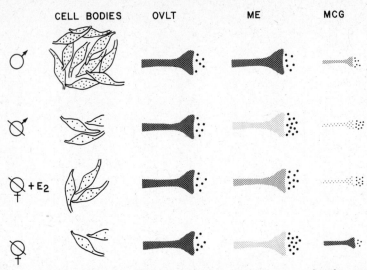

Figure 5. Schematic summary of the major effects of gonadectomy of male rats and estradiol treatment of gonadectomized female rats on the LHRH system. For each group, the relative number of and optical density (indicated by number of dots) of stain in LHRH cell bodies are shown, along with a representation of relative LHRH content in terminals (indicated by darkness of shading) and presumed relative rates of LHRH release (indicated by number of released vesicles), in three brain areas. From Shivers et al. (17). Reprinted by permission of S. Karger AG, Basel.

5.2.2   Effects of Estrogenic Treatment in Gonadectomized Female Rats

Estrogen replacement in gonadectomized females does not significantly alter the number of LHRH cells (Figure 2) or their distribution (Table 1). Estrogen replacement does, however, significantly shift the optical density of LHRH cells so that they are more darkly staining, presumably reflecting increased amounts of immunoreactive LHRH (Figure 3C,D). While estrogen replacement does not change the percentage of area in the OVLT covered by LHRH fibers, this hormone does significantly increase the percentage of area covered by LHRH fibers in the caudal aspect of the median eminence (17). In the midbrain central gray, estrogen replacement significantly *decreases* the number of LHRH fibers localized (Figure 4B). Taken together (Figure 5), these findings suggest that estrogen replacement increases the amount of immunoreactive staining in cell bodies and in fibers projecting to the median eminence but not to the OVLT. These increases can be interpreted as reflecting decreased LHRH release into portal blood, believed to be antecedent to decreases in circulating LH routinely measured following estrogen replacement in gonadectomized female rats (114). The finding of fewer LHRH fibers in the midbrain central gray following estrogen replacement can be interpreted as indicating increased release in this structure. The increased midbrain release of LHRH suggested in these studies is consistent with a role for LHRH in facilitation of lordotic responsiveness.

Since gonadal steroids have been repeatedly shown to exert powerful effects on LHRH regulation, and since cells that concentrate steroid have been located (116) in areas known from separate studies to contain LHRH-producing cells, the exact morphological relation of peptide-producing and steroid-concentrating cells presents an intriguing question. Studies in our laboratory have demonstrated, by combining immunocytochemistry for LHRH with autoradiography for ^{3}H-estrogen, cellular LHRH content and radioactive estrogen accumulation in the same tissue sections in the forebrain areas of ovariectomized rats. Of 435 LHRH cell nuclei examined in 240 tissue sections, radioactive estradiol was retained in only 1 LHRH cell nucleus (manuscript submitted). Results indicate that most neurons that produce LHRH do not concentrate estradiol, suggesting that steroid-concentrating interneurons may mediate some effects of estrogen on the LHRH signal. It remains a possibility that LHRH-producing cells could respond directly to steroids through a nongenomic mechanism.

6 WHAT IS THE LOCATION AND FUNCTION OF CELLS THAT RECEIVE LHRH?

The LHRH signal may be transmitted to other cells by three routes, each varying in the "privateness" and efficiency of the dispersal means —in blood, across synapses, and through cerebrospinal fluid.

6.1 Cells Receiving LHRH Dispersed by Blood

The location, identity, and function of only one group of LHRH target cells is known in any detail: the pituitary gonadotrophs receiving LHRH from fibers ending in the median eminence in proximity to portal blood vessels. The responses of these cells to the peptide are discussed in more detail in Section 7.1. The existence of receptors for LHRH in peripheral target organs, such as the ovary (117) and the testis (118), suggests the possibility that blood-borne LHRH signals may affect the activity of cells in these organs. However, given the short half-life of LHRH in blood (119, 120) and the low or undetectable levels of LHRH in the systemic circulation (121), a response of gonadal LHRH receptors to the peptide in the systemic circulation is unlikely. The possibility of a local synthesis of LHRH in the testis has been suggested (40).

6.2   Cells Receiving LHRH Across Synapses

Although LHRH fibers have been detected in a variety of brain regions, it is often difficult to determine at the light microscopic level whether the fibers terminate in a particular structure or pass through the structure without synapsing. If, however, LHRH fibers extend into a given structure and appear to stop there, it is likely that LHRH-releasing synapses are located there. We have seen such areas of LHRH fiber terminations in the lateral septum, OVLT, subfornical organ, corticomedial amygdala, hippocampus (only a few fibers present), superior colliculus (stratum opticum; only a few fibers present), and the midbrain central gray. Involvement of some of these structures in reproductive functions has been suggested. For instance, lesions of the lateral septum increase lordotic responsiveness in estrogen-treated rats (122). However, in general, the functional significance of LHRH terminals in most of these structures has not been identified. The evidence for a role of LHRH terminals in the midbrain central gray in facilitation of lordotic responsiveness represents the strongest case for a contribution to the reproductive effort mediated by contact between LHRH-producing cells and other neurons. This evidence was reviewed in more detail in Section 2.2.

6.3   Possibility that Cells Receive LHRH through Cerebrospinal Fluid

It is also possible that LHRH signals are transmitted to other cells via the cerebrospinal fluid. A relationship between LHRH fibers and the ventricular system has been emphasized by several investigators (45, 123, 124) and can be seen in our immunocytochemical studies. We have seen LHRH fibers in the OVLT, subfornical organ, subcommissural organ (only a few fibers present), choroid plexus of the lateral ventricle, subarachnoid space, and lining the ventral walls of the third ventricle and cerebral aqueduct (Shivers et al., in preparation). However, only conjectures about release into the cerebrospinal fluid can be made from morphological studies. Infusion of LHRH into the ventricular system rapidly elicits LH release from the pituitary (125). However, radioimmunoassay of the cerebrospinal fluid in rats (126) and sheep (127) has failed to detect measurable levels of this peptide.

7   HOW DO TARGET CELLS RECEIVE, ENCODE, AND TRANSMIT LHRH SIGNALS?

7.1   Pituitary Cells

Although our main focus in this chapter is the role of LHRH as a neural integrator of reproduction, it is important to understand the phenomenology and mechanism of action of LHRH on pituitary cells, since this may provide insight into effects of LHRH on nerve cells. Any model of the mechanism of action of LHRH on pituitary gonadotropes must account for several aspects of LHRH action. The peptide induces release of both LH and FSH. The responsiveness of the pituitary to LHRH is altered by circulating steroid levels (128). LHRH exerts a "self-priming" effect (129), that is, exposure of pituitaries to LHRH augments the response to additional exposure some 30–60 min later. But continuous exposure to LHRH decreases pituitary sensitivity to the peptide (77).

Conn et al. (130) have examined mechanisms by which LHRH stimulates release of LH from perfused hemipituitaries and have proposed a three-step mechanism. The first step is binding of LHRH to specific receptor sites on the plasma membrane. This binding leads to a "mobilization" of Ca^{2+} at (as yet unidentified) sites inside the cell. The relative contributions of Ca^{2+} mobilized from extracellular vs. intracellular stores in controversial, although a requirement for extracellular Ca^{2+} appears to be clear. The third step in the action of LHRH is release of LH and FSH. Adams and Nett (131) have emphasized actions of LHRH beyond stimulation of LH release. These investigators propose that following binding of LHRH to receptors and mobilization of Ca^{2+}, adenyl cyclase is activated to synthesize cyclic AMP, which then induces phosphorylation of nuclear, ribosomal, Golgi, and/or microfilament proteins. While the requirement for cAMP in the release of LH is unclear (130), the phosphorylation induced by cAMP may be involved in synthesis of LH (and perhaps LHRH receptors) or in the conversion of LH into a "readily releasable pool." In either model, alterations in responsiveness to LHRH might occur by changes in the number of receptors for LHRH in the plasma membrane (132). Such changes in number of LHRH receptors might at least partly explain the changes in responsiveness to the peptide induced by both steroids and LHRH. Finally, regarding the termination of LHRH action, the peptide is known to be internalized into gonadotrophs (133), where it is believed eventually to be degraded in lysozomes. In addition, peptidases that degrade unbound LHRH are known to exist in brain, pituitary, and blood (for a review, see ref. 134).

7.2 Nerve Cells

Very little is known about the phenomenology or mechanism of action of LHRH in the brain. Electrophysiological effects of microelectrophoresis of LHRH onto single nerve cells in the brain have recently been reviewed by Moss (135). Although little is known about the mechanisms by which LHRH modulates nerve cell firing rates, gonadal steroids have been reported to alter the percentage of neurons activated or inhibited by LHRH or its analogs (136).

While a major difficulty in determining mechanisms of action of LHRH on nerve cells is the heterogeneity of neurons in the brain, an LHRH-sensitive system of less complexity has been discovered by Jan et al. (137). (See Chapter 23.) In the lumbar sympathetic chain of the bullfrog, stimulation of preganglionic fibers produces a slow excitatory post-synaptic potential (epsp) lasting for 5–10 min. Jan et al. (137) have accumulated evidence that the transmitter released by such stimulation is LHRH or a similar peptide. LHRH and its agonist analogs duplicate the slow epsp, while numerous other peptides do not, though the physiological significance of this action is unknown (for review, see ref. 138). The presence of an LHRH-like peptide in the appropriate ganglia has been demonstrated by radioimmunoassay (137) and immunocytochemistry (139). This peptide disappears after sectioning of preganglionic fibers and is released from the ganglia by isotonic KCl, in a Ca^{2+}-dependent manner. Finally, the substance that displaces ^{125}I-LHRH from the antiserum is not destroyed by boiling but is destroyed by α-chymotrypsin (as is synthetic LHRH), and it has an apparent molecular weight of approximately 1000 daltons.

Further analysis of the effect of LHRH and preganglionic fiber stimulation on intracellular recorded ganglion cells demonstrated that in several respects LHRH duplicates the effect of preganglionic fiber stimulation (140). Responses to LHRH and nerve stimulation were associated with similar membrane conductance changes, and the amplitudes of the responses varied in parallel as membrane potential was shifted over a wide range. Both LHRH and nerve stimulation increased the excitability of the neurons recorded, and both altered other synaptic inputs in a parallel fashion. Finally, the response to both LHRH and preganglionic nerve stimulation was blocked by an LHRH analog antagonistic to LHRH action on the rat pituitary. The mechanisms by which LHRH may induce this slow synaptic potential are not known, although a decrease in K^+ conductance may partly explain the epsp. Whether similar slow synaptic potentials might be induced by LHRH in the brain has not been determined. Studies to date on the effect of microelectrophoretic application of LHRH to nerve cells in the brain have been designed to monitor alterations in the firing rate of extracellularly recorded neurons (135). Abrupt changes (latency of 1 sec or less) in the firing rate of neurons during the microelectrophoretic application of LHRH have been noted. However, it is unlikely that slow synaptic potential changes would be detectable in such studies.

8 OUTLOOK

Studies have been initiated to identify the sites, actions, and functional significance of extrapituitary LHRH release in the brain. Additional morphological work will be necessary—including cytochemical staining, receptor mapping, and retrograde tracing at the light and ultrastructural levels—to determine how the LHRH system is organized and to identify the cells that respond to LHRH release. Electrophysiological, pharmacological, and biochemical studies will be required to determine the biophysical properties of LHRH neurons as well as the nature of the response and the functional significance of the activity of cells that respond to LHRH.

REFERENCES

1. F. H. A. Marshall and F. B. Verney, *J. Physiol.* **86**, 327 (1936).
2. G. W. Harris, *Proc. R. Soc. London, Ser. B* **122**, 374 (1937).
3. H. O. Haterius and A. S. Derbyshire, *Am. J. Physiol.* **119**, 329 (1937).
4. G. W. Harris, *Neural Control of the Pituitary Gland*, Edward Arnold, London, 1955.
5. S. M. McCann, *Am. J. Physiol.* **202**, 395 (1962).
6. H. Matsuo, Y. Baba, R. M. G. Nair, A. Arimura, and A. V. Schally, *Biochem. Biophys. Res. Commun.* **43**, 1334 (1971).
7. Y. Baba, H. Matsuo, and A. V. Schally, *Biochem. Biophys. Res. Commun.* **44**, 459 (1971).
8. R. Burgus, H. Butcher, M. Amoss, N. Ling, M. Monahan, J. Rivier, R. Fellows, R. Blackwell, W. Vale, and R. Guillemin, *Proc. Natl. Acad. Sci. USA* **69**, 278, (1972).
9. K. Folkers, E. Lundanes, S. Fuchs, K. Tsuji, J. Leban, N. Sakura, M. Lebek, G. Rampold, and C. Y. Bowers, in W. Wuttke, A. Weindl, K. H. Voight, and R. R. Dries, Eds., *Brain and Pituitary Peptides*, S. Karger, Basel, 1980, p. 46.
10. R. L. Moss and S. M. McCann, *Science* **181**, 177 (1973).
11. D. W. Pfaff, *Science* **182**, 1148 (1973).
12. D. W. Pfaff, *Estrogens and Brain Function*, Springer-Verlag, New York, 1980.
13. R. L. Moss and M. M. Foreman, *Neuroendocrinology* **20**, 176 (1976).
14. P. Riskind and R. L. Moss, *Brain Res. Bull.* **4**, 203 (1979).
15. Y. Sakuma and D. W. Pfaff, *Nature (London)* **283**, 566 (1980).
16. Z. Liposits and G. Sétáó, *Neurosci. Lett.* **20**, 1 (1980).
17. B. D. Shivers, R. E. Harlan, J. I. Morrell, and D. W. Pfaff, *Neuroendocrinology* **36**, 1 (1983).
18. Y. Sakuma and D. W. Pfaff, *Am. J. Physiol.* **237**, R278 (1979).
19. Y. Sakuma and D. W. Pfaff, *Am. J. Physiol.* **237**, R285 (1979).
20. Y. Sakuma and D. W. Pfaff, *Exp. Neurol.* **70**, 269 (1980).
21. Y. Sakuma and D. W. Pfaff, *J. Neurophysiol.* **44**, 1002 (1980).
22. Y. Sakuma and D. W. Pfaff, *J. Neurophysiol.* **44**, 1012 (1980).
23. P. G. Davis, B. S. McEwen, and D. W. Pfaff, *Endocrinology* **104**, 898 (1979).
24. B. S. Rubin and R. J. Barfield, *Endocrinology* **106**, 504 (1980).
25. W. K. Samson, S. M. McCann, L. Chud, C. A. Dudley, and R. L. Moss, *Neuroendocrinology* **31**, 66 (1980).
26. A. J. Kastin, D. H. Coy, A. V. Schally, and J. E. Zadina, *Pharmacol. Biochem. Behav.* **13**, 913 (1980).
27. J. I. Morrell and D. W. Pfaff, *Am. Zool.* **18**, 447 (1978).
28. M. -F. Cheng, *J. Endocrinology* **74**, 37 (1977).
29. M. R. Alderete, R. R. Tokarz, and D. Crews, *Neuroendocrinology* **30**, 200 (1980).
30. D. B. Kelley, *Soc. Neurosci. Abstr.* **7**, 615 (1981).
31. J. A. King and R. P. Millar, *Science* **206**, 67 (1979).

32. R. L. Moss, C. A. Dudley, M. M. Foreman, and S. M. McCann, in M. Motta, P. G. Crosignani and L. Martini, Eds., *Hypothalamic Hormones*, Academic Press, London, 1975, p. 269.
33. E. L. Ryan and A. I. Frankel, *Biol. Reprod.* **19**, 971 (1978).
34. D. M. Dorsa and E. R. Smith, *Regul. Peptides* **1**, 147 (1980).
35. P. A. McDonald, *Neuroendocrinology* **28**, 151 (1979).
36. C. H. Doering, D. R. McGinnis, H. C. Kraemer, and D. A. Hamburg, Arch. Sex. Behav. **9**, 441 (1980).
37. C. H. Doering, B. C. McAdoo, H. C. Draemer, H. K. H. Brodie, N. J. Dessert, and D. A. Hamburg, in E. Usdin, D. A. Hamburg, and J. D. Barchas, Eds., *Neuroregulators and Psychiatric Disorders*, Oxford University Press, New York, 1977, p. 267.
38. T. Baram, Y. Koch, E. Hazum, and M. Fridkin, *Science* **198**, 300 (1977).
39. G. S. Khodr and T. M. Siler-Khodr, *Science* **207**, 315 (1980).
40. W. K. Paull, C. M. Turkelson, C. R. Thomas, and A. Arimura, *Science* **213**, 1263 (1981).
41. G. E. Hoffman, V. Melnyk, T. Hayes, C. Bennett-Clark, and E. Fowler, in D. E. Scott, G. P. Kozlowski, and A. Weindl, Eds., *Brain-Endocrine Interaction, Vol. III: Neural Hormones and Reproduction*, S. Karger, Basel, 1978, p. 67.
42. A. J. Silverman, L. C. Krey, and E. A. Zimmerman, *Biol. Reprod.* **20**, 98 (1979).
43. J. Barry, *Int. Rev. Cytol.* **60**, 179 (1979).
44. P. E. Marshall and P. C. Goldsmith, *Brain Res.* **193**, 353 (1980).
45. L. Jennes and W. E. Stumpf, *Cell Tissue Res.* **209**, 239 (1980).
46. B. D. Shivers, R. E. Harlan, J. I. Morrell, and D. W. Pfaff, *Abstr. Soc. Neurosci.* **7**, 20 (1981).
47. J. E. King, S. A. Tobett, L. Snavely, and A. A. Arimura, *Peptides* **1**, Suppl. 1, 85 (1980).
48. C. H. Rhodes, J. I. Morrell, and D. W. Pfaff, *J. Comp. Neurol.* **198**, 45 (1981).
49. T. Hokfelt, A. Ljungdahl, H. Steinhusch, A. Verhofstadt, G. Nilsson, E. Brodin, B. Pernow, and M. Goldstein, *Neuroscience* **3**, 517 (1978).
50. Y. N. Jan and L. Y. Jan, *Soc. Neurosci. Abstr.* **7**, 603 (1981).
51. L. P. Renaud, in S. Reichlin, R. J. Baldesserini, and J. B. Martin, *The Hypothalamus*, Raven Press, New York, 1978, p. 269.
52. R. M. Lechan, J. L. Nestler, S. Jacobson, and S. Reichlin, *Brain Res.* **195**, 13 (1980).
53. R. M. Lechan, J. L. Nestler, and S. Jacobson, *Abstr. Soc. Neurosci.* **7**, 333 (1981).
54. G. Fink and M. G. Jamieson, *J. Endocrinol.* **68**, 71 (1976).
55. R. L. Eskay, R. S. Mical, and J. C. Porter, *Endocrinology* **100**, 263 (1977).
56. J. W. Everett, *Physiol. Rev.* **44**, 373 (1964).
57. K. Kubo, S. P. Mennin, and R. A. Gorski, *Endocrinology* **96**, 492 (1975).
58. F. Kimura and M. Kawakami, *Neuroendocrinology* **27**, 74 (1978).
59. M. Kawakami and S. Ando, *Brain Res.* **191**, 99 (1980).
60. L. C. Krey and A. J. Silverman, *Brain Res.* **157**, 247 (1978).
61. R. I. Weiner, E. Pattov, B. Kerdelhué, and C. Kordon, *Endocrinology* **97**, 1597 (1975).
62. B. Halász, in W. F. Ganong and L. Martini, Eds., *Frontiers in Neuroendocrinology, 1969* Oxford University Press, 1969, p. 307.
63. R. P. Millar, C. Aehnelt, and G. Rossier, *Biochem. Biophys. Res. Comm.* **74**, 720 (1977).
64. G. Gillies and P. Lowry, *Nature (London)* **278**, 463 (1979).
65. M. J. Brownstein, J. T. Russell, and H. Gainer, *Science* **207**, 373 (1980).
66. P. C. Goldsmith and W. F. Ganong, *Brain Res.* **97**, 181 (1975).
67. A. J. Silverman and P. Desnoyers, *Cell Tissue Res.* **169**, 157 (1976).
68. G. P. Kozlowski, L. Chu, G. Hostetter, and B. Kerdelhué, *Peptides* **1**, 37 (1980).
69. A. Barnea, W. B. Neaves, G. Cho, and J. C. Porter, *J. Neurochem.* **30**, 937 (1978).
70. J. H. Schwartz, *Sci. Am.* **242**, 152 (1980).
71. J. Barry, M. P. Dubois, and P. Poulain, *Z. Zellforsch.* **146**, 351 (1973).

72. D. E. Hartter and V. D. Ramirez, *Endocrinology* **107**, 375 (1980).
73. S. V. Drouva, J. Epelbaum, M. Hery, L. Tapra-Arancibia, E. Laplante, and C. Kordon, *Neuroendocrinology* **32**, 155 (1981).
74. R. G. Dyer, S. Mansfield, and J. O. Yates, *Exp. Brain Res.* **39**, 453 (1980).
75. V. L. Gay and N. A. Sheth, *Endocrinology* **90**, 158 (1972).
76. D. J. Dierschke, A. N. Bhattacharya, L. E. Atkinson, and E. Knobil, *Endocrinology* **87**, 850 (1970).
77. P. E. Belchetz, T. M. Plant, Y. Nakai, E. J. Keogh, and E. Knobil, *Science* **202**, 631 (1978).
78. P. C. Carmel, S. Araki, and M. Ferin, *Endocrinology* **99**, 243 (1976).
79. J. E. Levine and V. D. Ramirez, *Endocrinology* **107**, 1782 (1980).
80. J. E. Levine, F. Peu, V. D. Ramirez, and G. L. Jackson, *Soc. Neurosci. Abstr.* **7**, 20 (1981).
81. R. A. Steiner, W. J. Bremner, and D. K. Clifton, *Biol. Reprod.* **24**, Suppl. 1, 26A (1981).
82. A. Coquelin, W. Craigen, and F. H. Bronson, *Biol. Reprod.* **24**, Suppl. 1, 69A (1981).
83. R. G. Dyer and L. C. Mayes, *Exp. Brain Res.* **33**, 583 (1978).
84. D. E. Hartter and V. D. Ramirez, *Soc. Neurosci. Abstr.* **7**, 506 (1981).
85. J. W. Everett, C. H. Sawyer, and J. E. Markee, *Endocrinology*, **44**, 234 (1949).
86. B. A. Cross, R. E. J. Dyball, R. G. Dyer, C. W. Jones, D. W. Lincoln, J. F. Morris, and B. T. Pickering, *Rec. Prog. Horm. Res.* **31**, 243 (1975).
87. W. C. Young, in W. C. Young, Ed., *Sex and Internal Secretions*, Vol. 2, Williams and Wilkins, Baltimore, 1961, p. 1173.
88. D. W. Pfaff and Y. Sakuma, *J. Physiol.* **288**, 203 (1979).
89. D. W. Pfaff and Y. Sakuma, *J. Physiol.* **288**, 189 (1979).
90. C. W. Malsbury and J. T. Daood, *Brain Res.* **159**, 451 (1978).
91. J. I. Morrell and D. W. Pfaff, *J. Histochem. Cytochem.* **29**, 894 (1981).
92. D. M. Quadagno, J. Shryne, and R. A. Gorski, *Horm. Behav.* **2**, 1 (1971).
93. T. C. Rainbow, P. G. Davis, M. McGinnis, and B. S. McEwen, *Soc. Neurosci. Abstr.* **6**, 862 (1980).
94. R. E. Harlan, B. D. Shivers, L. -M. Kow, and D. W. Pfaff, *Brain Res.* **238**, 153 (1982).
95. R. E. Harlan, B. D. Shivers, L. -M. Kow, and D. W. Pfaff, *Brain Res.* in press.
96. J. C. Hoffman, in *Handbook of Physiology, Section 7, Vol. 2, Part I: Endocrinology*, American Physiological Society, Washington, D.C., 1973, p. 57.
97. W. K. Whitten and A. K. Champlin, in *Handbook of Physiology, Section 7, Vol. 2, Part I: Endocrinology*, American Physiological Society , Washington, D.C., 1973, p. 109.
98. C. Aron, G. Asch, and J. Roos, *Int. Rev. Cytol.* **20**, 139 (1966).
99. J. W. Everett and C. H. Sawyer, *Endocrinology*, **47**, 198 (1950).
100. R. Sridaran and C. E. McCormack, *Biol. Reprod.* **20**, 705 (1979).
101. G. D. Gray, P. Södersten, D. Tallentire, and J. M. Davidson, *Neuroendocrinology* **25**, 174 (1978).
102. B. Shivers, R. Harlan, and R. L. Moss, *Fed. Proc.* **38**, 1108 (1979).
103. R. Y. Moore and V. B. Eichler, *Brain Res.* **42**, 201 (1972).
104. B. Ruzak and I. Zucker, *Physiol. Rev.* **59**, 449 (1979).
105. M. V. Sofroniew and A. Weindl, *Am. J. Anat.* **153**, 391 (1978).
106. L. Krulich and C. P. Fawcett, in S. M. McCann, Ed., *Endocrine Physiology II, Vol. 16: International Review of Physiology*, University Park Press, Baltimore, 1977, p. 35.
107. S. M. McCann, E. Vijayan, W. K. Samson, J. Koenig, and L. Krulich, in W. Wuttke, A. Weindl, K. H. Voigt, and R. -R. Dries, Eds., *Brain and Pituitary Peptides*, S. Karger, Basel, 1980, p. 223.
108. T. H. McNeill and J. R. Sladek, *Science* **200**, 70 (1978).
109. G. Alonso, M. Balmefrezol, and I. Assenmacher, *C. R. Soc. Biol.* **172**, 138 (1978).

110. K. Ajika, *J. Anat.* **128**, 331 (1979).

111. Y. Ibata, K. Watanabe, H. Kinoshita, S. Kubo, Y. Sano, S. Sin, E. Hashimera, and K. Imagawa, *Neurosci. Lett.* **11**, 181 (1979).

112. A. J. Silverman and J. R. Sladek, Jr., *Soc. Neurosci. Abstr.* **4**, 282 (1978).

113. L. Jennes, W. C. Beckman, Jr., R. Grzanna, and W. E. Stumpf, *J. Histochem. Cytochem.* **29**, 893 (1981).

114. G. Fink, *Ann. Rev. Physiol.* **41**, 571 (1979).

115. B. D. Shivers, R. E. Harlan, J. I. Morrell, and D. W. Pfaff, *J. Histochem. Cytochem.* **29**, 901 (1981).

116. D. Pfaff and M. Keiner, *J. Comp. Neurol.* **151**, 121 (1973).

117. R. N. Clayten, J. P. Harwood, and K. J. Catt, *Nature (London)* **282**, 90 (1979).

118. G. A. Bourne, S. Regiani, A. N. Payne, and J. C. Marshall, *J. Clin. Endocrinol. Metab.* **51**, 407 (1980).

119. A. Dupont, F. Labrie, G. Pelletier, R. Puviani, D. H. Coy, E. J. Coy, and A. V. Schally, *Neuroendocrinology*, **16**, 65 (1974).

120. B. Pimstone, S. Epstein, S. M. Hamilton, D. LeRoith, and S. Hendricks, *J. Clin. Endocrinol. Metab.* **44**, 356 (1977).

121. T. M. Nett and T. E. Adams, *Endocrinology*, **101**, 1135 (1977).

122. D. M. Nance, J. Shryne, and R. A. Gorski, *Horm. Behav.* **5**, 73 (1974).

123. A. Weindl and M. V. Sofroniew, in D. E. Scott, G. P. Kozlowski, and A. Weindl, Eds., *Brain-Endocrine Interaction Vol. III: Neural Hormones and Reproduction*, S. Karger, Basel, 1978, p. 117.

124. B. J. Burchanowski, K. M. Knigge, and L. A. Sternberger, *Proc. Natl. Acad. Sci. USA* **76**, 6671 (1979).

125. R. I. Weiner, J. Terkel, C. A. Blake, A. V. Schally, and C. H. Sawyer, *Neuroendocrinology* **10**, 261 (1972).

126. O. M. Cramer and C. A. Barraclough, *Endocrinology*, **96**, 913 (1975).

127. R. J. Coppings, P. V. Malven, and V. D. Ramirez, *Proc. Soc. Exp. Biol. Med.* **154**, 219 (1977).

128. M. S. Aiyer, G. Fink, and F. Grieg, *J. Endocrinol.* **60**, 47 (1973).

129. M. S. Aiyer, S. A. Chiappa, and G. Fink, *J. Endocrinol.* **62**, 573 (1974).

130. P. M. Conn, J. Marian, M. McMillian, J. Stern, D. Rogers, M. Hamby, A. Penne, and E. Grant, *Endocr. Rev.* **2**, 174 (1981).

131. T. E. Adams and T. M. Nett, *Biol. Reprod.* **21**, 1073 (1979).

132. K. R. Park, B. B. Saxena, and H. M. Gandy, *Acta Endocrinol.* **82**, 62 (1976).

133. E. Hazum, P. Cuatrecasas, J. Marian, and P. M. Conn, *Proc. Natl. Acad. Sci. USA* **77**, 6692 (1980).

134. K. Bauer, in W. Wuttke, A. Weindl, K. M. Voigt, and R. -R. Dries, Eds., *Brain and Pituitary Peptides*, S. Karger, Basel, 1980, p. 213.

135. R. L. Moss, *Ann. Rev. Physiol.* **41**, 617 (1979).

136. R. L. Moss and C. A. Dudley, *Brain Res.* **149**, 511 (1978).

137. Y. N. Jan, L. Y. Jan, and S. W. Kuffler, *Proc. Natl. Acad. Sci. USA* **76**, 1501 (1979).

138. S. W. Kuffler, *J. Exp. Biol.* **89**, 257 (1980).

139. L. Y. Jan, Y. N. Jan, and M. S. Brownfield, *Nature (London)* **288**, 380 (1980).

140. Y. N. Jan, L. Y. Jan, and S. W. Kuffler, *Proc. Natl. Acad. Sci. USA* **77**, 5008 (1980).

18

Central Nervous Control of Sex and Gonadotropin Release: Peptide and Nonpeptide Transmitter Interactions

GEORGE FINK

HELEN F. STANLEY

ALAN G. WATTS

Medical Research Council Brain Metabolism Unit
Department of Pharmacology
Edinburgh, Scotland

1 INTRODUCTION

Thirty-five years ago it was shown that ovulation in the rabbit could be blocked by intravenous injections of atropine within 15 sec or dibenamine within 1 min after coitus. This suggested that cholinergic and adrenergic mechanisms were involved in the reflex release of the ovulatory hormone, luteinizing hormone (LH) (1). Subsequent studies showed, however, that physiological concentrations of acetylcholine or the monoamines could not release LH by a direct action on the pituitary gland; it is now known that stimulation of LH release by the brain is mediated by the decapeptide, luteinizing hormone releasing hormone (LHRH) (2). Nonetheless, the early studies on the mechanisms of LH release in the rabbit established that nonpeptide transmitters were involved in the control of gonadotropin secretion, and consequently the control mechanism for gonadotropin secretion was the first and has remained perhaps the most important neuroendocrine model for investigating the interactions between peptide and nonpeptide neurotransmitters.

This area of research has always been controversial. Thus Markee et al. (3) concluded, on the basis of pituitary infusions, that adrenaline was the neurochemical mediator for gonadotropin release in the rabbit; however, the effect of adrenaline seems to have been due to the low pH of the vehicle (4). Swedish workers demonstrated the presence in the median eminence of a dense dopaminergic (DA) innervation (5, 6), and the studies they carried out with synthesis blockers to determine turnover led to the conclusion that dopamine inhibited gonadotropin release—a conclusion that conflicted with the findings of pharmacological studies (7). Even the more widely accepted view that a central noradrenergic (NA) system plays a key role in stimulating LHRH and thereby LH release has been challenged by the finding that lesions of the main NA projections to the hypothalamus have only a transient inhibitory effect on LH release and ovulation (8–10).

This chapter covers some aspects of the interactions between peptide and nonpeptide transmitters in the gonadotropin control mechanism that have not been reviewed in depth or in the same manner by other recent reviews of this subject (11–14). Although emphasis is placed on the control of gonadotropin secretion, the neural control of prolactin secretion is considered briefly because this hormone is involved in an important, though so far ill-defined, manner in gonadotropin control.

2 ANATOMICAL PATHWAYS

Detailed accounts of the anatomical pathways, especially peptidergic, relevant to gonadotropin control may be found in other chapters in this volume (see Chapters 27, 28, 33). A brief outline of the anatomy of nonpeptidergic neurons is necessary here to facilitate consideration of interactions between the relevant peptidergic and monoaminergic neurons.

2.1 Gamma Amino Butyric Acid (GABA)

GABAergic neurons may play a role in the control of prolactin and to a lesser extent gonadotropin release. Biochemical and immunohistochemical studies have shown the presence of relatively large amounts of both GABA and its synthesizing enzyme, glutamic acid decarboxylase (GAD), in the hypothalamus (15, 16). Deafferentation studies (17, 18, 19) have suggested that some of the GABAergic neurons have their origins within the hypothalamus. Vincent et al. (16) have shown GAD-positive cell bodies in the posterior hypothalamus and throughout nuclei in the hypothalamus. Tappaz et al. (20), using tritiated GABA and its structural analogs, and Vincent et al. (16), using immunohistofluorescence, have shown dense labeling within the external layer of the median eminence.

2.2 Monoaminergic Pathways

2.2.1 Serotonin (5HT)

The early histochemical work of Fuxe and coworkers (21, 22) showed that most of the serotonin (5HT) innervation of the brain originates from cell bodies in the raphe nuclei in the midbrain. This was confirmed by histofluorescence studies of the brain after lesioning 5HT pathways either surgically (23, 24) or cytotoxically (25, 26), by autoradiographic tracing of uptake of ^{3}H-5HT (27, 28), and by immunohistochemical studies (29, 30).

Within the hypothalamus 5HT innervation is dense (28, 31, 32); although most nuclei have some detectable 5HT, the suprachiasmatic nucleus (SCN) and arcuate (ARC) nuclei have the highest concentrations (33). Electrolytic lesions of the dorsal raphe nucleus lead to significant reductions of 5HT in several hypothalamic nuclei (34), as does deafferentation of the medial basal hypothalamus (MBH) (17). Recent work by Van de Kar and Lorens (35) has suggested that the hypothalamus is differentially innervated from the raphe nuclei, with the median raphe nucleus supplying the SCN, anterior hypothalamus, and medial preoptic area (MPOA), and both the median and dorsal raphe nuclei supplying the anteriolateral hypothalamus and ARC. On the basis of autoradiographic studies showing that various nuclei have ^{3}H-5HT-labeled cell bodies (27, 28, 31, 36), an intrinsic hypothalamic 5HT system has been suggested. However, as assessed by immunochemistry, the presence of cell bodies within the hypothalamus remains unconfirmed (29, 30).

2.2.2   Dopamine

Of the several DA neuronal systems of the brain (37, 38), three are of
immediate interest here: (i) The mesocortical system, with cell bodies
located in the ventral tegmentum and substantia nigra. Some of their
projections run to the amygdala (39, 40) and possibly to the SCN, ventromedial nucleus, and median eminence (41). (ii) The incerto-
hypothalamic system, cell bodies of which are found in the posterior
hypothalamus and zona incerta and in the periventricular nucleus (42,
43). These two cell systems supply their surrounding areas with short,
diffuse fibers (43). (iii) The tuberoinfundibular dopaminergic (TIDA) system, which, in terms of neuroendocrine interactions, is the best studied
(see below). Cell bodies are located in the ARC and periventricular nuclei (21, 44, 45), with projections to three areas: the neural lobe of the
pituitary (46), the intermediate lobe of the pituitary (47), and the median
eminence (45–51).

2.2.3   Noradrenaline

Noradrenergic neurons, like serotonergic neurons, have their cell bodies
in the brainstem (21, 52–58). Two groups of cell bodies supply the brain:
first, a system originating in the locus coeruleus and containing 43% of
the cell bodies of NA fibers in the brain (56), and second, neurons with
cell bodies originating in the lateral tegmentum. The hypothalamus receives the majority of its NA innervation from the lateral tegmental
group; only the supraoptic, dorsomedial, paraventricular, and periventricular nuclei receive fibers from the locus coeruleus (59, 60). Biochemical
(61, 62), histofluorescence (22, 44, 52, 63, 64), and immunohistochemical
data have shown that the hypothalamus contains a rich, diffuse NA innervation, with greatest concentrations in the retrochiasmatic area,
paraventricular, and dorsomedial nuclei. The median eminence also
contains some NA terminals, as shown by the existence of dopamine β-
hydroxylase (65). The principal innervation to the hypothalamus comes
by way of the principal NA bundle, which projects rostrally through the
dorsal mesencephalic tegmentum and zona incerta (56).

2.2.4   Adrenaline

Present in the ARC and median eminence is a considerable amount of
phenylethanolamine transferase activity, and, therefore, adrenaline.
Studies with hypothalamic deafferentation have shown that most of the
adrenergic fibers, including those that form a particularly dense plexus
in the paraventricular nucleus, are derived from cell bodies in the A1
(lateral reticular nucleus of medulla) area of the brainstem (17, 66).

2.2.5   Histamine

Histamine is present in the median eminence, ARC, and ventromedial and dorsomedial nuclei of the hypothalamus. The concentrations of this amine are unchanged by deafferentation, possibly because of the large number of mast cells in the region (17).

2.3   Acetylcholine

Acetylcholine (ACh) and its metabolic enzymes, choline acetyltransferase (CAT) and acetylcholinesterase (AChE), can all be visualized within the hypothalamus. Parent and Butcher (67) found appreciable amounts of AChE activity in the paraventricular and supraoptic nuclei, with lesser amounts in the ARC and ventromedial nuclei. Brownstein et al. (68) found very high concentrations of CAT activity in the median eminence. Both these observations were confirmed by Hoover et al. (69). Using tritiated and iodinated bungarotoxin and tritiated quinuclidinyl benzilate, Block and Billiar (70) were able to measure the concentrations of nicotinic and muscarinic receptors within the hypothalamus. They found an even spread of muscarinic receptors throughout various hypothalamic nuclei, but a greater concentration of nicotinic receptors in the SCN, preoptic, and dorsomedial nuclei than in other nuclei.

2.4   Synaptic Contacts

As expected, numerous axo-dendritic and axo-somatic synapses are found in the various nuclei of the hypothalamus. In the median eminence, however, ultrastructurally, there are no classical features of axo-axonic synapses. The processes of nerve terminals, glial cells, and tanacytes form an orderly array around the portal capillaries separated from the endothelial cells by a 2–6 μm wide perivascular space (71, 72).

3   FACTORS AFFECTING PEPTIDERGIC AND NONPEPTIDERGIC NEURONS AND INTERACTIONS BETWEEN THEM

Nonpeptidergic neurons could influence peptidergic neurons by affecting or controlling (i) the rate of firing of peptidergic neurons by postsynaptic excitatory or inhibitory mechanisms, (ii) the amount of peptide available for release by transsynaptic induction of the macromolecular machinery of peptide synthesis, storage, and release, and (iii) presynaptic junctions on the terminals of peptidergic neurons. The nonpeptidergic transmitter could also affect the action of the peptide on its target cell by effects on the peptide–receptor interactions.

Most studies carried out so far have been on the effect of nonpeptidergic (particularly monoaminergic) neurons on peptidergic neurons. Investigation of this type of interaction has been carried out mainly with the aid of pharmacological agents, albeit mostly with more than one action, that block the synthesis, uptake, degradation, and action of nonpeptide transmitters. Few agents of this type are available for the study of the effect of peptidergic on nonpeptidergic neurons, and so fewer data are available.

In addition to their effects on one another, peptidergic and nonpeptidergic neurons are also probably influenced by peripheral hormones, especially steroids. There is evidence that the levels of enzymes responsible for monoamine synthesis and metabolism are affected by steroids (73–80), and this is no doubt true of peptides as well (81–83). Studies of transcriptional control mechanisms and of translational and posttranslational events in peptidergic neurons are still in their infancy, but they promise to help in the unraveling of central neuroendocrine mechanisms.

4 GONADOTROPIN CONTROL IN SPECIFIC PHYSIOLOGICAL AND EXPERIMENTAL MODEL SYSTEMS

This section shows the way in which the structural and functional interactions described above play a key role in specific physiological systems central to reproductive processes and in experimental models that have been used to investigate the central control of gonadotropin secretion. Most of the data referred to have been obtained from studies in the female rat, but in principle many of these can be extrapolated to other species, including the human.

4.1 Sexual Differentiation of the Brain

The adult pattern of gonadotropin output and sexual behavior in a number of species is known to be dependent not on genetic sex but on the endocrine status of the animal during a critical period of development. Early studies on neonatal guinea pigs (84) and rats (85) showed that implantation of a testis into the female abolished cyclic gonadotropin output. Experiments carried out with pituitary grafts (86) suggested that the hypothalamus, rather than the pituitary, was masculinized by testicular hormones. Testosterone proved to be as effective as a testicular graft in masculinizing animals. The precise mechanisms by which testosterone causes these changes are unknown.

The MPOA and anterior hypothalamus are the major centers involved in the control of cyclicity. A number of approaches, including the use of tritiated steroid autoradiography (87), steroid implants (88), and morphological and electrophysiological techniques, have indicated that those regions of the brain that specifically bind androgens, including the MPOA and anterior hypothalamus, exhibit a number of sexually dimorphic features. Within these areas, the conversion of ^{3}H-estradiol has been shown to occur as a consequence of an aromatase enzyme system (89); this fact, together with the observations that estrogens are equally as potent as or more potent than testosterone in causing masculinization (90) and that antiestrogens are effective inhibitors of the process (91), suggests that an estrogen, rather than testosterone itself, renders the hypothalamus acyclic. It has been suggested that in addition to its probable role in masculinizing the brain in the male, estradiol may be essential for "feminizing" the female brain (92).

Although neurotransmitter involvement in control of the LH surge has been extensively studied in the adult rat (4.2 and 4.3), the role played by the indole and catecholamines in the process of sexual differentiation itself is still not understood. There is no information with regard to peptidergic influences on such differentiation. It is unlikely that it is the absolute level of any one transmitter or peptide hormone that is important in developmental changes, but rather the resulting net changes in input to sexually differentiating regions of the brain (see also Section 4.2).

4.2   Postnatal Development and Puberty

Neuronal systems before the critical period (postnatal day 5) for sexual differentiation are not fully developed or remain susceptible to differentiating forces. Ultrastructural studies show that in the rat, between days 4 and 11 after birth, there is an exponential increase in the presence of transmitter vesicles in nerve terminals of the median eminence, and this is followed by an exponential increase in secretory granules in the pars distalis (71). This increase in transmitter vesicles and secretory granules corresponds with an increase in monoamines and acetylcholine in the median eminence (93, 94) and a fivefold increase in the LHRH content of the hypothalamus (95, 96), and a correspondingly sharp increase in the pituitary contents of LH, FSH, and adrenocorticotropin (96).

The broad pattern that emerges is that peptide and nonpeptide transmitter systems begin to develop gradually late in the fetal life of the rat and then develop exponentially after the critical period for sexual differentiation. No major sex differences have been found in this pattern of development, and at present it seems that sexual differentiation is not due to transmitter content or receptor density of the brain but rather to the differences in the development of functional pathways. Sexual differentiation does, however, cause changes in transmitter development during "adolescence," puberty, and adulthood. Before puberty, the hypothalamic content of LHRH increases in parallel in the male and fe-

male; in the female, however, the increase stops at puberty, while in the
male hypothalamic LHRH continues to increase steeply well into adult
life (96). Neonatal administration of testosterone results in a pattern of
LHRH increase that lies between the male and female pattern. Sex differences in the pituitary and plasma concentrations of the gonadotropins are much more marked than in the hypothalamic content of LHRH
(96), and in the normal female the onset of puberty (vaginal opening
and first estrus) is preceded on the first proestrus by a spontaneous ovulatory surge of LH (97). In the androgenized female, vaginal opening is
significantly delayed and there is no evidence of ovulation or a preovulatory gonadotropin surge.

The mechanism that evokes the first spontaneous ovulatory surge of
gonadotropins (97) is broadly similar to that in the adult (see Section
4.3) with the exception that, in contrast with the adult, the rate of synthesis of LHRH and the gonadotropins is not able to keep up with release, and therefore at the time of the surge there is a significant drop
in the hypothalamic content of LHRH and the pituitary content of LH
and FSH. The hypothalamic-pituitary mechanisms for the production of
the surge are established long before puberty, and the rate-limiting step
is the maturation of the ovarian mechanism for the generation of a
surge of estradiol-17β, which triggers both a surge of LHRH and an increase in the responsiveness of the pituitary to LHRH (97, 98). Some of
the key evidence for the modulation of LHRH release by central
catecholaminergic systems is in fact based on studies in immature rats;
this evidence is discussed in detail in Section 4.3.

4.3   Control of the Spontaneous Ovulatory Gonadotropin Surge

4.3.1   Key Events in the Production of the Ovulatory
Gonadotropin Surge

Ovulation in the rat, as in all other spontaneously ovulating mammals,
is triggered by a spontaneous surge of LH, which in turn is preceded by
a significant increase in the plasma concentration of estradiol-17β and
is accompanied by an increased secretion of ovarian progesterone (Figure 1). The spontaneous surge of LH is brought about by a cascade (Figure 2) initiated by the increase in the plasma concentration of
estradiol-17β. The latter produces a relatively massive increase in the
responsiveness of the anterior pituitary gland to LHRH (99, 100) and
triggers a surge of LHRH (Figure 3; 101–103). The responsiveness of the
anterior pituitary gland to LHRH is increased further by the increased
secretion of ovarian progesterone (100, 104, 105) and the priming effect
of LHRH (106–108). The priming effect of LHRH probably serves to coordinate the surge of LHRH with the increase in pituitary responsiveness so that the two events reach a peak at about the same time,
thereby ensuring a relatively massive ovulatory surge of LH.

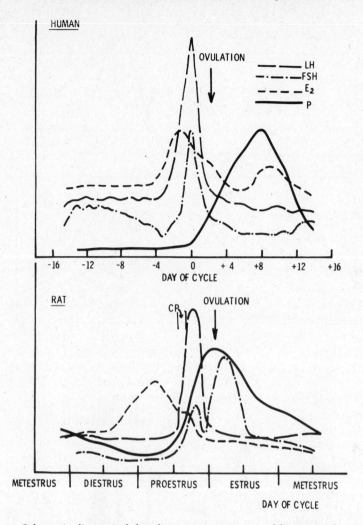

Figure 1. Schematic diagram of the plasma concentrations of luteinizing hormone (LH), follicle stimulating hormone (FSH), estradiol-17β (E₂), and progesterone (P) during the menstrual cycle of the human and estrous cycle of the rat. The critical period (CP) in the rat is the time before which administration of neural blocking agents will block the LH surge and ovulation (174). Reproduced with permission of Churchill Livingstone from Fink et al. (175).

Only flimsy data exist on the mechanism of action of estradiol-17β. The length of time between the first significant rise in plasma estradiol concentrations on diestrus and the LH surge (about 25–27 h) is compatible not only with the synthesis of new proteins but also with structural changes, possibly involving, for example, the establishment of new synapses. In the brain, estrogen increases progesterone receptors (109) and the firing rate of some of the neurons in the MPOA and anterior hypothalamus (110), and affects the activity of enzymes that synthesize

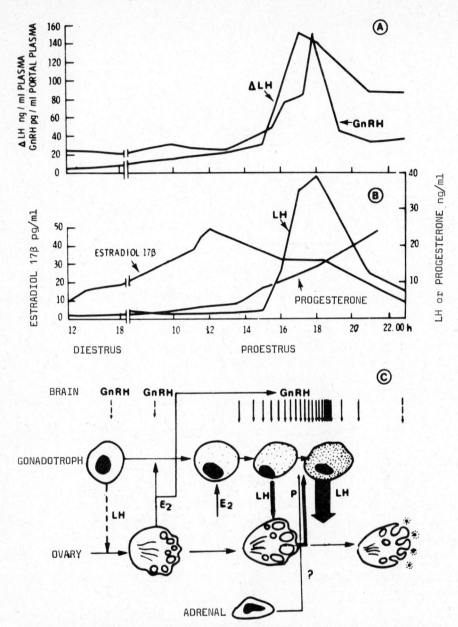

Figure 2. Cascade of events leading to the spontaneous ovulatory surge in Wistar rats. (A) Changes in pituitary responsiveness (curve labeled △LH) and mean concentrations of gonadotropin releasing hormone (GnRH = LHRH in this chapter) in hypophyseal portal plasma during diestrus and proestrus. △LH: mean maximal increments in peripheral plasma LH after intravenous injection of 50 ng GnRH/100 g body weight. (B) Mean peripheral plasma concentrations of estradiol-17β, progesterone, and LH. (C) Schematic interpretation of data in (A) and (B). Low (basal) secretion of FSH and LH stimulates growth of ovarian follicles, which secrete estradiol-17β (E$_2$). This ovarian signal (E$_2$) increases the

monoamines (Section 3.2.1). The "sensitizing" effect of estradiol on the anterior pituitary gland requires that the gland be exposed to at least some LHRH (111).

A large body of pharmacological data indicates that the stimulatory action of estradiol-17β and the LH surge do, at least acutely, depend upon the integrity of NA neurons, although recent data suggest that when the NA neurons are destroyed, a "bypass" mechanism for LH release may become operative (8–10).

4.3.2   The Role of Catecholaminergic Neurons in the LH Surge Mechanism

Direct evidence for a stimulatory role of a central NA mechanism in gonadotropin control has come from measurements of LHRH released into hypophyseal portal blood in immature female rats treated with pregnant mare serum gonadotropin (PMSG) (112). Female rats injected with PMSG on day 30 have a surge of LH on day 32 and ovulate on day 33. This surge of LH is triggered by a surge of LHRH, but unlike the spontaneous surge of LH, it is not preceded or accompanied by a major change in pituitary responsiveness to LHRH (97). Administration of α-methyl-p-tyrosine, diethyldithiocarbamate (DDC), or fusaric acid (inhibitors of dopamine-β-hydroxylase) inhibited the PMSG-induced surge of LHRH and LH. The administration of dihydroxyphenylserine (DOPS) reversed the inhibitory effect of DDC. In agreement with the effects of α-adrenoreceptor blockers on LH release in other model systems (113), phenoxybenzamine also inhibited the PMSG-induced surges of LH and LHRH.

The role of central DA neurons in the control of gonadotropin release has long been and remains controversial (12–14). In our studies on the PMSG-treated rat, we found that the LH and LHRH surges were significantly increased by pimozide and domperidone and decreased by haloperidol, effects that were reversed by apomorphine. Domperidone, when given before the "critical" period on proestrus, also greatly increased the height of the spontaneous surge of LH in the adult rat (112). Furthermore, 6-hydroxydopamine (6-OHDA)-induced lesions predominantly of

---

responsiveness of the pituitary gonadotrophs (increased stippling) to GnRH and also triggers the surge of GnRH. Pituitary responsiveness to GnRH is further increased by progesterone secreted from the ovary in response to the LH released during the early part of the LH surge and by the priming effect of GnRH. The priming effect of GnRH coordinates the surge of GnRH with increasing pituitary responsiveness so that the two events reach a peak at the same time. The conditions are thereby made optimal for a massive surge of LH. This cascade, which represents a form of positive feedback, is terminated by the rupture of ovarian follicles (ovulation). Reproduced with permission of the British Council from (176).

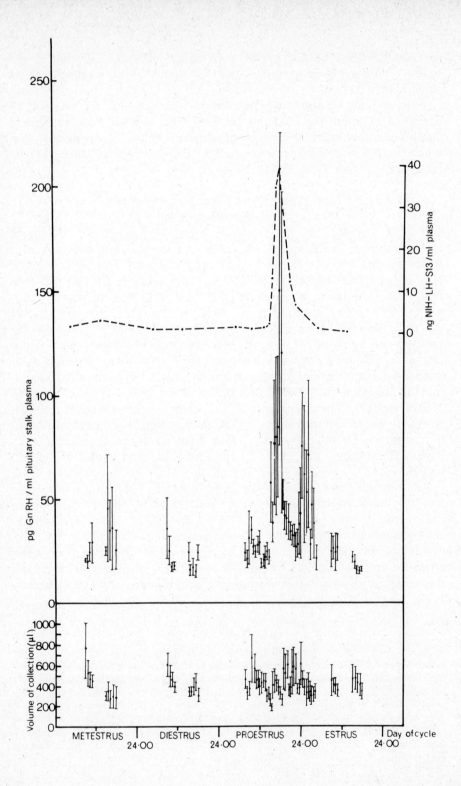

the DA terminals of the median eminence significantly increased the PMSG-induced surge of LHRH (114). Lesions of NA terminals in the dorsal hypothalamus, on the other hand, produced a reduction in the height of the PMSG-induced surges of LH and LHRH. The latter is consistent with the finding of Martinovic and McCann (115) that acute injections of 6-OHDA into the ventral NA tract blocked the spontaneous and steroid-induced surges of LH.

Lesions of the ascending NA systems do not necessarily lead to permanent loss of estrous cycles in the rat (8–10). However, in the study of Clifton and Sawyer (9), about 20% of the NA in the ME remained. The apparent conflict between the results of acute compared with long-term catecholaminergic lesions on the cyclical release of LH could be explained by invoking supersensitivity, the fact that the remaining NA fibers after a lesion might be sufficient to drive the system, or that in placing lesions, not only NA systems but also systems antagonistic to the NA systems are destroyed by the lesion (thus correcting the "imbalance") (14).

4.3.3 Effect of Prolactin

Hyperprolactinemia is frequently associated with infertility and amenorrhea (116), whether the hyperprolactinemia is due to suckling and lactation, a pituitary tumor, or intake of neuroleptic (dopamine receptor-blocking) drugs. Where and how prolactin and/or suckling stimuli exert their effects is not clear, although several possible mechanisms have been suggested. Evans et al. (116), for example, suggest that increased plasma prolactin concentration stimulates an increased turnover of hypothalamic DA (as part of a negative feedback loop—since DA inhibits prolactin secretion), which, in turn, inhibits the secretion of LH. While such a mechanism might explain the inhibition of gonadotropin secretion under some circumstances, it could not easily explain the amenorrhea that accompanies neuroleptic-induced hyperprolactinemia, since

---

Figure 3. Mean ($\pm$ SEM) plasma concentrations of GnRH (= LHRH in this chapter) and blood volume of 30 min collections of hypophyseal protal blood at different times of the estrous cycle. The mean concentrations of plasma LH are shown by the interrupted line. Studies with neural blocking agents (174, 178) suggested that a neural signal might occur each day. The above data show that if a daily neural signal does occur it it not expressed as a surge of LHRH except on proestrus, when the brain has been exposed to elevated plasma concentrations of estradiol-17β for about 25–27 h. A daily neural signal is expressed as a surge of LHRH, however, in long-term ovariectomized rats treated with high doses of estrogen (see Section 4.3.5). Infusion studies (107, 177) show that the portal plasma concentrations of LHRH shown here are of the order that would produce a surge of LH in proestrous rats. Reproduced with the permission of *Nature* from Sarkar et al. (101).

the neuroleptics block DA receptors. Our current understanding of the neurochemical anatomy of the hypothalamus is too poor to permit a clear view of how the systems that control prolactin and gonadotropin are linked.

4.3.4   Effect of the Endogenous Opiate System on Gonadotropin Release

Barraclough and Sawyer (117) were the first to show that gonadotropin release was blocked by morphine. The discovery of the endogenous opiates, the enkephalins and endorphins, led to renewed interest in the possible interactions between central opioid and neuroendocrine neurons. Several studies have shown that in a number of mammals, including humans, gonadotropin secretion is suppressed by morphine, enkephalin, or endorphin or their agonists, and is stimulated by the administration of morphine antagonists such as naloxone and naltrexone (118–124). Anti-β-endorphin and antidynorphin sera, when injected into the ARC or MBH, produced a significant increase in the plasma concentration of LH in immature female rats (125). The opiates and their agonists and antagonists do not significantly affect pituitary responsiveness to LHRH, and this suggests a hypothalamic site of action. However, whether the central opioid neurons act directly on LHRH neurons and/or indirectly by effects mediated by either catecholamine (126) or catechol-estrogen (127) systems remains to be established.

Since opiates stimulate prolactin release, the possibility has been raised that an opioid mechanism may be involved in the abnormal gonadotropin secretion that occurs in hyperprolactinemia (116).

4.3.5   Experimental Models for the Study of Acute Gonadotropin and Prolactin Release

Several steroid models have been developed in order to facilitate the study of the mechanisms that underlie the surge release of the gonadotropins and prolactin (128). Much of the data cited in Section 4.3.1 are based on a model in which rats are subjected to steroid manipulation, acutely before the presumptive day of proestrus. Many studies have been carried out on two models developed by Taleisnik and his associates, in which long-term ovariectomized rats are exposed to high doses of estrogen (129–131) or a single large dose of estrogen followed by an injection of progesterone (128, 131). The first model (I) produces, after two days, a diurnal afternoon surge of the gonadotropin and prolactin, while the second (II) produces a massive surge of LH, with a peak 5 h after the injection of progesterone. Although it is not certain that either model replicates the mechanism or even uses the same components of the mechanism of the spontaneous ovulatory surge of gonadotropin and prolactin, both models have been used extensively to study possible interactions between the LHRH and nonpeptidergic systems of the hypothalamus.

Importance of Serotonergic Neurons.   In model I, the diurnal rhythm of LH depends upon the integrity of the SCN (132, 133), is found only in female rats (130, 134), and is driven by a different neural mechanism from that of the pulsatile LH rhythm in ovariectomized rats (133). Because of the high concentration of 5HT terminals within the SCN, work has focused on the role of 5HT in driving this rhythm. Treatment with parachloro-phenylalanine (PCPA), a blocker of tryptophan hydroxylase that results in a massive depletion of brain 5HT, will completely block the LH surge (135). Injection of 5HTP (the immediate precursor of 5HT) into PCPA-treated animals during a "critical period" in the morning will restore the surge in the afternoon. However, lesions of the raphe nuclei, which supply the 5HT innervation to the SCN, do not completely inhibit the surge (136, 137). This suggests that the hypothalamus receives 5HT innervation from a source outside the raphe nuclei, or that PCPA also depletes a compound other than 5HT that is essential for the rhythm to occur (137), or both.

Estradiol itself did not alter the 5HT content of the SCN 48 h after injection in ovariectomized rats (138), but this does not exclude the possibility of changes in turnover. Estradiol did, however, produce an initial reduction in brain 5HT receptors before a localized increase in receptor number in the hypothalamus, MPOA, and amygdala (139).

In contrast with the diurnal release of LH, the surge of LH induced by estrogen-progesterone treatment (model II) seems to be unaffected by lesions of the raphe nuclei (140). Indeed, electrical stimulation of the raphe nuclei resulted in a reduction in the progesterone-induced LH surge. Waloch et al. (140) suggested that the raphe nuclei inhibited progesterone-induced LH release.

Like the estradiol-induced diurnal rhythm, progesterone exhibits a diurnal variation in efficacy to induce an LH surge (129, 141, 142). A possible role for the SCN and 5HT is shown by the loss of LH surges induced by progesterone after lesions of the SCN (141) and the facilitation of the surge by 5HTP treatment in response to an injection of progesterone at 0700 h, a time at which progesterone does not normally trigger a surge (143). Franks et al. (143) also showed that treatment with a serotonin antagonist at 1200 h blocked the progesterone-induced LH (but not FSH) surge later in the afternoon.

Different mechanisms subserve these two types of surges of LH. The estradiol-induced diurnal release of LH is accompanied by a surge of LHRH into the portal vessels (142) but no diurnal change in pituitary responsiveness to LHRH (130), although the pituitary response throughout the day is much greater than at proestrus. The progesterone-induced surge is not accompanied by any detectable surge of LHRH (142) and is therefore likely to be due mainly to the massive increase in pituitary responsiveness to LHRH (144) brought about by progesterone.

Catecholamines. Recent work (145–149) has suggested that both the content and turnover rate of NA and DA in discrete brain nuclei is changed by ovarian steroid manipulation. With regard to Model I, Honma and Wuttke (147) used α-methyl-*p*-tyrosine treatment to show that NA turnover increased from morning to afternoon in the MPOA and both the anterior and posterior mediobasal hypothalamus; similar results were seen two and three days after estrogen treatment (148, 150). Described changes in dopamine turnover are less conclusive (147, 150).

Estradiol rapidly lowers (143, 151) plasma LH concentrations in ovariectomized rats by inhibiting LHRH release. This mechanism may involve interactions with opioid neurons (152) and NA (149) but not with 5HT metabolism (A. G. Watts, unpublished data), which leads to a reduction in LHRH secretion.

Interactions between peptidergic and nonpeptidergic neurons in Model II present a confused picture. After the massive initial progesterone-induced surge of LH, no further LH surges occur (153, 154). The increase in NA turnover in hypothalamic regions found in the afternoon in Model I appear to be abolished by progesterone in Model II (150). Rance et al. (150) found elevated DA turnover rates in the MPOA, the ARC, and the median eminence. In conscious ovariectomized rats Leung et al. (154) showed that estradiol-progesterone treatment would decrease the inhibitory action of NA on the multiple unit electrical activity of the MPOA, the anterior hypothalamic area, and the diagonal band of Broca. This suggests that if the multiple unit activity represents the activity of LHRH neurons, estradiol-progesterone treatment decreases the efficacy of NA to inhibit LHRH neuronal firing rate. A similar reversal of NA effects on LH secretion as a result of estrogen-progesterone treatment, but not estrogen alone, was reported by Gallo and Drouva (155).

4.3.6 The Control of Pulsatile LH Release

Like most hormones, LH is released in a pulsatile manner. In the human, this is seen when the gonads are intact, but in the rat pulsatile LH release is seen most clearly after gonadectomy. Pulsatile LH release is almost certainly due to pulsatile release of LHRH (142, 156, 157). The role of monoamines in the generation of pulsatile LH release is, however, not clear, at least as assessed in long-term ovariectomized rats. Thus, while electrical stimulation of the raphe nuclei inhibits pulsatile LH release, an effect that can be reversed by PCPA (158), depletion of brain 5HT with PCPA did not change the character of pulsatile release

(159, 160). Pulsatile LH release is not affected by pimozide (161, 162) or α-methyl-p-tyrosine (163).

With respect to NA, most data show that this monoamine inhibits pulsatile LH release, in contrast with its stimulatory role in the preovulatory LH surge. Thus, pulsatile LH release was inhibited by intraventricular infusion of NA (155, 164), intravenous injection of the adrenoreceptor agonists clonidine, phenylephrine and to a lesser extent isoproterenol (164), and electrical stimulation of the ascending NA bundle (165). In conscious animals, intraventricular infusion of NA inhibited multiple unit activity of neurons within the diagonal band of Broca, the MPOA, and the anterior hypothalamus.

4.4 Senescence

After the period of normal regular estrous cycles and fertility, female rats undergo changes in reproductive patterns that eventually lead to cessation of reproductive function (166–168). Estrous cycles begin to lose regularity and are replaced by prolonged, persistent vaginal estrus (at around 10–12 months of age) and eventually by long periods of diestrus interrupted by occasional ovulatory activity (repetitive pseudopregnancy). The constant estrous (CE) smear pattern is accompanied by increased secretion of estrogens but decreased secretion of progestins, whereas in pseudopregnancy plasma estrogen concentrations are constant while plasma progestin increases (169). Lu et al. (169) showed that CE rats show no response to ovariectomy followed by estrogen-progesterone treatment; this is in contrast with the pseudopregnant state in which estrogen-progesterone stimulates LH release.

In the hypothalamus, transmitter function is altered. Although the hypothalamic content of LHRH is the same in females before and after the loss of regular cycles, levels fall in old anestrous rats (170). Hypothalamic 5HT concentrations are reduced in old CE rats (171), and drug treatments to the rostral hypothalamus (including the SCN) are most effective in inducing CE in young rats when 5HT levels are reduced to those found in elderly CE rats (171). Simpkins et al. (172) found depressed content and turnover rates of NA and DA with an increased turnover rate of 5HT, and Walker et al. (171) showed that CE occurred in 50–63% of young rats treated with α-methyl-p-tyrosine and diethyldithiocarbamate to the rostral hypothalamus. Estrous cycles could be reinitiated in aging female rats by L-Dopa or iproniazid (167, 173).

Taken together, these results suggest that modification of hypothalamic monoamines in the hypothalamus involving NA, DA, and especially 5HT lead to loss of rhythmical LH release and eventual anestrus. This loss of rhythm probably involves changes in the SCN, perhaps with 5HT depletion, as is suggested by the induction of CE in animals with SCN lesions (141) and PCPA treatment (171).

5 SUMMARY

Ultrastructural, immunohistochemical, and fluorescence histochemical studies have demonstrated that in the neuroendocrine brain there are several levels at which major interactions could occur between nonpeptidergic neurons and the neurons that release LHRH, the decapeptide that mediates central nervous control of gonadotropin secretion. However, in spite of the fact that pharmacological studies demonstrate that interactions do occur, especially between monoaminergic and LHRH neurons, the precise nature of the interactions is still not clear. The most clear-cut evidence is for the facilitating action of a central NA system in the production of the ovulatory surge of LHRH and thereby LH. Ovulatory surges of LH can occur, however, even when the hypothalamus has been largely depleted of its NA content by transection of the ascending NA projections from the brainstem. The role of DA neurons, especially of the TIDA system, remains controversial, but on balance the evidence suggests that DA inhibits LHRH and thereby LH release. In contrast to its facilitating action with respect to the ovulatory surge, NA reduces pulsatile LH release. Central 5HT neurons are important for the circadian pattern of LH (and therefore probably LHRH) release that can be produced by ovariectomy and estrogen treatment, but the relevance of this for the control of spontaneous LH in intact animals remains to be established. The ovulatory LH surge is blocked in hyperprolactinemia. Whether this is due to a direct action of prolactin or an interaction between the LHRH control system and the hypothalamic factors that inhibit (dopamine, GABA) or facilitate (TRH, vasoactive intestinal peptide, the enkephalins) prolactin release is not known, but the interactions between the control systems make it difficult to establish by pharmacological techniques the importance of peptidergic-nonpeptidergic interactions during sexual differentiation, development, and senescence, when the interactions are likely to be slow and subtle. The LHRH system also seems to be affected by other peptidergic systems, notably the opioids that inhibit LH release. The overall pattern of the control system is further complicated by the fact that gonadal and adrenal steroids have potent effects on the activity of both peptidergic and nonpeptidergic neurons.

Thus, although after more than five decades of intensive research we have a good understanding of the descriptive physiology of sexual differentation and gonadotropin secretion, the precise nature of the interactions between central transmitter systems important for gonadotropin control remains, as ever, a tantalizing but treacherous field of research.

ACKNOWLEDGMENTS

We are grateful to Norma Brearley, Jo Donnelly, and Celia Leitch for their careful preparation of this manuscript.

REFERENCES

1. C. H. Sawyer, J. E. Markee, and W. H. Hollinshead, *Endocrinology* **41**, 395 (1947).
2. A. V. Schally, A. Arimura, and A. J. Kastin, *Science* **179**, 341 (1973).
3. J. E. Markee, C. H. Sawyer, and W. H. Hollinshead, *Anat. Rec.* **97**, 398 (1947).
4. B. T. Donovan and G. W. Harris, *J. Physiol.* **132**, 577 (1956).
5. K. Fuxe and T. Hökfelt, in W. Bargmann and B. Scharrer, Eds., *Aspects of Neuroendocrinology*, Springer, Berlin, 1970, pp. 195–205.
6. K. Fuxe, T. Hökfelt, and O. Nillson, *Acta Endocrinol.* **69**, 625 (1972).
7. H. P. G. Schneider and S. M. McCann, in W. Bargmann and B. Scharrer, Eds., *Aspects of Neuroendocrinology*, Berlin, Springer, 1970, pp. 177–191.
8. D. K. Clifton, and C. H. Sawyer, *Neuroendocrinology* **28**, 442 (1979).
9. D. K. Clifton, and C. H. Sawyer, *Endocrinology* **106**, 1099 (1980).
10. G. Nicholson, G. Greeley, J. Humm, W. Youngblood, and J. S. Kizer, *Endocrinology* **103**, 559 (1978).
11. S. J. Ojeda and S. M. McCann, *Clin. Obstet. Gynecol.* **5**, 283 (1978).
12. G. Fink and L. B. Geffen, in R. Porter, Ed., *International Review of Physiology, Vol. 17: Neurophysiology III*, University Park Press, Baltimore, 1978, pp. 1–48.
13. R. I. Weiner and W. F. Ganong, *Physiol. Rev.* **58**, 905 (1978).
14. C. A. Barraclough and P. M. Wise, *Endocrinol. Rev.* **1**, 91 (1982).
15. M. L. Tappaz, M. J. Brownstein, and I. J. Kopin, *Brain Res.* **125**, 109 (1977).
16. S. R. Vincent, T. Hökfelt, and J -Y. Wu, *Neuroendocrinology* **34**, 117 (1982).
17. M. J. Brownstein, M. Palkovits, J. M. Saavedra, and J. S. Kizer, in L. Martini and W. F. Ganong, Eds., *Frontiers in Neuroendocrinology*, Raven Press, New York, 1976, pp. 1–23.
18. M. L. Tappaz and M. J. Brownstein, *Brain Res.* **132**, 95 (1977).
19. D. K. Meyer, W. H. Oertel, and M. J. Brownstein, *Brain Res.* **200**, 165 (1980).
20. M. Tappaz, M. Aguera, M. F. Belin, and E. F. Pujol, *Brain Res.* **186**, 379 (1980).
21. A. Dahlström and K. Fuxe, *Acta Physiol. Scand.* **62**, Suppl. 232 1 (1964).
22. K. Fuxe, *Acta Physiol. Scand.* **64**, Suppl. 247, 37 (1965).
23. U. Ungerstedt, *Acta Physiol. Scand. Suppl.* **367**, 1 (1971).
24. M. J. Kuhar, G. K. Aghajanian, and R. H. Roth, *Brain Res.* **44**, 165 (1972).
25. A. Björklund, A. Nobin, and U. Stenevi, *Z. Zellforsch. Mikrosk. Anat.* **145**, 479 (1973).
26. K. Fuxe and G. Jonsson, in E. Costa, G. L. Gessa, and M. Sandler, Eds., *Advances in Biochemical Pharmacology*, Vol. 10, Raven Press, New York, 1974, pp. 1–12.
27. V. Chan-Palay, *J. Comp. Neurol.* **176**, 467 (1977).
28. A. Parent, L. Descarries, and A. Beaudet, *Neuroscience* **6**, 115 (1981).
29. H. W. M. Steinbush, *Neuroscience* **6**, 557 (1981).
30. A. Consolazione and A. C. Cuello, in N. N. Osbourne, Ed., *Biology of Serotonergic Transmission*, Wiley, New York, 1982, pp. 29–61.
31. L. Descarries and A. Beaudet, in J. D. Vincent and C. Kordon, Eds., *Biologie cellulaire des processus neurosecretoires hypothalamiques*, Colloques Internationaux du CNRS, Vol. 80, Paris, 1978, pp. 135–153.
32. D. L. Kent and J. R. Sladek Jr., *J. Comp. Neurol.* **180**, 221 (1978).
33. J. M. Saavedra, M. Palkovits, M. J. Brownstein, and J. Axelrod, *Brain Res.* **77**, 157 (1974).
34. M. Palkovits, J. M. Saavedra, D. M. Jacobowitz, J. S. Kizer, L. Zaborsky, and M. J. Brownstein, *Brain Res.* **130**, 121 (1977).
35. L. D. Van de Kar and S. A. Lorens, *Brain Res.* **162**, 45 (1979).
36. A. Beaudet and L. Descarries, *Brain Res.* **160**, 231 (1979).
37. R. Y. Moore and F. E. Bloom, in W. M. Cowan, Z. W. Hall, and E. R. Kandel, Eds., *Annual Review of Neuroscience*, Vol. 1, Annual Reviews, Palo Alto, Calif., 1978, pp. 129–169.
38. M. Palkovits, *Neuroendocrinology* **33**, 123 (1981).

39.   J. H. Fallon and R. Y. Moore, *Anat. Rec.* **184**, 399 (1976).
40.   J. H. Fallon and R. Y. Moore, *Soc. Neurosci. Abstr.* **2**, 486 (1976).
41.   J. S. Kizer, M. Palkovits, and M. J. Brownstein, *Brain Res.* **108**, 363 (1976).
42.   O. Lindvall, A. Björklund, R. Y. Moore, and U. Stenevi, *Brain Res.* **81**, 325 (1974).
43.   A. Björklund, O. Lindvall, and A. Nobin, *Brain Res.* **89**, 29 (1975).
44.   T. Hökfelt, and K. Fuxe, in K. M. Knigge, E. E. Scott, and A. Weindl, Eds., *Median Eminence: Structure and Function*, S. Karger, Basel, 1972, pp. 181–223.
45.   A. Björklund, B. Falck, A. Nobin, and U. Stenevi, in F. Knowles and L. Vollrath, Eds., *Neurosecretion: The Final Neuroendocrine Pathway*, Springer, New York, 1973, p. 209–222.
46.   G. C. Smith and G. Fink, *Brain Res.* **43**, 37 (1972).
47.   A. Björklund, B. Falck, F. Hromek, C. Owman, and K. A. West, *Brain Res.* **17**, 1 (1970).
48.   G. Jonssen, K. Fuxe, and T. Hökfelt, *Brain Res.* **40**, 271 (1972).
49.   K. Ajika and T. Hökfelt, *Brain Res.* **57**, 97 (1973).
50.   A. Björklund, R. Y. Moore, A. Nobin, and U. Stenevi, *Brain Res.* **51**, 171 (1973).
51.   K. Ajika and T. Hökfelt, *Cell Tissue Res.* **158**, 15 (1975).
52.   N. E. Andén, A. Dahlström, K. Fuxe, K. Larsson, L. Olson, and U. Ungerstedt, *Acta Physiol. Scand.* **67**, 313 (1966).
53.   N. A. Hillarp, K. Fuxe, and A. Dahlström, *Pharmacol. Rev.* **18**, 727 (1966).
54.   L. Olsen and K. Fuxe, *Brain Res.* **43**, 289 (1972).
55.   M. Palkovits and D. M. Jacobowitz, *J. Comp. Neurol.* **157**, 29 (1974).
56.   L. W. Swanson and B. K. Hartman, *J. Comp. Neurol.* **163**, 467 (1975).
57.   J. C. Dupin, L. Descarries, and J. de Champlain, *Brain Res.* **103**, 588 (1976).
58.   O. Lindvall and A. Björklund, in I. Iversen, S. Iversen, and S. H. Snyder, Eds., *Handbook of Psychopharmacology*, Plenum Press, New York, 1978, pp. 139–231.
59.   M. Segal, V. Pickel, and F. Bloom, *Life Sci.* **13**, 817 (1973).
60.   B. E. Jones and R. Y. Moore, *Brain Res.* **127**, 23 (1977).
61.   M. Palkovits, M. Brownstein, and M. J. Saavedra, *Brain Res.* **77**, 137 (1974).
62.   D. H. G. Versteeg, J. van der Gugten, W. De Jong, and M. Palkovits, *Brain Res.* **113**, 563 (1976).
63.   K. Fuxe and T. Hökfelt, in L. Martini and W. F. Ganong, Eds., *Frontiers in Neuroendocrinology*, Oxford University Press, New York, 1969, pp. 47–96.
64.   D. M. Jacobowitz and M. Palkovits, *J. Comp. Neurol.* **157**, 13 (1974).
65.   K. Fuxe, T. Hökfelt, L. F. Agnati, O. Johansson, M. Goldstein, M. Perez de la Mora, L. Possani, R. Tapia, L. Teran, and R. Palacios, in M. A. Lipton, A. Dimascio, and K. F. Killam, Eds., *Psychopharmacology: A Generation of Progress*, Raven Press, New York, 1978, pp. 67–94.
66.   T. Hökfelt, K. Fuxe, M. Goldstein, and O. Johansson, *Brain Res.* **66**, 235 (1974).
67.   A. Parent and L. L. Butcher, *J. Comp. Neurol.* **170**, 205 (1976).
68.   M. J. Brownstein, R. D. Utiger, M. Palkovits, and J. S. Kizer, *Proc. Natl. Acad. Sci. USA.* **72**, 4177 (1975).
69.   D. B. Hoover, E. A. Muth, and D. M. Jacobowitz, *Brain Res.* **153**, 295 (1978).
70.   G. A. Block and R. B. Billiar, *Brain Res.* **212**, 152 (1981).
71.   G. Fink and G. C. Smith, *Z. Zellforsch.* **119**, 208 (1971).
72.   K. M. Knight, D. E. Scott, and A. Weindl, *Brain Endocrine Interaction*, S. Karger, Basel, 1972.
73.   E. E. Baetge, B. B. Kaplan, D. J. Reis, and T. H. Joh, *Proc. Natl. Acad. Sci. USA.* **78**, 1269 (1981).
74.   C. W. Beattie and L. F. Soyka, *Endocrinology* **93**, 1453 (1973).
75.   C. W. Beattie, C. H. Rodgers, and L. F. Soyka, *Endocrinology* **91**, 276 (1972).
76.   J. S. Kizer, M. Palkovits, J. Zivin, J. M. Brownstein, J. M. Saavedra, and I. J. Kopin, *Endocrinology* **95**, 799 (1974).

77. J. S. Kizer, E. Muth, and D. M. Jacobowitz, *Endocrinology* **98**, 886 (1976).
78. T. Lloyd, B. Boyd, M. A. Walega, B. J. Ebersole, and J. Weisz, *J. Neurochem.* **38**, 948 (1982).
79. I. Vernes, M. Varszegi, E. K. Toth, and G. Telegdy, *Neuroendocrinology* **28**, 386 (1978).
80. J. W. Simpkins, P. S. Kalra, and S. P. Kalra, *Neuroendocrinology* **31**, 177 (1980).
81. R. A. Maurer, *J. Biol. Chem.* **257**, 2133 (1982).
82. H. Kuhl, C. Rosniatowski, and H. D. Taubert, *Acta Endocrinol. Scand.* **87**, 476 (1978).
83. E. C. Griffiths and K. C. Hooper, *Acta Endocrinol. Scand.* **74**, 41 (1973).
84. E. Steinach, *Zentralblatt Physiol.* **27**, 717 (1913).
85. C. A. Pfeiffer, *Am. J. Anat.* **58**, 195 (1936).
86. G. W. Harris and D. Jacobsohn, *Proc. R. Soc. London Ser. B.* **139**, 263 (1952).
87. D. W. Pfaff, *Endocrinology* **82**, 1149 (1968).
88. L. W. Christensen and R. A. Gorski, *Brain Res.* **146**, 325 (1978).
89. F. Naftolin, K. J. Ryan, I. J. Davies, V. V. Reddy, F. Flores, Z. Petro, M. Kuhn, R. J. White, Y. Takaoka, and L. Wolin, *Rec. Prog. Horm. Res.* **31**, 295 (1975).
90. C. Doughty, J. E. Booth, P. G. McDonald, and R. F. Parrot, *J. Endocrinol.* **67**, 419 (1975).
91. P. G. McDonald and C. Doughty, *J. Endocrinol.* **55**, 455 (1972).
92. K. D. Dohler and J. L. Hancke, in G. Dörner and M. Kawakami, Eds., *Hormones and Brain Behaviour*, North Holland, Amsterdam, 1978, pp. 153–168.
93. G. C. Smith and R. W. Simpson, *Z. Zellforsch.* **104**, 541 (1970).
94. J. T. Coyle and S. J. Enna, *Brain Res.* **111**, 119 (1976).
95. S. Araki, C. D. Toran-Allerand, M. Ferin and R. L. Vande Wiele, *Endocrinology* **97**, 693 (1975).
96. S. A. Chiappa and G. Fink, *J. Endocrinol.* **72**, 211 (1977).
97. D. K. Sarkar and G. Fink, *J. Endocrinol.* **83**, 339 (1979).
98. S. R. Ojeda, W. W. Andrews, J. P. Advis, and S. Smith White, *Endocr. Rev.* **1**, 228 (1980).
99. M. S. Aiyer, G. Fink, and F. Greig, *J. Endocrinol.* **60**, 47 (1974).
100. M. S. Aiyer and G. Fink, *J. Endocrinol.* **62**, 553 (1974).
101. D. K. Sarkar, S. A. Chiappa, G. Fink, and N. M. Sherwood, *Nature* **264**, 461 (1976).
102. N. M. Sherwood, S. A. Chiappa, D. K. Sarkar, and G. Fink, *Endocrinology* **207**, 1410 (1980).
103. M. Ching, *Neuroendocrinology* **34**, 279 (1982).
104. G. Fink and S. R. Henderson, *J. Endocrinol.* **73**, 157 (1977).
105. J. L. Turgeon and D. W. Waring, *Endocrinology* **108**, 413 (1981).
106. M. S. Aiyer, S. A. Chiappa, and G. Fink, *J. Endocrinol.* **62**, 573 (1974).
107. G. Fink, S. A. Chiappa, and M. S. Aiyer, *J. Endocrinol.* **69**, 359 (1976).
108. A. Pickering and G. Fink, *J. Endocrinol.* **81**, 223 (1979).
109. N. J. Machusky and B. S. McEwen, *Nature* **274**, 276 (1978).
110. B. A. Cross and R. G. Dyer, *J. Physiol.* **222**, 25P (1972).
111. A. Speight, R. Popkin, A. G. Watts, and G. Fink, *J. Endocrinol.* **88**, 301 (1981).
112. D. K. Sarkar and G. Fink, *Endocrinology* **108**, 862 (1981).
113. P. S. Kalra, S. P. Kalra, L. Krulich, C. P. Fawcett, and S. M. McCann, *Endocrinology* **90**, 1168 (1972).
114. D. K. Sarkar, G. C. Smith, and G. Fink, *Brain Res.* **213**, 335 (1981).
115. J. V. Martinovic and S. M. McCann, *Endocrinology* **100**, 1206 (1977).
116. W. S. Evans, M. J. Cronin, and M. D. Thorner, in W. F. Ganong, and L. Martini, Eds., *Frontiers in Neuroendocrinology*, Vol. 7, Raven Press, New York, 1982, pp. 77–122.
117. C. A. Barraclough and C. H. Sawyer, *Endocrinology* **57**, 329 (1955).

118. T. J. Cicero, E. R. Meyer, R. D. Bell, and G. A. Koch, *Endocrinology* **98**, 367 (1976).
119. T. J. Cicero, T. M. Badger, C. E. Wilcox, R. D. Bell, and E. R. Meyer, *J. Pharmacol. Exp. Ther.* **203**, 548 (1977).
120. T. J. Cicero, B. A. Schainker, and E. R. Meyer, *Endocrinology* **104**, 1286 (1979).
121. J. F. Bruni, D. Van Vugt, S. Marshall and J. Meites, *Life Sci.* **21**, 461 (1977).
122. G. Delitala, L. Devilla, and L. Arata, *Acta Endocrinol.* **97**, 150 (1981).
123. P. Grossman, P. J. A. Moult, R. C. Gaillard, G. Delitala, W. A. Toff, L. H. Rees, and G. M. Besser, *Clin. Endocrinol.* **14**, 41 (1981).
124. J. F. Ropert, M. E. Quigley, and S. S. C. Yen, *J. Clin. Endocrinol. Metab.* **52**, 583 (1981).
125. R. Schulz, A. Wilhelm, K. M. Pirke, C. Gramsch, and A. Herz, *Nature* **294**, 757 (1981).
126. W. H. Rotsztejn, S. V. Drouva, E. Pattou, and C. Kordon, *Nature* **274**, 281 (1978).
127. J. Fishman, B. I. Norton, and E. F. Hahn, *Proc. Natl. Acad. Sci. USA* **77**, 2574 (1980).
128. G. Fink, *Ann. Rev. Physiol.* **41**, 571 (1979).
129. L. Caligaris, J. J. Astrada, and S. Taleisnik, *Endocrinology* **88**, 810 (1971).
130. S. R. Henderson, C. Baker, and G. Fink, *J. Endocrinol.* **73**, 455 (1977).
131. L. Caligaris, J. J. Astrada, and S. Taleisnik, *Acta Endocrinol.* **59**, 177 (1968).
132. M. Kamakami, J. Arita, and E. Yoshioka, *Endocrinology* **106**, 1087 (1980).
133. A. G. Watts and G. Fink, *J. Endocrinol.* **89**, 141 (1981).
134. J. D. Neill, *Endocrinology* **90**, 1154 (1972).
135. M. Héry, E. Laplante, and C. Kordon, *Endocrinology* **99**, 496 (1976).
136. M. Héry, E. Laplante, and C. Kordon, *Endocrinology* **102**, 1019 (1978).
137. C. W. Coen, M. Coombs, P. M. J. Wilson, E. M. Clement, and P. C. P. MacKinnon, *Neuroscience* **7**, Suppl., S.42 (1982).
138. W. R. Crowley, T. L. O'Donohue, E. A. Muth, and D. M. Jacobowitz, *Brain Res. Bull.* **4**, 571 (1978).
139. A. Biegon and B. S. McEwen, *J. Neurosci.* **2**, 199 (1982).
140. M. Waloch, D. Gilman, D. Whitmoyer, and C. H. Sawyer, *Brain Res.* **217**, 305 (1981).
141. K. Brown-Grant and G. Raisman, *Proc. R. Soc. Lond., Ser. B.* **198**, 279 (1977).
142. D. K. Sarkar and G. Fink, *J. Endocrinol.* **86**, 511 (1980).
143. S. Franks, J. McElhone, S. N. Young, I. Kraulis, and K. B. Ruf, *Endocrinology* **107**, 353 (1980).
144. M. S. Aiyer, M. C. Sood, and K. Brown-Grant, *J. Endocrinol.* **69**, 255 (1976).
145. A. Löfström, P. Eneroth, J.-A. Gustafsson, and P. Skett, *Endocrinology* **101**, 1559 (1977).
146. W. R. Crowley, T. L. O'Donohue, H. Wachslicht, and D. M. Jacobowitz, *Brain Res.* **154**, 345 (1978).
147. K. Honma and W. Wuttke, *Endocrinology* **106**, 1848 (1980).
148. P. M. Wise, N. Rance, and C. A. Barraclough, *Endocrinology* **108**, 2186 (1981).
149. W. R. Crowley, *Neuroendocrinology* **34**, 381 (1982).
150. N. Rance, P. M. Wise, M. K. Selmanoff, and C. A. Barraclough, *Endocrinology* **108**, 1795 (1981).
151. C. A. Blake, R. L. Norman, and C. H. Sawyer, *Neuroendocrinology* **16**, 22 (1974).
152. M. C. Freeman, K. C. Dupke, and C. M. Croteau, *Endocrinology* **99**, 223 (1976).
153. L. V. DePaulo and C. A. Barraclough, *Biol. Reprod.* **20**, 1173 (1979).
154. P. C. K. Leung, D. I. Whitmoyer, G. W. Arendash, and C. H. Sawyer, *Brain Res.* **226**, 143 (1981).
155. R. V. Gallo and S. V. Drouva, *Neuroendocrinology* **29**, 149 (1979).
156. G. A. Schuiling and H. P. Gnodde, *J. Endocrinol.* **70**, 97 (1976).
157. C. A. Blake, R. Sridaran, K. A. Elias, O. A. Ashiru, and M. E. Rush, *Neuroendocrinology* **30**, 45 (1980).
158. G. W. Arendash and R. V. Gallo, *Endocrinology* **102**, 1199 (1978).

159. R. V. Gallo, *Neuroendocrinology* **31**, 161 (1980).
160. D. D. Rasmussen, W. Jacobs, P. T. Kissinger, and P. V. Malven, *Brain Res.* **229**, 230 (1981).
161. R. F. Weick, *Neuroendocrinology* **26**, 108 (1978).
162. R. V. Gallo, *Neuroendocrinology* **30**, 122 (1980).
163. S. V. Drouva and R. V. Gallo, *Endocrinology* **99**, 651 (1976).
164. P. C. K. Leung, G. W. Arendash, D. I. Whitmoyer, R. A. Gorski, and C. H. Sawyer, *Neuroendocrinology* **34**, 207 (1982).
165. P. C. K. Leung, G. W. Arendash, D. I. Whitmoyer, R. A. Gorski, and C. H. Sawyer, *Endocrinology* **109**, 720 (1981).
166. H. H. Huang, R. W. Steger, J. F. Bruni, and J. Meites, *Endocrinology* **103**, 1855 (1978).
167. J. Meites, H. H. Huang, and J. W. Simpkins, in E. L. Schneider, Ed., *The Aging Reproductive System*, Raven Press, New York, 1978, pp. 213–236.
168. J. Meites, *Neuroendocrinology* **34**, 151 (1982).
169. J. K. H. Lu, D. A. Damassa, D. P. Gilman, H. L. Judd, and C. H. Sawyer, *Biol. Reprod.* **23**, 345 (1980).
170. J. Meites, R. W. Steger, and H. H. Huang, *Fed. Proc.* **39**, 3168 (1980).
171. R. F. Walker, R. L. Cooper, and P. S. Timiras, *Endocrinology* **107**, 249 (1980).
172. J. W. Simpkins, G. P. Mueller, H. H. Huang, and J. Meites, *Endocrinology* **100**, 1672 (1977).
173. S. K. Quadrei, G. S. Kledzik, and J. Meites, *Neuroendocrinology* **11**, 248 (1973).
174. J. W. Everett, Physiol. Rev., **44**, 373 (1964).
175. G. Fink, in J. Stallworthy and G. Bourne, Ed., *Recent Advances in Obstetrics and Gynaecology*, Churchill Livingstone, Edinburgh, 1977, pp. 3–34.
176. G. Fink, Br. Med. Bull., **35**, 155 (1979).
177. G. Fink, M. Aiyer, S. Chiappa, S. Henderson, M. Jamieson, V. Levy-Perez, A. Pickering, D. Sarkar, N. Sherwood, A. Speight, and A. Watts, in K. W. McKerns, Ed., *Hormonally Active Brain Peptides*, Plenum Press, New York, 1982, pp. 397–426.
178. J. W. Everett, *J. Endocrinol.* **75**, 3 (1977).

19

Identification and Localization of Neuropeptides in the Vertebrate Retina

NICHOLAS C. BRECHA

Center for Ulcer Research and Education
Veterans Administration Medical Center–Wadsworth
Los Angeles, California
and
Department of Medicine, Jules Stein Eye Institute,
and Brain Research Institute
University of California at Los Angeles School of Medicin

H. J. KARTEN

Department of Neurobiology and Behavior
and
Department of Psychiatry and Behavioral Sciences
State University of New York at Stony Brook

The presence of peptide activity in the retina was first reported more than 25 years ago by Duner et al. (1), who observed substance P biological activity in mammalian retinal extracts. But only recently has detailed documentation been presented of the presence and localization of peptide systems within the vertebrate retina (see reviews, refs. 2, 3). This renewed interest is no doubt a direct result of current general interest in nervous system and gut peptides as well as the attractiveness of the retina for detailed anatomical, physiological, and biochemical studies.

The vertebrate retina has proven to be amenable to detailed experimental study for several reasons. First, the morphology of the retina is well understood and is characterized by a clear and distinct laminar organization (Figure 1). Light microscopic studies have demonstrated that the retina contains a limited number of major cell types, which can be characterized both by the location of their soma in the retina and the

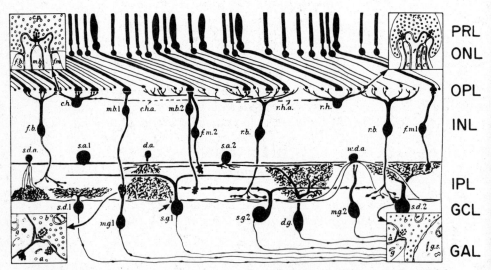

Figure 1. Schematic representation of the retina illustrating its basic organizational features which are described in the text. Photoreceptor cells (cp, cones; rs, rods) make synaptic contact with bipolar cells (fb, flat bipolar cell; mb1 and mb2, midget bipolar cells; fm2 and fm1, flat midget bipolar cells; rb, rod bipolar cells) and horizontal cells (ch, type A horizontal cell; rh, type B horizontal cell; cha, type A horizontal cell axon; rha, type B horizontal cell axon) in the outer plexiform layer (OPL). Bipolar cells in turn make synaptic contact with amacrine cells (sda, stratified diffuse amacrine cell; sa1 and sa2, unistratified amacrine cells; da, narrow field diffuse amacrine cell; wda, wide field diffuse amacrine cell), and ganglion cells (sd1 and sd2, stratified diffuse ganglion cells; mg1 and mg2, midget ganglion cells; sg1 and sg2, stratified ganglion cells; dg, diffuse ganglion cell) in the inner plexiform layer (IPL). Interplexiform, displaced amacrine, and displaced ganglion cells are not illustrated. A detailed description of this figure may be found in Boycott and Dowling (48). Modified from Boycott (62) with permission.

pattern of arborization of their processes (4). In addition, the synaptic organization and relationships of these neuronal cell types is known. Second, electrophysiological studies have characterized the responses of the retina as a whole and its major cell types to light stimulation (5). Finally, the retina is readily accessible to experimental manipulation and can easily be used *in situ, in vivo,* and *in vitro* for a variety of physiological, pharmacological and biochemical studies. All these factors combined provide the opportunity to assess better the functional role of presumed transmitter substances in visual processes and, more generally, to understand better what functional role or roles these substances play in neuronal processing within the nervous system.

In this chapter we review the evidence for the presence, localization, and possible functions of peptides in the retina.

1 ORGANIZATION OF THE RETINA

Several excellent reviews of the functional and morphological organization of the retina have been published (4, 6–8). The retina is a thin sheet of tissue characterized by a distinct laminar organization of its neurons and their processes. Naming from the distal retinal surface adjacent to the pigment epithelium to the proximal or vitreal retinal surface (Figure 1), the retinal layers are designated photoreceptor layer (PRL), outer nuclear layer (ONL), outer plexiform layer (OPL), inner nuclear layer (INL), inner plexiform layer (IPL), ganglion cell layer (GCL), and optic axon layer (GAL). The retina contains six major neuronal cell types: photoreceptor (rods and cones), bipolar, horizontal, amacrine, interplexiform, and ganglion. Identifying characteristics for each neuronal cell type are the location of its cell body within one of the nuclear layers and the distribution of its processes within one or both of the plexiform layers. In addition, glia cells, of which the majority are a specialized glia known as Müller cells, are located in the retina. Müller cells are distributed in a radial manner across the nuclear and plexiform layers perpendicular to the vitreal surface.

A simplified description of the essential organizational features of the retina as suggested by both morphological and physiological studies is one of parallel neuronal pathways consisting of photoreceptor, bipolar, and ganglion cells. Photoreceptor cells, which transduce light energy into biological signals, form synaptic contacts with bipolar cells in the OPL. Bipolar cells in turn form synaptic contacts within the IPL. Ganglion cells, with dendrites distributed in the IPL, give rise to the retinal projections upon the central visual nuclei via the optic nerve and tract. The information processing in these parallel retinal pathways is modified by interactions with (i) horizontal cells, which form synaptic connections with both photoreceptor and bipolar cells in the OPL, (ii) amacrine cells, which form synaptic connections with bipolar, amacrine, and ganglion cells within the IPL, and (iii) interplexiform cells, which form presynaptic contacts in the OPL and postsynaptic contacts in the IPL. Morphological studies have demonstrated that retinal neurons interconnect in a specific manner to form distinct neuronal pathways which have been demonstrated by physiological studies to undergo complex interactions in the processing of visual stimuli.

2   PRESENCE OF PEPTIDES IN THE VERTEBRATE RETINA

Bioassay, immunoassay, and immunohistochemical studies have firmly established the presence of peptide-like substances in the retinas of all vertebrate species studied to date (Table 1). Using these techniques, at least 10 neuropeptides have been described in the vertebrate retina. Undoubtedly, several more peptide-like substances will be reported in the retina in the near future, since there is currently a great interest in identifying new biologically active peptides in both the gut and nervous system. The best evidence to date suggests that several neuropeptides are present in the retina of any one species. However, not all of the neuropeptides found in the retina of one vertebrate species will necessarily be found in the retina of another vertebrate species. Moreover, as detailed below, both the retinal content of the peptide-like substances and the morphological appearance of the peptide-containing cells differ for each vertebrate species. To date, no study has fully characterized the amino acid composition or sequence of any of the immunoreactive peptide substances found in the retina. Until these peptide-like substances are fully identified, it is appropriate to refer to them using such modifiers as "like" or "immunoreactive."

2.1   Bioassay Studies

Bioassay studies first described substance P-like (SP) bioactivity in dog and bovine retinal extracts (1). This study, which utilized a guinea pig smooth muscle (ileum) preparation, demonstrated a high SP content in these retinas. A subsequent study using a similar smooth muscle preparation reported that SP bioactivity in bovine retinal extracts is low and that the majority of SP bioactivity is present in optic nerve extracts (9). Using a somatostatin bioassay system, recent studies have demonstrated that crude retinal extracts or immunoaffinity-purified retinal immunoreactive somatostatin-like (SRIF, somatotropin release inhibiting factor) extracts from either rat or human retina will inhibit in a dose-related manner the release of growth hormone from anterior pituitary cell cultures (10, 11). The inhibition of growth hormone release by retinal extracts is similar to the inhibition produced by synthetic

TABLE 1 Presence of Peptide-like Immunoreactivity in the Retina of Various Vertebrates, Based on Radioimmunoassay or Immunohistochemical Evidence or Both

Animal	SP	ENK	SRIF	NT	VIP	GLU	CCK	TRH	β-END	LRF
Fish										
Goldfish (*Carassius auratus*)	+	+	+	+		+	+			
File perch (*Damanichthys vacca*)	+	+		+						
Cohoe salmon	+	+								
Sturgeon poacher	+									
Plainfin midshipman (*Porichthys pacifica*)	+									
Surfsmelt (*Hypomesus pretisus*)	+									
Rockfish (*Sevastes caurinus*)	+	+								
Channel catfish		+								
Carp	+	+	+			+				
Amphibians										
Xenopus laevis	+									
Toad (*Bufo marinus*)	+		+							
Frog (*Rana pipiens*)	+	+	+	+		+			+	+
Bullfrog (*Rana catesbeiana*)	+		+					+		
Tiger salamander (*Ambysoma tigrinum*)	+	+								
Mudpuppy (*Necturus maculosus*)	+	+	+	+	+	+	+			
Reptiles										
Turtle (*Chrysemys scripta*)	+	+		+		+				
Lizard (*Anolis carolinensis*)	+	+								
Lizard (*Uta stansburiana*)	+									
Lizard (*Gecko gecko*)	+	+								
Birds										
Pigeon (*Columba livia*)	+	+	+	+	+	+				
Chicken (*Gallus domesticus*)	+	+	+	+	+	+				
Mammals										
Rat	+		+		+		+	+		
Rabbit	+		+		+			+		
Cat	+		+		+					

TABLE 1   *(Continued)*

Animal	SP	ENK	SRIF	NT	VIP	GLU	CCK	TRH	β-END	LRF
Cat	+		+		+					
Guinea pig		+								
New World monkey (*Saimira sciureus*)	+		+		+					
Old World monkey (*Macaca nemestrima*)	+		+		+					
(*Macaca facicularis*)	+		+		+					

somatostatin, supporting the suggestion that somatostatin is present in these retinas. To date, no other neuropeptides—such as enkephalin, cholecystokinin, or vasoactive intestinal polypeptide, which are present in the retina, as evidenced by immunoassay or immunohistochemical studies—have been tested in a biological assay system. These biological assay systems are important because they provide an independent corroboration of the presence of the peptide-like substance in the retina. Indeed, in lieu of actual isolation, characterization, and sequencing of the peptide-like substance, these biological assay studies are of critical importance in establishing the identity of the substance.

2.2   Immunoassay Studies

Using radioimmunoassay techniques, the presence of at least 10 neuropeptides has been described in the retinas of various vertebrate species (Table 1). Cholecystokinin-like (CCK), enkephalin-like (ENK), SP, SRIF, and thyrotropin releasing hormone-like (TRH) immunoreactivity are present in the retinas of several different vertebrate species, including the goldfish, frog, pigeon, rat, and monkey (2, 10–33). ENK immunoreactivity has been detected in nonmammalian but not in mammalian retinal extracts by radioimmunoassay (15, 19, 20), although a recent study reports the presence of ENK immunoreactivity in the guinea pig retina by immunohistochemistry (34). In addition, β-endorphin-like (β-END), glucagon-like (GLU), luteinizing releasing hormone-like (LRH), neurotensin-like (NT), and vasoactive intestinal polypeptide-like (VIP) immunoreactivity have been described in the retina of just one or two different vertebrate species (12, 13, 21, 31). For instance, β-END immunoreactivity has been reported in frog retina (21); GLU, NT, and VIP immunoreactivity have been reported in pigeon retina (12, 13; unpublished observations); and LRH imunoreactivity has been reported in goldfish and frog retina (unpublished observations).

The retinal content of immunoreactive peptides, including CCK, SP, and SRIF, ranges from very low to moderate in comparison with such peptide-rich regions of the central nervous system as the hypothalamus, basal ganglia, and brainstem (10, 16, 23, 27, 32, 33). For example, SRIF content in the retina is less than SRIF content in the optic tectum, hypothalamus, and brainstem (10, 11, 18, 24, 28, 31, 33, 35, 36) and comparable to the pineal, cerebellum, and substantia nigra (35, 36). It is noteworthy that a marked variance in the retinal content of immunoreactive peptides has been observed among vertebrate species. Some of the variability may be due to technical differences such as tissue preparation and extraction. But in some instances the wide variance in the reported retinal immunoreactive peptide content appears to be genuine in that several groups have independently obtained similar findings. For instance, retinal SP content differs between the bullfrog (218 $+$ 26.2 pg/mg wet wt) and monkey (7 $+$ 1.2 pg/mg wet wt) retinas (16), and retinal SRIF content differs among the goldfish (4 $+$ 1.8 pmol/mg protein), frog (390 $+$ 110 pg/mg protein), rat (0.621 $+$ 0.44) pg/mg protein), and rabbit (9.2 $+$ 1.8 pmol/mg protein) retinas (10, 16, 18, 24, 28, 30, 31, 33). The functional consequence of these differences is not known.

Gel filtration and high pressure liquid chromatographic techniques have been used to further characterize retinal peptide-like substances. To date, these techniques have provided evidence for the presence of CCK, ENK, SP, and SRIF peptides in the vertebrate retina (10, 17, 20, 32, 33).

Immunoreactive CCK extracted from the retina of a frog (*Rana pipiens*) coelutes with synthetic cholecystokinin-8 on Sephadex G-50 (26, 32). Other cholecystokinin-related peptides such as cholecystokinin-4 may also be present in this extract. In addition, acid extracts of frog retina contain a minor form of immunoreactive CCK that elutes between the bovine serum albumin standard and CCK-33 and CCK-39 (32). This observation suggests that a larger CCK-related peptide is present in the retina.

Chromatographic studies of immunoreactive ENK extracted from the chick retina have demonstrated that Met[5]-enkephalin coelutes with one of three ENK immunoreactive peaks on Sephadex G-50 (20). These studies suggest that other enkephalin-related peptides are present in addition to Met[5]-enkephalin. Whether these immunoreactive enkephalin-related peptides are similar to or identical with β-endorphin (20) or newly identified enkephalin-related peptides (37, 38) or precursors (39) such as Met[5]-enkephalin-Arg[6]-Phe[7] (37) and dynorphin (38) is unknown.

Immunoreactive SRIF extracted from goldfish and rat retinas coelutes with synthetic somatostatin on Sephadex G-50 or G-25 (10, 30, 33), suggesting the presence of somatostatin-14.second SRIF immunoreactive peak, larger than that of somatostatin-14, has been demonstrated in the goldfish retina (33). This observation suggests that a somatostatin-related peptide, perhaps somatostatin-28, is also present.

Retinal immunoreactive SP has been studied using high pressure liquid chromatography in several different vertebrate species (17). Immunoreactive SP from chick, rat, and monkey retinal extracts have a retention time identical with synthetic substance P by reverse phase–high pressure liquid chromatography. This observation suggests that retinal immunoreactive SP in these species corresponds to substance P. In addition, some immunoreactive SP from chick and all immunoreactive SP from bullfrog and carp retinal extracts have a shorter retention time than substance P by reverse phase–high pressure liquid chromatography. Retinal immunoreactive SP from these vertebrates does not appear to correspond to such peptides as bombesin, physalaemin, or eledoisin—suggesting the presence of a novel peptide or peptides in these retinas that cross-reacts with the substance P antiserum used in these studies.

In conclusion, both radioimmunoassay and chromatography studies have provided good evidence for the presence of several different neuropeptides within the retina. Radioimmunoassay studies have suggested that these retinal immunoreactive substances are similar to if not identical with known biologically active gut and nervous system peptides. Chromatography studies generally support this conclusion. In addition to the documentation of the presence of neuropeptides in the vertebrate retina, a great deal of information on the morphological localization of these substances has been obtained using immunohistochemical techniques.

2.3 Immunohistochemical Studies

Immunohistochemical studies have described the localization of nine neuropeptides including ENK, SP, SRIF, and VIP in both mammalian and nonmammalian retinas (Table 1) (2, 12–14, 17, 26, 32, 33, 40–45; unpublished observations). Neuropeptides in most cases are present only within amacrine cells, although there is now some good evidence for the presence of peptide-containing interplexiform and perhaps ganglion cells (2, 42; unpublished observations). An LRH immunoreactive retinal centrifugal system has recently been described in the teleost (46). Interestingly, each of these peptide-like substances usually is present in one or two morphologically distinct cell types (2, 3) although some exceptions have recently been described (Table 2) (42, 47). Moreover, and perhaps most important, each peptide-containing cell type is different in its morphology and histochemistry from other peptide-containing cell types. Recent studies of (i) the localization of SP immunoreactivity in several different vertebrate species and (ii) the localization of several peptides in the avian retina demonstrate these general observations; they are discussed below. Overall immunohistochemical studies suggest that each immunohistochemical cell type makes up a distinct and unique population of cells. These morphological observations imply that there is a distinct functional role for each of the peptide-containing cell populations in retinal processing.

TABLE 2 Localization of Substance P-like Immunoreactivity in the Retina of Various Vertebrates

Animal	GCL	IPL	INL	OPL	Cell Types
Fish					
Goldfish (*Carassius auratus*)	+	3	+		1
File perch (*Damanichthys vacca*)		1,5	+		1[a]
Cohoe salmon		1,5	+		1[a]
Sturgeon poacher		1	+		1
Plainfin midshipman (*Porichthys pacifica*)		1,5	+		1[a]
Surfsmelt (*Hypomesus pretisus*)		5	+		1
Rockfish (*Sevastes caurinus*)		1,2,4,5	+		1[a]
Carp		3	+		1
Amphibians					
Xenopus laevis	+	1,2,4,5	+		2[a]
Toad (*Bufo marinus*)	+	1,2,3,4,5	+		2[a]
Frog (*Rana pipiens*)		3,5	+		1[a]
Tiger salamander (*Ambysoma tigrinum*)		3,5	+		1[a]
Mudpuppy (*Necturus maculosus*)		1,5	+		1
Reptiles					
Turtle (*Chrysemys scripta*)		M[b]	+		1[a]
Lizard (*Anolis carolinensis*)		3	+		1
Lizard (*Uta stansburiana*)	+	3	+		1
Lizard (*Gecko gecko*)		1,3,5	+		1
Birds					
Pigeon (*Columba livia*)		3	+		1
Chicken (*Gallus domesticus*)		3	+		1
Mammals					
Rat		M[b]	+		1[a]
Rabbit	+	1,3,5	+	+	3[a]
Cat	+	3	+		1
New World monkey (*Saimira sciureus*)	+	1,3,5	+		2[a]
Old World monkey (*Macaca nemestrima*)	+	1,3,5	+	+	4[a]
(*Macaca facicularis*)		3	+	+	1[a]

[a] Possibly more cell types.
[b] M, multistratified.

2.3.1 Distribution of Substance P-like Immunoreactivity in the Vertebrate Retina

Recent studies have examined the localization of SP immunoreactivity in a variety of vertebrate species, including the goldfish, frog, mudpuppy, lizard, pigeon, rabbit, and monkey (Table 2) (2, 17, 42–44, 47; unpublished observations). Specific SP immunoreactivity may be present in amacrine, displaced amacrine, interplexiform, and perhaps ganglion cells. These immunoreactive cells and their processes are distributed throughout the retina, and usually their highest densities are within central retinal regions.

A single, seemingly distinct population of unistratified SP-containing amacrine cells are present in goldfish (*Carassius auratus*), lizard (*Uta stansburiana*), and pigeon (*Columba livia*) retinas (43, 44; unpublished observations) (Figure 2). In these species, SP-containing cells typically have a round shape and measure about 7–9 μm in diameter. These cells usually give rise to a single process, which descends to and ramifies within lamina 3 of the IPL. In each of these species, SP-containing cells are located at or near the border of the INL and IPL. There are some differences, however, in the immunohistochemical patterns observed in these retinas. In goldfish retina, SP immunoreactive cells are characterized by a medium-caliber primary process; in lizard and pigeon retinas, these cells are characterized by a fine-caliber primary process. In the *Uta* retina, SP processes are distributed in a broader band within the IPL than in either the goldfish or pigeon retina. Furthermore, SP-containing cells within the goldfish and lizard retinas are scattered throughout the retina, and to date no obvious regional differences have been described. In contrast, SP-containing amacrine cells in pigeon retina are distributed preferentially within peripheral and ventral retinal regions. These SP-containing amacrine cells resemble unistratified cell types depicted by Cajal (4) and by Boycott and Dowling (48) from their Golgi and reduced silver preparations.

In contrast with the relatively simple SP immunoreactive patterns in the goldfish, lizard and pigeon retinas are the SP immunoreactive patterns in the mudpuppy (*Necturus maculosus*), bullfrog (*Rana catesbeiana*), frog (*Rana pipiens*), toad (*Bufo marinus*), lizard (*Gecko gecko*),

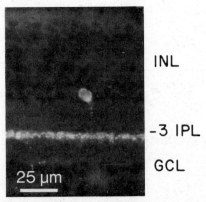

Figure 2.   Unistratified SP-containing amacrine cell in the *Uta stansburiana* retina. These cells give rise to a single process, which forms a broad of SP-containing processes in lamina 3 of the inner plexiform layer (IPL).

rabbit, and monkey (*Macaca nemestrima, Samimira sciureus*) retinas (Table 2; 17, 42, 47; unpublished observations). In these retinas the majority of SP immunoreactivity is distributed in the INL and IPL but is also present in the GCL. SP appears to be present in several distinct cell populations in several of these retinas (*vide infra*).

In mudpuppy retina, SP immunoreactivity appears to be present in amacrine cells, which may have bistratified processes (unpublished observation) (Figure 3). These SP-containing cells have a round shape and give rise to processes that are distributed predominantly to laminae 1 and 5 of the IPL. These immunoreactive cells are usually located in the INL at the border of the IPL and are present in all retinal regions. In contrast, in both the bullfrog and toad retina SP-containing cells are present in the INL and GCL, and their processes are distributed in several or all laminae of the IPL (17; unpublished observations). These observations suggest the presence of a minimum of two SP immunoreactive cell populations; amacrine cells and displaced amacrine cells and/or possibly ganglion cells. Because detailed immunohistochemical studies have not been conducted, it is not possible to suggest the number of distinct SP immunoreactive cell populations present in these retinas. These observations clearly demonstrate that SP immunoreactive cells may have bistratified or multistratified processes.

As described below, SP immunoreactivity may be present in several distinct retinal cell populations (Table 2).

In rabbit retina, SP immunoreactive somata are located in the INL and GCL and the majority of their processes are located in the IPL (Figure 4; 47). SP immunoreactive processes are distributed within laminae 1, 3, and 5 of the IPL, they are most prominent in lamina 5 (Figures 4A and 4B). An occasional SP immunoreactive process is also present in the OPL (Figure 4C). At least three distinct populations of retinal cells

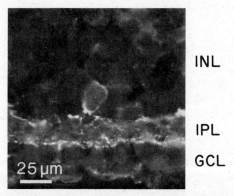

INL

IPL

GCL

25 µm

Figure 3. SP immunoreactivity in the mudpuppy retina. SP-containing somata are present in the inner nuclear layer (INL) at or near the inner plexiform layer (IPL) border. SP processes are usually distributed in the most distal and proximal portions of the IPL.

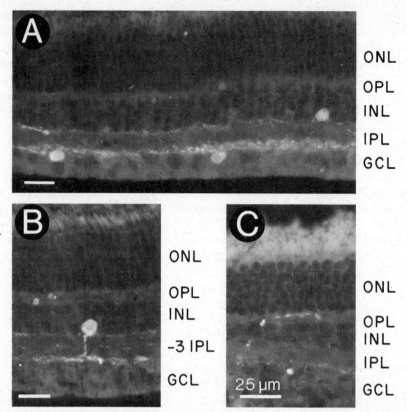

Figure 4. SP immunoreactivity in the rabbit retina. (A) SP immunoreactive amacrine and perhaps displaced amacrine cells or ganglion cells. SP-containing cells in the ganglion cell layer (GCL) typically give rise to processes that ramify only in lamina 5 of the inner plexiform layer (IPL). (B) Unistratified SP immunoreactive amacrine cell. This type of SP-containing amacrine cell gives rise to a single stout process, which ramifies in lamina 5 of the IPL. Note the laminar distribution of SP-containing processes in laminae 1, 3, and 5 of the IPL. (C) SP-containing process in the outer plexiform layer (OPL); peripheral retina.

contain SP. There are two populations of amacrine cells; one is located at the border of the INL and IPL and gives rise to a single stout process, which descends to and ramifies within lamina 5 of the IPL (Figure 4B). A second amacrine cell type gives rise to several fine-caliber processes which ramify in laminae 1, 3, and 5 of the IPL. Finally, SP-containing cells with somata located in the GCL give rise to several primary processes which ramify within lamina 5 of the IPL (Figure 4A). To date, no axon-like process has been observed to be associated with these cells; however, a few scattered SP-containing processes are present in the GAL, suggesting the existence of SP-containing ganglion cells. This suggestion is supported by a radioimmunoassay study describing SP immunoreactivity in rabbit optic nerve extracts (31).

In retinas of Old World monkeys (*Macaca nemestrima*) and New World monkeys, (*Samimira sciureus*), most SP immunoreactivity is present within somata located in the proximal INL, IPL, and GCL as well as processes located in the IPL (42). SP-containing processes are distributed within laminae 1, 3, and 5 of the IPL. These processes are most dense in lamina 3 of the Old World monkey retina and lamina 5 of the New World monkey retina. There are at least four distinct SP-containing retinal cell populations in the *Macaca nemestrima* retina (42). SP-containing amacrine cells whose somata are located at the border of the INL and IPL give rise to a single process which descends to and ramifies in lamina 3 of the IPL. A second SP-containing cell population, located within the IPL midway between the INL and GCL, gives rise to processes, from both ends of its somata, that only appear to ramify within lamina 3 of the IPL. These cells do not appear to give rise to an axon nor are they labeled by retrograde transport of horseradish peroxidase (HRP) following HRP injections into central visual nuclei (Hendrickson, personal communication). These observations suggest that these cells are interstitial amacrine cells rather than displaced ganglion cells. Finally, two other types of immunoreactive cells are located within the GCL; one of these SP-containing cell populations gives rise to one or more primary processes that ascend to and ramify in lamina 3 of the IPL. This type of cell is similar in appearance to the SP-containing amacrine cell located in the INL. A second cell type gives rise to several processes, which ramify within lamina 5 of the IPL. Whether these latter two cell populations are displaced amacrine cells or ganglion cells has yet to be established.

In both the rabbit and *Macaca* retina, a few immunoreactive processes are observed in the distal INL and in the OPL (Table 2); 42, 47; Figure 4C). These processes course radially through the INL and upon entering the OPL run tangential to the vitreal surface for a short distance. These immunoreactive processes do not appear to ramify into finer processes within either the INL or OPL (42). Although the somata giving rise to these processes have not been identified, their presence does imply the existence of SP-containing interplexiform cells.

Earlier reports of SP biological activity (9) and immunoreactivity (23, 27, 31) in optic nerve extracts and the presence of SP-containing cells in the GCL of the bullfrog, toad, rabbit, and monkey retina (17, 42, 47) suggest the existence of SP-containing ganglion cells. This suggestion can be directly tested by double-label experiments using retrograde transport techniques in combination with immunohistochemistry; such testing could provide a final identification and classification of these SP immunoreactive cells.

In conclusion, SP immunoreactivity is distributed in morphologically distinct retinal cell types in every vertebrate species studied to date. SP may be present in amacrine, displaced amacrine, interplexiform, and/or

ganglion cells. These general patterns of SP immunoreactivity as described above are representative of the patterns of CCK, ENK, GLU,
SRIF, and VIP immunoreactivity observed in other vertebrate retinas (2,
13, 14, 26, 32, 33, 40, 41, 45; unpublished observations).

2.3.2 Distribution of Peptide-like Immunoreactivity in the Avian Retina

Using the bird retina as a model system, detailed studies of the presence and distribution of peptide-like immunoreactivity have been conducted (2, 3, 12–14, 40, 41, 44).

The presence of ENK, GLU, NT, SP, SRIF, and VIP immunoreactivity
by radioimmunoassay within the avian retina has been reported (12–16,
20, 27). These studies indicate the presence of at least six neuropeptides
in the avian retina, which as described below, are present in selected
amacrine cell populations. These studies also indicate that both CCK
and TRH immunoreactivities are either absent or very low in the chick
retina (14, 15).

Immunohistochemical studies have identified six specific peptide-
containing amacrine cell populations in the pigeon retina (2, 3, 12, 13,
40, 41, 44). These studies have clearly established the presence of
unistratified SP and multistratified ENK, NT, and SRIF immunoreactive
cell populations. In addition, preliminary studies have suggested the
presence of at least two VIP-containing and three GLU-containing cell
populations. As described below, each of these immunoreactive substances is present in morphologically distinct amacrine cells, which differ from one another.

ENK immunoreactivity is present in what appears to be a specific
group of multistratified amacrine cells in both the pigeon and chicken
retina (40) (Figure 5). In central retina, these multistratified amacrine
cells are characterized by a single process, which descends to the border of the IPL before arborizing into several secondary processes. These
processes ramify in lamina 1 and give rise to processes that descend to
and ramify within laminae 3, 4, and 5 of the IPL. ENK immunoreactive
somata usually are located within the second and third tier of cells of
the proximal INL, are ovoid in shape, and measure about 7.5 μm in diameter. In the pigeon retina, ENK-containing amacrine cells are distributed within all retinal regions although their density is greatest in
central retinal regions.

Pigeon and chicken retinas also contain multistratified SRIF-containing and NT-containing amacrine cell populations (Figures 6 and 7; 13,
14). SRIF and NT immunoreactive cells like the ENK-containing amacrine cells give rise to a single process, which descends to lamina 1 of
the IPL before ramifying into several secondary processes. Some of
these secondary processes then descend to and ramify within laminae 3
and 4 of the IPL. The SRIF and NT immunoreactive cells both measure

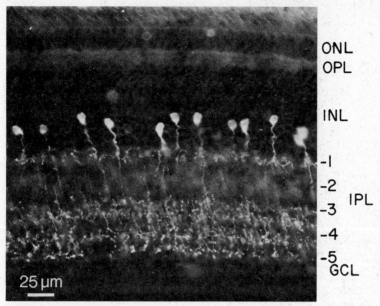

ONL
OPL

INL

-1
-2
-3 IPL
-4
-5
GCL

25 μm

Figure 5. ENK-containing amacrine cells located in the central retina of the pigeon. These cells give rise to multistratified processes that ramify in laminae 1, 3, 4, and 5 of the inner plexiform layer (IPL). Enkephalin antiserum used for this study was supplied by Dr. K.-J. Chang.

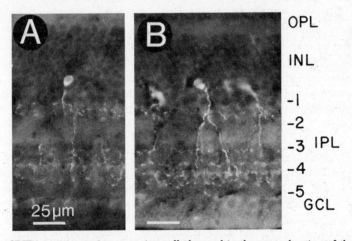

OPL

INL

-1
-2
-3 IPL
-4
-5
GCL

25 μm

Figure 6. SRIF immunoreactive amacrine cells located in the central retina of the pigeon. These cells give rise to multistratified processes that ramify in laminae 1, 3, and 4 of the inner plexiform layer (IPL). Somatostatin antisera used for this study was supplied by Drs. W. Vale and T. Yamada.

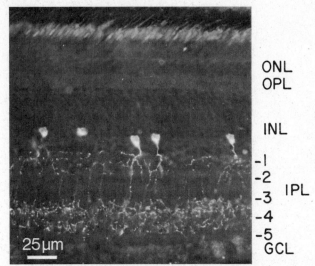

ONL
OPL

INL

-1
-2
-3 IPL
-4
-5
GCL

25µm

Figure 7. NT immunoreactive amacrine cells located in the central retina of the pigeon. These cells give rise to multistratified processes that ramify in laminae 1, 3, and 4 of the inner plexiform layer (IPL). Neurotensin antisera used in this study was supplied by Dr. M. Brown and Mr. J. Koeing.

about 7 µm in diameter, are located in the proximal INL, and are distributed in all retinal regions. The density of SRIF-containing and NT-containing cells is also greatest in central retinal regions.

ENK, SRIF, and NT immunoreactive amacrine cells are strikingly similar in appearance (Figures 5, 6, and 7). These multistratified cells have similar-sized somata, which usually give rise to a single primary process that descends to and ramifies in lamina 1 of the IPL. The secondary immunoreactive processes in lamina 1 in turn give rise to processes that descend to and ramify in more proximal regions of the IPL. However, on the basis of their histochemistry it is clear that the ENK-, SRIF-, and NT-containing amacrine cells constitute separate cell populations. That is, double-label immunohistochemical experiments have demonstrated that there is no overlap of staining of each cell type in the same section (2, 3, 13). In addition, there are fine morphological differences in the appearance of these immunoreactive cell types, especially in the arborization pattern of their processes within the proximal IPL (2, 3, 13).

Unistratified SP-containing amacrine cells are present in the pigeon retina (44). These cells give rise to a single process, which arborizes in lamina 3 of the IPL. Interestingly, their density is greatest in peripheral and ventral retinal regions, unlike the ENK-, NT- and SRIF-containing amacrine cells.

In the pigeon retina, VIP immunoreactivity is present within medium-sized somata, measuring about 12 µm in diameter and located at the border of the INL and IPL, and it is present in processes within laminae 1, 3, and 5 of the IPL (2, 41) (Figure 8). These processes are most prominent in lamina 3 and 5 of the IPL. VIP-containing amacrine cells typically give rise to a single process, which descends and ramifies in two bands at the border of laminae 2 and 3 and within lamina 5 of the IPL. An occasional VIP-containing cell has been observed to give rise to processes that ramify in lamina 1 of the IPL. Whether these cells also give rise to processes that ramify in more proximal regions of the IPL remains to be investigated. The pigeon retina may thus contain uni-, bi-, and/or tristratified VIP immunoreactive amacrine cells; further studies are needed to identify the exact number of different VIP-containing amacrine cell types.

GLU immunoreactivity is present in amacrine cells located in the INL and in processes that are most prominent in lamina 1 of the IPL and in the ora serrata (2, 12, 41; unpublished observations) (Figure 9). In central retina, the majority of GLU immunoreactive cells have a round shape, measure about 7 μm in diameter, and give rise to one, two, or three primary processes, which arborize in lamina 1 of the IPL (Figures 9A and 9B). Some of these processes give rise to secondary processes, which descend to and arborize in a thin band in lamina 3 of the IPL. A second GLU immunoreactive retinal cell population is present most prominently in ventral retinal regions. These cells have a round shape and a medium-to-large somata measuring about 18 μm. These cells are characterized by a single thick primary process, which courses tangential to the vitreal surface in lamina 1 of the IPL for a short distance be-

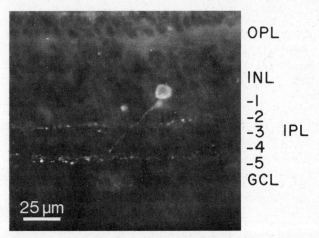

Figure 8. VIP immunoreactivity in the pigeon retina. VIP-containing cells, of which there are at least two types, may give rise to processes that may ramify in laminae 1, 3, and/or 5 of the inner plexiform layer (IPL). Vasoactive intestinal polypeptide antiserum used in this study was supplied by Dr. J. Walsh.

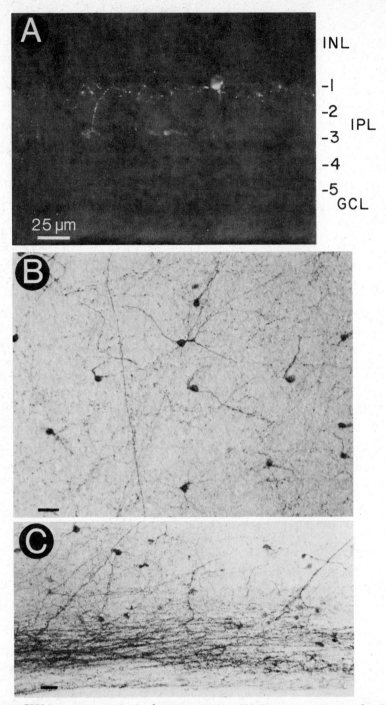

Figure 9. GLU immunoreactivity in the pigeon retina. (A) Transverse section of a GLU-containing amacrine cell located in central retinal regions. (B) Tangential section of GLU-containing amacrine cells located in central retinal regions. (C) Tangential section of peripheral retina including the ora serrata. Glucagon antiserum for this study was supplied by Dr. N. Track.

fore ramifying into many fine processes which are distributed to laminae 1, 3, and 5 of the IPL. One of these fine processes courses in lamina 1 directly to the edge of the retina, where it joins a fascicle of GLU immunoreactive processes (Figure 9C) within the ora serrata. A third population of GLU immunoreactive cells is present in peripheral retinal regions. These cells have medium-sized somata measuring about 12 μm and two or three primary processes which ramify in lamina 1 and perhaps deeper lamina of the IPL. Some of these processes also join the fascicle of GLU-containing processes, which appear to course through the ora serrata to encircle the retina. These observations suggest at least three types of GLU-containing cells; the majority of cells in central retinal regions appear to be unistratified or bistratified amacrine cells or both. The medium-to-large diameter immunoreactive cells located in ventral and peripheral retinal regions, however, differ slightly from traditionally described amacrine cells in that their processes course through the IPL sometimes over several hundred microns to peripheral retinal regions, where they form a fascicle of GLU-containing processes within the ora serrata. These cells may be similar to association amacrine cells in the passerine retina, described by Cajal (4).

2.4   Co-Occurrence of Peptide-like Immunoreactivity with "Conventional" Transmitters

In pigeon retina, in addition to peptide immunoreactive amacrine cell populations, other histochemically identified amacrine cells have been identified. These include catecholamine fluorescence (49), γ-aminobutyric acid (GABA)-, glycine-, choline-, and indoleamine-accumulating amacrine cells (50–54), and serotonin-, tyrosine hydroxylase-, and L-glutamate decarboxylase (GAD)-like immunoreactive amacrine cells (unpublished observations). A comparison of peptide immunoreactive amacrine cells with the choline- and indoleamine-accumulating (50, 53) and the serotonin-like immunoreactive amacrine cells suggest they do not occur with one another. That is, indoleamine-accumulating and serotonin-like immunoreactive amacrine cells give rise to a single primary process which descends to and ramifies in lamina 1 of the IPL. Processes in lamina 1, in turn give rise to fine processes, which descend to and ramify in lamina 5 of the IPL. These bistratified amacrine cells are clearly different from any of the peptide-containing amacrine cells described in the pigeon retina to date. Likewise the catecholamine fluorescence (49) and tyrosine hydroxylase-like immunoreactive amacrine cells give rise to processes that ramify predominantly in lamina 1 of the IPL. A few processes also ramify in laminae 3 and 5 of the IPL. These cells superficially resemble the GLU and VIP immunoreactive amacrine cells; however, (i) tyrosine hydroxylase immunoreactivity is not present in the ora serrata, and (ii) the number of tyrosine hydroxylase-containing amacrine cells is markedly less than the number of GLU-containing and VIP-containing amacrine cells (3). These observations suggest that tyrosine hydroxylase is not present in every cell that contains GLU or VIP. However, the possibility that tyrosine hydroxylase is present in a subset of GLU or VIP immunoreactive amacrine cells remains to be established. Whether neuropeptides are present within either glycine- and/or GABA accumulating (GAD-like immunoreactive) amacrine cell populations is unknown. Overall, these studies suggest that at least in bird retina, peptide immunoreactive amacrine cells are not likely to contain a second peptide or "conventional" transmitter substance. Thus in pigeon retina, on the basis of histochemical criteria at least 12 distinct populations of amacrine cells have been identified.

In conclusion, specific peptide-like immunoreactivity is present in at least six amacrine cell populations. On the basis of other histochemical data, several other amacrine cell populations are also present in the pigeon retina. The presence of these distinct populations suggests that each of these amacrine cell types plays a defined and perhaps unique role in retinal processing.

3 PHYSIOLOGICAL STUDIES OF PEPTIDE SYSTEMS IN THE VERTEBRATE RETINA

The exact functional role neuropeptides have in visual processes is unknown, although undoubtedly neuropeptides are important and critical in retinal function. This assumption is based upon their presence and widespread distribution in all vertebrate retinas and their localization to specific retinal cell populations. Recent physiological studies also suggest the importance of peptides in visual function.

3.1 Release Studies

Previous studies, using the teleost retina, have demonstrated that GABA is accumulated by selected pyriform amacrine cells (55) and released from these cells by K^+ stimulation in a Ca^{2+}-dependent manner (56). This K^+-stimulated, Ca^{2+}-dependent release of GABA is blocked by Met^5-enkephalin or Leu^5-enkephalin in a dose-related manner and by morphine (57). Moreover, naloxone blocks the suppressive action of Met^5-enkephalin (Figure 10). These data suggest that enkephalin or enkephalin-related peptides have a specific action on GABAergic amacrine cell systems in the teleost retina.

A K^+-stimulated, Ca^{2+}-dependent release of SP, SRIF, and TRH immunoreactivity from bullfrog retina has also been described (16).

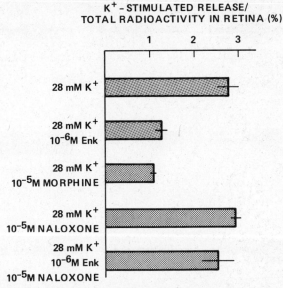

Figure 10. Effects of Met[5]-enkephalin or Leu[5]-enkephalin (Enk), morphine and naloxone on the K^+ stimulated, Ca^{2+} dependent release of ^3H-GABA from amacrine cells in the goldfish retina. This figure illustrates the inhibition of ^3H-GABA release by enkephalins and morphine and the prevention of this effect by the opiate antagonist naloxone. Modified from Djamgoz et al. (57) with permission.

3.2 Electrophysiological Studies

Electrophysiological studies have also provided some evidence for a functional role of enkephalin in the teleost retina (Figure 11) (57). D-Ala 2-Met 5-enkephalinamide (DALA), when applied by an atomizer system to an eyecup preparation at an estimated concentration of 0.1–1.0 μM, (i) enhanced spontaneous activity and the light-evoked response of ON-center ganglion cells, and (ii) inhibited the spontaneous activity and the light-evoked response of OFF-center ganglion cells. These effects were reversible and could be prevented by pretreatment of the retina with naloxone. Similar but irreversible effects on ganglion cell activity were observed following morphine application. The physiological actions of this enkephalin analog in the retina is consistent with histochemical observations demonstrating multistratified ENK-containing amacrine cells in the goldfish retina (58).

The effects of exogenously applied substance P on ganglion cell activity in the amphibian and teleost retina have been described (59, 60). Using iontophoretic techniques, substance P or the substance P 4–11 fragment has been shown to excite all ganglion cells sampled in the mudpuppy retina (59). In carp retina, in which synthetic substance P was applied by a nebulizer system, substance P was reported to excite

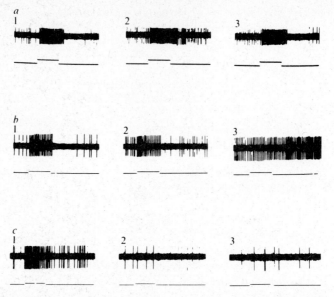

Figure 11. Extracellular recordings of ganglion cells from an isolated goldfish retina. *a*: (1) Control; (2) 1.0 *μM* DALA; (3) 5 min after application of 1.0 *μM* DALA. *b*: (1) Control; (2) 1.0 *μM* DALA; (3) 1.0 *μM* morphine sulfate. *c*: (1) Control; (2) 40 *μM* naloxone; (3) 1 *μM* DALA and 40 *μM* naloxone. These recordings demonstrate the increased spontaneous activity and light-evoked firing of ON-center ganglion cells or morphine following application of DALA and the inhibition of this effect by naloxone. Redrawn from Djamgoz et al. (57) with permission.

most ON- and ON-OFF-center ganglion cells (60). The localization of SP immunoreactivity to amacrine cells in mudpuppy and carp retinas (unpublished observations) and the excitatory action of this substance on ganglion cell discharge is consistent with the idea that substance P plays a functional role in the IPL.

3.3 Effects of Light Stimulation on Retinal Peptide Content

Retinal TRH content as measured by radioimmunoassay fluctuates with lighting conditions in the rat (29). TRH levels are highest during light periods and lowest during dark periods. Whether this light vs. dark difference is related to circadian rhythms must await a more rigorous analysis. A recent developmental study in the rat has shown that TRH immunoreactivity is not detectable in the retina before the eyes open, is low at eye opening (day 8), and is very high 30 days after eye opening (25). At somewhat later time periods, TRH immunoreactivity declines to more intermediate levels characteristic of the adult retina. Interestingly, the appearance of TRH immunoreactivity in the developing rat retina is prevented by maintaining the rat pups in the dark. These experiments

(25, 29) support the notion that the retinal content of TRH immunoreactivity is dependent upon light stimulation.

A recent abstract has described a light stimulated release of SP immunoreactivity from the rabbit retina (61).

In conclusion, both release and electrophysiological studies support the proposition that neuropeptides play specific roles, perhaps as neurotransmitters and/or neuromodulators, in the retina. Furthermore, in some cases light appears to have a marked effect on retinal peptide content.

4 SUMMARY

The presence of several peptide-like substances has been described in the vertebrate retina by bioassay, immunoassay, and immunohistochemistry. Radioimmunoassay and chromatographic studies have demonstrated that these substances are likely to be similar to if not identical with previously identified gut and nervous system peptides. Immunohistochemical studies have clearly demonstrated that these immunoreactive peptides are localized to distinct retinal cell types. It is noteworthy that most of the peptide-containing (and dopamine-containing) elements detected to date are amacrine cells. By the same token, it is somewhat disappointing that so little is known about the neurotransmitters used by photoreceptor, bipolar, and ganglion cells. These three cells, as mentioned earlier, are directly responsible for the transfer of visual information to the brain. Horizontal and amacrine cells contribute to the formation of "local circuits" within the retina, modulating and integrating the activities of bipolar and ganglion cells and helping to dictate the complicated receptive field properties of specific ganglion cells—properties that may explain the considerable processing of visual information that occurs in the retina. Although the architecture of the retina has always appeared extraordinarily simple, comprised of only six main cell types, the discovery of a variety of peptidergic neurons has shown the classical view to have been a markedly oversimplified one.

Further research is needed—including the chromatographic analysis, isolation, and characterization of these immunoreactive substances, the identification, characterization, and localization of peptide binding sites, and detailed light and electron microscopic analysis of peptide-containing cell populations—to clarify the functional role of peptides in the retina.

Studies to date have provided convincing evidence for the existence of distinct peptide-containing retinal cell populations within all vertebrate retinas. Certainly the localization of these substances to selected retinal cell populations supports the suggestion that peptides play a specific and unique role in retinal function. This role may be as a neuro-transmitter and/or neuromodulator. These substances may thus play a direct role in light-activated responsiveness of retinal cells, and perhaps they have a role in retinal adaption to light and dark conditions.

ACKNOWLEDGMENTS

We wish to express appreciation to Marianne Cilluffo for the help she gave in preparing this review and to Anita Boesman for typing the manuscript. We also thank Dr. C. Gall for her timely and helpful criticisms, without which this review would not have been completed. This review was supported by the National Eye Institute (EY 02146 to H. J. K., EY 04067 to N. B.) and AM 17328 to CURE–J. Walsh.

REFERENCES

1. H. Duner, U. S. von Euler, and B. Pernow, *Acta Physiol. Scand.* **31**, 113–118 (1954).
2. N. Brecha, in P. C. Emson, Ed., *Neurochemical Anatomy*, Raven Press, New York, 1983.
3. H. J. Karten and N. Brecha, in H. F. Bradford, Ed., *Neurotransmitter Interaction and Compartmentation*, Plenum Press, New York, 1982, pp. 719–733.
4. S. R. Cajal, *La Cellule* **9**, 17–257 (1893).
5. A. Kaneko, in W. M. Cowan, Z. W. Hall, E. R. Kandel, Eds., *Ann. Rev. Neurosci.*, Annual Review, Palo Alto, Calif., 1979, pp. 169–191.
6. W. K. Stell, in M. G. F. Fuortes, Ed., *Handbook of Sensory Physiology*, Vol. 7, Part II, Springer-Verlag, Berlin, 1972, pp. 111–213.
7. R. W. Rodieck, *The Vertebrate Retina*, W. H. Freeman, San Francisco, 1973.
8. B. B. Boycott, J. E. Dowling, S. L. Fisher, H. Kolb, and A. M. Laties, *Proc. R. Soc., Ser. B 191*, 353–368 (1975).
9. A. F. Winder and P. N. Patsalos, *Biochem. Soc. Trans.* **4**, 1260–1261 (1974).
10. O. P. Rorstad, M. J. Brownstein, and J. B. Martin, *Proc. Natl. Acad. Sci. USA* **76**, 3019–3023 (1979).
11. O. P. Rorstad, M. K. Senterman, K. M. Hoyte, and J. B. Martin, *Brain Res.* **199**, 488–492 (1980).
12. N. Brecha, M. Cilluffo, and T. Yamada, paper presented at the *4th International Symposium on Gastrointestinal Hormones*, Stockholm, June, 1982.
13. N. Brecha, H. J. Karten, and C. Schenker, *Neuroscience* **6**, 1329–1340 (1981).
14. M. Buckerfield, J. Oliver, I. W. Chubb, and I. G. Morgan, *Neuroscience* **6**, 639–695 (1981).
15. L. E. Eiden, M. C. Beinfeld, and R. L. Eskay, *Neurosci. Abstr.* **6**, 680 (1980).
16. R. L. Eskay, R. T. Long, and P. M. Iuvone, *Brain Res.* **196**, 554–559 (1980).
17. R. L. Eskay, J. F. Furness, and R. T. Long, *Science* **212**, 1049–1051 (1981).
18. P. Giraud, P. Gillioz, B. Conte-Devolx, and C. Oliver, *C.R. Acad. Sci., Paris* **288**, 127–129 (1979).
19. R. D. Howells, J. Groth, J. M. Hiller, and E. J. Simon, *J. Pharmacol. Exp. Ther.* **215**, 60–64 (1980).
20. J. Humbert, P. Pradelles, C. Gros, and F. Dray, *Neurosci. Lett.* **12**, 259–263 (1979).
21. I. M. D. Jackson, J. L. Bolaffi, and R. Guillemin, *Gen. Comp. Endocrinol.* **42**, 505–508 (1980).

22. I. M. Jackson and S. Reichlin, *Science* **198**, 414–415 (1977).
23. I. Kanazawa and T. Jessell, *Brain Res.* **117**, 362–367 (1976).
24. N. Lake and Y. C. Patel, *Brain Res.* **181**, 234–236 (1980).
25. E. Martino, H. Seo, A. Lernmark, and S. Refetoff, *Proc. Natl. Acad. Sci. USA* **77**, 4345–4348 (1980).
26. N. N. Osborne, D. A. Nicholas, A. C. Cuello, and G. J. Dockray, *Neurosci. Lett.* **26**, 31–35 (1981).
27. J. C. Reubi and T. M. Jessell, *J. Neurochem.* **31**, 359–361 (1978).
28. S. M. Sagar, O. P. Rorstad, D. M. Landis, and J. B. Martin, *Neurosci. Abstr.* **7**, 278 (1981).
29. J. M. Schaeffer, M. J. Brownstein, and J. Axelrod, *Proc. Natl. Acad. Sci. USA* **74**, 3579–3581 (1977).
30. B. Shapiro, S. Kronheim, and B. Pimstone, *Horm. Metab. Res.* **11**, 79–80 (1979).
31. W. G. Unger, J. M. Botler, D. E. Cole, S. R. Bloom, and G. P. McGregor, *Exp. Eye Res.* **32**, 797–801 (1981).
32. T. Yamada, N. Brecha, G. Rosenquist, and S. Basinger, *Peptides* **2**, *Suppl. 2*, 93–97 (1981).
33. T. Yamada, D. Marshak, S. Basinger, J. Walsh, J. Morley, and W. Stell, *Proc. Natl. Acad. Sci. USA* **77**, 1691–1695 (1980).
34. R. A. Altschuler, J. L. Mosinger, D. W. Hoffman, and M. Parakkal, *Proc. Natl. Acad. Sci. USA* **79**, 2398–2400 (1982).
35. M. Brownstein, A. Arimura, H. Sato, A. V. Schally, and J. S. Kizer, *Endocrinology* **96**, 1456–1461 (1975).
36. R. M. Kobayashi, M. Brown, and W. Vale, *Brain Res.* **126**, 584–588 (1977).
37. A. S. Stern, R. V. Lewis, S. Kimura, J. Rossier, L. D. Gerber, L. Brink, S. Stein, and S. Udenfriend, *Proc. Natl. Acad. Sci. USA* **76**, 6680–6683 (1979).
38. A. Goldstein, S. Tachibana, L. I. Lowney, M. Hunkapiller, and L. Hood, *Proc. Natl. Acad. Sci. USA* **76**, 6666–6670 (1979).
39. M. Comb, P. H. Seeburg, J. Adelman, L. Eiden, and E. Herbert, *Nature* **295**, 663–666 (1982).
40. N. Brecha, H. J. Karten, and C. Laverack, *Proc. Natl. Acad. Sci. USA* **76**, 3010–3014 (1979).
41. N. Brecha, H. J. Karten, and B. Davis, *Neurosci. Abstr.* **6**, 346 (1980).
42. N. Brecha, A. Hendrickson, I. Floren, and H. J. Karten, *Invest. Ophthalmol. Vis. Sci.*, **23**, 147–153 (1982).
43. N. Brecha, S. C. Sharma, and H. J. Karten, *Neuroscience* **6**, 2737–2746 (1981).
44. H. J. Karten and N. Brecha, *Nature* **283**, 87–88 (1980).
45. I. Loren, K. Tornqvist, and J. Alumets, *Cell Tissue Res.* **210**, 167–170 (1980).
46. H. Munz, B. Claas, W. E. Stumpf, and L. Jennes, *Cell Tissue Res.* **222**, 313–323 (1982).
47. E. V. Famiglietti Jr., N. C. Brecha, and H. J. Karten, *Neurosci. Abstr.* **6**, 212 (1980).
48. B. B. Boycott and J. E. Dowling, *Philos. Trans. R. Soc. London, Ser. B.* **255**, 109–184 (1969).
49. B. Ehinger, *Z. Zellforsch.* **82**, 577–588 (1967).
50. R. W. Baughman and C. R. Bader, *Brain Res.* **138**, 469–486 (1977).
51. J. Marshall and M. J. Voaden, *Invest. Ophthalmol.* **13**, 602–607 (1974).
52. S. Yazulla and N. Brecha, *Invest. Ophthalmol. Vis. Sci.* **19**, 1415–1426 (1980).
53. I. Floren, *Acta Ophthalmol. (Kobenhaun)* **57**, 198–210 (1979).
54. J. Marshall and M. Voaden, *Biochem. Soc. Trans.* **2**, 268–270 (1974).
55. R. E. Marc, W. K. Stell, D. Bok, and D. M. K. Lam, *J. Comp. Neurol.* **182**, 221–246 (1978).
56. D. M. K. Lam, R. E. Marc, P. V. Sarthy, C. A. Chin, Y. Y. T. Su, C. Brandon, and J.-Y. Wu, *Neurochemistry* **1**, 183–190 (1980).
57. M. B. A. Djamgoz, W. K. Stell, C.-A. Chin, and D. M. K. Lam, *Nature* **292**, 620–623 (1981).

58. W. K. Stell, K. S. Chohan, and N. Brecha, *Neurosci. Abstr.* **7**, 94 (1981).

59. E. Dick and R. F. Miller, *Neurosci. Lett.* **26**, 131–135 (1981).

60. R. D. Glickman, A. R. Adolph, and J. E. Dowling, *Brain Res.* **234**, 81–99 (1982).

61. C. Schenker and S. E. Leeman, *Neurosci. Abstr.* **7**, 60 (1981).

62. B. B. Boycott, in R. Bellairs and E. G. Gray, Eds., *Essays on the Nervous System*, Clarendon Press, Oxford, 1974, pp. 223–257.

PART
3

Methodologies for Study of Brain Peptides

20

Competitive Binding Assays

O. P. RORSTAD

Department of Medicine
University of Calgary
Calgary, Alberta, Canada

1   INTRODUCTION

Competitive binding assays (CBA) have contributed significantly to the
rapid progress of our understanding of brain peptides. These remarkably sensitive, specific, and widely available methods for peptide measurement have provided the experimental bases for major concepts that
are now generally accepted, such as the occurrence of particular
peptides in both the brain and gastrointestinal tract, the widespread anatomical distribution of peptides in the nervous system, and the heterogeneity of molecular forms of particular brain peptides.

The essential components of a CBA are (i) a molecular or cellular
preparation (antibody or receptor) that specifically binds the peptide of
interest, (ii) a standardized reference preparation of the peptide, (iii) a
radioactively labeled tracer that will compete with the reference peptide for binding, and (iv) a method to separate bound and free ligand.
CBAs of brain peptides include radioimmunoassays (RIA) and radioreceptor assays (RRA). In the case of an RIA the concentration of peptide
in an "unknown" sample is determined by quantitatively comparing the
capacity of the "unknown" and standard peptides to compete with the
radiolabeled tracer for binding to the antiserum. The general theory and
practice of CBAs are discussed in detail elsewhere (1–6), and therefore
this chapter is restricted to some particulars of methodology and validation of CBAs for brain peptides.

2   RADIOIMMUNOASSAY METHODOLOGY

2.1   Immunogenicity of Brain Peptides

Most brain peptides, being of less than 4000 daltons molecular weight,
would not be expected to induce a brisk immune response if used alone
for immunization. The vast majority of antisera to brain peptides have
been raised to a complex of the hapten peptide and a larger molecule.
One convenient approach has been to absorb the peptide noncovalently
onto a carrier molecule, for instance polyvinylpyrrolidone, used with luteinizing hormone releasing hormone (LHRH), glucagon, and vasoactive
intestinal polypeptide (VIP) (5, 7, 8); aluminum oxide, used with LHRH
(8); and methylated bovine serum albumin, used with somatostatin (9).
Although immunization with an adsorbed peptide has generated satisfactory antisera, it has the limitation of not permitting the investigator to
direct rationally the specificity of the antiserum to a desired sequence of
the peptide. In addition, antisera raised to nonspecifically adsorbed peptides, especially those of over 10 amino acids, have an increased likelihood of binding to more than one region of the peptide, as in the case of
two somatostatin antisera raised in this manner (35). Such heterogene-

ous specificities may be of practical value if the affinity constants and titers of antiserum binding to the different regions are sufficiently similar so that the RIA requires integrity of a major portion of the peptide or the entire peptide for recognition of the assayed material as immunologically identical to the peptide. On the other hand, heterogeneity of binding specificities increases the chance of cross-reactivity of the RIA with other molecules (often unknown) that are structurally related to the peptide.

The major advantages of covalent conjugation of a peptide to a carrier molecule are enhanced immunogenicity and the opportunity to predetermine the binding specificity of the antiserum by judicious selection of the conjugation reaction. For most brain peptides a synthetic or highly purified preparation is available for immunization. Although desirable, the use of a highly purified peptide as immunogen is not essential for generation of an adequate antiserum, as demonstrated by several RIAs developed with immunogens of incompletely purified preparations of gastrointestinal hormones or adrenocorticotrophic hormone (ACTH) (5, 10). If one has limited quantities of a purified peptide it is generally preferable to reserve it for use as an assay standard rather than use it as an immunogen, for which a less pure preparation may serve the purpose. Proteins commonly used for conjugation to peptides include bovine or human serum albumin, globulins, bovine thyroglobulin, and hemocyanin. Comparative studies of the success of inducing antisera and the titer of antisera with conjugated lysine vasopressin and neurotensin suggest that the largest molecular weight conjugates generally produce the best results (Table 1) (11, 12).

A variety of reagents have proved useful for conjugating peptides and proteins through particular functional groups (Table 2). The carbodiimides and glutaraldehyde have achieved the greatest popularity.

TABLE 1   Influence of Protein Conjugation on Antiserum Production by Rabbits[a]

Conjugated Protein[b]	Molecular Weight	Antibody Response %	Titer of Antiserum
A. Lysine Vasopressin (12)			
None		0	
Bovine serum albumin	66,000	0	
Human serum albumin	60,000	75	< 1: 10,000
Bovine thyroglobulin	670,000	100	> 1: 50,000
B. Neurotensin (11)			
Polyglutamic acid	90,000	16	< 1: 10
Poly(Glu^{60},Lys^{40})	40,000	66	< 1: 7500
Bovine thyroglobulin	670,000	100	< 1: 100,000
Keyhole limpet hemocyanin	2,000,000	100	< 1: 150,000

[a] Adapted from Carraway and Leeman (11) and Skowsky and Fisher (12).
[b] Carbodiimide was used for all conjugations.

TABLE 2 Selected Coupling Reagents Used with Brain Peptides

Functional Groups	Coupling Reagents	References
NH$_2$	Glutaraldehyde	
NH$_2$, COOH	Carbodiimides	
NH$_2$, tyrosine, histidine	Diazonium compounds	
	eg: bisdiazotized benzidine	16, 17
	p-diazonium phenylacetic acid	22
Histidine, tyrosine, NH$_2$	1,5-difluoro-2,4-dinitrobenzene	25
Tyrosine	2,4-dichloro-6-methoxy-1,3,5-triazine	23, 26

Carbodiimides, 1-ethyl-3-(3-dimethylaminopropyl)-carbodiimide being a frequently used representative of this class, will predominantly link carboxyl and amino groups via an amide bond (13). The coupling reaction can be directed to occur between specific desired peptide or protein functional groups by chemical modification of either peptide or protein. For example, Carraway and Leeman (11) methylated the carboxyl groups of neurotensin and modified the amino groups of carrier proteins with succinic anhydride prior to carbodiimide conjugation, thereby directing the coupling reaction to occur between the lysine amino group (Lys[6]) of neurotensin and the carboxyl groups of the proteins. Restriction of the peptide and carrier to contain either amino or carboxyl groups, but not both, reduces the number of peptide–peptide or carrier–carrier conjugates produced by carbodiimide. Succinylation not only increases the number of carboxyl groups on the protein but also introduces a spacer group between the protein and conjugated peptide. Antisera generated by the conjugate usually will recognize a region of the peptide removed at some distance from the site of conjugation, probably because of steric hindrance by the bulk of the carrier protein and alterations to the peptide structure introduced at the site of conjugation. By selective conjugation through Lys[6] of neurotensin, Carraway and Leeman were able to obtain antisera directed against the biologically important carboxyl terminal region. A potentially undesirable property of the carbodiimides is their reactivity with tyrosine residues to form O-aryl isourea derivatives (14). However, the phenolic group of tyrosine can be regenerated, if desired, by reaction with hydroxylamine, as has been done with the Tyr[2] of lysine vasopressin (12). The bifunctional reagent glutaraldehyde (15) achieves coupling via amino groups of the peptide and protein and, unlike carbodiimides, interposes itself as a carbon chain spacer group between the conjugated molecules.

Alternative approaches to conjugation may be used when the peptide does not contain either a free amino or carboxyl group or when coupling through other moieties of the peptide is desired (Table 2). As a first example, reagents are available that will conjugate peptides via tyrosine or histidine residues. Thyrotropin releasing hormone (TRH), which has no amino or carboxyl group, was coupled to a carrier protein via histidine by bisdiazotized benzidine, a bifunctional diazonium compound that reacts with tyrosine and histidine (16, 17) This reagent also served for LHRH, which contains neither terminal amino nor carboxyl group (8), and for the tyrosine-substituted analog [Tyr^{11}]somatostatin, producing in the latter instance an antiserum with specificity directed to the spatially removed N-terminus of somatostatin (18). A potential limitation of bifunctional reagents like bisdiazotized benzidine and glutaraldehyde is the generation of a number of peptide–peptide and carrier–carrier conjugates lacking appropriate immunogenicity.

A second alternative approach to the preparation of specific immunogenic conjugates involves synthesis of peptide analogs or derivatized peptides that contain amino or carboxyl groups which can be coupled to protein by carbodiimide or glutaraldehyde. Examples include: (i) N-Gly-[Glu^1]bombesin, [Lys^4]bombesin, or [Lys^{12}]bombesin which is used because bombesin has neither terminal carboxyl, terminal amino, nor tyrosine residues (19, 20). (ii) [Glu^1]LHRH and [Gly^{10}]LHRH (5, 8). (iii) The free acid of TRH, pGlu-His-Pro (21). (iv) TRH derivatized on histidine with p-diazonium phenylacetic acid (22). In addition, appropriate synthetic fragments of a peptide may be used for immunization so as to direct production of site-specific antisera (23). A variety of other reagents for chemical modification and conjugation are available and may prove useful under certain circumstances (5, 17, 24). Techniques of animal immunization—including selection of animal species, use of Freund's adjuvant, and inoculation schedules—are described elsewhere (1–6).

2.2 Properties of Antisera to Brain Peptides

Three major properties of antisera are titer, sensitivity, and site specificity, the last defining the region of the peptide that the antiserum recognizes. An antiserum produced against a purified peptide by conventional immunization techniques often recognizes a single determinant region, usually consisting of two to eight amino acid residues. Such specificity is remarkable considering that a conventional antiserum contains several heterogeneous immunoglobulin molecules. Some antisera are capable of distinguishing to a quantitatively useful extent between two naturally occurring peptides that differ only by a single amino acid, such as leucine and methionine enkephalin (27). The availability of synthetic analogs of brain peptides has made possible precise mapping of the peptide determinants required for binding of the antiserum, lending validity to the use of an antiserum as a "molecular probe." In some instances an antiserum recognizes two or more regions of a peptide. Although such heterogeneous binding functions could theoretically reside in a single polyfunctional antibody and therefore be inseparable, affini-

ty adsorption techniques have successfully separated certain populations of antibodies with different specificities (23). For example, a sheep
antiserum showed binding to both the N-terminal and central regions of
somatostatin. The antibodies directed against the central region bound
well to [Tyr¹]somatostatin immobilized on an insoluble matrix, Se-
pharose, whereas the antibodies that required N-terminus integrity did
not bind to the N-terminus-substituted analog, thereby remained in solution and provided a convenient separation of the two antibody populations (35).

The affinity constant of antiserum for peptide binding largely determines the sensitivity of an RIA. Manipulations of the RIA incubation
conditions, particularly the use of a nonequilibrium protocol, may improve assay sensitivity to variable extents (1–6). It is desirable that the
RIA be sensitive enough so that the assayed concentration of peptide in
an "unknown" sample of tissue extract or fluid is sufficient to fall near
the midpoint of the RIA standard curve where assay precision is maximal. In some instances, such as the RIA of cerebrospinal fluid peptides,
the measured concentration may be much lower than the midpoint of
the RIA standard curve. If this occurs, then one needs to carefully consider whether the RIA is valid and sufficiently precise for the purposes
intended.

2.3   Selection of a Radiolabeled Ligand

Methods for radioactively labeling peptides to high specific activity
have been essential to the development of RIA. Although rarely tritium
labeled peptides may serve as useful RIA tracers, such as [³H]enke-
phalin (specific activity 18–20 Ci/mmol) (28), the degree of specific activity of radiolabel required for optimal RIA sensitivity can usually only
be achieved with radioactive iodine (^{125}I or ^{131}I). In contrast with
[³H]enkephalin, the maximal theoretical specific activity of a peptide iodinated with one atom of ^{125}I per molecule of peptide is 2200 Ci/mmol.
Most investigators prefer ^{125}I to ^{131}I for peptide radioiodination because
of its longer half-life (60 days versus 8 days), greater isotopic abundance in commercial preparations, and lower energy emission (4).

2.3.1   Oxidative Iodination

An atom of radioactive iodine can be conveniently introduced onto tyrosine or histidine residues by oxidative iodination, using the reagent
chloramine T, or enzymatically with lactoperoxidase and hydrogen pe-
roxide. Exposure of a peptide to these conditions, especially chloramine
T, may potentially lead to oxidation of methionine, tryptophan, and cysteine residues and consequently to altered peptide structure and reduced immunoreactivity. Nevertheless, low concentration chloramine T

radioiodination has achieved widespread use and has proven satisfactory for a large number of RIAs of brain peptides. Radioiodination of a histidine compared with a tyrosine residue requires higher pH and concentration of chloramine T, which increases the risk of oxidative damage to the peptide. Chloramine T is very satisfactory for radioiodination of the histidine of TRH, a tripeptide, whereas in the case of secretin, a 27-amino-acid peptide containing one histidine and no tyrosine residues, a more gentle lactoperoxidase procedure produces a more satisfactory iodination (29). The reducing agent sodium metabisulfite is usually used to terminate chloramine T iodination, but in the case of peptides such as oxytocin, vasopressin, and somatostatin, which contain disulfide bonds that may be broken by reducing conditions, sodium metabisulfite may be omitted and the reaction stopped safely with excess albumin and buffer (5). Clearly, one must individualize the iodination methods to suit different peptides.

A new oxidizing reagent 1,3,4,6-tetrachloro-3α,6α-diphenyl-glycoluril (Iodogen) shows considerable promise, as indicated by its successful iodination of several polypeptide hormones (30). This water-insoluble agent is used while coated onto the walls of reaction vessels, thereby permitting separation of the oxidizing agent and labeled peptide by merely removing the liquid phase, containing peptide, after completion of the iodination.

2.3.2 Conjugation Labeling

Bolton and Hunter have provided an alternative to oxidative iodination whereby a previously radioiodinated molecule, ^{125}I 3-(p-hydroxyphenyl) propionic acid N-hydroxysuccinimide ester, is conjugated via an amide bond to amino groups on the peptide (31). This approach avoids oxidation of the peptide and obviates the need to synthetically introduce a tyrosine residue into naturally histidine- or tyrosine-deficient peptides in order for iodination to be possible. Conjugation labeling has been of great benefit to the RIA of cholecystokinin (CCK), a peptide that is sensitive to oxidation, probably because of its three methionine residues (32). The Bolton-Hunter method preserves both immunoreactivity and biological activity of CCK, thereby providing a radiolabel appropriate for both RIA and RRA (33). On the other hand, a disadvantage of conjugation labeling is that it adds a relatively large functional group, which in some peptides may cause substantial alterations in immunoreactivity.

2.3.3 Effects of Radioiodination on Immunoreactivity

One should recollect that even oxidative iodination introduces a very large atom into the peptide structure, potentially resulting in reduced immunoreactivity. In instances where a peptide does not contain a tyrosine residue, for example, substance P, somatostatin, or bombesin, analogs containing tyrosine substitutions commonly serve for iodination, thereby introducing an additional perturbation to the structure of the peptide to which one has raised antiserum. These structural alterations may be inconsequential if the site of iodination does not impinge on the antibody-binding region—label and standard will behave identically immunologically. On the other hand, if tyrosine substitution or iodination occurs at a region to which antibody normally binds, then the iodinated tracer may show low immunoreactivity (34). For example, one somatostatin antiserum requires integrity of residues Phe^{11} and Thr^{12} for binding. The antiserum will not bind the iodinated, tyrosine-substituted analog [^{125}I-Tyr^{11}]somatostatin whereas it binds well to [^{125}I-Tyr^{1}] somatostatin or ^{125}I-N-Tyr-somatostatin in which the alterations due to substitution and iodination are far removed from the binding site (35). Alteration of tracer immunoreactivity by substitution and iodination may prove of practical value in the case where an antiserum has more than one binding specificity. Another somatostatin antiserum shows binding specificity for both the N-terminal and the central molecular regions. The use of [^{125}I-Tyr^{1}]somatostatin or ^{125}I-N-Tyr-somatostatin as tracer results in an RIA with only central molecular specificity because the antibodies directed to the N-terminus cannot bind to the tracers that are substituted and iodinated at the N-terminus, whereas central-directed antibodies bind these tracers well. The use of [^{125}I-Tyr^{11}]somatostatin as tracer with this antiserum yields an RIA with N-terminal specificity, probably because the N-terminus specific antibodies are present in much higher titer than are the central specific antibodies in this antiserum, or possibly because substitution and iodination at Phe^{11} perturbs the central molecular antibody binding region (Figure 1; 35). Of practical significance is that the N-terminal-directed RIA is highly specific for

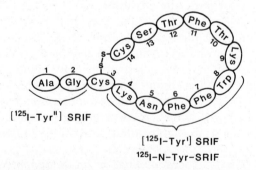

[^{125}I-Tyr^{11}] SRIF

[^{125}I-Tyr^{1}] SRIF
^{125}I-N-Tyr-SRIF

Figure 1. Binding specificities for a particular somatostatin antiserum (sheep B) are dependent upon which radiolabeled tracer one uses.[35] With [^{125}I-Tyr^{11}] SRIF, specificity is directed to the N-terminal region, whereas with ^{125}I-N-Tyr-SRIF or [^{125}I-Tyr^{1}] SRIF, central specificity is evident. Abbreviation: SRIF, somatotropin release inhibiting factor, somatostatin.

somatostatin-14 and shows low immunoreactivity with the larger N-terminus extended forms of somatostatin, such as somatostatin-28, whereas the centrally directed somatostatin RIA recognizes somatostatin-14
and somatostatin-28 equipotently because they share common antibody
binding sites. Other examples of modification of antiserum binding
specificity by selective use of radiolabeled tracers include RIAs of
physalaemin, angiotensin, and gastrin (36–38).

Nonradioactive tracers, such as enzymes or fluorescent probes covalently linked to peptides, have seen little use for competitive binding assay of brain peptides (39). Because of the large size of the indicator
group relative to iodine, greater influence on tracer immunoreactivity
may be expected. For instance, an enzyme immunoassay of somatostatin using somatostatin-alkaline phosphatase conjugate as the tracer
was considerably less sensitive than other reported RIAs for somatostatin (40).

2.4 The Reference Standard Peptide

Usually a synthetic preparation of peptide is available as an RIA reference standard. Although it is desirable to compare the immunoreactivity of synthetic and purified naturally occurring peptide, as Carraway
and Leeman did for their RIAs of neurotensin to check RIA "standard
peptide" validity, such comparisons are rarely reported in the literature
(11). Loss of RIA sensitivity may result from alterations to the standard
peptide during storage, such as uptake of water and modifications to
peptide functional groups. Since frequently an RIA "recognizes" different molecular weight forms of a peptide, it seems more appropriate and
accurate to express RIA data in molar units of peptide-like immunoreactivity rather than the more commonly used mass units.

2.5 Separation of Bound and Free Ligand

Separation of antibody-bound and free ligand is a fundamental RIA
step that one may accomplish in a variety of ways, including: (i) precipitation of the primary antibody by a second heterologous antibody with
specificity directed against the immunoglobulin class of the primary antibody, (ii) adsorption of free antigen to a solid phase material such as
charcoal, (iii) prebinding of the primary antibody to a solid phase such
as the walls of test tubes, and (iv) nonspecific organic solvent or
salting-out precipitation of the antibody-bound antigen, such as with alcohol or ammonium sulfate (1–6). Second-antibody and charcoal separation have seen the most use, but all methods are generally applicable to
the RIA of selected brain peptides. An alternative, promising method
uses the *Staphylococcus aureus* cell wall protein A, which binds to the
Fc portion of IgG from a variety of animal species (41). Separation of

bound and free antigen occurs rapidly by addition of killed *S. aureus* to the RIA followed by centrifugation. This procedure has advantages over the second antibody method of rapidity of reaction and applicability to antisera from several species, with the exception of sheep and goat antisera, to which protein A does not bind.

3   VALIDITY OF RADIOIMMUNOASSAYS

The issue of validity refers to whether the RIA measures what it is intended to measure. Validity can only be proved ultimately by demonstration of structural identity between the "unknown" assayed material and the peptide of interest. Although this rigorous criterion has been met in the cases of somatostatin and neurotensin, it is not practical for the vast majority of useful RIAs that have been developed. Establishment of validity most often results from accumulation of several pieces of evidence that together put the question "beyond reasonable doubt." Traditional pieces of evidence have been the exclusion of potential interference in the RIA and demonstration that the assayed material mimics the standard peptide under various immunological, chemical, physical, and biological tests of identity. Perhaps the major contribution toward validation of an RIA for a brain peptide is determination of the region of the peptide responsible for antibody binding. A region-specific RIA may be valid for the measurement of heterogeneous forms of peptides that share similar binding regions but have different physical-chemical or biological properties from the reference peptide.

3.1   Nonimmunological Interference

An RIA basically detects the presence of antigen in an "unknown" sample by a reduction of tracer binding to primary antibody. Any factors that interfere with antibody–tracer binding may potentially be measured incorrectly as antigen. Examples include: pH, ionic strength, denaturing agents such as urea, proteases, protease inhibitors, binding proteins, bacterostatic agents, and heparin (42–44).

3.1.1   Tracer Degradation

Tracer degradation during RIA is an underestimated, often subtle, problem that one can detect by appropriate quality control. Yalow and Straus have described in detail methods for detecting tracer degradation during RIA (42, 44). Irrespective of factors in the "unknown" sample, the "carrier" protein added to RIA incubation buffers to reduce nonspecific binding to glassware may itself cause a degree of tracer degradation, which may compromise the quality of the RIA. Gelatin, egg albumin, or serum significantly reduced tracer–antibody binding in an RIA for somatostatin, whereas purified bovine or human serum albumin was free of degrading activity (personal observation).

3.1.2 Extraction of Peptides

An ideal extraction procedure for RIA purposes should first completely solubilize the tissue or fluid content of the peptide without chemically modifying the peptide, and second, inactivate peptidases that may degrade the peptide or interfere in the RIA. Extraction conditions must be individualized for the peptide of interest; unfortunately, such methodological studies are largely empirical. The conditions used for discovery, original isolation or traditional extraction of a peptide, may not be the optimal methods for maximal extraction yield. For example, Ryder et al. (45) recently observed that alkaline aqueous extraction of CCK-like immunoreactivity from rat brain resulted in a twofold to fourfold greater yield than traditional neutral or acidic extraction methods. Investigators often include boiling, denaturants, or enzyme inhibitors in the extraction formula to inactivate peptidases. One should consider the extent to which higher-molecular-weight forms of peptide-like immunoreactivity are extracted under the conditions used, because these forms may have different solubilities or sensitivities to chemical or temperature degradation from smaller forms of the peptide. Quantitation of the recovery of added synthetic peptide subjected with the tissue or serum sample to the extraction procedure is a fundamental test of the efficiency of extraction and the stability of the peptide to the conditions used.

The RIA of peptides in serum or plasma presents particular problems due to peptidases, binding proteins, and other interfering factors. A detailed consideration of these problems is available elsewhere (5, 43, 46). Extraction of serum may eliminate interference, but on the other hand it may introduce some loss of peptide and it adds an additional step to the assay. RIA of peptides in unextracted serum is fraught with hazard, but where undertaken it has traditionally been accompanied with neutralization of peptidase activity and the use of antigen-free reference samples either occurring naturally or produced by chemical stripping of the sample, such as by charcoal or more specifically by affinity adsorption. In the case of tissue extracts, nonimmunological interference is usually avoided if the extract can be assayed in high dilution. If the tissue extract must be used in low dilution, it may be necessary to correct internally for RIA interference as for serum samples by preparing mock antigen-free extracts. Fortunately, RIA of peptides in cerebrospinal fluid is not accompanied by the formidable interference problems encountered with serum.

3.1.3 "Parallelism" of Standard and Unknown

Demonstration of parallel competitive binding curves for standard peptide and "unknown" is a prerequisite for a valid RIA, although it does
not alone establish validity. In the instance in which "unknown" serum
contains antibodies or proteins that bind the tracer, then a parallel
dose-response curve that mimics the presence of ligand can be obtained
in an RRA or a second antibody RIA (47) (The complex of tracer with
"unknown" antibody or binding protein will not be precipitated by the
second antibody). The assay will indicate spuriously high levels of ligand. The presence of interfering binding factors in serum may be
detected by direct assay of the serum for tracer binding or by RIA using
a different separation method, such as charcoal, alcohol, or ammonium
sulfate precipitation, which will yield results discrepant from those of
the second antibody RIA.

3.2 Immunological Cross-Reactivity

Certain families of peptides, such as the gastrin-CCK family (48, 49),
share structural homology and demonstrate well recognized cross-
reactivities in some RIAs. Strategies to maximize the specificity of RIAs
by rational preparation of immunogens and tracers have been discussed
above. If the cross-reactivity by peptide B in the RIA of peptide A is
known to be small, and the concentration of B in "unknown" samples
as determined by a specific independent assay for B is not sufficiently
high for it to be detectable in the RIA for A, then the cross-reactivity
may be ignored as not practically relevant. If the cross-reactivity of B in
the RIA of A is substantial, it may still be feasible to measure A by first
selectively removing B from the "unknown" samples by affinity adsorption, provided one has a specific antiserum to B. Alternatively, cross-reactive peptide B may be separated from peptide A by physical-chemical
means, such as gel filtration, before RIA for A, although these manipulations make for a tedious assay.

Several polypeptide hormones, such as insulin, growth hormone, gastrin, and calcitonin, show variation in their amino acid sequence among
different animal species. Heterologous RIAs, in which peptide in one
species is assayed using antiserum directed to another species' peptide,
have had varying degrees of success depending on whether the species'
peptides share identical antibody binding sites. In the relatively few
species for which the amino acid sequence of brain peptides has been
determined, conservation of structure appears to be common. Owing to
the small size of most brain peptides, major structural modifications
would have a high probability of affecting biological activity and therefore would be expected to be tolerated poorly during evolution. As a
note of caution, although heterologous RIAs for brain peptides are in

wide use, one should repeat the validation of an RIA for each different species being studied.

Fragments, or larger forms of a peptide within the same species, may cross-react in an RIA. Often these heterogeneous forms will be immuno-logically identical due to preservation of the binding site structure, for example somatostatins 14 and 28. On the other hand, they may be im-munologically nonidentical, usually detectable by having nonparallel competitive binding curves when compared with the standard peptide. The significance of peptide heterogeneity is considered in the chapters on specific peptides in this volume and in other sources (48, 49).

3.3 Validation by Independent Assay

Traditionally, to establish RIA validity one has had to confirm the RIA results by an independent assay method such as another RIA, a RRA, or bioassay. Accordingly, Carraway and Leeman applied an equivalen-cy criterion for validation of the RIA for neurotensin, whereby an equal concentration of peptide was detected by a variety of antisera with specificities for different regions of the peptide (11). When one encoun-ters a variety of heterogeneous, structurally related peptides with differ-ing immunoreactivities, receptor binding, and biological potencies, as is the case with some brain peptides, the equivalency criterion can no longer be a strict requirement of assay validity. RIAs, RRAs, and bioas-says may detect quite different peptide concentrations based on the dif-ferent properties of the heterogeneous peptides (50).

3.4 Validation by Physical-Chemical Characterization

The immunoreactive material detected by an RIA should exhibit, at least in part, similar physical-chemical properties to the standard pep-tide. One can choose from a variety of chromatographic and electropho-retic methods to compare unknown and standard. For example, neurotensin-like immunoreactivity extracted from rat brain elutes on gel filtration chromatography as a major peak in the region of synthetic neurotensin (51). Often, however, separation techniques reveal heteroge-neity of peptide-like immunoreactivity, presumably due to precursors, fragments, and cross-reactive peptides, as illustrated by the somatosta-tins and CCKs (9, 52).

3.5 Validation by Appropriate Physiological Responses

The criterion of validation by physiological response has seen less ap-plication to the RIA of brain peptides, for which the physiological stim-uli for release and the response parameters are less completely understood, than to traditional hormones in serum. If a stimulus is known to increase the concentration of a peptide in serum or other fluid, then a valid RIA should detect this response. For example, introduction of an alkaline solution into the duodenum of a dog should stimulate release of motilin, which is known to increase gastric motility. As part of the validation of their RIA for motilin, Dryburgh and Brown demonstrated a coincidental increase in serum concentration of motilin-like immunoreactivity and gastric motility after duodenal alkalinization (53; Figure 2).

3.6 Mapping of the Peptide Determinants for Antibody Binding

Determination by analog studies of the peptide regions that an RIA recognizes has assumed considerable importance as a validation step because of the molecular heterogeneity encountered with several brain

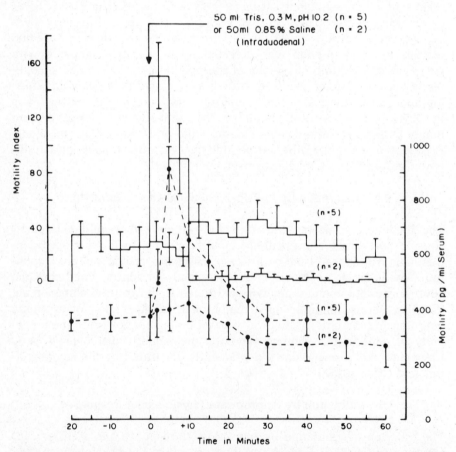

Figure 2. Gastric motility (solid lines) and serum motilin-like immunoreactivity (dashed lines) responses to intraduodenal infusion of alkaline buffer ($n=5$) or saline ($n=2$). The right hand vertical axis should read "motilin (pg/mL serum)." Reproduced with permission from Dryburgh and Brown (53).

peptides (54). The lengthy expression of RIA data as "sequence x-y of peptide A-like immunoreactivity" has little chance of being misleading but is not perfect. Because antibody binding occurs to a three-dimensional domain, a description of the peptide binding site in terms of a linear amino acid sequence may not accurately represent the binding determinants of the peptide. For example, the spatial orientation of a precursor peptide may completely mask a potential antibody binding region or alter its immunoreactivity compared with a smaller homologous peptide with a different conformation.

4 MONOCLONAL ANTIBODIES TO BRAIN PEPTIDES

The technique of generating monoclonal antibodies with homogeneous affinity and specificity using hybrid myeloma cells (hybridomas), developed initially by Köhler and Milstein (55), holds great promise for maximizing RIA specificity and reproducibility (56). Fundamentally, hybridomas are generated by fusion of clonal myeloma cells and spleen cells from an immunized animal followed by selection and maintenance of hybridomas that produce antibody with desired properties (Figure 3; ref. 57 discusses hybridoma techniques in detail). One great advantage of hybridoma technology over conventional immunization methods is that an impure antigen can be used as an immunogen to generate homogeneous antibody to a specific antigen, whereas conventionally one would obtain a heterogeneous mixture of antibodies that recognize multiple determinants. Monoclonal antibody techniques have had less impact on the study of brain peptides than on other areas of biology because pure synthetic peptides are available for immunization and have generated satisfactory antisera with a single antigenic specificity, as described above (58, 59). Nevertheless, a monoclonal antibody, although more work to generate, does possess homogeneous specificity, is available in unlimited supply, and should avoid potential cross-reactivity with structurally unrelated molecules. A monoclonal antibody to substance P has proved useful for RIA and produced a very clean immunofluorescence reaction to substance P-like immunoreactivity in tissue when compared with conventional antisera, probably because of the absence of unreactive immunoglobulins or the lack of cross-reactivity with nonspecific tissue antigens (58, 60). However, cross-reactivity of a site-specific monoclonal antibody with structurally related peptides still applies, as for conventional antisera (Figure 4; 58).

5 RADIORECEPTOR ASSAYS

Investigators have developed RRAs for several neuropeptides. A variety of binding preparations, including whole cells (33, 61), membrane fractions of broken cells (50, 62, 63), and soluble receptors may serve for

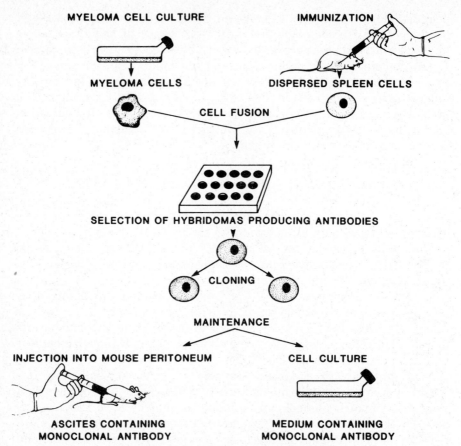

Figure 3. Generation of monoclonal antibodies.

RRA provided their binding affinities for peptide are sufficiently high to detect endogenous concentrations of peptide. The techniques of RRA introduce several variations in tracer preparations, incubation conditions, separation methods, and data analysis from those discussed for RIA (64–66). RRAs and RIAs for the same peptide may yield concordant or discrepant results depending on the presence and reactivity of structurally related peptides. For example, RRA and RIA of VIP detected similar concentrations of VIP-like peptides in the rat gastrointestinal tract (62), but RRA of opiate peptides using labeled enkephalin tracer detected a much higher concentration of RRA-reactive peptides in the rat brain than did an RIA for enkephalins (50). This discrepancy is explainable by the presence of nonenkephalin opiate peptides that bind to the receptor preparation but not to enkephalin antibodies.

In conclusion, a distinct advantage of RRAs over RIAs is that they have a greater probability of measuring substances that have biological relevance. Because receptor binding is considered to be an important

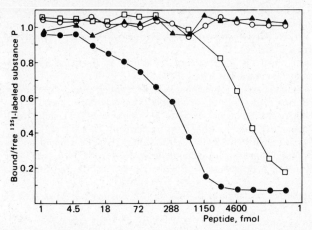

Figure 4. Radioimmunoassay for substance P using a monoclonal antibody. ● substance P; ▲ β-endorphin; ○ somatostatin; □ eleidosin. Cross-reactivity is evident with eleidosin, which shares with substance P the same tripeptide sequence at its carboxyl-terminal region. Reproduced with permission from Cuello et al. (58).

initial step toward eliciting a biological response to a peptide, the RRA provides information about the potential biological activity of the peptide material assayed. However, a caveat applies whereby the only biological activity implied for a substance detected by RRA is that which is capable of being mediated via the particular receptor used for RRA. A RIA, in contrast, does not necessarily yield information about biological activity because immunological reactivity does not bear any obligatory relationship to biological activity. Finally, most RRAs, when compared with traditional bioassays for peptides, have practical advantages of greater sensitivity, precision, convenience, and economy.

ACKNOWLEDGMENTS

I thank Drs. J. B. Martin and M. A. Arnold for providing selected somatostatin antisera for study and Dr. J. Rivier who kindly contributed alanine-substituted analogs of somatostatin used for site-specificity studies. Drs. D. Hanley, M. Huang, Y. Lefebvre, and K. Lederis provided helpful critical comments on the manuscript. I also thank Drs. A. C. Cuello, C. Milstein, and J. C. Brown for permission to reproduce figures from their publications.

REFERENCES

1. S. A. Berson and R. S. Yalow, Eds., *Methods in Investigative and Diagnostic Endocrinology*, Part I, Vol. 2, Elsevier, New York, 1973, p. 84.
2. W. M. Hunter, in D. M. Weir, Ed., *Handbook of Experimental Immunology*, 2nd ed., Blackwell, Oxford, 1973, p. 17.1.

3. W. D. Odell and W. H. Daughaday, Eds., *Principles of Competitive Protein-Binding Assays*, Lippincott, Philadelphia, 1971.
4. C. W. Parker, *Radioimmunoassay of Biologically Active Compounds*, Prentice-Hall, Englewood Cliffs, N.J., 1976.
5. B. M. Jaffe and H. R. Behrman, Eds., *Methods of Hormone Radioimmunoassay*, 2nd ed., Academic Press, New York, 1979.
6. H. Van Vunakis and J. J. Langone, Eds., *Immunochemical Techniques, Part A* (*Methods in Enzymology*, Vol. 70), Academic Press, New York, 1980.
7. N. Yanaihara, M. Sakagami, H. Sato, K. Yamamoto, T. Hashimoto, C. Yanaihara, Z. Ito, K. Yamaguchi, and K. Abe, *Gastroenterology* **72**, 803 (1977).
8. A. Arimura and A. V. Schally, in M. Motta, P. G. Crosignani and L. Martini, Eds., *Hypothalamic Hormones*, Academic Press, New York, 1975, p. 27.
9. O. P. Rorstad, J. Epelbaum, P. Brazeau, and J. B. Martin, *Endocrinology* **105**, 1083 (1979).
10. H. Yoshimi, S. Matsukura, S. Sueoka, M. Fukase, M. Yokota, Y. Hirata, and H. Imura, *Life Sci.* **22**, 2189 (1978).
11. R. Carraway and S. Leeman, *J. Biol. Chem.* **251**, 7035 (1976).
12. W. R. Skowsky and D. A. Fisher, *J. Lab. Clin. Med.* **80**, 134 (1972).
13. T. L. Goodfriend, L. Levine, and G. D. Fasman, *Science* **144**, 1344 (1964).
14. K. L. Carraway and D. E. Koshland Jr., *Biochim. Biophys. Acta* **160**, 272 (1968).
15. F. M. Richards and J. R. Knowles, *J. Mol. Biol.* **37**, 231 (1968).
16. R. M. Bassiri and R. D. Utiger, *Endocrinology* **90**, 722 (1972).
17. S. M. Beiser, V. P. Butler Jr., and B. F. Erlanger, in P. A. Miescher and H. J. Muller-Eberhard, Eds., *Textbook of Immunopathology*, Vol. 1, 2nd ed., Grune and Stratton, New York, 1976, p. 15.
18. W. Vale, N. Ling, J. Rivier, J. Villarreal, C. Rivier, C. Douglas, and M. Brown, *Metabolism* **25**, Suppl. 1, 1491 (1976).
19. M. Brown, R. Allen, J. Villarreal, J. Rivier, and W. Vale, *Life Sci.* **23**, 2721 (1978).
20. C. Yanaihara, A. Inoue, T. Mochizuki, J. Ozaki, H. Sato, and N. Yanaihara, *Biomed. Res.* **1**, 96 (1980).
21. T. J. Visser, R. Docter, and G. Hennemann, *Acta Endocrinol.* **77**, 417 (1974).
22. Y. Koch, T. Baram, and M. Fridkin, *FEBS Lett.* **63**, 295 (1976).
23. G. J. Dockray, *Regul. Peptides* **1**, 169 (1980).
24. V. Likhite and A. Sehon, in C. A. Williams and M. W. Chase, Eds., *Methods in Immunology and Immunochemistry*, Vol. 1, Academic Press, New York, 1967, p. 150.
25. T. J. Visser, W. Klootwijk, R. Docter, and G. Hennemann, *FEBS Lett.* **83**, 37 (1977).
26. K. L. Agarwal, S. Grudzinski, G. W. Kenner, N. H. Rogers, R. C. Sheppard, and J. E. McGuigan, *Experientia* **17**, 514 (1971).
27. R. J. Miller, K.-J. Chang, B. Cooper, and P. Cuatrecasas, *J. Biol. Chem.* **253**, 531 (1978).
28. S. Sullivan, H. Akil, S. J. Watson, and J. D. Barchas, *Commun. Psychopharmacol.* **1**, 605 (1977).
29. K. N. Holohan, R. F. Murphy, R. W. J. Flanagan, K. D. Buchanan, and D. T. Elmore, *Biochim. Biophys. Acta* **322**, 178 (1973).
30. W. G. Wood, C. Wachter, and P. C. Scriba, *Fresenius Z. Anal. Chem.* **301**, 119 (1980).
31. A. E. Bolton and W. M. Hunter, *Biochem. J.* **133**, 529 (1973).
32. J. F. Rehfeld, *J. Biol. Chem.* **253**, 4016 (1978).
33. H. Sankaran, C. W. Deveney, I. D. Goldfine, and J. A. Williams, *J. Biol. Chem.* **254**, 9349 (1979).
34. E. Straus. H.-J. Urbach, and R. S. Yalow, *Biochem. Biophys. Res. Commun.* **64**, 1036 (1975).
35. O. P. Rorstad, *J. Immunoassay* **4**, 49 (1983).
36. L. H. Lazarus, R. I. Linnoila, O. Hernandez, and R. P. Diaugustine, *Nature* **287**, 555 (1980).
37. J. Giese, M. D. Nielsen, and M. Jorgensen, *Nature New Biol.* **229**, 189 (1971).

38. J. F. Rehfeld, in S. R. Bloom, Ed., *Gut Hormones*, 1st ed., Churchill Livingstone, Edinburgh, 1978, p. 112.
39. R. F. Schall and H. J. Tenoso, *Clin. Chem.* **27**, 1157 (1981).
40. K. Nakagawa, T. Obara, M. Matsubara, and H. Horikawa, *Endocrinol. Jpn.* **25**, 197 (1978).
41. M. A. Frohman, L. A. Frohman, M. B. Goldman, and J. N. Goldman, *J. Lab. Clin. Med.* **93**, 614 (1979).
42. E. Straus and R. Yalow, in H. Gainer, Ed., *Peptides in Neurobiology*, Plenum Press, New York, 1977, p. 39.
43. M. G. Bryant, in S. R. Bloom, Ed., *Gut Hormones*, 1st ed., Churchill Livingstone, Edinburgh, 1978, p. 120.
44. R. S. Yalow and E. Straus, in G. B. J. Glass, Ed., *Gastrointestinal Hormones*, Raven Press, New York, 1980, p. 751.
45. S. W. Ryder, J. Eng, E. Straus, and R. S. Yalow, *Biochem. Biophys. Res. Commun.* **94**, 704 (1980).
46. Y. C. Patel, T. Wheatley, D. Fitz-Patrick, and G. Brock, *Endocrinology* **107**, 306 (1980).
47. D. Rodbard, *Endocrinology* **101**, 1180 (1977).
48. G. J. Dockray, in R. F. Beers Jr. and E. G. Bassett, Eds., *Polypeptide Hormones*, Raven Press, New York, 1980, p. 357.
49. J. F. Rehfeld, *Am. J. Physiol.* **240**, G255 (1981).
50. C. Gros, P. Pradelles, C. Rouget, O. Bepoldin, F. Dray, M. C. Fournie-Zaluski, B. P. Roques, H. Pollard, C. Llorens-Cortes, and J. C. Schwartz, *J. Neurochem.* **31**, 29 (1978).
51. R. Carraway and S. E. Leeman, *J. Biol. Chem.* **251**, 7045 (1976).
52. J. F. Rehfeld, *J. Biol. Chem.* **253**, 4022 (1978).
53. J. R. Dryburgh and J. C. Brown, *Gastroenterology* **68**, 1169 (1975).
54. J. F. Rehfeld, *Biomed. Res.* **1** Suppl., 73 (1980).
55. G. Köhler and C. Milstein, *Nature* **256**, 495 (1975).
56. B. A. Diamond, D. E. Yelton, and M. D. Scharff, *N. Engl. J. Med.* **304**, 1344 (1981).
57. R. H. Kennett, T. J. McKearn, and K. B. Bechtol, Eds., *Monoclonal Antibodies*, Plenum Press, New York, 1980.
58. A. C. Cuello, G. Galfre, and C. Milstein, *Proc. Natl. Acad. Sci. USA* **76**, 3532 (1979).
59. I. Gozes, D. Barry, R. Benoit, F-T. Liu, D. H. Katz, R. J. Milner, and F. E. Bloom, *Program of the 11th Meeting of the Society for Neuroscience*, 1981, p. 98. Abstract No. 32.8.
60. A. C. Cuello, G. Galfre, and C. Milstein, in G. Pepeu, M. J. Kuhar, and S. J. Enna, Eds., *Receptors for Neurotransmitters and Peptide Hormones*, Raven Press, New York, 1980, p. 349.
61. A. Faivre-Bauman, D. Gourdji and A. Tixier-Vidal, *Ann. Endocrinol.* **37**, 325 (1976).
62. J. Besson, M. Laburthe, D. Bataille, C. Dupont, and G. Rosselin, *Acta Endocrinol.* **87**, 799 (1978).
63. P. Kitabgi, C. Poustis, C. Granier, J. V. Rietschoten, J. Rivier, J.-L. Morgat, and P. Freychet, *Mol. Pharmacol.* **18**, 11 (1980).
64. J. Roth, *Metabolism* **22**, 1059 (1973).
65. J. Roth, in B. W. O'Malley and J. G. Hardman, Eds., *Hormone Action, Part B: Peptide Hormones (Methods in Enzymology, Vol. 37)*, Academic Press, New York, 1975, p. 66.
66. J. D. Gardner, *Gastroenterology* **76**, 202 (1979).

21

Immunocytochemistry

ROBERT ELDE

Department of Anatomy
University of Minnesota Medical School
Minneapolis, Minnesota

1 INTRODUCTION

The study of brain peptides by immunohistochemical methods has represented a significant portion of the total immunohistochemical literature of the past decade. Among other factors, this is likely to be due to the power of the technique in revealing details of previously anonymous neuronal circuits, as well as the remarkable increase in the number of brain peptides that have become chemically characterized. It is noteworthy that immunohistochemical studies have shown neuropeptides to be contained within discrete neurons and, moreover, within subcellular organelles of those neurons that are implicated in neurotransmitter synthesis, storage, and release.

The indirect immunofluorescence method of Coons (1) remained largely unmodified for nearly two decades and has been a productive technique for localization of neuropeptides. With rapid advances in immunobiology and neuroscience, a variety of modifications of the method have emerged. These refinements, along with recent developments in molecular biology, have elevated the issues raised by immunohistochemical studies to levels unimaginable just a few years ago. The purpose of this chapter is not a broad presentation of the varieties and details of existing immunohistochemical methods. Such information has been recently reviewed (2–4) and is available from numerous sources, including commercial concerns that produce reagents used in most of the major methods. Rather, this review is an attempt to outline unsettled issues that remain to haunt the immunohistochemist in making ultimate conclusions concerning the localization of brain peptides.

2 PRODUCTION OF ANTIBODIES TO NEUROPEPTIDES

Immunohistochemical studies of neuropeptides have until recently been accomplished with serum from animals immunized with hapten–protein complexes, with synthetic peptides serving as haptens. In most cases, the peptides have been covalently coupled to carrier proteins using bifunctional reagents such as glutaraldehyde or by formation of peptide bonds with water-soluble carbodiimides (5). In addition, adsorption of peptides onto charged proteins such as methylated serum albumin has been shown to produce an effective immunogen (6–8). These approaches have been criticized, in part because high titers of antibodies directed against the carrier proteins are concurrently generated. In some cases, antibodies to the carrier proteins give rise to nonspecific staining of neuronal or glial elements. But this problem is usually solved by immunoprecipitation of such undesirable antibodies before incubating the antiserum on the tissue section. Covalent coupling of peptides to carrier proteins is advantageous in that one can, to a certain extent, "engineer" the antipeptide-antibody population by selectively coupling the amino terminus of small peptides, such the enkephalins, to the carrier proteins, leaving the carboxy terminus exposed as a major antigenic determinant. Resultant antisera have often been found to display exquisite specificity for the carboxy terminus of the peptide and they fail to cross-react with carboxy-terminal extensions of the molecule (9, 10).

An additional criticism of antisera to peptides used for immunohistochemistry relates to the problem of the heterogeneity of antibodies with respect to their affinity for the peptide as well as the variety of determinants they may recognize on larger peptides. This problem is now surmountable with the advent of lymphocyte hybridoma technology and the production of monoclonal antibodies to a variety of neural antigens, including peptides (11).

Advances in peptide sequencing technology and in methods of complementary DNA hybridization with messenger RNA followed by nucleotide sequencing have rapidly provided information concerning the biosynthetic precursors of neuropeptides (see Miller, Baxter, and Eberhardt, Chapter 2 in this volume). This information has been used by immunohistochemists, in that investigators have produced antisera to fragments of biosynthetically related molecules (9). Such studies have suggested, for example, that Arg^6-Phe^7-Met-enkephalin and Met-enkephalin immunoreactivity coexist, for the most part, within certain enkephalinergic neurons. Recently, we have produced antisera to the "nonsomatostatin" portion of somatostatin 28 (i.e., the 1–14 component of somatostatin 28; see S. Reichlin, Chapter 29 in this volume). These sera recognize neuronal perikarya, fibers, and terminals with a distribution identical with those revealed with antisomatostatin. Similarly, the two antisera reveal identical populations of pancreatic delta cells (R. Sorenson and R. Elde, unpublished). Together, these findings suggest that the localizations obtained with the original antisera to enkephalins and somatostatin, respectively, are very likely to represent localizations of immunoreactive molecules closely related to the family of molecules that are cleavable from their respective biosynthetic precursors, since the antisera directed against the other fragments coincidentally localize the same cells.

3   PRIMARY ANTIBODY SPECIFICITY

The major issue related to the interpretation of results of immunohistochemical studies of neuropeptides centers on the specificity of the observed staining. The standard procedure used to verify staining specificity is the blocking of antigen binding sites by incubating the antiserum with an excess of the antigen for some time prior to application of the antiserum to the tissue section. Staining obtained with untreated antiserum is deemed to be "specific" (in a limited sense) if the blocked antiserum fails to reveal structures made visible with untreated, normal antiserum. As has been discussed in several instances (2–4, 12–14), these control maneuvers are absolutely essential, yet they do not establish that the staining observed with the untreated, normal antiserum represents molecules with an amino acid sequence identical with the peptide used as an immunogen.

On the one hand, it is prudent not to diminish the importance of the absorption control test. One must continue to apply rigorously such standards to all localizations reported. For example, if the staining observed has nothing to do with the antipeptide activity present in the antiserum but instead represents the binding of antibodies directed against the carrier protein, the results are of limited interest to the scientific community. Thus, one must continue to conduct absorption control experiments.

On the other hand, it must also be emphasized that discrepancies can be found in the immunohistochemical literature that in all probability must be related to differences in the specificity of the primary antisera that are not revealed in blocking studies. For example, some investigators have reported the occurrence of enkephalin immunoreactivity in the hippocampal formation (15, 16), whereas other investigators, using different antisera, have been unable to confirm the abundance of enkephalinergic fibers and cells within this brain region (17–21). Yet, in most other areas of the central and peripheral nervous system, neuronal elements revealed by a variety of enkephalin antisera are virtually identical. In all cases, absorption control studies have suggested that the staining, whether within the hippocampal formation or elsewhere, is specific in the limited sense described above. The disparate findings in the hippocampus outlined above might be explained by a recent biochemical and immunochemical study suggesting that the majority of the opioid peptides found in the hippocampal formation may arise from prodynorphin rather than proenkephalin (22; see also 23). Thus, it is clear that the absorption control test is not adequate to answer ultimate questions of specificity.

The absorption control idea has been modified, in some instances, to a solid-phase immunoaffinity system in order to differentially purify antibodies from an antiserum. Thus, Swaab and Pool (24) and Vandesande and Dierickx (25) removed antioxytocin activity from antivasopressin serum by passing the crude antiserum over an oxytocin–agarose matrix. Other modifications of this approach have also been reported in studies of the posterior pituitary peptides (26, 27). An analogous approach has been used to differentially localize Met- and Leu-enkephalin immunoreactive nerve fibers in the feline gut (28). Thus, antiserum directed principally against Met-enkephalin was "purified" by passing over a Leu-enkephalin agarose matrix and vice versa. The purified antisera were then shown to reveal somewhat separate populations of nerve fibers within the feline gut. These results, although technically convincing, are difficult to interpret in light of the amino acid sequence of the presumed biosynthetic precursor to the enkephalins (see 23), which suggests that copies of both enkephalins should be found within the same cellular elements. On the other hand, it may be that the Leu-enkephalin immunoreactivity reported to exist in the absence of Met-enkephalin may represent peptides of the recently characterized precursor "proenkephalin B" or "prodynorphin" (23). Yet another possibility exists that the cat, whose opioid peptides have not been chemically characterized, produces somewhat different versions of the opioid peptides.

On occasion, some investigators have argued that antisera used for immunohistochemistry should be tested for cross-reactivity under radioimmunoassay conditions. This approach provides very limited information regarding cross-reactivity in the immunohistochemical procedure since peptides in an aldehyde-fixed section of tissue have been altered in structure when compared with peptides extracted from fresh tissue. Aldehyde fixation of tissue also immobilizes peptides so that the antigen–antibody reaction has lost one degree of freedom, thereby altering the kinetics of the reaction compared with radioimmunoassay conditions. Thus, because of the above consideration, it is not clear that cross-reactivity in a radioimmunoassay is linearly related to cross-reactivity in an immunohistochemical procedure. Finally, a radioimmunoassay will only test for cross-reactions with the radiolabeled peptide. For example, suppose a rabbit was immunized with two structurally unrelated peptides, A and B. A radioimmunoassay using labeled peptide A would recognize peptide A and would allow one to determine cross-reactivity for analogs of peptide A, but peptide B would not compete with labeled peptide A for the antigen combining site. In contrast, an immunohistochemical procedure on tissue that contained both peptides would reveal both peptides in a nondifferential manner. Thus, radioimmunoassay procedures are useful for confirming the presence of a peptide in a tissue that is under immunohistochemical investigation (29), but they do not help to establish that all of the immunohistochemical staining observed in that region is due to that particular peptide.

The requirement for immunohistochemical specificity controls is an adequate model of the peptides as they occur immobilized and derivatized in a fixed tissue section. In a very few instances, such model systems are found in tissues themselves. For example, the rat posterior pituitary is known to contain arginine vasopressin and oxytocin, as in most mammals. The pig posterior pituitary, on the other hand, contains lysine vasopressin and oxytocin. If one is concerned about the specificity of an antiserum to arginine vasopressin, one can fix and process pituitaries from the rat and pig and conduct localizations upon those tissues, varying, for example, the concentration of primary antiserum. If the antiserum is specific for arginine vasopressin, one should be able to find a dilution of the antiserum that will allow localization of nerve terminals in the rat posterior pituitary, whereas the same dilution of antiserum should not stain terminals in the pig posterior pituitary (30). If such conditions are met, one can safely conclude that the antiserum *as employed in that particular immunohistochemical procedure* is specific for arginine vasopressin and is unable to recognize lysine vasopressin and oxytocin.

Similarly, genetic models—such as the Brattleboro rat, which does not synthesize arginine vasopressin—provide good systems in which to test the cross-reactivity of vasopressin antisera for oxytocin. Since its posterior pituitary contains no vasopressin but contain a near-normal content of oxytocin, dilutions of antivasopressin serum should be found that stain a normal rat pituitary but do not stain terminals in the Brattleboro pituitary (26, 27).

In some instances it is possible to find tissues that exclusively contain a molecule structurally related to the substance in question, but not that substance itself. For example, the intermediate lobe of the rodent pituitary synthesizes pro-opiomelanocortin and stores and releases β-endorphin. Although the Met-enkephalin sequence is buried within the sequence of these molecules, we have found the Met-enkephalin antisera we employ are unable to stain cells of the intermediate lobe of the pituitary, even though they brilliantly stain enkephalin-immunoreactive neurons and fibers in many brain regions (10). Thus, we cannot suggest that our Met-enkephalin antisera are absolutely specific for Met-enkephalin but rather that they do not cross-react with β-endorphin.

Unfortunately, such tissue models are not available for most of the neuropeptides one wishes to study. Therefore, it is of paramount importance to develop a model system for the investigation of the specificity of staining in immunohistochemical procedures for neuropeptides. The goals of such a model should include independent, multiple, physical-chemical methods to separate all brain peptides from the crudest possible extract, and, using the antiserum in question, to ascertain staining of molecular species on a solid phase, chemically analogous model of fixed tissue. Limited progress has been reported toward this goal (31, 32). Techniques that eventually yield such a model might include two-dimensional electrophoretic separation of peptides followed by transfer of the separated peptides onto a solid-phase support, or alternatively, separation of peptides by high performance liquid chromatography followed by immobilization on a solid-phase support. After immobilization, the antiserum should be used to immunochemically localize those peptides it recognizes, and the pattern of the stained peptides from the extracts should be compared with synthetic peptides as references. Such an approach will greatly expand our ability to discuss the specificity or lack of specificity for the peptide per se.

4 TISSUE PROCESSING

As we have previously discussed (2), problems of tissue fixation and processing techniques present serious constraints to immunohistochemical staining of neuropeptides. These problems are not too apparent in studies at the light microscopic level of resolution, but they are serious barriers to high-resolution localizations of neuropeptides at the electron microscopic level of analysis. This dilemma is largely attributable to the necessity for a trade-off between procedures for fixation and embedding that are robust enough to maintain the peptide *in situ* and preserve ultrastructural morphology and procedures that are yet gentle enough not to compromise the antigenicity of the neuropeptide. These limitations have for the most part prevented the application of the full power of electron microscopy to questions of the details of the localization of neuropeptides. Questions that have remained largely unanswered because of this include; Which subcellular organelles are responsible for storage and release of peptides from nerve terminals?, and What are the putative synaptic interactions among peptidergic neurons in discrete areas of neuropil? The technical problems have forced a compromise approach for most investigators, the so-called "pre-embedding" staining method, wherein the immunostaining procedure is conducted in a manner essentially identical to the procedure for light microscopy, after which the tissue is dehydrated, embedded in an epoxy resin, and sectioned on an ultramicrotome for viewing in the electron microscope. As previously discussed (2), results from these studies have provided a general understanding of ultrastructural features of peptidergic neurons, but diffusion of the antigen or the diaminobenzidine reaction product, or both, prevent conclusions to be formed concerning the storage and release compartments for peptides. Moreover, because these localizations are conducted on a tissue section several microns thick, it is extremely difficult or impossible to determine synaptic interactions among peptidergic neurons, which are directly discernible only by immunostaining of adjacent ultrathin sections.

Progress toward overcoming these limitations of ultrastructural immunocytochemistry has been made by the rapid, ultra-low temperature freezing and freeze-drying method of Coulter and colleagues (33). In this method, fresh brain is rapidly frozen by controlled contact with a liquid helium-chilled sapphire. After controlled sublimation of frozen water, the tissue is fixed by exposure to osmium tetroxide vapor and embedded in epoxy resin without exposure to water or to water and ethanol solutions. The latter have been shown to extract peptide immunoreactivity from tissue whether in a fresh or fixed state (34). Coulter has shown the utility of his approach for questions of coexistence of neuropeptides and interaction of peptidergic neurons by localizations of neuropeptides within adjacent ultrathin sections of posterior pituitary and, more recently, substantia gelatinosa of the spinal cord (35).

Although in its present state of development this work is not readily adaptable to the general neuropeptide laboratory, it holds good promise for future investigations. The success of the pre-embedding staining method has led investigators to improve fixation methods that continue to make this approach useful. Thus, several fixation methods (36–38) have been developed that significantly enhance the retention of peptides *in situ* during the pre-embedding immunohistochemical procedure, and these methods deserve further attention.

5   DETECTION SYSTEMS

The immunohistochemist now has a variety of ways to detect the binding of primary antibodies to neuropeptides in tissue sections (3, 4). Chronologically, the techniques that have proved most widely useful in immunohistochemical investigations of neuropeptides have been the indirect immunofluorescence method of Coons (1), the enzyme (peroxidase) labeled method of Nakane and Pierce (39), the four-step bridge method of Mason and colleagues (40), the peroxidase-antiperoxidase method of Sternberger and colleagues (41), the radiolabeled and gold-labeled antigen methods of Larsson and Schwartz (42, 43), and the avidin-biotin-peroxidase method of Hsu and colleagues (44). These methods are, for the most part, applicable at both the light and electron microscopic levels and are designed to amplify the localization through enzymatic or immunochemical means. A characteristic of each newly introduced modification of the techniques is the claim that it is more sensitive than previously described methods. Although these claims have usually been documented in the report characterizing the new system, few claims have stood up in more widespread, independent applications. This is said not to minimize the important contributions of the variety of immunohistochemical detection systems but to underscore the controversy that has developed among devotees of each of the several systems. Final analysis may well demonstrate insignificant differences in efficiency of these detection systems, and thus in the interim, the investigator might be wise to optimize conditions for reliable localizations with one of the methods, rather than half-heartedly test all options.

ACKNOWLEDGMENTS

I am grateful for assistance in manuscript preparation from Jeri Lu Mattson and for helpful discussion with immunohistochemically oriented colleagues in the Department of Anatomy, University of Minnesota. Studies in the author's laboratory were supported by USPHS grant DA02148.

REFERENCES

1. A. H. Coons, in J. F. Danielli, Ed., *General Cytochemical Methods*, Academic Press, New York, 1958.
2. R. Elde, H. D. Coulter, and V. Seybold, in J. L. Barker and T. G. Smith, Ed., *The Role of Peptides in Neuronal Function*, Marcel Dekker, New York, 1980, p. 1.
3. L. A. Sternberger, *Immunocytochemistry*, John Wiley, New York, 1979.
4. F. Vandesande, *J. Neurosci. Meth.* **1**, 3 (1979).
5. W. R. Skowsky and D. A. Fisher, *J. Lab. Clin. Med.* **80**, 134 (1972).
6. R. Benoit, N. Ling, S. Lavielle, P. Brazeau, and R. Guillemin, *Fed. Proc.* **39**, 488 (1980).
7. S. Cummings, R. Elde, J. Ells, and A. Lindall, *J. Neurosci.*, In press (1983).
8. B. J. Wilcox and V. S. Seybold, *Neurosci. Lett.* **29**, 105 (1982).
9. R. G. Williams and G. J. Dockray, *Brain Res.* **240**, 167 (1982).
10. P. Micevych and R. Elde, *J. Comp. Neurol.* **190**, 135 (1980).
11. A. C. Cuello, G. Galfre, and C. Milstein, *Proc. Natl. Acad. Sci. USA* **76**, 3532 (1979).
12. P. Petrusz, M. Sar, P. Ordronneau, and P. DiMeo, *J. Histochem. Cytochem.* **24**, 1110 (1976).
13. D. F. Swaab, C. W. Pool, and F. W. VanLeeuwen, *J. Histochem. Cytochem.* **25**, 388 (1977).
14. J. Rossier, *Neuroscience* **6**, 989 (1981).
15. C. Gall, N. Brecha, H. J. Karten, and K. -J. Chang, *J. Comp. Neurol.* **198**, 335 (1981).
16. M. Sar, W. E. Stumpf, R. J. Miller, K. -J. Chang, and P. Cuatrecasas, *J. Comp. Neurol.* **182**, 17 (1978).
17. R. P. Elde, T. Hökfelt, O. Johansson, and L. Terenius, *Neuroscience* **1**, 349 (1976).
18. S. Haber and R. Elde, *Neuroscience* **7**, 1049 (1982).
19. R. Simantov, M. J. Kuhar, G. R. Uhl, and S. H. Snyder, *Proc. Natl. Acad. Sci. USA* **74**, 2167 (1977).
20. J. K. Wamsley, W. S. Young, and M. J. Kuhar, *Brain Res.* **190**, 153 (1980).
21. S. J. Watson, H. Akil, S. Sullivan, and J. D. Barchas, *Life Sci.* **21**, 733 (1977).
22. C. Chavkin, J. McGinty, W. S. Shoemaker, and F. E. D. Bloom, *Soc. Neurosci. Abstr.* **8**, 479 (1982).
23. J. Rossier, *Nature* **298**, 221 (1982).
24. D. F. Swabb and C. W. Pool, *J. Endocrinol.* **66**, 263 (1975).
25. F. Vandesande and K. Dierickx, *Cell Tissue Res.* **164**, 153 (1975).
26. R. M. Buijs, D. F. Swaab, J. Dogterom, and F. W. van Leeuwen, *Cell. Tissue Res.* **186**, 423 (1978).
27. F. W. van Leeuwen and D. F. Swabb, *Cell Tissue Res.* **177**, 493 (1977).
28. L. -I. Larsson and K. Stengaard-Pedersen, *J. Neurosci.* **2**, 861 (1982).
29. N. Aronin, M. DiFiglia, A. S. Liotta, and J. B. Martin, *J. Neurosci.* **1**, 561 (1981).
30. R. Elde, Ph.D. Dissertation, University of Minnesota (1974).
31. L. -I. Larsson, *J. Histochem. Cytochem.* **29**, 408 (1981).

32. W. van Raamsdonk, C. W. Pool, and C. Heyting, *J. Immunol. Meth.* **17**, 337 (1977).
33. H. D. Coulter, R. P. Elde, and S. L. Unverzagt, *Peptides* **2**, Suppl. 1, 51 (1981).
34. H. D. Coulter and R. P. Elde, *J. Histochem. Cytochem.* **27**, 1293 (1979).
35. H. D. Coulter, *Soc. Neurosci. Abstr.* **8**, 808 (1982).
36. A. Berod, B. K. Hartman, and J. F. Pujol, *J. Histochem. Cytochem.* **29**, 844 (1981).
37. R. Murphy, A. M. Beardsley, J. B. Furness, M. Costa, and J. R. Oliver, *Regul. Peptides* **4**, 67 (1982).
38. P. Somogyi and H. Takogi, *Neuroscience* **7**, 1779 (1982).
39. P. K. Nakane and G. B. Pierce Jr., *J. Histochem. Cytochem.* **14**, 929 (1967).
40. T. E. Mason, R. F. Phifer, S. S. Spicer, R. A. Swallow, and R. B. Dreskin, *J. Histochem. Cytochem.* **17**, 563 (1969).
41. L. A. Sternberger, P. H. Hardy Jr., J. J. Cuculis, and H. G. Meyer, *J. Histochem. Cytochem.* **18**, 315 (1970).
42. L. -I. Larsson and T. W. Schwartz, *J. Histochem. Cytochem.* **25**, 1140 (1977).
43. L. -I. Larsson, *Nature* **282**, 743 (1979).
44. S. M. Hsu, L. Raine, and H. Fanger, *J. Histochem. Cytochem.* **29**, 577 (1981).

22

Neuroanatomical Techniques

MIKLÓS PALKOVITS

Laboratory of Cell Biology
National Institute of Mental Health
Bethesda, Maryland

1 INTRODUCTION

This chapter presents a view of neuroanatomical techniques relevant for studies of neuropeptides in the central nervous system. A number of techniques are available in the neuroanatomical arsenal, but only immunohistochemistry has the ability to visualize neuropeptides—or, more correctly, neuropeptide-like substances—in the brain. Section 2 is intended to summarize not the technical points but the usefulness of immunohistochemical techniques in combination with other neuroanatomical methods. A short guide is presented to indicate how neuropeptide-containing cells, pathways, and nerve terminals can be visualized, localized, and quantitated at the light and electron microscopic level.

Neuroanatomical techniques in neuropeptide research are not restricted only to immunohistochemistry, many of them are successfully applied to other neurobiological disciplines. These techniques are briefly discussed in Section 3.

Section 4 presents an overview of neuroanatomical techniques that may be applied directly or indirectly to neuropeptide research. Principles, probable applications, advantages, and disadvantages—but not technical details of the techniques—are summarized.*

Neuropeptide research is a typical interdisciplinary study; knowledge of the technical neuroanatomical repertoire is a requirement not only for morphologists but for neuroscientists. The goal of this chapter is to indicate the most appropriate neuroanatomical methods and combinations of methods for studying neuropeptides in the central nervous system.

2 NEUROANATOMICAL DEMONSTRATION OF NEUROPEPTIDE-CONTAINING NEURONS

At the present time, immunohistochemistry is the only technique available by which neuropeptides (neuropeptide-like immunoreactive substances) can be visualized in nerve cells. Methods have been developed that are sensitive enough to demonstrate peptides in each portion of the neuron (perikaryon, dendrites, nerve terminals) by light microscopy or in subcellular organelles by electron microscopy. The demonstration of neuropeptides in a given neuron, although highly important, is not the only possible morphological information that can be derived concerning a neuropeptide-containing cell. There are a wide range of neuroanatomical techniques that in combination with immunohistochemistry, provide further knowledge concerning the source, transport, and the destination of neuronal neuropeptides. Such combinations of techniques are summarized in the following pages.

*Valuable handbooks are available for methodical descriptions (1–3).

2.1 Cell Bodies

2.1.1 Visualization by Immunohistochemistry

Neuropeptides are synthetized in the perikarya. They are rapidly transported to the nerve terminals where they are stored until release. Therefore, in order to visualize peptides in cell bodies by immunohistochemistry, axonal transport should be blocked. Blocking agents that disrupt the microtubules are used for this purpose: colchicine, vinblastine, vincristine, podophyllotoxin, griseofulvin, maytansine, nocodasole. Colchicine is the most commonly used blocker: rats should be pretreated with colchicine (50 μg/100 g in 10 μL) intraventricularly. Surgical transection of nerve fibers also results in an accumulation of neuropeptides in the parent cells; such cells can be visualized 2–3 days after surgery.

2.1.2 Determination of the Number of Neuropeptide-Containing Cells

None of the immunohistochemical methods available completely satisfy the requirements of quantitative histology. The fixation, embedding, sectioning, staining procedures, the antibody method employed, the specificity of the antibody used (see Section 4.5.), and the method of microscopic visualization all influence the recognition of immunostained cells or of staining inside cell bodies. The combination of these factors may result in an observed relatively large variation of immunostained cell numbers. Therefore, absolute numbers of cells in certain brain areas or in the brain in toto, may refer only to a given brain examined, and the variation may reach $\pm$ 100% of this value. It is more practical if the relative number of neuropeptide-containing cells are calculated (see Section 4.7). In that case, cell numbers can be expressed as cells/section (this is the less accurate approach), or as cell/anatomical nucleus ratios. It is more informative if the ratio is calculated not as the number of cells but as the percentage of the total cell number in a particular nucleus. The most valuable parameter is the cell density (neuropeptide-containing cell/mm^2 or mm^3). The advantages of the calculation of cell density are that the results are comparable because the variation factors are minimized, the absolute cell number and other ratios can be calculated, data can be used in comparison with electron microscopic measurements (cell/synapse ratio, see Section 4.7.3), and the data allow quantitative evaluation in experimental conditions.

2.1.3 Cytological Parameters of Neuropeptide-Containing Neurons

Certain cell types can easily be recognized under the microscope (motoneurons, Purkinje cells, pyramidal cells); others should be characterized by their size, shape, or dendritic arborization. Routine immunohistochemistry, even in colchicine-pretreated animals, does not provide Golgi-like staining of cell bodies. For complete visualization of the whole perikaryon and dendrites, immunohistochemical staining can be intensified by metallic ions (see Section 4.5.1) or combined with Golgi or single cell staining techniques (see Section 4.1). The most commonly measured parameters are: diameters of the cells; eccentricity (elongation) of the cell (long axis/short axis ratio); shape (uni-, bi- or multipolar); type of dendritic arborization; orientation of cell body or dendrites in space in comparison with the three major planes or brain surface or ventricles. For technical details, see Section 4.7.

2.1.4 Topographical Localization of Neuropeptide-Containing Neurons

Three-dimensional topographical localization of neuropeptide-containing cells can be performed on serial sections of 10–15 μm thickness, by the "scanning technique" (see Section 4.7.4). The rostrocaudal planes and coordinates should be controlled during sectioning; the vertical (the top and the base of the brain sections) and mediolateral (midline = 0) coordinates can be determined under the microscope. The localization of the cells can be expressed either in the three-dimensional coordinates or by their topographical relation to major anatomical landmarks (ventricles, bundles) or their topography inside the nucleus. The scanning technique and the three-dimensional reconstruction can be performed manually or by semiautomatic or automatic (computer-controlled) devices (see Section 4.7.4).

Neurons that have been identified immunohistochemically may be filled up by intracellular staining techniques (see Section 4.1.1). In simultaneous or subsequent studies, cells and dendrites can be recognized, measured, and three-dimensionally reconstructed by a computer-microscope system (see Section 4.7.4). The territory occupied by dendrites of a single, neuropeptide-containing neuron can be calculated. These data are used for the calculation of synapse/cell ratio (number of axo-dendritic synapses/cell) or for demonstration of colocalization of different nerve terminals in a neuronal territory (see Section 4.7).

2.1.5 Coexistence of Neuropeptides in the Same Neuron

Most of the cell populations in the brain are heterogenous. An anatomically well-localized nucleus may contain more than one (sometimes more than 10) neuropeptide-containing neurons (4). In many cases, the total cells exhibiting different immunostaining is far higher then the total cell number of the nucleus, indicating that two or more neuropeptides may be located in the same cells. Increasing numbers of studies demonstrate transmitter amino acids plus biogenic amines, or different biogenic amines, or biogenic amines plus neuropeptides, or different neuropeptides in the same neurons (5). Such variations are not detailed here, but the techniques that allow investigation of this phenomenon are described. The coexistence of different neurotransmitter substances in the same neuron may be demonstrated by (i) Simultaneous staining on consecutive ("adjacent") thin (1–2 μm) or ultrathin serial sections: Ultrathin serial sections can be immunostained for electron microscopy by any of the postembedding staining methods (see Section 4.6.2). (ii) Sequential staining: after the first immunostaining (and photography of the staining pattern), the antiserum is eluted and the section is restained by the second antiserum (6). Both immunofluorescence and unlabeled enzyme antibody technique can be used. In the latter case the same enzyme but different substrates are applied, and the substrates appear in different colors in the section (see 4.5.2.). (iii) Simultaneous immunostaining of the same section based on the combination of two immunohistochemical methods, wherein different enzymes and substrates do not interfere with each other (see Section 4.5.2). For electron microscopy, the protein A–colloidal gold method seems to be most appropriate: different antigens may be recognized by labeling gold particles of different size (see Section 4.6.3).

2.2 Pathways

Only fragmented portions of neuropeptide-containing pathways may be recognized by immunohistochemistry. On serial sections, large bundles may be reconstructed by a mosaic-manner, but their arborization, collaterals, and fine destinations may be followed by a combination of techniques.

2.2.1 Biochemical Localization

This technique is indirect. The pathway will not be visualized under the microscope, but its existence can be proved by surgical lesioning followed by biochemical (radioimmunoassay) measurements of neuropeptides in microdissected brain areas (see Sections 4.8 and 4.9). Two experimental situations should be distinguished: (i) neuropeptide levels may be determined on brain regions that do not have cell bodies containing the neuropeptide that is to be measured; (ii) neuropeptide levels are determined on regions containing such cell bodies. In the first case, neuropeptide levels may be depleted secondarily to lesioning of cells or pathways followed by the degeneration of nerve terminals present in the area investigated. In the second case, neuropeptide levels may be depleted secondarily to the lack of necessary neuronal input to the neuropeptide-synthetizing cells. The two possibilities may occur together.

The biochemical localization of a neuropeptide-containing pathway is a sensitive technique. Its specificity depends on the specificity of the assay and the lesioning technique used (see Section 4.8.1). Small increases or decreases in neuropeptide concentrations in brain regions that are not visible or that are subjectively nondetectable under the microscope can be measured biochemically. In subsequent studies, multiple projections of certain pathways or the convergence of different pathways in a given brain area can be elucidated. The disadvantage of the technique is its indirect character. In combination with immunohistochemistry, or with immunohistochemistry plus nerve degeneration (see Section 4.5.3), this technique is a powerful tool in neuropeptide studies.

2.2.2   Immunohistochemical Localization

Neuropeptides are transported by fast axoplasmic flow from the cells to the nerve terminals, therefore the axon may contain only a small amount of peptide en route. Pathways, therefore, are not always immunostained or are not detectable on microscopic examination. By transecting fibers, accumulation in the proximal segment (connected with the cell body) and a total disappearance from the peripheral segment (disconnected from the cell) can be seen 2–7 days after the lesion.

2.3   Nerve Terminals

Neuropeptides in nerve terminals can be demonstrated by light and electron microscopic immunohistochemistry. By light microscopy, the innervation field of a certain cell group or pathway can be visualized. Demonstration of neuropeptides in nerve terminals (presynaptic boutons) requires an electron microscope (see Section 2.3.2).

2.3.1   Light Microscopic Localization

By the use of light microscopic immunohistochemistry, the following studies may be performed: (i) The area to which a particular cell group or pathway projects (see Section 4.7.4) can be localized. (ii) Neuropeptide-containing terminal fields for further electron microscopic studies can be visualized. (iii) Multiple innervation of a brain region by two or more neuropeptides can be demonstrated by an overlap of their terminal fields. (iv) In combination with lesioning of cell groups or pathways (see Section 4.8), the projections of these cells or pathways can be demonstrated by the disappearance of immunostaining from their projection fields; the rate of disappearance can be measured by radioimmunoassays in the same experiment or in a parallel experiment (one side of the brain can be used for biochemical studies, the other side for immunohistochemistry—if the existence of decussating fibers can be excluded in a preliminary study). (v) In combination with tract-tracing techniques (see Section 4.5.3), the innervation pattern of a particular neuropeptide containing neuron can be localized anatomically (see Section 2.3.3).

2.3.2 Electron Microscopic Demonstration of Neuropeptides.

Pre-embedding immunostaining allows the demonstration of one neuropeptide. With postembedding techniques, more than one neuropeptide can be demonstrated in the same section (see Section 4.6). By multiple staining, either nerve terminals stained with different antisera may be localized in synaptic contact with unstained cells or both presynaptic and postsynaptic elements can be immunostained simultaneously. By combining electron microscopic immunocytochemistry with other neuroanatomical techniques, not only the nerve terminals but their parent cells can be characterized (see Section 2.3.4).

Quantitative estimation of neuropeptide-containing nerve terminals is also possible but it is not a routine procedure at the present time. The number of immunostained boutons can be expressed by their surface or volume density ($n/1000$ μm^2 or μm^3). Since complete serial sections of neurons with dendritic trees are technically almost impossible, for counting of immunostained boutons a large number (200–300) of randomly taken electron micrographs are required (see Section 4.7.3). The ratio of the volume density of synaptic boutons and the cell density (taken from light microscopy) expresses the average synapse/cell ratio, that is, how many immunostained boutons may belong to one cell in a particular brain area.

2.3.3 Innervation Pattern of Neuropeptide-Containing Neurons (Neuronal Efferents)

The axonal projection of neuropeptide-containing cells can be studied by simultaneous application of tract-tracing techniques and immunohistochemistry or by using them in parallel experiments (see Section 4.5.3). To demonstrate the neuropeptide-containing cell and its projection field in the same animal, a combination of two techniques is needed:

1. Retrograde tracers (horseradish peroxidase or fluorescent dyes, see Sections 4.4.1 and 4.4.2) are injected into the presumed projection field of a cell or cell groups. The tracer substance is transported back and accumulated in the cell body, which may be characterized by immunostaining. Fluorescent dyes may be combined with immunofluorescence and horseradish peroxidase with unlabeled enzyme antibody methods (see Section 4.5.3). Retrograde autoradiography may also be combined with immunohistochemistry (see Section 4.5.3).

2. Anterograde tracing techniques may be used in combination with immunohistochemistry. Intracellular injection of dyes or horseradish peroxidase (see Section 4.1.2) or cellular uptake of labeled amino acids (see Section 4.3.2) makes it possible to visualize axons and projection fields in immunostained sections (see Section 4.5.3).

By combinations of three techniques, cell bodies, projecting fields, and afferents to the cell may be visualized in the same section (see Section 4.5.3). The possible triple combinations are: (i) double immunostaining and retrograde tracing (the cell body is immunostained by the first antiserum, the projection field is localized by retrograde tracing, the afferents are stained by the second antiserum); (ii) immunostaining, retrograde tracing, and nerve degeneration (the cell body is immunostained, the projection field is localized by retrograde tracing, the afferents are visualized by degenerating nerve terminals); (iii) immunostaining, retrograde tracing, and autoradiography (the cell body is immunostained, the projection field is localized by retrograde tracing, the afferents are labeled by anterograde autoradiography).

Since a single cell may project to more than one brain area and receives afferents from many cells, the triple combinations may not visualize the whole neuronal network but only a part of it. Further combinations employing multiple immunostaining plus multiple retrograde and anterograde tracing are also possible, but this is theoretical and not experimental practice today.

2.3.4 Nerve Terminals on Neuropeptide-Containing Neurons (Neuronal Afferents)

The demonstration of nerve terminals synapsing with perikarya or dendrites is the subject of electron microscopy. Therefore, combined characterization of neuronal afferents and target cells is possible by using either multiple immunocytochemistry (see Section 4.6.3) or immunocytochemistry in combination with other electron microscopic neuroanatomical techniques (see Section 4.6.4). The technically possible combinations are:

1. Immunocytochemistry plus nerve degeneration technique (see Section 4.6.4): the immunostained postsynaptic elements can be demonstrated in synaptic contact with degenerating presynaptic boutons.

2. Immunocytochemistry plus anterograde autoradiography (see Section 4.6.4): in this combination, the cells are immunostained and the afferents are labeled.

3. Immunocytochemistry plus anterograde horseradish peroxidase tracing (see Section 4.4.1): the cells are immunostained and the afferents contain HRP.

Afferents to a particular neuropeptide-containing cell or cell group can also be quantitated. By the calculation of synapse/cell ratio (see Section 4.7.3), the total number of nerve terminals synapsing with the perikarya or dendrites can be estimated. After selective lesioning of brain areas or pathways that presumably project to the cells investigated, or by labeling various brain areas, in subsequent studies the participation of labeled or lesioned areas in the innervation of immunostained cells can be expressed by their fraction of the total synapse/cell ratio (see Section 4.7.3).

3 APPLICATION OF NEUROANATOMY IN NONANATOMICAL NEUROPEPTIDE STUDIES

Immunohistochemistry is the most direct neuroanatomical technique for investigating brain neuropeptides. Several other neuroanatomical techniques are indirectly used in neuropeptide studies. These techniques may be applied as complementary studies or used as tools for nonanatomical techniques.

3.1 Post-Experimental Histological Validating Studies of the Brain

Before the immunohistochemical era, the contribution of neuroanatomy to neuropeptide studies was almost limited to the neurohistological or histochemical demonstration of neurons and their alterations in experimental or pathological conditions. Although a number of sensitive and specific methods have been developed and applied for neuropeptide studies, neurohistology and neuropathology remain important methods in the neuroanatomical repertoire.

3.1.1 Demonstration of Cytological Alterations

Cellular or subcellular changes in neurons; accumulation or disappearance of substances from the cells or nerve terminals during experimental or pathological conditions; degeneration of cells, cell groups or pathways due to drugs, lesions or diseases—all these are the subject of neurohistology. Hundreds of useful staining recipes have been accumulated that enable visualization of the above alterations. (Refer to histological handbooks for methods 7–9.)

The histological study may include investigating subcellular changes in the neurons by means of electron microscopy. The basic technical procedures for electron microscopic studies on the nervous system are summarized by Friedrich and Mugnaini (10) and Johnson (11). The electron microscopy of the central nervous system has been superbly demonstrated by Peters et al. (12).

3.1.2   Topographical Validating Studies After Brain Surgery

All chemical or surgical interventions on the brain should be studied histologically. Brain lesions (see Section 4.8.1), knife cuts, transection of pathways (see Section 4.8.2), injections, implantations, into the brain, microcannulations or recording (see Section 4.8.3) should be precisely localized. Therefore, serial sections from the target regions are needed. For topographical evaluation and the reproducibility of the experiment, the surgical intervention and its consequences (lesion, hemorrhage, ischemia) may be mapped on a stereotaxic atlas (see Section 4.8) or characterized by three-dimensional coordinates.

3.2   Stereotaxic Manipulations in the Brain

There are three major types of stereotaxic maneuvers: (i) lesioning of brain nuclei or pathways, (ii) intracerebral (or intracerebroventricular) application of substances, (iii) electrophysiological manipulations.

1. In neuropeptide studies, brain lesions or transections are employed for: (i) biochemical measurements demonstrating changes in neuropeptide levels in various brain regions following lesioning of other cell groups or transection of the neuronal afferents; (ii) immunohistochemical visualization of neuropeptide-containing pathways and projection fields by the demonstration of disappearance of neuropeptide from fibers and terminals, and its accumulation in cells proximal to the lesion; (iii) demonstration of degenerating nerve terminals on immunocytochemically characterized neurons; (iv) demonstration of neurophysiological and behavioral changes due to the lack of neuropeptides in certain brain regions, which may then be influenced by exogenous neuropeptide application; (v) demonstration of lack of known neurophysiological, neuroendocrine and neuropharmacological effects of exogenous neuropeptides secondary to the elimination of target neurons by lesioning; (vi) demonstration of neurohormonal effects of neuropeptides by alterations in the neuroendocrine axis following hypothalamic lesions, median eminence or pituitary stalk transections; (vii) demonstration of the neurotransmitter character of neuropeptides by recording electrophysiological parameters in neuroanatomical systems in animals with and without brain lesions. The technical details of brain lesioning and fiber-transections are summarized in Sections 4.8.1 and 4.8.2.

2. Intracerebral injections or implantations may be used in neuro-peptide studies for the following purposes: (i) to study the effect of drugs, exogenous neuropeptides or precursors on neuronal synthesis of neuropeptides; (ii) to alter the axonal transport of neuropeptides (block-ing axonal flow to visualize cell bodies; see Section 2.1); (iii) to demon-strate the axonal transport of neuropeptides by tract-tracing substances (see Section 4.4); (iv) to effect neuropeptide release from nerve termi-nals; (v) to demonstrate neuropeptides in nerve terminals by blocking their release (demonstration of accumulation) or by accelerating their release (demonstration of disappearance); (vi) to demonstrate axonal collaterals of neuropeptidergic neurons by injecting tract-tracing sub-stances into the brain and localizing them in combination with immuno-histochemistry (see Sections 4.5.3 and 4.6.3); (vii) to demonstrate axonal projection fields (efferents) of neuropeptide-containing neurons by intraneuronal injection or cellular uptake from local injection of antero-grade tracing substances in combination with immunohistochemistry (see Section 4.6.3); (viii) to demonstrate neurophysiological, neurophar-macological and neuroendocrine effects of exogenous neuropeptides by injections or implantation into neurons or neuronal cellgroups; (ix) to restore neuropeptide-related functions in brain-lesioned animals by ex-ogenous neuropeptide injections. Techniques and instruments used for microinjections and implantations are detailed in Section 4.8.3.

3. Electrophysiological studies can be utilized to: (i) demonstrate the neurotransmitter character of neuropeptides in neurons of certain brain areas; (ii) demonstrate the neurotransmitter nature of exogenous neuropeptides following intracellular injection; (iii) electrophysiological-ly map neuropeptidergic neuronal projections; (iv) localize antidromi-cally neuropeptide-containing cell bodies by excitation of their terminal fields. Neuropeptide release induced by single cell or field excitation *in vivo* or *in vitro* can be measured by radioimmunoassay or demonstrat-ed by immunocytochemistry. By the use of chronically implanted elec-trodes, a variety of neurobiological studies can be performed by electrical stimulation of certain brain areas in conscious animals. The combination of intracellular electrodes with micropipette, microinjection (and subsequent light and/or electron microscopic evaluation) and elec-trophysiological recording can provide functional characterization (and localization) of a single neuron in the brain (see Section 4.8.3).

3.3 Dissection of the Brain

Not only large brain regions but also small nuclei can be dissected. Technically, fresh, frozen, or fixed brains can all be used for microdis-section, but further studies depend on the treatment employed. Dissec-tion of cell groups from fixed brain serves for better orientation in electron microscopic techniques for recognition of small cell groups. Fresh brain samples are needed for *in vitro* and bioassay studies (see Section 3.3.2), and frozen brain sections are routinely used for neuropeptide biochemistry (see Section 3.3.1).

3.3.1 Dissection for Biochemical Studies

Large regions can be separated in fresh brain or dissected out from brain sections. When more than 2 mg tissue weight is dissected the procedure is called macrodissection and can be performed without a dissecting microscope. Dissection of smaller regions, or individual brain nuclei, requires a dissecting microscope (microdissection).

Either fresh or frozen sections can be used for neuropeptide biochemistry. Brains are cut by free hand, or with a tissue chopper, but fine serial sections can be cut only with a cryostat (see Section 4.9). Microdissection of rat brains is performed from 300 μm thick coronal sections with fine knives or micropunch needles (see Section 4.9). As small an area as 10 μm of brain tissue can be removed with a needle of 0.2 mm inside diameter. In rat brain, more than 220 nuclei can be recognized under a dissecting microscope and removed individually by micropunch.

The microdissected tissue may be homogenized and centrifuged, and the supernatant used for radioimmunoassay. Protein should be measured in 5–20 μL of the homogenates and neuropeptide concentrations expressed in ng/ mg protein.

Microdissection of brain nuclei is used in neuropeptide biochemistry for:

1. determining and mapping neuropeptide concentrations in the brain
2. measuring neuropeptide levels in animals with congenital, acquired or experimentally induced pathological conditions
3. measuring neuropeptide levels following various treatments and experimental conditions
4. measuring neuropeptide levels in neuronal pathway studies following brain lesions or transections of fibers (see Section 2.2.1)
5. measuring the concentrations of endogenous non-neuropeptide substances (enzymes, neurotransmitters) which may be related to brain neuropeptides (influence of exogenous neuropeptides on these substances)
6. receptor studies
7. measuring the synthesis of neuropeptides following precursor injections into the brain

8. biochemical analysis of neuropeptides and related substances (precursors, metabolic products, etc.) from brain areas where they are synthetized or stored

3.3.2   Dissection for In Vitro Studies

Living brain tissue is required for *in vitro* studies, therefore dissection is performed on fresh brains. Regions can be macrodissected from whole brain or brain sections. Brains are cut by free hand and nuclei are microdissected immediately (see Section 4.9). Fresh microdissected brain tissue can be used for many purposes.

Neuropeptides in Tissue Cultures. Diverse strategies are commonly used to culture nerve cells. They include organ cultures (whole brain areas or fragments), explants, monolayers, dissociated cells, reaggregates, and continuous cell lines. Fetal cells in tissue culture, being capable of cellular growth and morphological differentiation, provide an excellent system. If they are peptidergic neurons, they can synthesize and release peptides during culture. In general practice, large brain regions—mainly hypothalamus—or their fragments are dissected. The great advantage of the microdissection technique is that anatomically identified cell groups (i.e., nuclei) can be removed and cultured (13). Dispersed cell cultures are used for days. Fetal cells can be maintained in suspension or organ cultures for a considerable period of time; they preserve their identity and neuropeptide-synthesizing capacity for 2–6 weeks.

The tissue culturing technique may be applied to *in vitro* developmental studies using light and electron microscopic immunohistochemistry, electrophysiological studies on neuropeptide-containing cells, and in measuring the neuropeptide content, biosynthesis, and release from cultured cells, nuclei, larger brain fragments, or slices of regions.

Subcellular Distribution of Neuropeptides. Synaptosomes can be obtained by homogenization and differential sucrose sedimentation of brain nuclei. This subcellular compartment contains various brain-borne substances including neuropeptides. Their concentration and release from synaptosomes can be detected by radioimmunoassay.

In Vitro Neuropeptide Measurements. Biosynthesis of neuropeptides can be measured by *in vitro* systems. Brain fragments, slices, microdissected nuclei, or dispersed neurons are incubated with labeled amino acids (^{14}C-glutamic acid) and their incorporation into the *de novo* peptide can be detected by radioimmunoassay or autoradiography. Release of neuropeptides from incubated neurons or nuclei elicited by electrical or chemical stimulations can also be measured by radioimmunoassay.

4 NEUROANATOMICAL TECHNIQUES FOR DIRECT OR INDIRECT APPLICATIONS IN NEUROPEPTIDE STUDIES

This section contains brief summaries of neuroanatomical techniques that may be applied directly or in combination with others for peptide studies in the central nervous system. Each of these techniques constitutes an individual research field with its own literature, and many of them require the full time involvement not only of individuals but of entire research laboratories. The main purpose of this section is to provide the researcher who is not a neuroanatomist with a guide to the main principles, usefulness, and advantages of the modern neuroanatomical techniques that are suitable for neuropeptide studies. None of the techniques are described in detail, but the references provided, including chapters and review papers in recent books, should provide relevant information.

4.1 Neurohistological Staining

A great number of histological and histochemical stainings are available to visualize neuronal elements in the central nervous system. Descriptions of these procedures can be found in handbooks of histological techniques, such as Romeis (7), Gabe (8) or Bancroft and Stevens (9).

For general use to demonstrate simultaneously nerve fibers and cell bodies with distinctive colors, the Luxol Fast Blue–Cresyl Violet staining (14) is recommended. The staining is excellent for mapping cell groups, and controlling surgical interventions. Cresyl Violet staining alone is simpler, is also useful for mapping, but only for cell groups not fibers. It is widely used as a counterstain. To visualize neuronal pathways, including fine nerve fibers, silver and cupric impregnation techniques are available (7–9).

Light microscopic quantitative studies, semiautomatic or automatic evaluation of the histological picture, especially cell counting techniques, require sharp and constant color or density differences between cells (cell nuclei) and the background. The simplest and most reproducible staining for this purpose is still the classic hematoxylin staining or its variations (chrome-hematoxylin).

Most of the tract-tracing techniques and also immunohistochemistry requires counter-staining. Such counterstaining should be as simple as possible and without any influence on the specific procedure. Cresyl Violet, thionine, safranin, toluidine blue, neutral red, and light green are the most commonly used counterstains. Acridine Orange, Ethidium Bromide, Bisbenzimide, Nuclear Yellow, Neutral Red, Astrazone Red, and Safranin-O are used as fluorescent counterstains (15). For semithin sections of brains cut from blocks embedded for electron microscopy, Methylene Blue staining is widely used for orientation and recognition and localization of labeled cells or fibers.

Brain lesions or transections can be localized by one of the above mentioned stains. Small lesions, less than 100 μm in diameter, are difficult to find in sections; Cajal's gold chloride sublimate staining is recommended for this purpose (16).

4.1.1 Golgi Impregnation

The special advantage of the Golgi impregnation technique is that it displays individual nerve cells with their dendrites and axons. It is the most spectacular procedure for revealing the shape of neurons and understanding the geometry and organization of local neuronal patterns. The technique is widely used for classifying the various types of neurons at the light microscopic level. Since only a few percent of the neurons are impregnated, the technique does not permit quantitative analysis.

Since 1873, when Golgi described his procedure, a number of modifications of the original technique have been reported. They are summarized and detailed in a recent review by Millhouse (17).

The Golgi impregnation technique may be successfully combined with other techniques such as nerve degeneration (see Section 4.2.3), autoradiography (see Section 4.3.4), retrograde tracing techniques (see Section 4.4.4), or immunohistochemistry (see Section 4.5.3). All these combined strategies make it possible to recognize and identify afferent nerve terminals in contact with impregnated nerve cells.

The Golgi technique has also been adapted to electron microscopy (18, 19). Studies on impregnated ultrathin serial sections permit fine ultrastructural analysis of the synaptic relations of neurons recognized and localized by previous light microscopic impregnation. The large amount of silver chromate precipitation that normally fills impregnated neurons and does not permit fine structural examination can be removed by sodium thiosulfate (20) or a diluted solution of ammonia (21).

4.1.2 Intraneuronal Staining

The intracellular application of various substances allows examination of the location and dimensions of neuronal cell bodies, dendritic trees, and sometimes of axons and axon collaterals. The intracellular marking techniques are also useful for identifying recorded neurons in the brain.

Various materials can be applied intracellularly, such as fluorescent dyes (Procion Yellow, Lucifer Yellow, Ethidium Bromide), cobalt ion, tritiated glycine with subsequent autoradiography, and horseradish peroxidase. Until recently, Procion Yellow was the most widely used intracellular stain but Lucifer Yellow has proved to be about 100 times more fluorescent than Procion Yellow. The advantage of cobalt chloride is that both central and peripheral ends of cut axons can be filled. Horseradish peroxidase is less toxic than fluorescent dyes and its histological resolution is excellent. The horseradish peroxidase reaction product is electron-dense, therefore the ultrastructure of the injected neurons can be examined by electron microscope. Intracellular staining techniques in general have been described in detail by Kater and Nicholson (22), Tweedle (23), Kitai and Bishop (24), and Alheid et al. (25).

Two methods have been used to inject substances into the neurons: iontophoresis and pressure microinjections. The iontophoretic technique has proved to be the more popular for application of fluorescent dyes, and the microinjection technique is satisfactory for the application of horseradish peroxidase (see also Section 4.8.3).

4.2 Nerve Degeneration Methods

The experimental nerve degeneration technique has been widely used to recognize and localize the innervation fields of neurons or neuronal pathways in the central nervous system. The technique is based on an observation by Waller more than 130 years ago that the nerve terminal and axon distal to the lesion will degenerate upon transection of the axon or lesioning of the cell body. The degenerating fibers and terminal degeneration (also called Wallerian degeneration or anterograde or orthograde degeneration) can be demonstrated by selective silver impregnations at the light microscopic level (see Section 4.2.1); it can also be recognized under an electron microscope (see Section 4.2.2).

The main advantage of the technique is that monosynaptic connections between two brain areas can be visualized. In certain conditions the degeneration is not only anterograde but degeneration may occur in the perikarya in which axons have been lesioned (retrograde degeneration) or in cells in which neuronal afferents have degenerated (transneuronal degeneration). The degenerating cell bodies, however, can be easily recognized, thus the possible existence of retrograde or transneuronal degenerations can be taken into consideration. The recognized transneuronal degeneration itself is also a useful tool as it makes possible the identification of a two-neuronal pathway.

A further advantage of the technique is that it can be combined with Golgi impregnation (see Section 4.2.3), tract-tracing techniques (see Section 4.4.1), and immunohistochemistry (see Section 4.5.3), whereby several elements (afferent and efferent projections) of a neuronal system can be identified simultaneously.

4.2.1 Light Microscopy

The technique is based on the demonstration of anterograde degenerations, therefore it is most suitable to study efferent neuronal projections. The more selective and specific the type of the lesion employed to cause degeneration (see also Section 4.8.1), the more valuable the results. In the past 30 years, a number of silver impregnation methods have been reported; for details see reviews by Heimer (26) and de Olmos et al. (27). The important advantage of recent techniques is their ability to demonstrate fine degenerating axons and pathways for long distances (28) and the general pattern of degenerating nerve terminals (29).

The major difficulty of the nerve degeneration technique is the appropriate choice of the postoperative survival period, as impregnation is optimal only in a relatively short period of time after lesioning. This period, usually between one and four days, depends on a number of factors (the type and chemical character of the lesioned cells and fibers, the type of the lesion, the length of the pathway, etc.) that have to be determined before the experiment. Even though recent techniques provide a high-contrast image of degenerating particles, the nerve degeneration method is suitable for only approximate quantitation.

4.2.2 Electron Microscopy

In spite of the high resolution of recent light microscopic nerve degeneration techniques, which are capable of impregnating degenerating axon fragments and nerve terminals separately, the recognition of neuronal connections and identification of presynaptic and postsynaptic elements requires electron microscopic observations. Electron microscopy, however, cannot provide information regarding the topography of nerve fibers and terminals; therefore, it should be supplemented with light microscopic orientations. This can be done on semithin sections before the electron microscopic examinations, or silver impregnation sections can be subsequently prepared for electron microscopy (30).

The most common type of degenerating nerve terminals seen is referred to as electron-dense degeneration. This form is characterized by a darkening of the axoplasm with disintegrating organelles. During the early stage of degeneration the darkened synaptic bouton remains attached to the postsynaptic elements; later it detaches and is engulfed by glial cells. In some cases, presynaptic boutons show neurofilamentous hypertrophy (filamentous degeneration); others are characterized by an initial increase of electron opacity (pynocytotic degeneration) or a flocculent appearance of the axoplasm (flocculent degeneration). In all these three forms of degeneration the synaptic vesicles are disintegrating and their number are sharply depleted. These forms are characteristic for the early stage of degeneration (8–24 hours after lesioning) and later (24–72 hours) transform into the electron-dense degeneration. In the third period of the degeneration, the electron-dense bodies, axon-cytolysomes or multilocular bodies (electron-transparent boutons with aggregated synaptic vesicles and degenerating mitochondria) are phagocytized by glial cells, where they can still be found 5–7 days after lesion production.

Depending on the type of neurons, the form and speed of terminal degeneration are different, therefore the above detailed forms of degeneration may occur simultaneously. For further details see reviews of Mugnaini and Friedrich (30) and Záborszky et al. (31).

In addition to the demonstration of the presence of degenerating synapses, their number can be established. The number of degenerating terminals may be expressed either as number per unit area (density of the degeneration), as percentage of the total synaptic profiles, or as number of degenerating presynaptic boutons per cell. The participation of certain brain areas in the innervation of a particular cell groups can be quantitated in a quasi-mosaic manner by the determination of degenerating synapses per cell ratio after selective brain lesions (for further detail see Section 4.7).

4.2.3   In Combination with Other Techniques

The combination of nerve degeneration technique and Golgi impregnation at the electron microscopic level allows one to recognize both presynaptic and postsynaptic structures simultaneously. Degenerating presynaptic boutons, as a consequence of lesioning of afferent neurons, can be demonstrated in contact with silver impregnated nerve cells. Further combination of techniques is also possible: nerve degeneration plus Golgi impregnation plus horseradish peroxidase retrograde tracing (see Section 4.4.4); nerve degeneration plus immunohistochemistry (see Sections 4.5.3 and 4.6.4) can be successfully applied simultaneously.

4.3   Autoradiography

This technique has been in use for more than a century but it entered neurobiology only in the 1960s. The method has been applied in many fields of neurobiology: neuroanatomical localization of neurotransmitter binding sites at the cellular and subcellular level (see Section 4.3.1); autoradiographic tracing of axonal connections in the central nervous system (see Section 4.3.2); characterization of neurons according to their specific uptake, reuptake, and storage capacity (32); dry-mount and thaw-mount autoradiography, which have been frequently used to locate the cellular uptake and retention of steroid hormones, assuming that they are indicative of the presence of receptor systems for these hormones (33); examination of functional connections in brain areas based on the autoradiographic visualization of glucose metabolism in brain nuclei (see Section 4.3.3).

In each above application, the technique may be used under the electron microscope and may be evaluated by quantitative or semiquantitative methods (see Section 4.7). Autoradiography can be combined with histological, tract-tracing techniques and also with immunohistochemistry (see Sections 4.3.4 and 4.5.3).

The autoradiographic technique, in general, is based on the following steps: (i) labeling the system to be studied; (ii) preparation of brain sections (either for light or electron microscopy); (iii) covering tissue slides with radiosensitive emulsion; (iv) photographical development of the emulsion. In light microscopic studies, the developed sections are subsequently stained and coverslipped. In electron microscopy, the sections are stained with uranyl acetate and lead citrate previous to the development. For technical details and advice, see ref. 34.

4.3.1 Autoradiography in Receptor Studies

One approach to the study of the topographical distribution of neurotransmitter receptors in the brain is to use specific ligands for the receptors and visualize them at the light or electron microscopic level. Antibodies can be raised against the purified receptor protein and demonstrated by coupling them with horseradish peroxidase or a fluorescent or radioactive marker. Both *in vivo* and *in vitro* application of this method has been developed.

For *in vivo* experiments, animals are injected with radioactive ligand and killed, and the brain is removed, frozen and cut. The sections (3–6 μm thick) are then picked up on slides previously coated with a photographic emulsion. The emulsion is developed to display autoradiographic grains. For *in vitro* binding technique, tissue is removed, frozen, and cut, and thereafter sections are incubated with radioactive ligands, covered with emulsion-coated coverslips, and developed. The methods are explained in detail by Murrin (35) and Young and Kuhar (36).

4.3.2 Autoradiography as a Tract-Tracing Technique

The autoradiographic fiber-tracing method is based on the anterograde (from the cell body towards the nerve terminals) and in certain conditions on the retrograde transport of intracerebrally applied labeled amino acids. Amino acids are incorporated into proteins and transported via axonal flow. Fast-moving (100–400 mm/day) proteins—neurotransmitters belong to this category—are good markers for the demonstration of nerve terminals, since slow-moving proteins (1–20 mm/day) may outline the axons and their collaterals (37). The labeled substance is administered either directly into the perikarya or by infiltrating a certain brain area. The mode of application may be microinjection or microiontophoresis (see Section 4.8.3). Initially the use of ^{3}H-leucine was most common; now mainly ³H-proline is used, alone or in combination with ³H-leucine or ³H-lysine. ³⁵S-methionine is used when electrophoretic analysis of the labeled protein is performed; for labeling of cysteine-rich neurohypophyseal peptides, ³⁵S-cysteine has been used.

Light microscopic autoradiography can give considerable information about the origin of a pathway and its course, but identifying the nerve terminal area can be difficult. The latter is a subject for electron microscopic autoradiography.

The autoradiographic tract-tracing can be applied in animals whose protein synthesis is blocked by local injections of puromycin or by transection the pathway between two brain areas. In that case, the innervated area (and axons, proximal to the lesion) is unlabeled while labeled proteins accumulate at the ends of transected fibers. These kind of studies can provide significant information after unilateral lesioning by comparing ipsilateral and contralateral alterations.

For methodological details and application of autoradiography as a tract-tracing technique, see reviews by Cowan et al. (38) and by Edwards and Hendrickson (37).

In addition to the axonal transport of materials from the neuronal perikarya to the terminals, there is also a form of opposite transport from the terminals toward the cell body (retrograde transport). Various substances can be applied to demonstrate neuronal projections by retrograde tracing:

1.   Axon terminal uptake and retrograde transport of ³H-leucine plus ³H-lysine provide excellent labels both at light and electron microscopic levels (39).

2.   By intracerebral injections of radioactive labeled transmitters or related molecules, autoradiography may be useful in transmitter-specific retrograde labeling (40). Amino acid-containing pathways have been identified by retrograde labeling with ³H-aspartate, ³H-glycine and ³H-GABA. Similarly, aminergic (dopamine, noradrenaline, serotonin) and cholinergic (using ³H-choline) pathways have also been demonstrated. Although these techniques have yielded new information concerning the character of certain neuronal connections, the presence of unspecific labeling and the existence of a number of unknown factors involved in the uptake mechanism of nerve terminals must be kept in mind in evaluating the results of such experiments.

3.   For retrograde labeling, tritiated proteins may also be used, either individually or in combination with nonlabeled tracers for retrograde double-labeling. Labeled horseradish peroxidase, wheat germ agglutinin, bovine serum albumin, tetanus toxin, cholera toxin, nerve growth factor, dopamine-β-hydroxylase antibodies—all have proved useful as retrograde tracers.

A third form of tract-tracing exists: transsynaptic labeling. A small portion of the anterogradely transported radioactive materials (especially ^{3}H-proline) leaves the nerve terminals and is taken up by the second neuron. Proteins can be labeled *in vivo* with N-succinimidyl(2,3-^{3}H)-propionate, which can cross cell membranes and react with intraneuronal proteins (covalent labeling). Intra-axonal injection of this substance provides a tool to study both anterograde and retrograde transport of endogenous proteins (41).

In tract-tracing autoradiography, the observations are limited to only a single time-point. Recently, methods are reported that allow radioactivity to be monitored continuously while it is traveling along the axon (42).

Tract-tracing autoradiography is widely used in electron microscopy to demonstrate the presence of labels in the presynaptic boutons. Since the boutons remain labeled for a long period after injection, the electron microscopic autoradiograph can be used for quantitative estimations (see Section 4.7).

4.3.3 2-Deoxy-Glucose Technique

This technique was developed to measure the local rates of energy metabolism in particular brain regions (43). The method employs a labeled analog of glucose [2-deoxy-D-(^{14}C)glucose] to trace local cerebral glucose utilization in the brain by autoradiography. Because glucose is almost the sole substrate for brain oxidative metabolism, its utilization is related to oxygen consumption, which is the most direct parameter of energy metabolism in the neurons. Regional localization and concentration of radioactivity is achieved by the use of quantitative autoradiography. A computerized image-processing system has been developed: autoradiographs are scanned automatically by a scanning microdensitometer (for technical details, see refs. 44, 45).

The method has been utilized to map the functional organization of major systems in the brain (see refs. 44, 45) and to map functional pathways by surveying the metabolic rate of brain nuclei following selective lesions, transections of pathways, and drug treatments. Stimulation of brain regions or pathways also alters the rate of glucose utilization in the related brain regions; this can be recognized, mapped, and measured on autoradiographs.

4.3.4 Autoradiography in Combination with Other Techniques

The anterograde autoradiographic tracing in combination with retrograde tract-tracing methods is a useful tool for studying two-neuronal pathways (see Section 4.4.4). Autoradiography in combination with formaldehyde-induced fluorescence has been described for the localization of radioactively labeled substances (steroid hormones) in relation to monoamine neurons (46). Autoradiography in combination with immunohistochemistry is detailed in Section 4.5.3. This combination at the electron microscopic level (see Section 4.6.4) has the advantage that subcellular structures are well-preserved; both anterogradely labeled presynaptic boutons and immunostained postsynaptic sites can be readily recognized.

4.4   Tract-Tracing Techniques

Various methods for demonstrating neuronal pathways have become available in the past decade. Tract-tracing techniques in general include all neuroanatomical procedures by which the neuron and its projection can be visualized. According to this term, successful Golgi impregnation, single cell labeling, or immunohistochemistry can be considered among tract-tracing techniques (3), but because they are less effective in demonstrating long axonal projections, these techniques are discussed elsewhere in this chapter (see Sections 4.1 and 4.5). The nerve degeneration technique is also a powerful tool in pathway studies but it is not a tracing method (see Section 4.2). One of the main application of autoradiography is indeed tract-tracing; this is detailed in the autoradiography section (Section 4.3.2) because of its methodical procedure. Therefore, this section includes only those techniques wherein horseradish peroxidase, certain lectins (see Section 4.4.1), and dyes (see Section 4.4.2) or their combinations (see Section 4.4.3) are used for tracing. Tract-tracing techniques based on above labels can be combined with other neuroanatomical techniques; this approach is summarized in Section 4.4.4.

4.4.1   Horseradish Peroxidase Technique

Horseradish peroxidase (HRP) is a glycoprotein able to catalyze the oxidation of certain chromogens, thus resulting in a microscopically (in certain cases electron microscopically) detectable reaction product. HRP is picked up by nerve terminals and carried by retrograde transport to the cell bodies. Therefore, HRP histochemistry was introduced to neuroanatomy as a retrograde transport method for tracing neuronal afferents. HRP enters nerve terminals by pinocytosis. Inside nerve terminals it is found in synaptic vesicles, coated vesicles, and some tubular elements. From the nerve terminals HRP is transported inside various vesicular and tubular organelles through the axon into the cell body, where it is found in lysosomes.

HRP is initially taken up by nerve terminals and transported retrogradely towards the perikarya; it can also enter the collateral branches of the axons and reach the terminals of these axon collaterals by anterograde transport. Furthermore, it has been demonstrated that HRP can also be taken up by cell bodies or dendrites by endocytosis and can be carried down the axon to the nerve terminals by fast anterograde transport. Therefore, HRP histochemistry can also be used as an anterograde tract-tracing method for tracing neuronal efferents. (The third application of HRP histochemistry is single-cell staining by direct intracellular injection, see Section 4.1.2).

The uptake of HRP is coupled to the activity of nerve terminals, dendrites, or perikarya; it can be reduced by inhibition of synaptic activity and increased by stimulation.

The most common method is to apply HRP with the aid of pressure injection or electrophoresis (see Section 4.8.3). HRP can enter not only intact terminals but also the transected axons or the growth cones of regenerating axons. Labeling with HRP is actually increased where axons have been severed, and one of the disadvantages of the HRP tract-tracing technique is that the labeling of fibers passing through but not originating in the investigated area results in significant unexpected tracings. To increase the sensitivity of HRP tracing technique, one can apply HRP in pellets or slow-release gels (47).

The optimal survival time after HRP application depends on various factors (48); in most cases it is 24–48 h. The retrograde movement of HRP is estimated in a range of 50–120 mm/day. The anterograde transport is related to the fast axoplasmic flow; it is at least 300 mm/day (49). Colchicine and pentobarbital reversibly block anterograde transport by causing disruption of microtubules or of endoplasmic reticulum (49). Conjugates of HRP with cholera toxin or wheat germ agglutinin (see Section 4.4.3) are superior to free HRP as an anterogradely transported marker (50). For further details see reviews by Warr et al. (48) and Mesulam (51).

Several techniques are available for the visualization and localization of HRP in the brain. These procedures are based on a histochemical reaction: The tissue is incubated in a medium containing hydrogen peroxidase and chromogens; the chromogen is oxidized to a color product by the peroxidase-antiperoxidase system. The most commonly used chromogens are DAB (3,3'-diaminobenzidine tetrahydrochloride), a brown reaction product; TMB (3,3',5,5'-tetramethylbenzidine), a grayish blue reaction product in bright-field microscope and golden granules in dark-field microscope; o-dianisidine (3,3'-dimethoxybenzidine dihydrochloride), a brown reaction product; and BDHC (benzidine dihydrochloride), a blue reaction product. The DAB method is simple, reproducible, and has good visibility in dark-field illumination. The reaction product is osmiophilic, therefore it is suited for electron microscopy. The sensitivity is much less than that of the TMB method. The BDHC method provides fine reaction products, is successful in demonstrating axonal projections and collaterals, does not fade as easily as the other reaction products, but is less sensitive than the TMB method.

After a comparison of available techniques, Mesulam and Rosene (52) and Morrell et al. (53) concluded that the TMB method was significantly superior to the others in the number of labeled perikarya. The TMB procedure resulted in a more complete topography of neurons and filled the retrogradely labeled neurons with reaction product, giving a Golgi-like picture of the neuron.

The electron microscopic demonstration of HRP is most commonly accomplished by using the DAB method. (For technical details, see review by Hanker et al., 54). Silver intensification of the method is successfully applied to improve the detection of HRP product (55). The DAB method, however, is less sensitive than methods based on other chromogens. Recently, the TMB, BDHC, and *o*-tolidine reaction products were found to be suitable for electron microscopy. Eight methods for the electron microscopic demonstration of HRP have been compared by Carson and Mesulam (56). The largest distribution of reaction product was observed with the TMB method. The sensitivity of the method is excellent and the reaction products are electron-dense, showing a very distinctive crystalloid appearance.

4.4.2 Fluorescent Dyes

Fluorescent dyes constitute another group of substances that may be used for retrograde tract tracing. The fluorescent method is simple, fast, and sensitive. The main advantage of the technique is that each substance requires a particular wavelength of light for excitation and appears in a different color, so that double or triple labeling of the same cell is possible (57, 58). The technique is excellent for demonstrating neurons with divergent axon collaterals. Different dyes are injected into those brain regions to which the investigated cells presumably project. The existence of such projections can be proved by demonstrating the presence of two or more dyes in the same cells. The following dyes may be used (59): Evans Blue, DAPI (4'-6-diamidino-2-phenylindol), Primuline, Bisbenzimide, Nuclear Yellow, Propidium Iodide, True Blue, Granular Blue, Fast Blue. For technical details and further references see the summary by Kuypers (59).

4.4.3 Multiple Tract-Tracing

Beside horseradish peroxidase, other proteins are also applied as retrograde tracers, individually or in combination with HRP. These are lectins (mainly wheat germ agglutinin), bovine serum albumin, toxins (cholera or tetanus), and nerve growth factor. Wheat germ agglutinin, which is an excellent retrograde marker by itself, becomes superior in conjugation with HRP for studies of retrograde axonal transport (60). Conjugates of HRP with cholera toxin and wheat germ agglutinin have been reported as a superior anterograde marker (50). A desirable feature of lectins is that they do not undergo any transsynaptic transfer.

As has been detailed previously, fluorescent dyes are used in combination with each other for double and triple retrograde labeling. They may also be used in combination with HRP: simultaneous visualization of HRP and Nuclear Yellow in tissue sections for neuronal double labeling has been reported recently (61).

4.4.4 Tract-Tracing Techniques in Combination with Other Techniques

In addition to the combination of HRP and other retrograde tracers with each other, the HRP technique has been introduced in combination with other techniques for double or triple labeling of various components of neuronal circuits. Each double-labeling or triple-labeling combination has its specific advantages.

HRP Technique in Combination with Golgi Staining. Retrogradely transported HRP histochemistry has been successfully combined with Golgi impregnation for light and subsequent electron microscopic studies (62). The combined technique is useful in localizing and characterizing cell types in heterogenous cell populations or in multilayered structures which selectively project to another brain area. The projection is demonstrated by HRP retrograde labeling while the projecting neurons are visualized by Golgi staining and characterized on the basis of their size, shape, dendritic and local axonal patterns.

HRP Technique in Combination with Nerve Degeneration Technique (63). Both afferent and efferent connections of a neuron characterized by means of Golgi impregnation can be simultaneously visualized by the combination of nerve degeneration, HRP technique, and Golgi staining (64). By lesioning an area or pathway that possibly projects to the labeled cell, the afferent fibers (and, using electron microscopy, the presynaptic nerve terminals) and the efferents of the neuron can be localized by retrograde HRP tracing.

Tract-Tracing Technique in Combination with Autoradiography. In double tracer experiments, HRP is visualized histochemically and labeled substances are visualized autoradiographically. Successful applications of the following combinations have been reported (see 65 for details): (i) Retrograde double labeling procedures using HRP and tritiated HRP; HRP and enzymatically inactivated ^{3}H-apo-HRP (66); HRP and ^{3}H-wheat germ agglutinin (67); and HRP and labeled bovine serum albumin (65)—all of these combined techniques can be adapted to electron microscopy. (ii) HRP in combination with anterograde tracing—the anterograde projections from the area of the injection of tritiated amino acids or choline are revealed with autoradiography, whereas the cells of origin of the afferent projections to the injected area are retrogradely labeled by HRP (68). (iii) HRP in combination with 2-deoxyglucose technique (65).

Retrograde Tracing Techniques and Transmitter-Related Histochemistry. Studies have been reported combining HRP technique with histofluorescence (69, 70). These procedures are rather difficult, however, and the HRP is therefore replaced with fluorescent dyes. The simultaneous use of retrograde fluorescent tracers and formaldehyde-induced fluorescent technique has been reported for mapping monoaminergic projections and collateral arrangements (71). Another approach relying on the combination of retrograde tracing and immunohistochemistry is discussed in Section 4.5.3.

4.5   Light Microscopic Immunohistochemistry

Immunohistochemistry is increasingly employed as a powerful tool in neurobiology, including neuropeptide studies. The technique is based on an antigen-antibody reaction, which can be visualized on histological sections by labeling the antibody directly with marker compounds (direct method) or by employing an anti-immunoglobulin intermediary to couple the antibody to the marker compound (indirect method). Various techniques and several modifications of each have been developed to increase the specificity and sensitivity of the methods. All these aspects and technical details are not covered here but are treated extensively in Chapter 21 in this book and in extensive reviews (72–74). This section deals with details of combinations of immunohistochemical techniques (double immunolabeling, see Section 4.5.2) and combinations of immunohistochemistry with other neuroanatomical techniques (see Section 4.5.3). Electron microscopic immunohistochemistry is treated in a separate section (see Section 4.6).

Until 1980, antibodies used in immunohistochemistry were of polyclonal origin: raised in laboratory animals by the repeated injection of antigen. Recently, monoclonal antibodies produced by hybrid myelomas have been successfully applied in immunohistochemistry (75, 76). The use of monoclonal antibodies has two valuable advantages: they are highly specific and they are present in continous supply in unlimited quantity. The monoclonal antibody technique has been shown to be suitable for the application of indirect immunofluorescence and unlabeled antibody enzyme methods (75, 76). With the use of internally labeled monoclonal antibodies ("radioimmunohistochemistry"), autoradiography can be combined with immunohistochemistry for single- or double labeling, at both the light and electron microscopic levels (see Section 4.5.3).

The value of the immunohistochemical techniques is related to the accuracy, sensitivity, and specificity of the methods as well as the antisera (74, 77, 78). The *accuracy* of the technique depends on the careful preliminary standardization of all steps of the method used. The *sensitivity* of an immunohistochemical method is represented by the lowest staining intensity that can be distinguished from background. (The specificity of various methods is discussed in Section 4.5.1.) With long-term storage and repeated use of diluted antisera the sensitivity and reproducibility of the light microscopic immunohistochemical methods may be increased (79). The *specificity* of the techniques depends on the specificity of the method and the specificity of the antibodies. Both have to be controlled.

1. *The "method specificity."* Various procedures have been recommended to test the specificity of the immunohistochemical method: (i) Absence of labeling after replacement of the primary antiserum with normal, preimmune serum or other antisera; (ii) Absence of labeling after the omission of the secondary antiserum; (iii) Dilution-dependent staining with the primary antiserum: the gradual dilution of the antiserum should reduce the labeling until total disappearance.

2. *The "antibody specificity."* Antibodies recognize only a small site of the antigen molecule, therefore immunohistochemistry can be site-specific but not molecule-specific. The recognized site may occur in several other (precursor, related or even unrelated) molecules: all these can therefore cross-react with the antibody. The specificity may be tested by blocking of the antiserum by immunoabsorption with homologous antigen, or by the lack of blocking by heterologous antigens (immunohistological cross-reactivity test). Recently, a new technique ("gelatin gel model") has been reported for detecting the antibody specificity of immunohistochemical techniques (80).

Since immunohistochemical staining does not recognize the neuropeptide molecules but only antigenic determinants, peptide-like (but not peptide) immunoreactivity can be visualized under the microscope. To support the validity of the immunohistochemical localization, other relevant techniques such as bioassays, radioimmunoassays, and physiological experiments have to be performed.

4.5.1 Immunohistochemical Methods

Immunohistochemical methods are based on the visualization of the binding of antibody to specific tissues antigen. At the present time, the more sensitive indirect methods are used. In the indirect methods the antibody (primary antibody) is coupled to an intermediate (anti-immunoglobulin), called secondary antibody. This secondary antibody is goat or sheep antiserum prepared against the immunoglobulin of the animal used for producing the primary antibody and it is bonded with histological markers ("sandwich technique"). The indirect techniques can be divided into two groups depending on the type of bonding between the secondary antibody and markers: covalent bonding (labeled antibody methods) and immunologic bonding (unlabeled antibody methods). The labeled methods can be further divided according to the substance employed for labeling: fluorochrome labeled (fluorescein-conjugated antibody method) and immunoenzyme labeled (enzyme-conjugated antibody method) techniques.

Indirect Immunofluorescence (Fluorescein-Conjugated Antibody) Method. This method has been extensively used for the immunohistochemical localization of catecholamine synthetizing enzymes, but it has also wide applicability in neuropeptide studies. The most widely used fluorochromes are the fluorescein isothiocyanate (FITC), giving a green fluorescence, or rhodamine β isothiocyanate (RITC), giving an orange-red fluorescence. The method is simple, quick, very economical and relatively sensitive—about 10 times more sensitive than the direct method. The method can be combined with other neuroanatomical techniques (see Section 4.5.3). However, it cannot be adapted to electron microscopy, and the reaction products are not stable.

Enzyme-Conjugated Antibody Method. This is also a "sandwich technique" in which an enzyme is bonded with the anti-immunoglobulin and detected by a histochemical reaction. The most widely used enzyme is horseradish peroxidase, which forms a brown precipitate on the section after reacting with hydrogen peroxidase in the presence of 3,3'-diaminobenzidine (DAB). The sensitivity of this method is not better than that of immunofluorescence, but the background is lower, the tissue penetration is better, and the end-product is stable. The same preparation can be utilized for light and electron microscopy. The procedure is much more complicated and time-consuming than immunohisto-fluorescence.

Unlabeled Antibody Enzyme Methods. The anti-immunoglobulin and the label are immunologically bonded without the use of covalent bonding. This group includes the peroxidase-antiperoxidase (PAP) method (81). This is a simple, economical, highly sensitive procedure with low background staining. For light microscopy, paraffin, Vibratome, or frozen sections can be used. After completion of the immunolabeling procedure, the sections can be examined with either bright-field or dark-field illumination, and the method is easily adapted to electron microscopy. The DAB reaction product can be further intensified by silver nitrate (82) or nickel ammonium sulfate (83): the reaction products become intense black and they are very stable, therefore it is useful for dual PAP staining (see Section 4.5.2). This method can be combined with other techniques such as autoradiography and nerve degeneration (see Section 4.5.3). The main shortcoming of the method is that false positive results might be obtained. The primary antibody–tissue antigen binding depends on the titer and dilution of the primary antiserum, the time and temperature of the incubation, the accessibility of the antigen, and the tissue antigen concentration, which also depends on the fixation and embedding procedures.

Avidin-Biotin-Peroxidase Complex (ABC) Method (84, 85).   This is a superior technique to localize antigens in formalin-fixed tissues. Avidin is a glycoprotein that has an extraordinary affinity for biotin. The biotin covalently bound to immunoglobulin or peroxidase molecules has an ability to bind avidin molecules. The method involves application of biotin-labeled secondary antibody followed by the addition of avidin-biotin-peroxidase complex. The method is less time-consuming and much more sensitive than the PAP method.

4.5.2 Dual and Multiple Immunostainings

Dual or multiple immunostaining methods have been worked out for simultaneous localization of two or more antigens in the same section. Two types of procedures have been reported: (i) Simultaneous staining, based on the combination of two indirect immunohistochemical methods (86) or by combining the immunoperoxidase with immunofluorescence methods (87); the methods involve different enzymes and substrates without interfering with each other. (ii) Sequential stainings, in which the same enzyme but different substrates are used; after the localization of the first antigen, the antibody and the peroxidase are eluted except for the color reaction product (6), then the second antigen is localized using a substrate that develops a reaction product of a different color than that of the substrate employed in the first step. The double staining procedure can be applied to the enzyme-labeled antibody method (88), to the unlabeled antibody (PAP) method (89, 90) or to the avidin-biotin-peroxidase complex (ABC) method (91). In order to obtain two different colors, the peroxidase substrate 3,3′-diaminobenzidine (DAB) is used for brown reaction products and 4-Cl-1-naphthol for grayish-blue products. In a modification, α-naphthol-pyronin has been introduced instead of 4-Cl-1-naphthol, which gives red-purple end-products fine enough not only for demonstrating two different cell bodies but also nerve terminals (79). The other techniques are based on the color modification of the DAB reaction by metallic ions (83, 91). Nickel ions change DAB color from brown to blue-black, cobalt to dark blue, and copper to grayish blue.

The multiple staining procedures have the advantages of demonstrating as many as three antigens inside the same cell, or in different types of cells inside a heterogeneous cell group (brain nuclei), or in nerve fibers.

4.5.3 Immunohistochemistry in Combination with Other Techniques

Immunohistochemistry is successfully achieved in combination with other neuroanatomical techniques to chemically identify cells, pathways or nerve terminals which have been previously or simultaneously localized by other staining or labeling methods.

Immunostaining and Single-Cell Labeling. This type of combination is useful for visualizing immunostained nerve terminals, or a particular neuronal perikarya or dendrites stained with Golgi technique or intracellular staining (see Section 4.1). It is possible to impregnate a section previously subjected to immunohistochemistry (the thickness of the blocks is a limiting factor). Intracellular cell labeling can be followed by immunostaining (92).

Immunostaining in Combination with Autoradiography. A combined technique of autoradiography and immunohistochemistry has been described for the localization of radioactively labeled ligands (labeling of steroid hormone-concentrating neurons) and neuropeptides (93, 94) or biogenic amine synthesizing enzymes in the brain (93). *In vivo* and *in vitro* methods for simultaneous use of immunohistochemistry (PAP method) and ^{3}H-thymidine autoradiography have been used for studying developing systems in the embryonic and postnatal rat brain (95). A radioimmunocytochemical method has been developed for simultaneous localization of two antigen sites at both the light and electron microscope levels (96). Radiolabeled antigen is incubated with a surplus amount of antibody. One combining site of the antibody binds the labeled antigen while the other site is free to react with tissue-bound antigen. The method is advantageously combined with the immunoperoxidase method. Similarly, immunohistochemistry (PAP method) gives excellent double labeling in combination with autoradiographic detection of internally labeled monoclonal antibodies (75, 76).

Immunostaining in Combination with Tract-Tracing Techniques

1. Monoamines and neuropeptides on the same microscopic sections may be traced by combining fluorescence histochemistry with immunohistochemistry (97).

2. The use of immunofluorescence in combination with horseradish peroxidase retrograde transport allows transmitters to be characterized

in identified neurons (98). Photomicrographic localization of retrogradely labeled cells is followed by a subsequent immunostaining in the same section. For simultaneously visualizing retrogradely labeled cells, the HRP technique is combined with the PAP method. In this combination, the retrogradely transported HRP and the immunoperoxidase are visualized, using the same staining procedure but distinguishing them on the basis of their microscopic appearance (99–101). Wheat germ agglutinin as retrograde tracer has also been used combined with immunofluorescence (102).

3. The major disadvantage of HRP in combination with immunofluorescence is that HRP is sensitive to ultraviolet radiation and sections have to be analyzed with two different microscopes. The introduction of fluorescent dyes (see Section 4.4.2) offered a new approach as they are suitable for combination with immunohistochemistry. Both the retrogradely transported fluorescent dyes and the marker for the transmitter can be studied under the same microscope (103). Several dyes have been tested for combination with indirect immunofluorescence (104, 105). Propidium Iodide and Fast Blue are reported the best for such combination. For technical details, see Skirboll et al. (105). (The PAP method is also compatible with fluorescent dyes for the double labeling technique, but because of high-background labeling (106) it seems to be less useful than immunofluorescence.)

For triple labeling as immunofluorescence markers, two dyes—Fast Blue plus New Nuclear Yellow or Primuline plus New Nuclear Yellow—can be used with Rhodamine, or Propidium iodine plus New Nuclear Yellow can be used with fluorescein-isocyanide. The three simultaneously used substances can be distinguished either by their spectral characteristics or by their cellular compartmentalization (105). Another possibility for triple labeling is the combination of retrograde tracing with elution restaining immunohistochemistry using two different antisera (105).

4.6 Electron Microscopic Immunocytochemistry

Various electron microscopic approaches have been worked out for the visualization of intracellular antigenic sites. (Since subcellular rather than cellular distribution of immunolabeled substances can be recognized under the electron microscope, the use of the term "immunocytochemistry" is suggested for electron microscopic studies and "immunohistochemistry" for light microscopic studies.)

The light microscopic immunohistochemical methods, except for immunofluorescence, can be applied to electron microscopy. The unlabeled antibody enzyme method (PAP) is the most popularly used method for electron microscopy, but other techniques, such as the avidin-biotin-per-oxidase complex method (ABC) and a protein A-gold complex method, have already been introduced.

To demonstrate substances immunocytochemically, they can be immunostained either on thick sections of fixed brain before embedding and ultrathin sectioning (pre-embedding staining) or on ultrathin sections after embedding (post-embedding staining). Both techniques have their own advantages and pitfalls (see Sections 4.6.1 and 4.6.2). Since the PAP method, which is poorly adapted to post-embedding staining, has mainly been used in immunocytochemical practice, the first data on the subcellular distribution of neurotransmitters and neuropeptides in the brain have been reported using pre-embedding staining.

The specificity of electron microscopic immunocytochemistry, like that of light microscopic staining, depends on the specificity of the methods and the antigens (see Section 4.5). Detailed descriptions of the technical procedures or specificity are outside the scope of this chapter; good summary articles are available (72, 74, 107, 108).

4.6.1 Pre-embedding Immunostaining

The PAP method is widely used for pre-embedding immunostaining. The labeling procedure is performed before the embedding of the tissue. In this technique, the main problem is the penetration of the antibody into the tissue and through the cellular membranes. The fixation of the brain and its sectioning are crucial for good labeling. The commonly used fixative is a combination of 4% paraformaldehyde and 0.2% glutaraldehyde mixture in phosphate buffer. Recently another fixative (4% paraformaldehyde + 0.05% glutaraldehyde + 0.2% picric acid with pH 7.2–7.4) has been reported to give satisfactory penetration of antibodies and good preservation of fine structures (109). The fixative is used as primary fixative for the perfusion of the brain. After perfusion, brains are removed and postfixed in the same fixative for 1–3 h at 4°C. Brain regions to be investigated are cut out, washed, and frozen in liquid N_2 and thawed in buffer (109). Sections of 20–70 μm are cut on a Vibratome, washed, and immunostained. After the staining procedure the tissue is flat-embedded in Epon and the staining and general topography are checked under the light microscope. A small piece of the section containing the region to be studied by electron microscopy can be cut out under a dissecting microscope, fixed subsequently in 2% osmium tetroxide, re-embedded, and cut into ultrathin sections. At several intervals during ultrathin sectioning, the topography can be controlled in the block or in semithin sections under a light microscope. Ultrathin sections are mounted on copper grids and counterstained with uranyl acetate and lead citrate.

The main advantage of the pre-embedding technique is that it allows intense immunostaining and good preservation of fine structure. Membrane permeability is achieved by Vibratome sectioning and the freeze-thaw procedure, but unfortunately, these procedures alter the fine structure. A disadvantage of the technique is the possible dislocation of the antigen during the staining procedure, which results in less accurate localization of the labeled substance. The reaction products are relatively large in size and may cover ultrastructural details.

4.6.2 Post-embedding Immunostainings

Post-embedding staining directly upon ultrathin sections solves the problem of the penetration of antibody into the tissue. The structural preservation is excellent; however, the antigens lose their antigenic properties during dehydration or can be structurally altered by the embedding medium. Therefore, the immunoreactivity and specificity is less than with the pre-embedding staining. But post-embedding staining has the advantage that different immunostaining can be performed on serial ultrathin sections of the same brain area, even of a single cell.

Unlabeled Antibody Enzyme Method. The PAP technique has been adapted for post-embedding immunostaining. Several steps of the procedure are modified to increase the sensitivity and preserve the specificity of the technique. The most useful fixatives are a formaldehyde–picric acid combination or osmium tetroxide, with or without glutaraldehyde. Embedding in Araldite is recommended. The fixation may be performed by a freeze-drying technique followed by vacuum embedding in a water-free medium. Immunostaining is performed on ultrathin sections placed on nickel or gold grids. Pretreatment is suggested using either normal serum of the same species donating the link antiserum or preimmunization serum from the same animal in which the anti-immunoglobulin was produced. For technical details, see Sternberger (72).

Avidin-Biotin-Peroxidase Complex Method. The ABC method (84, 85) can be applied to post-embedding staining of glutaraldehyde fixed, Araldite embedded ultrathin sections on nickel grids (110). The staining intensity may be increased by osmium tetroxide, which also allows easier identification of stained cells in the section. The high affinity of avidin for biotin allows the use of relatively high dilutions of antisera, and the incubation time can be markedly reduced. The high background stain, however, is an important limitation of the technique at the present time.

Protein A–gold Complex (pAg) Method. An immunocolloid method for electron microscopy by using a complex of antibodies and colloidal gold particles has been introduced for cell surface antigen localization. Colloidal gold can be prepared as a sol of particles of either similar or heterogeneous (between 3–12 μm) diameter. Recently, the protein A–gold (pAg) method has been adapted to post-embedding staining performed on ultrathin sections of aldehyde-fixed and resin (Araldite, Epon)-embedded material on nickel or gold grids (111, 112). The method is simple and reliable for the ultrastructural detection of intracellular antigens. It is carried out in two steps: thin sections are incubated with specific antisera and the antigen-immunoglobulin complex is then visualized with a protein A–gold solution. The protein A can be labeled by both gold particles and fluorescein isothiocyanate (FITC), and this complex can be used as a second-step reagent for the visualization of cellular antigens in the light and electron microscopes (113).

The technique is a simple and short procedure, and it provides highly specific and sensitive labeling and good structural preservation. The binding is stable, and permits long-term storage. The gold particles are highly electron-dense, and they are easily detectable on the sections. Simultaneous localization of different antigens can be achieved on the same section by the use of gold particles of different size.

4.6.3   Multiple Labeling

Simultaneous electron microscopic localization of two or more antigens in the same neuron has not yet become a widely used procedure in neuroanatomical practice.

The pre-embedding staining methods do not allow the use of different stainings on consecutive sections. Simultaneous staining with a mixture of two primary antisera is possible and provides informative data (114), but its routine application requires further control investigations on the specificity of the method and the immunocytochemical cross-reactivity of the antigens used in a mixture.

The post-embedding staining methods provide two possible combinations:

1. Parallel immunostaining on consecutive serial sections. By complete ultrathin serial sectioning a single neuron can be cut into 25–40 sections. Theoretically, the same number of simultaneous immunostainings are possible.

2. Simultaneous staining with two or more antisera on the same ultrathin section may be accomplished with the use of the pAg method. Different antigens may be recognized by labeling of gold particles of different size (115).

The application of the above techniques is rather preliminary in neuropeptide studies in the central nervous system.

4.6.4 Electron Microscopic Immunostaining in Combination with Other Neuroanatomical Techniques

Combination with Single-Cell Staining. Ultrastructural analysis of an electrophysiologically identified single neuron is possible with a combined technique of intracellular staining and immunocytochemistry. Intracellular recording is followed by intracellular staining with Lucifer Yellow and stained by indirect RITC immunofluorescence (see Section 4.5.1). After light microscopic (and photographic) localization of the cell, ultrathin sections can be prepared for electron microscopy (116).

Combination with Nerve Degeneration Technique. To investigate neuronal inputs to an immunologically characterized neuron, the nerve degeneration technique (see Section 4.2) is combined with electron microscopic immunocytochemistry (117). The combined application of these two techniques enables presynaptic and postsynaptic structures to be characterized simultaneously. About 1–4 days after lesioning neurons or transecting neuronal pathways, degenerating nerve terminals are still found in synaptic contact with perikarya or dendrites that can be characterized by immunostaining. Nerve degeneration is without influence on immunostaining procedures, therefore both pre-embedding and post-embedding stainings can be used.

Combination with Autoradiography. The ability of certain labeled transmitters to be taken up specifically by nerve cells and transported by axons allows visualization by autoradiography of substances in nerve terminals that are in contact with immunoreactive cells or dendrites (118). Monoclonal antibodies labeled by ^{3}H-lysine can be localized on the immunoreactive sites on ultrathin sections by electron microscopic autoradiographic detection (75, 76).

Autoradiography based on specific uptake of tritiated monoamines in combination with immunocytochemistry in animals with brain lesions or pathway transection allows triple labeling. Under the electron microscope, immunostained and degenerating nerve terminals can be recognized in synaptic contact with labeled cells and dendrites (119).

4.7 Quantitative Neuroanatomical Methods

To deal adequately with quantitative histological techniques would mean writing an entire chapter or even book on that topic alone. Therefore, only principles, basic technical rules, and measurable parameters necessary to work out a strategy quantifying neuroanatomical data relating to neuropeptide studies are briefly summarized here.

The theoretical and practical problems of characterizing three-dimensional structures from their appearance in two-dimensional sections are treated in stereological handbooks (120, 121). Although most of the morphological techniques have developed their own automatic or computer-aided devices (122, 123), several quantitative histological parameters are still measured manually or are counted under the microscope.

4.7.1   Cell Numbers and Cell Density

The number of neuropeptide-containing cells can be expressed in the following ways:

1.   Cell number per section. Without unit or topographical relations this provides no more information than the subjective "few-moderate-lot" qualification.

2.   Surface density of cells (cell number/unit area, mainly expressed in mm^2). This can be calculated by cell counts on a measured surface area. The size of the surface area can be determined either by grids (insertion of a grid into the eyepieces of the microscope, microprojector projection of an image on a grid, or setting a transparent grid on the screen of a projecting microscope or an image analyzer) or by a planimeter (manual or automatic).

3.   Cell number per section profile of a brain nucleus. The section profile is measured by a planimeter, the cells are counted in it. Only those values are comparable which have been taken from sections characterized by topographical coordinates.

4.   Cell packing density (cell number/unit volume, mainly expressed in mm^3). This is one of the most useful parameters because it provides data comparable with quantitative electron microscopic data (see Section 4.7.3). The cell number is divided by the related volume, which can be calculated by multiplying the surface of the measured area by the section thickness. To avoid repeated calculation of the same cells in neighboring sections, a corrected section thickness has to be used (120, 121, 124, 125).

5.   The total number of neuropeptide-containing neurons in a particular brain nucleus. This number can be obtained in three ways: by counting each immunostained cell on complete serial sections of the nucleus, by calculating from the volume of the nucleus (determined by planimeter on serial sections) and the average of its cell-packing density, or by summarizing individual packing densities and volumes of each serial section of the nucleus.

6.   Neuropeptide-containing neurons as a percentage of the total cell number in a brain nucleus. This parameter is important especially in those brain nuclei which contain several types of neuropeptide-containing (or other chemically characterized) cells. In certain brain nuclei this

percentage exceeds 100%, indicating a coexistence of neuropeptides (or neuropeptides and neurotransmitters) in the same cells.

The percentage of neuropeptide-containing cells in a nucleus can be calculated by counting neuropeptide-containing cells and taking the total cell number of the nucleus from the literature, or by counting both the neuropeptide-containing and all other cells. Simple counting of cell numbers in a heterogeneous cell population can be achieved only when the size and the shape of the different cells are similar or almost equal. Otherwise, the larger cells have a higher probability of appearing in sections than the smaller cells. In heterogeneous populations, the number of each cell type can be calculated separately, using individually corrected section thicknesses for each cell type (see above, paragraph 5).

4.7.2 Density of Intracellular Substances

Manual optical densitometers, semiautomatic and automatic densitometers, and computer-aided image analyzer systems are available for determining substances (immunohistochemical reaction products, autoradiographic grains, tracing dyes or stainings) in nerve cells. Two major types of measurement can be distinguished, intracellular measurements (cellular density) and area measurements (field density). Cellular density is widely used to quantitate stainings and to count grains in the neurons (both at the light and electron microscopic levels); field density is used to numerically characterize nerve terminals (stained, labeled, or degenerated) in a particular brain area. In quantitating staining of brain areas, the measured data may be divided by the cell numbers in the investigated area or volume.

Semiautomatic and automatic densitometry is determined with a microspectrophotometer (microfluorimeter) equipped with microscope scanning stages (operated manually or by computer) and interfaced to an image analysis unit. Such equipment is commercially available from several companies (122, 126). The system can be adapted for analyzing various densities and particles on electron micrographs.

Computerized image-analysis systems have been developed for enumerating silver grains in autoradiographs (126, 127) but they can also automatically measure all types of particle density. The most modern systems are composed of a scanning microdensitometer, a computer, an image memory and display system, and monochrome or color monitors. The section (or photograph) is automatically scanned and the optimal density of each spot is digitized and stored in memory. Images can be reconstructed from the data in memory and utilized for microdensitometric analysis (127).

The automated multicolor fluorescence cytophotometer is equipped with different sets of interchangeable filters that enable the system to determine consecutively the content of several intracellular components (proteins, grains, immunostainings) in the same neuron. In the most modern technique, CYBEST (Cytobiological Electronic Screening System), the cytophotometry is combined with cytological pattern recognition (123).

4.7.3 Electron Microscopic Quantitative Methods

Two major types of techniques, densitometry and morphometry, can be adapted for analyzing electron micrographs. Both techniques are useful in neuropeptide studies. Electron-dense immunoreaction products, silver or gold grains, and degenerating nerve terminals can all be enumerated by scanning image analysis or by particle counting on manual grid sampling of electron micrographs. In morphometry, neuronal afferents to neuropeptide-containing neurons can be characterized by (i) measuring nerve terminal density or (ii) measuring synapse density or (iii) calculating synapse/cell ratio (see Section 2.3.4).

1.   The *density of nerve terminals*, (presynaptic boutons) is usually expressed as the number of boutons per unit area (1000 μm^2) or per unit volume (1000 μm^3). Several methods have been proposed to determine synaptic bouton density by measuring and counting the section profiles of boutons, which are geometrically irregular in shape and randomly oriented in space (120, 121, 128, 129). The validity of methods was considered, and finally a simple, less time-consuming and reproducible method, which does not require any special instrumentation, was introduced (128): Three parameters must be measured; first the total measured area of the electron micrographs (F) and second area occupied by synaptic profiles (f). The f/F ratio is the fraction of the surface occupied by synaptic boutons. f can be measured by a planimeter or by the point counting method. [In the point-counting method (see refs. 120, 121), a random grid or a systematic lattice is superimposed randomly on the electron micrographs and the points that fall over the synaptic bouton profiles are counted. Their total number divided by the total points on the grid gives the percentage of synaptic boutons in the measured area (f/F).] The third parameter to be measured is the number of synaptic profiles on the electron micrographs (n). The final equation: *the packing density of boutons* $= f/F{:}\beta\sqrt{f^3/n}$, which can be expressed as $n/1000$ μm^3. [β is a shape coefficient; its value is about 1.382 (129).]

2.   The *packing density of presynaptic boutons* includes all boutons independent of whether or not synaptic contact (cleft) is visible on the section. Since not all bouton-shape varicosities form synaptic contacts, or, contrariwise, since some boutons are apposed to more than one postsynaptic element, the bouton density may not equal the synapse density. By counting the number of synaptic boutons and measuring the

length of synaptic membranes and the total perimeter of the boutons, the actual number of synapses per unit area can be calculated (129).

3. The *synaptic bouton/cell ratio* represents the main goal of light and electron microscopic quantitative analysis of neuronal afferents to a single cell or to a brain nucleus. The synaptic bouton density divided by cell-packing density (see Section 4.7.1) gives the bouton/cell ratio, which expresses the average number of boutons terminating on a single neuron (128). The ratio is a useful measure for determining the number of nerve terminals arising from various brain regions to a particular neuron. In such studies, brain regions are lesioned or pathways are transected and the number of degenerating bouton/cell ratio is determined in the supposed innervating area. In consecutive experiments, afferents from various brain regions to the investigated neurons can be summarized in a mosaic-like manner. By the use of nerve degeneration in combination with immunocytochemistry, the number of projections from certain brain areas to a particular group of immunostained cells can be evaluated (see Sections 2.3.4 and 4.6.4).

4.7.4 Three-Dimensional Topography

This approach is particularly attractive for localizing and reconstructing cells and cell groups in a three-dimensional coordinate system.

1. For the three-dimensional reconstruction of neurons, single cells or cellular elements can be reconstructed by graphic techniques: vertical, lateral, or tilted projection techniques are used on serial sections or serial electron micrographs (130). A computer with an associated terminal screen and plotter is potentially a powerful tool for all kinds of three-dimensional reconstructions. It is possible to extrapolate the three-dimensional array of dendritic fields of neurons. The size and coordinates of the territory occupied by dendrites may provide important parameters, in combination with measurements of synaptic packing density in that territory, to determine neuronal imputs (axo-dendritic synaptic density) to a particular neuron, including its dendrites.

2. To measure the distribution pattern of identified (by histofluorescence or immunohistochemistry) nerve terminals, a two-dimensional quantitative method has been reported (131). Systematic (scanning) measurements by a semiautomatic device and reconstruction in a coordinate system allow the visualization of topographical relations of different immunostained nerve terminal fields to each other or to particular cells or cell groups.

3. Three-dimensional topography of cell groups (brain nuclei) can be outlined according to their packing density. Serial sections are cut and samples are taken at 50 or 70 μm distances. By superimposing a lattice of 50 or 70 μm squares on the projected section, the number of cells (or

cell nuclei or nucleoli) are counted in each square. The cell number/square ratio is classified into categories and marked by different symbols on a contact drawing of the section with the same lattice (132). Cell types in a heterogeneous population can be distinguished from each other according to their shape or size (or the shape or size of their nuclei) by a dot diagram technique (124). On the diagram, cells with small, large, round, or spherical nuclei can be easily separated (124, 132).

4.8 Neurosurgical Techniques

Several types of surgical interventions on the brain are routinely used in neurobiology for different purposes. Brain lesions, pathway transections, microinjections, implantations, cannulations, or electrophysiological recording of nerve cells or neuronal fields all constitute powerful tools of the neurosurgical repertoire. Since all the above techniques have been raised to a high level and in many cases single cells are their target, the knowledge of the fine anatomical topography of the brain became a basic requirement for not only anatomists but for all who adopt these techniques. Anatomically precise and reliable stereotaxic maps are available for the brain topography of birds (133–135); mouse (136); rat (137–142); opossum (143); guinea pig (144); rabbit (139, 145); goat, sheep, pig, cattle, and horse (135); cat (139, 146, 147); dog (148, 149); and primates (150–159). Several other stereotaxic maps illustrate not the whole brain but certain regions (see refs. 160 and 161 for reviews).

4.8.1 Brain Lesioning

Experimentally induced brain lesions have been used in several contexts (see Section 3.2). A variety of methods are available for producing localized damages of the nervous system. The production of fine and reproducible lesions is based on stereotaxic technique. Specific details of these methods have been recently reviewed by Moore (160).

Brain lesions can be produced by mechanical devices including needles, electrodes, and knives, or by other means such as heat, aspiration, ultrasound, and laser. Aspiration is particularly well suited to destruction of superficial brain structures. Surgical knife cuts are principally useful for transection of fiber bundles (see Section 4.8.2). The two most popular methods for producing discrete brain lesions are electrolytic and chemical lesions.

Electrolytic Lesions. This technique utilizes fine needle electrodes capable of discrete (as small as 0.2 mm in diameter) brain lesions by the aid of a stereotaxic apparatus. The size and the shape of lesions depends on the type of electrodes, the size and shape of their free, noninsulated tips, and the current applied. For further details, see ref. 160.

Chemical Lesions. Selective neurotoxin-induced brain lesions have been introduced as a tool in neurobiology during recent years. The advantage of chemical lesions is their relative selectivity.

1. Glutamate and its derivates. Monosodium glutamate rapidly destroys neurons in discrete brain areas (mainly used for lesioning of the hypothalamic arcuate nucleus) when administered subcutaneously to infant animals (162). Brain lesions characterized by intracellular edema and neuronal necrosis developed within a few hours after injection in a dose of 0.5 mg/g. Kainic acid, a glutamate analog, is much more powerful but less toxic than glutamate itself (163). It is a selective neurotoxin for neuronal perikarya and dendrites, sparing axons of passage and nerve terminals. Its selectivity depends on the dose and the type of administration (see ref. 160 for details). Some neurons are very sensitive while others may be totally resistant to any effects of kainic acid. Neurons seem to require a glutamate innervation to be affected by kainic acid. Ibotenic acid, a heterocyclic structural analog of monosodium glutamate, is less toxic than kainic acid and produces more discrete lesions in the area injected locally. It also destroys cell bodies and dendrites but not axons and nerve terminals (164). Neither monosodium glutamate nor its derivatives pass the blood-brain barrier; consequently, only structures outside the barrier can be affected by systemic administration of these substances. This fact, however, is rather an advantage than a pitfall in experimental brain lesioning strategy, since brain structures outside the barrier—such as the arcuate nucleus–median eminence, the organum vasculosum laminae terminalis-preoptic nuclei, the subfornical organ, the subcommissural organ-medial habenular nucleus, and the area postrema-nucleus of the solitary tract—can be lesioned selectively by subcutaneous injection of monosodium glutamate or kainic acid. The penetration of these substances through liquor–brain barrier is also poor; only regions close to the ventricle (e.g., hippocampus, dentate gyrus) could be affected by intraventricular injection. The most popular mode of administration of these substances is stereotaxic local microinjections into brain nuclei. By injection of kainic acid in a small volume (1 nmol/0.5 μl) into discrete brain regions, about 1.0–1.5 mm radius around the needle-tip can be lesioned (160).

2. Neurotoxic catecholamine and indolamine derivates. 6-Hydroxydopamine and 6-hydroxydopa injected intraventricularly deplete catecholamine levels in the brain. They pass the blood-brain barrier, therefore they can be administered parenterally. For increasing the specificity and selectivity of lesions induced by these substances, they can be injected locally into the brain, but in that case, several factors should be taken into consideration (160). The central indolamine neuron system can be lesioned by intraventricular or local injections of 5,6- or 5,7-dihydroxytryptamines.

3.   Selective lesion of hypothalamic ventromedial nucleus can be induced by injections of gold thioglucose (165) or bipiperidyl mustard (166). Lesioning of this area, like its electrolytic lesioning leads to obesity in rats and mice. Further studies are needed to prove the lesioning specificity and selectivity of these substances.

4.   Capsaicin treatment of newborn animals results in a rather selective degeneration of sensory nerve terminals in the brain stem and spinal cord (167). Capsaicin depletes substance P levels in these areas (168), but its substance specificity is relative because it also influences brain serotonin and somatostatin levels.

5.   The duodenal ulcerogenic drug cysteamine (2-mercaptoethylamine) produces a dramatic decline in the content of somatostatin both in the brain and the periphery (169). A single injection of cysteamine (300 mg/kg, subcutaneously) decreases somatostatin levels in both somatostatin-containing cell body and nerve terminal areas in the hypothalamus without affecting the levels of other neuropeptides (170a,b).

6.   Cobalt has been reported to be a neurotoxic agent. Injected locally into the brain, it destroys neuronal perikarya without lesioning fibers of passage or nerve terminals (171).

7.   Certain toxic lectins (ricin, abrin, modeccin) are taken up and transported retrogradely along the axons to the cells. Local injection of these toxins into nerves or nerve terminal areas may result in death of the parent cell, "suicide transport" (172).

4.8.2   Pathway Transections, Deafferentations

Neuronal pathways can be destroyed by electrolytic lesions but knife cuts are proving to be selective. For transecting of discrete fiber systems the knife is attached to the stereotaxic apparatus directly or through a versatile carrier (173). Larger bundles and pathways close to the brain surface can be transected by free hand under an operating microscope. Surgical isolation of larger brain regions from each other can be performed in the same way.

Surgical transections have become popular for tracing neuronal projections. In combination with nerve degeneration technique (see Section 4.2), the terminal pattern of a neuronal pathway can be visualized. By demonstrating the disappearance or accumulation of tracers (see Sections 4.3 and 4.4) or immunostaining (see Section 4.5) in the transected axons or cell body, the whole neuronal network can be mapped.

Knife cuts can be combined with other stereotaxic interventions (lesions, injections, electrophysiological recording) simultaneously or subsequently. The main goal of subsequent manipulations, so-called "two-step lesions," is that the possible effect of lesioning fibers of passage can be eliminated by the first cut (lesion), and a few days later (during which time fibers of passage have already degenerated) the second lesion (cut) destroys only the local neuronal elements in the lesioned area.

Knife cuts are also used for isolating whole brain areas (e.g., hypothalamus) from other parts of the brain. Those brain regions that are supplied by relatively straight perpendicular blood vessels from the brain surface can be totally isolated—deafferentated—by rotating knives without major ischemic damage (174, 175).

Several designs for microknives have been published:

1. Simple stainless steel knives. A straight, single or double-edged wire or blade is attached to the electrode carrier of the stereotaxic instrument. The edge of the knife may be tilted or L-shaped.

2. "Glass knives." Very fine (0.08 mm thick) knives can be fashioned from histological coverslips with a diamond stick (176). This type of knife may be moved down to the brain free hand, after making holes in the skull according to the exact coordinates. The shape and width of the knife employed depend upon the size and topography of pathways to be transected. Sharp penetration allows perfect separation of brain regions without much additional damage.

3. Rotatory knives. The most popular type of knife in this category was constructed by Halász and Pupp (174). One end of a stainless wire is ground to form a double-edged knife and it is bent to a bayonet shape. The wire itself is inserted into a stainless steel tube attached to the stereotaxic carrier. By the rotation of the knife a bell-shaped cut can be produced in the brain, and with an additional movement of the carrier a dome-shaped cut. By alterations of the shape of the edge of the knife, a wide variety of transections can be produced.

4. Retractable knives. This type of knife can transect fibers with the least additional damage. The knife is a flexible stainless steel wire that is retractable into the electrode tube. During penetration into the brain and during removal, the knife itself is in a withdrawn position in the electrode. The tip of the electrode tube is machined to provide an exit aperture which bends the wire and forces it to emerge at an angle (173, 175).

4.8.3 Microinjections, Implantations and Cannulation in the Brain

The delivery of substances into the brain by microinjection or implantation is a sophisticated technique often used in neuropeptide studies. The technique itself is a very general, non-neuroanatomical procedure, but its useful application for tracing, injecting, or recording from single neurons or localized cell groups requires the use of stereotaxic devices and neuroanatomical orientation in the brain. The history, literature, and practical aspects have been reviewed extensively (22, 23, 25, 177).

Pressure Microinjections. Microsyringes or micropipettes with various diameters on the tip are used: 0.5–1.0 μm for intracellular (177) and 1–10 μm (Hamilton fixed-needle syringes) for extracellular delivery of tracers. The injection unit is attached to a stereotaxic electrode carrier. Substances (0.2 μL or more by syringes, less than 0.2 μL by glass micropipettes) can be injected either manually or by hydraulic or pneumatic pressure (see 25, 177 for technical details).

Microiontophoresis and Cell Recording. By this technique substances are ejected extra- or intracellularly after establishing a suitable voltage gradient between the solution and the tissue. The micropipette is mounted to a micromanipulator and connected to a current source. Recently, high-resistance multibarreled micropipettes with protruding recording electrodes have been introduced. These electrodes have been successfully used for extracellular single-unit or intracellular recording with simultaneous extracellular or intracellular administration of substances by microiontophoresis, and for intracellular staining of single neurons for subsequent light or electron microscopic evaluation (25, 178, 179).

Microimplantations. Various carriers—agar, gum arabicum, silicone rubber, cocoa butter—are used to limit the diffusion of substances injected into the brain. Drugs, hormones, or crystallized dyes can be directly implanted in localized brain areas with stereotaxic instruments. Small tissue pellets from endocrine organs or microdissected brain regions can be implanted or reimplanted. No special instrumentation is required, only a micropipette with a precise stylet and a versatile stereotaxic carrier system.

Microcannulation. In neuropeptide studies, microcannulation has been extensively used for three main purposes: collecting cerebrospinal fluid from brain ventricles; collecting cerebral, but especially hypophyseal portal blood (180); and measuring *in vivo* synthesis and release of neuropeptides by push-pull perfusion systems. In this technique, cannulas are stereotaxically introduced into the brain for single or continuous cannulation when the cannula or its carrier are fixed outside on the skull. By means of a push-pull perfusion system, a stainless steel outer cannula fitted with a removable stylet is implanted into a localized region of the brain of conscious, freely moving animals (181). The particular brain region is continuously superfused with a trace amount of labeled substances. The newly synthetized and *in situ* released substances are collected in serial samples.

4.9 Brain Dissection Techniques

Concentrations of neuropeptides or their precursors or metabolic products can be measured in dissected brain areas by biochemical assays.
Regions of different size can be dissected from fresh or frozen brains or
even from living, anesthetized animals by stereotaxic surgery.

4.9.1 Macrodissection

Large brain regions (over about 2.0 mg wet weight) can be dissected
without a microscope. Brain regions are either separated from each other *in situ* or brains are sliced and regions are cut out with knives or
blades. The brains of larger animals can be sectioned free hand on a
rubber sheet: 10–15 mm thick coronal serial sections from fresh, 3–10
mm thick sections of frozen brain can be obtained. Rat brains can also
be sliced or dissected *in situ* into seven (182) or seventeen (183) major
regions.

4.9.2 Micropunch Technique (184)

The micropunch technique is carried out on frozen, fresh, or irradiated
(to avoid postmortem alterations) brain sections. The thickness of the
section depends on the technique used to cut the brains and the areas
to be removed. Most commonly, the sectioning of frozen brain is
performed in a cryostat at $-10°C$. The optimal section thickness has
been found to be 300 μm. The white matter and the ventricles can be
perceived on frozen sections. The orientation is further improved if the
brain tissue is stained prior to microdissection (185). With suitable
neuroanatomical knowledge, after a short period of practice the topography of several brain nuclei can be well recognized on serial coronal
sections of the brain even without any staining. Available for better orientation are microdissection maps for rat brain (186) and detailed
guides and maps for microdissection of individual nuclei from major
brain areas of rat, such as cerebral cortex (187), hypothalamus (188),
thalamus (189), limbic system (190), or lower brain stem (191). Microdissection of brain nuclei from other animals is aided by a number of excellent stereotaxic maps (see Section 4.8).

Special hollow needles of varying inner diameter (between 0.2 and
2.0 mm) are used for micropunch under a stereomicroscope or dissecting
microscope with 6 to 20-fold magnification. Fresh brain nuclei can be
removed from sections that have been placed on a black rubber plate
(large stopper). Frozen sections are placed on a histological slide and
kept frozen on a cold stage while being dissected. After micropunch, tissue pellets are blown out (or pushed out if a needle with stylet is used)

into a tube and homogenized by microhomogenizers or by sonication. Several brain areas can be punched from a single section, and more than 200 areas can be dissected from serial sections of the brain. Various procedures have been worked out to validate the microdissection by microscopic control of the topography of removed nuclei. General rules and principles, technical details, and practical advice for the micropunch technique have been recently summarized (192).

REFERENCES

1. W. J. H. Nauta and S. O. E. Ebbesson, Eds., *Contemporary Research Methods in Neuroanatomy*, Springer Verlag, Berlin, 1970.
2. R. T. Robertson, Ed., *Neuroanatomical Research Techniques*, Academic Press, New York, 1978.
3. L. Heimer and M. J. Robards, Eds., *Neuroanatomical Tract-Tracing Methods*. Plenum Press, New York, 1981.
4. M. Palkovits, in K. W. McKerns and V. Patic, Eds., *Hormonally Active Brain Peptides: Structures and Functions*, Plenum Press, New York, 1982, p. 279.
5. T. Hökfelt, J. M. Lundberg, M. Schultzberg, O. Johansson, A. Ljungdahl, and J. Rehfeld, in E. Costa and M. Trabucchi, Eds., *Neural Peptides and Neuronal Communication*, Raven Press, New York, 1980, p. 1.
6. G. Tramn, A. Pillez, and J. Leonardelli, *J. Histochem. Cytochem.* **26**, 322 (1978).
7. B. Romeis, *Mikroskopische Technik*, R. Oldenburg, Munich, 1968.
8. M. Gabe, *Histological Techniques*, Masson, Paris, and Springer-Verlag, New York, 1976.
9. J. D. Bancroft and A. Stevens, *Theory and Practice of Histological Techniques*, Churchill-Livingstone, Edinburgh, 1977.
10. V. L. Friedrich Jr., and E. Mugnaini, in L. Heimer and M. J. Robards, Eds., *Neuroanatomical Tract-Tracing Methods*, Plenum, New York, 1981, p. 345.
11. J. E. Johnson, Jr., in J. E. Johnson, Jr., Ed., *Current Trends in Morphological Techniques*, Vol. 1, CRC Press, Boca Raton, 1981, p. 213.
12. A. Peters, S. L. Palay, and H. deF. Webster, *The Fine Structure of the Nervous System: The Neurons and Supporting Cells*, W. B. Saunders, Philadelphia, 1976.
13. A. T. Gyévai and M. Palkovits, *Cell Biol. Int. Rev.* **5**, 773 (1981).
14. H. Klüver and E. Barrera, *J. Neuropath. Exp. Neurol.* **12**, 400 (1953).
15. L. C. Schmued, L. W. Swanson, and P. E. Sawchenko, *J. Histochem. Cytochem.* **30**, 123 (1982).
16. A. J. S. Summerlee, A. C. Paisley, and C. L. Goodall, *J. Neurosci. Methods* **5**, 7 (1982).
17. O. E. Millhouse, in L. Heimer and M. J. Robards, Eds., *Neuroanatomical Tract-Tracing Methods*, Plenum Press, New York, 1981, p. 311.
18. T. W. Blackstad, in L. Heimer and M. J. Robards, Eds., *Neuroanatomical Tract-Tracing Methods*, Plenum Press, New York, 1981, p. 407.
19. A. Peters, in J. E. Johnson Jr., Ed., *Current Trends in Morphological Techniques*, Vol. 1, CRC Press, Boca Raton, 1981, p. 187.
20. A. Fairén, A. Peters, and J. Saldanha, *J. Neurocytol.* **6**, 311 (1977).
21. H. Braak and E. Braak, *Neurosci. Lett.* **32**, 1 (1982).
22. S. B. Kater and C. Nicholson, Eds., *Intracellular Staining in Neurobiology*, Springer-Verlag, New York, 1973.

23. C. D. Tweedle, in R. T. Robertson, Ed., *Neuroanatomical Research Techniques*, Academic Press, New York, 1978, p. 141.

24. S. T. Kitai and G. A. Bishop, in L. Heimer and M. J. Robards, Eds., *Neuroanatomical Tract-Tracing Methods*, Plenum, New York, 1981, p. 263.

25. C. F. Alheid, S. B. Edwards, S. T. Kitai, M. R. Park, and R. C. Switzer III, in L. Heimer and M. J. Robards, Eds., *Neuroanatomical Tract-Tracing Methods*, Plenum Press, New York, 1981, p. 91.

26. L. Heimer, in W. J. H. Nauta and S. O. E. Ebbesson, Eds., *Contemporary Research Methods in Neuroanatomy*, Springer-Verlag, Berlin, 1970, p. 106.

27. J. S. de Olmos, S. O. E. Ebbesson, and L. Heimer, in L. Heimer and M. J. Robards, Eds., *Neuroanatomical Tract-Tracing Methods*, Plenum, New York, 1981, p. 117.

28. F. Gallyas, J. R. Wolff, H. Böttcher, and L. Záborszky, *Stain Technol.* **55**, 291 (1980).

29. F. Gallyas, J. R. Wolff, H. Böttcher, and L. Záborszky, *Stain Technol.* **55**, 299 (1980).

30. E. Mugnaini and V. L. Friedrich, in L. Heimer and M. J. Robards, Eds., *Neuroanatomical Tract-Tracing Methods*, Plenum Press, New York, 1981, p. 377.

31. L. Záborszky, Cs. Léránth, and M. Palkovits, *Brain Res. Bull.* **4**, 99 (1979).

32. A. Parent, L. Descarries, and A. Beaudet, *Neuroscience* **6**, 115 (1981).

33. W. E. Stumpf and M. Sar, in B. W. O'Malley and J. G. Hardman, Eds., *Methods in Enzymology*, Vol. 36, Part A, Academic Press, New York, 1975, p. 135.

34. V. Chan-Palay, in J. E. Johnson Jr., Ed., *Current Trends in Morphological Techniques*, Vol. 2, CRC Press, Boca Raton, 1981, p. 53.

35. L. C. Murrin, *Int. Rev. Neurobiol.* **22**, 111 (1981).

36. W. S. Young III and M. J. Kuhar, in J. E. Johnson Jr., Ed., *Current Trends in Morphological Techniques*, Vol. 3, CRC Press, Boca Raton, 1981, p. 119.

37. S. B. Edwards and A. Hendrickson, in L. Heimer and M. J. Robards, Eds., *Neuroanatomical Tract-Tracing Methods*, Plenum Press, New York, 1981, p. 171.

38. W. M. Cowan, S. I. Gottlieb, A. E. Hendrickson, J. L. Price, and T. A. Woolsey, *Brain Res.* **37**, 21 (1972).

39. J. Kiss, É. Mezey, and M. Palkovits, *Neuroscience* **6**, 2035 (1981).

40. P. Streit, *J. Comp. Neur.* **191**, 429 (1980).

41. D. J. Fink and H. Gainer, *J. Cell Biol.* **85**, 175 (1980).

42. B. Grafstein and D. S. Forman, *Physiol. Rev.* **60**, 1167 (1980).

43. L. Sokoloff, M. Reivich, C. Kennedy, M. H. Des Rosiers, C. S. Patlak, K. D. Pettigrew, O. Sakurada, and M. Shinohara, *J. Neurochem.* **28**, 897 (1977).

44. L. Sokoloff, *Int. Rev. Neurobiol.* **22**, 287 (1981).

45. P. J. Hand, in L. Heimer and M. J. Robards, Eds., *Neuroanatomical Tract-Tracing Methods*, Plenum Press, New York, 1981, p. 511.

46. L. D. Grant and W. E. Stumpf, *J. Histochem. Cytochem.* **29**, 175 (1981).

47. G. Griffin, L. R. Watkins, and D. J. Mayer, *Brain Res.* **168**, 595 (1979).

48. W. B. Warr, J. S. de Olmas, and L. Heimer, in L. Heimer and M. J. Robards, Eds., *Neuroanatomical Tract-Tracing Methods*, Plenum Press, New York, 1981, p. 207.

49. M.-M. Mesulam and E. J. Mufson, *Neuroscience* **5**, 1277 (1980).

50. J. Qu. Trojanowski, J. O. Gonatas, and N. K. Gonatas, *Brain Res.* **223**, 381 (1981).

51. M.-M. Mesulam, in J. E. Johnson Jr., Ed., *Current Trends in Morphological Techniques*, Vol. 1, CRC Press, Boca Raton, 1981, p. 1.

52. M.-M. Mesulam and D. L. Rosene, *J. Histochem. Cytochem.* **27**, 763 (1979).

53. J. I. Morrell, L. M. Greenberger, and D. W. Pfaff, *J. Histochem. Cytochem.* **29**, 903 (1981).

54. J. S. Hanker, L. C. Ellis Jr., A. Rustioni, K. A. Carson, A. Reiner, W. Eldred, and H. J. Karten, in J. E. Johnson Jr., Ed., *Current Trends in Morphological Techniques*, Vol. 1, CRC Press, Boca Raton, 1981, p. 55.

55. Z. S. Liposits, T. Görcs, F. Gallyas, B. Kosaras, and G. Sétáló, *Neurosci. Lett.* **31**, 7 (1982).

56. K. A. Carson and M.-M. Mesulam, *J. Histochem. Cytochem.* **30**, 425 (1982).
57. H. G. J. M. Kuypers, C. E. Catsman-Berrevoets, and R. E. Padt, *Neurosci. Lett.* **6**, 127 (1977).
58. J. de Olmos and L. Heimer, *Neurosci. Lett.* **19**, 7 (1980).
59. H. G. J. M. Kuypers, in L. Heimer and M. J. Robards, Eds., *Neuroanatomical Tract-Tracing Methods*, Plenum Press, New York, 1981, p. 299.
60. N. K. Gonatas, C. Harper, T. Mizutani, and J. O. Gonatas, *J. Histochem. Cytochem.* **27**, 728 (1979).
61. S. Katan, J. Gottschall, and W. Neuhuber, *Neurosci. Lett.* **28**, (2) (1982).
62. P. Somogyi and A. D. Smith, *Brain Res.* **178**, 3 (1979).
63. A. Blomqvist and J. Westman, *Brain Res.* **99**, 339 (1975).
64. P. Somogyi, A. J. Hodgson, and A. D. Smith, *Neuroscience* **4**, 1805 (1979).
65. O. Steward, in L. Heimer and M. J. Robards, Eds., *Neuroanatomical Tract-Tracing Methods*, Plenum Press, New York, 1981, p. 279.
66. N. L. Hayes and A. Rustioni, *Exp. Brain Res.* **41**, 89 (1981).
67. D. A. Steindler and J. M. Deniau, *Brain Res.* **196**, 228 (1980).
68. S. P. Hunt, P. Streit, H. Künzle, and M. Cuénod, *Brain Res.* **129**, 197 (1977).
69. B. Berger, J. Nguyen-Legros, and A. M. Thierry, *Neurosci. Lett.* **9**, 297 (1978).
70. W. W. Blessing, J. B. Furness, M. Costa, and J. P. Chalmers, *Neurosci. Lett.* **9**, 311 (1978).
71. B. Björklund and G. Skagerberg, *J. Neurosci. Methods* **1**, 261 (1979).
72. L. A. Sternberger, *Immunocytochemistry*, Prentice-Hall, Englewood Cliffs, N.J., 1974.
73. F. Vandesande, *J. Neurosci. Methods* **1**, 3 (1979).
74. V. M. Pickel, in L. Heimer and M. J. Robards, Eds., *Neuroanatomical Tract-Tracing Methods*, Plenum Press, New York, 1981, p. 483.
75. A. C. Cuello, C. Milstein, and J. V. Priestley, *Brain Res. Bull.* **5**, 575 (1980).
76. A. C. Cuello, J. V. Priestly, and C. Milstein, *Proc. Natl. Acad. Sci. USA* **79**, 665 (1982).
77. G. V. Childs, *J. Histochem. Cytochem.* **31**, 168 (1983).
78. P. Petrusz, *J. Histochem. Cytochem.* **31**, 177 (1983).
79. M. V. Sofroniew and U. Schrell, *J. Histochem. Cytochem.* **30**, 504 (1982).
80. J. Schipper and F. J. H. Tilders, *J. Histochem. Cytochem.* **31**, 12 (1983).
81. L. A. Sternberger, P. H. Hardy, J. J. Cuculis, and H. G. Meyer *J. Histochem. Cytochem.* **18**, 315 (1970).
82. F. Gallyas, T. Görcs, and I. Merchenthaler, *J. Histochem. Cytochem.* **30**, 183 (1982).
83. M. B. Hancock, *J. Histochem. Cytochem.* **30**, 578 (1982).
84. J. -L. Guesdon, T. Ternynck, and S. Avrameas, *J. Histochem. Cytochem.* **27**, 1131 (1979).
85. S. -M. Hsu, L. Raine, and H. Fanger, *J. Histochem. Cytochem.* **29**, 577 (1981).
86. G. T. Campbell and A. S. Bhatnagar, *J. Histochem. Cytochem.* **24**, 448 (1976).
87. J. Lechago, N. C. J. Sun, and W. M. Weinstein, *J. Histochem. Cytochem.* **27**, 1221 (1979).
88. P. K. Nakane, *J. Histochem. Cytochem.* **16**, 557 (1968).
89. F. Vandesande and K. Dierickx, *Cell Tissue Res.* **164**, 153 (1975).
90. L. A. Sternberger and S. A. Joseph, *J. Histochem. Cytochem.* **27**, 1424 (1979).
91. S. -M. Hsu and E. Soban, *J. Histochem. Cytochem.* **30**, 1079 (1982).
92. T. R. Reaves Jr. and J. N. Hayward, *Proc. Natl. Acad. Sci. USA* **76**, 6009 (1979).
93. M. Sar and W. E. Stumpf, *J. Histochem. Cytochem.* **29**, 161 (1981).
94. C. H. Rhodes, J. I. Morrell, and D. W. Pfaff, *Neuroendocrinology* **33**, 18 (1981).
95. J. M. Lauder, P. Petrusz, J. A. Wallace, A. Dinome, M. B. Wilkie, and K. McCarthy, *J. Histochem. Cytochem.* **30**, 788 (1982).
96. L. -I. Larsson and T. W. Schwartz, *J. Histochem. Cytochem.* **25**, 1140 (1977).

97. T. H. McNeill and J. R. Sladek Jr., *Science* **200**, 72 (1978).
98. A. Ljungdahl, T. Hökfelt, M. Goldstein, and D. Park, *Brain Res.* **84**, 313 (1975).
99. M. V. Sofroniew and U. Schrell, *Neurosci. Lett.* **19**, 257 (1980).
100. R. M. Bowker, H. W. M. Steinbusch, and J. D. Coulter, *Brain Res.* **211**, 412 (1981).
101. J. V. Priestley, P. Somogyi, and A. C. Cuello, *Brain Res.* **220**, 231 (1981).
102. D. M. Lechan, J. Nestler, and S. J. Jacobson, *J. Histochem. Cytochem.* **29**, 255 (1981).
103. T. Hökfelt, L. Terenius, H. G. J. M. Kuypers, and O. Dann, *Neurosci. Lett.* **14**, 55 (1979).
104. T. Hökfelt, G. Skagerberg, L. Skirboll, and A. Björklund, in A. Björklund, T. Hökfelt, and M. Y. Kuhar, Eds., *Handbook of Chemical Neuro-anatomy,* in press.
105. L. Skirboll, T. Hökfelt, H. G. J. M. Kuypers, M. Bentivoglio, C. Catsman-Berrevoets, M. Goldstein, H. Steinbusch, A. Verhofstad, S. Jeffcoate, O. Phillipson, G. Dockray, M. Brownstein, and G. Norell, *Neuroscience,* in press.
106. M. R. Brann and P. C. Emson, *Neurosci. Lett.* **16**, 61 (1980).
107. J. E. Vaughn, R. P. Barber, C. E. Ribak, and C. R. Houser, in J. E. Johnson Jr., Ed., *Current Trends in Morphological Techniques,* Vol. 3, CRC Press, Boca Raton, 1981, p. 33.
108. J. V. Priestley and A. C. Cuello, in A. C. Cuello, Ed., *Neuroimmunohistochemistry,* IBRO Handbook Series, Wiley, in press.
109. P. Somogyi and H. Takagi, *Neuroscience* **7**, 1779 (1982).
110. G. V. Childs and G. Unabia, *J. Histochem. Cytochem.* **30**, 1320 (1982).
111. J. Roth, M. Bendayan, and L. Orci, *J. Histochem. Cytochem.* **26**, 1074 (1978).
112. T. F. C. Batten and C. R. Hopkins, *Histochemistry* **60**, 317 (1979).
113. J. Roth, M. Bendayan, and L. Orci, *J. Histochem. Cytochem.* **28**, 55 (1980).
114. Cs. Léránth, M. Palkovits, and D. T. Krieger, *Neuroscience,* in press.
115. M. Bendayan, *J. Histochem. Cytochem.* **30**, 81 (1982).
116. T. A. Reaves Jr., G. R. Cummin, M. T. Libber, and J. N. Hayward, *Neurosci. Lett.* **29**, 195 (1982).
117. M. Palkovits, Cs. Léránth, J. Y. Jew, and T. H. Williams, *Proc. Natl. Acad. Sci. USA* **79**, 2705 (1982).
118. A. I. Basbaum, E. J. Glazer, and B. A. P. Lord, *J. Histochem. Cytochem.* **30**, 780 (1982).
119. J. Kiss and Cs. Léránth, in press.
120. R. T. DeHoff and F. N. Rhines, *Quantitative Microscopy,* McGraw-Hill, New York, 1968.
121. E. R. Weibel, *Stereological Methods, Vol. 1: Practical Methods for Biological Morphometry,* Academic Press, London, 1979.
122. T. A. Woolsey and M. L. Dierker, in R. T. Robertson, Ed., *Neuroanatomical Research Techniques,* Academic Press, New York, 1978, p. 47.
123. K. Hoshino, *J. Histochem. Cytochem.* **31**, 244 (1983).
124. M. Palkovits and J. Fischer, *Karyometric Investigations,* Akadémiai Kiadó, Budapest, 1968.
125. M. Palkovits, P. Magyar, and J. Szentágothai, *Brain Res.* **32**, 1 (1971).
126. R. J. Sklarew, *J. Histochem. Cytochem.* **30**, 49 (1982).
127. C. Goochee, W. Rasband, and L. Sokoloff, *Ann. Neurol.* **7**, 359 (1980).
128. M. Palkovits, *Brain Res.* **108**, 413 (1976).
129. T. M. Mayhew, *J. Neurocytol.* **8**, 121 (1979).
130. T. W. Blackstad, in L. Heimer and M. J. Robards, Eds., *Neuroanatomical Tract-Tracing Methods,* Plenum Press, New York, 1981, p. 43.
131. L. F. Agnati, K. Fuxe, T. Hökfelt, M. Goldstein, and S. L. Jeffcoate, *J. Histochem. Cytochem.* **25**, 1222 (1977).
132. M. Palkovits, *Acta Morph. Acad. Sci. Hung.* **23**, 283 (1975).
133. A. van Tienhoven and L. P. Juhász, *J. Comp. Neurol.* **118**, 185 (1972).

134. H. J. Karten and W. Hodos, *A Stereotaxic Atlas of the Brain of the Pigeon (Columba livia)*, Johns Hopkins Press, Baltimore, 1967.

135. T. Joshikawa, *Atlas of the Brains of Domestic Animals*, Tokyo and Pennsylvania State University Presses, University Park, Pa., 1968.

136. R. L. Sidman, J. B. Angevine Jr., and E. Taber Pierce, *Atlas of the Mouse Brain and Spinal Cord*, Harvard University Press, Cambridge, Mass., 1971.

137. J. de Groot, *The Rat Brain in Stereotaxic Coordinates*, North-Holland Medical Press, Amsterdam, 1963.

138. J. F. König and R. A. Klippel, *The Rat Brain: a Stereotaxic Atlas of the Forebrain and Lower Parts of the Brain Stem*, Williams and Wilkins, Baltimore, 1963.

139. E. Fifkova and J. Marsala, in J. Bures, M. Petráir, and J. Zachar, Eds., *Electrophysiological Methods in Biological Research*, Academic Press, New York, 1967, p. 653.

140. L. J. Pellegrino, A. S. Pellegrino, and A. J. Cushman, *A Stereotaxic Atlas of the Rat Brain*, 2nd ed., Plenum Press, New York, 1979.

141. E. L. Simson, A. P. Jones, and R. M. Gold, *Brain Res. Bull.* **6**, 297 (1981).

142. G. Paxinos and C. Watson, *The Rat Brain in Stereotaxic Coordinates*, Academic Press, Sydney, 1982.

143. E. Oswaldo-Cruz and C. E. Rocha-Miranda, *The Brain of the Opossum (Didelphis marsupialis): A Cytoarchitectonic Atlas in Stereotaxic Coordinates*, Inst. Biotisica Univ. Fed. do Rio de Janeiro, Rio de Janeiro, 1968.

144. T. J. Luparello, *Stereotaxic Atlas of the Forebrain of the Guinea Pig*, Williams and Wilkins, Baltimore, 1967.

145. M. Monnier and H. Gangloff, *Atlas for Stereotaxic Brain Research on the Conscious Rabbit*, Elsevier, Amsterdam, 1961.

146. R. S. Snider and W. T. Niemer, *A Stereotaxic Atlas of the Cat Brain*, University of Chicago Press, Chicago, 1961.

147. W. J. C. Verhaart, *A Stereotaxic Atlas of the Brain of the Cat*, Van Gorcum, Assen, 1964.

148. R. K. S. Lim, C. Liu, and R. Moffitt, *A Stereotaxic Atlas of the Dog's Brain*, Thomas, Springfield, Ill., 1960.

149. S. Dua-Sharma, S. Sharma, and H. L. Jacobs, *The Canine Brain in Stereotaxic Coordinates*, MIT Press, Cambridge, Mass., 1970.

150. J. Tigges and T. R. Shantha, *A Stereotaxic Brain Atlas of the Tree Shrew (Tupaia glis)*, Williams and Wilkins, Baltimore, 1969.

151. H. Stephan, G. Baron, and W. K. Schwerdtfeger, *The Brain of the Common Marmoset (Collithrix jacchus): A Stereotaxic Atlas*, Springer Verlag, Berlin, 1980.

152. J. A. Gergen and P. D. MacLean, *A Stereotaxic Atlas of the Squirrel Monkey's Brain (Saimiri sciureus)*, U.S. Public Health Service Publ. No. 933, Washington, D.C., 1962.

153. R. Emmers and K. Akert, *A Stereotaxic Atlas of the Brain of the Squirrel Monkey (Saimiri sciureus)*, University of Wisconsin Press, Madison, 1963.

154. E. Eidelberg and C. A. Saldias, *J. Comp. Neurol.* **115**, 103 (1960).

155. S. L. Manocha, R. T. Shantha, and G. H. Bourne, *A Stereotaxic Atlas of the Brain of the Cebus (Cebus apella) Monkey*, Oxford University Press, Oxford, 1968.

156. T. R. Shantha, S. L. Manocha, and G. H. Bourne, *A Stereotaxic Atlas of the Java Monkey Brain (Macaca irus)*, Williams and Wilkins, Baltimore, 1968.

157. R. S. Snider and J. C. Lee, *A Stereotaxic Atlas of the Monkey Brain (Macaca mulatta)*, University of Chicago Press, Chicago, 1961.

158. M. R. de Lucchi, B. J. Dennis, and W. R. Adey, *A Stereotaxic Atlas of the Chimpanese Brain (Pan satyrus)*, University of California Press, Berkeley–Los Angeles, 1965.

159. R. Davis and R. D. Huffman, *A Stereotaxic Atlas of the Brain of the Baboon (Papio)*, University of Texas Press, Austin, 1968.

160. R. Y. Moore, in L. Heimer and M. J. Robards, Eds., *Neuroanatomical Tract-Tracing Methods*, Plenum Press, New York, 1981, p. 55.
161. M. Palkovits, in T. C. Jones, Ed., *Monographs on Pathology of Laboratory Animals*, Springer Verlag, Berlin, 1983.
162. J. W. Olney, *Science* **164**, 719 (1969).
163. J. W. Olney, V. Rhee, and O. L. Ho, *Brain Res.* **77**, 507 (1974).
164. R. Schwarcz, T. Hökfelt, K. Fuxe, G. Jonsson, M. Goldstein, and L. Terenius, *Exp. Brain Res.* **37**, 199 (1979).
165. N. B. Marshall, R. J. Barrnett, and J. Mayer, *Proc. Soc. Exp. Biol. Med.* **90**, 240 (1955).
166. R. J. Rutman, F. S. Lewis, and W. D. Bloomer, *Science* **153**, 1000 (1966).
167. G. Jancsó and E. Kiraly, *J. Comp. Neurol.* **190**, 781 (1980).
168. R. Gamse, P. Holzer, and F. Lembeck, *Br. J. Pharmacol.* **68**, 207 (1980).
169. S. Szabo and S. Reichlin, *Endocrinology* **109**, 2255 (1981).
170. a) M. Palkovits, M. J. Brownstein, L. E. Eiden, M. C. Beinfeld, J. Russell, A. Arimura, and S. Szabo, *Brain Res.* **240**, 178 (1982). b) S. M. Sagar, D. Landry, W.J. Millard, T. M. Badger, M. A. Arnold, J. B. Martin, *J. Neurosci.* **2**, 225 (1982)
171. J. G. Malpeli and B. D. Burch, *Neurosci. Lett.* **32**, 29 (1982).
172. R. G. Wiley, W. W. Blessing, and D. J. Reis, *Science* **216**, 889 (1982).
173. C. W. Scouten, C. F. Cegavske, and L. Rozboril, *Physiol. Behav.* **26**, 1115 (1981).
174. B. Halász and L. Pupp, *Endocrinology* **77**, 553 (1965).
175. L. Voloschin, S. A. Joseph, and K. M. Knigge, *Neuroendocrinology* **3**, 387 (1968).
176. M. Palkovits, L. Tapia-Aroncibia, C. Kordon, and J. Epelbaum, *Brain Res.* **250**, 223 (1982).
177. C. D. Woody, C. E. Ribak, M. Sakai, H. Sakai, and B. Swartz, in J. E. Johnson Jr., Ed., *Current Trends in Morphological Techniques*, Vol. 2, CRC Press, Boca Raton, 1981, p. 219.
178. A. Dray, G. Marschall, and R. D. Pinnock, *J. Neurosci. Methods* **5**, 121 (1982).
179. J. T. Haskins and R. L. Moss, *Brain Res. Bull.* **7**, 479 (1981).
180. J. C. Porter and K. R. Smith, *Endocrinology* **81**, 1182 (1967).
181. J. E. Levine and V. R. Ramirez, *Endocrinology* **107**, 1782 (1980).
182. J. Glowinski and L. L. Iversen, *J. Neurochem.* **13**, 655 (1966).
183. W. H. Gispen, P. Schotman, and E. R. de Kloet, *Neuroendocrinology* **9**, 285 (1972).
184. M. Palkovits, *Brain Res.* **59**, 449 (1973).
185. R. E. Zigmond and Y. Ben-Ari, *J. Neurochem.* **26**, 1285 (1976).
186. M. Palkovits, *Guide and Map for the Isolated Removal of Individual Cell Groups from the Rat Brain*, Akadémiai Kiadó, Budapest, 1980 (Hungarian text).
187. M. Palkovits, L. Záborszky, M. J. Brownstein, M. I. K. Fekete, J. P. Herman, and B. Kanyicska, *Brain Res. Bull.* **4**, 593 (1979).
188. M. Palkovits, in W. E. Stumpf and L. D. Grant, Eds., *Topographical Neuroendocrinology*, S. Karger, Basel, 1975, p. 72.
189. M. J. Brownstein, R. M. Kobayashi, M. Palkovits, and J. M. Saavedra, *J. Neurochem.* **24**, 35 (1975).
190. M. Palkovits, J. M. Saavedra, R. M. Kobayashi, and M. J. Brownstein, *Brain Res.* **79**, 443 (1974).
191. M. Palkovits, M. J. Brownstein, and J. M. Saavedra, *Brain Res.* **80**, 237 (1974).
192. M. Palkovits and M. J. Brownstein, in A. C. Cuello, Ed., *Methods in the Neuroscience, Brain Microdissection Techniques*, International Brain Research Organization Handbook Series, Wiley, Chichester, 1983.

23

Electrophysiological Techniques

YUH NUNG JAN

LILY YEH JAN

Department of Physiology
School of Medicine
University of California, San Francisco

1   INTRODUCTION

The recent discovery of many bioactive peptides in the nervous system
constitutes a major development in neurobiology. These peptides are
contained in distinct neuronal pathways, and are often concentrated in
nerve terminals (1). The release of peptides upon stimulation of peptide-
containing pathways has been demonstrated in several cases (e.g., 2, 3).
Thus, peptides may play important roles in intercellular communication,
plausibly functioning as neurotransmitters (4–8), hormones (9), or tropic
factors (10). In this chapter, we focus on the possibility that peptides act
as neurotransmitters. This subject has been studied and reviewed extensively in recent years (4–8), and we do not attempt to review the
electrophysiological studies to date but instead concentrate on methodology and some general features that may be characteristic of peptide
actions.

1.1   Criteria for Transmitter: "Classic" Definition

To discuss the possible transmitter roles of peptides, it is important to
provide a definition for the term "transmitter." Until recently, transmitters were generally thought to operate in a stereotyped fashion, exemplified by acetylcholine at the vertebrate neuromuscular junction (11). A
transmitter substance is liberated by presynaptic nerve terminals. These
molecules diffuse across a narrow synaptic gap of several hundred ang-
stroms, and act upon the postsynaptic membrane. The effects of transmitters on the postsynaptic cell involve rapid changes, which usually
include an increase in the membrane conductance to one or more ions.
The liberated transmitters are promptly removed either by enzyme degradation or through a reuptake system into the presynaptic terminal.
This narrow definition of transmitter requires that its action be highly
localized to the synaptic regions and that the duration of the action be
brief, in the order of milliseconds. Such a "classical" transmitter action
is clearly distinct from the action of hormones. But from recent experiments on the central and peripheral nervous system, it becomes increasingly clear that putative transmitters may be capable of a wide
range of actions. In fact, the duration of action for many putative transmitters, including amines and perhaps most peptides, may be seconds,
minutes, or longer, and the distance between the release sites and their
targets may be as far as many micrometers (12–15). In other words, in
terms of the duration and range of action, there seems to be a continuum between the classical synaptic interaction and the action of hormones. To refer to substances with nonclassical transmitter actions,
some authors prefer to use terms other than "transmitters." The most
common is probably "modulator," but unfortunately, there is no consensus

on its definition and different authors use the term to mean different sets of properties (for discussions of various meanings of "modulator," see ref. 16).

1.2 Criteria for Transmitter: "Broad" Definition

Perhaps it is just as satisfactory to use the term "transmitter" in a less restricted manner. In this discussion we adopt a broad definition: a transmitter is a substance that is released from a presynaptic neuron to act on other postsynaptic cells. The terms "presynaptic" and "postsynaptic" are used without implying the existence of a narrow synaptic cleft between them. A transmitter may act on the postsynaptic cell by increasing its membrane conductance to certain ions, as occurs at the neuromuscular junction (11). Or a transmitter may exert effects by decreasing the membrane conductance, as has been found in the central and autonomic nervous system (see 17, 18). The membrane conductance involved may be voltage-dependent in such a way that the transmitter may alter the excitability of the postsynaptic cell without significantly affecting its membrane potential (for a review, see ref. 19). A transmitter may also act mainly by altering the response of the postsynaptic cell to other synaptic inputs (e.g., 20). In this chapter we focus our attention on transmitter-mediated changes that can be measured with electrophysiological methods. Biochemical changes such as calcium mobilization and altered adenylate cyclase activities are dealt with by Chang and Cuatrecasas in Chapter 25.

Given this broad definition of transmitter, the minimal criteria for a substance to qualify as a transmitter are:

1. The substance is present in the presynaptic cell.
2. The substance is released from the presynaptic cell upon stimulation and depolarization.
3. The substance produces physiological changes in the postsynaptic cell identical with those produced by stimulating the presynaptic cell.
4. Antagonists of the substance must also block the nerve-evoked response.

The last two criteria are usually examined in physiological experiments. In Section 2 we discuss the methods and approaches used with regard to their ability to reveal the physiological effects of peptides. In Section 3 we discuss some novel features of peptidergic transmission.

2   ELECTROPHYSIOLOGICAL METHODS AND APPROACHES USED IN STUDYING EFFECTS OF PEPTIDES

Electrophysiological techniques used in studying the effects of peptides are essentially the same as those used in studying other putative transmitters. Much of the information is obtained from intracellular studies. In this section we review the advantages and disadvantages of several different systems.

2.1   Studies of the Central Nervous System

Electrophysiological studies of the central nervous system have provided valuable information regarding the firing patterns of central neurons *in situ* and the effects of peptides on firing patterns (see 6, 16). However, the intact central nervous system imposes serious limitations on the types of electrophysiological experiments one can do. For instance, because of the lack of precise visual control, pharmacological agents usually cannot be delivered to the exact location desired. And because of the blood-brain barrier, the extracellular environment, such as the Ca^{2+} concentration, cannot be easily controlled. In general, it is exceedingly difficult to determine whether the effect of a putative transmitter such as a peptide is direct. With a few exceptions (see 6, 21) it has also been difficult to probe the cellular mechanisms of their actions.

2.1.1   Brain Slices

Some of the difficulties encountered in the electrophysiological studies of the intact central nervous system can be avoided by using brain slices. This technique has gained enormous popularity in recent years (for review, see refs. 22, 23). Tissue slices have been taken from many parts of the central nervous system (see 18, 22–24). In this method, a slice of brain a few hundred microns in thickness is maintained in a suitable chamber with an adequate supply of oxygenated artificial cerebrospinal fluid. Such a preparation offers several advantages. First, high quality, long-lasting intracellular recordings are relatively easy to make because of the mechanical stability and the possibility of using high-resistance electrodes to minimize damages caused by impalement. Further, the slice technique allows recording and drug applications under visual control. Unlike the situation in working with the intact central nervous system, where iontophoretic electrodes are usually coupled to the recording electrode in a multibarrel configuration, here the drug-delivery electrode can be physically separated from the recording electrode and positioned near various parts of the cells of interest. Another important advantage of the slice preparation is the absence of a blood-brain barrier. This makes it possible to change the chemical composition of the extracellular fluid. There are also disadvantages with the slice technique. A major potential problem is that slicing the brain may remove important nervous inputs from regions outside the slice. In the case of fast synaptic inputs, from a knowledge of anatomy one may have a fairly good idea about the possible omissions in the slice preparation. In cases where transmitters such as peptides may be released microns from the target in vivo, it may not be as obvious what is missing in the slice preparation. Nonetheless, valuable information has been obtained from studies of brain slices. Pharmacological experiments have been done using brain slices to analyze whether a peptide directly affects a particular neuron or affects it indirectly by acting on its presynaptic neurons (see 24–26). It is also feasible to examine the receptor-mediated ionic conductance changes (see 18, 22–24). In situations where the anatomy is favorable (see 27), it is conceivable that one will be able to compare physiological effects of a peptide with those induced by nerve stimulation.

There are several methods for applying peptides to brain slices. Bath application has the advantage of exposing all cells to peptides at a well-defined concentration, if no serious diffusion barriers exist in the tissue. But in cases where the peptidergic receptors desensitize readily, the gradual increase of peptide concentration during bath application may cause desensitization and consequently may elicit only a small peptide response. Desensitization is less of a problem when peptides are delivered in a brief pulse by pressure or by passing current. Possible artifacts associated with these methods are membrane potential changes associated with movement of the tissue during a pressure pulse or membrane effects associated with the transient increase in concentration of ions other than peptides during iontophoresis (e.g., hydrogen ions) (28). The best control for these is to show that the peptide-induced effects are blocked by specific antagonists. In cases where antagonists are not available, one must resort to the vehicle control or to a control showing that application of an inactive analog of the peptide does not produce an effect.

2.1.2 Cultured Neurons

For pharmacological experiments, dissociated neurons in culture offer the advantage of easy accessibility to the neuronal cell membrane. Peptides can be applied under visual control and there are no barriers to diffusion. A wide range of peptide actions have been reported (e.g., 29–32). Even in the absence of any obvious diffusion barrier, the action of thyrotropin releasing hormone (TRH) on anterior pituitary cells (32) and the action of substance P on cultured spinal cord neurons (30) turn out to be remarkably slow. Whether the slow action is intrinsic to the receptor-associated ionic conductance changes is not known. With the recent development of patch clamp, as described below, one may resolve this question by examining properties of individual receptor-mediated conductance changes of cultured neurons.

2.1.3 Patch Clamp

The ionic mechanisms underlying electrical excitability or chemical transmission often involve the opening and closing of ionic channels. From noise analysis, one deduces that individual channels have conductance in the range of 1 to 100 pS (10^{-12} to 10^{-10} Ω^{-1}) and that the average period during which a channel stays open is in the range of 1 to 100 msec (33). With a resolution of 10^{-9} to 10^{-8} Ω^{-1} for conventional recordings using micropipettes, it is impossible to observe directly the conductance change of a single channel, which is 10 to 100 times smaller than the background noise. A technical breakthrough has been made recently by Neher, Sakmann, and their colleagues (34, 35) which allows detection of currents flowing through individual channels within a small patch of membrane. By pressing a clean pipette with steep taper at the very end (and an opening of about 1 μm) against the cell membrane and applying a little suction, one causes direct contact between the cell membrane and the surface of the glass pipette. The resistance achieved with such a good seal is of the order of 10^{10}–$10^{11}\Omega$, or 10–100 GΩ (hence the name "gigaseal") (35). The high resistance of this seal ensures that most of the current originating in a small patch of membrane flows into the pipette, and from there into the current measurement circuitry. If one pulls the pipette away from the cell, a closed membrane vesicle will form at the tip of the pipette. It is possible to "pop" either the half of the vesicle inside the pipette or the half of the vesicle exposed at the tip of the pipette, leaving a patch of cell membrane with its intracellular or extracellular surface facing the content inside the pipette. This patch of membrane can be voltage-clamped so that there is a constant potential difference across it and the ionic composition on either side can be varied. Currents passing through a single channel are usually considerably above the background noise level so that the conductance of a single channel, the period of time during which a single channel remains open, and other kinetic parameters for processes such as desensitization and inactivation can be measured with great precision (36–40).

Alternatively, after the pipette has formed a "gigaseal" with the cell membrane of a small cell (diameter < 30 μm), one can break away the small patch membrane inside the pipette without breaking the gigaseal (35). This allows access to the interior of the cell from inside the pipette, permitting control of the chemical composition of the solution inside the cell. The cell is now clamped to the potential difference applied between the pipette and the bath ground electrode, and the total ionic currents induced pharmacologically or induced by a step in voltage can be measured. Although the background noise is somewhat larger with this arrangement compared with recordings from a small patch of membrane, relatively large single-channel currents, such as those induced by acetylcholine in muscles, are detectable (35).

A crucial requirement for the success of the patch clamp is a clean pipette, a clean solution and a clean cell surface. Cultured cells are ideal for this purpose. Neurons from the central or peripheral nervous system may also be used for patch clamp after the glial processes and connective tissues have been removed by enzyme treatments (35).

Each of the above approaches has its advantages and disadvantages. For instance, although cultured neurons can be subjected to the whole range of sophisticated pharmacological and biophysical analysis, there is always a question about the possible heterogeneity of cells in culture and a question whether the properties of cultured neurons are identical with neurons *in vivo*. By doing comparative studies on the same type of neuron *in vivo* and *in vitro*, one may be able to resolve these questions.

2.2 Studies of the Peripheral Nervous System

The use of simple model systems can circumvent many of the difficulties encountered in studying the effects of peptides in the central nervous system. Simple model systems have proved very useful in the past; for instance, the knowledge of synaptic transmission gained from studies of the frog neuromuscular junction (11) seems to apply to fast chemical transmission in general.

The study of peptidergic transmission may benefit from a similar strategy. A sufficiently simple preparation may permit a rigorous and detailed characterization of peptidergic transmission. Promising model systems are provided by the autonomic nervous system. A number of peptides have been found in the autonomic ganglia (41). Some have been shown to alter the membrane potential and membrane conductance of peripheral neurons. Where intracellular recordings have been made, the peptide-induced membrane potential changes all seem to have a slow time-course (e.g., 15, 42–45). Because of the simple anatomy and easy accessibility of the peripheral nervous system, it is a much easier arena than the central nervous system for testing whether a peptide fulfills the criteria for a transmitter. In several cases, peptides that are present in presynaptic terminals and can be released upon stimulation produce physiological responses similar to those induced by nerve stimulation (15, 42, 44). To give an example of the type of peptide actions found in the peripheral nervous system, we briefly describe two studies on the vertebrate sympathetic ganglia:

2.2.1   Inferior Mesenteric Ganglia of the Guinea Pig

Both substance P-like and enkephalin-like immunoreactivity have been
found in preganglionic fibers. A substance P-like peptide may be the
transmitter for a slow synaptic potential lasting for minutes in ganglion
cells because (i) the substance P-like material is present in the ganglia;
denervation causes its diminution in the ganglia and a concomitant accumulation in the proximal segment of the lumbar splanchnic nerve; (ii)
there is a calcium-dependent release of the substance P-like immunoreactivity when the ganglia are immersed in solutions with a high concentration of potassium; (iii) substance P acts directly on ganglion cells and
causes an increase in membrane resistance and a slow depolarization
(44). Enkephalins, unlike substance P, cause a prolonged presynaptic inhibition of both the release of acetylcholine (45) and a noncholinergic
slow synaptic potential (44). This effect is mimicked by stimulation of
preganglionic fibers. Naloxone antagonizes both the nerve-evoked and
the enkephalin-induced presynaptic inhibition. Presynaptic inhibitory
function has been ascribed to enkephalins in both central and peripheral nervous system. For example, opiates and enkephalins are thought to
act on nociceptive afferent terminals and reduce transmitter release
from these sensory neurons (46). The mammalian inferior mesenteric
ganglion appears to be an excellent model system for an in-depth study
of enkephalin actions.

2.2.2   Paravertebral Sympathetic Ganglia of the Frog

Frog sympathetic ganglia have been a favorite preparation of many
physiologists over the years (e.g., 13–17, 47–52). Neurons in these ganglia are divided into two groups according to their size and innervation
(Figure 1; 50). The large cells with fast-conducting axons are called B
cells. The smaller cells with more slowly conducting axons are called C
cells (51). A major attraction of this preparation is that in spite of the
structural simplicity, the ganglionic neurons exhibit four different types
of synaptic potentials with time courses ranging from milliseconds to
minutes (Figure 2; 48–51). One can therefore, study not only mechanisms
of fast and slow chemical transmission but also interactions between
different synaptic responses in these ganglia (13–17, 47–53). Of the four
types of synaptic potentials, three are mediated by acetylcholine: (i) the
nicotinic fast excitatory post-synaptic potential (epsp) (lasting for 30–50
msec) (48), (ii) the muscarinic slow inhibitory post-synaptic potential
(ipsp) (lasting 1–2 sec) (49, 50, 53), and (iii) the muscarinic slow epsp
(lasting 30–60 sec) (49, 50). The slowest synaptic potential, lasting for
minutes, was discovered by Nishi and Koketsu (49) and named the "late
slow epsp." Recently, it has been shown that the late slow epsp is prob-

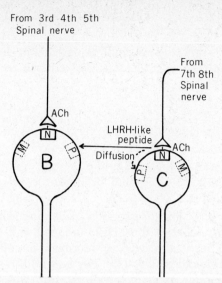

Figure 1. Scheme of innervation of neurons in 9th or 10th ganglia. Cholinergic axons for B neurons arise from the 3rd, 4th, and 5th spinal nerves; preganglionic fibers for C cells come through the 7th and 8th spinal nerves. LHRH-positive nerve terminals are present only on C cells. Most likely both the LHRH-like peptide and acetylcholine are contained and released from the same preganglionic fibers for C cells. N, nicotinic cholinergic receptors; M, muscarinic cholinergic receptors; P, peptidergic receptors. Of the three receptor types, the nicotinic cholinergic receptors have been localized. They are situated right in opposition to the synaptic boutons. (75). From L. Y. Jan and Y. N. Jan (15).

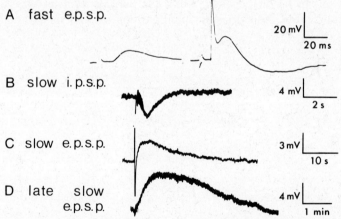

Figure 2. Four types of synaptic signals in the 10th sympathetic ganglion recorded with intracellular electrodes. (A) A single nerve stimulus initiates a subthreshold epsp (left); with stronger stimulation (right), a second, larger epsp produces an impulse. (B) Slow ipsp on stimulation of central portions of 7th and 8th spinal nerves (13 stimuli at 20/sec). The fast epsp was blocked by 1 μM dihydro β-erythroidine. (C) Four stimuli at 50/sec to sympathetic chain above the 7th ganglion result in a slow epsp lasting about 30 sec. The initial rapid deflections are four large conducted impulses. (D) Late slow epsp (300 sec duration) on stimulation of the 7th and 8th spinal nerves (50 stimuli at 10/sec). Note different time scales. No drugs were used in A, C, and D. Upstroke of impulse in A has been touched up. From Y. N. Jan et al. (54).

ably mediated by a peptide resembling luteinizing hormone releasing hormone (LHRH) (15, 54–56). The minimal criteria for transmitters are fulfilled in this case:

1. The LHRH-like material is present in preganglionic nerve terminals (54, 56).
2. There is release of the LHRH-like peptide following either nerve stimulation or high potassium treatment, a release that requires calcium (15, 54).
3. LHRH acts directly on ganglion cells and mimics the nerve-evoked response: Both the LHRH-induced and the nerve-evoked response are associated with an increase in membrane resistance and membrane excitability (55). Further, both responses varied in a parallel manner upon hyperpolarization and depolarization of the membrane potential (15, 55).
4. Antagonists of LHRH block both the LHRH-induced and nerve-evoked responses (55) (Figure 3).

Studies from model systems such as those mentioned above have revealed some novel features of peptidergic transmission. These features may turn out to be properties general for peptide transmitters. Some of these features and their possible implications are discussed in the next section.

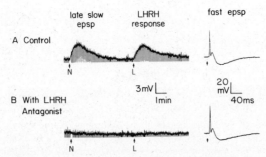

Figure 3. Effect of bath application of an antagonist of LHRH on the late slow epsp (*N*), the LHRH-induced response (*L*), and the cholinergic fast epsp. Applying an antagonist, [D-pGlu[1], D-Phe[2], D-Trp[3,6]]-LHRH, to the bathing medium to a final concentration of 10^{-5} *M* had no effect on the membrane potential, the membrane resistance, or the cholinergic fast epsp but completely blocked both the late slow epsp and the LHRH-induced response. From L. Y. Jan and Y. N. Jan (15).

3   SOME POSSIBLY GENERAL FEATURES OF PEPTIDERGIC TRANSMISSION

3.1   Diffusion of the Peptidergic Transmitters

A surprising observation made in the frog sympathetic ganglia is that the peptidergic synaptic boutons are localized only on C cells (56). As mentioned in Section 2.2.2, the sympathetic ganglia contain two types of neurons, B cells and C cells, interspersed in the 9th and 10th ganglia, the last two ganglia in the sympathetic chain. All the neurons have both cholinergic and peptidergic synaptic potentials. The cholinergic synaptic boutons on B cells arise from preganglionic fibers contained in the 3rd, 4th and 5th spinal nerves, and the synaptic boutons on C cells arise from preganglionic fibers contained in the 7th and 8th spinal nerves (15, 50) (Figure 1). Sectioning of the sympathetic chain rostal to the 7th ganglion removed all nerve terminals on B cells but did not eliminate the peptidergic synaptic response on B cells (15, 56). Therefore, B cells must be able to respond to LHRH-like peptide released from peptidergic terminals on C cells, which are microns away. This conclusion is supported by physiological experiments. Applying antagonists of LHRH onto a B cell during a nerve-evoked peptidergic response caused the slow potential to be truncated (15), indicating that for many seconds the peptide transmitters are still on or in the vicinity of the receptor (Figure 4).

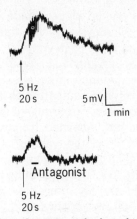

Figure 4.   Effect of an antagonist of LHRH on the late show epsp. After a late slow epsp was initiated by stimulating the 7th and 8th spinal nerves at 5 Hz for 20 sec pressure, application of [Ac-$\triangle^3$-Pro^1, pF-D-Phe^2, D-Trp^{3,6}]-LHRH, an antagonist of LHRH (1 lb/sq in., 25 sec), reduced both the amplitude and the duration of the late slow epsp. The antagonist by itself has no effect on the membrane potential of this cell. Notice that the spontaneously occurring action potentials during the late slow epsp were also eliminated. From L. Y. Jan and Y. N. Jan (15).

Is the long-range and long-lasting action of the peptidergic transmitters a general feature of peptidergic transmission? Although there is not much evidence for this hypothesis, the present data are compatible with it: (i) For a peptide to diffuse for a distance of a few cell diameters (tens of microns) takes several seconds (assuming free diffusion) or longer. Hence, a peptidergic response must take at least several seconds to reach its peak level if it is produced by peptides released within tens of microns from the postsynaptic cell membrane. In a number of autonomic ganglia where peptides are suspected of mediating some of the synaptic potentials, almost without exception those responses are slow in onset (hundreds of msec) and take seconds to reach their peak (15, 42–45, 55). (ii) If peptides can diffuse for microns before acting, they must be effective at very low concentrations. This requires that peptide receptors have relatively high affinity for the ligands. Indeed, the dissociation constants for peptidergic receptors were found to be in the range of 10^{-10}–10^{-9} M (e.g., 5, 6, 57–59), which is 10^3–10^4 times lower than that of classical transmitters such as acetylcholine and amino acids.

Suppose that, in general, peptide transmitters act in a range intermediate between the focal action of classical transmitters such as acetylcholine and the global actions of hormones, one can imagine that this feature can be used to achieve selective communication between neurons. One usually thinks of precise circuitry of synaptic contacts as the only means by which selective communications between neurons are achieved, especially in regions of the nervous system where several different types of neurons are interspersed. However, in situations where the speed of action is not crucial or perhaps a slower and prolonged influence is more desirable, conceivably the "presynaptic" neurons may terminate in the vicinity of the "postsynaptic" neurons without making synaptic contacts. Such an arrangement would work if the transmitter released can diffuse for a distance of several cell diameters before acting on receptors. Selective communication is possible if different neurons in a given region express different subsets of receptors on their surfaces, so that a transmitter released from the "presynaptic" cell influences only those neurons in the vicinity which have receptors for that transmitter. Intuitively this arrangement seems more economical and conceivably plasticity (i.e., an alteration in response characteristics), might occur merely by an alteration in the type of receptors expressed on the surface of the "postsynaptic" cell. For this type of interneuronal communication to be used extensively in the nervous system without cross-talks between parallel pathway, a necessary requirement is that many different molecules are used as transmitters. Perhaps this is one reason for the multiplicity of peptides implicated as neurotransmitters.

The distribution of the LHRH-like peptide in the frog sympathetic ganglia (56) raises an interesting point: Even in cases where presynaptic nerve terminals make close synaptic contacts on a postsynaptic cell, the action of transmitters released from the terminals may not be limited to cells with which synaptic contact is made. As described earlier in this section, the LHRH-like peptide is concentrated in boutons that make synaptic contacts on C cells. Electron microscopy reveals these synaptic contacts as typical axosomatic synapses in autonomic ganglia (60). The synaptic cleft is about 200 Å wide. There is a mixture of clear-core and dense-core vesicles inside the terminals. However, LHRH-like peptides released from this conventionally appearing synapse can diffuse and act on B cells tens of microns away (15, 56). This example illustrates that one cannot rely on morphology alone to identify all cells that are communicating with a given cell by means of transmitters. For clarification of this point it would be very important to know the receptor localization. For instance, opiate analgesics were found to inhibit substance P release from spinal trigeminal nuclei (2) and cultured sensory neurons (46). This led to the hypothesis that enkephalin-containing interneurons form presynaptic contacts on terminals of primary afferents and inhibit the release of substance P (2). The fact that no such axo-axonic synapses were found (61) was often taken as evidence against the possible actions of endogenous opiates on sensory afferents. However, if inactivation of enkephalins *in vivo* is slow, interaction of enkephalin-containing interneurons and of primary afferents may take place without close apposition of enkephalin-containing terminals to terminals of sensory fibers.

3.2 Peptides and Other Transmitters May Use the Same Ionic Mechanism in the Postsynaptic Cell

Adams and Brown (62) suggested that LHRH acts on the same voltage-sensitive potassium current (the M-current) in frog sympathetic neurons as muscarinic agonists. Although it is unlikely that LHRH affects only potassium currents (55), it is quite possible that both LHRH and muscarinic agonists act on the same channels. In fact, the muscarinic slow epsp was greatly reduced when it was initiated during the LHRH-induced or the nerve-evoked responses, even when currents were injected into the cell to counteract the effect of the peptide on the membrane potential (14, 15, 55, 63). Such interaction between peptidergic and muscarinic responses cannot be accounted for by changes in the membrane potential or resistance but may arise because both responses involve the same ionic channels (62, 63). In mammalian sympathetic ganglia, serotonin and substance P also elicit similar physiological responses in ganglion cells (42, 64). Whether they actually affect the same channels is not known.

Generally, do different transmitters act on the same effector mechanism postsynaptically? If a neuron is influenced by a number of different transmitter substances, conceivably several of them might share the same postsynaptic machinery so that a multiplicity of presynaptic inputs would not require a multiplicity of ionic channels, adenylate or guanylate cyclases, and so on. This possibility raises a note of caution against taking mimicry of physiological effects as the proof for a substance to be a transmitter. The case for it being a transmitter would be much strengthened if one can demonstrate that the natural transmitter and the transmitter candidate act on the same receptor by using specific antagonists or by doing cross-desensitization experiments.

3.3   Coexistence of Two Transmitters in the Same Neuron

The possibility of transmitter coexistence has received considerable attention recently (1, 65). Often a peptide and a "conventional" transmitter are found in the same neuron. For instance, substance P and serotonin are found in the same cell bodies in medullary raphe nuclei (66, 67). They are also found in the same dense-core vesicles in raphe nuclei and the dorsal horn of the spinal cord (68). There is also evidence that vasoactive intestinal peptide (VIP) and acetylcholine may be present in the same autonomic neurons innervating exocrine glands (69). In fact, there are enough such cases to suggest that perhaps as a rule rather than an exception all neurons contain and release more than one transmitter. In frog sympathetic ganglia, both acetylcholine and the LHRH-like peptide are contained in preganglionic C fibers arising from the 7th and 8th spinal nerves. By stimulating these C fibers at different strengths and recording from C cells, we usually see 3–5 different inputs which have different thresholds. As the stimulation strength is increased, each time a cholinergic fiber is recruited, initiating an additional cholinergic fast response, there is a corresponding increment in the peptidergic response. Thus, the threshold of cholinergic fibers correlates well with the threshold of peptidergic fibers, suggesting that the same preganglionic C fibers supply both cholinergic and peptidergic inputs (70).

The possibility that a neuron generally contains and releases more than one transmitter deserves special attention as one attempts to identify the neurotransmitter in a pathway. To give an example, there is good evidence that substance P is contained and released from pain-sensitive sensory neurons (4, 7). Substance P also causes slow depolarization of spinal cord neurons (71). These findings raised the possibility that substance P is the pain-mediating transmitter. There has been much debate concerning why the substance P-induced response is slow (71, 72). It is still possible that the substance P that is released from sensory afferents causes a slow depolarization in spinal cord neurons *in vivo* and that another, as yet unidentified, fast-acting transmitter is released together with substance P from sensory neurons. The development of specific antagonists of substance P would help in resolving these questions. Reports on substance P antagonists have begun to emerge (73). Antisera to peptides have also been used as antagonists, as in the case of VIP (69, 74).

4 CONCLUSION

That peptides are concentrated in nerve terminals and can be released upon nerve stimulation raises the possibility that peptides may function as transmitters. To understand the physiological effects of peptides and the type of signals transmitted by peptides, one often needs information from electrophysiological and pharmacological studies. The autonomic nervous system, because of its simple anatomy and easy accessibility, allows detailed studies of peptide actions. A hypothesis derived from such studies is that peptides probably function as transmitters and in general mediate responses of slow time-course. Part of the reason for the slowness of the responses could be a relatively long lifetime of peptides after they are released from the nerve terminals (75). With the recent development of brain slices, cultured neurons, and patch clamp, investigators may be able to test hypotheses formulated from studies of the peripheral nervous system in the central nervous system. Finally, we wish to stress the importance of the development of specific antagonists for peptides. Given the possibility that more than one transmitter may be released from a presynaptic neuron and that a particular ionic mechanism in the postsynaptic neuron may be activated by more than one transmitter substance, experiments using specific antagonists are necessary before one can ascribe a particular function to a peptide.

REFERENCES

1. T. Hökfelt, O. Johannson, A. Ljungdahl, J. M. Lundberg, and G. Nilsson, *Nature (London)* **284**, 515 (1980).
2. T. M. Jessell and L. L. Iversen, *Nature (London)* **268**, 549 (1977).
3. J. Fahrenkrug, U. Haglund, M. Jodal, O. Lundgren, L. Olbe, and O. B. S. de Muckadell, *J. Physiol.* **284**, 291 (1978).
4. R. A. Nicoll, C. Schenker, and S. E. Leeman, *Ann. Rev. Neurosci* **3**, 227 (1980).
5. S. H. Snyder, *Science* **209**, 976 (1980).
6. L. L. Iversen, R. A. Nicoll, and W. Vale, in *Neurobiology of Peptides*, Neurosci. Res. Prog. Bull. 16, No. 2, 1978, pp. 211–370.
7. M. Otsuka and T. Takahashi, *Ann. Rev. Pharmacol.* **17**, 425–439 (1977).
8. A. N. Starratt, *Trends Neurosci.* **2**, 15 (1979).
9. E. Scharrer and B. Scharrer, *Neuroendocrinology*, Columbia University Press, New York, 1963.
10. T. M. Jessel, R. E. Siegel, and G. D. Fischbach, *Proc. Natl. Acad. Sci., USA.* **76**, 5397 (1979).
11. B. Katz, *Nerve, Muscle, and Synapse*, McGraw-Hill, New York (1966).

12. G. Burstock and M. Costa, *Adrenergic Neurons: Their Organization, Function and Development in the Peripheral Nervous System,* John Wiley, New York, 1975.

13. K. Kuba and K. Koketsu, *Prog. Neurobiol.* **11**, 77 (1978).

14. S. W. Kuffler, *J. Exp. Biol.* **89**, 257 (1980).

15. L. Y. Jan and Y. N. Jan, *J. Physiol. (London)* **327**, 219 (1982).

16. J. W. Daly, B. J. Hoffer, and R. K. Dismukes, in *Mechanisms of Regulation of Neuronal Sensitivity,* Neurosci. Res. Prog. Bull. 18, No. 3, 1980, pp. 325–456.

17. F. F. Weight and J. Votava, *Science* **170**, 755 (1970).

18. J. Dodd, R. Dingledine, and J. S. Kelly, *Brain Res.* **207**, 109 (1981).

19. J. L. Barker, in L. L. Iversen, S. D. Iversen, and S. H. Snyder, Eds., *Handbook of Psychopharmacology,* Raven Press, 1981.

20. W. B. Stallcup and J. Patrick, *Proc. Natl. Acad. Sci. USA* **77**, 634 (1980).

21. I. Engberg and K. C. Marshall, *Neuroscience* **4**, 1583 (1979).

22. P. Andersen and I. A. Langmoen, *Q. Rev. Biophys.* **13**, 1 (1980).

23. R. Dingledine, J. Dodd, and J. S. Kelly, *J. Neurosci. Methods* **2**, 323 (1980).

24. R. A. Nicoll, B. E. Alger, and C. E. Jahr, *Proc. R. Soc. Lond., Ser. B* **210**, 133 (1980).

25. S. Jeftiniga, V. Miletić, and M. Randić, *Brain Res.* **213**, 231 (1981).

26. R. J. Valentino and R. Dingledine, *J. Neurosci.* **1**, 784 (1981).

27. W. D. Knowles and P. A. Schwartzkroin, *J. Neurosci.* **1**, 318 (1981).

28. D. L. Gruol, J. L. Barker, S. M. Paul, P. Marangos, and P. Skolnick, *Brain Res.* **183**, 247 (1980).

29. J. L. Barker, D. L. Gruol, L. Y. M. Huang, J. F. MacDonald, and T. G. Smith, *Neuropeptides* **1**, 63 (1980).

30. L. M. Nowak and R. L. MacDonald, *Brain Res.* **214**, 416 (1981).

31. P. S. Taraskevich and W. W. Douglas, *Neuroscience* **5**, 421 (1980).

32. S. Ozawa, *Brain Res.* **209**, 240 (1981).

33. E. Neher and C. F. Stevens, *Ann. Rev. Biophys. Bioeng.* **6**, 345 (1977).

34. E. Neher and B. Sakmann, *Nature* **260**, 799 (1976).

35. O. P. Hamill, A. Marty, E. Neher, B. Sakmann, and F. J. Sigworth, *Pflüger's Archiv.* **391**, 85–100 (1981).

36. B. Sakmann, J. Patlak, and E. Neher, *Nature* **286**, 71 (1980).

37. R. Horn, J. Patlak, and C. F. Stevens, *Nature* **291**, 426 (1981).

38. F. Conti and E. Neher, *Nature* **285**, 140 (1980).

39. A. Marty, *Nature* **291**, 497 (1981).

40. B. S. Pallotta, K. L. Magleby, and J. N. Barrett, *Nature* **293**, 471 (1981).

41. G. Burstock and T. Hökfelt, in *Non-Adrenergic, Non-Cholinergic Autonomic Neurotransmission Mechanism,* Neurosci. Res. Prog. Bull. 17, 1979, pp. 379–519.

42. K. Morita, R. A. North, and Y. Katayama, *Nature* **287**, 151 (1980).

43. Y. Katayama and R. A. North, *J. Physiol.* **303**, 315 (1980).

44. S. Konishi, A. Tsunoo, and M. Otsuka, *Proc. Jpn. Acad., Ser B* **55**, 525 (1979).

45. S. Konishi, A. Tsunoo, and M. Otsuka, *Nature* **294**, 80 (1981).

46. A. W. Mudge, S. E. Leeman, and G. D. Fischbach, *Proc. Natl. Acad. Sci. USA* **76**, 526 (1979).

47. J. N. Langley and L. A. Orbeli, *J. Physiol.* **41**, 450 (1910).

48. R. M. Eccles, *J. Physiol.* **130**, 572 (1955).

49. S. Nishi and K. Koketsu, *J. Neurophysiol.* **31**, 109 (1968).

50. S. B. Libet, S. Chichibu, and Tosaka, *J. Neurophysiol.* **31**, 383 (1968).

51. S. Nishi, H. Soeda, and K. Koketsu, *J. Cell Comp. Physiol.* **66**, 19 (1965).

52. B. Libet, in C. McC. Brooks, K. Koizumi, A. Sato, Eds., *Integrative Functions of the Autonomic Nervous System,* Elsevier/North-Holland, Biomedical Press, Amsterdam, 1979.

53. J. P. Horn and J. Dodd, *Nature* **292**, 625 (1981).

54. Y. N. Jan, L. Y. Jan, and S. W. Kuffler, *Proc. Natl. Acad. Sci., USA* **76**, 1501 (1979).

55. Y. N. Jan, L. Y. Jan, and S. W. Kuffler, *Proc. Natl. Acad. Sci., USA* **77**, 5008 (1980).

56. L. Y. Jan, and Y. N. Jan, and M. S. Brownfield, *Nature* **288**, 380 (1980).

57. T. W. Moody, C. B. Pert, J. Rivier, and M. R. Brown, *Proc. Natl. Acad. Sci USA* **75**, 5372 (1978).

58. D. P. Taylor and C. B. Pert, *Proc. Natl. Acad. Sci. USA* **76**, 660 (1979).

59. M. R. Hanley, B. E. B. Sandberg, C. M. Lee, L. L. Iversen, D. E. Brundish, and R. Wade, *Nature* **286**, 810 (1980).

60. J. Taxi, in R. Llinas and W. Precht, Eds., *Frog Neurobiology*, Springer-Verlag, New York, 1976.

61. S. P. Hunt, J. S. Kelly, and P. C. Emson, *Neuroscience* **5**, 1871 (1980).

62. P. R. Adams and D. A. Brown, *Br. J. Pharmacol.* **68**, 353 (1980).

63. T. J. Sejnowski and S. W. Kuffler, *Neurosci. Abstr.* **7**, 726 (1981).

64. J. D. Wood and C. J. Mayer, *J. Neurophysiol.* **42**, 582 (1979).

65. T. Hökfelt, J. M. Lundberg, M. Schultzberg, O. Johansson, A. Ljungdahl, and J. Rehfeld, in E. Costa and M. Trabucchi, Eds., *Neural Peptides and Neuronal Communication, Advances in Biochemical Psychopharmacology* Vol. 22, Raven Press, New York, 1980, pp. 1–24.

66. V. Chan-Palay, G. Jonsson, and S. L. Palay, *Proc. Natl. Acad. Sci. USA* **75**, 1582 (1978).

67. T. Hökfelt, A. Lungdahl, H. Steinbusch, A. Verhofstad, G. Nilsson, E. Brodin, B. Pernon, and M. Goldstein, *Neuroscience* **3**, 517 (1978).

68. G. Pelletier, H. W. M. Steinbusch, and A. A. J. Verhofstad, *Nature* **293**, 71 (1981).

69. J. M. Lundberg, A. Angaard, J. Fahrenkrug, T. Hökfelt, and V. Mutt, *Proc. Natl. Acad. Sci. USA* **77**, 1651 (1980).

70. Y. N. Jan and L. Y. Jan, *Neurosci. Abstr.* **7**, 603 (1981).

71. J. L. Henry, K. Krnjević, and M. E. Morris, *J. Physiol. Pharmacol.* **53**, 423 (1975).

72. P. G. Guyenet, E. A. Mroz, G. K. Aghajanian, and S. E. Leeman, *Neuropharmacology* **18**, 553 (1979).

73. S. Leander, R. Håkanson, S. Rosell, K. Folkers, F. Sundler, and K. Tornquist, *Nature* **294**, 467 (1981).

74. R. K. Goyal, S. Rattan, and S. I. Said, *Nature* **288**, 378 (1980).

75. L. M. Marshall, *Proc. Natl. Acad. Sci. USA* **78**, 1948 (1981).

24

Receptors and Second Messengers

KWEN-JEN CHANG

PEDRO CUATRECASAS

Department of Molecular Biology
Wellcome Research Laboratories
Research Triangle Park, North Carolina

1 INTRODUCTION

The wide distribution of neuropeptides in the central and peripheral nervous system and in the gastrointestinal tract as well as other non-neuronal systems have suggested their possible function as neuro-transmitters or neuromodulators in synapses as well as hormones in neuroendocrine, paracrine, and endocrine systems (1). Many peptides have now been found in cells or neurons that also contain classical neurotransmitters (2, 3). This new concept of cotransmission and its possible physiological implications is discussed first in this chapter. In the nervous system, the neuropeptide molecules, once released from the presynaptic storage vesicles, diffuse across the narrow synaptic cleft and act directly on the receptor sites located on postsynaptic mem-branes. In the paracrine system, the peptide molecules diffuse to and act on the adjacent target cells. In the neuroendocrine and endocrine systems, they enter the circulation and are carried to distant target tis-sues. In all cases, these molecules recognize the specific receptors on the plasma membranes of the target cells or neurons and form receptor-ligand complexes, which initiate a given sequence of events. Membrane ionic permeability may be altered, leading to a change in membrane ex-citability or intracellular calcium ion concentrations. Adenylate cyclase activity may be inhibited or stimulated and the intracellular level of cyclic AMP ultimately altered. Such changes eventually lead to a vari-ety of biological responses, the nature of which are dependent upon the particular system involved.

In this chapter we focus on receptor recognition and modulation and the possible immediate events following the initial ligand-receptor event, such as receptor mobility, crosslinking, aggregation, internaliza-tion, down-regulation, and the possible roles of these processes on mechanisms of action. The heterogenous properties of many neuro-peptide receptors are also discussed because of their significance for the differential regulation of given peptide fragments on multiple recep-tor subtypes (4–6).

2 COTRANSMISSION

The evidence to support cotransmission of peptides and amines has been recently demonstrated by immunohistochemical, biochemical, and physiological studies. The costorage and cosecretion of opioid peptides and catecholamines have been investigated extensively. Evidence for the enkephalins/amines dual function in neurons and cells of the amine-precursor-uptake-decarboxylation class include the following:

1. Using immunocytochemical or immunofluorescent studies, Leu-enkephalin-like material has been found in many of the 5-hydroxytryp-

tamine (5-HT) containing enterochromaffin cells of the gut (7) as well as in some chromaffin cells that are known to contain catecholamines, such as the adrenal medullary chromaffin cells (8), human pheochromocytoma cells (9), and type 1 cells of the carotid body (10). Coexistence is also present in noncatecholamine nerve terminals of the adrenal medulla and sympathetic ganglia as well as in small, intensely fluorescent cells and in a small number of principal ganglion cells and various peripheral ganglia (11). Electron microscopic examination of ultrathin slides indicate that enkephalin-like material in enterochromaffin cells of the gut is localized in secretory granular vesicles (7). In the human adrenal medulla and in pheochromocytoma, enkephalin-like immunoreactivity with a granular localization is observed in cells that can also be visualized using antisera specific for the catecholamine-synthesizing enzymes, dopamine-β-hydroxylase and phenylethanolamine-N-methyltransferase (9).

2. The coexistence of enkephalins and their precursor peptides with catecholamines is further substantiated by biochemical analyses of cell and tissue extracts (3). Parallel comigration of enkephalins with catecholamines and dopamine-β-hydroxylase-containing vesicles upon sucrose density gradient centrifugation has been described for preparations from the adrenal medulla (12, 13), splenic sympathetic nerves (14), and human pheochromocytoma (15). In bovine splenic nerves, enkephalins migrated exclusively with large dense-core noradrenergic vesicles on density gradient centrifugation (14).

3. Secretion of enkephalins with catecholamines was studied in parallel *in vitro* by using retrogradely perfused adrenal preparations (12, 16) or primary cultures of isolated adrenal medullary cells (17, 18). In these preparations, cholinergic agonists stimulate enkephalins, enkephalin precursors, and catecholamine release in a Ca^{2+}-dependent fashion. Ba^{2+} is also a potent secretagog for both peptides and catecholamines. High K^+ medium also stimulates the Ca^{2+}-dependent release of both catecholamines and peptides. In all cases, the ratios of cellular catecholamines to enkephalins are close to the ratio in the medium after stimulation with secretagogs. Veratridine can also stimulate the proportional secretion of enkephalins and catecholamines in chromaffin cells. The parallel secretion and the closeness of the ratio in cell and medium after stimulation of both neurohormones are further evidence for their storage within the same particles.

More than a dozen additional cases of amine-peptide or peptide-peptide multiple histochemical reactivity have also been reported (2, 19). Hökfelt and his colleagues (20) have reported the presence of vasoactive intestinal peptide (VIP) in cholinergic neurons and the presence of immunoreactive somatostatin (SS-IR) (immunoreactivity), Met-enkephaline-IR, and avian pancreatic-polypeptide-IR in apparently adrenergic sympathetic neurons. Substance P-IR has been shown to be present in

5-HT-containing neurons in median raphe nucleus (21). Cholecystokinin (CCK)-IR is present in a subpopulation of dopamine neurons in rats and humans (20). Although the physiological role of those multiple coneuro-transmitters or coneurohormones is obscure, there is evidence for the possible coordinative function for secretion and vasodilation of acetyl-choline (ACh) and VIP, respectively, in cat submandibular glands and nasal mucosa (22). VIP-IR is present in the salivary gland in many cell bodies of the postganglionic parasympathetic neurons and in their axons juxtaposed to the secretory cells, the ducts, and the blood vessels of the glands. In cat nasal mucosa, in the parasympathetic ganglion (sphenopalatine), previously assumed to contain only cholinergic cell bodies, it has been shown that 98.5% of the cell bodies display VIP-IR. Removal of the ganglion produces coordinate falls of 70–80% in the VIP-IR and choline acetyltransferase activity in the nasal mucosa. Stimulation of the preganglionic axons leads to release of VIP-IR into the venous flow during the period of vasodilation. Antiserum raised against VIP partially blocks the atropine-resistant vasodilation produced by para-sympathetic activity (22). VIP causes vasodilation and is more active than ACh, but not with regard to secretion of saliva. The vasodilation is atropine-resistant.

Although many neuropeptides may function as cotransmitters in con-ventional neurotransmitter systems, the replenishment and regulation of synthesis appear to be different. In primary cell cultures of isolated adrenal chromaffin cells, enkephalins or their precursor molecules are synthesized through *de novo* ribosomal protein synthesis. Radiolabeled tyrosine or methionine are incorporated into enkephalins (17) and large peptides containing the enkephalin sequence (23) in cultured chromaffin cells. Reserpine treatment depletes catecholamines and stimulates enkephalin synthesis and the incorporation of labeled amino acids into enkephalins (17), a process partially blocked by cycloheximide and acti-nomycin D. When the levels of enkephalins in the nerve vesicles were compared for the proximal, middle, and distal segments of the bovine splenic nerves, vesicular enkephalin content per mg protein did not sig-nificantly differ between the nerve segments (14). In contrast, noradren-aline content increased by 60% per mg protein (14). This observation suggested that enkephalins were synthesized on the ribosomes of the cell soma, packed into vesicles, and transported to the nerve terminal without local synthesis, processing, or reuptake in the nerve ending.

3   RECEPTOR RECOGNITION: HETEROGENEITY AND MODULATION

Among the nearly 20 different known brain peptides, at least 13 neuropeptides have been successfully labeled with either ^{3}H or ^{125}I to a high specific radioactivity. In most cases, successful receptor binding studies with these labeled peptides have been carried out in the presence of peptidase inhibitors such as bacitracin, phenylmethylsulfonyl fluoride, or trasylol or their combination to reduce the degradation of the labeled peptides. For these basic peptides, the inclusion of bovine serum albumin or myelin basic protein to diminish the nonspecific absorption to glassware has often been the key to success. Both rapid wash with filtration method and centrifugation have been used for the separation of receptor-bound ligand from free, unbound ligand. Filtration using Whatman glass fiber has been applied to [^{3}H]TRH (thyrotropin releasing hormone) (24), ^{125}I-bombesin (25), [^{3}H]angiotensin II (26) and [^{3}H]enkephalin (27, 28), ^{125}I-[Leu^8, [D-Trp^{22}, Try^{25}]somatostatin-28 (SS-28) (29), as well as ^{125}I-labeled metabolically stable enkephalin analogs (30–32). Millipore filters have been used for ^{125}I-VIP (33), [^{3}H]substance P (34), [^{3}H]angiotensin II (35), and [^{3}H]neurotensin (36, 37). The centrifugation method seems more popular and has been used in systems with ^{125}I-secretin (38, 39), ^{125}I-VIP (40), ^{125}I-[Tyr^1]Kallidin (41), [^{3}H]bradykinin (42), [^{2}H]LHRH (43), ^{125}I-[Bolton-Hunter]CCK-33 (44–47) ^{125}I-substance P (29, 48–50), ^{125}I-Angiotensin II (51), [^{3}H]angiotensin II (35), ^{125}I-neurotensin (52), ^{125}I-[Tyr^1]somatostatin-14 (SS-14) (53, 54), and ^{125}I-[Tyr^{11}] SS-14 (55). The specific receptor binding sites studied with the above labeled ligands follow the law of mass-action and involve high affinity and reversible binding kinetics. In most cases, the binding affinities of a series of compounds parallel the biological potency. However, detailed analyses of binding affinities have revealed multiple receptor characteristics for many neuropeptides.

The existence of multiple receptors for various neurotransmitters has been well established for many years (4, 5). Based primarily on pharmacological experiments, muscarinic and nicotinic cholinergic receptors, α and β adrenergic receptors, as well as H$_1$ and H$_2$ histaminergic receptors that have distinct functional manifestations and different anatomical localization have been well esta blished. During the past few years, biochemical studies—primarily receptor binding studies with isolated membranes or cells and highly radioactively labeled ligands—have provided information useful in understanding the multiplicity of various dopaminergic (D$_1$,D$_2$), β adrenergic (β_1, β_2), α adrenergic (α_1, α_2), serotonin (5-HT$_1$, 5HT$_2$), adenosine (A$_1$, A$_2$), benzodiazepine and muscarinic receptors. Similar multiplicity has been implicated for many neuropeptide receptors and is discussed categorically below.

Regulatory activities of ions and guanylnucleotide have been well established for many neurotransmitters and hormones (4). Guanosine triphosphate (GTP), a known obligatory cofactor for the hormonal activation of adenylate cyclase activity, often reduces selectively the binding affinity of agonists but not antagonists (or to a lesser extent) to their receptor binding sites. These selective effects have been described for dopaminergic (56), α and β adrenergic (57–60), muscarinic (61), 5-HT (62), and opiate receptors (63–66). Multiple neurotransmitter receptors can be differentiated by their association with adenylate cyclase and its regulation by nucleotides. GTP and GDP decrease the affinity of agonists for receptor binding sites, while GMP and adenine nucleotides are essentially inactive. 5-HT$_1$ but not 5-HT$_2$ (62) binding sites are regulated by GTP, fitting well with the fact that drug potencies at the 5-HT-sensitive adenylate cyclase correlate with their affinities for 5-HT$_1$ (but not 5-HT$_2$) receptors. α_2, but not α_1 sites are regulated by guanine nucleotides (58–60), which corresponds to a possible association of α_2 sites with the cyclase. Similarly, D-1 receptors are those linked to adenylate cyclase, and the binding of [^{3}H]dopamine agonists apparently associated with D-1 receptors is selectively regulated by guanine nucleotides, whereas ^{3}H-antagonist binding is not regulated by guanine nucleotides. Both binding sites appear to be on the same neuron (56). Similarly selective effects are also found with many simple ions. Such properties of many brain peptide receptors are summarized in the following subsections.

3.1 Opiate Receptors

Currently it is believed that there are at least five distinct opiate receptor subtypes (μ, δ, κ, ϵ, and σ receptors) based on pharmacological experiments, while four specific binding sites have been surmised to exist on the basis of receptor binding studies (6). μ, κ, and σ receptors were first proposed by Martin and colleagues (67, 68) to account for the distinct pharmacological actions of morphine, ketocyclazocine, and N-allylnormetazocine (SKF10047). Morphine was believed to behave as a prototypic μ agonist. Ketocyclazocine and ethylketocyclazocine (EKC) are prototypic agonists for κ receptors. The latter two drugs produced withdrawal symptoms different from those of morphine after chronic administration in dogs with chronic lesions of the spinal cord. Like morphine, they produced analgesia, but 20–30 times larger quantities of naloxone were required to antagonize their action. They neither precipitate abstinence nor suppress withdrawal symptoms in morphine-dependent animals, yet they suppress the cyclazocine-induced abstinence syndrome. SKF10047, a prototypic agonist for σ receptors, causes pupillary dilation, increases respiratory and pulse rates, induces canine delirium, and precipitates abstinence in morphine-dependent animals; these properties differ from those produced by μ and κ agonists. δ and ϵ receptors were proposed from studies on isolated mouse and rat vas deferens. Lord et al. (28) demonstrated that enkephalins were more potent than morphine in inhibiting the electrically evoked muscle contraction of mouse vas deferens; the receptor activity in this tissue was ascribed to the action of δ receptor, which distinguished it from the μ receptor system in which morphine is more potent than enkephalin. ϵ receptor was suggested by Schultz and colleagues (69) on the basis that the vas deferens of the rat (unlike the mouse) contained a receptor that was very much more sensitive to β-endorphin than to enkephalins and morphine.

Guinea pig ileum contains predominantly μ receptors since the intrinsic activity of μ receptors is much greater in this tissue. The presence of μ receptors has been confirmed by receptor binding studies using low concentrations of selective μ agonists such as [^{3}H]dihydromorphine and ^{125}I-FK33824, {[D-Ala^2, NMePhe^4, Met (O)^{5}ol]enkephalin}, as well as with selective μ antagonists such as [^{3}H]naloxone or naltrexone (6). For μ receptors, Met- and Leu-enkephalins exhibit relatively lower affinity ligands compared with morphine. Morphiceptin, a tetrapeptide fragment of β-casein, a major protein of milk, has been shown to be a highly specific peptide agonist for morphine (μ) receptors (70). In the receptor binding assay, morphiceptin has an affinity for morphine (μ) receptors that is at least a thousand times higher than its affinity for enkephalin (δ) receptors and benzomorphan binding sites (see below). In the guinea pig ileum, a model tissue for μ receptors, morphiceptin is as potent as morphine. In the mouse vas deferens, a model tissue for δ receptors, it is less active than morphine and 1/10,000 as active as [D-Ala^2, D-Leu^5]-enkephalin, a δ agonist. In the ϵ-receptor-containing rat vas deferens, it is virtually inactive. A peptide analog of enkephalin, [D-Ala^2, NMePhe^4, Gly^{5}ol]enkephalin, is similarly selective for μ receptors (71, 72). Naloxone and naltrexone are potent and relatively selecuive antagonists for μ receptors. Ten to 20 times greater concentrations are required to antagonize the δ, κ and ϵ agonists (73). Receptor binding studies have shown that μ receptors predominate in the hypothalamus and thalamus (32, 73). By *in vitro* autoradiography (74, 75), μ receptors can be differentially localized in layers I and IV of frontal cortex, in cluster areas of the corpus striatum, in the pyramidal cell layer of the hippocampus, in the thalamus and hypothalamus, inferior colliculi, the periaqueductal gray, the median raphe, and the interpeduncular nucleus. Interestingly, high concentrations of μ receptor are found in areas that are relevant to pain sensation or stimulatin-analgesia production, such as the substantia gelatinosa, the periaqueductal gray, the median raphe, the dorsomedial thalamus, and layer IV of the cortex. Such localizations, combined with the evidence from pharmacological studies that μ-selective drugs are more potent in analgesia than δ-selective drugs (76, 77), suggest that μ receptors mediate a major portion of the opiate-induced analgesia. Recently we have shown that morphiceptin, a highly specific μ agonist, produces analgesic and cataleptic activities in rat when injected into the brain, and this can be blocked by naloxone, suggesting that μ receptors also mediate the cataleptic activity of opiates in animals (77). The possible existence of the subcategories, μ_1 and μ_2 receptors, has been suggested by Pasternak and colleagues (78–80). They showed that the saturation binding curves of many labeled opioids, including naloxone, SKF10047, EKC, and enkephalin analogs, showed nonlinear Scatchard plots with a low number of high-affinity binding sites. These high-affinity sites can be irreversibly and selectively inhibited by naloxazone pretreatment both *in vivo* and *in vitro*. They postulated that the receptors sensitive to irreversible naloxazone inhibition are μ_1 receptors because the remaining μ receptors (presumably μ_2-receptors) still retain relatively high affinity for morphiceptin and other μ agonists compared with δ agonists (80, 81).

Delta receptors can be characterized selectively by using low concentrations of either ^{3}H-labeled or ^{125}I-labeled [D-Ala^2, D-Leu^5]enkephalin (31). Some crossover with μ receptor always occurs because of the relatively high content of μ receptor in brain and the slight cross-reactivity with μ receptors. This problem can now be largely overcome by using an unlabeled specific μ agonist such as morphiceptin (73) to "quench" the μ receptor. Several neuroblastoma cells containing relatively homogenous δ receptors have been identified (6). These cells are useful for studies of the molecular and cellular actions of opioids.

By *in vitro* autoradiography using ^{125}I-[D-Ala^2, D-Leu^5]enkephalin (75) in the presence of low concentration of FK33824 (to quench μ receptor), the δ receptor has been shown to be localized predominantly in layers II, III, and V of the cortex, the olfactory tubercle, the nucleus accumbens, the amygdala, and the pontine nuclei, and is diffusely localized in the hippocampus and corpus striatum. Many of the areas found to be rich in δ receptors are components of the limbic system that are associated with control of emotion and reward behavior. It is possible that δ receptors mediate the epileptic seizures observed with enkephalins and the euphoric and affective actions of opiates. Naloxone antagonizes the effects of δ agonists 20 times less effectively than those of μ agonists. Diprenorphine is about equally active against μ and δ agonists (73).

Ketocyclazocine and ethylketocyclazocine are prototypic κ agonists. Mouse vas deferens rendered tolerant to μ and δ agonists responds well to κ agonists without significant cross-tolerance (82, 83). However, after chronic treatment with κ agonnists, the mouse vas deferens develops tolerance to κ agonists but not to μ and δ agonists. It has been shown recently that dynorphin-1-13 displays cross-tolerance to κ agonists but not to μ and δ agonists, thus suggesting the dynorphin may be a specific κ agonist (83, 84), at least in isolated tissues.

It is now believed that the σ receptors may not really be opiate receptors (85–87). The typical σ agonists, SKF10047 and cyclazocine, produce mydriasis and delirium in dogs and hyperactivity in rats (68, 88). These effects are not antagonized by naloxone and may be related to the actions of phencyclidine since phencyclidine and SKF10047 produce similar effects in dogs with spinal cord transection (88). This suggestion is further supported by studies on stimulus-discriminative studies (89, 90). Rats trained to discriminate phencyclidine generalize to SKF10047. Thus, the putative σ activities may be indicative of nonopiate receptor-mediated actions inasmuch as the phencyclidine-like effects are also generally resistant to blockade by narcotic antagonists and reside with the (+) isomer of SKF10047 (90, 91). Furthermore, binding studies suggest that σ agonists share certain binding properties similar to those of phencyclidine, such as relative affinities and (+) stereospecificity, in addition to their opiate receptor activities (86, 87).

Among the above four opiate receptor subtypes (μ, δ, κ, and ϵ), the μ and δ receptors have achieved confirmation from receptor binding studies with labeled selective μ and δ ligands. The existence of a third biochemically identifiable opiate binding site in rat brain has recently been demonstrated by using [³H]diprenorphine after quenching the μ and δ receptors with morphiceptin and [D-Ala², D-Leu⁵]enkephalin (73). The order of ranking of potency for this site is cyclazocine, UM1072 > ethylketocyclazocine, N-allylnormetazocine > morphine, Fentanyl, FK33824 > enkaphalins and their analogs. These sites also bind oxilorphan and butorphanol with an affinity higher than for morphine and enkephalins. Naloxone and nalorphine bind to these sites with an affinity of about 15 nM, similar to that for δ receptors and one-twentieth that of μ receptors. These binding sites have been tentatively referred to as "benzomorphan binding sites" because most benzomorphan drugs in the chemical family of 6,7-benzomorphan-11-ol with bulky substitutions at the nitrogen atom (including cyclazocine, oxilorphan, ethylketocyclazocine, N-allylnormetazocine, and butorphanol) exhibit relatively high affinity.

It is very interesting that, in contrast to other enkephalins, β_h-endorphin binds to benzomorphan binding sites with a very high affinity (92). The apparent K_i value of β_h-endorphin for benzomorphan binding sites is 7.6 nM, which is about 8–12 times higher than its K_i value for morphine (μ) and enkephalin (δ) binding sites and about 100 times lower than that of enkephalins for benzomorphan binding sites. These data suggest that benzomorphan binding sites might be related to the ϵ receptor proposed for rat vas deferens, since β_h-endorphin is a potent opioid agonist in this tissue and enkephalins and morphine are only weakly active (93). Furthermore, ethylketocyclazocine behaves as a potent antagonist in the rat vas deferens (94).

Etorphine binds to both morphine (μ) and enkephalin (δ) binding sites with extremely high (and about equal) affinity (73). It binds to benzomorphan binding sites with about a twentieth of the affinity. The potent antagonist, diprenorphine, binds with about equally high affinity to all opiate binding sites. Naloxone and nalorphine have 15–50 times lower affinity for enkephalin (δ) and benzomorphan binding sites compared with morphine (μ) binding sites. Kosterlitz and colleagues (71) and Pfeiffer and Herz (95) have also claimed that a similar κ binding site can be identified by using [³H]ethylketocyclazocine. However, etorphine, which is believed to have no κ-agonist activity, has high affinity for this [³H]EKC binding site. β-Endorphin also shows high affinity compared with enkephalin and morphine. It remains to be established whether the benzomorphan or the so-called κ binding sites are the same as the κ receptor postulated by Martin. A binding site with similar κ-receptor characteristics has also been identified in human placenta membranes using [³H]EKC (96).

Using ^{125}I-labeled [D-Ala²]β_h-endorphin, we have reported the existence of nonopiate but β-endorphin-specific binding sites (97). A similar nonopiate but β-endorphin-specific binding activity has been described in a neuroblastoma cell line (N18TG2) by Hammonds and Li with the use of ³H-labeled β-endorphin (98).

Both μ and δ receptor are regulated by sodium ions and guanine nucleotides, which differentially reduces the binding affinities of agonists but not antagonists for binding (65). However, guanine triphosphate and GPP(NH)P are more effective in reducing the agonist affinity for μ receptors than for δ receptors (63–66). The report of differential binding properties, designated "type 1 and type 2," with regional variations and differential sensitivity to GTP, probably reflect μ (type 1) and δ (type 2) receptors, respectively (64).

While the heterogeneous properties of opiate receptors emerges from a large number of pharmacological, biochemical, and anatomical studies, the molecular basis for these differences in receptor subtypes still remains unknown. Lee and Smith (99) have proposed a model in which a single opiate receptor provides separate binding regions for enkephalin and opiate alkaloids. β-Endorphin interacts with both sites, thus exhibiting its high potency. A similar model has been proposed by Chavkin and Goldstein (100) for the dynorphin (K) receptor in the guinea pig ileum myenteric plexus. They proposed an N-terminal tetrapeptide pocket (message) and C-terminal potency-enhancing domain (address) for dynorphin receptors. Both would be responsible for the specificity and high potency of dynorphin. Recently, it has become possible to solubilize opiate receptors (101–104). Their eventual isolation and purification may help resolve the hypothesis of receptor multiplicity by providing distinguishing molecular properties such as size, subunit composition, and structure.

3.2   Cholecystokinin Receptors

Cholecystokinin (CCK-33) receptors have been identified with ^{125}I-labeled [Bolton-Hunter (B-H)]CCK-33 (44–47) in pancreatic and brain membranes (44–47, 105, 106). The binding is saturable, reversible and of high affinity. The peptide specificity of the binding is suggestive of a physiologically relevant receptor. [Leu¹⁵]gastrin-17-1, pentagastrin and CCK-4 are 500–2000 time more potent in binding to the brain than to pancreatic membranes (46). This indicates that the CCK receptors in the pancreas differ from those in the brain. Guanine nucleotides also regulate the CCK receptors. GTP and GPP(NH)P decrease [125]I-(B-H)CCK-33 binding to both pancreatic and brain membranes (46). GDP is slightly less active. By contrast, GMP and the adenine nucleotides, ATP, ADP, and AMP, were virtually inactive in reducing binding. But the relative and absolute potencies of GPP(NH)P and GTP differ in guinea pig brain and rat pancreas. The IC_{50} values for GPP(NH)P are 0.7 and 35 μM in pancreas and brain, respectively. GTP was half as potent as GPP(NH)P in decreasing [125]I-(B-H)CCK-33 receptor binding in pancreas, whereas GTP was only 1/16 as potent as GPP(NH)P in brain. These data thus suggest heterogeneity of CCK receptors.

Na[+], K[+], Li[+], lubidium, and cesium were similarly potent in reducing the binding, being twice as potent in brain membranes as in pancreatic membranes (46). Ca^{2+} and Mg^{2+} were roughly equipotent, doubling binding at 5 mM (46).

One of the most interesting aspects of CCK receptors is the ability of dibutyryl-cyclic GMP to compete with the binding of ^{125}I-CCK-33 (45, 105). This effect of dibutyryl-cyclic GMP and various cyclic nucleotides appears to parallel their potency in inhibiting amylase release induced by CCK-33 (45, 105).

3.3 Substance P Receptors

Substance P, labeled to a high specific radioactivity with ^{3}H, was recently shown by Hanley et al. (34) to bind specifically to rat brain membranes. Liang and Cascieri (48) prepared a biologically active ^{125}I-substance P derivative (^{125}I-SP) by conjugating substance P with [^{125}I]Bolton-Hunter reagent, and they showed specific high affinity binding to rat parotid cells and membranes. In both studies, physalaemin, the naturally occurring SP-related peptide, potently inhibits the binding of the radioactive labels. In rat brain membranes, the hexapeptide, the pyroglutamyl substance P-6-11, is more potent than the native peptide in competing for the binding of [^{3}H]SP, which is consistent with its potency in depolarizing motor neurons after application to newborn rat spinal cord. In contrast, in parotid acinar cells, this hexapeptide fragment had only 0.005-fold the potency of substance P, consistent with its lower potency in stimulating salivation (50). These differences in potencies of pyroglutamyl SP-6-11 in rat brain and parotid cells suggest the possible heterogeneity of substance P receptors.

Similar substance P receptors have also been reported in pancreatic acinar cells using either ^{125}I-labeled [Tyr[8]]SP or physalaemin (107). The specific binding of [^{3}H]substance P to phospholipids has also been reported (108, 109). The physiological significance of these binding sites remains obscure since the biologically related peptides, physalaemin, [Tyr[8]]SP and eladosin, all of which are potent analogs of substance P, do not inhibit the binding.

3.4   Neurotensin Receptors

Brain tissues contain specific binding sites of high affinity for ^{125}I-neurotensin (NT) (51, 110) and [3H]NT (36, 37). A similar high-specific binding of [3H]NT to a cell line derived from human colon carcinoma has also been reported (36). Neurotensin induces contraction of the logitudinal smooth muscle of the guinea pig ileum by stimulating the release of acetylcholine. The biological potency in this tissue correlates very well with the binding potency of neurotensin analogs in brain membranes. The binding studies reveal that the C-terminal hexapeptide (NT-8-13) possesses full receptor activity.

3.5   Angiotensin II Receptors

The angiotensin II receptors have been explored extensively in both the brain and peripheral tissues. ^{125}I-angiotensin II(A-II) binds specifically and reversibly to a high affinity binding site in brain (52), adrenal membrane (111), rabbit uterus (52), and primary cultured cells of fetal rat brain (112). [3H]A-II binding has been studied successfully with rabbit aorta membranes (113). Sodium cholate-solubilized angiotensin II receptors have been obtained from rabbit aorta membranes (113).

A large number of angiotensin II analogs have been synthesized. The replacement of phenalanine at 8-position by aliphatic amino acid yields a specific angiotensin antagonist. The angiotensin antagonist, [Sar^1 Leu^8] A-II was iodinated and found to bind specifically to angiotensin II receptors in calf cerebellar cortex, bovine adrenal, and rabbit uterus (114, 115).

Despite the fact that no definitive linkage between angiotensin II receptors and adenylate cyclase has been demonstrated, the angiotensin II binding to bovine adrenal cortex is regulated by nucleotides. The binding is greatly decreased by GTP, GDP, and GPP(NH)P at or below μM concentrations; other nucleotide triphosphates and GMP do not have effects on angiotensin II binding (111). It is noteworthy that the effect of guanyl nucleotides on the reduction of binding was much decreased in the presence of sodium ions.

Bennett and Snyder studied the binding of ^{125}I-labeled A-II and [Sar^1, Leu^8]A-II (the antagonist) to calf cerebellar cortex, adrenal cortex, and rabbit uterus (114, 115). The binding of ^{125}I-A-II to brain membranes and adrenal cortex is greatly increased, 25- or 2.5-fold, respectively, by increasing the sodium ion concentration from 10 mM to 140 mM; [125]I-[Sar^1, Leu^8]A-II is much less sensitive to changes in sodium ion concentrations. Unlike opiate and α adrenergic receptors, the influence of sodium ions upon angiotensin II receptors does not differentiate agonists from antagonists. The effect of Na$^+$ on the potency of antagonist analogs in competing for ^{125}I-[Sar^1, Leu^8]A-II binding does not correlate with their agonist or antagonist properties but is greatest for peptides with aspartic acid at position 1 in the peptide structure (114).

In brain membranes, increasing sodium concentrations accelerate the rate of association but decrease that of dissociation of ^{125}I-A-II. In contrast, in rabbit uterus homogenates, neither ^{125}I-A-II nor ^{125}I-[Sar^1, Leu^8] A-II binding is significantly altered by changes in the sodium ion concentration (115). The differential effect of Na$^+$ on the angiotensin II binding to brain membrane, adrenal cortex, and rabbit uterus tissue suggests the possible heterogeneity of angiotensin II receptors. This is further supported by the many similarities between brain and uterus receptor sites, and by the marked differences between these two tissue receptors compared with adrenal receptor sites. A detailed evaluation of 28 angiotensin analogs indicated that most angiotensin analogs tend to be one order of magnitude less potent in competing for binding to adrenal cortex membrane compared with uterine and cerebellar membranes. Angiotensin II contracts rat aortic strips. Comparison of the potencies of various peptides upon aortic-strip contraction with binding studies reveals that the correlations are much better for adrenal cortex than for brain and uterus, suggesting that the physiological angiotensin receptors in the aortic strip differ from the receptor sites studied in cerebellar and uterine tissues.

3.6 Bradykinin Receptors

[^{3}H]Bradykinin(BK) binds specifically to guinea pig ileum and rat uterus membranes (42). The binding is saturable and is inhibited by a series of peptide analogs related to bradykinin. Over the extensive group of peptides studied, contractile potencies in both ileum and uterus correlate well with the binding affinities for ileum and uterus membrane preparations. Several peptides differ in their uterine contractile effects. For example, [β-(2-thienyl)alanine$^{5,\ 8}$]BK is 10 times and 2 times more potent than bradykinin in contracting uterus and ileum, respectively, and it is similar to bradykinin in its ileal binding affinity. [Hydroxyproline^3]BK and Met-Lys-BK are less than half as potent as bradykinin in contracting and binding to the ileum but are equal to bradykinin in contracting rat uterus. This discrepancy suggests that ileal and uterine receptors may differ in their recognition sites.

Both monovalent and divalent cations regulate bradykinin receptor binding at physiological concentrations. Sodium ions reduce binding to 20% at about 80 mM. Lithium is similar to sodium. K$^+$ appears to be half as potent. Ca^{2+} lowers binding by 50% at 5 mM, and Mg^{2+} is less effective. The guanine nucleotides and the nonmetabolized analogs have no effect on bradykinin binding at 1 mM.

3.7 Somatostatin Receptors

Somatostatin receptors in pituitary cells in culture have been identified and characterized by using ^{125}I-[Tyr^1]somatostatin(SS)-14 (116). Similar somatostatin receptors in rat brain have also been characterized by ^{125}I-[Tyr^{11}]SS-14 (55), [Tyr^1]SS-14 (53, 116), or ^{125}I-[Leu^8, D-Trp^{22}, Tyr^{25}]SS-28 (29). Reubi *et al.* (29) found that SS-28 competes better with ^{125}I-[Leu^8, D-Try^{22}, Tyr^{25}]SS-28 for binding to brain membranes than does SS-14. Srikant and Patel (117) observed that SS-28 exhibited 3.2-fold greater affinity for the binding sites of ^{125}I-[Tyr^{11}]SS-14 in the pituitary, whereas in the hypothalamus and cortex, it exhibited threefold and sixfold lower affinity, respectively. This receptor binding affinity of the peptide correlates well with its reported threefold to 14-fold higher potency for growth hormone suppression in cultured rat anterior pituitary cells. This differential potency of somatostatin cannot be explained by differences in metabolism since somatostatin remains intact in the experimental binding conditions. The differential potency of SS-28 in pituitary and brain together with its different potency for competing with the binding of ^{125}I-[Tyr^{11}]SS-14 and ^{125}I-[Leu^8, D-Try^{21}, Tyr^{25}]SS-28 suggest the existence of multiple receptors for somatostatin, at least in brain.

4 RECEPTOR REGULATION BY LIGAND: DESENSITIZATION

The phenomenon of diminished response during or subsequent to the initial action of a ligand is commonly referred to as desensitization, tachyphylaxis, tolerance, refractoriness, or subsensitivity. This desensitization process has long been observed in a wide variety of cellular systems. Desensitization can be specific or nonspecific and acute or chronic. Specific desensitization is often attributed to events at the level of the receptor itself and nonspecific desensitization to postreceptor events. Acute desensitization develops rapidly and is usually rapidly reversible. Chronic desensitization develops slowly, is frequently slowly reversible, and is often accompanied by true receptor loss (down regulation) rather than the diminished receptor function that is typical of acute desensitization.

Cells and neurons can respond to changes in ambient ligand concentration by regulatory changes in receptor function. Receptors can be altered in a number of ways upon interacting with ligand. Down regulation, the reduction in receptor number in response to ligand, is increasingly recognized as an important regulatory mechanism for many peptide hormone systems (118, 119). This process often involves receptor clustering in specific membrane regions termed "coated pits" (the membrane analog of galactic black holes), from which selective endocytosis occurs with subsequent degradation or delivery to lysosomes or other intracellular organelles (120). This is described in more detail in Section 7. Conformational changes in the binding site itself can lead to increased affinity and prolonged receptor occupancy (121–124). Receptor transformation to a low affinity state has also been postulated (124). In addition, cryptic receptors and receptor shedding can also occur. Little information regarding these processes is available for brain peptides, and we will focus our attention on opiate receptor systems.

Chronic treatment with opiates leads to the development of tolerance and dependence. Some receptor binding studies, employing different approaches, have suggested that neither receptor number nor affinity are grossly altered and that the main adaptive responses to chronic opiate actions do not occur at the level of receptor recognition site but rather at a more distal process (125). The development of a nonspecific supersensitivity to neurotransmitters that have opposing effects has been postulated (126). Other hypotheses include the proposition that rebound increases in the release of neurotransmitters can occur (127).

The development of selective tolerance has recently been demonstrated in the mouse vas deferens, which contains μ, δ, and κ receptors (82, 83, 128). Animals treated chronically with [D-Ala^2, D-Leu^5]enkephalin (a δ agonist) or sulphentanyl (a μ agonist) or EKC (a κ agonist), through the use of osmotic minipumps, demonstrate that chronic treatment with [D-Ala^2, D-Leu^5]enkephalin results in a high degree of tolerance to δ agonists but not to μ or κ agonists, and that sulphentanyl treatment results in selective tolerance to μ agonists with little change in sensitivity to δ and κ agonists. Similarly, chronic EKC treatment leads to selective tolerance for κ agonists and dynorphin. These findings suggest that very specific changes occur at the receptor level.

With a neuroblastoma cell line containing a relatively homogenous enkephalin (δ) receptor, we have been able to show a specific loss (down regulation) of enkephalin receptors after treatment with an opioid peptide (129, 130). This effect is dependent on time, temperature, and dose. It appears to be specific to opioid peptides. Leu-, Met-, [D-Ala^2, D-Leu^5]enkephalin, [D-Ala^2, Met^5]-enkephalinamide, and β_h-endorphin show similar activities in inducing enkephalin receptor down regulation. Neither classical opiate agonists nor antagonists induce significant down regulation, but these can specifically block the down-regulation effect of the opioid peptides. The reason for previous failures in demonstrating the receptor alteration *in vivo* after chronic opiate treatment might be that peptides have not been used. It remains to be shown whether the opioid peptide-induced down regulation can be demonstrated *in vivo* for some or all opiate receptor subtypes.

Direct binding studies of neuroblastoma cells with ^{125}I-[D-Ala^2, D-Leu^5]-enkephalin would appear to indicate that neither receptors nor ligand are internalized since virtually all (>90%) initially cell-associated (or bound) labeled ligands can be dissociated as intact molecules (30). Using rhodamine-conjugated [D-Ala^2, Lys^6]Leu-enkephalin and video-intensified fluorescence microscopy (described below), the fluorescent enkephalin receptors form clusters on the cell surface and do not appear to be internalized (131). The receptor-bound fluorescent ligands can also be dissociated nearly completely by washing the cells. However, recent studies show that, under conditions optimal for receptor down regulation (129), monolayer cells accumulate [^{3}H][D-Ala^2,D-Leu^5] enkephalin in excess of their surface receptor number (130). This uptake and the down regulation can be inhibited by opiate antagonists (132). Metabolic inhibitors sodium azide and 2-4-dinitrophenol inhibited the uptake and down regulation without interefering with cell surface receptor binding (130). The lysosomotrophic amines chloroquine and methylamine inhibited the dissociation of cell associated [^{3}H][D-Ala^2,D-leu^5]enkephalin but did not affect receptor down regulation (130). These findings suggest that receptor recycling occurs, ligand is internalized and enkephalin-receptor down regulation has some mechanistic features in common with other receptor systems known to exhibit receptor-mediated endocytosis (described below).

5   RECEPTOR MOBILILITY AND CLUSTERING

The mobility of cell-surface macromolecules in intact, livin has been studied by using the fluore scence photobleaching recovery method (FPR) (133–135). A focused laser beam bleaches a small area of a cell that is tagged with a specific, fluorescently labeled ligand. The rate of recovery of fluorescence in this region reflects the diffusion of the bleached molecules into that area, in a manner related to the diffusion constant of the labeled molecules. Measurement by the FPR method shows that lipid-like molecules diffuse rapidly with a diffusion constant about 10^{-8} cm^2/sec, whereas proteins move more slowly (i.e., about 4×10^{-10} cm^2/sec). Elson and Reidler (133) first showed that membrane receptors for rhodamine-labeled concanavalin A and bungarotoxin on myoblasts are rapidly mobile within the plane of the membrane at 37°C. The synthesis of highly fluorescent derivatives of the peptide hormones insulin, epidermal growth factor (EGF) (135), and nerve growth factor (NGF) (136) has allowed similar examination ot the mobility of these receptors in cultured cells. The receptors of the fibroblast cell line 3T3 labeled with rhodamine-insulin or rhodamine-EGF, and of cultured embryonal sensory ganglia cells labeled with rhodamine-NGF, have diffusion constants at 37°C (about 4×10^{-10} cm^2/sec) consistent with rapidly mobile, integral membrane proteins.

The ligand–receptor complex can be visualized directly using a fluorescently labeled ligand with a video-intensifying camera attached to a fluorescent microscope, called video-intensified fluorescence (VIF)

(137, 138). VIF permits considerable enhancement of the microscopic images at low levels of light intensity and has been used to visualize the pattern and mobility of receptors for EGF (137), insulin (137), α_2-macroglobulin (138), chemotactic peptide (139), NGF (136), gonadotropin releasing hormone (140), and enkephalins (131, 141, 142). The general characteristics of interaction of a variety of fluorescently labeled ligands with cells *in vitro* are similar. Initially, those complexes are labeled diffusely and they remain so for long periods at 4°C. However, at physiological temperatures (37°C) aggregates appear on the cell surface, forming fluorescent patches or clusters. The fluorescent patches or clusters are formed in a manner dependent upon time and temperature. Many of these large "patches," observed at 37°, actually represent endocytosed ligand.

N4TG1 is a tissue culture line of mouse neuroblastoma cells that has been shown to have a single, homogeneous, delta-type enkephalin receptor (31). When these cells are incubated with rhodamine-enkephalin and the distribution of the ligand–receptor complex is observed directly by VIF, the cells incubated at 4°C reveal only diffuse fluorescence that appears to remain stable over the cell surface. Upon warming to 37°C, visible patches of specific binding form slowly and appear maximal at about 40 min. While cluster formation is not affected by inhibitors of energy metabolism, sulphydryl and disulfide reagents can block cluster formation (141). Once clusters are formed, these agents cannot disperse the clusters so long as the ligand is present (142). Dithiothreitol can disperse the agonist but not antagonist-induced clusters in the absence of ligand (142). These data suggest that cluster formation may be related to sulphydryl and disulphide links between receptor molecules.

Although the evidence from the fluorescence studies suggest that freely mobile hormone or peptide receptors are induced to aggregate by seemingly monovalent ligands, more sensitive techniques show that in some instances a small number of the surface receptors may be preaggregated. For example, by transmission electron microscopy it was found that ferritin-labeled insulin and ferritin-EGF were found to preexist as receptor microaggregates (2–10 receptors/aggregate) in isolated adipocytes (143) and fibroblasts (144, 145). These preformed surface clusters are too small to be seen with existing fluorescence techniques and appear as diffuse labeling.

Cholinergic receptors in myoblasts have also been shown to preexist in a clustered state although they can be further induced upon innervation (146, 147). The possibility cannot be neglected that many neurotransmitter receptors in synaptic membrane may already exist in a clustered state. The large clusters induced by enkephalin are maintained for long periods of time even after the ligand has been removed (141, 142). Similarly stable cholinergic receptor clusters in myotubes have also been observed (147).

6   RECEPTOR CROSSLINKING AND AGGREGATION IN BIOLOGICAL ACTIONS

For some receptor ligand systems, receptor crosslinking and aggregation appear to be essential for triggering biological responses. The most convincing evidence for such a mechanism has been obtained for immunoglobulin-E(IgE)-receptor-mediated histamine release (148–151), EGF-mediated mitogenesis (152), and insulin-receptor-mediated glucose transport (153, 154). It has been shown that a series of divalent antigens can activate basophils to release histamine, whereas the monovalent compounds cannot. Anti-IgE-receptor antibodies cause histamine release; Fab[1] fragments bind to the IgE receptor but are inactive, whereas crosslinking the Fab[1]-receptor complanti-Fab[1] restores the antibody-induced activity.

Studies with fluorescently labeled insulin and EGF show that binding leads to receptor aggregation. Multivalent ligands such as plant lectins (wheat germ agglutinin, concanavalin A) (155) and antibodies to the insulin receptor (156), which presumably can crosslink receptors, can trigger biological effects even though these ligands bind to the receptor at a site different from the insulin binding sites. Kahn et al. (156) showed that the insulin-like activity of antireceptor antibodies is dependent upon their valence. Monovalent Fab fragments were inactive but antagonized the effect of insulin or antireceptor antibody. The insulin-like effect of Fab fragments was restored by crosslinking with bivalent anti-Fab antibody.

Furthermore, under certain conditions bivalent but not monovalent antibodies directed to insulin and EGF can dramatically enhance the activities of very low concentrations of these hormones in fibroblasts (157). A biologically inactive analog of EGF (cyanogen bromide-cleaved EGF) has been described which retains its ability to bind but does not induce aggregation of receptors. Addition of bivalent anti-EGF antibodies restores both the bioactivity and the morphological crosslinking (patch formation) of this derivative toward that observed with the native hormone (152).

Enkephalin receptors in neuroblastoma cells can form large visual clusters (131, 141, 142). Enkephalins and opiate agonists inhibit the adenylate cyclase activity of this neuroblastoma cell line (142). Sulphydryl and disulfide reagents inhibit the gross visual cluster formation of enkephalin receptors but do not interfere with the inhibitory effect of opioids and enkephalin on adenylate cyclase, thus suggesting that the inhibitory effects of opioids on adenylate cyclase occur before and are independent of the formation of gross visual clusters. However, we have recently demonstrated that the dimer analog of oxymorphone and enkephalin exhibit slightly greater affinity than the corresponding monomer analogs for the receptors in membranes, and they exhibit much greater activity in the guinea pig ileum (158). Others have reported that the dimer, N^{α}, N^{ϵ}-bis[D-Ala; Met^5]enkephalin is four times more potent in analgesic activity than [D-Ala^2, Met^5]enkephalin amide in the rat after central injection (159). A superactive enkephalin–tobacco mosaic virus conjugate has also been reported (160). The data suggest that aggregation or crosslinking of opiate receptors by the dimers may be important for the enhanced biological responses of opioids. The acute inhibitory effect of opioids on adenylate cyclase activity can occur when the receptor is in a "grossly" diffuse state rather than in the visual clustered pattern. Therefore, if microaggregation is involved in these effects (which is very possible) it must be submicroscopic, perhaps involving only dimerization or limited crosslinking reactions. Two adenylate cyclase stimulatory hormones, gonadotropin (161) and thyrotropin (TSH) (162), also induce the clustering of their surface receptors. In both cases, the binding of hormones to the receptor causes prompt stimulation of adenylate cyclase prior to the formation of *visible* clusters. Bivalent antibody against TSH receptors isolated from serum of patients with Graves's disease mimics TSH action and activates thyroid adenylate cyclase (163). These data again suggest that receptor microclusters, which may be too small to be detected by fluorescence microscopy, rather than visible patches, play a role in the activation of adenylate cyclase.

While all the above evidence indicates that perturbation of the receptor by crosslinking can trigger or enhance a biological response, physiological activation of the receptor by natural ligands may still occur through entirely different mechanisms.

7 RECEPTOR MEDIATED LIGAND INTERNALIZATION AND RECEPTOR DOWN REGULATION

Surface aggregation or clustering of peptide hormone receptors ultimately results in internalization of the complex by endocytosis. Receptor-mediated endocytosis is a process that directs the uptake or transport of a variety of serum proteins. This process has been studied extensively for ligands such as low density lipoproteins (LDL) (120), EGF (137, 164) α-2-macroglobulin (136, 165), asialoglycoprotein (166), insulin (137), and chemotactic peptide (139). One of the best-studied systems in which internalization of receptors serves as a selective transport mechanism is that for LDL. The receptor-mediated endocytosis of LDL coordinates the transport of cholesterol from plasma into the cells (120). The ligand initially binds to cell surface receptors and becomes localized to coated pits. Coated pits are invaginated regions of cell membranes surrounded by an electron-dense cage that is composed primarily of clathrin, a high-molecular-weight protein (167). Coated pits rapidly pinch off to form small, thin-walled vesicles, devoid of a clathrin coat, which contain ligand that is presumed to be complexed with its receptor (118, 165, 166). The small, thin-walled endocytic vesicles are initially located below the plasma membrane. They rapidly migrate to the Golgi region of the cell, in the process becoming larger and irregularly shaped. Presumably, this occurs by fusion with each other or with other intracellular vesicles. In the Golgi region, they appear to interact with elements of the Golgi or GERL (Golgi apparatus–endoplasmic reticulum–lysosomes) (118, 165, 166). Soon after their arrival at the Golgi region of the cell, internalized ligand is found in large, sometimes multivesicular vesicles that morphologically resemble secondary lysosomes (118, 165, 166). These structures, however, do not stain for acid hydrolases and are therefore probably not secondary lysosomes (165, 166). Only after longer times is acid hydrolase found in ligand-containing vesicles (165, 166). The protein of LDL is hydrolyzed to amino acids, and the cholesterol esters are hydrolyzed and release cholesterol, which crosses the lysosomal membrane and enters the cytoplasmic component. LDL receptors that enter cells in coated vesicles can be very rapidly recycled, and they are not destroyed. In fact, morphological and kinetic studies indicate that the whole pathway of insertion of receptor clustering in coated pits, internalization, and recycling occurs continuously whether or not LDL is present (120, 168).

Highly fluorescent rhodamine derivatives of insulin and EGF have been used to study the patterns and the mobility of receptors on fibroblastic cells (137, 138). It has been found that both insulin and EGF receptors are initially distributed uniformly at 4°C, and they quickly form patches that are subsequently internalized into endocytic vesicles within cells through coated pits. In some cases, ligands can be internalized by noncoated invaginations. The internalization step is found to be temperature-dependent and requires metabolic energy. In the case of EGF, the internalization of hormone–receptor complexes is related to receptor down regulation and degradation of EGF and the receptor (119). The majority of internalized receptor is degraded in lysosomes and there is an excellent correlation between this process and down regulation of surface receptor (119). In the case of insulin, it appears that the internalization of the hormone–receptor complex may mediate the degradation of insulin molecules; most internalized receptors escape degradation and are recycled to the plasma membranes (169–171), although this appears to depeninsulin molecu found with tetramethylrhodamine-labeled *N*-formyl Nle-Leu-Phe-Nle-Tyr-Lys in monocytes (172), which is a potent membrane chemoattractant for human neutrophils (139). In this system, diffused membrane fluorescence is seen initially at 4°C. However, in contrast with insulin and EGF, it is followed by very rapid (minutes) aggregation and internalization of the fluorescent peptide at 37°.

Nerve growth factor is a large polypeptide hormone that enters cells at the tip of the axon and migrates in retrograde fashion to the cell body in an intact form through receptor-mediated endocytosis (136). Recent studies with rhodamine conjugate of NGF and cultured neuronal cells have indicated that the receptors are initially distributed uniformly at 4°C, and that at 37°C they form clusters that are subsequently internalized in 60 min.

Among the large number of adenylate cyclase stimulatory hormones, the relationship between activation, desensitization, and cluster formation has only been carefully examined for gonadotropins. Exposure of ovarian tissue to leuteotropin or human chorionic gonadotropin, both of which bind to the same receptors, causes prompt stimulation of adenylate cyclase, followed by a slower desensitization of the enzyme to any renewed hormonal challenge (173, 174). Clustered leuteotropin–receptor complexes are internalized into cultured granulosa cells, where they are translocated to lysosomes and ultimately degraded (161, 175–177). The process of desensitization is apparent after 2–3 h of exposure to chorionic gonadotropin in granulosa cultures, and it persists for several days under these conditions. By morphological criteria, most of the hormone–receptor complexes remain at the cell surface during these early incubation periods. Thus, the process of receptor internalization and degradation may not account for the immediate loss of adenylate cyclase activation, since desensitization of the enzyme precedes the massive loss of specific receptors (176). The refractoriness may, therefore, be the result of cluster formation, which reduces the efficiency of hormone–receptor coupling to adenylate cyclase. The more prolonged desensitization event may indeed be directly attributable to the slower, more protracted loss of receptors occurring at later times. Similar phenomena have been described for the β adrenergic system (178), which also exerts its effect through activation of adenylate cyclase.

Although submicroscopic crosslinking of surface receptors may be an important mechanism for the immediate effects produced by certain ligands, the possibility exists that the delayed alterations (e.g., mitogenesis) in cellular metabolism may be a result of internalization or subsequent degradation of the ligand or receptors (179).

8   RECEPTOR-MEDIATED ALTERATION IN ADENYLATE CYCLASE ACTIVITY

Like many hormones, many neuropeptides have been shown to be associated with adenylate cyclase, a plasma membrane-bound enzyme that catalyzes the formation of the intracellular second messenger, cyclic AMP (cAMP). Cholecystokinin, secretin, VIP, TRH, vasopressin, and oxytocin can stimulate adenylate cyclase activity and raise the intracellular levels of cAMP. Enkephalins have been shown to inhibit this enzyme activity (142, 180–183). Possible molecular mechanisms of how hormones activate and enkephalins inhibit adenylate cyclase are discussed briefly below.

It is now well established that hormone-dependent adenylate cyclase activity is dependent on at least three independent protein macromolecules (184): The receptor for ligand or hormone recognition, the catalytic unit of adenylate cyclase, and the GTP regulatory unit which is associated with the catalytic unit and interacts with the receptor unit. The receptor recognition site faces the outside of the cell whereas the catalytic unit and the GTP regulatory unit are located in the cytoplasmic face. The binding of ligand is a necessary but insufficient biochemical condition to activate the system. The supply of GTP to the GTP regulatory unit is required in parallel to induce enzyme activation. The simultaneous occupancy of the receptor by the agonist and the regulatory unit by GTP is required to transform the adenylate cyclase system from an inactive state to an activated state. Hormone receptors are believed in most cases to be membrane entities separate from adenylate cyclase and the GTP regulatory protein. Stimulatory hormones or peptides increase the mobility of the receptor–hormone complex and promote the receptor–receptor interaction (i.e., aggregation and cluster formation as described above) or modulate the interaction between receptors and the GTP binding regulatory protein (185, 186). This interaction favors exchange of bound GDP for GTP at a regulatory site, which in turn leads to activation of the catalytic unit of adenylate cyclase. This activation is terminated by hydrolysis of GTP at the regulatory site as suggested by Cassel and Selinger (185).

Recently, Blume et al. (183) have shown that inhibition of the adenylate cyclase in neuroblastoma-glioma hybrid by opiate agonists and enkephalin requires both GTP and sodium ions, the two components also known to regulate the binding affinity of agonists. Koski and Klee (187) recently reported that enkephalins and opiates stimulate plasma membrane-bound GTPase activities in this same cell line. This stimulatory activity of a series of opioids on GTPase seems to correlate with their potencies in inhibiting adenylate cyclase. Both activities require sodium ions. Opioids do not inhibit adenylate cyclase activity when measured in the presence of concentrations exceeding 10 μM of the nonhydrolyzable GTP analog, GPP(NH)P. Under this condition, an enzyme-GPP(NH)P complex is formed that is not susceptible to hydrolysis, and thus GTPase would not be expected to affect adenylate cyclase activity. In conjunction with the model for the hormonal stimulation of adenylate cyclase proposed by Cassel and Selinger, Koski and Klee proposed that opioids act through their receptors to catalyze the GTP hydrolysis reaction and thereby reduce adenylate cyclase activity.

9 ROLE OF CA²⁺ AND CALMODULIN

The general role of Ca^{2+} in mediating the excitation-contraction coupling and stimulation-secretion coupling is well established. The excitation of a neuron or a cell by agents (i.e., excitatory neuropeptides) or by
electrical activity such as depolarization and hyperpolarization may
lead to an alteration in intracellular Ca^{2+} concentration, which in turn
can modulate a large number of metabolic events. The ability of opiates
and endorphins to inhibit the synaptosomal Ca^{2+}-uptake is well documented (188). Many of these Ca^{2+}-dependent biological processes are
now known to be mediated by a Ca^{2+}-binding protein called calmodulin
(189, 190). Calmodulin is found in many, if not most, eukaryotic cells. It
is a small (MW 16,790), heat- and acid-stable protein whose amino acid
sequence has been conserved throughout evolution. Calmodulin can
bind the antipsychotic tranquilizers, phenothiazines, in the presence of
Ca^{2+}. This protein regulates a large number of Ca-dependent enzymes,
including cyclic nucleotides phosphodiesterase, brain adenylate cyclase,
the ATPase and Ca^{2+} pump of the erythrocyte plasma membrane, myosin light chain kinases, brain membrane kinases, phosphorylase b kinase, and NAD kinase in plants. Calmodulin may also play an important
role in the regulation of the processes of assembly and disassembly of
microtubules by its control of protein kinase activities and may exert an
indirect influence upon a wide variety of cellular processes.

Calmodulin may be considered as a special kind of Ca^{2+}-receptor. Its
regulation of enzyme activity has generally been found to require Ca^{2+}
and results in enhanced enzyme activity. The control process occurs in
two stages: binding of Ca^{2+} to calmodulin, accompanied by conformational changes, followed by the binding of the calmodulin-Ca^{2+} complex
to an enzyme. The enzyme in turn undergoes a conformational change
(189), which in all cases known so far is accompanied by an increase in
activity.

The important role of Ca^{2+} in neuronal functions is suggested by the
high content of calmodulin in brain (189, 190). A variety of calmodulin-
binding proteins have been isolated from brain (189, 190). These include
calmodulin-dependent enzymes that are not necessarily specific to the
neuron systems such as cyclic nucleotide phosphodiesterases, myosin
light-chain kinase, adenylate cyclase, and the synaptic plasma membrane ATPase (189, 190).

In brain extracts, a protein that appears to be specific for the nervous system and acts as an inhibitor of the activation of cyclic
neucleotide phosphodiesterase by calmodulin is found to be the major
soluble calmodulin-binding protein (191–194). This protein also inhibits
other calmodulin-dependent enzyme activations (189). This calmodulin-
binding protein is composed of two subunits, a large MW 61,000 polypeptide that interacts with calmodulin in a Ca^{2+}-dependent fashion (191,

194) and a small MW 15,000 polypeptide subunit that binds Ca^{2+} (194). On the basis of its high affinity for Ca^{2+} ($K_d < 10^{-6} M$) and its nervous tissue localization, it was called calcineurin (195). Although its function is still unknown, it may play a role in the regulation of free Ca^{2+} in neurons and thereby modulate the release and action of neurotransmitters at the synaptic level.

Calmodulin can also regulate the Ca^{2+}-dependent phosphorylation of specific neuronal proteins. Phosphorylation has been proposed to be an important aspect of the postsynaptic actions of neurotransmitters (196). One neuronal protein composed of two subunits, designated protein Ia and Ib, is found in synaptic vesicles and postsynaptic densities and is a substrate for cyclic AMP-dependent phosphorylation (196–198). In the intact synaptosomes, this same protein can also be phosphorylated, probably at different sites, by a Ca^{2+}-dependent kinase stimulated by agents known to induce membrane depolarization and increased cellular levels of Ca^{2+} (199, 200). Proteins with similar molecular weights were shown to be phosphorylated by a Ca^{2+}-dependent, calmodulin-dependent kinase associated with synaptosomal membranes (201, 202). The involvement of calmodulin and calcineurin in synaptic actions can also be inferred from their localization at postsynaptic densities together with the specific neuronal protein I and enzymes of cyclic nucloetide metabolism (203).

Finally, many enzymes regulated by calmodulin-Ca^{2+} complexes or calmodulin-Ca^{2+}-dependent kinases can be substrates for cAMP-dependent kinases as well. Thus, these two major second-messenger systems are functionally coupled and integrated at the level of phosphorylation. The two systems are also coupled quite directly at the level of calmodulin-Ca^{2+} regulation of phosphodiesterase and adenulate cyclase activities.

REFERENCES

1. S. H. Snyder, *Science* **209**, 976 (1980).
2. T. Hökfelt, O. Johansson, Å. Ljungdahl, J. M. Lundberg, and M. Schultzberg, *Nature* **284**, 515 (1980).
3. K. -J. Chang, S. P. Wilson, and O. H. Viveros, in F. Izumi, Ed., *Synthesis, Storage and Secretion of Adrenal Catecholamines: Dynamic Integration of Functions*, Pergamon Press, Oxford, 1982.
4. S. H. Snyder and R. R. Goodman, *J. Neurochem.* **35**, 5 (1980).
5. S. H. Snyder, R. F. Bruns, J. W. Daly, and R. B. Innis, *Fed. Proc.* **40**, 142 (1981).
6. K. -J. Chang and P. Cuatrecasas, *Fed. Proc.* **40**, 2729 (1981).
7. J. Alumets, R. Häkanson, F. Sundler, and K. -J. Chang, *Histochem.* **56**, 187 (1978).
8. J. Schultzberg, T. Hökfelt, L. Terenius, L. G. Elfrin, J. M. Lundberg, J. Brandt, R. Elde, and M. Goldstein, *Neuroscience* **3**, 1169 (1978).
9. J. M. Lundberg, B. Hamberger, M. Schultzberg, T. Hökfelt, P. O. Granberg, S. Efendic, L. Terenius, M. Goldstein, and R. Luft, *Proc. Natl. Acad. Sci. USA* **76**, 4079 (1979).

10. J. Wharton, J. M. Polak, A. G. E. Pearse, G. P. McGregor, M. G. Bryant, S. R. Bloom, P. C. Emson, G. E. Bisgard, and J. A. Will, *Nature* **284**, 269 (1980).

11. T. Hökfelt, M. Schultzberg, R. Elde, G. Nilsson, L. Terenius, S. Said, and M. Goldstein, *Acta Pharmacol. Toxicol.* **43**, 79 (1978).

12. O. H. Viveros, E. J. Diliberto, Jr., E. Hazum, and K. -J. Chang, *Mol. Pharmacol.* **16**, 1101 (1979).

13. O. H. Viveros, E. J. Diliberto, Jr., E. Hazum, and K. -J. Chang, in E. Costa and M. Trobucchi, Eds., *Neural Peptides and Neural Communication*, Raven Press, New York, 1980, p. 191.

14. S. P. Wilson, R. L. Klein, K. -J. Chang, M. S. Gusparis, O. H. Viveros, and W. -H. Yang, *Nature* **288**, 707 (1980).

15. S. P. Wilson, L. X. Cubeddu, K. -J. Chang, and O. H. Viveros, *Neuropeptides* **1**, 273 (1981).

16. D. L. Kilpatrick, R. V. Lewis, S. Stein, and S. Udenfriend, *Proc. Natl. Acad. Sci. USA* **77**, 7473 (1980).

17. S. P. Wilson, K. -J. Chang, and O. H. Viveros, *Proc. Natl. Acad. Sci. USA* **77**, 4364 (1980).

18. J. Rossier, D. M. Dean, B. G. Livett, and S. Udenfriend, *Life Sci.* **28**, 781 (1981).

19. T. Hökfelt, J. M. Lundberg, M. Schultzberg, O. Johansson, Å. Ljungdahl, and J. Rehfeld, in E. Costa and M. Trabuchi, Eds., *Neural Peptides and Neuronal Communication*, Raven Press, New York, 1980, p. 1.

20. T. Hökfelt, L. G. Elfvin, R. Elde, M. Schultzberg, M. Goldstein, and R. Luft, *Proc. Natl. Acad. Sci. USA* **74**, 3587 (1977).

21. V. Chan-Palay, G. Jonsson, and S. L. Palay, *Proc. Natl. Acad. Sci. USA* **75**, 1582 (1978).

22. J. M. Lundberg, *Acta Physiol. Scand. Suppl.* **496**, 1 (1981).

23. J. Rossier, J. M. Trifaro, R. V. Lewis, R. W. H. Lee, A. Stern, S. Kimura, S. Stein, and S. Udenfriend, *Proc. Natl. Acad. Sci. USA* **77**, 6889 (1980).

24. D. R. Burg and S. H. Snyder, *Brain Res.* **93**, 309 (1975).

25. T. W. Moody, C. B. Pert, J. Rivier, and M. R. Brown, *Proc. Natl. Acad. Sci. USA* **75**, 5372 (1978).

26. M. A. Devynick and P. Meyer, *Am. J. Med.* **61**, 758 (1976).

27. S. R. Childers, I. Creese, A. M. Snowman, and S. H. Snyder, *Eur. J. Pharmacol.* **55**, 11 (1979).

28. J. A. H. Lord, A. A. Waterfield, J. Hughes, and H. W. Kosterlitz, *Nature* **267**, 495 (1977).

29. J. C. Reubi, M. H. Perrin, J. E. Rivier, and W. Vale, *Life Sci.* **28**, 2191 (1981).

30. K. -J. Chang, R. J. Miller, and P. Cuatrecasas, *Mol. Pharmacol.* **14**, 961 (1978).

31. K. -J. Chang and P. Cuatrecasas, *J. Biol. Chem.* **254**, 2610 (1979).

32. K. -J. Chang, B. R. Cooper, E. Hazum, and P. Cuatrecasas, *Mol. Pharmacol.* **16**, 91 (1979).

33. D. Desbuquois, M. H. Laudat, and P. H. Laudat, *Biochem. Biophys. Res. Comm.* **53** (4), 1187 (1973).

34. M. R. Hanley, B. E. B. Sandberg, C. M. Lee, L. L. Iverson, D. E. Brundish, and R. Wade, *Nature* **286**, 810 (1980).

35. H. Glossmann, A. J. Baukal, and K. J. Catt, *J. Biol. Chem.* **249**, 825 (1974).

36. P. Kitabgi, C. Poustis, C. Granier, J. VanRietschoten, J. Rivier, J. L. Morgat, and P. Freychet, *Mol. Pharmacol.* **18**, 11 (1980).

37. P. Kitabgi, R. Carraway, J. Van Rietschoten, C. Granier, J. L. Morgat, A. Menez, S. Leeman, and P. Freychet, *Proc. Natl. Acad. Sci. USA* **74**, 1846 (1977).

38. J. D. Gardner, T. P. Conlon, H. C. Breyerman, and A. VanZon, *Gastroenterology* **73**, 52 (1977).

39. J. D. Gardner, A. J. Rottman, S. Natarajan, and M. Bodanszky, *Biochim. Biophys. Acta* **583**, 491 (1979).

40. J. P. Christophe, T. P. Conlon, and J. D. Gardner, *J. Biol. Chem.* **251**, 4629 (1976).

41. C. E. Odya, T. L. Goodfriend, and C. Pena, *Biochem. Pharm.* **29**, 175 (1980).
42. R. B. Innis, D. C. Manning, J. M. Steward, and S. H. Snyder, *Proc. Natl. Acad. Sci. USA* **78**, 2630 (1981).
43. B. S. Conne, M. L. Aubert, and P. C. Sizonenko, *Biochem. Biophys. Res. Comm.* **90**, 1249 (1979).
44. H. Sankaran, I. D. Goldfine, C. W. Deveney, K. Y. Wong, and J. A. Williams, *J. Biol. Chem.* **255**, 1849 (1980).
45. R. T. Jensen, G. F. Lemp, and J. D. Gardner, *Proc. Natl. Acad. Sci. USA* **77**, 2079 (1980).
46. R. B. Innis and S. H. Snyder, *Proc. Natl. Acad. Sci. USA* **77**, 6917 (1980).
47. R. W. Steigerwalt and J. A. Williams, *Endocrinology* **109**, 1746 (1981).
48. T. Liang and M. A. Cascieri, *Biochem. Biophys. Res. Comm.* **96**, 1793 (1980).
49. R. T. Jensen and J. D. Gardner, *Proc. Natl. Acad. Sci. USA* **76**, 5679 (1979).
50. T. Liang and M. A. Cascieri, *J. Neurosci.* **1**, 1133 (1981).
51. G. R. Uhl, J. P. Bennett Jr., and S. H. Snyder, *Brain Res.* **130**, 299 (1977).
52. J. P. Bennett Jr. and S. H. Snyder, *J. Biol. Chem.* **251**, 7423 (1976).
53. J. W. Kebabian and D. B. Calne, *Nature* **277**, 92 (1979).
54. L. Tapia-Arancibia, J. Epelbaum, A. Enjalbert, and C. Kordon, *Eur. J. Pharmacol.* **71**, 523 (1981).
55. C. B. Srikant and Y. C. Patel, *Proc. Natl. Acad. Sci. USA* **78**, 3930 (1981).
56. I. Creese, D. R. Sibley, S. Leff, and M. Hamblin, *Fed. Proc.* **40**, 147 (1981).
57. R. J. Lefkowitz, *Fed. Proc.* **37**, 123 (1978).
58. D. C. U'Prichard and S. H. Snyder, *J. Biol. Chem.* **253**, 3444 (1978).
59. D. C. U'Prichard and S. H. Snyder, *Life Sci.* **24**, 79 (1979).
60. D. C. U'Prichard, D. A. Greenberg, and S. H. Snyder, *Mol. Pharmacol.* **13**, 454 (1977).
61. E. J. Ehlert, N. R. Roeske, and H. Yamamura, *Fed. Proc.* **40**, 153 (1981).
62. S. J. Peroutka, R. M. Lebovitz, and S. H. Snyder, *Mol. Pharmacol.* **16**, 700 (1979).
63. R. S. Zukin and A. R. Gintzler, *Brain Res.* **186**, 486 (1980).
64. C. B. Pert and D. Taylor, in E. Way, Ed., *Endogenous and Exogenous Opiate Agonists and Antagonists*, Pergamon Press, Elmsfor, N.Y., 1980, p. 87.
65. S. R. Childers and D. Taylor, *J. Neurochem.* **34**, 583 (1980).
66. K. -J. Chang, E. Hazum, A. Killian, and P. Cuatrecasas, *Mol. Pharmacol.* **20**, 1 (1981).
67. W. R. Martin, C. G. Eades, J. A. Thompson, R. E. Huppler, and P. E. Gilbert, *J. Pharmacol. Exp. Ther.* **197**, 517 (1976).
68. P. E. Gilbert and W. R. Martin, *J. Pharmacol. Exp. Ther.* **198**, 66 (1976).
69. R. Schultz, E. Faase, M. Wuster, and A. Herz, *Life Sci.* **24**, 843 (1979).
70. K. -J. Chang, A. Killian, E. Hazum, P. Cuatrecasas, and K. -J. Chang, *Science* **212**, 75 (1981).
71. H. W. Kosterlitz, S. J. Paterson, and L. E. Robson, *Br. J. Pharmacol.* **73**, 939 (1981).
72. B. K. Handa, A. C. Lane, J. A. H. Lord, B. A. Morgan, M. J. Rance, and C. F. C. Smith, *Eur. J. Pharmacol.* **70**, 531 (1981).
73. K. -J. Chang, E. Hazum, and P. Cuatrecasas, *Proc. Natl. Acad. Sci. USA* **78**, 4141 (1981).
74. W. S. Young and M. J. Kuhar, *Brain Res.* **179**, 255 (1979).
75. R. R. Goodman, S. H. Snyder, M. J. Kuhar, and W. S. Young, *Proc. Natl. Acad. Sci. USA* **77**, 6239 (1980).
76. A. Herz, J. Blasig, H. M. Emrich, C. Cording, S. Piree, A. Kölling, and D. V. Zerssen, *Adv. Biochem. Psychopharmacol.* **18**, 333 (1978).
77. K. -J. Chang, P. Cuatrecasas, E. T. Wei, and J. -K. Chang, *Life Sci.* **30**, 1547 (1982).
78. G. W. Pasternak, *Neurology* **31**, 1311 (1981).
79. A. Z. Zhang and G. W. Pasternak, *Life Sci.* **29**, 843 (1981).
80. B. L. Wolozin and G. W. Pasternak, *Proc. Natl. Acad. Sci. USA* **78**, 6181 (1981).
81. A. Z. Zhang, J. K. Chang, and G. W. Pasternak, *Life Sci.* **28**, 2829 (1981).

82. M. Wüster, R. Schulz, and A. Herz, *Eur. J. Pharmacol.* **62**, 235 (1980).
83. M. Wüster, P. Rubini, and R. Schulz, *Life Sci.* **29**, 1219 (1981).
84. C. Chavkin and A. Goldstein, *Nature (London)* **291**, 591 (1981).
85. R. S. Zukin and S. R. Zukin, *Life Sci.* **29**, 2681 (1981).
86. R. S. Zukin and S. R. Zukin, *Mol. Pharm.* **20**, 246 (1981).
87. R. W. McLawhon, R. E. West, Jr., R. J. Miller, and G. Dawson, *Proc. Natl. Acad. Sci. USA* **78**, 4309 (1981).
88. D. B. Vaupel and D. R. Jasinski, *Fed. Proc.* **38**, 435 (1979).
89. S. G. Holtzman, *J. Pharmacol. Exp. Ther.* **214**, 619 (1981).
90. S. Herling and J. H. Woods, *Life Sci.* **28**, 1571 (1981).
91. K. T. Brady, R. L. Balster, and E. L. May, *Science* **215**, 178 (1982).
92. K. -J. Chang and P. Cuatrecasas, in Takagi, Ed., *Advances in Endogenous and Exogenous Opioids*, Pergamon Press, Oxford, 1982.
93. F. Huidobro, J. P. Huidoboro-Toro, and H. Miranda, *Br. J. Pharmacol.* **70**, 519 (1980).
94. M. G. C. Gillian, H. W. Kosterlitz, and J. Mognan, *Br. J. Pharmacol.* **72**, 13 (1981).
95. A. Pfeiffer and A. Herz, *Biochem. Biophys. Res. Comm.* **101**, 38 (1981).
96. G. Porthé, A. Valette, and J. Cros, *Biochem. Biophys, Res. Comm.* **101**, 1 (1981).
97. E. Hazum, K. -J. Chang, and P. Cuatrecasas, *Science* **205**, 1033 (1979).
98. R. G. Hammonds Jr., and C. H. Li, *Proc. Natl. Acad. Sci. USA* **78**, 6764 (1981).
99. N. M. Lee and A. P. Smith, *Life Sci.* **26**, 1459 (1980).
100. C. Chavkin and A. Goldstein, *Proc. Natl. Acad. Sci. USA* **78**, 6543 (1981).
101. J. M. Bidlack and L. G. Abood, *Life Sci.* **27**, 331 (1980).
102. W. F. Simonds, G. Koski, R. A. Streaty, L. M. Hjelmeland, and W. A. Klee, *Proc. Natl. Acad. Sci. USA* **77**, 4623 (1980).
103. U. T. Rüegg, J. M. Hiller, and E. J. Simon, *Eur. J. Pharmacol.* **64**, 367 (1980).
104. T. M. Cho, C. Yamato, J. S. Cho, and H. H. Loh, *Life Sci.* **28**, 2651 (1981).
105. R. B. Innis and S. H. Snyder, *Europ. J. Pharmacol.* **65**, 123 (1980).
106. A. Saito, H. Sankaran, I. D. Goldfine, and J. A. Williams, *Science* **208**, 1155 (1980).
107. L. Sjödin, E. Brodin, G. Nilsson, and T. P. Conlon, *Acta Physiol. Scand.* **109**, 97 (1980).
108. Y. Nakata, Y. Kusaka, T. Segawa, H. Yajima, and K. Kitagawa, *Life Sci.* **22**, 259 (1977).
109. Y. Nakata, Y. Kusaka, H. Yajima, K. Kitagawa, and T. Segawa, *Arch. Pharmacol.* **314**, 211 (1980).
110. L. H. Lazarus, M. R. Brown, and M. H. Perrin, *Neuroendocrinology* **16**, 625 (1977).
111. H. Glossmann, A. Baukal, and K. J. Catt, *J. Biol. Chem.* **249**, 664 (1974).
112. M. K. Raizada, J. W. Yang, M. I. Phillips, and R. E. Fellows, *Brain Res.* **207**, 343 (1981).
113. M. A. Devynik, M. -G. Pernollet, P. Meyer, S. Fermandjian, and F. M. Bumpus, *Nature* **249**, 67 (1974).
114. J. P. Bennett Jr. and S. H. Snyder, *Europ. J. Pharmac.* **67**, 1 (1980).
115. J. B. Bennett Jr. and S. H. Snyder, *Europ. J. Pharmac.* **67**, 11 (1980).
116. A. Schonbrunn and A. H. Tashjian Jr., *J. Biol. Chem.* **253**, 6473 (1978).
117. C. B. Srikant and Y. C. Patel, *Nature* **294**, 259 (1981).
118. I. H. Pastan and M. C. Willingham, *Science* **214**, 504 (1981).
119. A. C. King and P. Cuatrecasas, *New Engl. J. Med.* **305**, 77 (1981).
120. J. L. Goldstein, R. G. W. Anderson, and M. S. Brown, *Nature (London)* **279**, 679 (1979).
121. B. Katz and S. Thesleff, *J. Phsiol. (London)* **138**, 63 (1957).
122. T. Heidmann and J. P. Changeux, *Eur. J. Biochem.* **94**, 255 (1979).
123. T. Heidmann and J. P. Changeux, *Annu. Rev. Biochem.* **47**, 317 (1978).
124. R. S. Kent, A. DeLean, and R. J. Lefkowitz, *Mol. Pharmacol.* **17**, 14 (1980).
125. A. Herz, R. Schulz, and M. Wüster, in G. Pepeu, M. J. Kuhar, and S. J. Enna, Eds., *Receptors for Neurotransmitters and Peptide Hormones*, Raven Press, New York, 1980, p. 329.

126. A. Herz, R. Schulz, and J. Bläsig, R. F. Beers Jr., and E. G. Bassett, Eds., *Mechanisms of Pain and Analgesic Compounds*, Raven Press, New York, 1979, p. 383.
127. H. O. J. Collier, in R. F. Beers Jr., and E. G. Bassett, Eds., *Mechanisms of Pain and Analgesic Compounds*, Raven Press, New York, 1979, p. 389.
128. R. Schulz, M. Wüster, H. Krenss, and A. Herz, *Nature* **285**, 242 (1980).
129. K. -J. Chang, R. W. Eckel, and S. G. Blanchard, *Nature* **296**, 446 (1982).
130. S. G. Blanchard, K. -J. Chang and P. Cuatrecasas, *J. Biol. Chem.* **258**, 1092 (1983).
131. E. Hazum, K. -J. Chang, and P. Cuatrecasas, *Science* **206**, 1077 (1979).
132. S. G. Blanchard, K. -J. Chang and P. Cuatrecasas, *Life Sci.* **31**, 1311 (1982).
133. E. L. Elson and J. A. Reidler, *J. Supramol. Struct.* **12**, 481 (1979).
134. D. L. Taylor and Y. L. Wang, *Nature* **284**, 405 (1980).
135. Y. Schechter, J. Schlessinger, S. Jacogs, K. -J. Chang, and P. Cuatrecasas, *Proc. Natl. Acad. Sci. USA* **75**, 2135 (1978).
136. A. Levy, Y. Schechter, E. J. Neufeld, and J. Schlessinger, *Proc. Natl. Acad. Sci. USA* **77**, 3469 (1980).
137. J. Schlessinger, Y. Shechter, M. C. Willingham, and I. Pastan, *Proc. Natl. Acad. Sci. USA* **75**, 2659 (1978).
138. F. R. Maxfield, J. Schlessinger, Y. Shechter, I. Pastan, and M. C. Willingham, *Cell* **14**, 805 (1978).
139. J. E. Niedel, I. Kahane, and P. Cuatrecasas, *Science* **205**, 1412 (1979).
140. E. Hazum, P. Cuatrecasas, J. Marian, and P. M. Conn, *Proc. Natl. Acad. Sci. USA* **77**, 6692 (1980).
141. E. Hazum, K. -J. Chang, and P. Cuatrecasas, *Nature* **282**, 626 (1979).
142. E. Hazum, K. -J. Chang, and P. Cuatrecasas, *Proc. Natl. Acad. Sci. USA* **77**, 3038 (1980).
143. L. Jarett and R. M. Smith, *J. Supramol. Struct.* **6**, 45 (1977).
144. H. T. Haigler, J. A. McKanna, and S. Cohen, *J. Cell Biol.* **81**, 382 (1979).
145. J. A. McKanna, H. T. Haigler, and S. Cohen, *Proc. Natl. Acad. Sci. USA* **76**, 5689 (1979).
146. H. C. Fertuck and M. M. Salpeter, *J. Cell Biol.* **69**, 144 (1976).
147. E. Frank and G. D. Fischbach, *J. Cell Biol.* **83**, 143 (1979).
148. K. Ishizaka, T. Ishizaka, *Ann. N.Y. Acad. Sci.* **190**, 443 (1971).
149. R. P. Sirganian, W. A. Hook, and B. R. Levine, *Immunochemistry* **12**, 149 (1975).
150. D. M. Segal, J. D. Taurog, and H. Hetzger, *Proc. Natl. Acad. Sci. USA* **12**, 549 (1978).
151. C. Isersky, J. D. Taurog, G. Poy, and H. Hetzger, *J. Immunol.* **12**, 549 (1978).
152. Y. Shechter, L. Hernaez, J. Schlessinger, and P. Cuatrecasas, *Nature* **278**, 835 (1979).
153. C. R. Kahn, K. Baird, J. S. Flier, and D. B. Jarrett, *J. Clin. Invest.* **60**, 1094 (1977).
154. S. Jacobs, K. -J. Chang, and P. Cuatrecasas, *Science* **200**, 1283 (1978).
155. P. Cuatrecasas and G. P. E. Tell, *Proc. Natl. Acad. Sci. USA* **70**, 485 (1973).
156. C. R. Kahn, K. L. Baird, D. B. Jarrett, and J. S. Flier, *Proc. Natl. Acad. Sci. USA* **75**, 4209 (1978).
157. Y. Shechter, K. -J. Chang, S. Jacobs, and P. Cuatrecasas, *Proc. Natl. Acad. Sci. USA* **76**, 2720 (1979).
158. E. Hazum, K. -J. Chang, H. J. Leighton, O. W. Lever Jr., and P. Cuatrecasas, *Biochem. Biophys. Res. Comm.* **104**, 347 (1982).
159. D. H. Coy, A. J. Kastin, M. J. Walker, R. F. McGivern, and C. A. Sandman, *Biochem. Biophys. Res. Commun.* **83**, 977 (1978).
160. V. M. Kriwackzek, R. Schwyer, M. G. C. Gillian, S. J. Paterson, and H. W. Kosterlitz, *Peptides* **2**, 89 (1981).
161. M. Conti, J. P. Harwood, M. L. Dufau, and K. J. Catt, *Mol. Pharmacol.* **13**, 1024 (1977).
162. A. Avivi, D. Tramontano, F. S. Ambesi-Impiomato, and J. Schlessinger, *Science* **214**, 1237 (1981).
163. S. A. Mehdi and J. P. Kriss, *Endocrinology* **103**, 296 (1978).

164. H. T. Haigler, J. A. McKanna, and S. Cohen, *J. Cell Biol.* **81**, 382 (1979).
165. M. C. Willingham and I. Pastan, *Cell* **21**, 67 (1980).
166. D. A. Wall, G. Wilson, and A. L. Hubbard, *Cell* **21**, 79 (1980).
167. B. M. F. Pearse, *J. Mol. Biol.* **97**, 93 (1975).
168. M. S. Brown and J. L. Goldstein, *Proc. Natl. Acad. Sci. USA* **76**, 330 (1979).
169. S. Terris and D. F. Steiner, in *Insulin Receptor Turnover and Down Regulation*, B. Brandenburg and A. Wollmer, Eds., Proceedings of the 2nd International Symposium, Aachen, Walter De Gruyter, Berlin, 1980, p. 277.
170. B. C. Reed and M. D. Lane, *Proc. Natl. Acad. Sci. USA* **77**, 285 (1980).
171. M. Krupp and M. D. Lane, *J. Biol. Chem.* **256**, 1689 (1981).
172. J. B. Weinberg, J. J. Muscato, and J. E. Niedel, *J. Clin. Invest.* **68**, 621 (1981).
173. M. Hunzicker-Dunn and L. Birnbaumer, *Endocrinology* **99**, 211 (1976).
174. S. A. Lamprecht, U. Zor, Y. Solomon, Y. Koch, K. Ahrén, and H. R. Lindner, *J. Cyclic Nucleotide Res.* **3**, 69 (1977).
175. M. Ascoli and D. Puett, *FEBS Lett.* **75**, 77 (1977).
176. A. Amsterdam, A. Nimrod, S. A. Lamprecht, and H. R. Burstein Lindner, *Am. J. Physiol.* **236**, E129 (1979).
177. M. Ascoli and D. Puett, *J. Biol. Chem.* **253**, 4892 (1978).
178. L. J. Pike and R. J. Lefkowitz, *Biochem. Biophys. Acta* **632**, 354 (1980).
179. C. F. Fox, M. Wrann, P. Linsley, and R. Vale, *J. Supramol. Struct.* **12**, 517 (1980).
180. A. Lampert, M. Nirenberg, and W. A. Klee, *Proc. Natl. Acad. Sci. USA* **73**, 3165 (1976).
181. S. K. Sharma, W. A. Klee, and M. Nirenberg, *Proc. Nat. Acad. Sci. USA* **72**, 3092 (1975).
182. J. Traber, K. Fischer, S. Latzin, and B. Hamprecht, *Nature* **253**, 120 (1975).
183. A. J. Blume, D. Lichtshtein, and G. Boone, *Proc. Natl. Acad. Sci. USA* **76**, 5626 (1979).
184. E. M. Ross and A. G. Gilman, *Ann. Rev. Biochem.* **49**, 533 (1980).
185. D. Cassel and Z. Selinger, *Proc. Natl. Acad. Sci. USA* **75**, 4155 (1978).
186. P. M. Lad, T. B. Nielson, S. Preston, and M. C. Rodbell, *J. Biol. Chem.* **255**, 988 (1980).
187. G. Koski and W. A. Klee, *Proc. Natl. Acad. Sci. USA* **78**, 4185 (1981).
188. D. B. Chapman and E. L. Way, *Ann. Rev. Pharmacol. Toxicol.* **20**, 553 (1980).
189. C. B. Klee, T. H., Crouch, and P. G. Richman, *Ann. Rev. Biochem.* **49**, 489 (1980).
190. W. Y. Cheung, *J. Cyclic Nucleotide Res.* **7**, 71 (1981).
191. C. B. Klee and M. H. Krinks, *Biochemistry* **17**, 120 (1978).
192. R. W. Wallace, T. J. Lynch, E. A. Tallant, and W. Y. Cheung, *Arch. Biochem. Biophys.* **187**, 328 (1978).
193. R. W. Wallace, T. J. Lynch, E. A. Tallant, and W. Y. Cheung, *J. Biol. Chem.* **254**, 377 (1979).
194. R. K. Sharma, R. Desai, D. M. Waisman, and J. H. Wang, *J. Biol. Chem.* **254**, 4276 (1979).
195. C. B. Klee, T. H. Crouch, and M. H. Krinks, *Proc. Natl. Acad. Sci. USA* **76**, 6270 (1979).
196. P. Greengard, *Fed. Proc.* **38**, 2208 (1979).
197. W. Sieghart, J. Forn, R. Schwarcz, J. T. Coyle, and P. Greengard, *Brain Res.* **16**, 345 (1978).
198. T. Ueda and P. Greengard, *J. Biol. Chem.* **252**, 5155 (1977).
199. B. K. Krueger, J. Forn, and P. Greengard, *J. Biol. Chem.* **252**, 2764 (1977).
200. I. Uno, T. Ueda, and P. Greengard, *J. Biol. Chem.* **252**, 5164 (1977).
201. H. Schulman and P. Greengard, *Proc. Natl. Acad. Sci. USA* **75**, 5432 (1978).
202. R. J. DeLorenzo, S. D. Freedman, W. B. Yohe, and S. C. Maurer, *Proc. Natl. Acad. Sci. USA* **76**, 1838 (1979).
203. D. J. Grab, K. Berzins, R. S. Cohen, and P. Siekevitz, *J. Biol. Chem.* **254**, 8690 (1979).

PART

4

Specific Neuropeptides

25

Oxytocin, Vasopressin, and Neurophysins

EARL A. ZIMMERMAN
College of Physicians and Surgeons
Columbia University
New York, New York

1   INTRODUCTION

The hypothalamo-neurohypophysial system has served as an important model of the peptidergic neurons for nearly half a century (1). Many important new concepts came from pioneering work on the magnocellular system, which secretes the hormones oxytocin and vasopressin and their associated neurophysin proteins into the general circulation. These studies demonstrated biosynthesis of the hormones by perikaryal ribosomal mechanisms, rapid axonal transport in granules, exocytosis at nerve terminals in posterior pituitary gland, and stimulus-secretion coupling (2–4). Nature's design of the system also offered some advantages for such studies over other hypothalamic peptidergic neurosecretory systems producing releasing and inhibiting factors that exert control over anterior pituitary function. Some of these attributes included storage of large amounts of the hormones in the posterior pituitary, which provided more material for chemical analysis, and the presence of the sulfur-rich neurophysins in the large granules containing the hormones, which facilitated anatomical studies by their reactivity to Gomori stains (3). Electrophysiological and lesioning studies were encouraged by the clustering of the large cell bodies of origin in the supraoptic nuclei (SON) and paraventricular nuclei (PVN) in the hypothalamus, and by the long axonal connection to the posterior pituitary neurosecretory site some distance away. These and other advantages, including early development of bioassays, resulted in greater progress in characterizing this peptidergic system. Even at this moment, many of the concepts concerning the nature of other peptide-producing neurons are extrapolated from what has been learned about the magnocellular system.

This chapter is primarily concerned with an explosion of new data obtained in the past 10 years by immunohistochemical methods. There is a strong suggestion that oxytocin and vasopressin are also produced in other, probably smaller neurons, which project to many other sites in the brain and spinal cord. It appears that the term "magnocellular system" with regard to oxytocin and vasopressin pertains mainly to the posterior pituitary connections. As has been established for most other peptide-containing neurons to date, these other vasopressin (suprachiasmatic nucleus and PVN) and oxytocin (PVN) neurons appear to be smaller ("parvocellular"). Pathways from these structures to other regions of the brain and spinal cord suggest many behavioral and autonomic functions for these peptides in the central nervous system.

2   THE CLASSIC MAGNOCELLULAR SYSTEM

2.1   Hormones in the Supraoptic Nuclei (SON) and Paraventricular Nuclei (PVN)

Studies with Gomori stains (aldehyde fuchsin, chrome-alum-hematoxylin) had shown that the large neurons of both SON and PVN contained a neurosecretory material transported through their axonal tracts to the posterior pituitary gland (1). Although bioassays had demonstrated oxytocin and vasopressin activity in both regions, the relative contributions of these hormones from the respective nuclei was debated (5). Until recently, one opinion favored the PVN as an oxytocin nucleus and the SON the major source of vasopressin (5). Immunohistochemical studies revealed approximately equal numbers of both types of neurons in both nuclei, although twice as many of both types are found in the SON (6). Electrophysiological studies revealed characteristic electrical activity for each of the two types of neurons in both nuclei (2). However, there may yet be some division of labor between these nuclei, as bilateral lesions of PVN appear to abolish the suckling response (J. Haldar, G. Nilaver, and E. A. Zimmerman, unpublished). How to interpret these preliminary results is not yet certain, since such lesions may interfere with regulatory afferent inputs from the brainstem or with reciprocal connections between PVN and brainstem relays (7).

2.2   Magnocellular Accessory Nuclei

It has been shown recently that additional "accessory" magnocellular nuclei in the hypothalamus and nearby regions contain oxytocin or vasopressin and project to the posterior pituitary gland (8, 9) (see Table 1). In addition, a few smaller neurons widely distributed in PVN also send fibers to the posterior pituitary (Table 1). By comparison, retrograde tracing studies from the median eminence suggested that most of the cells that project to the portal capillary bed are parvocellular neurons in medial and dorsal PVN (7–10). Electrophysiological studies suggest that some of the cells in PVN projecting to the median eminence are vasopressinergic by their phasic activity pattern, and that some project to both this secretory region and the posterior pituitary (11). If there are medial parvocellular PVN cells, they might contain neurotensin (12) or vasopressin. Branching of PVN vasopressin neurons has been noted (13). Similar recording studies have shown common projections of a few PVN neurons to the neurohypophysis and medulla (14), although simultaneous dye tracing studies suggest that they are generally separate (15).

2.3   Neurophysins as Markers

Studies with species-specific antiserum to the two respective neurophysins in ox, human, and monkey confirmed that these 10,000 dalton "carrier" proteins are localized to the same neurons containing the respective (1000 dalton) hormones (6). Furthermore, neurophysin was not found in the neurons lacking vasopressin in the ventral SON and parts of PVN in homozygous Brattleboro rats with diabetes insipidus (DI rat) (16). This finding supports the data from biosynthetic studies which suggest that both moieties come from a larger common precursor (see Chapter 3) that is absent in the DI rat (4). The neurophysins have been

TABLE 1 Neurosecretory Projections Containing Oxytocin or Vasopressin[a]

Terminal Field	Origin	Peptide	Method	References
Posterior pituitary gland	Magnocellular			
	anterior commissural	OT,NP	IHC,HRP	7, 55, 56
	medial magnocellular	OT	IHC dye	7
	medial and lateral paraventricular	OT,VP	IHC,HRP, dye	7, 8, 57
	accessory:	OT,VP		
	circularis		HRP,IHC	8, 57
	forebrain bundle			
	bed stria terminalis		Dye	9
	preoptic			
	zona incerta			
	substantia innominata			
	Parvocellular			
	PVN, some of all 5 divisions	?	Dye	7
Median eminence	Parvocellular PVN			
	medial (most)	?VP	HRP,dye	7–10
	dorsal (fewer)			
Organum vasculosum	Rostral magnocellular	NPS,OT,VP	IHC	58
	Suprachiasmatic	VP	IHC	38, 39

[a] Abbreviations: OT, oxytocin; NP, neurophysin; IHC, immunohistochemistry; HRP, horseradish peroxidase; VP, vasopressin; PVN, paraventricular nucleus.

extremely useful for a great number of experimental approaches to this system. Their large numbers of cystine residues permit labeling with ^{35}S-cystine to a high degree of specific activity for studies of biosynthesis and active transport (4). Their presence together with the hormones in the intra-axonal granules and their cosecretion into the general circulation provided evidence for an exocytotic mechanism of secretion (3). Radioimmunoassay of a specific neurophysin in human and monkey peripheral plasma was found to be stimulated by estrogens. Although this neurophysin was known to be localized in oxytocin cells by immunohistochemistry, owing to difficulties with the assay for oxytocin (17) it was only recently shown that oxytocin is secreted under the same conditions. Another neurophysin in primates colocalized with vasopressin and was secreted in response to nicotine and to physiological events associated with vasopressin secretion. Specific neurophysins were also found to be released with oxytocin and vasopressin in ox and ovine species (17).

2.4 Problems in Immunohistochemistry

The neurophysins also served as important additional markers for immunohistochemistry, since their colocalization with the hormones was more compelling evidence that the neurons actually produced the peptide hormones and did not take it up from elsewhere, and it indicated that the peptides were the substances in question and did not represent shared immunologic determinants with some other unidentified substances (18). These are extremely important considerations in interpreting immunohistochemical data. At present there is little colocalization data for most of the 30 or more peptides studied in brain except for this system and the ACTH/β-endorphin system (see Chapter 26). Furthermore, very few investigators have fully characterized the determinants of their antibodies to a given peptide in immunohistochemical procedures, which may explain some of the variable results obtained. There is now a strong movement in the field to develop libraries of antibodies to different determinants of the same peptide or parts of its precursor or products by immunizing with peptide fragments, or by selecting them by hybridoma techniques (19). This promises to bring immunohistochemistry closer to real chemistry than its present state permits.

Other considerations are also important for interpretation of immunohistochemical studies of this system. One has to do with difficulties that arise in reacting with the peptides compared with the neurophysins in extrahypothalamic sites (see Section 5.3). Another involves the dispute about the presence of extragranular hormone (20). By electron microscopic immunohistochemistry several investigators have observed extragranular in addition to intragranular hormone and neurophysin. At the present time it is not certain whether the extragranular reactions represent true cellular localization of the peptides or are due to granule destruction or dispersion of reaction products.

3 VASOPRESSIN PROJECTIONS TO THE HYPOPHYSIAL PORTAL SYSTEM: ANOTHER NEUROSECRETORY PATHWAY

3.1 The Pathway

Ten years ago neurophysin was first detected around portal capillaries in the zona externa of the median eminence (3). It was subsequently shown that the known increase in Gomori-positive material in the zona externa in response to adrenalectomy was associated with increases in vasopressin together with its neurophysin (21). Oxytocin projections were not observed to change with adrenalectomy. Subsequently, it was found that the PVN rather than the SON was the source of these projections (21). Retrograde tracing studies from terminals in the median eminence vs. posterior pituitary gland suggest that it is probably the smaller cells in PVN which contribute to this projection to the median eminence (7–10). The vasopressin-containing granules are also smaller (approximately 100 nm) (21) in terminals in zona externa compared with those in the posterior pituitary gland (120–180 nm). Recent tracing studies of ascending norepinephrine afferents indicate a different innervation of the two neurosecretory systems as well (22). The magnocellular neurons receive their main input from the A1 group (lateral reticular nucleus of medulla), while the parvocellular group is directly innervated from the A2 (nucleus solitarius) group. Depletion of norepinephrine causes a loss of vasopressin in the zona externa, but not in the posterior pituitary of normal rats, suggesting selective tonic inhibition of the median eminence system (23).

3.2 Vasopressin and ACTH

These anatomical observations together with the demonstration of very high concentrations of vasopressin in hypophysial portal blood, which is known to release ACTH (21), reopened the old controversy about vasopressin as a corticotropin releasing factor (CRF). Experiments in which antiserum to vasopressin blocked the activity of CRF preparations suggested that the hormone may be the major CRF (24). But ACTH and adrenal responses are relatively (not totally) normal in DI rats, and another more potent CRF which is not vasopressin has been repeatedly reported (24). This issue will probably soon be fully resolved since one potent CRF has now been isolated and synthesized (25).

3.3 Glucocorticoids and the Median Eminence System

The marked increase in zona externa vasopressin that occurs with adrenalectomy is inhibited by administration of glucocorticoid but not mineralocorticoids in the rat (26). Furthermore, adrenalectomy selectively increases RNA turnover (27) and the biosynthesis of vasopressin in this system (28). Whether the apparent inhibitory feedback of glucocorticoids occurs within cells at the PVN level or is indirect via effects on other neurons is not known. It is also not known if adrenalectomy is actually associated with increased secretion of vasopressin into the pituitary portal blood as occurs in the systemic circulation (17). It can be argued that increased content might be due to decreased release. Another point as yet not fully resolved is whether the PVN is the source of most of the portal vein vasopressin, or if it arises from neurohypophysis by retrograde flow (29). Stimulation of the PVN in cats caused release of both systemic vasopressin and ACTH, while SON activation resulted in the release of vasopressin and possibly some decline in ACTH (30). Although these results support the concept of a separate PVN–median eminence system in the regulation of ACTH, they are clouded by a possible inhibitory substance activated by SON stimulation. These issues may be resolved by measuring vasopressin in the portal blood of normal and adrenalectomized rats bearing bilateral PVN lesions.

The capacity of fibers of the PVN–median eminence system to sprout was recently discovered in the course of investigating whether the PVN projections to median eminence in rats were unilateral, as in monkeys, or bilateral (31). It was hypothesized that sprouting might account for the relatively long time course of increases in vasopressin in the zona externa after adrenalectomy. The pathway was studied by orthograde tracing with horseradish peroxidase (HRP) and by immunocytochemistry in normal, adrenalectomized, and chronic unilateral PVN-lesioned rats with and without prior adrenalectomy. We found that the system was unilateral in all cases except in those rats that received both adrenalectomy and the unilateral PVN lesion. The vasopressin-neurophysin fibers disappeared in the ipsilateral zona externa, a few days after the lesion in adrenalectomized animals. By 22 days the fibers had begun to grow across from the normal to the deficient zona externa, and by 26 days both sides were filled with terminals. These results suggest that sprouting contributes to increases in zona externa vasopressin in response to adrenalectomy only in rats with PVN lesions. They also suggest that the ability of this system to sprout is influenced greatly by the adrenal gland, probably glucocorticoid. Glucocorticoids are reported to inhibit sprouting in the hippocampus after lesions (32) and to prevent neurite outgrowth in cultured adrenal medullary cells (33). Neuronal outgrowth to blood vessels is well-known after transection of fibers of the magnocellular system in the pituitary stalk (34). The experiments described above, however, involve a different paradigm involving outgrowth of the normal system to supply a deficient target. It may be similar to the innervation of the vasopressin-deficient median eminence of the DI rat by third ventricular transplants of normal fetal magnocellular neurons (35).

4   VASOPRESSIN IN THE SUPRACHIASMATIC NUCLEUS

4.1   Vasopressin Within the Nucleus

Discovery of vasopressin and its neurophysin in the parvocellular neurons of the suprachiasmatic nucleus (SCN) was initially surprising (3) since this hormone was thought to reside only in magnocellular neurons (Figure 1). These cells have now been reported in many mammals, including humans (36). Suspicion that it represented cross-reactivity with arginine vasotocin, or some other substance was dispelled by the finding that staining was absent in the DI rat. In addition, a monoclonal antibody to vasopressin (19) and a rabbit antiserum (36) visualized vasopressin and not vasotocin. Oxytocin and its neurophysin are not found in these vasopressin cells, which tend to lie in the dorsal and medial parts of the major portion of the nucleus, although they are found throughout its entire rostrocaudal extent (37). Many fine reactive fibers form axosomatic contacts with neurons in the nucleus, and others can be traced dorsally out of the region.

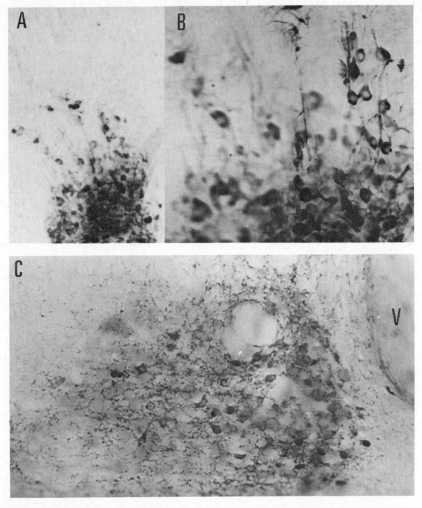

Figure. 1 Localization of vasopressin in coronal sections of rat hypothalamus by immunoperoxidase technique employing a monoclonal antibody: (A) Magnocellular neurons and fibers in supraoptic nucleus; (B) higher magnifications of (A); (C) parvocellular neurons and a dense plexus of fibers containing vasopressin in rostral suprachiasmatic nucleus. Same magnification as (B) V,ventricle. (From A. Hou-Yu, D. Englehardt, W. H. Sawyer, G. Nilaver, and E. A. Zimmerman, *J. Histochem Cytochem.*, 30, 1249 (1982) with permission.)

4.2 Projections Out of the Nucleus

The projections of vasopressin fibers from the SCN have not been entirely clarified, since they are hard to separate from those arising from the PVN. Some authors suggest that most forebrain structures are innervated from the SCN (38), while others consider its contributions to be more limited including the OVLT, (organum vasculosum lamina terminalis), the lateral septum and lateral habenula, and a few other sites (39) (see Table 2). Fibers originating in the SCN are also reported to project to the midbrain (38), which may explain why it is possible to abolish medullary neurophysin fibers but not those in midbrain after PVN lesions (G. Nilaver and E. A. Zimmerman, unpublished). Further studies after selective SCN and PVN lesions should help resolve these issues about fiber origin.

The basal part of the SCN contains many vasoactive intestinal polypeptide (VIP)-reactive neurons (37, 40). VIP and vasopressin fibers with-

TABLE 2   Extrahypothalamic Projections of Oxytocin, Vasopressin, Neurophysin Fibers by Immunohistochemistry[a]

Terminal Field	Origin	Peptide	Reference
Forebrain			
cortex	PVN	VP,OT,NP	19, 39, 46, 57, 59
medial septal	PVN	VP,OT	38, 39
lateral septal	SCN,PVN	VP	39, 44, 57
diagonal band	SCN,PVN	VP,NP	38, 43
amygdala			
medial	PVN	VP,OT,NP	39, 43
	SCN	VP	9
central, lateral, basal	PVN	VP,OT	38, 39, 57
medial-dorsal thalamus	SCN	VP	36, 38, 39
lateral habenular	SCN	VP	36, 38, 39, 44
ventral hippocampus	PVN	VP,OT	38, 39, 44
subcommissural organ	SCN	VP	39
Brainstem			
substantia migra	PVN	OT,VP,OTNP	38, 46, 57
mesencephalic grey	SCN	VP	38
	PVN	OT,NP	38, 43, 57
dorsal raphe	SCN	VP	38
	PVN	OT	38, 43
parabrachial	PVN	OT,VP,NP	7, 38, 43
locus coeruleus	PVN	NP	43
raphe magnus	PVN	OT,VP	38
tractus solitarius	PVN	OT,VP,NP	7, 38, 43, 46, 57
dorsal motor vagus	PVN	OT,VP,NP	7, 38, 43, 46, 57
ambiguus	PVN	OT,VP	38, 39, 57
lateral reticular	PVN	OT,VP	38
commissural	PVN	OT,VP,NP	38, 46
Spinal cord			
lamina I (dorsal horn)	PVN	OT,VP,NP	7, 38, 46, 57
lamina X (central grey)	PVN	OT,VP,NP	7, 38, 43, 45, 47, 57
		VPNP > OTNP	47
intermediolateral grey	PVN	OT,NP	7, 38, 43, 57, 45
		VPNP,OTNP	47

[a] Abbreviations: see Table 1; SCN, suprachiasmatic nucleus.

in the SCN form overlapping dense plexuses throughout much of the nucleus. VIP containing terminals form axodendritic contacts with other neurons in the nucleus (37). Some axons cross the chiasm to innervate the SCN nucleus on the contralateral side. A dense VIP-containing fiber projection can be traced from the SCN to the PVN, which appears to terminate along its ventral border (37). It is likely, but not yet directly proved, that SCN neurons shown to project to PVN by orthograde (37) and retrograde (41) techniques contain VIP. It is not known whether any contain vasopressin.

4.3   Role in Circadian Rhythm?

What role any of these peptides have in the known ability of the SCN to generate circadian rhythms is not known. In terms of vasopressin, available data does not support a critical role, since DI rats have normal circadian changes in adrenal function (24), drinking behavior, locomotor activity, and pineal N-acetyltransferase levels (37). In a recent report that documented a diurnal rhythm in cerebrospinal fluid vasopressin but which is not present in the peripheral circulation of cats, it was speculated that the SCN may secrete vasopressin into the ventricular system (42). VIP remains to be investigated as a participant in adrenal rhythms, possibly by its connections with vasopressin or CRF neurons originating in PVN and projecting to the hypophysial portal system in the median eminence.

5   EXTRAHYPOTHALAMIC PROJECTIONS

5.1   Projections

One of the major events of the past five years was the demonstration of extrahypothalamic fibers containing neurophysin which extend as far caudally as the spinal cord (7, 43). Their existence was suggested by preceding anatomical studies using orthograde and retrograde tracing methods (43). A very complex and widespread pattern of distribution of apparent oxytocin and vasopressin pathways is beginning to emerge, as reviewed in Table 2. Additional proposed termination areas are not included in the table since it is not clear whether these are fibers of passage or of termination. Other pathways, including those innervating other hypothalamic regions such as the preoptic area or the supramammillary nuclei, have also not been included. It seems certain that many more will be found.

There are many anatomical and biochemical issues to be resolved concerning these pathways before a solid basis can be provided for physiological studies. In most cases the nature of apparent terminal fields by light microscopy is not known. There is only one electron microscopic immunocytochemical study which demonstrates the presence and nature of vasopressin (lateral septum, habenula, medial amygdala) and oxytocin (medial amygdala) in vesicles in terminals which appear to make axodendritic synapses (44). Other reported sites may involve fibers of passage or endings on other structures, such as blood vessels (39).

5.2 Cells of Origin

Studies of the location of the neurons of origin and their trajectory are only beginning. It is not resolved whether the vasopressin fibers in the forebrain arise from the SCN, the PVN, or both (Table 2). Projections of PVN to lateral septum, amygdala, midbrain periaqueductal gray (11), and medulla have been confirmed by electrophysiological methods (14). The caudal pathways to brainstem and spinal cord have been studied more extensively by anatomical methods (7, 17, 22, 45–48). By combined retrograde dye methods from spinal cord and medulla with immunohistochemistry, most of the labeled PVN cells were shown to be located in parvocellular neurons, although some were found in posterior magnocellular neurons (7, 15). Spinal cord projecting neurons were present in the dorsal, lateral, and ventral aspect of the medial parvocellular divisions of PVN. Those ending in the medulla were localized to the latter two regions. About 15% of labeled cells projected to both regions. About twice as many peptide-identified cell bodies projected to cord than medulla, and the ratio of vasopressin to oxytocin neurons was 2:1 in the former case and 4:1 in the latter. A similar study of the medullary projection also found a 4:1 ratio in PVN, with a tendency for the labeled neurons to be small and localized in the caudal part of PVN, generally medial, but with some dorsal as well (48). Labeled cells ranged in size from 12–26 μm. Vasopressin or oxytocin labeled cells accounted for only about 10% of those retrogradely labeled in both studies, indicating that other substances will probably be found in these pathways, such as somatostatin or biogenic amines (7).

5.3 Biochemical Characterization

The chemical nature of the oxytocin and vasopressin in extra-hypothalamic sites remains to be fully established. Colocalization of specific neurophysins with the respective peptides remains to be done in most cases. In spinal cord, preliminary data suggests that the central descending pathway contains more vasopressin-neurophysin and vasopressin, and the dorsolateral pathway more oxytocin-neurophysin and oxytocin (47). By radioimmunoassay of extracts of dissected regions of rat, larger amounts of vasopressin than oxytocin were found in forebrain areas (septum and thalamus), while the reverse was found in medulla, which generally supports immunocytochemical data (49). We found significant concentrations of bioassayable oxytocin in the spinal cord of rats (J. Haldar, G. Nilaver, and E. A. Zimmerman, unpublished). However, we have encountered greater difficulty in visualizing the peptides as compared with the neurophysins in extrahypothalamic sites even in thick vibratome sections where the fibers are more readily seen. Although this may prove to be inept immunohistochemical visualization of the peptides, it still raises the possibility of different processing of the precursors in these extrahypothalamic projections. It has been shown that ^{35}S-cystine incorporated into neurophysin in the PVN is actively transported to the spinal cord in the rat (50). However, no definitive information was obtained concerning the associated peptides in this study. Additional chemical characterization of the extrahypothalamic system is needed in spinal cord and other sites.

6 POSSIBLE FUNCTIONAL ASPECTS

Despite incomplete data, it seems likely that the extensive oxytocin and vasopressin pathways in the central nervous system might have a wide variety of functions, some of which are listed in Table 3. Possible roles in memory and pain regulation are discussed in Chapters 13 and 17. It is possible that the tripeptide, Pro-Leu-Gly-amide (melanocyte-stimulating hormone inhibiting factor, MIF) may be derived from oxytocin fibers such as those in caudate. Such fibers might serve as the anatomical basis of the observations that MIF can ameliorate experimental Parkinsonism (51) or tardive dyskinesia (52). It remains to be proved whether MIF exists in brain and whether it is generated in oxytocin neurons.

One of the more compelling possibilities concerns the likely participation of the descending PVN system in the regulation of both sympathetic and parasympathetic nervous systems, as pointed out by Swanson and colleagues (7, 53). In the spinal cord of the rat, the innervations of the intermediolateral gray preganglionic neurons by PVN is highly organized to T1–T3, T9–T11 and T13–L2 (45). The T9–T11 preganglionics innervate adrenal gland and kidney (7), organs that are also targets of ACTH and vasopressin. These organs, in turn, influence PVN secretion via glucocorticoids or changes in osmolality. The parasympathetic system is also innervated by the PVN, for example the nucleus of the solitary tract. This nucleus receives visceral sensory information, via cranial nerves IX and X, about blood pressure and volume (aortic baroreceptors, carotid body chemoreceptors, and atrial stretch receptors) which also project to PVN to regulate vasopressin secretion (7). Among other functions, the PVN may maintain tonic inhibitory control over heart rate by its projections to the solitary region where it may regulate the carotid sinus reflex (7). Recent iontophoretic studies sug-

TABLE 3

Pathway Nuclear Origin	Termination	Peptide	Function
Supraoptic	Posterior pituitary	Vasopressin	Kidney: antidiuresis; Systemic arteries: blood pressure
		Oxytocin	Lactating breast: milk ejection Pregnant uterus: contraction
Paraventricular	Posterior pituitary	Vasopressin	Same as above
		Oxytocin	Same as above
Paraventricular	Median Eminence Portal System	Vasopressin	Anterior pituitary: stimulate ACTH
Suprachiasmatic	Forebrain, itself	Vasopressin	?Diurnal rhythm in CSF vasopressin
Paraventricular	Forebrain	Vasopressin Oxytocin	Memory, alertness
Paraventricular	Brainstem/spinal cord	Oxytocin	Regulate autonomic centers: both parasympathetic and sympathetic: heart rate, blood pressure, ?kidney and adrenal sympathetic tone
		Vasopressin	Inhibit pain. Regulate capillary permeability via locus coeruleus?
Paraventricular	Cerebral arteries	Oxytocin	Regulates blood flow?

gest that oxytocin inhibits neurons in the caudal medulla (54). Connections of the PVN to the locus coeruleus have also been postulated to affect capillary permeability via norepinephrine in response to changes in blood pressure or osmolality (53).

REFERENCES

1. E. Scharrer and B. Scharrer, *Recent Prog. Horm. Res.* **10**, 183 (1954).
2. B. A. Cross, R. E. Dyball, R. G. Dyer, C. W. Jones, D. W. Lincoln, J. F. Morris, and B. T. Pickering, *Recent Prog. Horm. Res.* **31**, 243 (1975).
3. E. A. Zimmerman in L. Martini and W. F. Ganong, Eds., *Frontiers in Neuro-endocrinology*, Vol. 4, Raven Press, New York, 1976, p. 25.
4. M. J. Brownstein, J. T. Russell, and H. Gainer, *Science* **207**, 373 (1980).
5. E. A. Zimmerman, A. G. Robinson, M. K. Husain, M. Acosta, A. G. Frantz, and W. H. Sawyer, *Endocrinology* **95**, 931 (1974).
6. R. Defendini and E. A. Zimmerman, in S. Reichlin, R. J. Baldessarini, and J. B. Martin, Eds., *The Hypothalamus*, Raven Press, New York, 1978, p. 137.

7. L. W. Swanson and P. E. Sawchenko, *Neuroendocrinology* **31**, 410 (1980).
8. S. J. Wiegand and J. L. Price, *J. Comp. Neurol.* **191**, 1 (1980).
9. J. Kelly and L. W. Swanson, *Brain Res.* **197**, 1 (1980).
10. W. H. Armstrong and G. I. Hatton, *Brain Res. Bull.* **5**, 473 (1980).
11. Q. J. Pittman, H. W. Blume, and L. P. Renaud, *Brain Res.* **215**, 15 (1981).
12. D. Kahn, G. M. Abrams, E. A. Zimmerman, R. Carraway, and S. Leeman, *Endocrinology* **107**, 47 (1980).
13. M. V. Sofroniew and W. Glasmann, *Neuroscience* **6**, 619 (1981).
14. L. Zerihun and M. Harris, *Neurosci. Lett.* **23**, 157 (1981).
15. L. W. Swanson and H. G. J. M. Kuypers, *J. Comp. Neurol.* **194**, 555 (1980).
16. H. W. Sokol, E. A. Zimmerman, W. H. Sawyer, and A. G. Robinson, *Endocrinology* **98**, 1176 (1976).
17. A. G. Robinson, J. G. Verbalis, J. A. Amico, and S. M. Seif, *Int. Rev. Physiol., Endocr. Physiol. III* **24**, 1 (1981).
18. E. A. Zimmerman, L. Krupp, D. L. Hoffman, E. Matthew, and G. Nilaver, *Peptides* **1**, Suppl. 1, 3 (1980).
19. A. Hou-Yu, D. Engelhardt, W. H. Sawyer, G. Nilaver, and E. A. Zimmerman, *J. Histochem. Cytochem.*, **30**, 1249 (1982).
20. B. Krisch, *Cell Tissue Res.* **197**, 95 (1979).
21. E. A. Zimmerman, M. A. Stillman, L. D. Recht, J. L. Antunes, P. W. Carmel, and P. C. Goldsmith, *Ann. N.Y. Acad. Sci.* **297**, 405 (1977).
22. P. E. Sawchenko and L. W. Swanson, *Science* **214**, 347 (1981).
23. V. Seybold, R. Elde, and T. Hökfelt, *Endocrinology* **108**, 1803 (1981).
24. G. Gillies and P. J. Lowry, in W. F. Ganong and L. Martini, Eds., *Frontiers in Neuroendocrinology*, Vol. 7, Raven Press, New York, 1982, p. 45.
25. W. Vale, J. Spiess, C. Rivier, and J. Rivier, *Science* **213**, 1394 (1981).
26. A. J. Silverman, D. L. Hoffman, C. Gadde, L. C. Krey, and E. A. Zimmerman, *Neuroendocrinology* **32**, 129 (1981).
27. A. J. Silverman, C. A. Gadde, and E. A. Zimmerman, *Neuroendocrinology* **30**, 285 (1980).
28. J. T. Russell, M. J. Brownstein, and H. Gainer, *Brain Res.* **201**, 227 (1980).
29. L. D. Recht, D. L. Hoffman, J. Haldar, A. J. Silverman, and E. A. Zimmerman, *Neuroendocrinology* **33**, 88 (1981).
30. A. Dornhorst, D. E. Carlson, S. M. Seif, A. G. Robinson, E. A. Zimmerman, and D. S. Gann, *Endocrinology* **108**, 1420 (1981).
31. A. J. Silverman, C. Moodhe, and E. A. Zimmerman, *Soc. Neurosci. Abstr.* **7**, No. 107.7 (1981).
32. S. W. Scheff, L. S. Benardo, and C. W. Cotman, *Exp. Neurol.* **68**, 195 (1980).
33. K. Unsicker, B. Krisch, U. Otten, and H. Thoenen, *Proc. Natl. Acad. Sci. USA* **75**, 3498 (1978).
34. J. L. Antunes, P. W. Carmel, E. A. Zimmerman, and M. Ferin, *Ann. Neurol.* **5**, 462 (1979).
35. D. Gash and J. R. Sladek Jr., *Peptides* **1**, 11 (1980).
36. M. V. Sofroniew and A. Weindl, *J. Comp. Neurol.* **193**, 659 (1980).
37. J. P. Card, N. Brecha, H. J. Karten, and R. Y. Moore, *J. Neurosci.* **1**, 1289 (1981).
38. M. V. Sofroniew, *J. Histochem. Cytochem.* **28**, 475 (1980).
39. R. M. Buijs, *Cell Tissue Res.* **192**, 423 (1978).
40. K. Sims, D. L. Hoffman, S. I. Said, and E. A. Zimmerman, *Brain Res.* **86**, 165 (1980).
41. A. J. Silverman, D. L. Hoffman, and E. A. Zimmerman, *Brain Res. Bull.* **6**, 47 (1981).
42. S. M. Reppert, H. G. Artman, S. Swaminathan, and D. A. Fisher, *Science* **213**, 1256 (1981).
43. L. W. Swanson, *Brain Res.* **128**, 346 (1977).
44. R. M. Buijs and D. F. Swaab, *Cell Tissue Res.* **204**, 355 (1979).
45. L. W. Swanson and S. McKellar, *J. Comp. Neurol.* **168**, 87 (1979).

46. G. Nilaver, E. A. Zimmerman, J. Wilkins, J. Michaels, D. Hoffman, and A. J. Silverman, *Neuroendocrinology* **30**, 150 (1980).
47. G. Nilaver, J. Mulhern, and E. A. Zimmerman, *Ann. N.Y. Acad. Sci.*, **394**, 759 (1982).
48. M. V. Sofroniew and U. Schrell, *Neurosci. Lett.* **22**, 211 (1981).
49. J. Dogterom, F. G. M. Snijdewint, and R. M. Buijs, *Neurosci. Lett.* **9**, 341 (1978).
50. E. A. Zimmerman, M. J. Brownstein, and H. Gainer, *Neurology* **32**, A107 (1982) (abstr.).
51. A. Barbeau, M. Roy, and A. J. Kastin, *Canad. Med. Assoc. J.* **114**, 120 (1976).
52. S. Chiu, C. S. Paulose, and R. K. Mishra, *Science*, **214**, 1261 (1981).
53. L. W. Swanson and B. K. Hartman, *Neurosci. Lett.* **16**, 55 (1980).
54. R. Morris, T. E. Salt, M. V. Sofroniew, and R. G. Hill, *Neurosci.* **18**, 163 (1980).
55. W. E. Armstrong, S. Warach, G. I. Hatton, and T. H. McNeill, *Neuroscience* **5**, 1931 (1980).
56. C. H. Rhodes, J. I. Morrell, and D. W. Pfaff, *J. Comp. Neurol.* **198**, 45 (1981).
57. E. A. Zimmerman, in J. B. Martin, S. Reichlin, and K. L. Bick, Eds., *Neurosecretion and Brain Peptides*, Raven Press, New York, 1981, p. 63.
58. J. L. Antunes, P. W. Carmel, and E. A. Zimmerman, *Brain Res.* **137**, 1 (1977).

26

Pro-Opiomelanocortin-Related
and Other Pituitary Hormones
in the Central Nervous System

ANTHONY S. LIOTTA

DOROTHY T. KRIEGER

Division of Endocrinology
Department of Medicine
Mount Sinai School of Medicine
New York, New York

1 INTRODUCTION

In higher vertebrates, peptides and proteins resembling the hormones of the anterior and intermediate pituitary lobe are present in the central nervous system as well as in several peripheral sites. Preliminary evidence indicates that at least some pituitary-like hormones are also present in simple invertebrates, and even in unicellular organisms. Such findings are not compatible with the traditional view that the pituitary is the sole site of synthesis of pituitary hormones, but rather indicate that these molecules existed long before the evolution of the pituitary gland. The presence of the same or similar peptides at multiple sites within an organism also implies that they serve different, albeit not necessarily mutually exclusive, functions at these sites.

The major portion of this chapter focuses on adrenocorticotropin (ACTH), β-endorphin, and related peptides in brain, their anatomical distribution, and their possible functional significance in view of the greater amount of data available for these pituitary-like hormones than others.

The physical proximity of the pituitary to the brain, the very high concentrations of these peptides in the pituitary relative to the brain, and the possible existence of vascular and neural routes that can transport pituitary hormones to the brain require more careful consideration of all available data than the data for most other messenger peptides reputed to be present in multiple tissue sites (e.g., the coexistence of similar peptides in gastrointestinal tract and brain). The presence of a peptide in a given tissue cannot be taken as evidence that the peptide is synthesized there, or even that it is transported there to serve a physiological function—it may merely represent contamination.

2 PROCESSING OF PITUITARY PRO-OPIOMELANOCORTIN (POMC): THE COMMON PRECURSOR OF ADRENOCORTICOTROPIN-RELATED AND β-ENDORPHIN-RELATED PEPTIDES

A knowledge of the chemical forms of pituitary-derived ACTH, β-endorphin, and related peptides and of the manner in which they are synthesized will aid in the study of ACTH- and β-endorphin-related peptides present in the brain. Both anterior and intermediate lobe pituitary corticotrophic cells synthesize a similar or identical glycoprotein molecule (or molecules) containing within it the complete sequences of ACTH and β-lipotropin, as well as a large glycopeptide that comprises the amino terminus of the molecule (Figure 1; refs. 1–9). This precursor molecule has been termed "pro-opiomelanocortin" (POMC) to indicate some of the putative biological activities derived from it (4). Pulse-chase

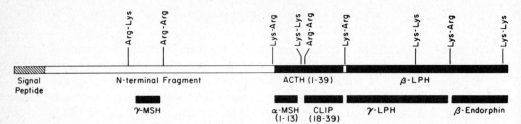

Figure 1. Structure of prepro-opiomelanocortin. Indicated are the major peptide products derived posttranslationally from the POMC common precursor protein in anterior and intermediate pituitary gland corticotrophic cells. ACTH-(1-39) and β-lipotropin are generated by proteolytic cleavages at Lys-Arg dipeptide "spacer" sequences. Likewise, γ-lipotropin and β-endorphin can be generated from β-lipotropin by cleavage of an internal Lys-Arg sequence. Although all pairs of basic amino acids are shown, Lys-Lys and Arg-Lys sequences do not appear to be major cleavage sites.

The generation of α-MSH from ACTH ultimately requires a cleavage at Val[13]-Gly[14]; it is likely that the cleavage is between the α-amino and the α-carbon of the glycine residue, thus producing the C-terminal Val-amide group of α-MSH.

The sequences of α-endorphin and γ-endorphin (not shown) are contained within the β-endorphin sequence [β-endorphin-(1-16) and -(1-17), respectively] and would require cathepsin D-like activity and a carboxypeptidase activity to generate them as free peptides. See Chapter 2 for more details.

studies have unequivocally demonstrated the precursor nature of POMC and established the major intermediates and products in the POMC processing pathways in rodent anterior and intermediate pituitary lobes (see refs. 1–3 for reviews). Molecular cloning of DNA complementary to pituitary POMC mRNA and genomic DNA fragments encoding POMC, followed by nucleotide sequencing of the cDNAs, have established not only the primary amino acid sequence (including the "signal" sequence) of POMC in human, cow, and rat (partial sequence) but also the noncoding sequences of the mRNAs and the structural organization of the POMC genes (10–18; see also Peng Loh and Gainer, Chapter 2 in this volume). The overall posttranslational processing of POMC, however, differs in the two pituitary lobes.

2.1   Anterior Lobe

In anterior pituitary corticotrophs, ACTH-(1-39), β-lipotropin, and an N-terminal glycopeptide (comprising approximately 75% of the N-terminal non-ACTH, non-β-lipotropin region of POMC and referred to as 16K fragment to indicate its apparent molecular weight of 16,000 daltons) appear to be major secretory products. Some of the β-lipotropin molecules are further processed to γ-lipotropin (comprising the N-terminal portion of β-lipotropin) and β-endorphin (comprising the C-terminal portion of β-lipotropin) (see Figure 1).

In addition, ACTH-(1-38), des-acetyl α-melanotropin (α-MSH), des-Tyr¹-β-endorphin, α- and γ-endorphin (contained within the N-terminal sequence of β-endorphin) and C-terminal fragments of β-endorphin appear to be minor products of POMC processing (19–21; Liotta and Krieger, unpublished observations).

2.2 Intermediate Lobe

In the intermediate lobe, the initial proteolytic cleavages of POMC appear to be the same as in anterior pituitary corticotrophs; however, relatively little intact β-lipotropin is stored in this tissue. β-lipotropin (β-LPH) is efficiently cleaved to γ-LPH and β-endorphin. β-endorphin is then α-N-acetylated and, on a slower time scale, C-terminally trimmed, yielding α-N-acetyl β-endorphin-(1-27) and α-N-acetyl β-endorphin-(1-26). The α-N-acetylated forms of β-endorphin, β-endorphin-(1-27), and β-endorphin-(1-26) appear to be the major β-endorphin-related peptide products in rat intermediate lobe cells (22–26). The extent of α-N-acetylation appears to be species specific, the rat intermediate pituitary lobe exhibiting the highest relative degree of acetylation of β-endorphin-related peptides (24). In contrast, no detectable α-N-acetylated or C-terminally trimmed forms are formed in anterior lobe; the low levels of such peptides in anterior pituitary reported by some investigators are most likely due to intermediate lobe cell contamination of anterior pituitary tissue. In analogy to β-endorphin, ACTH serves as a biosynthetic intermediate in intermediate lobe cells; it is α-N-acetylated and proteolytically cleaved to yield α-MSH [α-N-acetyl ACTH-(1-13)-amide] and ACTH-(18-39)-related peptides (1–3). A significant portion of porcine and rat intermediate lobe α-MSH has been identified as α-N,O-diacetylserine¹-α-MSH (27, 28). α- and γ-endorphin-like peptides are also present in the intermediate pituitary lobe. It is not clear how they are formed in the POMC processing pathway, but β-endorphin may not be an obligatory intermediate in their formation (20, 29).

POMC synthesized by both pituitary lobes exhibits size and charge heterogeneity, owing at least in part to several cotranslational/posttranslational covalent modifications such as glycosylation (30–32), phosphorylation (33–35), and sulfation (36), which occur in both cell types.

It is not known whether quantitative differences in the extent of any of these covalent modifications have a function in the differential processing of POMC in anterior and intermediate pituitary lobes (wherein the same proteolytic enzyme or enzymes could exhibit altered substrate specificies and, as a result of such modifications, yield different final products). Irrespective of the functional significance of these modifications, the chromatographic and electrophoretic heterogeneity they introduce can be used as "fingerprints" in characterizing extrapituitary

POMC-like material; if extrapituitary material exhibits the same behavior, presumptive evidence is obtained that not only is the same or a very similar POMC gene (or genes) expressed in these tissues, but the same covalent modifications occur.

PITUITARY-LIKE HORMONES PRESENT IN THE MAMMALIAN CENTRAL NERVOUS SYSTEM

3.1 Adrenocorticotropin-like and Endorphin-like Peptides

Immunoreactive and bioreactive α-melanotropin (α-MSH), ACTH, and β-endorphin-like material are present in the brains of all mammalian (and amphibian) species tested. Based on biological assays and chromatographic behavior, Guillemin and colleagues (37, 38) speculated that the MSH- and ACTH-like material they detected in extracts of pig and dog hypothalami might have a neurosecretory function of diencephalic origin. Contamination of hypothalamic tissue with stalk or pituitary tissue could not be ruled out in these studies (see refs. 39, 40 for historical reviews).

Our group (41, 42) reported that immunoreactive and bioreactive ACTH is present in the brains of intact and hypophysectomized rats; immunoreactive ACTH exhibited size heterogeneity. The hypothalamus contained the highest concentrations of ACTH-like material; several of the limbic system structures contained significant amounts of this material, with low concentrations detected in midbrain, pons, medulla, striatum, and cortex. Several subsequent studies verified these findings and reported on the presence of β-LPH-, α-MSH-, β-endorphin-, and γ-MSH-like peptides (see Figure 1) in the brains of several mammalian species, including the human (43–55). The regional distribution of these peptides was similar to that originally reported for ACTH-like material.

The brain content of these peptides has been reported to be in the range of 1/50–1/1000 the content of the whole pituitary gland. Some of the variability in the brain content reported by different groups is most assuredly due to the specificity of the antisera employed, the methods of animal sacrifice, and the tissue extraction procedures employed. If these peptides originate in the brain, only a small number of cells localized to the mediobasal hypothalamus appear to synthesize them. Thus the comparative data for brain and pituitary content are somewhat misleading. The actual cellular concentration in the two tissues may be very similar (see Sections 4 and 5).

3.2 Other Pituitary Hormones

Immunoreactive and bioreactive growth hormone (GH), prolactin, thyrotropin (TSH), and luteinizing hormone (LH)-like material are present in the mammalian brain (45, 56–63). Gel filtration and polyacrylamide gel electrophoretic characterization revealed that the major portion of the immunoreactive material present in brain tissue exhibited the same behavior as the corresponding authentic pituitary hormones. In the rat brain, the highest concentration of immunoreactive GH-like material is present in the amygdaloid nucleus, followed by the hypothalamus, caudate nucleus, thalamus, hippocampus, and cortex. The highest concentration of LH-like material is present in the hypothalamus, with decreasing concentrations in the amygdala, septum, preoptic area, caudate nucleus, hippocampus, and thalamus. A similar distribution has been reported for immunoreactive TSH (62). The brain content of LH-, TSH-, and GH-like material is approximately two to three orders of magnitude lower than the pituitary content of the authentic hormones. The presence of pituitary-like hormones in the cerebrospinal fluid (64–66) is briefly discussed in Section 4.2.3.

4 DISTRIBUTION OF PITUITARY-LIKE HORMONES IN THE CENTRAL NERVOUS SYSTEM

4.1 POMC-Related Peptides

Extensive immunocytochemical mapping studies utilizing antisera raised to several of the pituitary POMC-derived peptides (ACTH, α-MSH, β-lipotropin, β-endorphin, α- and γ-endorphin, and 16K fragment) have shown that such immunoreactive material has a widespread intraneuronal distribution throughout the mammalian brain. The distribution of the major reactive cell bodies, the hypothalamic and extrahypothalamic fiber pathways, and structures they appear to innervate are strikingly similar irrespective of the POMC-derived immunoreactive peptide or the mammalian species studied (e.g., monkey compared with rat).

The similar distribution pattern of the various immunoreactive POMC-derived peptides suggested, in analogy to pituitary, that all these activities are synthesized as part of a common precursor molecule and cosequestered within the same cells. (As noted in Chapter 21, immunocytochemical detection cannot distinguish between the presence of the multiple antigenic determinants within an intact precursor molecule or individual processed moieties.) Consistent with this hypothesis, several studies have demonstrated the presence in human (67, 68), rat (69–72), and sheep (73) of multiple immunoreactive POMC-related species within the same perikarya (in the mediobasal hypothalamus) and fibers, using sequential immunocytochemical staining of the same tissue sections, or staining of serial tissue sections with different antisera. Pelletier (74, 75) has shown that immunoreactive 16K fragment, ACTH, and β-lipotropin are contained within the same dense core granules, in the same hypothalamic cell bodies and fibers.

These results are therefore analogous to the ultrastructural localization of POMC-derived peptides to the same secretory granules of pituitary corticotrophic cells (76) and suggest that a similar biosynthetic and
"packaging" pathway exists in the brain. A general description of the
putative POMC-like neuronal network follows, compiled from studies
performed in the rat and monkey in which β-endorphin, ACTH, or α-
MSH antisera were employed.

4.1.1   Cell Bodies

Most or all immunoreactive perikarya appear to be localized to the
mediobasal hypothalamus. Specifically, postive cells are found throughout the rostrocaudal extent of the arcuate nucleus, extending laterally
along the floor of the hypothalamus; cells encircle and penetrate the lateral subdivision of the ventromedial nucleus; some cells are found in
the region of the ventral premammillary bodies (these cells are collectively referred to as the "arcuate nuclear region"). There is general
agreement in the literature as to the existence of these cell bodies (77–92).
    A second set of immunostainable α-MSH cell bodies have been de-
scribed within the dorsolateral aspects of the rat hypothalamus (93–95),
extending beyond the confines described for the above cells. Such cells
do not immunostain with β-endorphin or β-lipotropin antisera. Watson
and Akil (93) have postulated that two separate α-MSH neuronal systems may exist, the dorsolateral hypothalamic system synthesizing an
α-MSH-like species not derived from a POMC-like precursor or, if derived from a POMC-like precursor, involving rapid turnover of the other
POMC products or preferential storage of the α-MSH-like material.
These findings have not been extensively confirmed to date and should
at present be considered preliminary findings requiring further verification. If such cells exist, they contribute only a minor percentage to the
total brain content of α-MSH-like material and give rise to only a small
percentage of immunostainable α-MSH-like fibers (see Section 4.1.2).
    ACTH, β-endorphin, and 16K fragment immunostainable cell bodies
have been reported to be present in the supraoptic (SON) and
paraventricular (PVN) nuclei (96) of the hypothalamic magnocellular
system. Subsequent studies could not confirm this finding (79, 97) or
have indicated that such staining could not be abolished by preabsorption of the antiserum with ACTH or β-lipotropin (77, 84).
    Salih et al. (98) reported β-endorphin immunostainable non-neuronal
and neuronal cells in the brains of intact and hypophysectomized rats.
The positive non-neuronal cells included some ependymal cells of the
third ventricle and some cells of the choroid plexus. Immunostainable
β-endorphin cell bodies were also reported to be present in the hypothalamus, amygdala, hippocampus, thalamus, and cortex. This diffuse
localization of positive cell bodies has not been confirmed by any other

laboratories (with regard to the possible synthesis of POMC-like material in amygdala, see Section 6.1).

Leranth et al. (99), utilizing both light and electron microscopic immunocytochemical techniques, detected immunoreactive ACTH perikarya and dendrites in projection neurons of rat cerebellar nuclei. Immunoreactive β-endorphin perikarya were also detected in several divisions of the rat brainstem (80). These latter positive cell bodies were diffusely stained throughout the cytoplasm, in distinction to the granular appearance of reaction product present in the basal hypothalamic positive cell bodies. Staining of these cell bodies could only be completely abolished by preabsorption of antisera with synthetic β-endorphin, in the case of two of four β-endorphin antisera employed. The authors suggest caution in attributing specific staining of these cells, given the diffuse nature of the staining and the preabsorption anomalies.

4.1.2   Fiber Projections

Utilizing antisera raised to ACTH, α-MSH, β-endorphin, β-lipotropin, and 16K fragment, there is general agreement that immunostainable POMC fibers have a widespread distribution throughout the brain. Dense networks of positive fibers are present in the hypothalamus, preoptic area, mesencephalic gray, and at the level of the anterior commissure. Within the hypothalamus, most nuclei are innervated; within the mediobasal hypothalamus, fibers arising from cell bodies in the arcuate nuclear region course ventrally and terminate in the median eminence. Fibers also terminate within the arcuate nucleus, establishing contact with nonreactive (possibly dopaminergic) neurons.

Fibers, presumably originating from cell bodies in the arcuate nuclear region, leave the hypothalamus and innervate other brain structures, one such pathway coursing just ventral to the anterior commissure, projecting around its rostral and caudal aspects, and continuing dorsally, innervating the dorsal aspects of the bed nucleus of the stria terminalis, lateral septum, and the thalamic paraventricular and periventricular nuclei. Other fibers present in the medial, dorsal, and paraventricular thalamus arise from another fiber plexus, which courses in a rostral and dorsal path to the preoptic region and the hypothalamic periventricular nucleus, before reaching the thalamus. Both of these networks are believed to give off fibers that innervate the amygdala. The periaqueductal gray (PAG) region contains a rich supply of fibers, some of which course through the PAG and innervate the reticular formation. Fibers are present in the inferior colliculus and surrounding regions. Within the pons, fibers are present in the nucleus locus coeruleus and nucleus reticularis pontis oralis, nucleus reticularis tegmenti pontis, and nucleus reticularis pontalis caudalis. Another fiber bundle leaves the caudal aspect of the arcuate nuclear region and travels in a caudal and dorsal direction, innervating structures in the brainstem. The fiber networks innervating the thalamic nuclei may continue caudally also, innervating brainstem structures.

Sawchenko et al. (79) and Knigge and Joseph (78), confirming the heavy innervation of the hypothalamic paraventricular nucleus (PVN) noted in most previous studies, also reported that the dorsal and medial parvocellular regions of this nucleus are heavily innervated; ACTH staining was much less intense in the magnocellular division of the PVN. Utilizing a combined technique composed of ACTH immunocytochemistry and retrograde transport of true blue stain injected into the PVN, it could be shown that the ACTH-stained fibers and terminals present in the PVN arose from perikarya located in the arcuate nuclear area (79).

Knigge and Joseph (100) have described an ACTH immunoreactive fiber system which originates from the reactive perikarya in the basal hypothalamus and projects to the pituitary neural lobe, following the supraoptic-hypophyseal fiber tract through the zona interna of the median eminence. There has been no confirmation of this latter report.

4.2   Other Pituitary Hormones

4.2.1   Cell Bodies

Cell bodies containing immunostainable prolactin-like material, localized following colchicine treatment, are restricted to the hypothalamus and located in the region of the arcuate, ventromedial, and ventral premammillary bodies; a small number of positive cells are also present within the supraoptic and paraventricular nuclei. The staining of these perikarya was intensified following hypophysectomy (101, 102).

4.2.2   Fiber Pathways

Utilizing immunocytochemical techniques, prolactin-like material has been detected in networks of neuronal fibers and terminals of the rat hypothalamus and preoptic area (101, 102). Within the hypothalamus, immunostained beaded fibers are present in the periventricular nucleus, dorsomedial nucleus, ventromedial nucleus, arcuate nucleus, the subependymal and inner layers of the median eminence, the suprachiasmatic nucleus, and the supraoptic nucleus. Other areas containing immunostainable fibers include the paraventricular rotundocellular nucleus of the thalamus, medial amygdaloid nucleus, the supramammillary commissure, and the locus coeruleus. The staining pattern was the same in both male and female rats.

Toubeau et al. (103) reported on the presence of two different types of immunostainable prolactin-positive hypothalamic perikarya: those that contain prolactin-like material only, and those that stain positively for both prolactin and ACTH-like material. Both cell types were present in brains from colchicine-treated rats; no cells were detectable that stained for ACTH only. [These data must be viewed with caution, since the prolactin antiserum employed was raised to a preparation of purified rat prolactin (NIAMDD), which contains low levels of other peptides and proteins, including POMC-derived peptides; this same prolactin preparation was used to perform the immunocytochemical absorption controls. It is therefore possible that at least some of the prolactin-like material detected was related to POMC-derived peptides (e.g., β-endorphin, which shares sequence homology with rat growth hormone and would thus explain the dual localization reported).]

Lechan et al. (104), utilizing immunocytochemical methodology, reported on the presence of *human* growth hormone (hGH)-like material in *rat* brain. An antiserum raised to purified hGH was employed. This antiserum was preabsorbed with purified human β-lipotropin, because initial studies revealed that the antiserum also stained the POMC-like neuronal system, indicating that the antiserum also contained antibodies directed to the β-lipotropin sequence (indicating that the original hGH preparation probably contained human β-lipotropin as a contaminant). Immunostainable neuronal fibers were present in the zona externa of the median eminence, the lateral septum, and the organum vasculosum of the lamina terminalis. Following intraventricular colchicine treatment, immunostainable cell bodies were detected in several hypothalamic regions: in the anterior periventricular nucleus; in parvocellular neurons of the paraventricular nucleus; and in basal regions of the lateral hypothalamus, extending into the anterior and preoptic regions of the hypothalamus. The same staining patterns were obtained when brains from hypophysectomized rats were studied. Preabsorption of the antiserum with purified hGH, "core peptide" (hGH fragments 20–64 and 135–167, joined by a disulfide bridge), hGH (1–134) and (147–191), all abolished the staining reaction. However, rat GH (rGH) did not block the staining reaction, indicating that the antiserum was not reacting with rGH-like material previously reported to be present in rat brain. It is noteworthy that the anatomical localization of immunostainable hGH-like material is very different from that described for rGH-like material in rat brain.

4.2.3   Cerebrospinal Fluid (CSF)

POMC-related peptides are present in CSF. The source of these peptides is controversial (see refs. 64 and 65 for a review). However, available evidence indicates that at least some portion of these peptides are of brain origin, since: (i) electrical stimulation of the periaqueductal gray area in humans results in marked increases in ventricular CSF levels of immunoreactive ACTH and β-endorphin, with no change in plasma concentrations; (ii) immunoreactive peptides persist in CSF following hypophysectomy; and (iii) no correlation exists between plasma and CSF levels. For example, Nakao et al. (66) reported that although plasma levels of immunoreactive ACTH and β-endorphin decreased following surgical removal of pituitary adenomas (pituitary left intact) in five patients with Cushing's disease, such levels actually increased in CSF.

All the other anterior pituitary hormones are also present in CSF, and the source of these peptides is likewise controversial (see ref. 64 for a review).

5 ORIGIN OF PITUITARY-LIKE PEPTIDES PRESENT IN BRAIN

The presence of substances in brain which physicochemically resemble the pituitary hormones cannot be taken as evidence that they are synthesized within the central nervous system. Such material may be synthesized in the brain, may be transported there from the pituitary, or may be derived from both sources. (The demonstration of brain synthesis of pituitary-like hormones does not militate against the possibility that pituitary hormones may be transported to the brain under normal physiological conditions. Likewise, the demonstration that peptides can be transported from the pituitary to the brain does not preclude their synthesis within the central nervous system.)

If POMC-like material in brain is derived from both these sources, it is highly unlikely that material from each of the sources would subserve the same functions; this implies that the chemical forms of the peptides from each site might be different, reacting with their own unique receptors, or that they are functionally or physically differentially compartmentalized (thus avoiding "specificity spillover"), or both.

5.1 Anatomical Evidence

5.1.1 Transport Theories

Bergland and Page (105) have presented convincing anatomical evidence that pituitary secretions have the *theoretical potential* to be transported directly to the brain. This hypothesis was based on extensive three-dimensional scanning electron microscopic studies of gold palladium-coated methacrylate casts of the entire complex network of capillaries, arteries, and veins that supply and drain the primate (Rhesus monkey) pituitary gland. Other vertebrate species were studied as well (106–108). On the basis of these studies, in which they demonstrated that the volumetric capacity of the adenohypophyseal veins was small compared with the afferent vascular connections of the anterior pituitary, the authors suggested that some of the adenohypophyseal venous blood could return to the neurohypophysis by way of portal vessels connecting the adenohypophysis and neurohypophysis. They further proposed that blood could leave the neurohypophysis by seven potential routes, five of which are directed toward the brain. It was further suggested that blood could be preferentially directed toward brain or the systemic circulation by means of a "neurohypophyseal vascular switching" mechanism, wherein local vasodilatation or vasoconstriction of specific regions of this vascular system, or both, could specifically direct blood rich in anterior pituitary hormones toward the brain. (For a complete description of Bergland and Page's anatomical findings and a historical overview of pituitary-brain morphological relationships, see refs. 105, 106).

Crucial to the anatomical argument for anterior pituitary-to-brain blood flow was the suggestion that the adenohypophyseal veins were inadequate to drain all blood from the anterior lobe to the cavernous sinus. In this regard, Palkovits and Mezey (109) have suggested that one should not compare the capacity of the portal vessels to the adenohypophyseal veins but to that portion of the hypophyseal arteries that supplies the pituitary gland; in such a comparison, the venous drainage does not appear inadequate.

5.1.2 CNS Distribution of ACTH As a Function of Brain Size

Yalow and colleagues (110, 111) have concluded that the pituitary is probably the sole site of ACTH synthesis in mammals. On the basis of analyses of rat, rabbit, dog, monkey, and human brains, they concluded that the extent to which immunoreactive ACTH was distributed within these brains was a function of brain size, not anatomical loci. The presence and concentration of immunoreactive ACTH in a given brain region was reported to be directly proportional to its absolute distance from the pituitary gland in both small and large brains. Immunoreactive ACTH was detected throughout the rat brain, but could be detected only in the hypothalamus of the larger brains. Since they reported that their commercially "hypophysectomized" rats obtained from one vendor contained functionally active pituitary remnants, they questioned the reports of others. In their studies, analyses of brain ACTH content were performed on animals possessing intact pituitaries. Inexplicably, they did not test their own hypothesis by analyzing the brains from their "hypophysectomized" rats or from rats derived from laboratories that ensure total hypophysectomy by routinely destroying any residual pituitary, pituitary stalk, and median eminence by application of formaldehyde at the time of surgery; according to their theory, these maneuvers would result in the complete disappearance of brain ACTH.

Other investigators (40, 44, 112) have shown that immunoreactive brain ACTH persists in rats shown to be completely hypophysectomized by the following criteria: (i) undetectable plasma levels under basal and stress conditions (<15 pg/mL); (ii) adrenal and testicular atrophy; and (iii) undetectable ACTH levels in sella turcica scrapings (indicating absence of functional pituitary remnants).

The major conclusion of the Yalow group's study, that ACTH distribution (and hence other POMC-derived peptides) in brain is a function of brain size, has not been verified by any other laboratory (e.g., immunoreactive ACTH is widespread in monkey and human brain; see refs. 54 and 90).

5.2 Physiological Evidence

Page (113) has recently made direct measurements of the direction of pituitary blood flow to determine if pituitary-to-brain blood flow indeed occurs, under conditions that do not have the potential to severely alter the normal pressure relationships within the region under study (e.g., surgical intervention, catheterization of portal vessels, intrapituitary injections, etc.). No evidence for direct blood flow from the pituitary to the brain was obtained. No blood flowing up the pituitary stalk (from the posterior lobe) entered the median eminence. No blood flowed from the adenohypophysis to the neurohypophysis; instead, blood within the adenohypophysis drained directly to the cavernous sinus by way of the adenohypophyseal branches of the confluent pituitary veins. This direct evidence puts into question the significance of previous observations.

Bergland et al. (114) compared plasma immunoreactive ACTH concentrations in blood obtained simultaneously from the sagittal sinus, carotid artery, and jugular vein of three normal and one hypophysectomized sheep, just before and at timed intervals following electrically induced seizures. They reasoned that the direction of blood flow from the pituitary could be determined by comparing the relative concentrations of immunoreactive ACTH in blood obtained from these three sampling sites above and below the pituitary gland; if blood flows upward to the brain, the concentration within the sagittal sinus should be highest. The sagittal sinus concentrations were highest in most of the postseizure samples obtained from the sheep with intact pituitaries. Immunoreactive ACTH (in lower concentrations) was also present in the sagittal sinus blood of the hypophysectomized sheep. However, an experimental manipulation performed on the hypophysectomized sheep could have significantly reduced the ability of the brain to secrete ACTH-like material in this animal. The entire median eminence was removed to assure complete removal of the pituitary and pituitary stalk. Since immunostainable ACTH terminals are present in the median eminence, damage was inflicted upon the neuronal POMC-like system. Specifically, an anatomical locus from which brain-synthesized ACTH-like material could enter the hypothalamic vasculature was removed. The experimental design therefore appears inappropriate to address the question at hand.

In another study, Dias et al. (115) reported that 10 and 30 min after electroconvulsive shock there was a 30–50% reduction in the concentration of immunoreactive β-endorphin in the rat hypothalamus and the remainder of the brain, while no changes were noted in the pituitary gland or trunk plasma. It is therefore possible that a significant amount of immunoreactive ACTH measured in sagittal sinus was of brain origin.

Mezey et al. (116) measured the regional distribution of radioactivity in rat brain following intrapituitary insertion of a tritium-labeled ACTH-(4-9) analog. Thirty minutes after intrapituitary injection, about 10% of the administered dose was present in brain. This radioactivity was differentially distributed in discrete brain regions. Although the hypothalamus contained the highest concentration of radioactivity, neither the distribution within the hypothalamus nor in other brain regions corresponded to the regional localization of endogenous ACTH-like material. Furthermore, the finding of radioactivity in the hypothalamic tissue gives no indication of its ultrastructural localization (i.e., whether intraneuronally localized).

Dorsa et al. (117) showed that intrapituitary injection of neurotensin significantly decreased rat colonic temperature, suggesting that neurotensin was transported to brain to affect its function (believed to be a central effect of neurotensin). However, the physiological significance of this experiment is questionable; a dose-response effect was observed between 10 μg and 50 μg doses of neurotensin. Since even 10 μg exceeds the endogenous total rat brain content of neurotensin by at least two orders of magnitude, only an extremely small percentage of the injected peptide must have reached its target(s) in the brain, indicating a rather inefficient mode of delivery.

Oliver et al. (118) demonstrated that rat pituitary portal blood (obtained via a cannulated portal vessel) contained anterior pituitary hormones at concentrations approximately 100 times those present in peripheral arterial blood and were greatly diminished following hypophysectomy. These findings were taken as evidence for retrograde blood flow in the pituitary stalk. The authors cautioned that the surgical intervention necessary to obtain the blood samples could have artifactually changed the blood flow within the portal vessels.

In contrast, Wardlaw et al. (119) measured immunoreactive β-endorphin in pituitary portal blood of intact and hypophysectomized monkeys following pituitary stalk section and found no difference in levels when blood was collected from the sectioned vessels still attached to the median eminence. In both cases, immunoreactive β-endorphin concentrations were 100 times greater than simultaneous peripheral concentrations. These results indicate that the β-endorphin-like material was of brain origin.

Lastly, because material present in the portal circulation can be of hypothalamic or pituitary origin (as well as of peripheral origin, given the lack of a blood-brain barrier in this region), one cannot conclusively determine the origin of a given constituent by determining its concentration in portal blood. The immunocytochemical data clearly indicate that some ACTH and β-endorphin immunostainable fibers originating from the arcuate nuclear region of the hypothalamus terminate in the median eminence; hence the morphological basis for release of POMC-like peptides of brain origin into the portal circulation.

6 EVIDENCE FOR BRAIN SYNTHESIS OF PITUITARY-LIKE HORMONES

6.1 Indirect Evidence

6.1.1 POMC-Related Peptides

Effect of Hypophysectomy. If the pituitary were the sole source of POMC-like peptides present in brain, then complete hypophysectomy would deplete the central nervous system of these substances. However, as previously noted, these pituitary-like peptides persist in the brain after hypophysectomy.

Immunocytochemical studies noted essentially no change in the regional distribution of immunostainable ACTH, α-MSH, β-lipotropin, and β-endorphin after hypophysectomy. At the light microscopic level, such staining still displayed the "beaded" appearance in axons and the granular appearance in perikarya; at the electron microscopic level, the predominant staining still occurred in dense core vesicles in perikarya, axons and nerve endings. Only one study reported a major decrease (90%) in immunoassayable β-endorphin in total rat brain content 90 days following hypophysectomy. In this report (120), values cited for the immunoreactive β-endorphin content of normal rat brain are more than tenfold higher than values reported by almost all other investigators. In this study, rats were sacrificed by microwave irradiation, and it was suggested that the higher values obtained by this method indicated that "degradation of β-endorphin in brain is triggered immediately after death in decapitated rats and is a very rapid event." Our own observations (Liotta and Krieger, unpublished data), suggest that under certain conditions microwave irradiation causes peptides and proteins of pituitary origin to become associated with brain tissue (in some cases the pituitary literally "explodes").

Effect of Inhibition of Axonal Transport. Colchicine and vinblastine inhibit (usually incompletely) the release of secretory proteins, and in neurons they inhibit axoplasmic transport of secretory granules from cell bodies to terminals. These compounds do not have a pronounced effect on the protein-synthesizing apparatus of neurons. Therefore, if intraneuronal POMC-like peptides are of brain origin, colchicine or vinblastine pretreatment should cause an intracellular buildup of POMC-like peptides in the perikarya that synthesize them. This is precisely the result obtained in all immunocytochemical studies utilizing antisera to pituitary POMC-derived peptides. Cell bodies in the arcuate nuclear region become intensely stained, while fiber and terminal staining is reduced. In fact, in almost all of the previously cited immunocytochemical studies, colchicine or vinblastine pretreatment was necessary in order to visualize these POMC-like cell bodies; most investigators specifically state that few or no cell bodies were detected in the control sections. Our laboratory also investigated this phenomenon in a quantitative manner, by performing β-endorphin and ACTH radioimmunoassays of specific rat brain regions two days after intraventricular administration of 40 μg colchicine. Immunoreactive ACTH and β-endorphin concentrations increased approximately twofold in the arcuate nucleus (the location of putative POMC-synthesizing cell bodies) and were markedly reduced in all other brain regions; immunoreactive levels in the median eminence (in which there are abundant terminals thought to originate from the arcuate nucleus) were approximately 20% of control levels (40). It is inconceivable that these results could be obtained if such immunoreactive material originated in the pituitary gland.

Effects of Hypothalamic Lesions. If the arcuate nucleus region were the major site of synthesis of ACTH- and β-lipotropin-like peptides present within hypothalamic and extrahypothalamic brain regions, then destruction of this region should greatly decrease the brain content of such material. Such destruction of the arcuate nucleus in the rat by neonatal monosodium glutamate administration (which produces brain lesions restricted largely to neurons of the arcuate nucleus and retina) resulted in a highly significant decrease in the concentrations of immunoassayable ACTH, β-endorphin, and α-MSH in most brain regions studied (approximately 50–90%) without altering pituitary levels (121). (Complete elimination of POMC-related peptides from brain should not have been expected, since immunocytochemical analysis revealed that some positive immunostainable cell bodies were present in the mediobasal hypothalamus, lateral to the arcuate nucleus, consistent with the radioimmunoassay data.) In addition, no significant change in immunoassayable ACTH or β-endorphin occurred in the frontal cortex of the MSG-treated rat brains (121); reduction in the concentrations in the amygdala, although statistically significant, showed the least reduction of the other brain regions studied (121). Such immunoreactive material could, of course, originate from the few positive cell bodies in the mediobasal hypothalamus that survived the MSG treatment. Alternatively, such material may be synthesized within the amygdala and cortex; Civelli and colleagues (122a, 122b) detected very low levels of POMC-like mRNA in these structures. Contrary to a possible extrahypothalamic site of production of POMC-related peptides, complete surgical isolation of the entire hypothalamus resulted in the complete loss of immunostainable ACTH, α-MSH, and β-lipotropin outside the hypothalamic island (123, 124). Electrolytic or surgical destruction of the arcuate nuclear region produced essentially the same results (125, 126). Unilateral electrolytic lesions, which were shown to destroy immunostainable β-lipotropin cell bodies on one side of the brain, resulted in a significant reduction of immunostainable ACTH and β-lipotropin fibers on the ipsilateral side of the brain as well as reducing its immunoassayable β-lipotropin brain content (69).

Surgical isolation (deafferentation) of the arcuate nucleus produced similar reductions in immunoassayable α-MSH throughout the brain, except that no significant reduction was observed within the arcuate nuclear island, indicating that no significant retrograde degeneration of neurons within the island occurred (123). One immunocytochemical study (127) noted an apparent increase in content of immunoreactive ACTH in arcuate nucleus cell bodies 10 days after surgical deafferentation of the rat basal hypothalamus (i.e., increased staining intensity) and "sprouting of new fibers throughout the island." Of interest is the finding that there was little reduction in immunoassayable α-MSH concentrations in the hippocampus in either the MSG or arcuate nucleus surgical isolation study (123, 128). Since immunocytochemical studies utilizing antisera raised to POMC-derived peptides other than α-MSH have not reported positive fibers in the hippocampus, it is possible that such hippocampal α-MSH-like material arises from the previously described immunostainable α-MSH-containing cell bodies detected in the dorsolateral regions of the hypothalamus (see Section 4.1.1).

These data, taken together, are consistent with the hypothesis that neuronal cell bodies located in the hypothalamus (the majority in the arcuate nuclear region) synthesize POMC-related peptides and send axonal projections to many hypothalamic and extrahypothalamic brain regions.

Demonstration of In Vitro Release of POMC-like Peptides from Hypothalamic Tissue. In order for neuronal POMC-like derived peptides to have physiological relevance as neurotransmitters or modulators of neuronal function, they must, of course, be releasable from neuronal sites.

In most cases (exceptions include some neurons of the retina, which do not exhibit action potentials), secretion of classical neurotransmitters (e.g., acetylcholine, catecholamines) from nerve terminals is initiated by action potentials that depolarize the nerve terminals, resulting in a calcium-dependent release (129) of the vesicle-stored transmitter. While immunocytochemical studies at the ultrastructural level have shown that POMC-related material is largely sequestered in granules in neuronal cell bodies, axons, and terminals (in analogy to the established neurotransmitters), the presence of such material in morphologically appropriate structures cannot be taken as *a priori* evidence that such material is releasable by mechanisms similar to those operative in the secretion of the established neurotransmitters.

Several studies have demonstrated that immunoreactive α-MSH and β-endorphin are released from hypothalamic tissue incubated *in vitro* (40, 130–132). Subcellular fractionation of hypothalamic tissue reveals that a major fraction of immunoreactive α-MSH and β-endorphin is present in synaptosomes; some of this immunoreactive material is released during *in vitro* incubation (134–137). Potassium or electrical membrane depolarization of intact hypothalamic tissue or synaptosomal-enriched preparations causes a calcium-dependent stimulated release of these peptides (130–137). Veratridine, a more specific neuronal depolarizing agent that acts by increasing Na^+ permeability of membrane (sodium influx depolarization), also stimulates the release of immunoreactive α-MSH from hypothalamic tissue in a Ca^{2+}-dependent manner; this effect is blocked by tetradotoxin, a specific blocker of Na^+ influx (131). Because synaptosomes are thought to be predominantly derived from presynaptic nerve terminals, these findings taken together suggest that at least some portion of tissue immunoreactive α-MSH and β-endorphin is selectively released from prejunctional nerve terminals *in vivo*. The *in vitro* nature of these studies may not reflect the *in vivo* capacity of the tissue to synthesize and release POMC-related peptides. For example, Fink et al. (138) have suggested that as much as 80% of total hypothalamic thyrotropin releasing hormone (TRH) content is released into the pituitary portal circulation in one hour.

6.1.2 Other Pituitary Hormones

Immunoreactive GH, TSH, prolactin, and LH persist in the brains of hypophysectomized rats. Following hypophysectomy, there is a significant transient reduction in the concentrations of immunoreactive GH and TSH in rat amygdala, hypothalamus, and thalamus; no changes were noted in caudate, hippocampus, or cortex (45, 56). At 28 and 48 days post hypophysectomy, the concentrations in the former three brain regions were more than twice the control levels.

Since brain GH-like material appears to be regulated by somatostatin (56) and since Baker et al. (139) have shown marked changes in rat me-

dian eminence immunostainable somatostatin following hypophysectomy, it is possible that the transient decrease of immunoreactive GH
noted in some regions of the rat brain following hypophysectomy is secondary to altered brain somatostatin levels (56).

Dispersed cells from amygdala, thalamus, hypothalamus, and cortex,
obtained from brains of intact and hypophysectomized rats and
maintained in tissue culture, release GH-like and TSH-like material into
the medium for several weeks (45, 62). No independent demonstration
was provided that any of this material was synthesized during the incubation. The majority of rat hypothalamic LH-like material is present in
synaptosomes (140, 141). Consistent with these reports, DeVito and
Hedge (63) have recently shown that release of immunoreactive TSH-
sized material from hypothalamic tissue, obtained from intact, thyroidectomized, and hypophysectomized rats, is stimulated by depolarizing
concentrations of K^+ or veratridine (calcium-dependent). Moreover,
concentrations of TRH that are effective in stimulating pituitary
TSH release were ineffective in releasing TSH-like material from hypothalamic tissue.

Brain and pituitary LH-like material exhibits a sexually dimorphic
pattern in the rat. Pituitary LH content is significantly greater in the
male; in brain, LH-like material content is significantly lower in the
male rat. This sex difference is obliterated after gonadectomy and is
reestablished upon sex steroid replacement therapy (140, 141). Ovariectomy is associated with an increase in pituitary LH levels but a decrease in hypothalamic levels of LH-like material (140).

Pituitary and plasma TSH exhibit a diurnal variation that is dependent on the light-dark cycle employed; brain TSH-like material exhibits
a diurnal variation independent of the light-dark cycle imposed (61).

6.2   Direct Evidence for De Novo Synthesis of POMC-Related Peptides by Hypothalamic Neurons

Several approaches can be used to demonstrate that a tissue can synthesize a particular protein (in this case, that the brain has the capacity
to synthesize POMC-related material). Two such methods have been
utilized to provide such evidence.

6.2.1   Incorporation of Radiolabeled Amino Acids into POMC-, ACTH-, and β-endorphin-related Peptides

Adult bovine (142) and neonatal rat hypothalamic tissue (143),
maintained in tissue culture, incorporate radiolabeled amino acids into
multiple molecular species that are specifically bound by affinity-purified antisera to ACTH and β-endorphin. Radiolabeled high-molecular-
weight material containing both ACTH and β-endorphin antigenic
determinants within the same molecules (shown by sequential use of

the immobilized antisera) can be detected in both cell and media extracts. Sephadex G-75 gel filtration revealed that the majority of this material eluted with the K_{av} of authentic POMC extracted from bovine anterior pituitaries. Further characterization of this POMC-like material revealed: (i) apparent size heterogeneity in both NaDodSO$_4$ polyacrylamide gel electrophoresis and gel filtration systems; (ii) the presence of carbohydrate moieties, as inferred from its ability to specifically bind to and be eluted from concanavalin A; (iii) a β-endorphin-(1–9)-like fragment generated by trypsinization; and (iv) a complex isoelectric focusing profile (144). Comparative analyses showed that the brain POMC-like material was physicochemically similar to pituitary POMC with respect to the foregoing chromatographic and electrophoretic behavior. In contrast, no radiolabeled products specifically reactive with either the ACTH or the β-endorphin antisera were detected when equal masses of parietal and frontal cortical tissue were similarly incubated.

In other studies utilizing cultures of rat neonatal hypothalamic neurons exhibiting extensive outgrowth of processes, [^{35}S]-methionine was incorporated into POMC-like molecules as well as into several smaller molecular species containing either the ACTH or β-endorphin antigenic determinants (but not both). α-MSH-sized and β-endorphin-sized moieties predominated, with lesser amounts of β-LPH- and ACTH-(1–39)-like material det ected (143). The synthesis of these multiple-size classes of immunoreactive ACTH and β-endorphin is consistent with a precursor–product relationship between the POMC-like material and the smaller forms. Comparative in vitro biosynthesis studies revealed the hypothalamic POMC-like material to be indistinguishable from POMC synthesized by rat anterior and intermediate lobe cells with respect to several physicochemical criteria. NaDodSO$_4$ polyacrylamide gel electrophoresis partially resolved POMC-like material from all three tissues into two predominant forms, exhibiting apparent MW of 33,000 $+$ 1000 and 36,000 $+$ 600. Both forms specifically bound to concanavalin A and yielded similar tryptic maps of [^{35}S]-methionine-containing fragments, indicating that both forms contain carbohydrate and possess similar primary sequences, at least with respect to the methionine-containing tryptic fragments.

Partial confirmation of these findings has been reported by Kendall et al. (145). They demonstrated [^{35}S]-methionine incorporation into immunoreactive ACTH-like material by mouse hypothalamic tissue maintained in organ culture. The majority of such material exhibited the approximate molecular weight of ACTH-(1–39) ($M_r \simeq 4500$) in a NaDodSO$_4$polyacrylamide gel electrophoresis system. Also detected was a high-molecular-weight (apparent MW $\simeq$ 37,000) peak of immunoreactive ACTH, presumably representing POMC-like material.

Although the neonatal rat hypothalamic cell culture noted above represents a more morphologically correct preparation than the bovine cell preparation, in view of the extensive outgrowth of processes in the former, the rather formidable *in situ* morphological and organizational complexity of the brain limits the type of information that one can obtain from *in vitro* cell preparations. Our laboratory has collaborated in preliminary *in vivo* biosynthetic studies of brain POMC (146). Rats were cannulated in the posterior periarcuate region; radiolabeled amino acids were infused for 15 min and animals sacrificed 2 h later. The arcuate region (site of putative POMC perikarya) and some of its CNS projection areas (both fibers of passage and terminals; POA, lateral septum) were separately extracted and analyzed for POMC and derived peptides by a sequential physicochemical characterization scheme (including sequential immunoadsorption, reverse phase HPLC and tryptic mapping). POMC-like material, as well as a peptide behaving identically with authentic rat β-endorphin, was detected in several brain regions. The ratio of POMC to β-endorphin was highest in the arcuate region and decreased in other brain areas as a function of the distance from the arcuate region, consistent with the notion that POMC is processed to smaller moieties during axonal transport. In the median eminence (site of terminal fields) only β-endorphin-sized and α-MSH-sized peptides were detected. These results are in agreement with the finding in fresh rat tissue extracts that a higher percentage of total immunoreactive ACTH is associated with high-molecular-weight material in the mediobasal hypothalamus (containing cell bodies) than in preoptic area (fiber projections) (147). In a similar experiment in which radiolabeled amino acids were infused for 8 h prior to sacrifice, POMC-like material, immunoreactive β-endorphin exhibiting the reverse phase HPLC retention time of authentic rat β-endorphin, as well as immunoreactive α-MSH exhibiting the retention time of des-acetyl α-MSH were detected in several brain regions (Liotta, McKelvy, Advis, Krause, and Krieger, submitted for publication). No evidence was obtained that any of these peptides were significantly α-N-acetylated. This *in vivo* labeling technique appears to be a valid method for studying the biosynthesis of POMC-like material in the arcuate nucleus, its axonal transport and processing, and factors that regulate the synthesis and release of this material *in situ*.

6.2.2 Detection and Quantification of POMC-like mRNA in Brain Tissue

Herbert and associates (122a, 122b) used a 144-base-pair DNA probe complementary to the portion of mouse pituitary POMC that codes for a 48-amino-acid segment of β-lipotropin, including most of the β-endorphin sequence. Northern blot analysis detected specific hybridizing POMC-like mRNA species in total poly(A) RNA prepared from rat hypothalamus, amygdala, and cortex (Figure 2). The hypothalamic POMC-like mRNA was shown to be the same size (about 1100 bases long) as

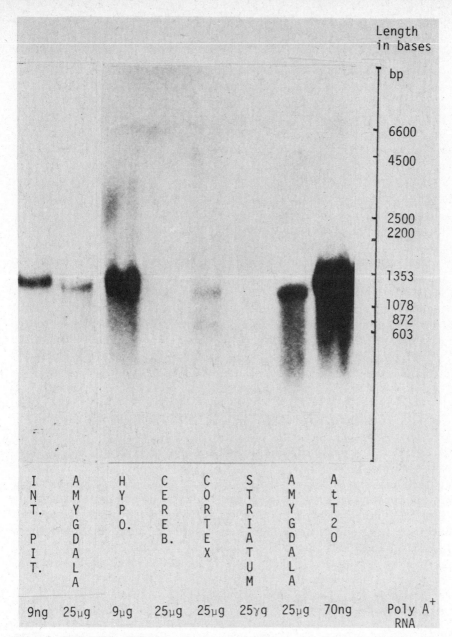

								Length in bases
								bp
								— 6600
								— 4500
								— 2500
								— 2200
								— 1353
								— 1078
								— 872
								— 603

I N T. P I T.	A M Y G D A L A	H Y P O.	C E R E B.	C O R T E X	S T R I A T U M	A M Y G D A L A	A t T 2 0	
9ng	25μg	9μg	25μg	25μg	25γq	25μg	70ng	Poly A⁺ RNA

Figure 2. POMC -like mRNA in rat brain. Poly(A) RNA extracted from rat pituitary intermediate lobe, various regions of rat brain, and a mouse anterior pituitary tumor cell line (AtT20) was electrophoretically separated according to size on an agarose gel, and the fractionated RNA was transferred to a nitrocellulose sheet. Nick-translated DNA complementary to a portion of mouse POMC (144-nucleotide sequence containing the entire complementary sequence encoding β-endorphin) was used as the hybridization probe, as described (122b). Autoradiography was performed for 6 h on the right side of the blot and for 24 h on the left side of the blot. *INT. PIT.*, pituitary intermediate lobe; *HYPO.*, hypothalamus; *CEREB.*, cerebellum.

rat anterior and intermediate lobe POMC mRNA; amygdalar and cortical POMC-like mRNA was shorter (about 1000 bases long). Solution hybridization analysis of rat brain and pituitary total poly(A)RNA was
performed to quantify the mRNA levels. Expressed as pg POMC mRNA
per μg total poly(A)RNA, the hypothalamus contains approximately 4%
and the amygdala approximately 0.5% of the POMC mRNA level in the
rat anterior lobe; the cortex contains less than 10% the POMC-like
mRNA level of the amygdala. Considering that the average weight of
hypothalamic tissue used to prepare RNA was 50 mg, and the fact that
the rat arcuate nucleus and surrounding tissue weighs only a few mg,
the hypothalamic POMC-like mRNA concentration reported is probably
a significant underestimate of its true concentration in the restricted region of the hypothalamus where the gene is thought to be expressed.

The significance of the shorter POMC-like mRNA in amygdala and
cortex cannot be determined from these experiments. The authors speculate that it could represent a second POMC gene (the pituitary and hypothalamus both expressing the same gene) or the same gene with a
shorter 3'-poly(A) tail. These results, however, do not provide definitive
data about the identity of the hypothalamic POMC-like mRNA with the
POMC gene (or genes) expressed in the pituitary; molecular cloning and
sequencing of the brain POMC-like mRNA will be required.

7 ONTOGENY OF PITUITARY PEPTIDES IN BRAIN

7.1 POMC-Related Peptides in CNS

Immunoreactive POMC-related material is present in hypothalamic cells
of the developing rat fetus four days before its detection in the anterior
pituitary lobe and five days before detection in the intermediate lobe.
Schwartzberg and Nakane (148), using antisera raised to β-endorphin,
ACTH, γ-lipotropin, and 16K fragment, reported that positively stained
cells were first detected in the ventral diencephalon of 12-day-old (day
E12) embryos; cells were conclusively identified as neurons by day 13
of gestation. By day E15, positively stained fibers had projected to the
roof of the diencephalon and mesencephalon; some of these fibers made
contact with capillaries within the basal hypothalamus. The fiber distribution became more widespread from embryonic day E13 through the
first week of neonatal life. Both the location of the reactive cell bodies
and the fiber pathways they establish are consistent with the previously
described distribution in the adult rat. Positively stained cells in the anterior and intermediate pituitary lobes were first detected on days E16
and E17, respectively, of fetal life. This is consistent with reports in
which immunoreactive β-endorphin was detected in discrete regions of
day E13 rat brain, with increasing concentrations noted in all brain re-

gions examined (save the striatum) between embryonic day E16 and postnatal day 25 (149).

As previously noted, the positive perikarya do not reside in a discrete hypothalamic nucleus (i.e., arcuate nucleus). Schwartzberg and Nakane (148) postulate that since the immunoreactive POMC-positive cells arise as a uniform band of cells before the arcuate nucleus is formed, "neurons containing ACTH-related peptides probably arise separately from the main mass of cells to become partly embedded inside and partly outside the arcuate nucleus in the adult." They also note that the POMC-like neuronal system is the earliest appearing peptidergic neuronal system demonstrated to date.

Haynes et al. (150) have reported that immunoreactive β-endorphin is transiently expressed in several cell types of the rat spinal cord, from embryonic day E14 to postnatal day 28.

7.2 Other Anterior Pituitary Hormones

Hojvat et al. (151) reported that immunoreactive growth hormone and thyrotropin are present in the fetal rat brain before they are detectable in the fetal pituitary. Both these immunoreactive species were detected at 10 days of gestation, whereas immunoreactive growth hormone and thyrotropin were first detected in the pituitary at E12 and E15 days, respectively. These data are consistent with a brain site of synthesis for these immunoreactive species. Such material appears even to precede the appearance of POMC-like peptides in the fetal brain, although it should be appreciated that these ontogenic studies should be considered preliminary, requiring verification and further characterization of immunoreactive species present.

8 EFFECTS OF ENDOCRINE PERTURBATIONS ON POMC-RELATED PEPTIDES

If the brain POMC-like neuronal network shares any regulatory mechanisms in common with the pituitary gland, or functionally interacts with it, then procedures known to alter pituitary-adrenal function might be associated with alterations in the brain content of these peptides.

8.1 Hypophysectomy

Hypophysectomy is sometimes associated with increased or decreased levels of immunoreactive POMC-derived peptides in some brain regions. Within a given study, levels in some brain regions are unaffected or increased following hypophysectomy, while other regions are associated with decreased immunoreactive concentrations (e.g., see refs. 46, 51).

Such alterations may indicate an "endocrine perturbation" of the brain POMC system. O'Donahue et al. (51) have reported a 38–69% decrease in immunoassayable α-MSH in several rat brain regions known to be rich in α-MSH-immunostainable fibers and terminals four weeks after hypophysectomy, while no change in α-MSH concentrations occurred in the arcuate nucleus (rich in POMC-like cell bodies). The authors suggested that the removal of the pituitary could have increased the turnover of brain α-MSH-like material in terminal fields and decreased the transport of peptide from perikarya to terminals, possibly due to a "deficit . . . of a feedback inhibitory component . . ." Such a postulate is not without endocrine precedent. An example of this is the well-known transient marked decrease in concentrations of anterior pituitary POMC-derived peptides (and increased plasma concentrations) that occurs shortly after bilateral adrenalectomy and that is later followed by significantly increased pituitary concentrations of these peptides (112, 152, 153). In this case, either increased or decreased concentrations of pituitary POMC-derived peptides would be observed, compared with control animals, as a function of the post-adrenalectomy sampling time.

Although specific effects on brain POMC-like peptides following hypophysectomy could be secondary to reduced concentrations of circulating glucocorticoids, this is unlikely since adrenalectomy has little effect on the brain levels of this material (see Section 8.4). Communication between brain and pituitary POMC systems could be mediated by a factor or factors released by the pituitary and transported to the hypothalamus via the portal circulation or could be due to an interaction of the brain POMC neuronal system and the corticotropin-releasing factor (CRF) neuronal system. Immunostainable CRF fibers have been detected in close proximity to the arcuate nucleus (154, 155). In addition, POMC-like neurons project to the paraventricular nucleus, a region containing positive CRF perikarya. The anatomical proximity of these two peptidergic systems thus appears to permit functional interactions. Recently, immunoassayable rat hypothalamic CRF has been shown to initially decrease following hypophysectomy, only to increase about sevenfold two weeks after hypophysectomy (156).

8.2 Effect of Gonadal Hormones

Total hypothalamic immunoreactive β-endorphin concentrations in rats do not change during the estrous cycle (157), although Barden et al. (158) have detected decreased levels in the arcuate nucleus and increased levels in the median eminence and suprachiasmatic nucleus, during the proestrous stage of the cycle. Hypothalamic immunoreactive β-endorphin levels are significantly increased in pregnant rats compared with nonpregnant control rats (41.6 ± 2.2 vs. 32.7 ± 1 ng/mg protein) (157). Although neither orchiectomy nor ovariectomy was associated with any changes of immunoreactive β-endorphin in rat hypothalamus or other brain regions (157, 159), estradiol treatment of ovariectomized rats resulted in significantly decreased immunoreactive levels in hypothalamus, thalamus, and midbrain. When progesterone was coadministered with estradiol, no significant decreases were noted in the thalamus or midbrain. Marked variations of hypophyseal portal blood (obtained by complete transection of pituitary stalk) immunoreactive β-endorphin concentrations are reported to occur at different stages of the menstrual cycle in rhesus monkeys; levels were undetectable during menstruation (<133 pg/mL) and were high in follicular and luteal stages (737 $\pm$ 256 and 1675 $\pm$ 1108 pg/mL, respectively) (157). Peripheral serum estrogen levels were high during the follicular and luteal stages and undetectable (<100 pg/mL) at menstruation.

Immunoreactive β-endorphin could not be detected (133 pg/mL) in the portal blood of rhesus or pigtail monkeys 4 to 12 months after ovariectomy (160). None of the other POMC-related peptides were measured in these studies.

8.3 Effect of Thyroid Hormones

Contradictory results have been reported on the effects of thyroid status on hypothalamic β-endorphin concentrations (159, 161).

8.4 Effect of Adrenal Steroids

Most studies have shown that neither short-term nor long-term adrenalectomy nor glucocorticoid pretreatment significantly altered rat hypothalami or whole-brain immunoreactive ACTH, α-MSH, or β-endorphin content (44, 112, 163). One group of investigators reported a significant increase in immunoreactive β-endorphin (in rat hypothalamus, midbrain, and hindbrain regions) one month after adrenalectomy (159); to date, this report has not been confirmed. Van Dijk et al. (162) have reported a transient decrease in the hippocampal concentration of immunoreactive ACTH at 3 days but not at 14 days following adrenalectomy; this decrease was observed in both intact and hypophysectomized rats. Glucocorticoid treatment of adrenalectomized rats failed to prevent this transient reduction in hippocampal levels.

8.5 Effect of Stress

Foot-shock stress caused a significant decrease in the immunoreactive β-endorphin levels in the rat hypothalamus and periventricular nucleus (163–165). Immobilization stress (2 h daily for 7 days) was associated with a highly significant increase in plasma ACTH and corticosterone levels and a statistically significant decrease in anterior pituitary ACTH content, while no changes occurred in the immunoreactive ACTH concentrations of median eminence or mediobasal hypothalamus (112). Acute (but not chronic) immobilization stress resulted in a significant reduction in immunoreactive α-MSH in the hypothalamic arcuate nuclear area, as well as in brain regions shown to be rich in immunostainable α-MSH fibers (166).

9 EFFECT OF AGING ON POMC-RELATED PEPTIDES IN BRAIN

Aging in the rat is associated with a decrease in the concentrations of POMC-related peptides in discrete brain regions (167–171). Immunoreactive β-endorphin, ACTH, α-MSH, and γ-LPH concentrations in the hypothalamus, preoptic area, and thalamus are decreased about 30–50% in 26–28-month-old female rats compared with 4-month-old (mature) control female rats (167). Barden et al. (169) found an approximately 50% decrease in immunoreactive β-endorphin concentrations in all brain regions studied except the median eminence, where there was no significant change between young (3 months) and old (24 months) male rats.

Barnea et al. (170) have shown that aging is not associated with any changes in the molecular weight profiles of immunoreactive ACTH in the mediobasal hypothalamus or preoptic area and have proposed that an overall reduction in the biosynthesis of brain POMC-like material occurs, with no change in the manner in which such precursor-like material is processed.

Decreased brain levels of a given constituent cannot be taken as *a priori* evidence of a decreased rate of synthesis because observed content is a function of several processes, including the relative rates of synthesis, release, reuptake, and activities of specific degradative enzymes. In this regard, it has been suggested that the reduction in concentrations of hypothalamic β-endorphin-like material in old rats may indicate an increased metabolism of β-endorphin in this brain region. This might account for the increased prolactin and decreased gonadotropin secretion observed in old rats (168).

Aging is consistently associated with decreased activities of catecholaminergic neurons in specific brain regions, including the mediobasal hypothalamus, the presumed site of neuronal POMC-like material synthesis. ACTH- and β-endorphin-related peptides are reported to modulate catecholaminergic transmission. Although a causal relationship has not been shown, the observed age-related declines in several brain functions thought to be influenced by these peptides (e.g., learning, short-term memory, sexual activity, food intake) may be a direct result of decreased neuronal POMC or catecholaminergic function. This raises the question whether replacement therapy, by administration of centrally acting catecholamine agonists or ACTH- and β-endorphin-related peptides, may improve some of the age-related deficits.

10   CNS RECEPTORS FOR PITUITARY HORMONES

10.1   Receptors for POMC-Derived Peptides

Pharmacological actions of β-endorphin and N-terminal fragments derived from it are at least partially mediated by interaction with opiate receptors. Opiate receptors are asymmetrically distributed in the central nervous system (and at peripheral sites). In general, a good correlation exists between the neuroanatomical distribution of opioid peptides and receptor localization (see Chapter 34), presumptive evidence that indeed such peptides serve as the natural ligands for these receptors. Receptor binding studies and the diversity of chemical, pharmacological, and behavioral responses elicited by different opioid peptides and model narcotic analgesics, as well as the multitude of actions elicited by a given opioid (especially as a function of the site of application in the central nervous system), strongly suggest the existence of multiple classes of receptors (mediating different functions) (172–176) that possess differential anatomical distribution. At least four classes of opiate receptors have been proposed: mu (comprised of N_1 and N_2), sigma, kappa, and delta. Three specific types of experimental findings form the basis for the multiple effects attributed to centrally administered β-endorphin: (a) β-endorphin binds to μ and δ receptors with nearly equal affinity; (b) μ and δ receptors are thought to mediate different physiological responses; and (c) μ and δ receptors are differentially localized in the central nervous system. Thus, in any given brain region the differential occupation of these receptors by β-endorphin may elicit a specific integrated response. Moreover, differences in the absolute dissociation rate constants (if they exist) would eventually lead to preferential occupation of only one receptor type, perhaps resulting in modulation of the initial response.

Although ACTH, N-terminal fragments of ACTH, des-acetyl α-MSH, α-MSH, β-endorphin and γ-endorphin, and their des-Tyr[1] derivatives, have been shown to influence specific intracellular biochemical reactions, alter the turnover of catecholamines in specific brain regions, and exert profound behavioral effects via opiate and nonopiate receptor-mediated mechanisms (des-Tyr[1] forms of endorphins do not bind to opiate receptors), no specific receptors for these peptides have been demonstrated in the central nervous system.

Specific binding of ACTH to rat brain structures has been detected only in the zona externa of the median eminence and possibly in the ventral region of the arcuate nucleus (177). The latter study utilized an autoradiographic procedure at the light microscopic level to detect binding of systemically administered [^{125}I]-ACTH-(1–24). [About 1 μg of labeled ACTH-(1–24) was utilized, probably resulting in an initial plasma ACTH concentration more than a thousandfold greater than normal physiological levels; it could not be determined in this experiment whether the binding observed was indeed to neuronal structures. In addition, since the labeled ACTH was administered intravenously, only structures outside the blood-brain barrier (circumventricular organs) that contained binding sites would be expected to be labeled.]

Although ACTH and N-terminal fragments thereof have been shown to displace [³H]-morphine and [³H]-naloxone from brain membranes and to inhibit the electrically evoked contractions of mouse vas deferens (naloxone reversible), and although a molecular model has been proposed to explain the direct interaction of ACTH with opiate receptors, the relative potencies of ACTH and N-terminal fragments in these systems are 2–4 orders of magnitude lower than for morphine, naloxone, β-endorphin, or Met-enkephalin (178–181). It has been suggested that such low-affinity binding to opiate receptors does not account for the opiate-like effects of ACTH-related peptides. Witter (182) suggests that it is more likely that high-affinity binding sites mediate the opiate-related actions of ACTH-related peptides; he postulates a separate class of ACTH receptors to mediate the non-opiate-related actions of ACTH and ACTH fragments on behavior modification. The relatively low concentrations of ACTH-related peptides necessary to elicit some of these responses predicts that such putative receptors are of high affinity and low capacity and hence will require labeled ligands possessing very high specific activities (greater than can normally be obtained utilizing tritiated ligands) to demonstrate their existence. (With respect to the existence of receptors for the intact ACTH molecule, it should be borne in mind that ACTH detected in neurons may represent solely a biosynthetic intermediate in the formation of α-MSH-related peptides and hence may not have a physiological role at all in brain. One would not then expect receptors for such a ligand to be present in the CNS.)

The lack of demonstration of receptors for des-Tyr¹ α- and γ-endorphins may also be due to the presence of very high-affinity, low-capacity receptors. Consistent with this hypothesis are the findings that (i) endogenous brain levels of α- and γ-endorphin-related peptides are much lower than those of the β-endorphin-related peptides (183, 184), and (ii) intraventricular injection of only 0.3 ng of des-Tyr¹ γ-endorphin facilitates the extinction of active avoidance and attenuates passive avoidance behavior in the rat (185). Alternatively, the CNS active forms of ACTH and α- and γ-endorphin related peptides may be formed extracellularly (and hence may represent shortened forms of these peptides). If this is the case, then the lack of demonstration of receptors would be a consequence of using inappropriate ligands.

10.2 Other Pituitary Hormones

Specific prolactin-binding sites have been demonstrated in the hypothalamus of several mammalian species (186, 187); injection into the intact animal of radiolabeled prolactin in the presence and absence of

excess unlabeled prolactin, followed by light microscopic autoradiographic detection, localized specific binding only to ependymal cells of
the choroid plexus (186). (Since such binding occurs in the circumventricular region, lacking the blood-brain barrier, both pituitary prolactin and prolactin-like material synthesized by the brain—if indeed such
synthesis occurs—would have access to such binding sites.)

DiCarlo and Muccioli (188) demonstrated that specific binding in the
rat hypothalamus decreased in the lactating rat (vs. nonlactating control) as well as in other hyperprolactinemic states. Specific prolactin
binding also decreased in liver, adrenal, and ovarian membranes prepared from the same animals. Low but specific prolactin binding was
demonstrated in cerebellum, pons-medulla area, and cortex. In contrast
to results in hypothalamus and peripheral tissues, no significant decrease in binding capacity of these tissues was noted during lactation
or induced hyperprolactinemia.

11   PROCESSING OF POMC-LIKE MATERIAL IN BRAIN

Although POMC-like related peptides in brain have been subjected to
moderate physicochemical characterization, to date there has been no
unequivocal demonstration that any of these peptides is structurally
identical to its pituitary counterpart. Neither has there been any definitive proof provided that the smaller immunoreactive ACTH- and β-lipo-
tropin-related peptides found in brain are, in fact, posttranslationally
derived from the POMC-like material present in brain. However, the
data summarized in the preceding section are consistent with the synthesis in brain of ACTH-related and β-endorphin-related products via
sequential cleavage of a large common precursor molecule (or molecules) that shares extensive sequence homology with pituitary POMC.
Consistent with identical structures, rat hypothalamic β-endorphin has
the same amino acid composition as rat pituitary β-endorphin (Liotta
and Krieger, unpublished results).

In analogy with studies conducted in the anterior and intermediate
pituitary lobes, the major peptide species detected in brain tissue probably reflect the major products of the brain POMC-like system. Using
such an approach, the major processing pathway in brain appears to resemble that demonstrated for the intermediate lobe of the pituitary, in
that immunoreactive α-MSH, CLIP, ACTH-(1–39) and β-endorphin-sized
peptides appear to be the major ACTH- and β- lipotropin-related peptides present in brain (40, 52–54, 93, 147, 189, 190). Within a species,
brain POMC-like material exhibits size and charge heterogeneity qualitatively similar to pituitary POMC (143, 144, 146), strongly suggesting
that similar or identical cotranslational and posttranslational modifications of pituitary POMC also occur in the brain.

A controversy exists with regard to possible acetylation of β-endorphin-sized and α-MSH-sized peptides in brain. Two research groups have reported that rat hypothalamic or whole brain α-MSH-like material is composed of approximately equal amounts of des-acetyl α-MSH and authentic α-MSH (α-N-acetyl ACTH amide) (49, 191). On the basis of these findings and pharmacological studies (intraventricular injection) performed in the rat with synthetic des-acetyl α-MSH and α-MSH, O'Donohue et al. (192) concluded that N-acetylation of brain des-acetyl α-MSH (and β-endorphin—see below) may be a physiological regulatory mechanism for modulating the behavioral activities of brain POMC-derived peptides. (α-MSH is much more potent than the des-acetyl form in eliciting "excessive grooming behavior," whereas des-acetyl α-MSH can block opiate-induced analgesia by blocking binding of opiates to opiate receptors. Authentic α-MSH is inactive in this regard.)

These authors have also recently reported on the presence and distribution, in rat brain, of acetyl transferase activity capable of α-N-acetylating synthetic des-acetyl α-MSH. They suggest that a specific α-MSH acetyltransferase exists in rat brain and may have a physiological role in regulating the activity of "α-MSH" in brain (193).

Zakarian and Smyth (194) have reported that all of the α-N-acetyl β-endorphin-derived peptides synthesized in rat intermediate pituitary lobe cells (acetylated forms of β-endorphin, β-endorphin-(1–27), and β-endorphin-(1–26); see Section 2), as well as their unacetylated forms, are also present in rat brain, with different brain regions containing significantly different proportions of t hese peptides. The hypothalamus, amygdala, and midbrain contain mostly unacetylated β-endorphin and β-endorphin-(1–26), whereas the hippocampus, colliculi, and brainstem extracts examined contained major peaks of α-N-acetyl forms of β-endorphin-(1–27) and β-endorphin-(1–26). They postulated two distinct processing mechanisms in rat brain analogous with the different pathways present in anterior and intermediate pituitary cells, the former pathway producing opiate active products and the latter producing species devoid of opiate-like activity (α-N-acetylation of Tyr[1] or removal of Tyr[1] results in a loss of affinity for opiate receptors) (see Chapter 34).

In contrast, others (189, 195, 196) have reported that most or all of rat brain α-MSH- and β-endorphin-sized peptides are present in the des-acetyl forms. Evans et al. (196), while detecting α-MSH and des-acetyl α-MSH in rat intermediate pituitary lobe, detected a single immunoreactive peak which exhibited the retention time of des-acetyl α-MSH by reverse phase HPLC in extracts of both hypothalamus and midbrain. Weber et al. (195), using a β-endorphin antiserum that requires the presence of the α-N-acetyl group for recognition, calculated that less than 2% of whole brain β-endorphin-sized material was α-N-acetylated; no α-N-acetylated peptides at all could be detected in hypophysectomized rats (suggesting pituitary α-MSH contamination of brains obtained from intact rats). Furthermore, immunocytochemical analysis of rat brain using this specific antiserum (affinity-purified) was negative. These latter findings are in accord with the previously cited *in situ* brain labeling experiment (see Section 7.2) in which ^{35}S-labeled des-acetyl α-MSH-like and β-endorphin-like peptides (but no acetylated peptides) were detected in rat brain tissue following an 8-h infusion of [^{35}S]-methionine into the hypothalamic arcuate nuclear region.

12   POSSIBLE PHYSIOLOGICAL FUNCTIONS OF PITUITARY PEPTIDES IN BRAIN

The extensive POMC-like neuronal network present in both hypothalamic and extrahypothalamic regions of the brain suggests that this system can influence both brain and pituitary function. In most cases, the study of effects of POMC-derived peptides on brain and pituitary function have been performed by the administration of synthetic peptides directly into the brain; that such effects are physiologically relevant is inferred in many cases. It is of historical interest that α-MSH, ACTH, and fragments thereof were shown to exert direct effects on the CNS many years before similar peptides were demonstrated to be present in brain or synthesized there.

12.1   Regulation of Pituitary Function

The inverse relationship noted between portal blood immunoreactive β-endorphin levels (thought to be of hypothalamic origin—see Section 8.2) and peripheral serum estrogen levels, and the decreased hypothalamic content of immunoreactive β-endorphin following estradiol treatment of ovariectomized rats, have led Wardlaw and colleagues (157, 160) to suggest that estrogens are normal physiological regulators of the brain POMC-like system, by acting to stimulate release of β-endorphin-like material from the hypothalamus. Exogenous opioids, including β-endorphin, inhibit gonadotropin secretion in the rat and human (197, 198), while naloxone causes an increase in release of LH (199, 200). Available evidence indicates that endogenous opioids are involved in the inhibition of release of follicle-stimulating hormone (FSH) and LH from the anterior pituitary at the level of the hypothalamus, perhaps by inhibiting gonadotropin releasing hormone (GnRH) release (either directly or by influencing neurotransmitters involved in its release) (201–203), thus suggesting that the hypothalamic β-endorphin system may have a physiological role in the control of gonadotropin secretion (157, 204).

Naloxone administration is known to decrease plasma prolactin levels (204–206), while intraventricular β-endorphin administration stimulates prolactin release from the anterior pituitary (207–210), not by a direct effect on the pituitary (207). β-endorphin has been shown to decrease median eminence and total hypothalamic dopamine turnover *in vivo* and *in vitro* (mechanisms appear to include both decreased release and increased uptake of dopamine by dopaminergic neurons) (204, 207–209, 211–214). Thus, the majority of these authors have concluded that hypothalamic β-endorphin participates in the regulation of prolactin secretion. Since prolactin secretion is known to be under the tonic inhibitory control of dopamine, β-endorphin can increase prolactin secretion by inhibiting the release of tuberoinfundibular dopamine.

Intraventricular administration of α-MSH increases the turnover of dopamine in the tuberoinfundibular dopaminergic system (215), stimulates the release of LH, and suppresses the release of prolactin from the anterior pituitary (216–218). α-MSH has no direct influence on the *in vitro* release of prolactin from pituitary tissue (216). α-MSH thus has an opposite effect to that of β-endorphin on the release of hypothalamic dopamine and pituitary prolactin and luteinizing hormone. These results suggest that hypothalamic α-MSH-like material has a physiological role in the regulation of these pituitary hormones. Since α-MSH and β-endorphin exert opposite effects on pituitary hormone release, modulation of release by the neuronal POMC-like system would require additional factors. For instance, the ratio of β-endorphin to α-MSH-like peptides released by these neurons may be variable (not in a coordinated fixed ratio), putative receptors for these peptides may be differentially up- or down-regulated, or pituitary β-endorphin and α-MSH-related peptides may gain access to such receptors. It is known that several other neuropeptides present in the hypothalamus affect prolactin and gonadotropin release and that α-MSH and β-endorphin affect the turnover of several other neurotransmitters present in the hypothalamus and other brain regions (219–226). All systems may function in a complex integrated fashion to regulate the synthesis and release of particular pituitary hormones.

Available data indicate a complex opioid regulatory control of pituitary secretion of ACTH-related peptides, dependent in part on the nature of the opioid, its dose, and duration of administration. Intraventricular administration of β-endorphin causes an increase in rat plasma corticosterone levels, which is blocked by naloxone; naloxone injected alone causes a significant decrease in plasma corticosterone levels (227). Pertinent to this point is the finding that morphine and opioid peptides stimulate the *in vitro* release of CRF-like activity by hypothalamic tissue in a naloxone-reversible manner (228). The pharmacological nature of available studies makes interpretation of such data difficult, especially in view of the existence of multiple classes of opiate receptors (some of which are naloxone-insensitive), the type and variable doses of opioids and naloxone employed, and the observations that ACTH- and β-endorphin-related peptides dramatically affect CNS neurotransmitter function in hypothalamic and extrahypothalamic regions. In addition, several studies have shown opposite or no effects on corticotrophic function by ACTH- and β-endorphin-related peptides.

12.2 Effects on Central Nervous System

Central administration of ACTH- and β-endorphin-related peptides exerts effects on the major mammalian homeostatic systems. Many of these actions are discussed in Chapters 5 through 14, and will only be briefly mentioned here.

12.2.1 Behavior

ACTH, α-MSH, and short N-terminal fragments of ACTH (which are also contained within the β-lipotropin sequence and the "γ-MSH" sequence residing within the N-terminus of POMC) have a short-term effect on the facilitation of learning and memory processes, possibly by temporarily increasing motivation; electrophysiological evidence implicates the limbic system and midbrain structures in mediating these behavioral effects. In humans, ACTH-(4-10) appears to facilitate short-term visual attention and memory and to improve attention and short-term memory. These activities could not be reversed by opiate antagonists. Such clinical trials in humans have been performed using a potent, long-lasting analog of ACTH-(4-9) (see 229–231 for reviews on CNS behavioral and biochemical effects of neuropeptides).

β-endorphin, α-endorphin, γ-endorphin, and des-Tyr[1] γ-endorphin also exert profound effects on behavior. Some of the effects of β-endorphin are mediated by the opiate receptors, since they can be blocked by opiate antagonists (e.g., the "excessive grooming" syndrome). β-endorphin and α-endorphin elicit behavioral effects similar to ACTH-(4-10). α-endorphin is the more potent peptide; in some respects its actions mimic those of the psychostimulants. γ-endorphin and des-Tyr[1]-γ-endorphin have effects opposite to those of α and β-endorphin, displaying classic neuroleptic activities, the des-Tyr[1] form being more potent than the intact γ-endorphin molecule. None of these latter behavioral responses is mediated by opiate receptors, since opiate antagonists cannot block these activities. Further evidence for this contention is provided by the fact that des-Tyr[1] β-endorphin has no affinity for any known class of opiate receptors and the observation that β-endorphin, the most potent analgesic peptide of the group, is the least potent in modifying these behavioral activities of des-Tyr[1] β-endorphin (see refs. 229, 230 for extensive reviews). De Wied (232) has suggested that the opposite behavioral effects elicited by exogenously administered α-endorphin (psychostimulant-like) and des-Tyr[1] γ-endorphin (neuroleptic-like) indicate that a balance between γ- and α-type endorphins is involved in the control of normal brain function. From this group's laboratory (231) has also come preliminary evidence that synthetic γ-MSH has opposite effects to those of ACTH-related peptides on some brain functions and interferes with some of the β-endorphin-induced effects.

Based on behavioral (hyperactive) and analgesic responses produced by injection of morphine into the periaqueductal gray matter, and the reversal only of the latter response by naloxone, Jacquet and colleagues have proposed a dual receptor mechanism for naloxone-insensitive opiate-related effects of ACTH (and fragments thereof) (233–237). β-endorphin and ACTH were proposed to be the natural ligands for the naloxone-sensitive and naloxone-insensitive receptors, respectively. It was further suggested that since the hyperactive effects noted were similar to those associated with morphine withdrawal, occupation of the putative ACTH receptor by "residual" morphine—rather than the absence of morphine—is the cause of the abstinence syndrome (233). If this dual receptor theory is correct, it is also quite possible that the withdrawal syndrome is mediated by endogenous ACTH-like ligands. Cross-tolerance between β-endorphin and morphine has been shown. Since ACTH-related and β-endorphin-related products would be expected to be released from neural elements in equimolar concentrations, the effective contribution of ACTH binding would be increased in a "β-endorphin-tolerant" individual.

More recently, Jaquet and Abrams (238) have shown that insertion of ACTH-(1-24), ACTH-(4-10), or α-MSH into the region of the locus coeruleus of the rat brainstem results in a rapid, dose-dependent onset of postural asymmetry and motor disorder, resembling human dystonia. This syndrome was not naloxone-reversible, nor could it be elicited by morphine. Since the locus coeruleus is composed mainly of noradrenergic neurons (and is shown by immunocytochemistry to contain POMC-like fibers) and is thought to be involved in Parkinson's disease, the authors suggest that endogenous brain-derived ACTH-related peptides may have a normal physiological role "in modulating posture and movement in this region of the brain stem." These findings are also in keeping with the hypothesis of multiple ACTH-like receptors, located in specific brain regions and modulating different physiological processes.

12.2.2 Neurotransmission

ACTH, ACTH fragments, α-MSH, β-endorphin, and β-endorphin fragments have been shown to modulate the activities of several central neurotransmitters (norepinephrine, dopamine, serotonin, acetylcholine, γ-aminobutyric acid) in specific brain regions (211, 215, 219–226, 239–252). ACTH- and β-endorphin-related peptides have been shown to exert opposite effects in some cases. For example, as noted above, α-MSH appears to increase the turnover of dopamine in the tuberoinfundibular dopaminergic system, β-endorphin inhibits the release of dopamine (251, 252), and ACTH and β-endorphin have opposite effects on hippocampal acetylcholine content (250). The overall actions of POMC-derived peptides may be mediated by modulation of neurotransmission. For example, a dopaminergic system has been implicted in ACTH-induced excessive grooming (253); the grooming response is suppressed when the dopamine antagonist haloperidol is administered (254).

12.2.3   Other Effects

ACTH and β-endorphin differentially affect sexual activity in rodents. β-endorphin has been implicated in feeding behavior, blood pressure, and temperature regulation. ACTH-related peptides induce hyperalgesia, while β-endorphin induces analgesia. (See specific chapters on the effects of neuropeptides in homeostatic systems.)

12.2.4   Mechanism of Action

In brain, ACTH-related and β-endorphin-related peptides have been shown to affect protein and RNA synthesis, adenylate cyclase activity, phosphorylation and dephosphorylation of specific membrane proteins, activation of acyl cholesterol hydrolase and triacyl glycerol lipase activities, and modulation of the turnover of membrane phosphoinositides (255–265). ACTH-(1-24) has been shown to specifically release a 41,000 dalton protein from rat brain synaptosomal plasma membrane preparations (266).

ACTH-induced adrenal steroidogenesis is associated with specific protein synthesis, phosphorylation, and dephosphorylation of specific adrenal proteins (some of which are clearly cAMP-dependent) and increases in adrenal polyphosphoinositides (267–269). Hence brain ACTH and related peptides act in brain via mechanisms similar to those thought to mediate ACTH-induced adrenal steroidogenesis. Specific phosphorylation-dephosphorylation reactions are known to represent a basic mechanism whereby both classical hormones and neurotransmitters control cellular functions (see ref. 270 for a review); differential effects on common intracellular kinases and phosphatases may represent at least one mechanism whereby brain ACTH- and β-endorphin-related peptides affect neurotransmitter function in an interactive manner.

12.3   Other Hormones

To date, there are no definitive studies concerning the role of other pituitary-like hormones in brain. The large literature dealing with prolactin effects on CNS neurotransmitters has been assumed to reflect that of pituitary-derived prolactin. Should brain synthesis be demonstrated, this will require evaluation.

13   POMC-LIKE PEPTIDES IN MAMMALIAN NON-CNS, NONPITUITARY SITES

In addition to the presence of POMC-like material in the central nervous system, material similar to POMC-derived peptides has been reported in the mammalian (including human) gastrointestinal tract (271–287), male reproductive tract (288–290), placenta (291–295), and lymphocytes (296, 297). Most of these studies have utilized immunocytochemical or radioimmunological techniques with further chromatographic or electrophoretic characterization of the immunoreactive species detected. One report (271) of POMC-derived peptides in human gut tissue also utilized an affinity chromatographic step, suggesting that the apparent presence of these peptides was not due to radioimmunological artifact (111). In addition, cultured human placental cells have been shown to synthesize substances physicochemically similar to human pituitary POMC and its derived peptides; one component of β-endorphin-sized material appears to be identical to authentic human β-endorphin (298, 299).

Only one POMC gene appears to exist in the human genome (30). Therefore, if POMC-like peptides are synthesized at extrapituitary sites in the human, the gene encoding pituitary POMC must be expressed at these extrapituitary sites. In this regard, Herbert and Uhler (300) have detected two POMC genes located on different chromosomes, in the mouse genome. One of these genes appears to be a pseudogene. These investigators conclude that "since the mouse has only one functional POMC gene, differential tissue expression of POMC appears to be related to different processing enzymes in each tissue."

14   PITUITARY-LIKE PEPTIDES IN INVERTEBRATES

14.1   Presence of ACTH-Related and Endorphin-Related Material in Invertebrates

Using immunocytochemical techniques, Fritsch et al. (301) have detected β-endorphin-like material in the cerebral ganglion of the sea squid *Ciona intestinalis*. Boer et al. (302) have detected immunoreactive ACTH-like material in two electrotonically coupled giant neurons in the pond snail *Lymnaea stagnalis*. Immunocytochemical localization of α-endorphin-like material is present in neurons of caterpillars (303, 304), and α-endorphin-like and β-endorphin-like material is present in neurons and other cell types of earthworms (305, 306). Royden et al. (307) have recently immunocytochemically localized ACTH-like material to the nervous and reproductive systems in *Drosophila melanogaster*. Using a DNA probe complementary to mouse ACTH, specific hybridization to *Drosophila* DNA restriction fragments was observed when moderately stringent conditions of hybridization were employed.

14.2   Presence of ACTH-like and β-Endorphin-like Peptides in a Unicellular Eukaryote

ACTH- and β-endorphin-like peptides have been detected in acid extracts of the unicellular eukaryote *Tetrahymena pyriformis* (308). Multiple size classes of immunoreactive ACTH and β-endorphin were revealed upon gel filtration. One form of immunoreactive ACTH-sized material exhibited ACTH bioreactivity, with a mean immunoreactive–bioreactive ratio of 1:5. A major peak of opiate radioreceptor activity was detected that exhibited an apparent molecular weight similar to authentic human β-endorphin. Reverse phase high pressure liquid chromatography revealed the presence of at least three partially resolved immunoreactive β-endorphin peaks exhibiting retention times similar to those of synthetic human and camel β-endorphin. Material in the apparent MW range 67,000–31,000 containing both ACTH and β-endorphin antigenic determinants was also present, suggestive of a common precursor molecule (or molecules), in analogy with POMC.

14.3   Other Pituitary Peptides

Immunocytochemically, human prolactin-like material has been detected in the cerebral ganglion of a species of sea squid (301).

15   EVOLUTIONARY PERSPECTIVE

The synthesis of similar or identical secretory peptides at multiple sites within an organism and their widespread phylogenetic occurrence is exemplified by the findings reported here for POMC-like peptides. The possibility that these peptides (hormonal peptides and proteins) existed at least at the level of the unicellular eukaryote, and possibly at the prokaryotic level (309) (see also Chapters 5 and 36) should not be surprising. Rather, the previously held view that a given hormone is synthesized within an organism solely by a unique cell type, located in an endocrine gland (and, by extrapolation, that an individual hormone evolved at the time its endocrine gland came into existence) is, in retrospect, quite simplistic. This notion, of course, required the messenger molecule (and possibly the target gland receptor or receptors) to evolve simultaneously with the endocrine gland itself. It rather seems more realistic that preexisting messenger molecules (and preexisting receptors) would be utilized whenever possible or would evolve from them. (See ref. 310 for a review.)

Additionally, the expression of POMC or any other secretory peptide or protein at multiple sites within an organism may indicate that the systems that synthesize the same peptides are functionally interrelated. Evidence for possible functional interaction of the CNS, pituitary corticotrophic cells, immune system, and germ-cell systems has recently been briefly discussed (311). Not mentioned in that review are the report that human immunoglobulins specifically bind (via the F_c portion of Ig) to human anterior pituitary corticotrophs, but to no other pituitary cell type (312), the demonstration that the heavy chain of the human IgG class shares sequence homologies with both ACTH and β-endorphin (313), or the report that β-endorphin binds to terminal complexes of human complement (314).

In some respects, the designation "neuropeptides" or "brain peptides" may be misleading. The central nervous system neurons clearly synthesize many secretory peptides that are involved in brain function, but these peptides are not exclusive to the brain. Instead, the brain, along with the other tissue systems, probably utilizes genes that existed before the evolution of the nervous system.

REFERENCES

1. B. A. Eipper and R. E. Mains, *Endocr. Rev.* **1**, 1 (1980).
2. E. Herbert, J. Roberts, M. Phillips, R. Allen, M. Hinman, M. Budarf, P. Policastro, and P. Rosa, in L. Martini and W. F. Ganong, Eds., *Frontiers in Neuroendocrinology*, Vol. 6, Raven Press, New York, 1980, p. 67.
3. M. Chretien and N. G. Seidah, *Mol. Cell. Biochem.* **34**, 101 (1981).
4. M. Chretien, S. Benjannet, F. Gossard, C. Gianoulakis, P. Crine, M. Lis, and N. G. Seidah, *Can. J. Biochem.* **57**, 1111 (1979).
5. A. S. Liotta, T. Suda, and D. T. Krieger, *Proc. Natl. Acad. Sci. USA* **75**, 2950 (1978).
6. T. Kita, A. Inove, S. Nakanishi, and S. Numa, *Eur. J. Biochem.* **93**, 213(1979).
7. J. L. Roberts, M. Phillips, P. A. Rosa, and E. Herbert, *Biochemistry* **17**, 3609 (1978).
8. M. Rubinstein, S. Stein, and S. Udenfriend, *Proc. Natl. Acad. Sci. USA* **75**, 669 (1978).
9. B. A. Eipper and R. E. Mains, *J. Biol. Chem.* **253**, 5732 (1978).
10. S. Nakanishi, A. Inoue, T. Kita, M. Nakamura, A. C. Y. Chang, S. N. Cohen, and S. Numa, *Nature* **278**, 423 (1979).
11. J. L. Roberts, P. H. Seeburg, J. Shine, E. Herbert, J. D. Baxter, and H. M. Goodman, *Proc. Natl. Acad. Sci. USA* **76**, 2153 (1979).
12. A. C. Y. Chang, M. Cochet, and S. N. Cohen, *Proc. Natl. Acad. Sci. USA* **77**, 4890 (1980).
13. J. Drouin and H. M. Goodman, *Nature* **288**, 610 (1980).
14. S. Nakanishi, Y. Teranishi, M. Noda, M. Notake, Y. Watanabe, H. Kakidani, H. Jingami, and S. Numa, *Nature* **287**, 752 (1980).
15. S. Nakanishi, Y. Terenishi, Y. Watanabe, M. Notake, M. Noda, H. Kakidani, H. Jingami, and S. Numa, *Eur. J. Biochem.* **115**, 429 (1981).
16. H. Takahashi, Y. Teranishi, S. Nakanishi, and S. Numa, *FEBS Lett.* **135**, 97 (1981).
17. P. L. Whitfeld, P. H. Seeburg, and J. Shine, *DNA* **1**, 133 (1982).
18. M. Cochet, A. C. Y. Chang, and S. N. Cohen, *Nature* **297**, 335 (1982).

19. P. L. Brubaker, H. P. J. Bennett, A. C. Baird, and S. Solomon, *Biochem. Biophys. Res. Commun.* **96**, 1441 (1980).

20. A. S. Liotta, P. Falaschi, and D. T. Krieger, *Program of the 64th Meeting of the Endocrine Society*, San Francisco, Calif., June 16–18, 1982, Abstr. 221.

21. J. Verhoef, J. G. Loeber, J. P. H. Burbach, W. H. Gispen, A. Witter, and D. de Wied, *Life Sci.* **26**, 851 (1980).

22. A. S. Liotta, H. Yamaguchi, and D. T. Krieger, *J. Neurosci.* **1**, 585 (1981).

23. B. A. Eipper and R. E. Mains, *J. Biol. Chem.* **256**, 5689 (1981).

24. E. Weber, C. J. Evans, J. -K. Chang, and J. D. Barchas, *J. Neurochem.* **38**, 436 (1982).

25. D. G. Smyth and S. Zakarin, *Nature* **288**, 613 (1981).

26. H. Akil, Y. Veda, H. L. Lin, and S. J. Watson, *Neuropeptides* **1**, 429 (1981).

27. D. I. Buckley, R. A. Houghten, and J. Ramachandran, *Int. J. Peptide Protein Res.* **17**, 508 (1981).

28. D. Rudman, R. K. Chaula, and B. M. Hollins, *J. Biol. Chem.* **254**, 10102 (1979).

29. D. M. Dorsa, M. B. Chapman, and D. G. Baskin, *Peptides* **3**, 455 (1982).

30. D. Owerbach, W. J. Rutter, J. L. Roberts, P. Whitfeld, J. Shine, P. H. Seeburg, and T. B. Shows, *Somatic Cell Genet.* **3**, 359 (1981).

31. M. A. Phillips, M. L. Budarf, and E. Herbert, *Biochemistry* **201**, 1666 (1981).

32. N. G. Seidah and M. Chretien, *Proc. Natl. Acad. Sci. USA* **78**, 4236 (1981).

33. H. P. J. Bennett, C. A. Browne, and S. Solomon, *Proc. Natl. Acad. Sci. USA* **78**, 4713 (1981).

34a. H. P. J. Bennett, C. A. Browne, and S. Solomon, *Biochemistry* **20**, 4530 (1981).

34b. C. A. Browne, H. P. J. Bennett, and S. Solomon, *Biochemistry* **20**, 4538 (1981).

35. B. A. Eipper and R. E. Mains, *J. Biol. Chem.* **257**, 4907 (1982).

36. H. Hoshina, G. Hortin, and I. Boime, *Science* **217**, 63 (1982).

37. R. Guillemin, A. V. Schally, H. L. Lipscomb, R. N. Andersen, and J. M. Long, *Endocrinology* **70**, 471 (1962).

38. A. V. Schally, H. S. Lipscomb, J. M. Long, W. E. Dear, and R. Guillemin, *Endocrinology* **70**, 478 (1962).

39. D. T. Krieger and A. S. Liotta, *Science* **205**, 366 (1979).

40. D. T. Krieger, A. S. Liotta, M. J. Brownstein, and E. A. Zimmerman, *Recent Prog. Horm. Res.* **36**, 277 (1980).

41. D. T. Krieger, A. S. Liotta, M. J. Brownstein, *Proc. Natl. Acad. Sci. USA* **74**, 648 (1977).

42. D. T. Krieger, A. S. Liotta, and M. J. Brownstein, *Brain Res.* **128**, 575 (1977).

43. D. T. Krieger, A. S. Liotta, T. Suda, M. Palkovits, and M. J. Brownstein, *Biochem. Biophys. Res. Commun.* **76**, 930 (1977).

44. E. Orwoll, J. W. Kendall, L. Lamorena, and R. McGilvra, *Endocrinology* **102**, 697 (1979).

45. S. T. Pacold, L. Kirsteins, S. Hojvat, A. M. Lawrence, and T. C. Hagen, *Science* **199**, 804 (1978).

46. C. Oliver and J. C. Porter, *Endocrinology* **102**, 697 (1978).

47. S. Matsukura, H. Yoshimi, S. Sueoka, K. Kataoko, T. Uno, and N. Ohgushi, *Brain Res.* **159**, 228 (1978).

48. J. Rossier, T. M. Vargo, S. Minick, N. Ling, F. E. Bloom, and R. Guillemin, *Proc. Natl. Acad. Sci. USA* **74**, 5162 (1977).

49. Y. -P. Loh, R. L. Eskay, and M. Brownstein, *Biochem. Biophys. Res. Commun.* **94**, 916 (1980).

50. F. LaBella, G. Queen, and L. Senshyn, *Biochem. Biophys. Res. Commun.* **75**, 350 (1977).

51. T. L. O'Donahue, G. E. Holmquist, and D. M. Jacobowitz, *Neurosci. Lett.* **14**, 271 (1979).

52. C. Gramsch, G. Kleber, V. Hollt, A. Pasi, P. Mehraein, and A. Herz, *Brain Res.* **192**, 109 (1980).

53. M. M. Wilkes, W. B. Watkins, R. D. Stewart, and S. S. C. Yen, *Neuroendocrinology* **30**, 113 (1980).
54. G. Kleber, C. Gramsch, V. Hollt, P. Mehraein, A. Pasi, and A. Herz, *Neuroendocrinology* **31**, 39 (1980).
55. T. Shibasaki, N. Ling, R. Guillemin, M. Silver, and F. Bloom, *Regul. Peptides* **2**, 43 (1981).
56. S. Hojvat, G. Baker, L. Kirstins, and A. M. Lawrence, *Brain Res.* **239**, 543 (1982).
57. N. Emanuele, E. Connick, T. Howell, J. Anderson, S. Hojvat, G. Baker, J. Souchek, L. Kirsteins, and A. M. Lawrence, *Biol. Reprod.* **25**, 321 (1981).
58. G. Hostetter, R. V. Gallo, and M. S. Brownfield, *Neuroendocrinology* **33**, 241 (1981).
59. J. L. Bakke and N. Lawrence, *Neuroendocrinology* **2**, 315 (1967).
60. S. A. Joseph and K. M. Knigge, *Am. J. Physiol.* **226**, 630 (1974).
61. J. E. Ottenweller and G. A. Hedge, *Endocrinology* **111**, 515 (1982).
62. S. Hojvat, G. Baker, L. Kirsteins, and A. M. Lawrence, *Neuroendocrinology* **34**, 327 (1982).
63. W. J. DeVito and G. A. Hedge, *Endocrinology* **111**, 1406 (1982).
64. R. M. Post, P. Gold, D. R. Rubinov, J. C. Ballenger, W. E. Bunner Jr., and F. K. Goodwin, *Life Sci* **31**, 1 (1982).
65. Y. Hosobuchi, in R. Collu et al., Eds., *Brain Peptides and Hormones*, Raven Press, New York, 1982, p. 197.
66. K. Nakao, S. Oki, I. Tanaka, K. Horii, Y. Nakai, T. Furui, M. Fukushima, A. Kuwayama, N. Kageyama, and H. Imura, *J. Clin. Invest.* **66**, 1383 (1980).
67. C. Bugnon, B. Bloch, D. Lenys, and D. Fellmann, *Cell Tissue Res.* **199**, 177 (1979).
68. B. Bloch, C. Bugnon, D. Fellman, and D. Lenys, *Neurosci. Lett.* **10**, 147 (1978).
69. S. J. Watson, C. W. Richard III, and J. D. Barchas, *Science* **200**, 1180 (1978).
70. B. Bloch, C. Bugnon, D. Fellmann, D. Lenys, and A. Gouget, *Cell Tissue Res.* **204**, 1 (1979).
71. C. Bugnon, B. Bloch, D. Lenys, A. Gouget, and D. Fellmann, *Neurosci. Lett.* **14**, 43 (1979).
72. S. Hisano, H. Kawano, T. Nishiyama, and S. Daikoku, *Cell Tissue Res.* **224**, 303 (1982).
73. G. Nilaver, E. A. Zimmerman, R. Defendini, A. S. Liotta, D. T. Krieger, and M. J. Brownstein, *J. Cell Biol.* **81**, 50 (1979).
74. G. Pelletier, *J. Histochem. Cytochem.* **27**, 1046 (1979).
75. G. Pelletier, *Neurosci. Lett.* **16**, 85 (1980).
76. G. Pelletier, R. Leclerc, F. Labrie, J. Cote, M. Chretien, and M. Lis, *Endocrinology* **100**, 770 (1977).
77. G. Pelletier and R. Leclerc, *Endocrinology* **104**, 1426 (1979).
78. K. M. Knigge and S. A. Joseph, *Brain Res.* **239**, 655 (1982).
79. P. E. Sawchenko, L. W. Swanson, and S. A. Joseph, *Brain Res.* **232**, 365 (1982).
80. J. C. W. Finley, P. Lindstrom, and P. Petrusz, *Neuroendocrinology* **33**, 28 (1981).
81. D. M. Jacobowitz and T. L. O'Donohue, *Proc. Natl. Acad. Sci. USA* **75**, 6300 (1978).
82. F. Bloom, E. Battenberg, J. Rossier, N. Ling, and R. Guillemin, *Proc. Natl. Acad. Sci. USA* **75**, 1591 (1978).
83. D. Dube, J. C. Lissitzky, R. Leclerc, and G. Pelletier, *Endocrinology* **102**, 1283 (1978).
84. S. J. Watson, J. D. Barchas, and C. H. Li, *Proc. Natl. Acad. Sci. USA* **74**, 5155 (1977).
85. M. W. Sofroniew, *Am. J. Anat.* **154**, 283 (1979).
86. D. Dube, J. Cote, and G. Pelletier, *Neurosci. Lett.* **12**, 171 (1979).
87. G. Pelletier and L. Desy, *Cell Tissue Res.* **196**, 525 (1979).
88. G. Pelletier and D. Dube, *Am. J. Anat.* **150**, 201 (1977).
89. L. Desey and G. Pelletier, *Brain Res.* **154**, 377 (1978).
90. G. M. Abrams, G. Nilaver, D. Hoffman, E. A. Zimmerman, M. Ferin, D. T. Krieger, and A. S. Liotta, *Neurology* **30**, 1106 (1980).

91. G. Pelletier, L. Desy, J. C. Lissitszky, F. Labrie, and C. H. Li, *Life Sci.* **22**, 1799 (1978).
92. E. A. Zimmerman, A. Liotta, and D. T. Krieger, *Cell Tissue Res.* **186**, 393 (1978).
93. S. J. Watson and H. Akil, *Brain Res.* **182**, 217 (1980).
94. S. J. Watson and H. Akil, *Eur. J. Pharmacol.* **58**, 101 (1979).
95. J. Guy, H. Vaudry, and G. Pelletier, *Brain Res.* **220**, 199 (1981).
96. W. B. Watkins, *Cell Tissue Res.* **207**, 65 (1980).
97. C. S. Leranth, T. H. Williams, M. Chretien, and M. Palkovits, *Cell Tissue Res.* **210**, 11 (1980).
98. H. Salih, A. E. Panerai, and H. G. Friesen, *Life Sci.* **24**, 111 (1979).
99. C. Leranth, T. H. Williams, J. Hamori, and M. Chretien, *Neuroscience* **6**, 481 (1981).
100. K. M. Knigge and S. A. Joseph, *Cell Tissue Res.* **215**, 333 (1981).
101. K. Fuxe, T. Hökfelt, P. Eneroth, J. Gustafsson, and P. Skett, *Science* **196**, 899 (1977).
102. G. Toubeau, J. Desclin, M. Parmentier, and J. L. Pasteels, *J. Endocrinol.* **83**, 261 (1979).
103. G. Toubeau, J. Desclin, M. Parmentier, and J. L. Pasteels, *Neuroendocrinology* **29**, 344 (1979).
104. R. M. Lechan, J. L. Nestler, and M. E. Molitch, *Endocrinology* **109**, 1950 (1981).
105. R. M. Bergland and R. B. Page, *Endocrinology* **102**, 1325 (1978).
106. R. M. Bergland and R. B. Page, *Science* **204**, 18 (1979).
107. R. B. Page, B. L. Munger, and R. M. Bergland, *Am. J. Anat.* **146**, 273 (1976).
108. R. B. Page and R. M. Bergland, *Am. J. Anat.* **148**, 345 (1977).
109. M. Palkovits and E. Mezey, in L. H. Rees and T. B. van Wimersma Greidanus, Eds., *Frontiers of Hormone Research, ACTH and Lipotropin in Health and Disease*, Vol. 8: S. Karger, Basel, 1981, p. 122.
110. R. Moldow and R. S. Yalow, *Proc. Natl. Acad. Sci. USA* **75**, 994 (1978).
111. R. S. Yalow and J. Eng, *Peptides* **2**, 17 (1981).
112. D. T. Krieger, A. S. Liotta, H. Hauser, and M. J. Brownstein, *Endocrinology* **105**, 737 (1979).
113. R. B. Page, *Endocrinology* **112**, 157 (1983).
114. R. Bergland, H. Blume, A. Hamilton, P. Monica, and R. Paterson, *Science* **210**, 541 (1980).
115. R. N. Dias, M. L. S. Perry, M. A. Carrasco, and I. Izquierdo, *Behav. Neural Biol.* **32**, 265 (1981).
116. E. Mezey, M. Palkovits, E. R. deKoet, J. Verhoef, and D. de Wied, *Life Sci.* **22**, 831 (1978).
117. D. M. Dorsa, E. R. de Kloet, E. Mezey, and D. de Wied, *Endocrinology* **104**, 1663 (1979).
118. C. Oliver, R. S. Mical, and J. C. Porter, *Endocrinology* **101**, 598 (1977).
119. S. L. Wardlaw, W. B. Wehrenberg, M. Ferin, P. W. Carmel, and A. G. Frantz, *Endocrinology* **106**, 1323 (1980).
120. N. Ogawa, A. E. Panaeri, S. Lee, S. Forsbach, H. Havhick, and H. G. Friesen, *Life Sci.* **25**, 317 (1979).
121. D. T. Krieger, A. S. Liotta, G. Nicholsen, and J. S. Kizer, *Nature* **278**, 562 (1979).
122a. O. Civelli, N. Birnberg, and E. Herbert, *J. Biol. Chem.* **257**, 6783 (1982).
122b. E. Herbert, N. Birnberg, J. -C. Lissitsky, O. Civelli, and M. Uhler, *Trends Neurosci.* **12**, 16 (1981).
123. R. L. Eskay, P. Giraud, C. Oliver, and M. J. Brownstein, *Brain Res.* **178**, 55 (1979).
124. G. Pelletier, A. LeClerc, M. J. Saavedra, M. J. Brownstein, H. Vaudry, L. Ferland, and F. Labrie, *Brain Res.* **192**, 433 (1980).
125. T. L. O'Donohue, R. L. Miller, and D. M. Jacobowitz, *Brain Res.* **176**, 101 (1979).
126. B. Kerdelhue, C. L. Bethea, N. Ling, M. Chretien, and R. I. Weiner, *Brain Res.*, **231**, 85 (1982).

127. P. M. Scott and K. M. Knigge, *Cell Tissue Res.* **219**, 393 (1981).
128. R. L. Eskay, M. J. Brownstein, and R. T. Long, *Science* **205**, 827 (1979).
129. M. P. Blaunstein, E. M. Johnson, and P. Needleman, *Proc. Natl. Acad. Sci. USA* **69**, 2237 (1972).
130. I. Vermes, G. H. Mulder, F. Berkenbosch, and F. J. H. Tilders, *Brain Res.* **211**, 248 (1981).
131. T. L. O'Donohue, C. G. Charlton, N. B. Thoa, C. J. Helke, T. W. Moody, A. Pert, A. Williams, R. L. Miller, and D. M. Jacobowitz, *Peptides* **2**, 93 (1981).
132. H. Osborne, R. Przewlocki, V. Hollt, and A. Herz, *Eur. J. Pharmacol.* **55**, 425 (1979).
133. F. Monnet, J. -C. Reubi, A. Eberle, and W. Lichtensteiger, *Neuroendocrinology* **33**, 284 (1982).
134. J. Fukata, Y. Nakai, and H. Imura, *Neurosci. Lett.* **19**, 79 (1980).
135. J. Fukuta, Y. Nakai, K. Takahishi, and H. Imura, *Brain Res.* **195**, 489 (1980).
136. V. Warberg, C. Oliver, A. Barnea, C. R. Parker, Jr., and J. C. Porter, *Brain Res.* **175**, 247 (1979).
137. Y. P. Loh, L. Zucker, H. Verpaget, and Tj. B. van Wimersma Greidanus, *J. Neurosci. Res.* **4**, 147 (1979).
138. G. Fink, Y. Koch, N. B. Akoya, *Brain Res.* **243**, 186 (1982).
139. B. L. Baker and Y. Y. Yen, *Proc. Soc. Exp. Biol. Med.* **151**, 599 (1976).
140. N. Emanuele, R. Oslapas, E. Connick, L. Kirsteins, and A. M. Lawrence, *Neuroendocrinology* **33**, 12 (1981).
141. N. Emanuele, J. Anderson, T. Howell, E. Andersen, S. Lipov, E. Connick, L. Kirsteins, and A. M. Lawrence, *Program of the 63rd Meeting of the Endocrine Society*, 1981, Abstr. 612.
142. A. S. Liotta, D. Gildersleeve, M. J. Brownstein, and D. T. Krieger, *Proc. Natl. Acad. Sci. USA* **76**, 1448 (1979).
143. A. S. Liotta, C. Loudes, J. F. McKelvy, and D. T. Krieger, *Proc. Natl. Acad. Sci. USA* **77**, 1880 (1980).
144. A. S. Liotta and D. T. Krieger, *Mol. Cell. Endocrinol* **16**, 221 (1979).
145. J. W. Kendall, E. S. Orwoll, and R. Allen, in E. Shark, G. B. Makara, Zs. Aces, and E. Endroczi, Eds., *Advances in Physiological Sciences*, Vol. 13, Pergamon Press, Akademia Kiado, Budapest, 1981, p. 167.
146. J. P. Advis, J. E. Krause, and J. F. McKelvy, *Program of the 64th Meeting of the Endocrine Society*, San Francisco, Calif., June 16–18, 1982, Abstr. 601.
147. A. Barnea, G. Cho, N. S. Pilotte, and J. C. Porter, *Endocrinology* **108**, 150 (1981).
148. D. G. Schwartzberg and P. K. Nakane, *Endocrinology* **100**, 855 (1982).
149. A. Bayon, W. J. Shoemaker, F. E. Bloom, A. Mauss, and R. Guillemin, *Brain Res.* **179**, 93 (1979).
150. L. W. Haynes, D. G. Smyth, and S. Zakarian, *Brain Res.* **232**, 115 (1982).
151. S. Hojvat, N. Emanuele, G. Baker, E. Connick, L. Kirsteins, and A. M. Lawrence, *Devel. Brain Res.* **4**, 427 (1982).
152. J. R. Hodges and M. T. Jones, *J. Physiol.* **173**, 190 (1964).
153. M. Moriarty and G. C. Moriarty, *Endocrinology* **96**, 1419 (1975).
154. C. Bugnon, D. Fellman, A. Gouget, and J. Cardot, *Neurosci. Lett.* **30**, 25 (1982).
155. W. K. Paull, J. Scholer, A. Arimura, C. A. Meyers, J. K. Chang, D. Chang, and M. Shimizu, *Peptides* **1**, 183 (1982).
156. R. L. Moldow and A. J. Fischman, *Peptides* **1**, 143 (1982).
157. S. L. Wardlaw, L. Thoron, and A. G. Frantz, *Brain Res.* **245**, 327 (1982).
158. N. Barden, Y. Merand, D. Roulfan, M. Garon, and A. Dupont, *Brain Res.* **204**, 441 (1981).
159. S. Lee, A. R. Panerai, D. Ballabarba, and H. G. Friesen, *Endocrinology* **107**, 245 (1980).
160. W. B. Wehrenberg, S. L. Wardlaw, A. G. Frantz, and M. Ferin, *Endocrinology* **111**, 879 (1982).

161. S. R. Gambert, T. C. Garthwaite, C. H. Pontzer, and T. C. Hagen, *Horm. Metab. Res.* **12**, 345 (1981).

162. A. M. A. van Dijk, Tj. B. van Wimersma Greidanus, J. P. H. Burbach, E. R. de Kloet, and D. de Wied, *J. Endocrinol.* **88**, 243 (1981).

163. J. Rossier, E. D. French, C. Rivier, N. Ling, R. Guillemin, and F. E. Bloom, *Nature* **270**, 618 (1977).

164. M. J. Millan, R. Przewlocki, M. Herliez, C. Gramsch, V. Hollt, and A. Herz, *Brain Res.* **208**, 325 (1981).

165. R. Przewlocki, M. J. Milan, C. Gramsch, M. H. Millan, and A. Herz, *Brain Res.* **242**, 107 (1982).

166. T. Torda, T. L. O'Donohue, J. Saavedra, and D. M. Jacobowitz, *Soc. Neurosci.* **6**, 622 (1980).

167. A. Barnea, G. Cho, and J. C. Porter, *Brain Res.* **232**, 345 (1982).

168. L. J. Forman, W. E. Sonnrag, D. A. van Vogt, and J. Meites, *Neurobiol. Aging* **2**, 281 (1981).

169. N. Barden, A. Dupont, F. Labrie, Y. Merand, D. Rouleau, H. Vaudry, and J. R. Boissier, *Brain Res.* **208**, 209 (1981).

170. A. Barnea, G. Cho, and J. C. Porter, *Brain Res.* **232**, 355 (1982).

171. S. R. Gambert, T. L. Garthwaite, C. H. Pontzer, and T. C. Hagen, *Neuroendocrinology* **31**, 252 (1980).

172. M. W. Adler, *Life Sci.* **28**, 1543 (1981).

173. R. S. Zukin and S. R. Zukin, *Life Sci.* **29**, 2681 (1981).

174. W. R. Martin, *Life Sci.* **28**, 1547 (1981).

175. B. L. Wolozin and G. W. Pasternak, *Proc. Natl. Acad. Sci. USA* **78**, 6181 (1981).

176. R. R. Goodman, S. H. Snyder, M. J. Kuhar, and S. W. Young III., *Proc. Natl. Acad. Sci. USA* **77**, 6239 (1980).

177. M. van Houten, M. N. Khan, R. J. Khan, and P. I. Posner, *Endocrinology* **108**, 2385 (1981).

178. L. Terenius, *J. Pharm. Pharmacol.* **27**, 450 (1975).

179. L. Terenius, W. H. Gispen, and D. de Wied, *Eur. J. Pharmacol.* **33**, 395 (1975).

180. C. R. Snell and P. H. Snell, *FEBS Lett.* **137**, 209 (1982).

181. G. J. J. Plomp and J. M. van Ree, *Br. J. Pharmacol.* **64**, 223 (1978).

182. A. Witter, *Receptors for Neurotransmitters and Peptide Hormones*, G. Peteu, M. J. Kuhar, and S. J. Enna, Eds., Raven Press, New York, 1980, p. 407.

183. J. Verhoef, V. M Wiegant, and D. de Wied, *Brain Res.* **231**, 454 (1982).

184. D. M. Dorsa, L. A. Majumdar, and M. B. Chapman, *Peptides* **2**, 71 (1981).

185. D. de Wied, G. L. Kovacs, B. Bohus, J. M. van Ree, and H. M. Greven, *Eur. J. Pharmacol.* **49**, 427 (1978).

186. R. J. Walsh, B. I. Posner, B. M. Kopriwa, and J. R. Bower, *Science* **201**, 1041 (1978).

187. R. DiCarlo and G. Muccioli, *Life Sci.* **28**, 2299 (1981).

188. R. DiCarlo and G. Muccioli, *Brain Res.* **230**, 445 (1981).

189. A. I. Smith, A. B. Keith, J. A. Edwardson, J. A. Biggins, and J. R. McDermott, *Neurosci. Lett.* **31**, 133 (1982).

190. S. Zakarian and D. G. Smyth, *Proc. Natl. Acad. Sci. USA* **76**, 5972 (1979).

191. T. L. O'Donohue, G. E. Handelmann, T. Chaconas, R. L. Miller, and D. M. Jacobowitz, *Peptides* **2**, 333 (1981).

192. T. L. O'Donohue, G. E. Handelmann, R. L. Miller, and D. M. Jacobowitz, *Science* **215**, 1125 (1982).

193. T. L. O'Donohue and M. C. Chappell, *Peptides* **3**, 69 (1982).

194. S. Zakarian and D. G. Smyth, *Nature* **296**, 250 (1982).

195. E. Weber, C. J. Evans, and J. D. Barchas, *Biochem. Biophys. Res. Commun.* **103**, 982 (1981).

196. C. J. Evans, R. Lorenz, E. Weber, and J. D. Barchas, *Biochem. Biophys. Res. Commun.* **106**, 910 (1982).

197. J. Meites, J. F. Bruni, D. A. van Vugt, and A. F. Smith, *Life Sci.* **24**, 1325 (1979).
198. R. L. Reid, J. D. Hoff, S. S. C. Yen, and C. H. Li, *J. Clin. Endocrinol. Metab.* **52**, 1179 (1981).
199. M. E. Quigley and S. S. C. Yen, *J. Clin. Endocrinol. Metab.* **51**, 179 (1980).
200. J. Blankstein, F. I. Reyes, J. S. D. Winter, and C. Faiman, *Clin. Endocrinol.* **14**, 287 (1981).
201. F. Kinoshita, Y. Nakai, H. Katakami, Y. Kato, H. Yamijima, and H. Imura, *Life Sci.* **27**, 843 (1980).
202. M. S. Blank, A. E. Panerai, and H. G. Friesen, *Science* **203**, 1129 (1979).
203. T. J. Cicero, B. A. Schanker, and E. R. Meyer, *Endocrinology* **104**, 1286 (1979).
204. M. Gold, D. Redmond, Jr., and R. Donabedian, *Endocrinology* **105**, 284 (1979).
205. J. F. Bruni, D. van Vugt, S. Marshall, and J. Meites, *Life Sci.* **21**, 461 (1977).
206. C. J. Shaar, R. C. A. Fredrickson, N. B. Dininger, and L. Jackson, *Life Sci.* **21**, 853 (1977).
207. C. Rivier, W. Vale, N. Ling, M. Brown, and R. Guillemin, *Endocrinology* **100**, 238 (1977).
208. A. Dupont, L. Cusan, F. Labrie, D. H. Coy, and C. H. Li, *Biochem. Biophys. Res. Commun.* **75**, 76 (1977).
209. L. Grandison and A. Guidotti, *Nature* **270**, 357 (1977).
210. G. R. van Loon, E. B. De Souza, and S. H. Shin, *Neuroendocrinology* **31**, 292 (1981).
211. G. R. van Loon, D. Ho, C. Kim, *Endocrinology* **106**, 76 (1980).
212. S. N. Deyo, R. M. Swift, and R. J. Miller, *Proc. Natl. Acad. Sci. USA* **76**, 3006 (1979).
213. S. R. George and G. R. van Loon, *Brain Res.* **248**, 293 (1982).
214. M. M. Wilkes and S. S. C. Yen, *Life Sci.* **27**, 1387 (1980).
215. W. Lichtensteiger and F. Monnet, *Life Sci.* **25**, 2079 (1979).
216. O. Khorram, H. Mizunuma, and S. M. McCann, *Neuroendocrinology* **34**, 433 (1982).
217. S. Alde and M. E. Celis, *Neuroendocrinology* **31**, 116 (1980).
218. P. D. Gluckman, C. Marti-Henneberg, S. Leisti, S. L. Kaplan, and M. M. Grumbach, *Life Sci.* **27**, 1429 (1980).
219. P. L. Wood, D. L. Cheney, E. Costa, *J. Pharmacol. Exp. Ther.* **209**, 97 (1979).
220. G. R. van Loon and E. B. de Souza, *Life Sci.* **23**, 971 (1978).
221. L. J. Botticelli and R. J. Wurtman, *Life Sci.* **24**, 1799 (1979).
222. G. Nistico, R. M. Di Giorgio, D. Rotiroti, F. Naccari, and A. Calatoni, *Res. Commun. Chem. Pathol. Pharmacol.* **26**, 469 (1979).
223. F. Moroni, D. L. Cheney, and E. Costa, *Neuropharmacology* **17**, 191 (1978).
224. P. M. Iuvone, J. Morasco, R. L. Delaney, and A. J. Dunn, *Brain Res.* **139**, 131 (1978).
225. M. Segal, *Neuropharmacology* **15**, 329 (1976).
226. B. E. Leonard, W. F. Kafoe, A. J. Thody, and S. Shuster, *J. Neurosci. Res.* **2**, 39 (1976).
227. J. L. Haracz, A. S. Bloom, R. I. H. Wang, and L.-F. Tseng, *Neuroendocrinology* **33**, 170 (1981).
228. J. C. Buckingham, *Neuroendocrinology* **35**, 111 (1982).
229. D. de Wied and J. M. van Ree, *Life Sci.* **31**, 709 (1982).
230. R. de Kloet and D. de Wied, in L. Martini and W. F. Ganong, Eds., *Frontiers in Neuroendocrinology*, Vol. 6, Raven Press, New York, 1980, p. 157.
231. D. de Wied, *Trends Neurosci.* **2**, 79 (1979).
232. J. M. van Ree, B. Bohus, K. M. Csontos, W. L. H. L. Gispen, H. M. Greven, F. P. Wijkamp, F. A. Opmeer, G. A. de Rotte, Tj. B. van Wimersma Greidanus, A. Witter, and D. de Wied, in D. Evered and G. Lawrenson, Eds., *Peptides of the Pars Intermedia*, Pitman Press, London, 1981, p. 263.
233. Y. F. Jacquet, *Science* **201**, 1032 (1978).
234. Y. F. Jacquet and A. Lajtha, *Science* **185**, 1055 (1974).
235. V. A. Lewis and G. F. Gebhart, *Brain Res.* **124**, 283 (1977).

236. Y. F. Jacquet, W. A. Klee, K. C. Rice, I. Iijima, and J. Minamikawa, *Science* **198**, 842 (1977).
237. Y. F. Jacquet and G. Wolf, *Brain Res.* **219**, 214 (1981).
238. Y. F. Jacquet and G. M. Abrams, *Science* **218**, 175 (1982).
239. G. R. van Loon and C. Kim, *Life Sci.* **23**, 961 (1978).
240. F. Moroni, D. C. Cheney, and E. Costa, *Nature* **267**, 267 (1977).
241. P. L. Wood, D. Malthe-Sorenssen, D. L. Cheney, and E. Costa, *Life Sci.* **22**, 673 (1978).
242. S. Berney and O. Hornykiewicz, *Commun. Psychopharmacol.* **6**, 597 (1977).
243. A. Arbilla and S. Z. Langer, *Nature* **271**, 559 (1978).
244. H. H. Loh, D. A. Brase, S. Sampath-Khanna, J. B. Mar, E. L. Way, and C. H. Li, *Nature* **264**, 567 (1976).
245. M. A. Spirtes, R. M. Kostrzewa, and A. J. Kastin, *Pharmacol. Biochem. Behav.* **3**, 1011 (1975).
246. D. H. Versteeg and R. J. Wurtman, *Brain Res.* **93**, 552 (1975).
247. S. S. Mosko and B. L. Jacobs, *Brain Res.* **89**, 368 (1975).
248. D. H. G. Versteeg, *Brain Res.* **49**, 483 (1973).
249. R. L. Delaney, N. R. Kramarcy, and A. J. Dunn, *Brain Res*, **231**, 117 (1982).
250. L. J. Botticelli and R. J. Wurtman, *Nature* **289**, 75 (1981).
251. W. Lichtensteiger and R. Lienhart, *Nature* **266**, 635 (1977).
252. W. Lichtensteiger, R. Lienhart, and H. G. Kopp, *Psychoneuroendocrinology* **2**, 237 (1977).
253. V. M. Wiegant, A. R. Cools, and W. A. Gispen, *Eur. J. Pharmacol.* **41**, 343 (1977).
254. R. L. Delaney, A. J. Dunn, and R. Tintner, *Horm. Behav.* **11**, 348 (1978).
255. A. J. Dunn and N. B. Gildersleeve, *Pharmacol. Biochem. Behav.* **13**, 823 (1980).
256. A. J. Dunn and P. Schotman, *Pharmacol. Ther.* **12**, 353 (1981).
257. R. Natsuki, R. J. Hitzmann, and H. H. Loh, *Res. Commun. Chem. Pathol. Pharmacol.* **24**, 233 (1979).
258. T. Motomatsu, M. Lis, N. Seidah, and M. Chretien, *Biochem. Biophys. Res. Commun.* **77**, 442 (1977).
259. Y. H. Ehrlich, L. G. Davis, P. Keen, and F. G. Brunngraber, *Life Sci.* **26**, 1765 (1980).
260. V. M. Wiegant, A. J. Dunn, P. Schotman, and W. H. Gispen, *Brain Res.* **165**, 565 (1979).
261. H. Zwiers, V. M. Wiegant, P. Schotman, and W. H. Gispen, *Neurochem. Res.* **3**, 455 (1978).
262. P. Schotman, J. Allaart, and W. H. Gispen, *Brain Res.* **219**, 121 (1981).
263. J. Jolles, H. Zwiers, C. J. van Dongen, P. Schotman, K. W. A. Wirtz, and W. H. Gispen, *Nature* **286**, 623 (1980).
264. D. Rudman, *Endocrinology* **103**, 1556 (1978).
265. J. Arnaud, O. Nobili, and J. Boyer, *Biochim. Biophys. Acta* **617**, 524 (1980).
266. V. J. Aloyo, H. Zwiers, and W. H. Gispen, *J. Neurochem.* **38**, 871 (1982).
267. R. V. Farese, M. A. Sabir, and R. E. Larson, *J. Biol. Chem.* **255**, 7232 (1980).
268. T. M. Koroscil and S. Gallan, *J. Biol. Chem.* **255**, 6276 (1980).
269. A. Dazord, D. Gallet de Santerre, and J. M. Saez, *Biochem. Biophys. Res. Commun.* **98**, 885 (1981).
270. P. Cohen, *Nature* **296**, 613 (1982).
271. I. Tanaka, Y. Nakai, K. Nakao, S. Oki, N. Masaki, H. Ohtsuki, and H. Imura, *J. Clin. Endocrinol. Metab.* **54**, 392 (1982).
272. G. E. Feurle, U. Weber, and V. Helmstaedter, *Biochem. Biophys. Res. Commun.* **95**, 1656 (1980).
273. G. E. Feurle, U. Weber, and V. Helmstaedter, *Life Sci.* **27**, 467 (1980).
274. J.-A. E. T. Fox and J. Kraicer, *Life Sci.* **28**, 2127 (1981).
275. O. Vuoteenaho, O. Vakkuri, and J. Leppaluoto, *Life Sci.* **27**, 57 (1980).

276. L.-I. Larsson, *Lancet*, 24, 31, 1321 (1977).

277. L.-I. Larsson, *Histochemistry* **55**, 225 (1978).

278. R. Sanchez-Franco, Y. C. Patel, and S. Reichlin, *Endocrinology* **108**, 2235 (1981).

279. L.-I. Larsson, *J. Histochem. Cytochem.* **28**, 133 (1980).

280. E. S. Orwoll and J. W. Kendall, *Endocrinology* **107**, 438 (1980).

281. R. Graf, *Histochemistry* **73**, 233 (1981).

282. L.-I. Larsson, *Proc. Natl. Acad. Sci. USA* **78**, 2990 (1981).

283. J. F. Bruni, W. B. Watkins, and S. S. C. Yen, *J. Clin. Endocrinol. Metab.* **49**, 649 (1979).

284. L.-I. Larsson, *Nature* **282**, 743 (1979).

285. L.-I. Larsson, *Histochemistry* **58**, 3 (1978).

286. L.-I. Larsson, *Life Sci.* **25**, 1565 (1979).

287. D. G. Smyth and S. Zakarian, *Life Sci.* **31**, 1887 (1982).

288. B. Sharp, A. E. Pekary, N. V. Meyer, and D. J. M. Hershman, *Biochem. Biophys. Res. Commun.* **95**, 618 (1980).

289. B. Sharp and A. E. Pekary, *J. Clin. Endocrinol. Metab.* **52**, 586 (1981).

290. S. D. Tong, D. Phillips, N. Halmi, A. S. Liotta, A. Margioris, C. W. Bardin, and D. T. Krieger, *Endocrinology* **110**, 2204 (1982).

291. F. Fraioli, A. R. Genazzani, *Gynecol. Obstet. Invest.* **11**, 37 (1980).

292. L. H. Rees, C. W. Burke, T. Chard, S. W. Evans, and A. T. Letchworth, *Nature* **254**, 620 (1975).

293. A. S. Liotta, R. Osathanondh, K. J. Ryan, and D. T. Krieger, *Endocrinology* **101**, 1552 (1977).

294. Y. Nakai, K. Nakao, S. Oki, and H. Imura, *Life Sci.* **23**, 2013 (1978).

295. E. D. Odagiri, B. J. Sherrell, C. D. Mount, W. E. Nicholson, and D. N. Orth, *Proc. Natl. Acad. Sci. USA* **76**, 2027 (1979).

296. J. E. Blalock and E. M. Smith, *Proc. Natl. Acad. Sci. USA* **77**, 5972 (1980).

297. E. M. Smith and J. E. Blalock, *Proc. Natl. Acad. Sci. USA* **78**, 7530 (1981).

298. A. S. Liotta and D. T. Krieger, *Endocrinology* **106**, 1504 (1980).

299. A. S. Liotta, R. Houghten, and D. T. Krieger, *Nature* **295**, 593 (1982).

300. E. Herbert and M. Uhler, *Cell* **30**, 1 (1982).

301. H. A. R. Fritsch, S. Van Noorden, and A. G. E. Pearse, *Cell Tissue Res.* **223**, 369 (1982).

302. H. H. Boer, L. P. C. Schot, E. W. Roubos, A. Maat, J. C. Lodder, D. Reichelt, and D. F. Swaab, *Cell Tissue Res.* **202**, 231 (1979).

303. C. Remy, J. Girardie, and M. P. Dubois, *Gen. Comp. Endocrinol.* **37**, 93 (1979).

304. C. Remy, J. Girardie, and M. P. Dubois, *C.R.H. Acad. Sci.* **286**(D), 651 (1978).

305. C. Remy and M. P. Dubois, *Experientia* **35**, 137 (1979).

306. J. Alumets, R. Hakanson, F. Sundler, and J. Thorell, *Nature* **279**, 805 (1979).

307. C. S. Royden, P. H. O'Farrell, E. Herbert, M. Uhler, Y. N. Jan, and L. Y. Jan, *Program of the 8th Society for Neuroscience Meeting*, 1982, Abstr. 2036.

308. D. LeRoith, A. S. Liotta, J. Shiloach, M. E. Lewis, C. B. Pert, and D. T. Krieger, *Proc. Natl. Acad. Sci. USA* **79**, 2086 (1982).

309. J. Roth, D. LeRoith, J. Shiloach, J. L. Rozensweig, M. A. Lesniak, and J. Havrankova, *N. Engl. J. Med.* **9**, 523 (1982).

310. H. D. Niall, *Ann. Rev. Physiol.* **44**, 615 (1982).

311. E. S Golub, *Nature* **299**, 483 (1982).

312. A. Poupland, G.-F. Bottazzo, D. Doniachi, and I. M. Roitt, *Nature* **261**, 142 (1976).

313. J. H. Julliard, T. Shibasaki, N. Ling, and R. Guillemin, *Science* **208**, 183 (1980).

314. L. Schweigerer, S. Bhakdi, and H. Teschemacher, *Nature* **296**, 572 (1982).

27

Thyrotropin Releasing Hormone (TRH)

IVOR M. D. JACKSON

RONALD M. LECHAN

Division of Endocrinology
Department of Medicine
New England Medical Center
Tufts University School of Medicine
Boston, Massachusetts

Work described from the authors' laboratory was supported in part by NIH grants AM 21863 and AM 31074.

1 INTRODUCTION

It had been recognized since the early 1950s that the hypothalamus
exerted an important influence on the regulation of the mammalian pituitary-thyroid axis, but it was not until 1969 that we entered the modern
era of neuroendocrinology, after the isolation of thyrotropin-releasing
hormone (TRH) from ovine and porcine hypothalamic tissue and the
elucidation of its chemical structure as a tripeptide amide (pGlu-His-
Pro-NH$_2$) (1). This discovery, made virtually simultaneously in the laboratories of Guillemin and Schally, ended almost overnight two decades
of skepticism about the authenticity of Harris's portal-vessel chemotransmitter hypothesis (2). Subsequently, three other hypophysiotropic
hormones, luteinizing hormone-releasing hormone (LHRH), growth hormone release-inhibitory hormone (somatostatin), and most recently, corticotropin releasing factor (CRF) (3) have been characterized and
recognized to be members of a family of neural peptides now numbering in excess of 30 (4). The availability of TRH in pure form led to the
development of specific radioimmunoassays for this substance and the
appreciation that TRH, identical with the substance present in the hypothalamus, also occurs in extrahypothalamic brain regions as well as
outside the CNS altogether (1). Although hypothalamic TRH, transported to the anterior pituitary via the portal vessel circulation, acts on the
thyrotrope in a classical hormonal (endocrine) sense to cause the release of thyroid stimulating hormone (TSH), much evidence suggests
that the TRH found in extrapituitary locations has a role in neurotransmission (neurocrine function) and in cell-to-cell regulation (paracrine function). In this report, the anatomical distribution of TRH is reviewed along with a consideration of its functional significance in
humans and other species.

2 HYPOPHYSIOTROPIC EFFECTS OF TRH

2.1 TSH Secretion

TRH stimulates release of pituitary TSH (thyrotropin) following attachment to high affinity receptors on the thyrotrope, activation of adenyl
cyclase, and the subsequent generation of cyclic adenosine 5′ monophosphate (cAMP) (5). The secretion of TSH is primarily regulated by
the negative feedback suppression of thyroid hormone at the level of
the thyrotrope, while TRH functions as the principal determinant of the

"set-point" of this function (6). In hypothyroidism the TSH response is much increased while in states of thyroid hormone excess the TSH response is suppressed (5, 6). Such effects have been useful in the diagnostic evaluation of patients with disorders of thyroid function (7). Two other hypothalamic factors, dopamine (DA) (8) and somatostatin (9) have inhibitory effects on TSH secretion at the level of the thyrotrope and may function as physiologic thyrotropin inhibitory factors; they reduce the degree of TSH release induced by TRH. The TSH response to TRH may also be enhanced by sex hormones but suppressed by cortisol and growth hormone (GH). While the steroids appear to have a direct effect on the thyrotrope, GH probably acts indirectly by enhancing hypothalamic somatostatin secretion via a short-loop feedback effect (10).

Following i.v. administration of TRH to normal human subjects, a peak rise in serum TSH is obtained in 15 to 30 min (5, 7). In the rat a significant rise can be observed within 2 min (1). The minimal dose required to produce a TSH response in humans is around 15 μg, and a dose-response is obtained with increasing doses up to 400 μg, after which no further increase is achieved (11). TRH is also effective orally, but doses 20 to 40 times higher are needed to produce an equivalent effect on the thyrotrope, presumably a reflection of impaired absorption or breakdown in the gastrointestinal tract or liver. In normal euthyroid subjects, women tend to show a greater response to TRH than men, and in men, though not in women, there is a decline in the TSH response with increasing age (11, 12).

2.2   Prolactin Secretion

TRH administration causes prolactin (PRL) secretion from the normal mammalian pituitary through direct stimulation of the lactotropes via the adenyl cyclase system. In humans the peak rise (a doubling or more of the basal value) occurs at 15 to 30 min. Despite its efficacy in stimulating the lactotrope, TRH does not appear to play an important role in the physiologic control of PRL secretion (13, 14), which is primarily regulated by the inhibitory effects of hypothalamic DA. However, inappropriate lactation, occasionally with elevated PRL levels, can be found in patients with primary hypothyroidism (15). The cause of the galactorrhea could be due to increased TRH receptor number on the lactotrope, increased TRH secretion, or diminished DA or other prolactin inhibitory factor (PIF) secretion. The galactorrhea usually responds to thyroid replacement.

2.3   GH Secretion

While TRH does not stimulate GH release from the normal rat pituitary *in vivo*, TRH does release GH *in vitro*, as well as from a pituitary transplanted under the kidney capsule of hypophysectomized rats. Furthermore, in rats with surgical separation of the anterior pituitary from the hypothalamus, a direct GH-releasing effect of TRH can be obtained (16). These GH responses in the rat are reminiscent of the "paradoxic" GH responses reported in humans with certain pathophysiologic disorders such as renal failure, liver disease, anorexia nervosa, and depression—conditions that have in common an altered neurotransmitter milieu or some "functional" disturbance or disconnection of the brain-hypothalamo-pituitary axis (17). Under special circumstances, TRH can be shown to have an inhibitory effect on GH secretion. It prevents the normal sleep-induced rise in blood GH in normal humans (18) and the pentobarbital-stimulated GH release in normal rats following intraventricular injection (19). These findings taken together suggest that TRH has a predominant effect on the CNS to inhibit GH release from the pituitary; however, when the central aminergic and/or peptidergic pathways are disrupted, the normally weaker stimulatory effect on the adenohypophysis becomes manifest.

3 ANATOMICAL LOCALIZATION

3.1 Hypothalamic-Pituitary Distribution

The highest concentration of TRH within the mammalian hypothalamus lies in the median eminence (ME) region with levels in excess of 3.5 ng/mg tissue in the rat (20) (Table 1). On immunohistochemistry, the densest concentration of TRH is found in the external zone of the ME juxtaposed to portal capillaries (Figure 1), consistent with its hypophysiotropic role. Studies by Brownstein et al. (21), utilizing a technique that allows discrete nuclei to be microdissected from rat brain, showed that TRH was present in high concentration within the hypothalamic "thyrotrophic area," a region localized to the paraventricular nucleus (PVN) (22). Further, immunohistochemical studies have demonstrated a dense concentration of TRH perikarya in the parvocellular division of the PVN (Figure 2), the likely source for the nerve terminals staining for TRH in the ME. However, other regions of the hypothalamus, including the suprachiasmatic preoptic nucleus, the dorsomedial nucleus, perifornical region and basolateral hypothalamus are also richly endowed with cells staining for TRH (23).

Ablation of the "thyrotrophic area" of the hypothalamus induces hypothyroidism in the rat (24), but the TRH levels in the hypothalamus of such lesioned animals were as much as 35% of the values found in the controls. The persistence of significant TRH levels in the hypothalamus following such a lesion suggests that TRH in hypothalamic regions outside the "thyrotrophic area" subserves a functional role (neurotransmission?) other than hypophysiotropic regulation; this phenomenon also

TABLE 1 TRH Distribution in Rat Brain[a]

	Brain Stem	Cerebellum	Diencephalon	Olfactory Lobe	Cerebral Cortex
Extra-hypothalamic Brain	5[b] [4–5][c]	2 [1–3]	6 [3–12]	6 [5–8]	2 [1–3]
	Dorsal hypothalamus	Ventral hypothalamus	Stalk median eminence	Posterior pituitary	Anterior pituitary
Hypothalamic-Pituitary Complex	49 [41–61]	64 [23–106]	3570 [920–7600]	155 [150–160]	10 [8–11]

[a] From Jackson and Reichlin (20). TRH in pg/mg tissue.
[b] Mean concentration.
[c] Range of values.

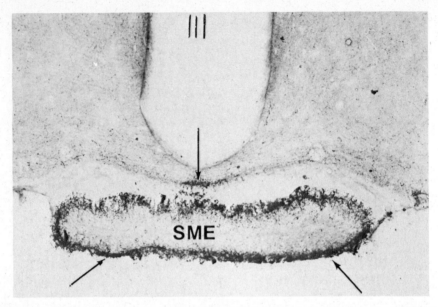

Figure 1. Coronal section (60 μm) through the stalk median eminence region (*SME*) of the rat showing immunohistochemical staining for TRH using the peroxidase-antiperoxidase (PAP) technique. Abundance of intensely dark staining reaction product is present in the external layer of the SME (lower arrows) localized in a network of nerve fibers in juxtaposition to the portal vessel capillaries. TRH staining is also observed in the posterior median eminence (upper arrow), 111, third ventricle. Initial magnification ×156.

provides a possible explanation for the fact that depression of baseline thyroid function after such a procedure is never as severe as that occurring after hypophysectomy.

TRH is also found in the posterior pituitary of the rat, its concentration there being exceeded in the CNS only by that of the hypothalamus (Table 1). Networks of TRH-positive fibers, terminating in grapelike swellings (23; Figure 3), have been observed extending into the posterior pituitary (25). Hypothalamic lesions lead to almost total depletion of posterior lobe TRH (Figure 4) and are consistent with the presence of a separate tubero-infundibular system. *In vitro* studies have shown that neural lobe TRH, presumably localized in nerve terminals, can be released by a K+ depolarization stimulus that is calcium dependent (26), findings in keeping with a neurosecretory role for TRH in this region. A function for TRH in the regulation of the neurohypophysis is supported by evidence that TRH can affect vasopressin secretion (27). Additionally, posterior lobe TRH could reach the anterior pituitary through vascular channels (28) and influence anterior pituitary secretion by this means, as has been proposed for the DA present in the neural lobe (29).

Significant levels of TRH are also to be found in the rat anterior pituitary (Table 1 and Figure 4). On electron microscopy, TRH has been

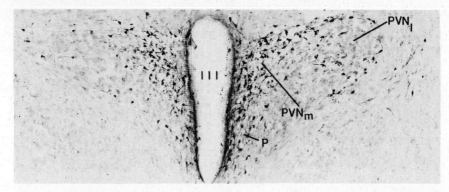

Figure 2. Coronal section (60 μm) through the rat hypothalamus at the level of the paraventricular nucleus (*PVN*) showing immunohistochemical staining for TRH (PAP technique). Numerous perikarya staining for TRH are present in the medial parvocellular division of the PVN (*PVNm*) and periventricular nucleus (*P*) on either side of third ventricle (111). A small number of parvocellular neurons staining for TRH are present in the lateral magnocellular division of the PVN (*PVN$_l$*). Initial magnification ×156.

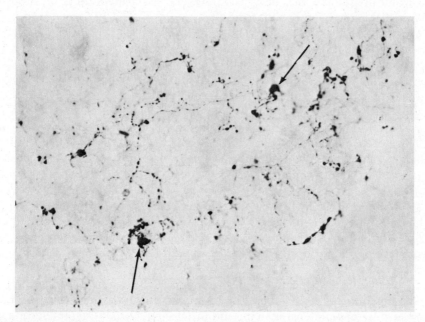

Figure 3. Coronal section (60 μm) through the rat neurohypophysis showing immunohistochemical staining for TRH (PAP technique). Note the branching axons containing irregularly sized beaded material terminating in larger grapelike clusters (arrows). Initial magnification ×500.

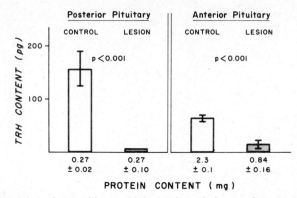

Figure 4. Effect of an electrical lesion of the rat hypothalamic "thyrotrophic" area on the content of TRH in the posterior and anterior pituitary. In the lesioned animals the posterior pituitary was almost wholly depleted of TRH. About 25% of basal TRH persisted in the anterior pituitary, which was shrunken in size in comparison with the posterior lobe, otherwise unchanged. Bars represent means $\pm$ SEM $N = 6$. Adapted from Jackson and Reichlin (24).

found as secretory granules in both the thyrotropes and lactotropes (30); although it would seem likely that adenohypophysial TRH is derived from the hypothalamus, the possibility that the tripeptide is of endogenous origin has been postulated (30).

3.2   Extrahypothalamic Nervous System Distribution

Significant concentrations of TRH are found throughout the CNS of the rat (20) (Table 1). Although such concentrations are small when compared with the levels in the hypothalamus, quantitatively over 70% of total brain TRH is found outside this region (1). The regions of the rat CNS most richly endowed with TRH are the thalamus, brain stem, olfactory lobe, and spinal cord. Extrahypothalamic brain tissue from normal human adults (killed in traffic accidents) also contains significant concentrations of TRH, especially in the thalamus and cerebral cortex (31). Since lesions of the thyrotrophic area (24) or deafferentation (32) of the rat hypothalamus leaves the extrahypothalamic brain content of TRH undisturbed, it appears that TRH in the extrahypothalamic nervous system is not derived from the hypothalamus and that *in situ* synthesis occurs.

On immunohistochemistry, networks of TRH-staining nerve terminals have been observed in several motor nuclei of the brain stem as well as in the intermediolateral column and in terminals around motoneurons of the spinal cord (Figure 5). Further, it has recently been reported that a TRH-like and a substance P-like peptide occur together in cell bodies of serotonin neurons located in the lower medulla oblongata (33). Treatment with specific serotonin neurotoxins causes loss of both serotonin

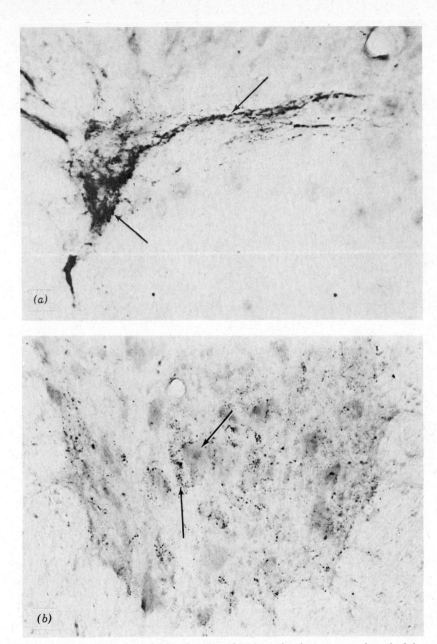

Figure 5. Immunohistochemical localization of TRH in the thoracic spinal cord of the rat utilizing the peroxidase-antiperoxidase (PAP) technique. (A) The intermediolateral column contains a dense accumulation of TRH reaction product (lower arrow); beaded fibers (upper arrow) can be seen arching medially towards the central canal. (B) The ventral horn contains a fine network of beaded TRH immunoreactive fibers in close association with α motoneurons. The lower arrow indicates darkly staining TRH reaction product concentrated in juxtaposition to a single α motoneuron (upper arrow). The rabbit antiserum was raised in this laboratory and utilized at a titer of 1:750. Original magnification ×500.

and TRH immunoreactive nerve terminals in the ventral horn, suggesting the coexistence of a neuropeptide and monoamine in the same nerve ending as well as their derivation from higher centers. Although the association of TRH, substance P, and serotonin contravenes the dictum "one neuron, one neurotransmitter" (mistakenly termed Dale's Principle), such a coexistence may turn out to be widespread for other peptides and neurotransmitters. Within the medulla oblongata TRH has been localized particularly to the nucleus tractus solitarius, nucleus ambiguus, and dorsal motor nucleus of the vagus—a distribution consistent with involvement of TRH in the regulation of the autonomic nervous system (34; see also Section 8).

In extracts of whole fetal rat and human cerebellum, the concentrations of TRH are high (35) but show a precipitous decline in the adult (36). However, in recent studies Pacheco et al. (37) have shown that TRH is unequally distributed within the adult rat cerebellum and that it is highly concentrated in the paraflocculi, flocculi, and nodules and deep cerebellar nuclei, but meager in the cerebellar hemispheres and vermis, which constitute the bulk of the cerebellar mass—a distribution that accounts for the low levels of TRH reported in the cerebellum as a whole.

4 CHARACTERIZATION OF TRH IN THE CNS

The presence of substantial quantities of TRH in the extrahypothalamic nervous system supports the view that TRH has a neuronal function in these locations. However, Youngblood et al. (38) have reported that the immunoreactive (IR)-TRH in extrahypothalamic regions is not identical with the tripeptide amide. This issue was of much importance since a neurocrine hypothesis to explain the effects of TRH in these regions would be undermined if the IR-TRH located there was not authentic. However, extracts of hypothalamus, extrahypothalamic brain and spinal cord, when subjected to high performance liquid chromatography (HPLC) following purification on affinity chromatography (39), have shown identity of the tissue TRH from all sites with synthetic TRH (Figure 6) as well as appropriate biological activity. Other groups (40, 41) have reported similar findings, and it has been suggested that Youngblood's discordant results reflect poor tissue extraction or interference in the TRH assay by the thin-layer gels (42).

5 REGULATION OF TRH SECRETION IN BRAIN TISSUE

It is believed that the hypothalamic peptidergic neuron is regulated by neurotransmitters largely of the monoaminergic variety and that the

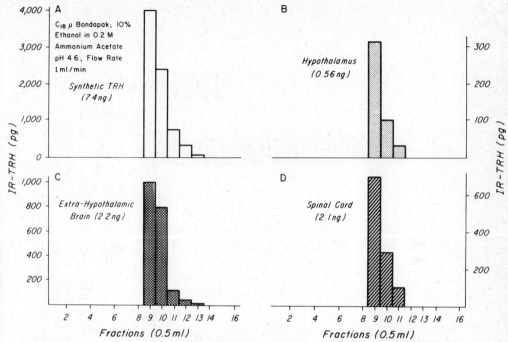

Figure 6. Characterization of immunoreactive (IR)-TRH present in the hypothalamus, brain, and spinal cord on high performance liquid chromatography (HPLC) following affinity chromatographic purification. The numbers in parenthesis represent the quantity of IR-TRH injected onto the column. Note different scales for IR-TRH. The retention time for neuronal tissue TRH was identical with that of synthetic TRH. From Jackson (39).

peptidergic neuron acts as a "neuroendocrine transducer" converting neural information from the brain into chemical information (43). Neuropharmacologic studies in the rat suggest that pituitary TSH secretion is under central α-adrenergic control (44), and at least in one physiologic system, there is evidence in favor of direct α-adrenergic regulation of hypothalamic TRH secretion. Acute cold exposure to the rat predictably gives rise to a sharp elevation in the serum TSH level. This TSH increase can be prevented either by pretreatment with α-adrenergic blockers (44) or by passive immunization with anti-TRH serum (Figure 7) which presumably neutralizes the noradrenergic stimulated TRH in pituitary portal blood. However, direct studies of TRH release from hypothalamic fragments *in vitro* have been contradictory. Norepinephrine (NE) (45, 46) dopamine (DA) (47), serotonin (5HT) (48), and histamine (49) have each been reported by different workers to stimulate TRH release, and in one study, DA was reported to cause release of TRH from hypothalamic but not septal synaptosomes (50).

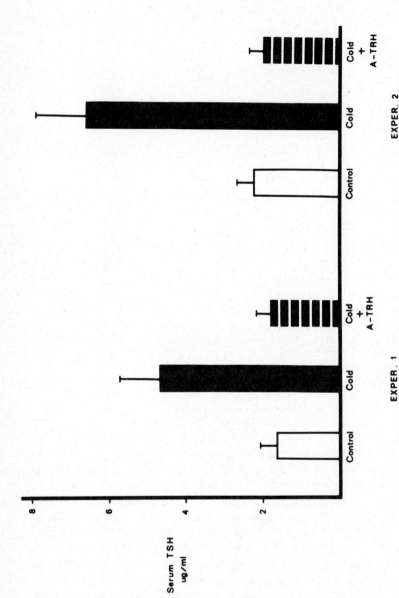

Figure 7. Effect of passive immunization with anti-TRH on the TSH rise in the rat following exposure to 4°C for 2 h. Prior treatment with antiserum abolished the TSH rise. The control animals are kept at room temperature. Bars represent mean ± SEM. $N = 4$ per group. The experiment was undertaken on two separate occasions. From Mueller and Jackson, unpublished.

Depletion of monoamines by specific neuropharmacologic probes has not consistently led to changes in the hypothalamic or regional brain content of TRH (51). However, large doses of amphetamine, which are thought to enhance central dopaminergic transmission, have been reported to lower TRH levels in the striatum by 50% but produce no changes in the hypothalamus or other brain regions (52). On the other hand, hemisection of the striatum leads to a significant increase in striatal TRH levels hypothesized as resulting from loss of an inhibitory interneuron system such as gamma-aminobutyric acid (GABA) (52). In this context it is of interest that the brains of patients dying of Huntington's disease—a degenerative neurologic disorder in which altered GABA metabolism has been postulated—contain significantly increased levels of TRH in the basal ganglia (53).

In contrast with these studies in the adult rat, in the neonate during the first 2–3 weeks of life, when marked ontogenetic changes in brain TRH concentration are occurring (54), catecholamine effects on the CNS content of TRH can be readily demonstrated. Administration of FLA 63 (code name for a DA β-hydroxylase inhibitor), which depletes the CNS of NE, causes a marked reduction in TRH levels throughout the brain. However, administration of alpha methyl paratyrosine (αMPT), which inhibits tyrosine hydroxylase, the rate limiting enzyme for catecholamine biosynthesis, and causes depletion of DA in addition to NE, restores TRH levels to normal. These changes in CNS tissue content of TRH induced by the catecholamines (NE stimulatory and DA inhibitory) suggest that in the neonatal rat brain both NE and DA are involved in the regulation of TRH secretion or biosynthesis, and that the direction of action of these two neurotransmitters is opposite (55).

Although thyroid hormone clearly regulates pituitary TSH secretion by direct negative feedback, an effect on TRH secretion has not been demonstrated. Roti et al. (56) have reported a depletion of hypothalamic TRH content following thyroidectomy and subsequent repletion on thyroid replacement. The same workers also found that the hypothalamic repletion of TRH requires TSH as well as thyroid hormone, for thyroid hormone by itself was ineffective in hypophysectomized animals. Interestingly, neither thyroidectomy nor hypophysectomy in this study were reported to affect extrahypothalamic brain TRH content—indicating that TRH within the hypothalamus is under different regulatory control. Studies in a number of other laboratories (1), however, have been unable to demonstrate a consistent effect of thyroid status on hypothalamic TRH content. TRH function can be regulated by thyroid hormone in other ways, for example, by "down regulation" of pituitary TRH receptors (57) or by enhancing the rate of degradation in portal blood (58). Thyroid hormone has also been reported to increase hypothalamic somatostatin secretion, which in turn has been shown to inhibit TRH release from hypothalamic fragments (46).

6   METABOLISM OF TRH

TRH is subject to rapid enzymatic breakdown in tissues and body fluids, a process that leads to the formation of several fragments (59) previously thought to be physiologically inert. However, studies by Peterkofsky and Battaini (60) have shown that TRH is converted to a biologically active cyclized metabolite histidyl proline diketopiperazine (His-Pro DKP), the formation of which may be enhanced by TSH and other pituitary hormones. His-Pro DKP, but not TRH, has been shown to inhibit DA uptake in rat brain striatal synaptosomes through effects on Na+, K+ ATPase. In addition, it is more effective than the tripeptide in suppresing appetite, elevating cerebellar cyclic guanosine monophosphate (cGMP), and antagonizing ethanol narcosis (60). However, it has been reported to possess prolactin inhibitory factor (PIF) activity (61) and to cause hypothermia (60), whereas TRH promotes PRL release (PRF activity) and causes hyperthermia (62). His-Pro DKP is widely distributed throughout the rat brain in concentrations greater than TRH (63). These findings have led to the suggestion the TRH in some instances can be a pro-hormone for its own metabolite, and the reported effect of TSH on TRH breakdown theoretically provides a means by which the pituitary gland could "feed back" to the hypothalamus to regulate its own function. However, an effect of His-Pro DKP on PRL secretion has not been confirmed by some workers (64). Further, studies undertaken in our laboratory by Abe have shown that although His-Pro DKP is readily measurable in the hypophysial portal vessel circulation, there is no gradient towards jugular venous His-Pro DKP; in addition, electrical stimulation of the median eminence does not alter the levels of His-Pro DKP in the portal circulation despite leading to a sharp rise in the concentration of TRH. These observations do not suggest a role for His-Pro DKP as a hypothalamic releasing factor. Additionally, although immunoreactive His-Pro DKP in the CNS is identical with synthetic His-Pro DKP, its regional distribution is unlike that of TRH. The dichotomy between TRH and His-Pro DKP in the CNS, portal blood, and systemic circulation raises the possibility that TRH does not solely account for the production of His-Pro DKP (65).

Although the initial studies suggested that the deamidated TRH (TRH-OH) present in low concentrations in rat brain (66) is biologically inactive, a recent report has indicated that it may be more active than TRH in producing "wet shakes" in rats (67)—symptoms similar to those produced by opiate withdrawtal.

7   BIOSYNTHESIS

TRH biosynthesis has been demonstrated in organ cultures of guinea pig hypothalamus (68) and newt forebrain. Earlier claims of a non-ribosomal, enzymatic synthesis have not been confirmed (see ref. 1 for a review). In frog brain, which contains high concentrations of TRH (20), Rupnow et al. (69) have described a macromolecule that yields TRH on chemical and enzymatic treatment. These workers have proposed that TRH is a posttranslational product, derived from a macromolecular precursor, which presumably arises by ribosomal synthesis. Further studies are required to support this hypothesis. More recently, in the rat CNS, the simultaneous occurrence of TRH in all neurons containing human growth hormone (hGH)-like material has been found (70). This observation raises the possibility that the hGH-like material forms part of a precursor hormone from which TRH is derived.

Since the antigenic determinants for all antibodies directed against the TRH tripeptide reside in the N-terminal pyroglutamyl ring and C-terminal amide, a TRH precursor cannot be identified by immunoradiometric means in a cell-free mRNA translation system. An approach to circumvent this problem currently being undertaken by a number of workers (71) involves synthesis of an oligodeoxynucleotide probe, deduced from the presumed TRH sequence [Gln-His-Pro-Gly (72)] within the hypothesized precursor, in order to prime the sequence of cDNA. Hybridization to RNA can subsequently allow prediction of the amino acid sequence of the precursor molecule. With this methodology a chemically synthesized oligonucleotide probe has been used to obtain mRNA sequences corresponding to somatostatin precursors (73).

8 EXTRAPITUITARY EFFECTS OF TRH IN THE CNS

Despite the fact that TRH crosses the blood brain-barrier poorly (74), CNS effects are obtained following systemic administration. In the rat, TRH reverses the narcotic depression induced by barbiturate and ethanol administration and causes enhanced motor activity in the hypophysectomized mouse pretreated with pargyline, a monoamine oxidase inhibitor, and then given L-Dopa [an animal model used for testing antidepressant drugs (75)]. However, a beneficial effect of TRH in human depression is controversial, though a trend towards mild euphoria in normal subjects and an increased sense of well being in the alcohol withdrawal syndrome does seem to occur (76).

How may TRH give rise to these biologic effects? Neurophysiologic studies show that TRH directly affects the electrical activity of single neurons or influences the excitatory or depressant effects induced by the neurotransmitters norepinephrine (NE) and acetylcholine (ACh) (77). Additionally, TRH has been reported to potentiate the excitatory effect of ACh on cerebral cortical neurons, enhance cerebral NE turnover, magnify the behavioral changes consequent on increased 5-OH tryptamine (5 HT) accumulation in rats, and produce alteration of rotational activity in the rat (believed to be a dopamine-mediated action). Thus, TRH may directly or indirectly influence the action of the established neurotransmitters NE, DA, 5HT, and ACh (75). Evidence of specificity of action is demonstrated by the effect of TRH in modulating the turnover of ACh in selected brain regions in comparison with other neuropeptides (78). Recently, Sobue et al. (79) have reported a beneficial effect of TRH on the ataxia and eye movement abnormalities of patients with spinocerebellar degeneration. These workers have postulated as the mechanism of action an improvement of abnormal NE metabolism in the cerebellum and brain stem, as suggested from their studies in the mutant ataxic mouse.

Recent studies by Brown and Taché (80) have emphasized the role of neural peptides in the CNS regulation of visceral functions through effects on sympathetic and parasympathetic outflow. Intraventricular injection of TRH in the rat causes an acute tachycardia and hypertension (possibly due to enhanced adrenal catecholamine release) as well as increased gastric acid secretion and colonic motility. The transient rise (or fall) in blood pressure and sensation of urinary urgency which frequently occur following i.v. administration in humans most likely also reflect direct central effects of the tripeptide.

The neurophysiological and neuropharmacological studies have led to the hypothesis that TRH forms an endogenous brain ergotropic or analeptic system (81) somewhat analogous to the endorphins (opioid peptides) present in the CNS. It has been proposed that the development of stable TRH analogs may have a role in treating narcotic depression and psychiatric disorders. Of interest, TRH does interact with the endorphin system, having been shown to antagonize certain behavioral effects of the opioid peptides, though not the analgesia (81, 82). Naloxone, a specific opioid antagonist, improves blood pressure and survival in experimental endotoxic, hemorrhagic, and spinal shock in experimental animals, suggesting an endorphin component to these conditions. TRH also reverses the hemodynamic disturbances in such shock, possibly through its effects on the autonomic nervous system (34), and it may be preferable to naloxone since the latter might exacerbate the concomitant traumatic pain (83). TRH has also been reported to improve neurologic recovery after spinal trauma in cats (84). These animal studies point to a potential therapeutic role for TRH in states of shock and spinal cord injury in humans.

9   TRH AS A CANDIDATE NEUROTRANSMITTER

The location of TRH in several cranial nerve nuclei of the brain stem and motor nuclei of the spinal cord (25) suggests a physiological role for this endogenous peptide, particularly in the motor side of the nervous system. Pharmacologic studies in animals as well as humans lend credence to such a view (75) and have led to the consideration that TRH might function as a neurotransmitter (1) in addition to its hypophysiotropic effects at the level of the adenohypophysis. Based on studies with the established neurotransmitters (catecholamines, 5-HT, and ACh), certain criteria have been established to define a neurotransmitter (85). These include: (i) localization within presynaptic nerve terminals; (ii) release upon nerve stimulation; (iii) attachment to specific post-synaptic receptors; (iv) induction of biological effects identical with those achieved by direct nerve stimulation ("synaptic mimicry"); (v) termination of effects by inactivation and re-uptake mechanisms; and (vi) capacity of the nerve cell to synthesize the material. TRH has been shown to fulfill most of these criteria, at least in certain systems.

By immunocytochemistry, TRH has been localized to nerve terminals (23), and depolarizing stimuli cause a release from hypothalamic synaptosomal preparations or fragments (26). High-affinity receptors for TRH have been identified in the extrahypothalamic brain (86), and enzymes active in metabolizing TRH in the CNS have been identified though their function has not been established. Synthesis of TRH in vertebrate neuronal tissue has been reported (68), and recently re-uptake of TRH by rat cerebellar slices has been described (87). It is possible that in some areas of the CNS, TRH functions as an "orthodox" neurotransmitter, while in other regions, it "modulates" the effects of the conventional neurotransmitters (85).

10 DISTRIBUTION AND FUNCTION OF TRH IN EXTRANEURONAL LOCATIONS

10.1 Pancreas and Gastrointestinal Tract

TRH is present in the gastrointestinal tract and pancreas of the rat. Within the pancreas, it has been localized to the islets of Langerhans (Figure 8). Ontogenic studies show the pancreas to contain much higher levels of TRH than the hypothalamus during the early neonatal period (54), but the concentrations in the pancreas and gastrointestinal tract subsequently decline with age (cf. cerebellum) while hypothalamic and overall brain levels gradually increase (Figure 9). The role of TRH in the neonatal pancreas is not known, but it has been shown to enhance arginine-induced glucagon release in the adult dog (88). Streptozotocin treatment, which destroys the insulin-secreting cells, markedly lowers islet TRH levels while increasing the levels of islet somatostatin (89). Since pancreatic somatostatin may be of physiological importance in the regulation of islet hormones, and because TRH tends to oppose somatostatin action in other systems, it has been postulated that TRH could serve a similar antagonistic role in the control of islet cell secretion (89).

The factors controlling pancreatic TRH in the neonatal rat have recently been studied by Engler et al. (55) and evidence has been provid-

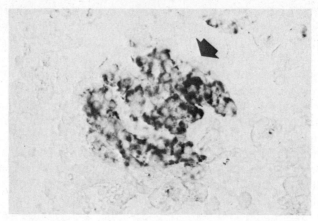

Figure 8. Immunoperoxidase staining of TRH in a 10 μm section of a day 2 neonatal rat pancreas. Reaction product is contained within the majority of cells in an islet of Langerhans (arrow). Original magnification ×400.

ed that brain catecholamines regulate the content of TRH, possibly through the sympathetic nervous system. Lowering brain NE by FLA 63 markedly reduces pancreatic TRH, whereas depletion of DA, in addition to NE, following αMPT administration significantly increases pancreatic TRH content. These findings demonstrate brain regulation of a neural peptide located in an extraneural site.

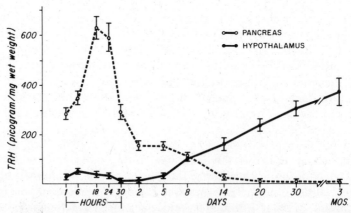

Figure 9. Ontogeny of TRH in the pancreas and hypothalamus of the rat. The TRH levels in the pancreas show a rise during the first 24 h postnatally to around 600 pg/mg tissue (a concentration about twice that present in the adult rat hypothalamus) before gradually declining to very low concentrations. Conversely, only meager amounts of TRH can be found in the hypothalamus at birth but the levels gradually increase with maturity. From Engler et al. (54).

TRH induces contractility of isolated segments of guinea pig duodenum (90), indicating that TRH can influence bowel motility by peripheral as well as central mechanisms (91). In humans, TRH has been reported to inhibit pentagastrin-stimulated acid secretion as well as to retard glucose and xylose absorption from the gut (92). The human and animal data are consistent with a physiological role for TRH in the regulation of gastrointestinal function. TRH also inhibits pancreatic enzyme secretion in the human (93), an effect consistent with direct action on the exocrine pancreas. In this regard TRH immunohistochemical staining of the luminal surface of the acinar cell has recently been demonstrated in the neonatal rat (94). It is proposed that TRH, secreted by the islet cells, reaches the pancreatic ductules, where it becomes localized to the luminal surface of the acinar cells, and at this site acts to regulate the exocrine secretion.

The occurrence of TRH in the CNS as well as the pancreas and gastrointestinal tract is similar to that observed for other neural peptides, suggesting that TRH is part of a diffuse neuroendocrine system (DNES) and that outside the confines of the nervous system, it is localized in "neuroendocrine programmed" cells derived from embryonic epiblast, or one of its principal descendants, that have migrated to the endoderm during embryonic development (95).

10.2   Other Tissues

TRH has been reported in the reproductive system of the male rat including the prostate, testis, epididymis and seminal vesicles (96). A role for TRH in gonadal function has not been determined. TRH has also been found in the human placenta—a tissue that shares a common embryologic origin with neuroectodermal structures (97). The functional role of placental TRH is unknown; it does not appear to regulate the release of either human placental lactogen (hPL) or human chorionic gonadotropin (hCG).

11   TRH IN BODY FLUIDS

Although it has been proposed that measurement of TRH and other hypothalamic releasing hormones in the systemic circulation might be used as a direct index of hypothalamic function, the wide anatomic distribution of the tripeptide and dilution of portal vessel blood in the systemic circulation makes it unlikely that measurement of TRH levels in body fluids can be used to impute dysfunction in the hypothalamus. The only exception to this view would be direct assay of pituitary portal vessel blood, and this circulation is inaccessible in the intact mammal.

There are considerable difficulties in measuring TRH in the systemic circulation because of rapid degradation by proteolytic enzymes, and its presence in human peripheral blood is controversial, with some workers finding levels that are low or undetectable and others detecting significant quantities of TRH-like immunoreactivity (1). In recent studies Mallik et al. (98) describe the presence of a TRH-like material in human peripheral blood ($\simeq$ 80 pg/mL), similar to the tripeptide amide on the basis of immunologic, chromatographic, and enzymatic studies. The levels were unaltered by variation in thyroid status. The concentration described cannot be reconciled at this time with a known central or peripheral source. However, the neonatal rat not only has high levels of authentic TRH in the peripheral circulation (54) but also low-plasma TRH-degrading activity (99). Human cord blood has also been reported to have reduced TRH degradative activity (100). TRH levels in the neonatal rat appear to emanate from extraneuronal structures, probably the pancreas and gastrointestinal tract, since encephalectomy at this time does not affect the concentrations (54). These findings point to the hazard of making interpretations about hypothalamic function on the basis of levels of TRH in the peripheral circulation, as the material measured cannot be assumed to be derived from the hypothalamus or even the brain.

Immunoreactive TRH (IR-TRH) has also been reported in human and rat urine, but again the nature of the material is controversial (1). Large quantities of TRH-like material have been found in human urine (101), but the origin of this immunoreactive substance was not determined by the authors. TRH has been detected in human lumbar CSF obtained from normal subjects as well as in cisternal fluid obtained from patients undergoing neuroradiologic examination (74). Whether this TRH-IR comes from hypothalamus, brain, or spinal cord is unknown. In the rhesus monkey, IR-TRH, identical with synthetic TRH on HPLC, is present in CSF taken from the cisterna magna, and shows a diurnal variation with maximal concentration occurring in the afternoon (102).

12   PHYLOGENETIC DISTRIBUTION OF TRH

The tripeptide amide, identical to that isolated from the mammalian hypothalamus, is distributed throughout the nervous system of vertebrate species (20). Although its role in regulating TSH secretion in mammals is clear, TRH is unable to activate thyroid function in amphibia and fish (Table 2), despite being present in the hypothalamus and brain of these species in concentrations far exceeding that found in the mammals (20). There is some evidence that TRH may release PRL and α MSH in amphibia but the physiologic significance of these effects is not clear (103). TRH in close association with 5HT (cf. mammalian medulla oblongata) is also found in extraordinarily high concentrations in the skin of the

TABLE 2   Hypophysiotropic Effects of TRH in Vertebrates[a]

Class	TSH	PRL	GH	Other
Mammalia	Stimulates	Stimulates	Stimulates release in certain pathologic states in man	Stimulates ACTH release in Cushing's disease in man
Aves	Stimulates	Stimulates (*in vitro* but ? not *in vivo*)	Stimulates	—[b]
Amphibia	No effect	Stimulates	—	Stimulates α MSH release
Pisces	No effect or ? inhibits	—	—	—

[a] For further details, see refs. 17, 103.
[b] Unknown.

frog (*Rana pipiens*) (104), a tissue derived from (or programmed by) primitive neuroectoderm, and which is also a rich source of other peptides structurally related to neural peptides located in mammalian brain and gut (103). TRH secretion from the amphibian skin is under dual neurotransmitter control, with stimulatory noradrenergic and inhibitory dopaminergic components (105). The stomach of the American alligator (*Alligator mississippiensis*) contains substantial levels of authentic TRH. Fasting induces a marked increase in gastric but not hypothalamic content of TRH, suggesting a physiologic role for TRH in the gastric function of this vertebrate (106).

TRH is also to be found in whole brain of the larval lamprey, in the head end of amphioxus, and in the circumesophageal ganglia of the invertebrate snail (20). As the lamprey lacks TSH and the amphioxus and snail lack a pituitary, the TSH regulating function of TRH in mammals provides an example of an organism acquiring a new function for a preexisting chemical. The ancient origins of TRH are further emphasized by the presence of an immunoreactive substance in the alfalfa plant resembling TRH (107). In the frog skin and snail ganglia, TRH appears to function generally in maintaining homeostasis by regulating salt and water metabolism (108). We speculate that the primitive role of TRH in neuronal tissue is concerned with neuronal function and only late in evolution did the pituitary "co-opt" TRH as a releasing hormone for TSH secretion (20).

13   CONCLUSIONS

Regulation of anterior pituitary hormone secretion is only a small aspect of the overall biological function that has been proposed for TRH, yet its hypophysiotropic effect on the pituitary thyrotrope is the only physiological role for the tripeptide that has been established. TRH is widely distributed throughout the extrahypothalamic brain and spinal cord, and much evidence suggests that the tripeptide amide functions in these regions as a neurotransmitter or neuromodulator. In this respect, TRH resembles its "sister" hypothalamic releasing hormones, luteinizing hormone releasing hormone (LHRH) and somatostatin. All three substances are part of a family of neural peptides (4, 103), which includes the endorphins, substance P, neurotensin and many others and has a distribution outside the confines of the CNS, especially in the gastrointestinal tract and pancreas. The function of TRH in the gut and pancreas as well as other "ectopic" sites is not established, but preliminary studies suggest a modulating role in endocrine and exocrine pancreatic secretion as well as in gut motility. The tripeptide is found in high concentration throughout the brain of lower vertebrates despite an inability to stimulate TSH secretion in species lower than aves. It appears that the primitive role of "TRH" is concerned with some aspect of homeostatic, neuronal, or metabolic function, and not with regulating the pituitary-thyroid axis.

REFERENCES

1.   I. M. D. Jackson and S. Reichlin, in R. Collu, A. Barbeau, J. R. Ducharme, and J. G. Rochefort, Eds., *Central Nervous System Effects of Hypothalamic Hormones and Other Peptides*, Raven Press, New York, 1979, p. 3.
2.   N. Wade, *The Nobel Duel*, Anchor Press/Doubleday, New York, 1981.
3.   W. Vale, J. Spiess, C. Rivier, and J. Rivier, *Science* 213, 1394 (1981).
4.   T. Hökfelt, O. Johansson, A. Ljungdahl, J. M. Lundberg, and M. Schultzberg, *Nature* 284, 515 (1980).
5.   J. M. Hershman, *N. Engl. J. Med.* 290, 886 (1974).
6.   S. Reichlin, J. B. Martin, and I. M. D. Jackson, in S. L. Jeffcoate and J. S. M. Hutchinson, Eds., *The Endocrine Hypothalamus*, Academic Press, New York, 1978, p. 230.
7.   C. T. Sawin, *Pharmacol. Ther., C.* 1, 351 (1976).
8.   M. F. Scanlon, D. R. Weightman, D. J. Shale, B. Mora, M. Heath, M. H. Snow, M. Lewis, and R. Hall, *Clin. Endocrinol.* 10, 7 (1979).
9.   P. Tanjasiri, X. Kozbur, and W. H. Florsheim, *Life Sci.* 19, (1976).
10.   M. Berelowitz, S. L. Firestone, and L. A. Frohman, *Endocrinol.* 109, 714 (1981).
11.   P. J. Snyder and R. D. Utiger, *J. Clin. Endocrinol. Metab.* 34, 380 (1972).
12.   H. G. Burger and Y. C. Patel, *Clin. Endocrinol. Metab.* 6, 83 (1977).
13.   K. M. Gautvik, A. H. Tashjian Jr., I .A. Kourides, B. D. Weintraub, C. T. Graeber, F. Maloof, K. Suzuki, and J. E. Zuckerman, *N. Engl. J. Med.* 290, 1162 (1974).
14.   A. C. Harris, D. Christianson, M. S. Smith, S. L. Fang, L. E. Braverman, and A. G. Vagenakis, *J. Clin. Invest.* 61, 441 (1978).
15.   M. O. Thorner, *Clin. Endocrinol. Metab.* 6, 201 (1977).

16. E. E. Müller, F. Salerno, D. Cocchi, V. Locatelli, and A. E. Panerai, *Clin. Endocrinol.* **11**, 645 (1979).

17. I. M. D. Jackson, *N. Engl. J. Med.* **306**, 145 (1982).

18. K. Chihara, Y. Kato, K. Maeda, H. Abe, M. Furomoto, and H. Imura, *J. Clin. Endocrinol. Metab.* **44**, 1094 (1977).

19. M. Brown and W. Vale, *Endocrinology* **97**, 1151 (1975).

20. I. M. D. Jackson and S. Reichlin, *Endocrinology* **95**, 854 (1974).

21. M. J. Brownstein, M. Palkovits, J. M. Saavedra, R. M. Bassiri, and R. D. Utiger, *Science* **185**, 267 (1974).

22. T. Aizawa and M. A. Greer, *Endocrinology* **109**, 1731 (1981).

23. R. M. Lechan and I. M. D. Jackson, *Endocrinology,* **111**, 55 (1982).

24. I. M. D. Jackson and S. Reichlin, *Nature* **267**, 853 (1977).

25. T. Hökfelt, K. Fuxe, O. Johansson, S. Jeffcoate, and N. White, *Neurosci. Lett.* **1**, 133 (1975).

26. A. Lackoff and I. M. D. Jackson, *Neurosci. Lett.* **27**, 177 (1981).

27. J. R. Sowers, J. M. Hershman, W. R. Skowsky, and H. E. Carlson, *Horm. Res.* **7**, 232 (1976).

28. R. M. Bergland and R. B. Page, *Science* **204**, 18 (1979).

29. L. L. Peters, M. T. Hefer, and N. Ben-Jonathan, *Science* **213**, 659 (1981).

30. G. V. Childs (Moriarty), D. E. Cole, M. Kubek, R. B. Tobin, and J. F. Wilber, *J. Histochem. Cytochem.* **6**, 901 (1978).

31. Y. Koch and E. Okon, *Int. Rev. Exp. Path.* **19**, 45 (1979).

32. M. J. Brownstein, R. D. Utiger, M. Palkovits, and J. S. Kizer, *Proc. Natl. Acad. Sci. USA* **72**, 4177 (1975).

33. T. Hökfelt, J. M. Lundberg, M. Schultzberg, O. Johansson, A. Ljungdahl, and J. Rehfeld, in E. Costa, M. Trabucchi, Eds., *Neural Peptides and Neuronal Communication,* Raven Press, New York, 1980, pp. 1–23.

34. M. R. Brown, *Life Sci.* **28**, 1789 (1981).

35. A. J. Winters, R. L. Eskay, and J. C. Porter, *J. Clin. Endocrinol. Metab.* **39**, 960 (1974).

36. C. R. Parker Jr., *J. Neurochem.* **37**, 1266 (1981).

37. M. F. Pacheco, J. F. McKelvy, D. J. Woodward, C. Loudes, P. Joseph-Bravo, L. Krulich, and W. S. T. Griffin, *Peptides* **2**, 277 (1981).

38. W. W. Youngblood, M. A. Lipton, and J. S. Kizer, *Brain Res.* **151**, 99 (1978).

39. I. M. D. Jackson, *Brain Res.* **201**, 245 (1980).

40. S. Kellokumpu, O. Vuolteenaho, and J. Leppaluoto, *Life Sci.* **26**, 475 (1980).

41. E. Spindel and R. J. Wurtman, *Brain Res.* **201**, 279 (1980).

42. M. S. Kreider, A. Winokur, and R. D. Utiger, *Brain Res.* **171**, 161 (1979).

43. R. J. Wurtman, *Neurosci. Res. Prog. Bull.* **9**, 172 (1979).

44. E. Montoya, J. F. Wilber, and M. Lorincz, *J. Lab. Clin. Med.* **93**, 887 (1979).

45. Y. Grimm and S. Reichlin, *Endocrinology* **93**, 626 (1973).

46. Y. Hirooka, C. S. Hollander, S. Suzuki, P. Ferdinand, and S. I. Juan, *Proc. Natl. Acad. Sci. USA* **9**, 4509 (1978).

47. K. Maeda and L. A. Frohman, *Endocrinology* **106**, 1837 (1980).

48. P. Joseph-Bravo, J. L. Charli, J. M. Palacios, and C. Kordon, *Endocrinology* **104**, 801 (1979).

49. Y. F. Chen and V. D. Ramirez, *Endocrinology* **108**, 2359 (1981).

50. J. M. Schaeffer, J. Axelrod, and M. J. Brownstein, *Brain Res.* **138**, 571 (1977).

51. F. Kardon, R. J. Marcus, A. Winokur, and R. D. Utiger, *Endocrinology* **100**, 1604 (1977).

52. E. R. Spindel, D. J. Pettibone, and R. J. Wurtman, *Brain Res.* **216**, 323 (1981).

53. E. R. Spindel, R. J. Wurtman, and E. D. Bird, *N. Engl. J. Med.* **303**, 1235 (1980).

54. D. Engler, M. F. Scanlon, and I. M. D. Jackson, *J. Clin. Invest.* **67**, 800 (1981).

55. D. Engler, D. Chad, and I. M. D. Jackson, *J. Clin. Invest.,* **69**, 1310 (1982).

56. E. Roti, D. Christianson, A. R. C. Harris, L. E. Braverman, and A. G. Vagenakis, *Endocrinology* **103**, 1662 (1978).

57. P. M. Hinkle, M. H. Perrone, and A. Schonbrunn, *Endocrinology* **108**, 199 (1981).

58. I. M. D. Jackson, P. D. Papapetrou, and S. Reichlin, *Endocrinology* **104**, 1292 (1979).

59. E. G. Griffiths and V. A. D. Webster, *Lancet* **1**, 836 (1981).

60. A. Peterkofsky and A. Battaini, *Neuropeptides* **1**, 105 (1980).

61. K. Bauer, K. J. Graff, A. Faivre-Bauman, S. Beier, A. Tixier-Vidal, and H. Kleinkauf, *Nature* **274**, 174 (1978).

62. M. Brown, J. Rivier, and W. Vale, *Life Sci.* **20**, 1681 (1977).

63. T. Yanagisawa, C. Prasad, and A. Peterkofsky, *J. Biol. Chem.* **235**, 10,290 (1980).

64. C. H. Emerson, S. Alex, L. E. Braverman, and M. S. Safran, *Endocrinology* **109**, 1375 (1981).

65. I. M. D. Jackson, Program of the 64th Annual Meeting of the Endocrine Society, San Francisco, Calif., June 16–18, 1982.

66. C. H. Emerson, W. Vogel, and B. L. Currie, *Endocrinology* **107**, 443 (1980).

67. G. Boschi, N. Launay, and R. Rips, *Neurosci. Lett.* **16**, 209 (1980).

68. J. F. McKelvy, M. Sheridan, S. Joseph, C. H. Phelps, and S. Perrie, *Endocrinology* **97**, 908 (1975).

69. J. H. Rupnow, P. M. Hinkle, and J. E. Dixon, *Biochem. Biophys. Res. Commun.* **89**, 721 (1979).

70. R. M. Lechan, M. E. Molitch, and I. M. D. Jackson, *Endocrinology* **112**, 877 (1983).

71. J. E. Dixon, W. L. Taylor, P. C. Andrews, C. D. Minth, P. M. Hinkle, and J. H. Rupnow, *Eur. J. Cell. Biol.* **22**, 792 (1980).

72. G. Suchanek and G. Kreil, *Proc. Natl. Acad. Sci. USA* **74**, 975 (1977).

73. W. L. Taylor, K. J. Collier, R. J. Deschenes, H. L. Weith, and J. E. Dixon, *Proc. Natl. Acad. Sci. USA* **78**, 6694 (1981).

74. I. M. D. Jackson, in J. H. Wood, Ed., *Neurobiology of Cerebrospinal Fluid*, Plenum Press, New York, 1980, pp. 625–650.

75. G. G. Yarbrough, *Prog. Neurobiology* **12**, 291 (1979).

76. A. J. Prange Jr., C. B. Nemeroff, P. T. Loosen, G. Bissette, A. J. Osbahr III, I. C. Wilson, and M. A. Lipton, in R. Collu, A. Barbeau, J. R. Ducharme, J. G. Rochefort, Eds., *Central Nervous System Effects of Hypothalamic Hormones and Other Peptides*, 1979, pp. 75–96.

77. A. Winokur and A. L. Beckman, *Brain Res.* **150**, 205 (1978).

78. D. Malthe-Sorenssen, P. L. Wood, D. L. Cheney, and E. Costa, *J. Neurochem.* **31**, 685 (1978).

79. I. Sobue, H. Yamamoto, M. Konagaya, M. Iida, and T. Takayanagi, *Lancet* **1**, 418 (1980).

80. M. Brown and Y. Taché, *Fed. Proc.* **40**, 2565 (1981).

81. G. Metcalf and P. W. Dettmar, *Lancet* **1**, 586 (1981).

82. J. W. Holaday, L. F. Tseng, H. H. Loh, and C. H. Li, *Life Sci.* **22**, 1537 (1978).

83. J. W. Holaday, R. J. D'Amato, and A. I. Faden, *Science* **213**, 216 (1981).

84. A. I. Faden, T. P. Jacobs, and J. W. Holaday, *N. Engl. J. Med.* **305**, 1063 (1981).

85. J. R. Cooper, F. E. Bloom, and R. H. Roth, Eds., *The Biochemical Basis of Neuropharmacology*, 3rd Ed., Oxford University Press, New York, 1978, p. 259.

86. N. Ogawa, Y. Yamawaki, H. Kuroda, T. Ofuji, E. Itoga, and S. Kito, *Brain Res.* **205**, 169 (1981).

87. M. F. Pacheco, D. J. Woodward, J. F. McKelvy, and W. S. T. Griffin, *Peptides* **2**, 283 (1981).

88. J. E. Morley, S. R. Levin, M. Pehlvanian, R. Adachi, A. E. Pekary, and J. M. Hershman, *Endocrinology* **104**, 137 (1979).

89. E. Martino, A. Lernmark, H. Seo, D. R. Steiner, and S. Refetoff, *Proc. Natl. Acad. Sci. USA* **75**, 4265 (1978).

90. K. Furukawa, T. Nomoto, and T. Tonoue, *Eur. J. Pharmacol.* **64**, 279 (1980).

91. J. R. Smith, T. R. LaHann, R. M. Chestnut, M. A. Carino, and A. Horita, *Science* **196**, 660 (1976).

92. L. Dolva, K. F. Hanssen, A. Berstad, and H. M. M. Frey, *Clin. Endocrinol.* **10**, 281 (1979).

93. L. Gullo and G. Labo, *Gastroenterology* **80**, 735 (1981).

94. D. Engler and R. M. Lechan, Program of the 64th Annual Meeting of the Endocrine Society, San Francisco, Calif., June 16–18, 1982.

95. A. G. E. Pearse and T. Takor Takor, Fed. Proc. **38**, 2288 (1979).

96. A. E. Pekary, N. V. Meyer, C. Vaillant, and J. M. Hershman, *Biochem. Biophys. Res. Commun.* **95**, 993 (1980).

97. G. Shambaugh III, M. Kubek, and J. F. Wilber, *J. Clin. Endocrinol. Metab.* **48**, 483 (1979).

98. T. Mallik, V. Richards, J. Seibel, C. Prasad, and J. Wilber, *Endocrinology* **106** (suppl), 233 (1980).

99. J. T. Neary, J. D. Kieffer, C. Nakamura, H. Mover, M. Soodak, and F. Maloof, *Endocrinology* **103**, 1849 (1978).

100. J. T. Neary, C. Nakamua, I. J. Cavies, M. Soodak, and F. Maloof, *J. Clin. Invest.* **62**, 1 (1978).

101. L. Bhandaru and C. H. Emerson, *J. Clin. Endocrinol. Metab.* **51**, 410 (1980).

102. M. Berelowitz, M. J. Perlow, H. J. Hoffman, and L. A. Frohman, *Endocrinology* **109**, 2102 (1981).

103. I. M. D. Jackson, "The Releasing Factors of the Hypothalamus", in E. J. W. Barrington, Ed., *Hormones and Evolution*, Academic Press, London, 1979, pp. 723–789.

104. G. P. Mueller, L. Alpert, S. Reichlin, and I. M. D. Jackson, *Endocrinology* **106**, 1 (1980).

105. J. L. Bolaffi, V. Lance, and I. M. D. Jackson, *Endocrinology* **108**, Suppl., 133 (1981).

106. J. L. Bolaffi and I. M. D. Jackson, *Endocrinology*, **110**:842 (1982).

107. I. M. D. Jackson, *Endocrinology* **108**, 344 (1981).

108. Y. Grimm-Jorgensen and C. L. Voute, *Gen. Comp. Endocrinol.* **37**, 482 (1979).

28

Leuteinizing Hormone Releasing Hormone (LHRH)

L. C. KREY

Rockefeller University
New York, New York

A. J. SILVERMAN

Department of Anatomy
College of Physicians and Surgeons
Columbia University
New York, New York

The purification, identification, and synthesis of the decapeptide luteinizing hormone releasing hormone (LHRH, also GnRH for gonadotropin releasing hormone) by Guillemin and Schally and their coworkers (1–3) can now be viewed as an important transition point in the history of the study of the neuroendocrinology of reproduction. On one hand, the identification of the LHRH molecule was the culmination of the research efforts of Hohlweg, Harris, McCann, Everett, and Sawyer during the previous five decades—research that implicated the central nervous system in the control of luteinizing hormone (LH) and follicle stimulating hormone (FSH) secretion by the adenohypophysis and suggested that this control was mediated by the discharge of neurohormone(s) into the hypophysial portal capillaries. On the other hand, the availability of the synthetic decapeptide has also led to the development of reagents (bioactive LHRH tracers, LHRH agonists/antagonists, antisera to LHRH) which have provided tools for garnering important new information about the organization of the LHRH networks in the brain and the intra- and intercellular mechanisms underlying LHRH synthesis, storage, secretion and action. In this chapter we review the recent advances in our understanding of the neuroanatomy and physiology of the LHRH-containing neurons and the influences that they exert on brain and pituitary function.

1   ANATOMY OF LHRH-CONTAINING NEURONS

Our understanding of the distribution of LHRH-containing neuronal networks in the central nervous system derives primarily from studies in which LHRH has been identified immunologically with antisera generated against LHRH-protein conjugates. As a result, the validity of the conclusions of these studies depends on the demonstration that this immunologic reactivity is associated with a molecule identical to LHRH as determined by current biochemical purification procedures and bioassay techniques. Such tests have been conducted on LHRH in a variety of vertebrate species, and it has been found that for rat and frog/toad (generalized to mammalian and amphibian), hypothalamic immunoactivity corresponds to the LHRH decapeptide (4). However, this was not the case for the LH releasing activity in the hypothalami of the bird, reptile, amphibian, and fish species examined. Presumably slight modifications in the amino acid composition of the releasing factor in these species results in a different migratory pattern in the chromatography systems utilized (4). Such findings indicate that caution is necessary when examining any report of LHRH distribution. This is especially so when considering extrahypothalamic LHRH, for there is no assurance that this immunoreactive material is identical with that present in the hypothalamus. In fact, in one instance, LHRH immunoreactivity in frog sympathetic ganglia (5) does not comigrate with synthetic LHRH in high pressure liquid chromatography systems and thus differs from the immunoreactivity seen in the frog hypothalamus (6). Taken together, the foregoing underscores the necessity for careful analyses of immunoreactive LHRH. With this in mind, the term LHRH in the ensuing portions of this chapter should be qualified as "LHRH-like immunoreactivity" until the rigorous separation and bioassay procedures have been performed to identify its biochemical characteristics and makeup.

Antisera to LHRH have been primarily used in two procedures to characterize the distribution of the decapeptide in the brain. In the first, the antisera are used in radioimmunoassays to quantify LHRH levels in microdissected brain regions (7). Such an approach has provided nucleus-by-nucleus descriptions of LHRH concentrations in the hypothalamus and elsewhere and has been used to characterize alterations in LHRH levels following either neurophysiological or endocrine manipulations (8, 9, 10). In spite of the above, this approach has one major drawback: it provides no information on the intracellular compartment in which the LHRH is stored–neuron perikarya, dendrites, fibers *en passage*, or synaptic terminals. Such a cellular profile can be provided by the second procedure utilizing antisera to LHRH for immunocytochemical analysis of LHRH in brain sections. Moreover, immunocytochemical studies have shown that LHRH-containing structures are scattered within a variety of brain regions with little reference to cytoarchitectonic boundaries, the only exception being the ganglionic arrangement of LHRH cells and fibers within the nervus terminalis (11).

LHRH was first localized immunocytochemically in sections of the guinea pig brain by Barry and colleagues (12, 13). In many early studies the demonstration of LHRH cell bodies, as compared with axons and terminals, was rare (see ref. 14 for a review). However, with the examination of brain regions outside of the classical hypothalamic hypophysiotropic area, the development of various fixatives and tissue preparative techniques that preserve antigenicity, the selection of appropriate animal models, and the generation of antisera directed against different portions of the LHRH molecule, there are now a substantial number of studies that describe the distribution of LHRH cells and their processes in a variety of species, including humans. Figure 1 is a diagrammatic representation of the distribution of cells and fibers in the rat brain (15, 16). Studies in other species are summarized in Table 1. Despite the variety of antisera and preparative procedures used in the study of these species, there are some underlying consistencies. The distribution of LHRH perikarya appears similar, the largest numbers being present in an apparent "continuum" from the septal nuclei and diagonal band of Broca through the preoptic region and extending into the anterior hypothalamic area. Although there has been controversy in the literature concerning the presence of LHRH cells in the medial basal hypothala-

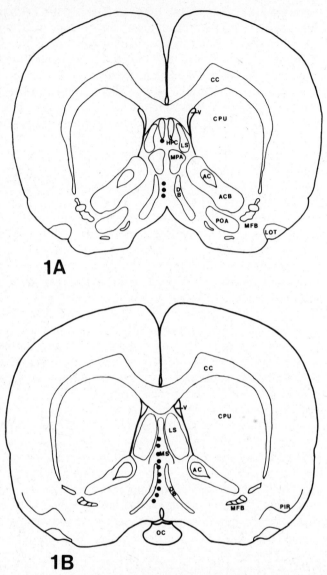

1A

1B

Figure 1. Distribution of LHRH cells (closed circles) and fibers (dashed lines) in the rat brain. Panels A–D are coronal sections from the level of the diagonal band of Broca (*DB*) to the suprachiasmatic nuclei (*SC*), regions richest in LHRH neurons. Figure 1E is a parasagittal section close to midline that illustrates the distribution of LHRH cells in this plane. Figure 1F shows the distribution of fiber pathways that contain immunoreactive axons.

Abbreviations: *AAA*, anterior amygdaloid nucleus; *AC*, anterior commissure; *ACA*, anterior communicating artery; *ACB*, nucleus accumbens; *AH*, anterior hypothalamic area; *AR*, arcuate nucleus; *BNST*, bed nucleus of the stria terminalis; *CC*, corpus callosum; *CPU*, caudate/putamen; *DB*, diagonal band; *F*, fornix; *HM*, medial habenula; *HPC*, hippocampal formation; *IC*, internal capsule; *IP*, interpeducular nucleus; *LOT*, lateral olfactory tract; *LS*

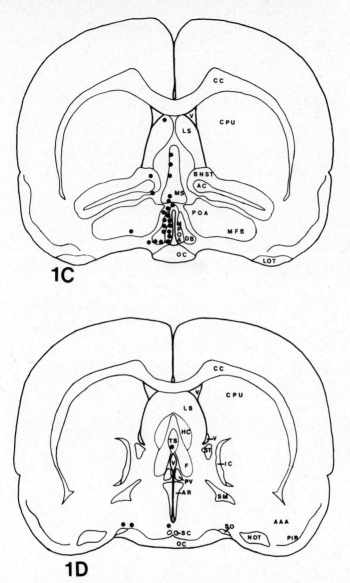

lateral septum; *ME*, median eminence; *MFB*, medial forebrain bundle; *MM*, medial mammillary nucleus; *MOT*, medial olfactory tract; *MPA* or *MPOA*, medial preoptic area; *MS*, medial septum; *NOT*, nucleus of the olfactory tract; *OC*, optic chiasm; *PIR*, piriform cortex; *POA*, preoptic area; *PV*, paraventricular nucleus of the hypothalamus; *SC*, suprachiasmatic nucleus; *SM*, stria medularis; *SO*, supraoptic nucleus; *ST*, stria terminalis; *TS*, triangular septal nucleus; *V*, ventricle.

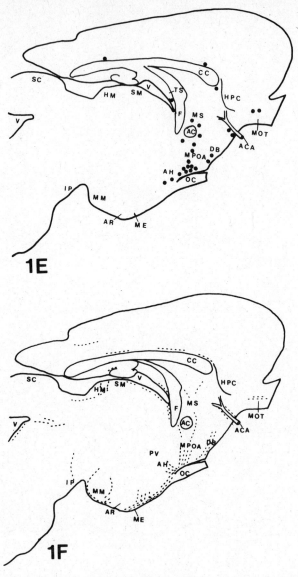

Figure 1. *(Continued)*

mus, that is the arcuate or infundibular nuclei, there is now unequivocal
evidence that such cells do exist in a large number of species, including
humans. Their numbers, or at least their detectability, vary amongst
species. The presence of cells in this region in the rat and mouse remains in question. The original demonstration of LHRH cells in the
mouse (17) might have been due to extracellular staining, and subse-

TABLE 1 Immunocytochemical Localization of LHRH-Containing Perikarya in Several Mammalian Species

Species	C	OB	NT	H	A	S	POA/AHA	MBH	M	Refs
Human	−	−	−	−	−	++	++	++	0	73, 74, 77
Baboon	−	−	−	−	−	++	++	++	0	78
Macaque	−	−	+	−	+	++	++	+++	0	41, 70
New World	−	−	+	+	−	++	++	++	+	14, 79, 80
Prosimians	−	−	+	−	−	0	+++	0	0	81
Sheep	−	−	−	−	−	+	++	++	−	56, 82
Cow	−	−	−	−	−	0	0	++	−	83
Horse	−	−	−	−	−	−	+	++	−	84
Cat	−	−	−	−	−	−	++	0	0	85
Dog	−	−	+	−	−	+	++	++	+	85
Rabbit	−	−	++	−	+	++	++	++	+	86
Guinea pig	−	0	++	0	+	++	++	*	+	12, 13, 18, 35
Rat	+	0	++	+	−	++	++	**	0	14, 21, 25–27
Mouse	−	−	+	−	−	++	++	**	0	17, 19, 20, 76
Hamster	+	++	+	+	0	++	++	+	0	36, 40, 42

Abbreviations: C=cortex; OB=olfactory bulbs; NT=nervus terminalis; H=hippocampal formation
A=Amgydala; S=septum; POA/AHA=preoptic/anterior hypothalamic area; MBH=medial preoptic area; M=midbrain.
Key: −, region not studied; 0, region has been reported not to contain LHRH positive structures; +, ++, +++, increasing numbers of LHRH cells in these regions; *, controversial.

quent demonstrations might have been due to contaminating antibodies
to ACTH (18–20). Recently King et al. (21) demonstrated a few LHRH
cells in the cell-poor zone between the arcuate and ventromedial nuclei
of the rat, and Toran-Allerand (22) has been able to show LHRH cells
in cultures derived from neonatal mouse medial basal hypothalami. Experimental procedures such as neonatal monosodium glutamate treatment (23) and surgical isolations of the medial basal hypothalamus (10,
24–27) indicate that if LHRH cells are present in the arcuate nucleus of
the rat and mouse they do not represent the major source of LHRH fibers to the median eminence. This contrasts with findings in the guinea
pig (18, 28, 29) and in the rhesus monkey (30, 31).

It is possible that the differences in the detectability of LHRH
amongst species (32, 33) can be explained by differences in the processing of a precursor protein (or proteins) (34). If LHRH were buried within
a larger protein it might not interact with antibodies until uncovered by
a local degrading enzyme. Alternatively, the immunoreactivity of the
precursor may play a crucial role in the detection of cellular LHRH.
Such a protein may react with an antiserum directed against one portion of the neurohormone but not with others directed against different
portions.

As mentioned above, investigators frequently describe the distribution of LHRH cell bodies as being present in a "continuum" from the
septal nuclei through the anterior hypothalamic region. The designation
"continuum" may well be a misrepresentation. Both telencephalic and
diencephalic components of the central nervous system are included in
these areas, and cells originate from different areas of the neuroep?theli-
um. In addition, the cells in these areas have different efferent projections (see Figure 1). This is perhaps best illustrated in the guinea pig
(35) and hamster (36). In the former, LHRH neurons in the septum project to the epithalamus via the stria medullaris and from there to the
midbrain interpeduncular nucleus via the fasciculus retroflexus. In contrast, cells within the preoptic/pericommissural region send axons that
terminate in the circumventricular organs of the organum vasculosum of
the lamina terminalis (OVLT), the subfornical organ, median eminence,
and neural lobe. These axons also project in a diffuse manner across
the hypothalamus toward the mammillary peduncle to enter the midbrain. Although the above description most likely does not represent a
complete listing of the projections of all of these cells, it does serve to
emphasize that the apparent continuum is composed of several cell
groups ordered by their efferent output rather than by cytoarchitectonic
boundaries.

In addition to the cells described above, there are LHRH-containing
neurons in other regions of the central nervous system. LHRH perikarya
have been observed in the hippocampus of hamster (36), mouse (37),
and rat (16) (Figure 1). LHRH cells are also present in the prepiriform

(36) and cingulate cortex (16; see Figures 1, 2). This latter observation is interesting since LHRH immunoreactivity in this region has been reported to be in the form of a large, precursor molecule (38). Observations by Witkin and Silverman (unpublished) suggest that these cortical cells send axons to the surface of the brain, where they appear to enter the subarachnoid space.

LHRH cells and fibers have also been observed in the main and accessory olfactory bulbs. Fibers have been seen in mouse (39) and rat (Witkin, unpublished observations); cell bodies have also been described in the hamster (37, 40) and rat (Witkin, unpublished observations). LHRH cell bodies are also present with the nervus terminalis (11, 40–42). This structure consists of a series of ganglia on the ventromedial surface of the brain from the olfactory bulb to the olfactory tubercle; these ganglia are external to the pia mater. Additional cells and fibers associated with the nervus terminalis are seen coursing peripherally with the olfactory and vomeronasal nerves and centrally with the anterior cerebral artery into the olfactory tubercle and ventral septum. The cells and fibers of this structure are exposed both to the CSF in the arachnoid space and to the cerebral blood supply. Indeed, there are many instances in which LHRH-containing structures, particularly axons, are in close contact with ventricular or vascular structures.

LHRH neurons have been seen in the amygdala (14, 42) and they probably contribute to the LHRH fibers observed in this area. Other origins for LHRH fibers in this limbic structure have also been proposed (14, 29, 43).

The foregoing description plus the information in Table 1 and Figure 1 summarize our knowledge of the similarities and differences in the distribution of LHRH cells among mammals (for reviews, see refs. 14, 44, 45). The description is still incomplete because investigators have not examined the entire central nervous system in any species. Future studies should be performed on tissue prepared to preserve maximal levels of antigenicity. Where feasible, studies should be carried out in animals pretreated with colchicine to block axonal transport of immunoreactive material. Ideally, antisera should be developed that react with the LHRH precursor or precursors to obtain a complete picture of the distribution of the cells that synthesize this molecule. Alternatively, the isolation of the mRNA responsible for the precursor synthesis and the development of radioactive complementary DNA probes (46) should allow us to determine if all LHRH perikarya synthesize the neurohormone in the same fashion either among species or over the range of developmental ages and physiological conditions within a species.

In general, less work has been done on the distribution of LHRH neurons and fibers in inframammalian species (see 14). However, what work has been done suggests that LHRH cells are localized in similar brain regions as observed in mammals. In both frogs (*Rana, Xenopus*)

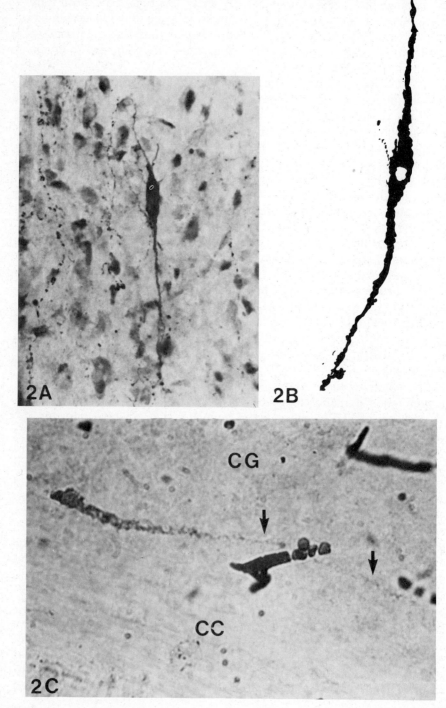

and toads (*Bufo*), LHRH cells have been observed in septal nuclei, near the preoptic recess, and in some cases in the infundibular area (47–50). Axons were also observed projecting to the median eminence and neural lobe. In the trout (*Salmo gairdneri*, 52) cells were observed on both sides of the ventriculus communis and in the area dorsalis pars medialis of the telencephalon with a diffuse projection of the pituitary stalk. In the platyfish (*Xiphophorus maculatus*, 53), cells were observed in the ventral telencephalon and the nucleus lateralis tuberis with axons projecting directly to gonadotrophs in the pars distalis. The latter observation has been confirmed at the ultrastructural level (53). A few avian species have also been studied. In the mallard duck (*Anas platyrhynchos*) LHRH cells were observed in the dorsolateral arcuate (54), in the periventricular preoptic nucleus, and in the infundibular area (55). Hoffman et al. (56) have also observed LHRH cells in the medial basal hypothalamus of the chicken and pheasant as well as in the medioseptal region, preoptic area, parolfactory region, and the olfactory bulb. In the latter two instances the LHRH immunoreactivity may actually be associated with the nervus terminalis.

Recently, immunocytochemical procedures have used tissues that have been sectioned and stained prior to or without embedding (15, 16, 21, 36, 41, 57). Such procedures avoid alcohol dehydration which removes the majority of immunoreactive material (58). As can be seen in Figure 3A–C, one obtains a more complete picture of the LHRH neuron with these procedures. Regardless of the location within the central nervous system the cell is fusiform or round, depending on the plane of section, and measures 8 to 12 μm diameter across the nucleus. Most cells have one or two dendrites; in the latter case they extend from opposite poles of the perikaryon. Occasional multipolar cells have also been observed. Dendrites are either unbranched or have a few branches occurring at about 50 μm or more from the cell body. These dendrites are up to 250 μm in length in the rat (15) and 2 mm in the macaque (41). Furthermore, these dendrites frequently extend outside of the nuclear region that contains the perikaryon. Since one must assume that synaptic input to the LHRH neuron can occur anywhere along the length of the dendrite, this observation should be remembered when interpreting the results of lesion, recording, stimulation or iontophoretic studies. For example, there may be circumstances in which an LHRH perikaryon re-

---

Figure 2. Illustrations of LHRH neurons. (A) Medial preoptic area neuron from the rhesus monkey. This is a 75 μm thick section counterstained with cresyl violet. The cell lies close to the third ventricle and has at least three dendrites. Beaded processes in the picture are axons. (B) Camera lucida drawing of another medial preoptic area neuron in the rhesus monkey from tissue prepared as in (A) Bar scale, 10μm. (C) LHRH neuron in the cingulate cortex (*CG*) of the rat. The arrows indicate the long dendritic process that is passing out of the plane of focus. *CC*, corpus callosum.

sides in an area poor in norepinephrine terminals but has dendrites that project into a zone rich in monoamines. Clearly, the nature of the synaptic input to LHRH neurons must await detailed studies in which double labels are used (59, 60).

LHRH axons have also been visualized in numerous immunocytochemical studies using cryostat or paraffin sections (see 14, 44, 45). In general, the LHRH reaction product has a beaded appearance. Whether

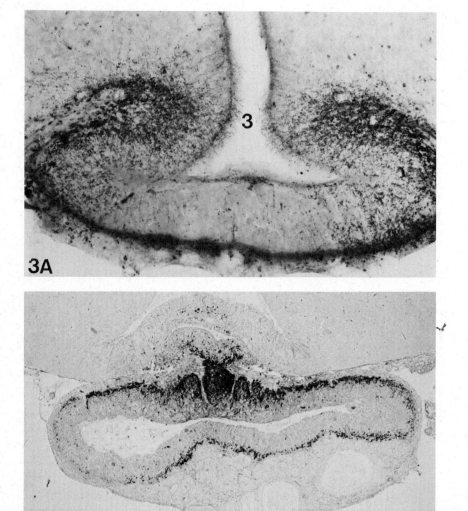

Figure 3. The median eminences of three species showing the differences in the distribution of LHRH axons. (A) Rat (50 μm section). (B) Guinea pig (6 μm section). (C) Rhesus monkey (75 μm section; dark field).

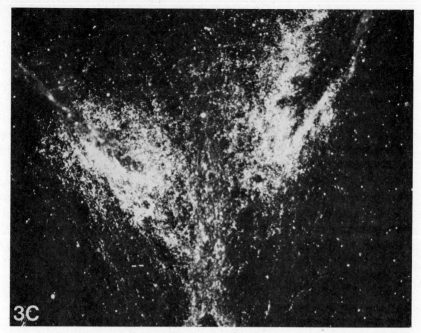

Figure 3. *(Continued)*

or not this beading has a functional significance is not known at this time.

2 ULTRASTRUCTURE STUDIES

Studies on the ultrastructure of the median eminence have shown that LHRH immunoreactivity is confined to membrane-bound granules within axon profiles and neurosecretory terminals (58, 61–63). In the guinea pig, granules within the axon profiles appeared to be larger (90–110 nm) than those in the terminals abutting on the perivascular space (40–60 nm) (62). A similar diversity of granule size has been reported in the human (63); granules in the cell body measured 60–130 nm while those in nerve terminals in the median eminence were 40–80 nm. The ultrastructure of LHRH terminals has also been studied in other circumventricular organs, such as the OVLT (64, 65) and in the lateral portion of the subfornical organ (66). Positive granules in the range of 110 nm have been noted in axon profiles in these structures.

Serial section, ultrastructural immunocytochemistry has also been used to demonstrate the presence of a second peptide within the LHRH-containing granules. This peptide reacts with an antiserum that recognizes the 17–39 fragment of ACTH (67, 68). This dual localization has been reported for LHRH neurons in the preoptic area and terminals in the median eminence of the guinea pig (67, 68).

The distribution of LHRH terminals within the median eminence (and neural lobe) appears to vary somwhat from species to species. Some of these differences are illustrated in the photomicrographs in Figure 3. In the rat and mouse, LHRH terminals are concentrated laterally over the tuberoinfundibular sulci (14, 45, 69). By contrast, LHRH terminals are more evenly distributed throughout the median eminence of the guinea pig but are concentrated in the dorsomedial aspect of the infundibular stalk (12, 13, 18). In the rhesus monkey, LHRH fibers converge on the caudal aspect of the tuber cinereum and, after entering the median eminence, diverge to form swirls around the portal capillaries throughout the structure (41, 70). In addition, in the rhesus monkey the entire infundibular stalk and neurohypophysis receive an LHRH innervation (38, 46). The exact distribution for other species can be found in the references in Table 1. The differences amongst species may be due in part to the organization of portal capillaries within the median eminence and in part to the differences in the contributions from the various cell groups of origin that project to the median eminence.

The exact numbers of LHRH-containing perikarya is still a matter of some debate. However, recent studies using unembedded tissue would place the numbers within the entire brain between 500 and 2000. Those that project to the median eminence may well be very few. When horseradish peroxidase or wheat germ agglutinin are applied to the median eminence of the rat, the cells labeled by the retrograde transport of the proteins in the area corresponding to LHRH cells (ventral preoptic area) only number about 30 (71). Thus, it is possible that the small number of LHRH neurons in this area is real and not a false negative artifact of immunological procedures. Such a conclusion must await the use of dual localization of retrogradely transported material from the terminal and immunocytochemical demonstration of LHRH (59).

Immunocytochemical studies have also been conducted to explore the ontogeny of LHRH neuron networks. Although LHRH can be measured by radioimmunoassay in the human brain by 32 days postconception (72), LHRH neurons have only been observed in the hypothalamus by the 9th week of gestation (73). By the 13th week perikarya are "concentrated in the mediobasal, premammillary and anterior hypothalamus (lamina terminalis and rostral commissural region) and their axons contribute to the tuberoinfundibular tract" (74). By the 16th week the extrahypothalamic projections to the septum and midbrain are also evident (74).

LHRH cells and fibers have been seen by immunocytochemistry before parturition in rat fetuses (15, 75). Fibers appear first in the organum vasculosum lamina terminalis (OVLT) on fetal day 18–19 and in the median eminence one to two days later. The time differential observed in the rat might be due to differences in the distances over which the axons must grow from the cells of origin in the ventral preoptic area. Alternatively, axons lacking sufficient immunoreactive material to be detected may be present in both regions, but the neurohormone is delivered to the terminals at different times in ontogeny. In the mouse, in contrast, LHRH fibers were observed simultaneously in the OVLT and median eminence on the 17th day of gestation (76).

The development of the LHRH neuronal networks of the fetal guinea pig has been also studied. Initial observations on late gestational animals were made by Barry and his collaborators (33) and a careful quantitative study for the entire gestational period (68 days) was carried out by Silverman and coworkers (34). In this species LHRH neurons and both hypothalamic and extrahypothalamic axons were readily visible after the 25th embryonic day (day E25). By day E28, LHRH could be found in the neurons and axons of the nervus terminalis throughout its peripheral, intracranial, and central portions. This corresponds to the onset of appearance of LH in cells of the pars distalis. No LHRH-containing structures were seen in the hypothalamus until day E30. At this time LHRH cells were observed in the septal nuclei, preoptic area, and arcuate nucleus of both males and females and fibers were seen in the median eminence. Between days E30 and birth there is a progressive "filling in" of the fiber tracts that project from the cell groups mentioned above; however, the majority of hypothalamic and extrahypothalamic fiber tracts are evident by day E40. As in the rat, it is uncertain if all of the axons have grown out at this early stage of development but contain no neurohormone, or if the axons grow to their targets over the entire time period of gestation and contain neurohormone as they grow.

Although the major aspects of the ontogeny of the LHRH systems described above were progressive, there were fluctuations among LHRH cell numbers in the arcuate nucleus throughout gestation (34). The number of LHRH cells was highest in the female on day E40 and in the male on day E45. In both sexes there was a subsequent drop in the number of detectable cells. This decline could have been due to natural cell death or to a major biochemical change in the intracellular processing of the LHRH precursor. An answer to this question must await the availability of the precursor protein and antibodies directed against it.

3 PHYSIOLOGY OF LHRH ACTION

Synthetic LHRH and antisera to LHRH have been incorporated into a wide variety of experimental approaches; neurochemical or electrolytic lesions with and without LHRH replacement (87–89); passive immuniza-

tion with LHRH antisera (87, 90); and radioimmunoassay determination
of LHRH levels in portal blood (91, 92). These studies have confirmed
that the secretion of LHRH into the portal vasculature is sufficient to
account for most alterations in LH and FSH secretion even when one
gonadotropin is "selectively" released. However, there may be two exceptions: both estrogen-induced LH release in the rhesus monkey and
the periovulatory discharge of FSH late on proestrous evening in the rat
appear to be able to occur independently of concurrent LHRH stimulation (93, 94). Nonetheless, both of these secretory phenomena depend on
prior exposure to LHRH.

The activation of gonadotropin secretion by LHRH appears to be mediated by a three-step mechanism (95). Initially, LHRH binds to a high-
affinity receptor in the gonadotroph membrane, and this results in the
"mobilization" of Ca^{2+} within the cell. It is this Ca^{2+} mobilization that
stimulates hormone release. Cyclic nucleotides do not appear to be involved in LHRH action (95). Although LHRH-complexes are internalized
in the gonadotroph, this process also does not appear to be essential for
the action of the decapeptide (96). That LHRH–receptor interactions are
important for bioactivity has been demonstrated with LHRH analogues
—only those agonists or antagonists that bind to the receptor effectively
can trigger gonadotropin release or inhibit LHRH-induced release, respectively (97, 98). Several analogs have been radiolabeled and used in
studies to quantify pituitary receptor levels in different endocrine states
(99). These studies have provided evidence that LHRH receptor levels
are influenced by at least three hormones. Estrogen increases receptor
levels (100, 101) whereas androgens and LHRH itself depress receptor
levels (99). This latter control would appear to be related to the internalization of the LHRH-receptor complex and most likely accounts for
the loss of hypophysial LHRH receptor and responsiveness to LHRH
observed following chronic treatment with high doses of the decapeptide or its analogs (87, 99, 102).

Radiolabeled LHRH analogs have also been used to look for LHRH
receptors in tissues other than the adenohypohysis. Such receptors are
present in rather high concentrations in the gonads (99, 102). Considering the absence of bioactive LHRH in the peripheral circulation, it
would appear unlikely that these receptors are influenced by LHRH released by the brain. Curiously, the gonads also contain cells which
make a peptide (or peptides) that crossreacts with various antisera to
LHRH (102, 103); whether this peptide is actually LHRH is open to question. Since LHRH will modulate gonadotropin-induced alterations in gonadal cell function that are associated with steroid biosynthesis (102),
the gonadal LHRH-like peptides and receptors may play an important
role in ovarian and testicular function.

In contrast to the foregoing, only very low levels of LHRH receptors
have been detected in grossly dissected regions of the brain (99). Such

negative data may be attributed to the possibility that the receptors are concentrated in small target regions or that neuronal LHRH receptors differ from those in the hypophysis and thus do not bind the analogs used in the studies. There is evidence to suggest this latter hypothesis: LHRH analogs display agonist–antagonist response patterns for the induction of lordosis behavior that differ markedly from those observed for the stimulation of gonadotropin release (104, 105). Clearly, reexamination of the brain for LHRH receptors is an important direction for future studies. The presence of LHRH in nerve terminals in various regions of the brain suggests that this peptide may be released at synapses. Thus, the demonstration of LHRH receptors at these sites would be an important piece of information in establishing the decapeptide as a neurotransmitter. These future studies should employ radiolabeled LHRH analogs which influence *neuronal* function. Such tracers could localize "hot-spots" of high-receptor density if they are incorporated into autoradiographic procedures similar to those used for cholinergic and aminergic receptors (106).

4 PHYSIOLOGY OF LHRH NEURONS

In this final section we review the recent information concerning the physiology of LHRH neurons, their activity patterns and the biosynthesis and packaging of LHRH. Discussion of the hormonal, environmental, and neuronal factors that influence LHRH neuron activity are brief.

Like other brain peptides, LHRH appears to be synthesized via ribosomal mechanisms. Studies by McKelvy and coworkers (107) have shown that the incorporation of radiolabeled proline and tyrosine into LHRH takes place primarily in cell fractions containing ribosomes and can be suppressed by puromycin and cyclohexamine, compounds known to inhibit ribosomal protein synthesis. Also consistent with this schema are the observations that LHRH is initially synthesized as a portion of a larger molecule (34, 38). The prohormone (or prohormones) that crossreacts with several antisera to synthetic LHRH, appears to colocalize with LHRH-containing perikarya in the anterior hypothalamus, whereas the decapeptide is the primary form in the nerve terminals in the median eminence (34). The cleavage of the prohormone to the decapeptide is, no doubt, accomplished by peptidases present in the hypothalamus. However, the intracellular site of this cleavage is open to question. Does it take place completely inside the secretory vesicle or is it completed following the release of vesicular contents?

Brain peptidases not only generate bioactive LHRH in the median eminence but, in concert with pituitary peptidases, degrade the decapeptide after it is secreted. There appear to be at least two primary peptidases that accomplish this degradation; these peptidases cleave

the molecule between glycine[6]–leucine[7] and proline[9]–glycine[10] ethylamide
(108, 109). This information has led to the development of LHRH analogs with amino acid substitutions at the above positions to prevent
degradation. Such analogs are appreciably more bioactive than the native decapeptide (97, 98). Because they do not bind to the peptidases,
the analogs are often used as tracers to label LHRH receptors (99).

At present, there is little information concerning the neurosecretory
process for LHRH. However, there is currently little doubt that this
event occurs episodically, thereby eventuating in the intermittent release of LH and FSH by the pituitary gland (87, 110–114). The evidence
for such a pattern of LHRH release is direct in that periodic elevations
of LHRH have been measured in portal blood (91, 115) and indirect in
that only intermittent LHRH replacement therapies restore episodic LH
secretion profiles following the interruption of endogenous LHRH release (87, 89). In general, the frequency of the LHRH discharges is, within each species, quantitatively similar to that of other intermittent brain
activities, such as REM sleep and the release of other pituitary hormones (111).

Recently, Knobil (87) reported that the frequency of episodic LHRH
release is an important factor that determines the secretory output of
the pituitary gland. They found that brief LHRH infusions to rhesus
monkeys most effectively stimulated LH and FSH release when administered at a frequency that mimicked that of endogenous LHRH release.
When LHRH infusions were administered at either higher or lower frequencies, they were appreciably less potent. The low-frequency treatments eventuated in high FSH : LH ratios in the blood, a fact related to
the relatively long half-life of FSH in the circulation.

The neuronal mechanisms that establish the frequency of episodic
LHRH release are presently unknown. Neurons in the arcuate nucleus
of the rhesus monkey display sudden brief increases in activity that occur concurrently with LHRH release (116). Whether these are LHRH
neurons or inputs to LHRH neurons is not known. Additional studies in
the rat and rhesus monkey have reported that episodic gonadotropin secretion persists after the transsection of all neuronal inputs to the arcuate nucleus region with a Halasz knife (30, 117). Such observations
suggest that the rhythm for LHRH is not dependent on neuron inputs to
this region. However, the arcuate nucleus of an intact animal does not
function as an "isolated island" but rather receives and processes numerous inputs from other brain regions. Thus, the observation that episodic LH, and thus LHRH, release can be disrupted by the administration of neuropharmacologic agonists and antagonists for a variety of
neurotransmitters (110, 118) indicates that this secretory phenomenon is
normally regulated by numerous neuronal mechanisms.

The episodic pattern of LHRH secretion is influenced by a wide variety of internal and environmental stimuli that are processed by the cen-

tral nervous system. In primates, evidences of episodic LHRH release can be observed immediately after birth but disappear rapidly only to reappear some time later at the time of puberty onset (119). In adult members of these and other mammalian orders, gonadotropin secretion is influenced by numerous environmental inputs, such as somatosensory stimuli [e.g., coital and suckling stimuli (120, 121)], photic cues [e.g., seasonal anestrus (122, 123)], and light-entrained circadian patterns of release (124). In addition, gonadal hormones modulate gonadotropin secretion; in several instances, these hormonal influences have been shown to result in alterations in LHRH levels in portal blood (91, 92, 125).

There are three ways in which LHRH secretion can change in response to the foregoing environmental and hormonal inputs: the quantity of LHRH released during each episodic discharge can vary; the frequency of episodic discharges can change; or, LHRH secretion can be shut down completely. There is some evidence for each of these possibilities. The size of the LHRH discharges in the portal blood of castrated rhesus monkeys has been observed to be greater than in intact controls (91). Although there are no reported instances of frequency shifts in LHRH patterns in portal blood, there are numerous examples of alterations in the frequency of episodic LH discharges. Such shifts are seen during rodent and human reproductive cycles (112, 113, 126–128) and following androgen administration or withdrawal in males (114, 122). Finally, although it would be difficult to verify a total absence of LHRH release, there are physiological and pathologic conditions in which episodic LHRH release appears to be absent or of such a low level as to be insufficient to evoke gonadotropin release. These circumstances include seasonal anestrus in lower mammals (122), childhood in primates (119), and the amenorrheas of anorexia nervosa (119, 127) and hypothalamic hypogonadotropism (130). The identification of the neurophysiologic and neurochemical mechanisms that account for these modulations in the activity of the LHRH neurons will be one of the more interesting problems for neuroendocrine research in the next decade.

REFERENCES

1. M. Amoss, R. Burgus, R. Blackwell, W. Vale, R. Fellows, and R. Guillemin, *Biochem. Biophys. Res. Commun.* **44**, 205 (1971).
2. A. V. Schally, A. Arimura, Y. Baba, R. M. G. Nair, H. Matsuo, T. W. Redding, L. Debeljuk, and W. F. White, *Biochem. Biophys. Res. Commun.* **43**, (1971).
3. H. Matsuo, Y. Baba, R. M. C. Nau, A. Arimura, and A. V. Schally, *Biochem. Biophys. Res. Comm.* **43**, 1374 (1971).
4. J. A. King and R. P. Miller, *Endocrinology* **106**, 707 (1980).
5. Y. N. Jan, L. Y. Jan, and S. W. Kuffler, *Proc. Natl. Acad. Sci. USA* **76**, 1501 (1979).
6. L. E. Eiden and R. L. Eskay, *Neuropeptides* **1**, 29 (1980).

7. M. K. Selmanoff, P. M. Wise, and C. A. Barraclough, *Brain Res.* **192**, 421 (1980).
8. S. M. McCann, S. Taleisnik, and H. M. Friedman, *Proc. Soc. Exp. Biol. (N.Y.)* **104**, 432 (1960).
9. R. I. Weiner, E. Pattou, B. Kerdelhue, and C. Kordon, *Endocrinology* **97**, 1597 (1975).
10. P. M. Wise, N. Rance, M. Selmanoff, and C. A. Barraclough, *Endocrinology* **108**, 2179 (1981).
11. M. Schwanzel-Fukuda and A. J. Silverman, *J. Comp. Neurol.* **191**, 213 (1980).
12. J. Barry, M. P. DuBois, and P. Poulain, *Z. Zellforsch.* **146**, 351 (1973).
13. J. Barry, M. P. DuBois, P. Poulain, and J. Leonardelli, *C. R. Acad. Sci., Paris,* **276**, 3191 (1973).
14. J. Barry, *Int. Rev. Cytol.* **60**, 221 (1979).
15. C. M. Paden and A. J. Silverman, *Soc. Neurosci.* **5**, 464 (1979).
16. J. W. Witkin, C. M. Paden, and A. J. Silverman, *Neuroendocrinology* **35**, 429 (1983).
17. E. A. Zimmerman, K. G. Hsu, M. Ferin, and G. P. Kozlowski, *Endocrinology* **95**, 1 (1974).
18. A. J. Silverman, *Endocrinology* **99**, 30 (1976).
19. G. E. Hoffman, K. M. Knigge, J. A. Moyinibian, V. Melnyk, and A. Arimura, *Neuroscience* **3**, 219 (1978).
20. C. J. Clayton and G. E. Hoffman, *Am. J. Anat.* **165**, 139 (1979).
21. J. C. King, S. A. Tobet, F. L. Snavely, and A. A. Arimura, *Peptides* **1**, 85 (1980).
22. C. D. Toran-Allerand, *Brain Res.* **149**, 257 (1978).
23. C. B. Nemeroff, R. J. Konkol, G. Bissette, W. Youngblood, J. B. Martin, P. Brazeau, M. S. Rone, A. J. Prange, G. Breese, and J. S. Kizer, *Endocrinology* **101**, 613 (1977).
24. M. Brownstein, A. Arimura, A. V. Schally, M. Palkovits, and J. S. Karger, *Endocrinology* **98**, 662 (1976).
25. Y. Ibata, H. Watanabe, H. Kinoshita, S. Kubo, and Y. Sano, *Cell Tissue Res.* **198**, 381 (1979).
26. I. Merchenthaler, G. Kovacs, G. Lovasz, and G. Setalo, *Brain Res.* **198**, 63 (1980).
27. H. Kawano and S. Saikoku, *Neuroendocrinology* **32**, 179 (1981).
28. L. C. Krey and A. J. Silverman, *Brain Res.* **157**, 247 (1978).
29. L. C. Krey and A. J. Silverman, *Brain Res.* **229**, 429 (1981).
30. L. C. Krey, W. R. Butler, and E. Knobil, *Endocrinology* **96**, 1073 (1975).
31. T. M. Plant, L. C. Krey, J. Moossy, J. J. McCormack, D. L. Hess, and E. Knobil, *Endocrinology* **102**, 52 (1978).
32. G. E. Hoffman, V. Melnyk, T. Hayes, C. Bennett-Clarke, and E. Fowler, In: D. E. Scott, A. Weindl and G. P. Kozlowki, Eds., *3rd International Brain-Endocrine Interaction: Neuroendocrine Control of Reproduction,* S. Karger, Basel, 1978, pp. 67.
33. M. Schwanzel-Fukuda, J. A. Robinson, and A. J. Silverman, *Brain Res. Bull.* **7**, 293 (1981).
34. R. P. Millar, C. Aehnelt, and G. Rossier, *Biochem. Biophys. Res. Comm.* **74**, 720 (1977).
35. A. J. Silverman and L. C. Krey, *Brain Res.* **157**, 233 (1978).
36. L. Jennes and W. E. Stumpf, *Cell Tissue Res.* **209**, 239 (1980).
37. G. E. Hoffman and S. Wray, *Soc. Neurosci. Abstr.* **7**, 98 (1981).
38. J. P. Gautron, E. Pattou, and C. Kordon, *Mol. Cell. Endocrinol.* **24**, 1 (1981).
39. A. J. Silverman and E. A. Zimmerman, in D. E. Scott, G. P. Kozlowski, and A. Weindl, Eds. *Neural Hormones and Reproduction,* S. Karger, Basel, 1978, pp. 83.
40. L. Jennes and W. E. Stumpf, *Neuroendocrinol. Lett.* **2**, 241 (1980).
41. H. S. Phillips, G. Hostetter, B. Kerdelhue, and G. P. Koslowki, *Brain Res.* **193**, 574 (1980).
42. A. J. Silverman, J. L. Antunes, G. M. Abrams, G. Nilaver, R. Thau, J. A. Robinson, M. Ferin, and L. C. Krey, *J. Comp. Neurol.* **211**, 309 (1982).
43. J. Leonardelli and P. Poulain, *Brain Res.* **124**, 538 (1977).
44. L. A. Sternberger and G. E. Hoffman, *Neuroendocrinology* **25**, 111 (1978).
45. A. J. Silverman, L. C. Krey, and E. A. Zimmerman, *Biol. Reprod.* **20**, 98 (1979).

46. R. Pochet, H. Brocas, G. Vassart, G. Toubeau, and S. Seo, *Brain Res.* **211**, 433 (1981).
47. L. C. Alpert, J. R. Brawer, I. M. D. Jackson, and S. Reichlin, *Endocrinology* **98**, 910 (1976).
48. J. Doerr-Schott and M. P. Dubois, *Cell Tissue Res.* **172**, 477 (1976).
49. J. Doerr, *Cell Tissue Res.* **172**, 477 (1976).
50. H. J. Goos, P. J. M. Lightenberg, and P. G. W. T. van Oordt, *Cell Tissue Res.* **168**, 333 (1976).
51. H. J. Goos and O. Murathanoglu, *Cell Tissue Res.* **181**, 163 (1977).
52. M. P. Shreibman, L. R. Halpern, H. J. Goos, and H. Margolis-Kazon, *J. Exp. Zool.* **210**, 153 (1979).
53. H. Margolis-Kazon, J. Peute, M. Schreibman, and L. R. Halpern, *J. Exp. Zool.* **215**, 99 (1981).
54. T. H. MacNeill, G. P. Kozlowski, J. H. Abet, and E. A. Zimmerman, *Endocrinology* **99**, 1323 (1976).
55. N. Bons, B. Kerdlehue, and D. Assenmacher, *Cell Tissue Res.* **188**, 99 (1978).
56. G. E. Hoffman, V. Melnyk, T. Hayes, C. Bennett-Clarke, and E. Fowler, in D. E. Scott, G. P. Kozlowski and A. Weindl, Eds., *Neural Hormones and Reproduction*, S. Karger, Basel, 1978, p. 67.
57. B. J. Burchanowski, K. M. Knigge, and L. A. Sternberger, *Proc. Natl. Acad. Sci. USA* **76**, 6671 (1979).
58. P. C. Goldsmith and W. F. Ganong, *Brain Res.* **97**, 181 (1975).
59. R. M. Bowker, H. W. M. Steinbusch, and J. D. Coulter, *Brain Res.* **211**, 412 (1981).
60. E. A. Nunez, M. D. Gershon, and A. J. Silverman, *J. Histochem. Cytochem.* **29**, 1136 (1981).
61. G. Pelletier, F. Labrie, R. Puviani, A. Arimura, and A. V. Schally, *Endocrinology* **95**, 314 (1974).
62. A. J. Silverman and P. Desnoyers, *Cell Tissue Res.* **169**, 157 (1976).
63. G. Bugnon, B. Bloch, D. Lenys, and D. Fellmann, *Brain Res.* **137**, 175 (1977).
64. M. Mazzuca, *Neurosci. Lett.* **5**, 123 (1977).
65. G. Pelletier, R. LeClerc, D. Dube, A. Arimura, and A. V. Schally, *Neurosci. Lett.* **4**, 27 (1977).
66. B. Krisch and H. Leonhardt, *Cell Tissue Res.* **210**, 33 (1980).
67. G. Tramu, J. Leondardelli, and M. P. Dubois, *Neurosci. Lett.* **6**, 305 (1977).
68. J. C. Beauvillain, G. Tramu, and M. P. Dubois, *Cell Tissue Res.* **218**, 1 (1981).
69. D. S. Gross, *Endocrinology* **98**, 1408 (1976).
70. A. J. Silverman, J. L. Antunes, M. Ferin, and E. A. Zimmerman, *Endocrinology* **101**, 134 (1977).
71. S. J. Wiegand and J. L. Price, *J. Comp. Neurol.* **192**, 1 (1980).
72. A. J. Winters, R. L. Eskay, and J. C. Roster, *J. Clin. Endocrinol. Metab.* **39**, 960 (1974).
73. L. Paulin, M. P. Dubois, J. Barry, and P. M. Dubois, *Cell Tissue Res.* **182**, 341 (1977).
74. C. Bugnon, B. Bloch, and D. Fellman, *J. Steroid Biochem.* **8**, 565 (1977).
75. K. Watanabe, *Endocrinology* **106**, 139 (1980).
76. D. S. Gross and B. L. Baker, *Am. J. Anat.* **148**, 195 (1977).
77. J. Barry, *Neurosci. Lett.* **3**, 287 (1976).
78. P. E. Marshall and P. C. Goldsmith, *Brain Res.* **193**, 353 (1980).
79. J. Barry and B. Carette, *Cell Tissue Res.* **164**, 163 (1975).
80. J. Barry, C. Girod, and M. P. Dubois, *Bull. Assoc. Anat.* **59**, 103 (197).
81. J. Barry, *Cell Tissue Res.* **208**, 327 (1980).
82. J. Polkowska, M. P. Dubois, and E. Domanski, *Cell Tissue Res.* **208**, 327 (1980).
83. W. L. Dees and N. H. McArthur, *Anat. Rec.* **200**, 281 (1981).
84. W. L. Dees, A. M. Sorensen Jr., W. M. Kemp, and N. H. McArthur, *Brain Res.* **208**, 123 (1981).
85. J. Barry and M. P. Dubois, *Neuroendocrinology* **18**, 290 (1975).

86. J. Barry, *Neurosci. Lett.* **2**, 201 (1976).
87. E. Knobil, *Recent Prog. Horm. Res.* **36**, 53 (1980).
88. C. A. Barraclough, P. M. Wise, J. Turgeon, D. Shander, L. DePaulo, and N. Rance, *Biol. Reprod.* **20**, 86 (1979).
89. G. A. Schuiling and H. P. Gnodde, *J. Endocrinol.* **70**, 97 (1976).
90. Y. Koch, in V. James, Ed., *Endocrinology*, Excerpta Medica, Amsterdam, 1976, p. 375.
91. P. W. Carmel, S. Araki, and M. Ferin, *Endocrinology* **99**, 243 (1976).
92. D. K. Sarkar and G. Fink, *J. Endocrinol.* **86**, 511 (1980).
93. L. Wildt, A. Hausler, J. S. Hutchison, G. Marshall, and E. Knobil, *Endocrinology* **108**, 2011 (1981).
94. C. A. Blake and R. P. Kelch, *Endocrinology* **109**, 2175 (1982).
95. P. M. Conn, J. Marian, M. McMillian, J. Stern, D. Rogers, M. Hamby, A. Penna, and E. Grant, *Endocr. Rev.* **2**, 174 (1981).
96. P. M. Conn, R. G. Smith, and D. C. Rogers, *J. Biol. Chem.* **256**, 1098 (1981).
97. M. H. Perrin, J. E. Rivier, and W. W. Vale, *Endocrinology* **106**, 1289 (1980).
98. R. N. Clayton and K. J. Catt, *Endocrinology* **106**, 1154 (1980).
99. R. N. Clayton and K. J. Catt, *Endocr. Rev.* **2**, 186 (1981).
100. G. E. Moss, M. E. Crowder, and T. M. Nett, *Biol. Reprod.* **25**, 938 (1981).
101. T. E. Adams, R. L. Norman, and H. G. Spies, *Science* **213**, 1388 (1981).
102. A. J. W. Hseuh and P. B. C. Jones, *Endocr. Rev.* **2**, 437 (1981).
103. W. F. Paull, C. W. Turkelson, C. R. Thomas, and A. Arimura, *Science* **213**, 1263 (1981).
104. A. Kastin, D. H. Coy, A. V. Schally, and J. E. Zadina, *Pharmacol. Biochem. Behav.* **13**, 913 (1980).
105. Y. Sakuma and D. W. Pfaff, *Neuroendocrinology* **36**, 218, (1983).
106. T. C. Rainbow, W. B. Bleisch, A. Biegon, and B. S. McEwen, *J. Neurosci. Methods* **5**, 127 (1982).
107. J. F. McKelvy, C-J. Lin, L. Chan, P. Joseph-Bravo, J. L. Charli, M. Pacheco, M. Paulo, J. Neale, and J. Barker, in A. M. Gotto Jr., E. J. Peck Jr., and A. E. Boyd III, Eds., *Brain Peptides: A New Endocrinology*, Elsevier, Amsterdam, 1979, p. 183.
108. Y. Koch, T. Baram, P. Chobsieng, and M. Fridkin, *Biochem. Biophys. Res. Commun.* **61**, 95 (1974).
109. E. C. Griffiths, J. A. Kelly, R. Forbes, S. L. Jeffcoate, N. White, R. D. G. Milner, and T. J. Visser, in A. M. Gotto Jr., E. J. Peck Jr., and A. E. Boyd III, Eds., *Brain Peptides: A New Endocrinology*, Elsevier, Amsterdam, 1979, p. 183.
110. R. V. Gallo, *Neuroendocrinology* **30**, 122 (1980).
111. P. V. Malven, *Neuroendocrinology* **19**, 81 (1975).
112. R. J. Santen and C. W. Bardin, *J. Clin. Invest.* **52**, 2617 (1973).
113. S. S. C. Yen, C. C. Tsai, F. Naftolin, G. Vandenburg, and L. Ajabor, *J. Clin. Endocrinol. Metab.* **34**, 671 (1972).
114. R. J. Santen, *J. Clin. Invest.* **56**, 1555 (1975).
115. J. E. Levine, F. Pau, V. D. Ramirez, and G. L. Jackson, *Soc. Neurosci.* **11**, 10 (1981).
116. E. Knobil, *Biol. Reprod.* **24**, 44 (1981).
117. C. A. Blake and C. H. Sawyer, *Endocrinology* **94**, 730 (1974).
118. T. M. Plant, Y. Nakai, P. Belchetz, E. Keogh, and E. Knobil, *Endocrinology* **102**, 1015 (1978).
119. L. C. Krey, in G. M. Brown, S. H. Koslow, and S. Reichlin, Eds., *Neuroendocrinology of Psychiatric Disorder*, Raven Press, New York, 1983, in press.
120. R. C. Tsou, R. A. Dailey, C. S. McLanahan, A. D. Parent, G. T. Tindall, and J. D. Neill, *Endocrinology* **101**, 534 (1977).
121. T. M. Plant, E. Schallenberger, D. L. Hess, J. T. McCormack, and E. Knobil, *Biol. Reprod.* **23**, 760 (1980).
122. G. A. Lincoln and R. V. Short, *Recent Prog. Horm. Res.* **36**, 1 (1980).

123. S. J. Legan, F. J. Karsch, and D. L. Foster, *Endocrinology* **101**, 1818 (1977).
124. J. W. Everett, *J. Endocrinol.* **75**, 1P (1977).
125. R. L. Eskay, R. S. Mical, and J. C. Porter, *Endocrinology* **100**, 263 (1977).
126. R. V. Gallo, *Biol. Reprod.* **24**, 771 (1981).
127. C. H. Rahe, R. E. Owens, J. L. Fleeger, H. J. Newton, and P. G. Harms, *Endocrinology* **107**, 498 (1980).
128. D. T. Baird, *Biol. Reprod.* **18**, 359 (1978).
129. R. Vigersky, in G. M. Brown, S. H. Koslow, and S. Reichlin, Eds., *Neuroendocrinology of Psychiatric Disorder*, Raven Press, New York, in press (1983).
130. G. Leyendecker, L. Wildt, and M. Hansman, *J. Clin. Endocrinol. Metab.* **51**, 1214 (1980).

29

Somatostatin

SEYMOUR REICHLIN

Endocrine Division
Department of Medicine
Tufts University School of Medicine
New England Medical Center
Boston, Massachusetts

Work from the author's laboratory alluded to in this chapter was supported by USPHS Grants No. AM16684, T32AM07039

1   INTRODUCTION

The term somatostatin (somatotropin release inhibiting factor, SRIF) was first applied to a specific cyclic peptide containing 14 amino acids isolated from ovine hypothalamus on the basis of its potent effects in inhibiting the release of growth hormone (GH, somatotropin) from rat pituitary cells in dispersed culture (1). Subsequent work has considerably expanded the initially simple concept of somatostatin as a tetradecapeptide primarily involved in the regulation of GH secretion. Somatostatin-like peptides are now seen to constitute a family of related molecules including the originally identified somatostatin (designated somatostatin-14), amino-terminal-extended somatostatin (somatostatin-28), and still larger forms, which range in molecular weight according to location and species from 11,500 to 15,700 daltons (Table 1). When the larger forms of somatostatin were first recognized, it was reasonable to consider them to be prohormones, but more recent studies have shown that under some circumstances somatostatin-28 and even the larger forms can be secreted as such and possess biological activity, thus suggesting that these larger forms can constitute both prohormone and hormone. All mammalian and most submammalian somatostatin-like molecules include a sequence identical with the originally described tetradecapeptide, but in at least one lower animal, the catfish, relatively large differences in sequence have been detected, and recombinant DNA studies show the existence of more than one gene coding for somatostatin. These aspects are dealt with further in Sections 3 and 5 on the phylogeny and biosynthesis of somatostatin. The original name, somatostatin, is somewhat inappropriate because this compound is distributed widely in cells throughout the nervous system and in many extraneural tissues where it exerts effects on a wide range of structures, including neurons, epithelia, and endocrine and exocrine glands.

In this chapter I have been fortunate in being able to refer to several reviews that help in organizing the enormous literature that has accumulated since 1973 (2–12).

TABLE 1 The Established Structures of Somatostatin and Somatostatin-Related Peptides[a]

Peptide	Amino acid sequence
Mammalian hypothalamic	Ala Gly Cys Lys Asn Phe Phe Trp Lys Thr Phe Thr Ser Cys
Catfish islet	Asp Asn Thr Val Arg Ser Lys Pro Leu Ala Pro Arg Glu Arg Lys – – – – – – – – – – – – – –
Anglerfish islet I	Ala Ala Ser Gly Gly Pro Leu Leu Ala Pro Arg Glu Arg Lys – – – – – – – – – – – – – –
Anglerfish islet II	Ser Val Asp Ser Thr Asn Leu Pro Pro Arg Glu Arg Lys – – – – – – Tyr – – Gly – – – –
Porcine 28	Ser Ala Asn Ser Asn Pro Ala Met Ala Pro Arg Glu Arg Lys – – – – – – – – – – – – – –
Rat MTC	Ser Ala Asn Ser Asn Pro Ala Met Ala Pro Arg Glu Arg Lys – – – – – – – – – – – – – –

[a] Amino acid sequences of the COOH-terminal regions of various somatostatin precursors. Sequences enclosed in box are homologous regions of the N-extended somatostatin-28. The dashes represent homologous amino acids in somatostatin-14. From Goodman et al. (29).

2 HISTORY

Krulich and his collaborators discovered growth hormone release inhibitory factors during the course of efforts to assay GH releasing factor from rat hypothalamus (13). These authors demonstrated that hypothalamic extracts contained regionally localized GH releasing and inhibitory factors, and they proposed the hypothesis that the secretion of GH was regulated by the interaction of the two kinds of chemical factors, both under the control of the nervous system. This hypothesis has since been well substantiated by more specific methods.

At about the same time that Krulich was studying GH release inhibiting factors in rat hypothalamic extracts, Hellman and Lernmark found that extracts of pigeon pancreatic islets inhibited release of insulin from mouse islets incubated *in vitro* (14). The efforts of these two laboratories was to converge later in the chemical identification of somatostatin in both tissues. Krulich's work attracted little attention, in part because inhibitory effects could be rationalized as being caused by nonspecific toxic factors, because the material was not isolated and chemically characterized, and because there were not, at the time, well worked out models for control of anterior pituitary secretion that involved an interplay between excitatory and inhibitory hypophysiotropic factors.

Growth hormone release inhibitory factor was rediscovered during another unsuccessful search for GH releasing factors in hypothalamic extracts, this time in the laboratory of Guillemin by a team of workers who were studying side fractions from ovine extracts used previously to isolate thyrotropin releasing hormone (TRH) and luteinizing hormone releasing hormone (1). Schally and colleagues then showed that an identical compound was present in porcine hypothalamic extracts, and they made the additional observation that another hypothalamic fraction had GH release inhibitory properties (15). This material is now recognized to be one of the larger somatostatin forms. High points in further elucidation of somatostatin chemistry are the demonstration of an identical tetradecapeptide in porcine intestinal extract by Schally and colleagues (16), the proof of an identical sequence in pigeon pancreas by Speiss and colleagues (17), the isolation from pig intestine of the N-terminal-extended somatostatin-28 and the elucidation of its sequence by Pradayrol and colleagues (18), the isolation of larger forms (19–24) that can be broken down to smaller somatostatin-like peptides (25), and the elucidation by recombinant DNA techniques of the sequence of somatostatin and its prohormones derived from angler fish islets (26, 27), catfish islets (28), and rat medullary thyroid carcinoma (29).

By bioassay techniques, Vale and colleagues demonstrated that nonhypothalamic brain tissues contained substances with GH release inhibitory factors (30), but the specificity of these findings were not established until the development of the first of many specific radioimmunoassays for somatostatin by Arimura and colleagues (31) and by the use of immunohistochemical staining techniques that utilize antisera developed against synthetic peptide. Subsequently, both radioimmunoassay and immunohistochemistry have shown that this peptide is widely distributed (see below) and that, for the most part, somatostatin produces biological effects on tissues in which it is normally present.

Important further steps in somatostatin research were the finding by Vale and colleagues that this compound inhibited TSH release (cf 2) and by Koerker and colleagues that it inhibited pancreatic secretion of insulin and glucagon (cf 2–4). When immunohistochemical study established the presence of somatostatin in a subpopulation of pancreatic islet cells, it became evident that this peptide might exert paracrine secretory control on the pancreas (see below). This paracrine model was then extended to the control of gastrointestinal secretions when it was established that somatostatin was present in both epithelial and neural elements in the gut and that it suppressed most gut secretions. A giant step was the demonstration of the presence of somatostatin in many nerve cells throughout the brain, even in areas unrelated to pituitary regulation, and the demonstration of its effect on neuronal function have suggested for somatostatin a role in nervous system function of considerable importance. In a word, somatostatin is a quintessential gut-brain peptide.

3 PHYLOGENETIC DISTRIBUTION

The literature dealing with the phylogeny of somatostatin reads like the passenger list of Noah's Ark (30, 32–34). Immunoreactive somatostatin-like molecules have been identified in tissues (brain, pancreas, intestine, or all three) from representatives of all vertebrate classes, including mammals, birds, reptiles, amphibians, teleost fish, cartilagenous fish, cyclostomes (lamprey eel and hagfish); from a protochordate, the sea squirt *Ciona intestinalis*—which possesses both intestinal and cerebral ganglion immunoreactive (IR)-somatostatin-containing cells—and from the brain cells of at least one protostomian, an insect, *Locust migratorius*. Most recently, immunoreactive somatostatin-like material has been isolated from a unicellular organism, *Tetrahymena pyriformis*, a protozoan. Somatostatin structure has been adduced by classical sequence analysis of peptide isolated from ovine (1) and porcine hypothalamus (15), porcine intestine (18), pigeon pancreas (17), angler fish (35), and catfish pancreas (36). Grimm-Jorgensen has recently reported that endolymph of snail contains IR-somatostatin, which does not behave chromatographically like the mammalian tetradecapeptide (37).

The occurrence of similar or identical molecules in species of such different complexity of function does not mean that the same function is expressed in all organisms. Rather, the same molecule probably serves different functions and is under different controlling inputs depending upon the functional requirement. This theme has been elegantly elaborated by Roth and collaborators (38). A similar case is espoused below in describing the multiple functions of somatostatin in higher organisms.

The claim that a protozoan contains somatostatin is perhaps the most interesting of all because it suggests that this molecule and its controlling gene or genes evolved before the evolutionary appearance of differentiated cell-to-cell and nerve-to-cell communication. The evidence favoring the presence of somatostatin in protozoa consists of parallel displacement by binding curves, identical chromatography, competitive binding in a receptor assay, and biological evidence of inhibition of GH release (34). I have also detected in tetrahymena extracts an IR-somatostatin that is identical with somatostatin-14 on Biogel P-10 chromatography (unpublished).

All of the somatostatin-like materials that have been structurally characterized thus far are highly conserved (Table 1).

The amino acid sequence of all mammalian somatostatin-14 and somatostatin-28 molecules are identical. At least two different genes coding for angler fish somatostatin have been identified (26, 27). One of the genes codes for terminal sequences identical with mammalian somatostatin (designated somatostatin I). This gene may in fact be polymorphic or it may be reduplicated, the duplicate expressing minor differences in the coding sequence. The second gene product, designated somatostatin II differs by two amino acids at positions 7 and 10. Only somatostatin I is expressed in normal islet tissue (39). Catfish islet cell somatostatin contains 22 amino acids, only seven of which are identical with the mammalian tetradecaptide (36), but there also is a normally unexpressed gene coding for somatostatin-14 (revealed by recombinant DNA techniques) in catfish islet cells (28). It has been pointed out that the peptide urotensin II, a dodecapeptide product of the caudal neurosecretory system of fishes, is homologous with mammalian somatostatin-14, positions 1, 2, 7, 8, and 9 being identical (40). The 7–9 sequence homology is especially important because it corresponds to the sequence responsible for somatostatin biological action in some assay systems. It is also a common site of antibody specificity. Even more instructive from an evolutionary point of view than sequence analysis of phenotypic somatostatin is the record left in the genotype. According to the recent studies of Goodman et al. (29), which compared rat medullary thyroid carcinoma somatostatin with angler fish somatostatin, 35 of the 42 nucleotides (83%) coding for somatostatin-14 are conserved: "Within the coding sequence for somatostatin-28, 22 of the 28 amino acids (79%) and 58 of the 84 nucleotides (69%) are maintained. The six amino acid substitutions between fish and rat somatostatin-28 sequence appear to be conservative in nature."

The sequence of N-terminal-extended somatostatin is less well conserved among species, and the untranslated regions even less so. Based on recombinant DNA techniques, there thus appear in nature at least five different genes coding for somatostatin—one in mammals, two or three in angler fish islets, two in catfish islets—occurring in animals that diverged in evolution at least 400 million years ago. Based on chromatography of cell-free translation products, Shields et al. report the existence of eight different prosomatostatins (41). Gene sequences (or their expressed products) coding for somatostatin obtained from different tissues of the same animal may also be different (42).

The fact that the phenotype of somatostatin-14 is so well conserved (and even the somatostatin-28, in part) suggests that throughout global history, the specific configuration of somatostatin-14 has endowed an evolutionary advantage on the animal organism.

4 ANATOMICAL DISTRIBUTION

Somatostatin is widely distributed in cells throughout the body of vertebrates, but, as noted by Guillemin, it does not inhibit the secretion of everything and anything (43). The peptide is found in most, but not all, organs and displays specific and selective functions depending upon its location.

Within the nervous system, somatostatinergic neurons form part of the tuberoinfundibular system that terminates in the median eminence. In this region they function in anterior pituitary regulation (44–52). In addition, somatostatinergic neurons terminate in the neurohypophysis (53, 54), where they have been postulated to modulate secretion of vasopressin and oxytocin; they are located in several defined long tracts, particularly in the limbic system; they are part of local short-range control systems especially in the cortex and hippocampus; they project caudally from the hypothalamus to brain stem and spinal cord (55); and they make up one or more classes of sensory fibers located in spinal, sympathetic, and vagus nerves (56–58), the retina (59–61), and the auditory system (62).

Outside the nervous system, somatostatin is distributed in specific secretory cells of the gut (2–5, 8–11, 20, 63–68), the pancreatic islets (2, 4, 9, 11, 69–73), the salivary glands (74), and the urinary excretory system (75, 76).

In all peptidergic neuronal systems that have been studied, somatostatin has been shown to be localized to nerve endings in secretory granules (77–79), to be released in response to depolarizing stimuli (see below), to be degraded by locally present enzymes (80, 81), and to bind to specific receptors, both pituitary (82) and neural (83). In the case of pituitary regulation it thus qualifies as a neurohormone, that is, a secretion from nerve cells that is released into the blood; in the nervous system it qualifies as a neurotransmitter or neuromodulator. Outside the brain, somatostatin can serve as a paracrine regulator and in some instances as a true hormone, and as a "lumone"—defined as a regulatory factor acting after secretion into the lumen of the gut (cf 83).

4.1   Tuberoinfundular System

4.1   Nervous System

Somatostatin cells and fibers are found in most parts of the hypothalamus and limbic system, with many terminating in the median eminence. To define those neurons related specifically to the tuberoinfundibular hypophysiotropic system, it is important to determine the site of origin of tuberoinfundular neurons in general and to determine which of these correspond to the somatostatinergic system. As defined by retrograde labeling of neuron cell bodies after median eminence injection of tracers (85, 86), the principal source of fibers projecting to the median eminence is a layer several cells thick located in the anterior periventricular nucleus in a position immediately under the ependymal lining. Analogous periventricular cells also form the medial division (parvocellular division) of the paraventricular nucleus. Both regions are rich in somatostatin-containing nerve cells. From the anterior periventricular nucleus somatostatin-containing fibers sweep laterally through the hypothalamus at the level of the suprachiasmatic nucleus and are reassembled posteriorly into a condensed bundle that enters the median eminence through its anterior margin. Small contributions to the median eminence come from the dorsal arcuate nucleus. It has not been determined with certainty where the somatostatinergic neurons terminating in the neurohypophysis originate. They do not arise in the supraoptic nucleus nor in the magnocellular portion of the paraventricular nucleus. The most important possibility is the parvocellular division of the paraventricular nucleus (46–49, 51, 52).

Among other nuclei containing somatostatinergic fibers or cells, the failure to find retrograde labeling of tracer allows one to exclude the following nuclei as being components of the tuberoinfundular system: suprachiasmatic, ventromedial, anterior hypothalamic, lateral hypothalamic, preoptic, olfactory tubercle, cerebral cortex, and hippocampus (85, 86). The relationship of the amygdala to the tuberoinfundular system is not clear. Lechan and colleagues found no evidence of retrograde labeling of this structure after median eminence application of horseradish peroxidase (HRP) (85), but Crowley and Terry (50) found that lesions of the medial-basal amygdala brought about reduction of median eminence immunoreactive somatostatin, and Layton and colleagues found that electrical stimulation of the amygdala produced orthodromic responses in 23% of tuberoinfundular neurons (87). Electrical stimulation of the medial amygdala of the rat brought about inhibition of GH secretion, a response compatible with a somatostatin-mediated effect. The essential problem then is whether at least some components of amygdala project directly to the median eminence or are important as interconnecting elements in the limbic system.

Immunohistochemical findings of peptide distribution in the brain are fully confirmed by immunoassays of hypothalamic nuclei punched out by the Palkovits technique (45) and by study of changes in concentration of somatostatin in the median eminence after selective lesions of the anterior periventricular–median eminence projections (44, 88–90). The decrease in median eminence somatostatin following lesions of the anterior periventricular nucleus or section of the periventricular–median eminence projection by the Halasz technique (88, 89) leads to predictable alterations in endocrine function, that is, increased GH and increased thyroid stimulating hormone (TSH) levels in peripheral blood (90).

4.1.2 Limbic System

According to Krisch (49), somatostatinergic fibers originating in the periventricular region (in addition to their projections to the median eminence) also project in short-distance trajectories to certain hypothalamic nuclei: the preoptic nucleus, suprachiasmatic nucleus, ventromedial nucleus, arcuate nucleus, and ventral premammillary nucleus. In long-distance trajectories they project rostrally to lamina terminalis (hence to subfornical organ), the organum vasculosum lamina terminalis (OVLT), olfactory tubercle, dorsal part of the stria terminalis, thence to amygdala and to the interstitial nucleus of the stria terminalis. Other long-distance projections from the periventricular nuclei are an ascending projection to the ventral amygdala–hypothalamic pathway of the stria terminalis, to the corticomedial amygdala, and to the caudal parts of the arcuate and ventral premammillary nuclei. Other limbic structures reported to contain somatostatinergic fibers are the dorsomedial accumbens nucleus, lateral septum (stria hypothalamic tract), bed nucleus of the anterior commissure, precommissural division of the stria terminalis, all divisions of the amygdaloid-nuclear complex, the medial corticohypothalamic tract, and the preoptic-hypothalamic division of the precommissural nucleus (51).

4.1.3 Brain Stem and Spinal Cord

Periventricular hypothalamic somatostatinergic fibers also project caudally into the brain stem and spinal cord (55). They travel through three main pathways: along the stria medullaris thalami, through the fasciculus retroflexus into the interpeduncular nucleus, and via the periventricular gray and the bundle of Schutz into the midbrain tegmentum. In these sites they interdigitate with somatostatin fibers arising from peripheral sensory inputs and from an intrinsic system of somatostatin cells in the central grey.

4.1.4 Sensory Systems

The descending hypothalamic somatostatin fibers of periventricular origin interdigitate within the spinal cord in "basketlike terminals" (55) with the terminals of somatostatinergic sensory afferents (spinal sensory, cranial sensory, and visceral-autonomic). They also interact with terminals of an intrinsic system of somatostatin fibers arising from within the spinal cord and brain stem.

Hökfelt and collaborators were the first to show that some spinal sensory ganglia cells were immunoreactive with antisomatostatin sera and that these fibers projected centrally to terminate in the substantia gelatinosa (Lissauer's tract, lamina II) of the dorsal entry zone (56, 57). The axons are distinct from a second class of afferent peptidergic neurons, the substance P system, although both are small, unmyelinated, and classified as type B, a category generally associated with perception of pain and temperature. Krisch has recently asserted (55) that sensory ganglia do not contain immunoreactive somatostatin, but her claim is controverted by Hökfelt's finding that the dorsal root entry zone is markedly depleted of somatostatin by section of the dorsal root, and by several studies by radioimmunoassay of dorsal ganglia—including those from my laboratory that both characterized the immunoreactive material chromatographically and demonstrated anterograde axoplasmic transport (91), those of Kessler and Black (92) who have shown that these cells are regulated by nerve growth factor, and by Mudge et al. who demonstrated immunoreactive somatostatin generation by chick dorsal ganglia in culture (93).

Sensory somatostatin fibers analogous to spinal afferents whose perikarya are located in sensory ganglia are those associated with the trigeminal nerve Gasserian ganglion (55) projecting distally to the face, centrally to the sensory root of the trigeminal, and presumably the central sensory projections of the hypoglossal nerve reported by Krisch (55) to terminate in the region of the nucleus praepositus hypoglossi and the solitary complex.

Ganglia associated with the autonomic nervous system also contain somatostatin-positive cells. These include the superior cervical, celiac, and superior mesenteric [of the guinea pig and rat (57, 58, 94)]. Since many of these cells also contain catecholamine-synthesizing enzymes and catecholamines (58, 94), it is likely that they are at least in part motor-efferent fibers. But the findings by Krisch (55) of immunoreactive somatostatin *terminals* in the region intermediolateralis (the site of origin of preganglionic sympathetic fibers) raises the question whether some of the somatostatin perikarya in the sympathetic ganglia are part of an afferent system conveyed in sympathetic nerves. Somatostatin has also been identified in two groups of parasympathetic ganglia: sacral ganglia (of the cat) that project centrally to the Lissauer tract of the sacral cord and nearby structures (95), and in the nodose ganglion of the vagus [in the rat (96)] distributed centrally to the nucleus of the tractus solitarius and peripherally to the gut, heart, and pancreas.

Krisch (55) also reports that somatostatin fibers project into the main portions of the auditory nerve (nucleus dorsalis lemnisci lateralis, and nucleus corporis trapezoidei). Somatostatin is demonstrable in the cochlea (62), but I am not aware of any work showing its presence in the sensory cells of the vestibular organ.

Immunoreactive somatostatin is also found in the retina (59–61), localized by immunofluorescence to four types of cell processes in the inner plexiform layer, including amacrine cells (60, 61, 96, 97), and is also found in the optic nerve, optic tectum (of the cow), and at several levels of the visual system of rats, mice, and guinea pigs, including the lateral geniculate nucleus, pretectal area, superior colliculus, and visual cortex (97). Whether retinal somatostatin-containing cells project centrally is not clear. Rorstad and colleagues found an increase in retinal somatostatin of the rat one year after surgical section of the optic nerve (59), a finding best interpreted to indicate that this system is entirely intrinsic to the retina.

With the possible exception of the retina, the data summarized above make it abundantly clear that somotostatinergic fibers projecting to the neuroaxis are involved in virtually all sensory systems. Further, the finding of somatostatin in at least one class of retinal cells implies a function of this peptide in vision.

In addition to the descending termini and segmental spinal sensory nerves as sources of brain stem and spinal afferents, several workers have adduced evidence for the presence of an intrinsic system of somatostatin fibers within the cord as well. Immunoreactive perikarya are found (in the tree shrew *Tupaia* by Burnweit and Forssmann, 98) in the substantia intermedia centralis of the lateral column (lamina X and the medial part of lamina VII) and an even more extensive distribution in cat spinal cord by Tessler et al. (99). Isolation of segments of cord by spinal root section and knife cuts above and below the site of study show that about two-thirds of regional somatostatin comes from outside the cord and from descending pathways but the rest arise from within the segments of the cord itself (99).

These local segmental signals interact upon the same second-order sensory afferents as those derived from local sensory inputs and with somatostatinergic fibers from long tracts descending from the hypothalamus many centimeters or even meters away.

The physiological meaning of this rich spinal innervation has not been elucidated, nor has the role of somatostatin in perception been clarified.

4.1.5   Cerebral Cortex

All parts of the cerebral cortex, including pyriform cortex and cingulate gyrus, contain cell bodies of somatostatinergic neurons which are located mainly, but not exclusively, in layers II, III, and VI (100). These cells can be pyramidal, bipolar, or multipolar (Bennett-Clarke et al., 52). Although concentrations in the cortex are the lowest of any part of the central nervous system, the total bulk of cortex (as compared with other parts of the brain) means that this portion of the brain, in the aggregate, contains the largest fraction of total brain somatostatin (20). None of the somatostatin in the cerebral cortex comes from the periventricular nucleus as shown by lesion experiments (88, 89). Cells of the frontal cortex differ morphologically from those of the hypothalamus, those of the cortex containing granules approximately 65 nm, compared with hypothalamic granules of 90–120 nm (100). The existence of an intrinsic (presumably intraneuronal) system of cerebral cortical nerve cells separate from the hypothalamus is further established by studies in which the cerebral mantle of fetal rats is grown in dispersed cell culture. These cells synthesize somatostatin over time (101) and release somatostatin as determined by modifications of the electrolyte and neurotransmitter milieu (See below).

4.1.6   Circumventricular Organs

The system of ependyma-derived neurohemal organs arranged around the third ventricle (subfornical organ, pineal, subcommissural organ, median eminence, and organum vasculosum of the lamina terminalis) and in the floor of the fourth ventricle (area postrema) all contain nerve terminals of somatostatinergic neurons (44, 50, 102). Their function is unknown.

4.2   Gastrointestinal Tract

4.2.1   Pancreas

Following the demonstration that somatostatin inhibited glucagon and insulin secretion, it was essential to determine whether these effects were part of a normal local control mechanism. The most crucial bit of evidence required to answer this question was to determine whether somatostatin is normally present in any cells of the pancreas. This question has been answered most emphatically in the affirmative (2–5, 8, 9, 11, 69–72). Somatostatin is present in a population of cells in the pancreas (in the "D" cell as well as in nerve endings), is synthesized by islet cells in culture, and contains mRNA coding for somatostatin. Somatostatin is found in D cells of even the most primitive of species. In rats and horses these cells are distributed primarily in the periphery, but in humans and guinea pigs D cells are scattered throughout. Regardless of the distribution within the islets, the most important aspect of the D cell is its anatomical relationship to the other islet cells. Occasionally somatostatin cells are separated from adjacent alpha and beta cells by gap junctions but most commonly they are related by a common contact with the continuous interstitial space of the islet and by fingerlike projections of the somatostatin-secreting cells that can interdigitate with several other cells. In some species, there is a local "portal" circulation that brings about local regional perfusion of somatostatin secreted from the D cells through a microvascular system to come into contact with the other islet cells.

4.2.2 Stomach and Intestine

Somatostatin-contain ing epithelial cells are present in digestive tracts of all species of animals (63–64, 67, 103). In humans, concentration decreases in a gradient from stomach to lower colon; within the stomach there is an especially high localization of somatostatin-containing epithelial cells in the antral region.

Somatostatin-secreting epithelial cells are found deep in the crypts of stomach and intestine and are of the category recognized as having a small process directly opening out on the gut lumen, which contains microvilli (103, 104). It is commonly thought that the presence of microvilli projecting into the lumen provides the means by which changes in luminal content, particularly hydrogen ion and certain nutrients, can regulate somatostatin secretion. The cells do not secrete through the small portion that communicates directly with the lumen but are presumed to release their products laterally into the interstitial space of the gut wall, whence they enter the venous blood draining the intestine; peptide is also released into the gut lumen. As in the case of the islet cell, it is reasonable to believe that the paracrine effects of somatostatin are exerted by release of the peptide into the interstitial space where it can come into contact with receptors located on membranes of other gut epithelia; that is, with gastrin-, gut glucagon-, secretin-, and cholecystokinin-secreting cells, all of which are influenced by somatostatin. An additional mechanism has been proposed by Larsson, who has shown that somatostatin-containing gut D cells possess a long ramifying process that puts each cell in contact with many other secretory cells (104).

In addition to somatostatin-containing epithelial cells, the gut is innervated by separate systems of peptidergic neurons located in both the submucosal and the myenteric plexus (105). Cell bodies of the intrinsic system are located in the submucosal plexus and the nerve endings come into contact with the interstitial space. The vagus nerve contributes an extrinsic somatostatinergic nerve fiber system as well. Because gut somatostatin content is unaltered by ligation of the nerve input to the intestine (or by transplantation), it has been concluded that the intrinsic system is the more important contributor to somatostatin nerve fiber activity in the gut.

As a general rule, the brain somatostatin neural system has no direct effect on the somatostatin system outside of the central nervous system. Lesions of the hypothalamus have no effect on pancreatic somatostatin (53).

Limited studies have been made of the electrophysiological effects of somatostatin on the intrinsic nerves of the gut. Only a small proportion of neurons of the myenteric plexus of the guinea pig responds to direct application of this peptide—some were depolarized and some were hyperpolarized (106). Most striking was the variability of the response. Tachyphylaxis was readily demonstrated, and the mode of exposure (perfusion, ejection, iontophoresis) changed the pattern and reproducibility of responses. These effects are to be compared with those of the central nervous system (see below).

It is not known at this time how the many somatostatin-containing elements of the gut—epithelia, nerve endings from vagus, and the intrinsic plexus—interact for physiological control of the gut.

4.3   Other Visceral Distribution

Somatostatin-immunoreactive D-type cells have been identified in salivary gland (73, 107); saliva contains somatostatin and this peptide causes decreased salivary flow following systemic injection (107).

Some of the parafollicular cells of the human thyroid (cells of origin of calcitonin) contain somatostatin, and others appear to contain calcitonin alone (108, 109). Somatostatin is synthesized by medullary thyroid carcinoma cells (29, 110, 111). In some studies, but not all, somatostatin appears to inhibit the secretion of calcitonin (cf 112). If this is part of a normal control system, it may be postulated that the somatostatin diffuses outside of the cell, is released from the cell, and diffuses into the interstitial space where it comes into contact with somatostatin receptors on the cell membrane. This kind of control has been called *autocrine* regulation.

Immunoreactive somatostatin has been identified in collecting tubules of the kidney of the toad and in virtually all cells of toad bladder (76), but efforts to show the presence of somatostatin in mammalian kidney have given contradictory findings. Our group found no immunoassayable somatostatin in extracts of rat kidney (20), whereas Kronheim et al. found it (113). Subsequently, I have again tried to identify somatostatin in rat kidney but without success. On the other hand, we found that human kidney contains immunoreactive somatostatin corresponding in molecular size to somatostatin-14 (Reichlin, Bollinger, Goodman, and Forrest, unpublished). A role for somatostatin in renal function is suggested by the finding in the dog that this peptide interferes with the antidiuretic action of vasopressin (114). In toad bladder, this system has been studied in detail by Forrest and collaborators, who have shown that somatostatin has no direct effect on toad bladder function by itself but does interfere with the action of antidiuretic hormone (75). Somatostatin is found in the urine (115) and inhibits stimulated renin release (116–118).

5 BIOSYNTHESIS, PROCESSING, AND TRANSPORT IN NEURONS

Molecular biological aspects of somatostatin biosynthesis have been alluded to in Section 3. The amino acid sequence of preprosomatostatin has been elucidated in several tissues and it is widely assumed that sequential processing of the peptide to smaller forms (corresponding to somatostatin-14, somatostatin-28, and larger molecular forms (prohormone, preprohormone) takes place within the endoplasmic reticulum and is translocated in the Golgi apparatus for processing and assemblage into granule form (cf 119). In epithelial cells the granules are thence transported to the plasma membrane for exocytic secretion; in neurons the granules are transported from cell bodies to nerve terminals for subsequent release. The transport of somatostatin in granules within the brain has been well documented in studies of effects of section of the tuberoinfundibular axonal projections (which depletes the median eminence) (88–90), by intraventricular injections of colchicine (Lechan, unpublished), and in ligation studies of the sciatic nerve of the rat (91). Transport rate of the mobile fraction in sciatic nerve is approximately 400 mm per 24 h, thus corresponding to the fast transport rate characteristic of secretion granules in neurosecretory fibers of the neurohypophysis and in the sympathetic nerves. Only 20% of the somatostatin in sciatic nerve appears to be in the rapidly mobile fraction. Content of somatostatin in sensory ganglia of the sciatic nerve is estimated to turn over between 9 and 18 times in 24 h (91).

Factors regulating somatostatin biosynthesis in the nervous system are poorly understood. As outlined in sections dealing with pituitary regulation, GH and thyroid hormones influence the content of somatostatin in the hypothalamus, although altered release has not been differentiated from altered synthesis. Our group has found that thyroid hormone effects on somatostatin are not limited to the hypothalamus, as shown by impaired axoplasmic transport in the sciatic nerve of hypothyroid rats (Rasool, Bradley, and Reichlin, unpublished), and Kessler and Black reported that the time of appearance of somatostatinergic sensory neurons was accelerated by the administration of nerve growth factor (as was that of substance P) (92). Neither finding adequately deals with more fundamental aspects of regulation of somatostatin synthesis. Our group has recently found that restriction of phenylalanine (an amino acid constituent of somatostatin) from tissue culture media favors the accumulation of somatostatin-14 over that of larger forms (120).

The relative amounts of the several forms of somatostatin secreted may have functional importance. All forms of somatostatin have growth hormone release inhibitory properties (23), and somatostatin-28 has further been shown to be even more potent as a pancreatic (121) and growth hormone (122) release inhibitory peptide than somatostatin-14.

The relative potency of the three different forms of somatostatin as neuromodulators has not been fully determined but Brown et al. (123) have recently reported that intraventricularly administered somatostatin-28 is much more potent than SRIF-14 in inhibiting bombesin-induced hyperglycemia. It must be concluded that all three forms of somatostatin are secreted as such, and each can be regarded as a hormone although the larger forms may be regarded as prohormones as well. In this respect, somatostatin resembles another gut-brain peptide, gastrin, which is secreted as "big" gastrin (34 amino acid residues, and "small" gastrin (17 amino acid residues), both with biological activity.

6   FUNCTION OF SOMATOSTATIN IN PITUITARY AND GUT REGULATION

6.1   Anterior Pituitary

6.1.1   Growth Hormone Secretion

The physiological relevance of somatostatin secretion for growth hormone regulation has been demonstrated in several ways. Lesions of the somatostatinergic tuberoinfundular tract leads to depletion of median eminence somatostatin and to increased basal levels of GH (and of TSH, see below) (90). Contrariwise, electrical stimulation of the anterior periventricular area in the rat corresponding to the cells of origin of the principal hypothalamic-median eminence projection leads to inhibition of GH secretion (124, 125), and appropriately, to increased release of somatostatin into the hypophysial-portal vessels (126). That somatostatin is involved in regulation of GH release under normal circumstances is shown in studies in which endogenous somatostatin is neutralized by administration of antisera to the peptide. Acute release of GH (127, 128) and reversal of the characteristic inhibition of GH release caused by physical stress (127, 129) and by starvation (130) are observed.

Somatostatin secretion also appears to be at least one of the factors mediating short-loop feedback control of GH secretion. GH deficiency (as produced by hypophysectomy) leads to decrease in somatostatin content of the median eminence, a change reversed by GH administration (131–134). Exposure of the hypothalamus to growth hormone, either by addition to incubated hypothalamic blocks (134, 135) or via

intracerebroventricular injection, brings about somatostatin release
(136), an effect mirrored in the suppression of GH release that follows
intraventricular GH injection (137). Growth hormone may be effective in
somatostatin regulation in two different ways, the first as a direct regulator, as outlined above, and the second through somatomedin C, a
well-characterized peptide of hepatic origin the production of which is
regulated by GH and which is the mediator of GH effects on the muscu-
loskeletal system. Exposure of hypothalamic blocks to somatomedin C
stimulated somatostatin release (138), and intraventricular injection of
somatomedin C in the rat inhibited GH secretion (137). Intraventricular
injection of somatostatin elevates GH release (139), an effect possibly
explained by the suppression of endogenous somatostatin.

Extensive studies have been carried out in an attempt to elucidate
the role of altered hypothalamic somatostatin secretion as the mediator
of the effects on GH release of neurotransmitters and neuropeptides.
These studies are summarized in Tables 2 and 3. Of factors reported to
stimulate somatostatin release from the hypothalamus, only melatonin
and neurotensin also inhibit GH secretion. Several factors reported to
stimulate somatostatin release from the hypothalamus paradoxically
stimulate the release of GH as well. These are glucagon, norepinephrine, and dopamine. Of factors reported to *inhibit* somatostatin secretion γ-amino butyric acid (GABA) appropriately leads to increased GH
release. Cholinergic stimuli, reported to release GH, have given contradictory results when tested for their effects on somatostatin release,
both inhibition and stimulation having been reported. Serotonin, which
clearly has a role in stimulating GH release in whole animals, has no
effect on somatostatin secretion. Opiates also bring about GH release,
but they either have no effect on somatostatin secretion or inhibit it.

Some of the discrepancies cited above signify that the predominant
influence on GH secretion of a given transmitter or peptide may be mediated by altered secretion of GH releasing factor rather than of
somatostatin secretion, but other discrepancies are probably caused by
the inherent limitations of the assay systems used. On the basis of all
findings cited above, it seems quite certain that somatostatin is involved in the regulation of GH in both basal and stimulated state and is
presumed to interact with GH releasing factor for GH regulation (see
Chap. 39). Unfortunately, most of the relevant research on this subject
has been carried out in the rat whose GH regulatory system differs
from that of primates, including humans; the details of this system remain to be worked out in other species of animals.

6.1.2 *Regulation of TSH Secretion*

Elucidation of the role of somatostatin in regulation of TSH release has
followed much the same logical sequence of development as that of GH
regulation. Somatostatin inhibits release of TSH from isolated pituitary

TABLE 2   Factors Reported to Influence Somatostatin Secretion from Hypothalamus and Cerebral Cortical Preparations[a]

Hormonal Changes

GH deficiency

↓	Hoffman and Baker, 1977, immunohistochemistry median eminence (131)
↓	Fernandez-Durango et al., 1978, hypothalamic content (133)
↓	Patel, 1979, hypothalamic content (240)

GH

↑	Hoffman and Baker, 1977, immunohistochemistry median eminence (131)
↑	Sheppard et al., 1978, hypothalamic fragment release (135)
↑	Patel, 1979, hypothalamic content (240)
↑	Pimstone et al., 1979, hypothalamic fragment release (5)
↑	Molitch and Hlivyak, 1980, content of hypothalamus (241)
↑	Chihara et al., 1981, portal vessels (136)
↑	Berelowitz et al., 1981, content and release from MBH fragment (134)

Somatomedin C

↑	Berelowitz et al., 1981, release from MBH fragment (138)

Thyroidectomy

↔	Fernandez-Durango et al., 1978, hypothalamic content (133)
↔	Gillioz et al., 1979, portal blood (242)
↓	Berelowitz et al., 1980, content and release from MBH fragment (150)

Thyroid hormone

↔	Fernandez-Durango et al., 1978, hypothalamic content (133)
↔	Gillioz et al., 1979, portal blood (242)
↑	Berelowitz et al., 1980, content and release from MBH (150)

Neurotransmitters

Catechol depletion

↓	Turkelson et al., 1979, portal vessel (243)

Dopamine

↑	Wakabayashi et al., 1977, synaptosome release (190)
↑	Negro-Villar et al., 1978 (244)
↑	Chihara et al., 1979, portal vessel (245)
↑ cortex ↓ hypo	Bennet et al., 1979, synaptosome release (191)
↑	Maeda and Frohman, 1980, hypothalamic fragment release (246)
↑	Ojeda et al., 1980, hypothalamic fragment release (194)
↔	Terry et al., 1980, hypothalamic fragment release (195)
↑	Berelowitz et al., 1980 hypothalamic fragment release (150)

Norepinephrine

↑	Negro-Villar et al., 1978, hypothalamic fragment release (244)
↑	Chihara et al., 1979, portal (245)
↑	Turkelson et al., 1979, portal blood (243)
↑ cortex ↓ hypo	Bennet et al., 1979, synaptosome release (191)
↔	Terry et al., 1980, hypothalamic fragment release (195)
↔	Maeda and Frohman, 1980, hypothalamic fragment release (246)
↔	Robbins et al., 1982, cortical neuron release (193)

Serotonin

↔	Chihara et al., 1979, portal blood (245)
↔	Turkelson et al., 1979, portal blood (243)
↑ cortex ↓ hypo	Bennet et al., 1979 (191)
↔	Maeda and Frohman, 1980, hypothalamic fragment release (246)
↓	Richardson et al., 1981, hypothalamic fragment release (247)

Acetylcholine

↑	Chihara et al., 1979, portal blood (245)
↔	Terry et al., 1980, hypothalamic fragment release (195)
↓	Richardson et al., 1980, hypothalamic fragment release (248)
↑	Robbins et al., 1982, cortical neuron release (193)

TABLE 2 (*Continued*)

GABA
- ↑   Turkelson et al., 1979, portal blood (243)
- ↓   Gamse et al., 1980, hypothalamic cells release (192)
- ↔   Terry et al., 1980, hypothalamic fragments (195)
- ↓   Robbins et al., 1982, cortical neuron release (193)

Peptides

Glucagon
- ↑   Abe et al., 1978, portal (249)
- ↔   Epelbaum et al., 1979, MBH fragment release (250)
- ↑   Shimatsu et al., 1981, hypothalamic fragment release (251)

VIP
- ↓   Epelbaum et al., 1979, MBH fragment release (250)
- ↓   Epelbaum et al., 1980, MBH fragments (252)
- ↓   Shimatsu et al., 1981, hypothalamic fragment release (251)
- ↑   Hermansen, 1980 (253)

Secretin
- ↓   Epelbaum et al., 1979, hypothalamic fragment release (250)

Substance P
- ↑   Sheppard et al., 1978, hypothalamic fragment release (135)
- ↔   Epelbaum et al., 1979, hypothalamic fragments (250)
- ↔   Maeda and Frohman, 1980, hypothalamic fragment release (246)
- ↑   Hermansen, 1980 (253)
- ↔   Abe et al., 1981, portal blood (254)

Opiates
- ↔   Sheppard et al., 1979, hypothalamic fragment release (255)
- ↓   Epelbaum et al., 1980, hypothalamic fragments (252)
- ↔   Abe et al., 1981, portal blood (254)
- ↓   Drouva et al., 1981, hypothalamic fragments (256)

Neurotensin
- ↑   Sheppard et al., 1979, hypothalamic fragments (255)
- ↑   Maeda and Frohman, 1980, hypothalamic fragments (246)
- ↑   Berelowitz et al., 1981, hypothalamic fragments (257)
- ↑   Abe et al., 1981, portal blood (254)

CCK-8 and CCK-4
- ↔   Shimatsu et al., 1981, hypothalamic fragment release (251)
- ↑   Hermansen, 1980 (253)

Bombesin
- ↑   Abe et al., 1981, portal blood (258)
- ↔   Hermansen, 1980 (253)

Metabolic Factors

Glucose
- ↑   Negro-Villar et al., 1980, MBH fragment release (259)

Cyclic AMP
- ↔   Maeda and Frohman, 1980, hypothalamic fragment release (246)
- ↑   Robbins et al., 1982, cortical neuron release (193)

Prostaglandins
- ↔   Ojeda et al., 1980, hypothalamic fragment release (194)
- ↔   Terry et al., 1980, hypothalamic fragment release (195)

Miscellaneous

Melatonin
- ↔   Terry et al., 1980, hypothalamic fragments (195)
- ↑   Richardson et al., 1980 (248)

---

[a] References cited showing effect on content only give no direct evidence of modified release.

Key: ↑, increased release; ↓, decreased release; ↔, unaltered release.

TABLE 3 Comparison of Factors Influencing Somatostatin, GH Release, and TSH Release

	GH Secretion	TSH Secretion
Increased Somatostatin Secretion		
Anterior periventricular stimulation	↓	↓
Hormonal changes		
GH administration	↓	↓
somatomedin C	↓	?
thyroid hormone excess	↑	↓
Neurotransmitters		
dopamine	↑	↓
norepinephrine	↑	↑
melatonin	↓	↓↑
acetylcholine	↑	?
Peptides		
glucagon	↑	?
neurotensin	↓	?
bombesin		?
Decreased Somatostatin Secretion		
Hormonal changes		
thyroid hormone deficiency	↓	↑
Neurotransmitters		
catechol depletion	↓	↓
serotonin	↑	↓↑
GABA	↑	↓
Peptides		
VIP	↑	↔
secretin	↑	?
Unaltered Somatostatin Secretion		
Neurotransmitters		
dopamine	↑	↓
norepinephrine	↑	↑
serotonin	↑	↓↑
acetylcholine	↑	?
melatonin	↓	↓
Peptides		
glucagon	↑	?
substance P	?	↔
endorphins	↑	↓
TRH	↓	?
cholecystokinin	?	?

Key: ↑, Elevated; ↓, decreased; ↔, no change; ↓↑, both increase and decreases have been reported; ?, no data available, or inadequate studies.

preparations (140), and reduces basal TSH levels in rats (141, 142) and humans (143). The effect is readily observed in the hypothyroid state (144) and after TRH stimulation (145, 146). Administration of antisomatostatin antibody potentiates the TSH response to cold exposure (147) or to TRH administration (in the rat) (148). These results clearly indicate that at the level of the pituitary, secretion of TSH is regulated by the interplay of TRH and somatostatin as well as by thyroid hormone (cf 149). In addition, thyroid hormone appears to modulate somatostatin secretion by the hypothalamus. Berelowitz and coworkers report that hypothyroid rats show reduced hypothalamic somatostatin, that release of the peptide *in vitro* is reduced, and that release is stimulated from hypothalami of normal rats *in vitro* by exposure to triiodothyronine (T3) (150). Portal vessel somatostatin concentration is less than normal in hypothyroid rats (151). The effects of somatostatin on anterior pituitary secretion are summarized in Table 4.

6.2   Gastrointestinal Tract

6.2.1   Pancreatic Islet Regulation

The role of somatostatin in the function of the pancreas has been reviewed in detail by Gerich (4, 9) and by Miller (11). Intravenous infusion of somatostatin in all vertebrate species inhibits secretion of insulin and glucagon. Neutralization of circulating somatostatin by intravenous injection of antisomatostatin sera does not modify secretion of either insulin or glucagon, but exposure of *isolated* islets to

---

TABLE 4   Actions of Somatostatin on Anterior Pituitary Secretion[a]

Growth Hormone

Inhibition of responses to prostaglandins, potassium, dibutyryl cAMP, theophylline, electrical stimulation of the hypothalamus, pentobarbital, chlorpromazine, isoproterenol, L-dopa, arginine, exercise, sleep, meals, insulin-induced hypoglycemia

Thyrotropin

Inhibition of responses to potassium, prostaglandins, theophylline, dibutyryl cAMP, basal levels in normal, basal levels in hypothyroidism, response to TRH

Prolactin

No effect on basal levels or on TRH-induced secretion in normal humans, inhibition of basal and TRH-induced release *in vitro*, diminution of circulating levels in certain patients with acromegaly.

Adrenocorticotropin

No effect on secretion *in vitro*, in normal humans given metyrapone, nor in insulin-induced hypoglycemia, but suppression in Addison's disease.

Gonadotropins

No effect on LH or FSH

---

[a] Adapted from table 3 of Gerich (7).

antisomatostatin does increase the secretion of both glucagon and insulin. These findings taken together indicate that somatostatin probably exerts a moderating effect on both tonic and stimulated secretion of glucagon and insulin and that these effects are mediated by local paracrine influences acting within the islet cell complex rather than by way of circulating hormone.

Although the factors that stimulate somatostatin release from the pancreas (whole preparations of pancreas, or isolated islet incubates or cultures) have been reasonably well characterized, the way in which the peptide interacts with the other islet cell secretions for overall control of islet function is still not clear. Some idea of the complexity of islet peptide interaction is given in Table 5. In the case of two of the islet peptides somatostatin appears to be part of a closed negative feedback control loop: glucagon, which stimulates somatostatin secretion, in turn is an inhibitor of glucagon release, and somatostatin itself (as inferred from studies in which a nonimmunoreactive analog was used) inhibits its own secretion (152). Insulin does not have an acute effect on

TABLE 5 Summary of Pancreatic Islet Cell Regulatory Factors[a]

	Somatostatin	Insulin	Glucagon
Substrates			
glucose	↑	↑	↓
amino acids	↑	↑	↑
Neurotransmitters			
acetycholine (muscarinic receptors)	↑	↑	↑
adrenergic α-1	↓		
adrenergic α-2	↓	↓	?↑
adrenergic β-2 (NE, E)	↑	↑	↑
dopamine	↓		
GABA	↓	↔	
Neuropeptides			
somatostatin	↓	↓	↓
insulin	↓?	?	?
glucagon	↑	?	?
pancreatic polypeptide	?	?	?
VIP	↑	↑	↑
secretin	↑		
substance P	↑	↓↑	↑
CCK	↑	↑	↑
gastrin	↑		
bombesin	↔	↑	↑
neurotensin	↑	↓↑	↑
endorphins	↓	↑↓	↑
prostaglandin E2 cyclic nucleotides	↑	↑↓	↑

[a] Adapted from S. Reichlin (7) and from Schally et al. (15).
Key: ↑, Increase; ↓, decrease; ↔, no change; ↑↓, conflicting reports.

somatostatin secretion. However, because beta cell destruction (by al-
loxan or streptozotocin) leads to increased secretion and increased content of pancreatic somatostatin, and because anti-insulin antisera
stimulates somatostatin release from islets in high glucose media, it is
likely that insulin is tonically suppressive to somatostatin secretion. If
such is the case, this secretory response cannot be construed as simply
being part of a negative feedback control loop. Other examples of stimuli that release somatostatin in a direction inappropriate to its postulated function as a local feedback regulator are the effects of arginine,
leucine, VIP, acetylcholine, alpha-2 adrenergic agonists, and CCK, all
factors that simultaneously stimulate the release of insulin and of glucagon as well. Somatostatin release is stimulated by glucose, which releases insulin but inhibits glucagon release. Peptides and adrenergic
agents presumably act on somatostatin regulation through the mediation
of cyclic adenosine 3′ 5′ monophosphate (cyclic AMP or cAMP) as inferred from studies of the effects of phosphodiesterase inhibitors. Because of the numerous examples of shifts in somatostatin secretion that
are not compatible with local feedback control, we must consider that
the islet cells operate as integrated functional units, with somatostatin
sometimes acting as a specific feedback element and sometimes as a
negative modulatory influence.

As mentioned above, in that form of experimental diabetes caused
by beta-cell destruction, somatostatin secretion is enhanced, but in other experimental models of diabetes one may find either increased or decreased function. The role of D cell abnormality in human diabetes is
not established, and there have been no clearly documented abnormalities of somatostatin secretion in Type I or Type II diabetes.

The rarely occurring somatostatin-secreting tumors illuminate the biological effects of this peptide. As outlined by Gerich (9), seven cases
have been reported up to 1981, all but one of which was malignant and
all but one of which originated in the pancreas. Physiological changes
attributed to these tumors are generally those expected from known effects of long-term somatostatin infusion: mild diabetes (due to suppression of both insulin and glucagon), suppressed GH release in response
to provocative stimuli, and a moderate degree of gut malabsorption. At
least five cases had cholelithiasis. This association may be fortuitous,
but it is more likely that somatostatin-induced cholestasis [demonstra-
ble in short-term infusion studies (153, 154)], could lead to biliary cholesterol concentrations favoring stone formation.

6.2.2 Gastrointestinal Tract

In keeping with its wide distribution throughout the gastrointestinal
tract in specialized epithelial cells (D cells), in intrinsic nerve plexuses,
and in autonomic nerves, somatostatin exerts an extraordinary range of

physiological effects on the gut. This very extensive literature has been reviewed recently (7, 12, 155–157) and is summarized in Tables 5, 6, and 7. Virtually every aspect of gut function is modulated by somatostatin. Although the predominant effect of somatostatin is presumed to be mediated by its paracrine mode, the peptide may influence gut function as a true hormone by way of the peripheral circulation—as has been shown for lipid digestion (158) and, by way of intralumenal secretion, as has been documented by Uvnas-Wallenstein (159).

Most physiological effects of somatostatin on gut function are attributable to direct actions of somatostatin on target cells, but in some instances observed effects are due to inhibition of an intervening factor. For example, impairment of gastric emptying by somatostatin may be due, in part, to inhibition of secretion of motilin, a hormone that stimulates gastric emptying of solid food.

Somatostatin inhibits virtually all exocrine gut secretions, including those of the stomach, small intestine, and pancreas. It impairs motility of stomach, possibly of the small intestine, and gallbladder, reduces intestinal absorption of all classes of nutrients including water, reduces blood flow to the intestine and possibly to the stomach, and inhibits cell proliferation in the stomach mucosa, even that induced by gastrin. The secretion of somatostatin is in turn modulated by virtually all of the factors that it influences.

A complete picture has not as yet emerged to explain how the secretion of somatostatin is integrated with other gut regulators, peptide hormones, neurotransmitters, and substrates to bring about the orderly

---

TABLE 6 Effects of Somatostatin on Gastrointestinal Function[a]

Gut Hormone Secretion

Inhibition of secretion of gastrin, pancreozymin, vasoactive active intestinal peptide, gut glucagon, motilin, gastric inhibitory peptide, pancreatic polypeptide, secretin secretion

Exocrine Secretion

Inhibition of gastric acid, pepsin and intrinsic factor, pancreatic bicarbonate, pancreatic enzyme secretion, colonic fluid, bile

Motor Activity

Inhibition of gastric emptying, gallbladder contraction, and small intestinal segmentation

Absorption

Decreases rate of absorption of calcium, glucose, galactose, glycerol, fructose, xylose, lactose, amino acids, triglycerides, water

Blood Flow to Gut

Decreases mesenteric blood flow, increases vascular resistance

Trophic Function

Decreases cell proliferation

Oral Ingestion of Somatostatin

Reduces gastric acid secretion

[a] Adapted from Table 4 of Gerich (9), with additions.

TABLE 7 Factors Modifying Somatostatin Secretion by the Gut[a]

Nutrients	
glucose	↔
amino acids	↑
lipids	↑
HCl	↑
mixed meal	↑
Neurotransmitters	
dopamine	↑
acetylcholine	↑
Peptides	
glucagon	↑
VIP	?
secretin	↑
substance P	↓
opiates	↓
gastrin (or pentagastrin)	↑
bombesin	↑
insulin	↓
calcitonin	↑
pancreatic polypeptide	↓
neurotensin	↔
cyclic nucleotides	↑

[a] Modified from Reichlin, [7] with additions, from Chayvialle et al. (239) and Y. C. Patel (240).

Key: ↑, elevated; ↓, decreased; ↔, no change; ?, no data available or studies are inadequate.

progression of classically recognized aspects of gut function: ingestion, propulsion, digestion, absorption, and assimilation. The most convincing analysis of these relationships is that of Schusdziarra and colleagues, who make a strong case that "somatostatin might play a physiological role in the regulation of the rate at which ingested nutrients enter the circulation" (160). The crucial findings that provide the underpinnings of this view are that somatostatin administered intravenously or by mouth reduces the postprandial rise in plasma triglycerides after a meat meal in dogs as well as the normal increases in enteroglucagon and gastrin. Further, intravenous administration of antisomatostatin leads to abnormally high postprandial levels of triglycerides, gastrin, and the pancreatic polypeptide (158). From the results of studies using antisera, they conclude that somatostatin is acting as a true hormone rather than through its paracrine effects.

Somatostatin may also serve as part of a negative feedback loop regulating gastrin and gastrin-stimulated acid secretion. Food ingestion stimulates acid production (through gastrin-mediated and vagal-muscarinic-mediated reflexes). The acidified stomach antrum is then believed (on the basis of classical experiments) to secrete a factor inhibitory to gastrin secretion—acid is one such factor, somatostatin may be another. In this context, somatostatin may be, in the words of Thomas, "the long lost antral chalone" (161). A chalone is, by definition, an inhibitory hormone. Therapeutic benefit in treatment of gastrointestinal hemorrhage has been reported by several groups (162, 163).

6.2.3 Cytoprotection in the Gastrointestinal Tract

Administration of somatostatin has been shown to reduce the toxic effects of several kinds of chemicals on gut, liver, and pancreas. These include prevention of duodenal ulcers in the rat caused by administration of several thiols including cysteamine and proprionitrile (164), adrenal cortical necrosis in the rat caused by cysteamine (165), bile-induced acute hemorrhagic pancreatitis in the dog (166), and phalloidin-induced hepatotoxicity in the rat (167). The mechanisms of prevention of toxicity have not been fully established, and might indeed be different in different kinds of injury. Cysteamine-induced ulcer is associated with severe and rapid depletion of the content of stomach, duodenal, and hypothalamic radioimmunoassayable somatostatin, leading to the suggestion that loss of the local or paracrine modulating effects of somatostatin on gastric secretion might be the mediating factor (168). However, protective doses of somatostatin do not influence acid secretion substantially (164), and depletion of somatostatin is not sufficient alone to cause ulcer, since vagotomy and bromocriptine prevent ulcer formation in cysteamine-treated rats who nevertheless show expected depletion of gut somatostatin (169).

Although there may be individual local protective factors specific to each tissue that are influenced by somatostatin, an alternative view, set forth by Szabo and Usadel (170), is that somatostatin may exert a relatively nonspecific local effect in preventing tissue injury, by a mechanism that has been termed cytoprotection. The concept of cytoprotection was introduced by Robert and colleagues (171) to describe the property of many prostaglandins to protect the mucosa of the stomach and the intestine from becoming inflamed and *necrotic* when this mucosa is exposed to noxious agents. This property is separate from and unrelated to inhibition of gastric secretion (172).

7 MECHANISMS OF ACTION OF SOMATOSTATIN

7.1 Binding

Somatostatin-binding sites have been identified by competitive binding assays in rat pituitary cells (82, 83, 173), in plasma membranes isolated from bovine pituitaries (174), in whole brain synaptosome membranes

(83, 175–177), and in isolated rat islet cells (177). Technical problems involved in measurement have been defined by Srikant and Patel (83) and include the necessity to use an analog of somatostatin that contains a tyrosine substituent (for radioiodination) and the problem of degradation by the membrane. The latter problem is important in carrying out comparative studies of a structure-function since the stability of the analog will influence the observed parameters of binding. According to Schonbrunn and Tashjian (82), rat pituitary tumor cells ($GH_4 C_1$ strain) have a single class of high-affinity binding sites ($K_d = 6 \times 10^{10}\,M^{-1}$ at 37°C), and a maximum binding capacity of 13,000 receptor sites per cell. Membranes derived from rat cerebral cortex also show a single high-affinity site ($K_d = 1.25 \times 10^{10}\,M^{-1}$) and have a maximum binding capacity (B_{max}) of 0.155×10^{-12} mole/mg (175). Cell function modulation by alteration in somatostatin receptor population is emerging as a possible mode of cell control. Schonbrunn and Tashjian have shown that exposure of rat pituitary tumor cells to TRH acutely increases the number, but not the affinity, of the somatostatin receptor but that chronic exposure for 4–72 h causes decrease in somatostatin receptor numbers (173). Exposure to cortisol also causes a decrease in somatostatin receptor numbers but by different mechanisms (178). Glucose concentration was shown by Mehler and colleagues (177) to regulate the number of somatostatin receptors on islet cells. These workers postulated that the change is due to the appearance on the cell membrane of a larger number of secretion vesicles which they have previously shown to have a higher affinity than the membranes themselves. In detailed analysis of structure-function relationships, Srikant and Patel (176) find that pituitary somatostatin receptors, as compared with brain receptors, behave differently toward several analogs, from which they have inferred that there may be more than one class of somatostatin receptor. In contrast to several other peptide systems studied previously, such as the endogenous opiates, the concentration of somatostatin in various parts of the brain is not closely correlated with receptor concentrations in the same areas (83).

7.2   Receptor Functions

Efforts to define a general mechanism to explain the action of somatostatin on a wide variety of cell types has been disappointing (see Gerich, 4, for a review). Most studies have been directed at pancreatic islet and pituitary somatotrope cells, virtually nothing being known about the biochemical-physiological basis of the action of somatostatin on neurons.

In pituitary cells, somatostatin exerts prompt and striking inhibition of secretion of GH and TSH; in pancreas somatostatin inhibits insulin and glucagon. This effect is not mediated through changes in cyclic nucleotides. Although the concentration of cyclic AMP (cAMP) is reduced in both pituitary and pancreas by exposure to somatostatin, the stimulatory effects on hormone secretion of cAMP or of agents that increase intracellular concentration of cAMP are also reduced by somatostatin. It has been concluded therefore that somatostatin acts "downstream" from cAMP to inhibit secretion.

Somatostatin reduces membrane permeability to calcium, and the inhibitory actions of somatostatin on hormone release are partially or completely reversed by exposure to A23187, an ionophore that opens calcium channels in both the external membrane and membranes of intracellular organelles. These findings have generally been interpreted to mean that somatostatin acts to block calcium-mediated intracellular activation.

A recent study by Pace and Tarvin has provided even more insight into the way somatostatin may act to inhibit islet cell function (179). The crucial new finding in their work is that somatostatin, in addition to inhibiting Ca^{2+} uptake by islet cells, also increases the permeability of cells to K^+ (as inferred from [86]rubidium washout). Since chemical agents that interfere with outward K^+ flux from islet cells (quinine and tetraethylammonium) block somatostatin effects on both insulin secretory response and the electrophysiological effects of high glucose on islet cells, these workers postulate that "SRIF may activate P_k as its primary mode of action, an event that may be sufficient to reduce the accumulation of intracellular Ca^{2+} thereby disrupting glucose-induced stimulus-secretion coupling."

The understanding of somatostatin effects on insulin secretion is further complicated by the finding that the two phases of insulin response to glucose administration (immediate and prolonged) are differentially influenced by somatostatin. The initial phase is extremely sensitive to somatostatin inhibition, whereas the later effects require much more hormone (180). Findings of this type and other evidence of dissociated responses to somatostatin further supports the suggestion that there may be more than one type of somatostatin receptor on secretory cells.

8 NEURAL FUNCTIONS OF SOMATOSTATIN

8.1 Regulation of Secretion

Depolarization of somatostatinergic nerve cells is uniformly followed by secretion of somatostatin in all preparations in which it has been studied. These include hypothalamic fragments (181–186), neurohypophysis (181, 186), cerebral cortical slices (183, 187), spinal cord (188), dispersed cerebral cortical cells in tissue culture (189), chick sensory ganglia cells in tissue culture (93), and synaptosomes (190, 191, 192). Depolarization-induced response is dependent upon the presence in the media of Ca^{2+}

and is blocked by agents that interfere with calcium entry, including Ba^{2+} and verapamil. It is clear that membrane control of somatostatin release is mediated in the same way as other neurotransmitter release processes (cf 183). Release of somatostatin is induced by veratridine, an agent that holds Na^+ channels in an open configuration (184, 189) and is blocked by the sodium channel blocker tetrodotoxin (189).

Electrical stimulation of neurohypophysis *in vitro* (181) and stimulation of the anterior periventricular area (124) leads to somatostatin release, presumably due to neuronal membrane depolarization.

The extensive list of neurotransmitters and neuropeptides that will activate somatostatin release from various neural preparations are listed in Table 2. In our own studies, the most consistent effects on cerebral cortical cells were obtained by acetylcholine, which shows a dose-related activation of somatostatin release, an effect blocked by the addition of atropine (193), indicating that it is the muscarinic form of the receptor that is being activated. The most convincing inhibitory effects were exerted by GABA, which suppressed somatostatin release. Picrotoxin, a GABA antagonist, reversed GABA effects, and, in fact, by itself produced a marked increase in somatostatin release. Gamse et al. have reported similar findings in hypothalamic cell cultures treated with GABA (192).

Influence of neuropeptides on somatostatin release is also summarized in Table 2. Most work has been carried out on hypothalamic preparations. The most consistent changes reported are increased somatostatin release after exposure to GH, glucagon, and neurotensin; inhibition of release has been reported to occur after exposure to VIP and secretin. Little is known about peptide effects on somatostatin secretion by extrahypothalamic neural tissues. Yet to be determined is whether somatostatinergic neurons in different regions are regulated in the same way by neuropeptides and neurotransmitters.

Mechanisms (including possible second messengers) by which somatostatin release is modified by neurotransmitters and neuropeptides have not been elucidated. We have found that relatively high concentrations of dibutyryl cAMP will release somatostatin from cerebral cortical cells in cultures (193), but Maeda and Frohman (184) reported no changes in release from hypothalamic fragments, and prostaglandins E_2, $E_{2\alpha}$ have been reported ineffective in modifying hypothalamic somatostatin release (194, 195, 197).

8.2 Degradation of Somatostatin

Elucidation of the mechanisms of enzyme degradation of somatostatin is relevant to understanding the role of local inactivation in control of activity of the peptide, and to the development of longer acting analogs resistant to proteolysis. This topic has been summarized (80, 81, 119).

Somatostatin is quickly broken down, by both soluble and particulate fractions of tissue, and by plasma. In plasma an active metabolite is formed (196). The best characterized enzymes responsible for this effect are endopeptidases, including cathepsin M and lysosomal cathepsin D. The latter enzyme from brain attacks the -Phe-Phe- bond in position 6-7. Digestion also takes place, but more slowly at the -Trp-Lys- bond, and this region of vulnerability can be modified by substituting D-Trp in position 8, a change which makes the molecule longer acting and increases its biological potency. Activity of both cathepsin D and pepsin are blocked by pepstatin. Regulation of hepatic degradation of somatostatin has been studied by Conlon et al. (197). Somatostatin degradation in blood is reduced by high concentrations of EDTA and aprotinin. That aprotinin is active suggests that plasmin-like activity is responsible for plasma breakdown, but the fact that this agent is not sufficient to block all degradation indicates that other enzymes are involved. Brain-degrading activity is present in both particulate and supernatant fractions of all regions of brain, although the activity is greatest in the supernatant fraction (81). There is little difference in total activity in various regions of the brain, but in the regions studied (81), activity in the cerebellum is the greatest, and, surprisingly, that of the hypothalamus is the least.

As in the case of other degrading systems found at the site of somatostatin action, little is known about factors regulating its breakdown other than thyroid status (198) or of their anatomical localization at the ultrastructural level.

8.3   Electrophysiological Effects

The earliest reports dealing with somatostatin effects on electrical activity of neurons indicated that in anesthetized cats or rats, "application of somatostatin by microiontophoresis decreases the spontaneous or glutamate evoked excitability of a proportion of neurons in the spinal cord, cerebral and cerebellar cortices and hypothalamus" (see Renaud, ref. 199, for a summary). This action, which somewhat resembles that of GABA, was not blocked by the GABA antagonists, picrotoxin or bicuculline. When iontophoresed onto cat spinal lamina V (the site of termination of dorsal root sensory nerves), spontaneous activity was depressed (Randic and Miletic, 200), and when perfused into isolated frog spinal cord, there followed, "a small but immediate hyperpolarization in ventral root fibers, an action that shows desensitization and tachyphylaxis, enhancement of synaptic transmission between dorsal and ventral roots with considerable delay, and persistence after exposure to the peptide, and expression of glutamate-evoked but not GABA-evoked responses" (quoted by Renaud, 199). Hyperpolarization of hippocampal pyramidal cells *in vitro* by somatostatin was reported by Pittman and Siggins (201).

Many of the more recent papers on somatostatin action report that this agent has an excitatory action on spontaneous activity. This has been reported for several brain areas, including cortex for rat (202, 203), in cerebral cortex of unanesthetized rabbits (204), in hippocampal slices (205), and in dispersed neuron cultures derived from mouse spinal cord (206) or rat cerebral cortex (207, 208). In the dispersed systems, application of somatostatin produced in some cells but not all, a number of effects including depolarization of neuronal membranes, enhancement of membrane excitability, increase in synaptic activity, and enhanced postsynaptic potentials.

Several unusual characteristics of the response to somatostatin may explain the discrepant reports in the literature. Delfs and Dichter (personal communication) find that there is a "rapid and dramatic diminution in the amount of polarizing or excitatory response with successive application of somatostatin", there is "an unusual dose-response relationship including an inverted U-shaped dose-response curve for membrane depolarization", and "different doses can result in qualitatively different responses with low concentrations tending to cause excitation and higher concentrations tending to cause inhibition of neuronal firing, and that a previous exposure to somatostatin can qualitatively alter the response to subsequent doses". These authors go on to postulate "the existence of two physiologically different receptors for somatostatin on cortical neurons." Similarly, variable responses to somatostatin are elicited from neurons of the myenteric plexus of guinea pig ileum (106).

8.4   Effect of Somatostatin on Neurotransmitter Secretion

Somatostatin has been reported mainly to inhibit release of neurotransmitters. This has been shown to be true for acetylcholine release from intestine (209, 210), norepinephrine release from hypothalamus (211) and from adrenal medullary cells (212), and TRH release from rat hypothalamus (213). On the other hand, somatostatin is reported to stimulate release of acetylcholine from rat hippocampal synaptosomes (214), norepinephrine release from cortex (215), and serotonin release from several brain areas (216). Somatostatin administered intracerebroventricularly is reported to increase concentrations of dopamine in several brain areas and 5-hydroxytryptamine (5-HT) in the limbic system (217), and to increase acetylcholine turnover rate in diencephalon and hippocampus (218).

8.5   Effects on Behavior

Many different behavioral changes have been noted to follow the intracerebroventricular injection of somatostatin. These have been summarized (219–222). Somatostatin under most but not all conditions causes an increased excitability of cerebral cortex. Intraventricular injection of antisomatostatin reduces the severity and duration of strychnine induced seizures (223). When given into the ventricles or into hippocampus, somatostatin "has a general arousal effect, reducing both slow-wave and paradoxical sleep, and in higher "pharmacological" doses (1–10 μg) it produces signs of pathological irritation such as hyperkinesia, stereotypic behavior, muscle tremor and rigidity, catatonia and finally, tonic-clonic seizures" (Ioffe et al, 204). The term catatonia is in reality of misnomer and more properly should be referred to as catalepsy, a response similar to that observed after intracerebral injection of β-endorphin. Somatostatin-induced effects (unlike those of endorphins) are not reversed by naloxone and hence are presumed to act through nonopiate mechanisms. Other behaviors that have been observed after central administration are decreased sleep, excessive grooming and exploring, arrest of ongoing behaviors, motor incoordination, and analgesia. These findings are most compatible with reports of increased firing of neurons after local exposure to the peptide (see above), and they indicate that somatostatin most likely exerts important neural effects in many regions of the brain, including motor cortex, hippocampus, and limbic system.

8.6   Somatostatin in Cerebrospinal Fluid

As might be expected from the wide distribution of somatostatin-secreting cells throughout the brain, and their proximity to the ventricles and subarachnoid space, this peptide is secreted into the cerebrospinal fluid (CSF). In the first studies of somatostatin CSF published from my laboratory (224), mean levels in normals were 35.4 pg/mL based on seven cases. A much larger series of cases, numbering 39 volunteers, all obtained between 8 and 9 a.m., gave a mean of 62.8 ± 6.38 SEM (225). Similar values have been reported by Kronheim et al. (226) and Wass et al. (227), and somewhat higher values in the study of Sørensen et al. (228). The peptide is relatively stable in cerebrospinal fluid, showing only a modest decline in immunoreactivity over time.

In an attempt to determine the site of entry of somatostatin into the CSF, comparisons have been made of the concentration of immunoreactive somatostatin in the first ml with that of later fractions. In the studies by Sørensen et al. (228) there was no difference in content in the eleventh ml as compared with the first ml. In our own studies, comparisons were made of the 29th ml with a pool of the 1–12 ml (225). Mean values were slightly but significantly higher in the later samples. The site of somatostatin release into the CSF is anatomically diffuse and not restricted to the hypothalamus, but a detailed profile of levels remains to be established. At the very least, these findings make it important for workers to measure defined samples when making comparisons of clinical states. Berelowitz et al. (229) have recently shown that CSF somatostatin concentration in the monkey varies with a distinct circadian rhythm, with maximum excursion of $\pm$ 10% of the mean value, the lowest values observed during the day. The functional significance of this variation is not known. It is not correlated with GH regulation (as judged by known patterns of diurnal GH secretion), nor is it correlated with the known alerting functions of somatostatin, since values are lowest during lighted hours. Acromegalic patients have normal CSF somatostatin levels (224, 227).

Published reports differ somewhat in their analysis of the molecular forms of somatostatin demonstrable in CSF. Our own studies, based on Biogel P10 chromatography, indicate that forms with the characteristics of somatostatin-14, somatostatin-28, and 11,500 daltons are present in human CSF, in proportion to the forms secreted into the media of cerebral cells in tissue culture or in extracts of cortical cells (230).

9 PATHOLOGICAL ALTERATIONS OF SOMATOSTATIN IN BRAIN DISEASE

9.1 Organic Brain Diseases

In view of its wide distribution and important physiological effects, studies of brain somatostatin secretion in various forms of brain disorder are of obvious importance. However, the limited approaches that are available to clinical investigators and problems of determining local secretion rates in functionally relevant brain regions make meaningful studies of this problem difficult. Hence, available studies have utilized the less satisfactory measurement of tissue concentrations in autopsy material or have used measurements of CSF. Somatostatin concentration in brains of patients with Alzheimer's disease and Alzheimer's senile dementia was reported to be markedly reduced in all regions tested; hippocampus, frontal cortex, parietal cortex, and superior temporal gyrus (231). Only acetylcholinergic neurons are similarly involved, other transmitter–containing neurons including dopaminergic, noradrenergic, serotonergic, and GABAergic being well maintained.

In another study (232), similar but less striking changes were reported for cerebral cortex, hippocampus, amygdala, and temporal cortex. The validity of using postmortem brains for analysis was established by Cooper et al. (233), who found little variations in concentration of somatostatin (or substance P) in brain tissue removed at different time periods up to 24 h and then stored. This is in contrast with the rapid degradation of somatostatin in incubated extracts, and it suggests that in whole brain, somatostatin is stored in a compartmented site where it is protected from peptidases. As pointed out by Bird (234), these studies do not exclude the occurrence of very early changes during the first two hours. Concentrations of somatostatin in several regions of the human brain have been reported by Patel et al. (224) and Cooper et al. (233). I measured somatostatin concentrations in the hypothalamus (exclusive of median eminence) of 20 patients with Huntington's disease and compared values obtained with those of 19 patients dying of noncerebral disorders, using samples prepared by Dr. Edward Bird (234). Choreic patients had significantly higher concentrations. This observation is made more meaningful by the recent report of Aronin et al in which somatostatin was shown to be increased in the basal ganglia in Huntington's disease.[234a]

Another brain disorder in which elevated somatostatin levels were determined in virtually all anatomical regions is the fetal alcohol syndrome in rats. Guyetsky, Jacobson, and Reichlin (unpublished) have found that rats born of alcohol fed mothers had significantly higher absolute and relative amounts of somatostatin in their brains, and that the defect persisted for more than a month after birth.

In collaboration with Paul Kornblith, I measured immunoreactive somatostatin in 17 cultured cell lines derived from glioblastoma, medulloblastoma, neuroma, meningioma, craniopharyngioma, astrocytoma, hemangioma, chordoma, and neuroblastoma. None showed any immunoreactivity. The only human brain tumor to have shown immunoreactive somatostatin that I am aware of was that of a case of hamartoma of the hypothalamus reported by Hochman et al. (235).

9.2 Somatostatin in Cerebrospinal Fluid in Neurological Disorders

Pathological increases in somatostatin concentration were observed in patients with a variety of structural CNS diseases including brain tumor, spinal cord compression, and metabolic encephalopathy, changes interpreted as indicating nerve cell damage, and possibly secretion by the tumor (224; Urosa and Reichlin, unpublished).

Decreased CSF somatostatin was reported in patients with multiple sclerosis in relapse (236). The difference from normal was quite small and, as noted above, values in the normals were considerably higher than those reported by several other authors.

9.3 Cerebrospinal Fluid in Psychiatric Disorders

In recent studies by Rubinow and collaborators (225), CSF somatostatin was found to be significantly reduced in patients with unipolar depression, and values returned to normal with recovery. Insufficient information is available to determine the significance of these findings. Are they indicative of a phase shift (values in monkeys as noted above are lowest during lighted hours), or a marker of state abnormality, or part of the mechanisms responsible for depression? Manic patients show CSF somatostatin levels indistinguishable from normal. Rubinow and colleagues (225) have also shown that administration of zimelidine (a serotonin agonist) raises CSF somatostatin, and that carbamazepine, an anticonvulsant with antidepressant properties, lowers CSF somatostatin. The mechanisms of action of these agents is unknown.

9.4 Potential for Therapeutic Use of Somatostatin

Intravenous somatostatin in humans was reported by Gerich to have a mild tranquilizing action (4). Specific effects on extrapyramidal motor dysfunction and on paroxysmal EEG were sought by Dupont et al. (239), who administered the peptide intravenously. No psychological changes of any kind were noted. These authors point out the obvious fact that entry of the peptide into the brain is uncertain. The use of agents that enter the brain will be required before an adequate answer can be given to the question of therapeutic use in humans.

REFERENCES

1. P. Brazeau, W. Vale, R. Burgus, N. Ling, M. Butcher, J. Rivier, and R. Guillemin, *Science* **179**, 77 (1973).
2. W. Vale, C. Rivier, and M. Brown, *Annu. Rev. Physiol.* **39**, 527 (1977).
3. J. E. Gerich, S. Raptis, and J. Rosenthal, Eds., *Somatostatin Symp. Metab.* **28**, 1129–1469 (1978).
4. J. E. Gerich, "Somatostatin," in M. Brownlee, Ed., *Handbook of Diabetes Mellitus*, Vol. 1, Garland STPM Press, New York, 1980, p. 297–354.
5. B. L. Pimstone, M. Sheppard, B. Shapiro, S. Kronheim, A. Hudson, S. Hendricks, and K. Waligora, *Fed. Proc.* **38**, 2330 (1979).
6. S. M. McCann, L. Krulich, A. Negro-Vilar, S. R. Ojeda, and E. Vijayan, *Adv. Biochem. Psychopharmacol.* **22**, 131 (1980).
7. S. Reichlin, *Adv. Biochem. Psychopharmacol.* **28**, 573 (1981).
8. J. E. Morley, *Endocr. Rev.* **2**, 396 (1981).
9. J. E. Gerich, *Am. J. Med.* **70**, 619 (1981).
10. A. Arimura and J. B. Fishback, *Neuroendocrinology* **33**, 246 (1981).
11. R. E. Miller, *Endocr. Rev.* **2**, 471 (1981).
12. I. S. Gottesman, L. J. Mandarino, and J. E. Gerich, in M. Cohen and P. Foa, Eds., *Special Topics in Endocrinology and Metabolism*, Vol. 4, 1982, in press.
13. L. Krulich, A. P. S. Dhariwal, and S. M. McCann, *Endocrinology* **83**, 783 (1968).
14. B. Hellman and A. Lernmark, *Endocrinology* **84**, 1484 (1969).
15. A. Schally, A. DuPont, A. Arimura, T. Redding, N. Nishi, G. L. Linthicum, and D. H. Schlesinger, *Biochemistry* **15**, 50 (1976).
16. A. V. Schally, A. DuPont, A. Arimura, T. W. Redding, N. Nishi, G. L. Linthicum, and D. H. Schlesinger, *Biochemistry* **15**, 509 (1976).
17. J. Speiss, J. E. Rivier, J. A. Rodkey, C. D. Bennett, and W. Vale, *Proc. Natl. Acad. Sci. USA* **76**, 2974 (1979).
18. L. Pradayrol, H. Jörnvall, V. Mutt, and A. Ribet, *FEBS Lett.* **109**, 55 (1980).
19. R. P. Miller, *J. Endocrin.* **77**, 429 (1977).

20.   Y. C. Patel and S. Reichlin, *Endocrinology* **102**, 523 (1978).
21.   J. Spiess and W. Vale, *Metabolism* **27**, Suppl. 1, 1175 (1978).
22.   J. Conlon, E. Zyznar, W. Vale, and R. Unger, *FEBS Lett.* **94**, 327 (1978).
23.   O. P. Rorstad, J. Epelbaum, P. Brazeau, and J. B. Martin, *Endocrinology* **105**, 1083 (1979).
24.   Y. C. Patel, T. Wheatley, and C. Ning, *Endocrinology* **109**, 1943 (1981).
25.   M. Lauber, M. Camier, and P. Cohen, *Proc. Natl. Acad. Sci. USA* **76**, 6004 (1979).
26.   R. H. Goodman, J. W. Jacobs, W. W. Chin, P. K. Lund, P. C. Dee, and J. F. Habener, *Proc. Natl. Acad. Sci. USA* **77**, 5869 (1980).
27.   P. Hobart, R. Crawford, L. P. Shen, R. Pictet, and W. J. Rutter, *Nature* **288**, 137 (1980).
28.   W. L. Taylor, K. J. Collier, R. J. Deschenes, H. L. Weith, and J. E. Dixon, *Proc. Natl. Acad. Sci. USA* **78**, 6694 (1981).
29.   R. H. Goodman, J. W. Jacobs, P. C. Dee, and J. R. Habener, *J. Biol. Chem.* **257**, 1156 (1982).
30.   W. Vale, N. Ling, J. Rivier, J. Villarreal, C. Rivier, M. Brown, and C. Douglas, *Metabolism* **25**, Suppl. 1, 1491 (1976).
31.   A. Arimura, H. Sato, D. Coy, and A. V. Schally, *Proc. Soc. Exp. Biol. Med.* 784 (1975).
32.   S. Falkmer, R. Elde, C. Hellerstrom, and B. Petersson, *Metabolism* **27**, Suppl. 1, 1193 (1978).
33.   I. M. D. Jackson, Am. Zool. **18**, 385 (1978).
34.   D. LeRoith, M. Berelowitz, M. Szabo, L. A. Frohman, H. Von Schenk, R. H. Unger, J. Shiloach, and J. Roth. *Diabetes* 30: (supplement 1) 179, 1981.
35.   B. D. Noe, J. Speiss, J. E. Rivier, W. Vale, *Endocrinology* **105**, 1410 (1979).
36.   H. Oyama, R. A. Bradshaw, O. J. Bates, and A. Permutt, *J. Biol. Chem.* **225**, 2251 (1980).
37.   Grimm-Jorgensen, *Y. Gen Comp. Endocrinol.* **35**, 387, 1978.
38.   J. Roth, D. LeRoith, J. Shiloach, J. L. Rosenzweig, M. A. Lesniak, and J. Havrankova, *N. Engl. J. Med.* **306**, 523 (1982).
39.   B. D. Noe, *J. Biol. Chem.* **256**, 9397 (1981).
40.   D. Pearson, J. E. Shively, B. R. Clark, I. L. Geschwind, M. Barkley, R. S. Nishioka, and H. A. Bern, *Proc. Natl. Acad. Sci. USA* **77**, 5021 (1980).
41.   D. Shields, T. G. Warren, R. F. Green, S. E. Roth, M. J. Brenner, in D. H. Rich and E. Gross, Eds., *Peptides: Synthesis, Structure, Function*, Pierce Chemical Co., 1981, pp. 471–479.
42.   R. H. Goodman, P. K. Lund, F. H. Barnett, and J. F. Habener, *J. Biol. Chem.* **25**, 1499 (1981).
43.   R. Guillemin, *Neurosci. Res. Program Bull.* **16**, 1 (1978).
44.   M. Brownstein, A. Arimura, H. Sato, A. V. Schally, and J. S. Kizer, *Endocrinology* **96**, 1456 (1975).
45.   M. Palkovits, M. J. Brownstein, A. Arimura, H. Sato, V. Schally, and J. S. Kizer, *Brain Res.* **109**, 430 (1976).
46.   L. C. Alpert, J. R. Brawer, Y. C. Patel, and S. Reichlin, *Endocrinology* **98**, 255 (1976).
47.   K. M. Knigge, S. A. Joseph, and G. E. Hoffman, "Organization of LRF- and SRIF-neurons in the endocrine hypothalamus," in S. Reichlin, R. J. Baldessarini, and J. B. Martin, Eds., *The Hypothalamus*, Raven Press, New York, 1978, p. 49–67.
48.   T. Hökfelt, R. Elde, K. Fuxe, O. Johansson, H. Ljungdahl, M. Goldstein, R. Luft, S. Efendic, G. Nilsson, L. Terenius, D. Ganten, S. L. Jeffcoate, J. Rehfeld, S. Said, M. Perez de la Mora, L. Possani, R. Tapia, L. Teran, and R. Palacios, in S. Reichlin, R. J. Baldessarini, and J. B. Martin, Eds., *The Hypothalamus*, Raven Press, New York, 1978, p. 69–135.
49.   B. Krisch, *Cell Tissue Res.* **195**, 499 (1978).
50.   W. R. Crowley and L. C. Terry, *Brain Res.* **200**, 283 (1980).

51. G. Pelletier, Prog. Histochem. Cytochem. **12**, 1 (1980).
52. C. Bennett-Clarke, M. A. Romagnano, and S. A. Joseph, *Brain Res.* **188**, 473 (1980).
53. Y. C. Patel, K. Hoyte, and J. B. Martin, *Endocrinology* **105**, 712 (1979).
54. F. W. van Leeuwen, C. de Raay, D. F. Swaab, and B. Fisser, *Cell Tissue Res.* **202**, 189 (1979).
55. B. Krisch, *Cell Tissue Res.* **217**, 531 (1981).
56. T. Hökfelt, R. Elde, O. Johansson, R. Luft, and A. Arimura, *Neurosci. Lett.* **1**, 231 (1975).
57. J. N. Lundberg, T. Hökfelt, G. Nilsson, L. Terenius, J. Rehfeld, R. Elde, and S. Said, *Acta Physiol. Scand.* **104**, 499 (1978).
58. T. Hökfelt, O. Johansson, A. Ljungdahl, J. M. Lundberg, and M. Schultzbert, *Nature* **284**, 515 (1980).
59. O. P. Rorstad, M. J. Brownstein, and J. B. Martin, *Proc. Natl. Acad. Sci. USA* **76**, 3019 (1979).
60. B. Krisch and H. Leonhardt, *Cell Tissue Res.* **204**, 127 (1979).
61. T. Yamada, D. Marshak, S. Basinger, J. Walsh, J. Morley, and W. Stell, *Proc. Natl. Acad. Sci. USA* **77**, 1691 (1980).
62. K. Takatsuki, S. Shiosaka, M. Sakanaka, S. Inagaki, E. Senba, H. Takagi, and M. Tohyama, *Brain Res.* **213**, 211 (1981).
63. C. Rufener, M. Dubois, F. Mallaisse-Lagae, and L. Orci, *Diabetologia* **11**, 321 (1975).
64. V. Helmstaedter, G. Feurle, and W. Forssmann, *Cell Tissue Res.* **177**, 29 (1977).
65. W. Forssman, V. Helmstaedter, J. Metz, G. Muhlmann, and G. Feurle, *Metabolism* **27**, Suppl. 1, 1179 (1978).
66. C. McIntosh, R. Arnold, E. Bothe, H. Becker, J. Kobberling, and W. Creutzfeld, *Metabolism* **27**, Suppl. 1, 1317 (1978).
67. J. A. Chayvialle, M. Miyata, P. L. Rayford, and J. C. Thompson, *Gastroenterology* **79**, 837 (1980).
68. M. Costa, J. B. Furness, I. J. Smith, B. Davies, and J. Oliver, *Neuroscience* **5**, 841 (1980).
69. M. Dubois, *Proc. Natl. Acad. Sci. USA* **72**, 1340 (1975).
70. L. Orci, D. Baetens, and C. Rufener, *Horm. Metab. Res.* **7**, 400 (1975).
71. P. Goldsmith, J. Rose, A. Arimura, and W. Ganong, *Endocrinology* **97**, 1061 (1975).
72. J. Polak, L. Grimelius, A. Pearse, S. Bloom, and A. Arimura, *Lancet* **1**, 1220 (1975).
73. V. Schusdziarra, E. Ipp, V. Harris, R. E. Dobbs, P. Raskin, L. Orci, and R. H. Unger, *Metabolism* **28**, 1227 (1978).
74. C. Girod, M. P. Dubois, and N. Durand, *Histochemistry* **69**, 137 (1980).
75. J. N. Forrest, Jr., S. Reichlin, and D. B. P. Goodman, *Proc. Natl. Acad. Sci. USA* **77**, 4984 (1980).
76. J. L. Bolaffi, S. Reichlin, D. B. P. Goodman, and J. N. Forrest Jr., *Science* **210**, 644 (1980).
77. G. Pelletier, F. Labrie, A. Arimura, and A. V. Schally, *Amer. J. Anat.* **140**, 445 (1974).
78. J. Epelbaum, P. Brazeau, D. Tsang, J. Brawer, and J. B. Martin, *Brain Res.* **126**, 309 (1977).
79. M. Berelowitz, J. Matthews, B. L. Pimstone, S. Kronheim, and H. Sacks, *Metabolism* **27**, Suppl. 1, 1171 (1978).
80. E. C. Griffiths, S. L. Jeffcoate, and D. T. Holland, *Acta Endocrinol. (KBH)* **85**, 1 (1977).
81. N. Marks, in W. F. Ganong and L. Martini, Eds., *Frontiers in Neuroendocrinology*, Vol. 5, Raven Press, 1978, p. 329–377.
82. A. Schonbrunn and A. H. Tashjian Jr., *J. Biol. Chem.* **253**, 6473 (1978).
83. C. B. Srikant and Y. C. Patel, *Proc. Natl. Acad. Sci. USA* **78**, 3930 (1981).
84. S. Reichlin, in F. E. Bloom, Ed., *Peptides: Integrators of Cell and Tissue Function*. Soc. Gen. Physiol. Series, Vol. 35, Raven Press, New York, 1980, p. 235.
85. R. N. Lechan, J. Nestler, S. Jacobson, and S. Reichlin, *Brain Res.* **195**, 13 (1980).

86. R. M. Lechan, J. L. Nestler, and S. Jacobson, *Brain Res.*, **245**, 1, 1982.
87. B. S. Layton, S. Lafontaine, and L. P. Renaud, *Neuroendocrinology* **33**, 235 (1981).
88. M. J. Brownstein, A. Arimura, R. Fernandez-Durango, A. V. Schally, M. Palkovits, and J. S. Kizer, *Endocrinology* **100**, 246 (1977).
89. J. Epelbaum, J. O. Willoughby, P. Brazeau, and J. B. Martin, *Endocrinology* **101**, 1495 (1977).
90. V. Critchlow, R. W. Rice, K. Abe, and W. Vale, *Endocrinology* **103**, 817 (1978).
91. C. G. Rasool, A. L. Schwartz, J. A. Bollinger, S. Reichlin, and W. G. Bradley, *Endocrinology* **108**, 996 (1981).
92. J. A. Kessler and I. B. Black, *Proc. Natl. Acad. Sci. USA* **78**, 4644 (1981).
93. A. W. Mudge, G. D. Fishbach, and S. E. Leeman, *Soc. Neurosci. Abstr.* **3**, 1304 (1977).
94. T. Hökfelt, L. G. Elfvin, R. Elde, M. Schultzberg, M. Goldstein, and R. Luft, *Proc. Natl. Acad. Sci. USA* **74**, 3587 (1977).
95. I. Lowe, D. Blais, O. Ronnekleiv, C. Morgan, I. Nadelhaft, and W. de Groat, *Soc. Neurosci. Abstr.* **7**, 101 (1981).
96. E. F. Eriksen and L. I. Larsson, *Peptides* **2**, 153 (1981).
97. L. K. Laemle, S. C. Feldman, and E. Lichtenstein, *Soc. Neurosci. Abstr.* **7**, 761 (1981).
98. C. Burnweit and W. G. Forssmann, *Cell Tissue Res.* **200**, 83 (1979).
99. A. Tessler, M. E. Goldberger, M. Murray, B. T. Himes, and R. Artymyshyn, *Soc. Neurosci. Abstr.* **6**, 173 (1980).
100. B. Krisch, *Cell Tissue Res.* **212**, 457 (1980).
101. J. Delfs, R. Robbins, J. L. Connolly, M. Dichter, and S. Reichlin, *Nature* **283**, 676 (1980).
102. B. Krisch and H. Leonhardt, *Cell Tissue Res.* **210**, 33 (1980).
103. R. Arnold and P. G. Lankisch, *Clin. Gastroenterol.* **9**, 733 (1980).
104. L. I. Larsson, in *Clin. Gastroenterol.* **9**, 485 (1980).
105. F. Sundler, R. Håkanson, and S. Leander, *Clin. Gastroenterol.* **9**, 517 (1980).
106. Y. Katayama and R. A. North, *J. Physiol.* **303**, 315 (1980).
107. J. Molnar, A. Arimura, and A. Kastin, *Fed. Proc.* **35**, 782 (1976).
108. S. VanNoorden, J. Polak, and A. Pearse, *Histochemistry* **53**, 243 (1977).
109. Y. Yamada, S. Ito, Y. Matsubara, and S. Kobayashi, Tohoku *J. Exp. Med.* **122**, 87 (1977).
110. F. Sundler, J. Alumets, R. Håkanson, L. Bjorklund, and O. Ljungberg, *Am. J. Pathol.* **88**, 381 (1977).
111. R. S. Birnbaum, M. Muszynski, and B. A. Roos, *Cancer Res.* **40**, 4192 (1980).
112. A. Gordin, B. Lamberg, R. Pelkonen, and S. Almqvist, *Clin. Endocrinol.* **8**, 289 (1978).
113. S. Kronheim, M. Berelowitz, and B. L. Pimstone, *Clin. Endocrinol.* **5**, 619 (1976).
114. I. Reid and J. Rose, *Endocrinology* **100**, 782 (1977).
115. S. Kronheim, M. Berelowitz, and B. Pimstone, *Clin. Endocrinol.* **7**, 343 (1977).
116. A. Gomez-Pan, M. Snow, D. Piercy, V. Robson, R. Wilkinson, R. Hall, C. Evered, G. M. Besser, A. V. Schally, A. Kastin, and D. Coy, *J. Clin. Endocrinol. Metab.* **43**, 240 (1976).
117. J. Rosenthal, F. Escobar-Jimenez, S. Raptis, and E. Pfeiffer, *Lancet* **1**, 772 (1976).
118. J. Rosenthal, F. Escobar-Jimenez, and S. Raptis, *Clin. Endocrinol.* **6**, 455 (1977).
119. B. S. Chertow, *Endocr. Reviews* **2**, 137 (1981).
120. R. Robbins, Program of the 64th Annual Meeting of the Endocrine Society, San Francisco, Calif., 1982, p. 138.
121. L. Mandarino, D. Stenner, W. Blanchard, S. Nissen, J. Gerich, N. Ling, P. Brazeau, P. Bohlen, F. Esch, and R. Guillemin, *Nature* **291**, 76 (1981).
122. C. A. Meyers, W. A. Murphy, T. W. Redding, D. H. Coy, and A. V. Schally, *Proc. Natl. Acad. Sci. USA* **77**, 6171 (1980).

123. M. Brown, J. Rivier, and W. Vale, *Endocrinology* **108**, 2391 (1981).

124. J. B. Martin, P. Brazeau, G. S. Tannenbaum, J. O. Willoughby, J. Epelbaum, L. C. Terry, and D. Durand, in S. Reichlin, R. J. Baldessarini, and J. B. Martin, Eds., *The Hypothalamus*, Raven Press, New York, 1978, p. 329–358.

125. L. C. Terry and J. B. Martin, *Endocrinology* **109**, 622 (1981).

126. K. Chihara, A. Arimura, C. Kubli-Garfias, and A. V. Schally, *Endocrinology* **105**, 1416 (1979).

127. A. Arimura, W. Smith, and A. V. Schally, *Endocrinology* **98**, 540 (1976).

128. L. Ferland, F. Labrie, M. Jobin, A. Arimura, and A. Schally, *Biochem. Biophys. Res. Commun.* **68**, 149 (1976).

129. L. C. Terry, J. O. Willoughby, P. Brazeau, J. B. Martin, and Y. C. Patel, *Science* **192**, 565 (1976).

130. G. Tannenbaum, J. Epelbaum, E. Colle, P. Brazeau, and J. Martin, *Endocrinology* **102**, 1909 (1978).

131. D. Hoffman and B. Baker, *Proc. Soc. Exp. Biol. Med.* **156**, 265 (1977).

132. I. Wakabayashi, R. Demura, M. Kanda, H. Demura, and K. Shizume, *Endocrinol. Jpn.* **23**, 439 (1976).

133. R. Fernandez-Durango, A. Arimura, J. Fishback, and A. Schally, *Proc. Soc. Exp. Biol. Med.* **157**, 235 (1978).

134. M. Berelowitz, S. L. Firestone, and L. A. Frohman, *Endocrinology* **109**, 714 (1981).

135. M. C. Sheppard, S. Kronheim, and B. L. Pimstone, *Clin. Endocrinol.* **9**, 583 (1978).

136. K. Chihara, N. Minamitani, H. Kaji, A. Arimura, and T. Fujita, *Endocrinology* **109**, 2279 (1981).

137. M. E. Molitch, H. Abe, J. J. Van Wyk, and L. E. Underwood, Program of the 64th Annual Meeting of the Endocrine Society, San Francisco, Calif., 1982, p. 126.

138. M. Berelowitz, M. Szabo, L. A. Frohman, S. L. Firestone, L. Chu, and R. L. Hintz, *Science* **212**, 1279 (1981).

139. M. D. Lumpkin, N. Negro-Vilar, and S. M. McCann, *Science* **211**, 1072 (1981).

140. W. Vale, C. Rivier, P. Brazeau, and R. Guillemin, *Endocrinology* **95**, 968 (1975).

141. P. Tanjasiri, X. Kozbur, and W. Florsheim, *Life Sci.* **19**, 657 (1976).

142. K. Chihara, A. Arimura, M. Chihara, and A. V. Schally, *Endocrinology* **103**, 1916 (1978).

143. J. Weeke, A. Hansen, and K. Lundbaek, *J. Clin. Endocrinol. Metab.* **41**, 168 (1975).

144. C. Lucke, B. Hoffken, and A. von zur Muhlen, *J. Clin. Endocrinol. Metab.* **41**, 1082 (1975).

145. T. Siler, S. Yen, W. Vale, and R. Guillemin, *J. Clin. Endocrinol. Metab.* **38**, 742 (1974).

146. J. Weeke, A. Hansen, and K. Lundbaek, *Scand. J. Clin. Lab. Invest.* **33**, 101 (1974).

147. A. Gordin, A. Arimura, and A. V. Schally, *Proc. Soc. Exp. Biol. Med.* **153**, 319 (1976).

148. A. Arimura and A. V. Schally, *Endocrinology* **98**, 1069 (1976).

149. S. Reichlin, J. B. Martin, and I. M. D. Jackson, in S. L. Jeffcoate and J. S. M. Hutchinson, Eds., *The Endocrine Hypothalamus*, Academic Press, London, 1978, p. 230–269.

150. M. Berelowitz, K. Maeda, S. Harris, and L. A. Frohman, *Endocrinology* **107**, 24 (1980).

151. H. Abe, R. Robbins, and S. Reichlin, Program of the 64th Meeting of the Endocrine Society, San Francisco, Calif., 1982, p. 309.

152. E. Ipp, J. Rivier, R. E. Dobbs, M. Brown, W. Vale, and R. H. Unger, *Endocrinology* **104**, 1270 (1979).

153. I. Holm, L. Thulin, H. Samnegard, S. Efendic, and G. Tyden, *Acta Physiol. Scand.* **104**, 241 (1978).

154. G. L. Ricci and J. Fevery, *Gastroenterology* **81**, 552 (1981).

155. S. Raptis, W. Schlegel, and E. E. Pfeiffer, in S. R. Brown, Ed., *Gut Hormones*, Churchill Livingstone, Edinburgh, 1978, p. 446–452.

156. R. Arnold and P. G. Lankisch, *Clin. Gastroenterol.* **9**, 733 (1980).

157. F. Sundler, R. Håkanson, and S. Leander, *Clin. Gastroenterol.* **9**, 517 (1980).

158. V. Schusdziarra, E. Zyznar, D. Rouiller, G. Boden, J. C. Brown, A. Arimura, and R. H. Unger, *Science* **207**, 530 (1980).

159. K. Uvnas-Wallenstein, *Clin. Gastroenterol.* **9**, 545 (1980).

160. V. Schusdziarra, D. Rouiller, and R. H. Unger, *Life Sci.* **24**, 1595 (1979).

161. W. E. G. Thomas, *Med. Hypotheses* **6**, 919 (1980).

162. H. Bauer and G. F. Schmidt, *Z. Gastroenterol.* **18**, 314 (1980).

163. L. Kayassah, K. Gyr, U. Keller, and G. A. Stalder, *Z. Gastroenterol.* **18**, 342 (1980).

164. U. Schwedes, K. Usadel, and S. Szabo, *Eur. J. Pharmacol.* **44**, 195 (1977).

165. D. J. McComb, K. Kovacs, H. C. Horner, G. T. Gallagher, U. Schwedes, K. H. Usadel, and S. Szabo, Exp. Mol. Pathol. **35**, 422 (1981).

166. U. Schwedes, P. H. Althoff, I. Klempa, U. Leuschner, L. Mothes, S. Raptis, J. Wdowinski, and K. H. Usadel, *Horm. Metab. Res.* **11**, 655 (1979).

167. J. M. Wdowinski, U. Schwedes, H. Faulstich, H. Dancygier, U. Leuschner, W. H. Siede, K. Hubner, K. Schöffling, and K. H. Usadel, *Res. Exp. Med.* **178**, 155 (1981).

168. S. Szabo and S. Reichlin, *Endocrinology* **109**, 2255 (1981).

169. S. Szabo and S. Reichlin, Abstract, 4th International Symposium on Gastrointestinal Hormones, Stockholm, Sweden, 20–23 June, 1982.

170. S. Szabo and K. H. Usadel, *Experientia* **38**, 254 (1982).

171. A. Robert, J. E. Nezamis, C. Lancaster, and A. J. Hancher, *Gastroenterology* **77**, 433 (1979).

172. A. Robert, *Gastroenterology* **77**, 761 (1979).

173. A. Schonbrunn and A. H. Tashjian Jr., *J. Biol. Chem.* **255**, 190 (1980).

174. J. W. Leitner, R. M. Rifkin, A. Maman, and K. E. Sussman, *Biochem. Biophys. Res. Com.* **87**, 919 (1979).

175. J. C. Reubi, M. H. Perrin, J. E. Rivier, and W. Vale, *Life Sci.* **28**, 2191 (1981).

176. C. B. Srikant and Y. C. Patel, *Endocrinology* **108**, 341 (1981).

177. P. S. Mehler, A. L. Sussman, A. Maman, J. W. Leitner, and K. E. Sussman, *J. Clin. Invest.* **66**, 1334 (1980).

178. A. Schonbrunn, *Endocrinology* **110**, 1147 (1982).

179. C. S. Pace and J. T. Tarvin, *Diabetes* **30**, 836 (1981).

180. D. L. Curry and L. L. Bennett, *Proc. Natl. Acad. Sci. USA* **73**, 248 (1976).

181. Y. C. Patel, H. H. Zingg, and J. J. Dreifuss, *Metabolism* **27**, 1243 (1978).

182. M. Berelowitz, S. Kronheim, B. Pimstone, and M. Sheppard, *J. Neurochem.* **31**, 1537 (1978).

183. L. L. Iversen, S. D. Iversen, F. Bloom, C. Douglas, M. Brown, and M. Vale, *Nature* **273**, 161 (1978).

184. K. Maeda and L. A. Frohman, *Endocrinology* **106**, 1837 (1980).

185. L. L. Iverson, C. M. Lee, R. F. Gilbert, S. Hunt, and P. C. Emson, *Proc. R. Soc. Lond., Ser., B* **210**, 91 (1980).

186. Y. C. Patel, H. H. Zingg, and J. J. Dreifuss, *Nature* **267**, 852 (1977).

187. S. L. Lee, V. Havlicek, A. E. Panerai, and H. G. Freisen, *Experientia* **35**, 351 (1979).

188. M. Sheppard, S. Kronheim, C. Adams, and B. Pimstone, *Neurosci. Lett.* **15**, 65 (1979).

189. R. J. Robbins, R. E. Sutton, and S. Reichlin, *Endocrinology* **110**, 496 (1982).

190. I. Wakabayashi, Y. Miyazawa, M. Kanda, N. Miki, R. Demura, H. Demura, and K. Shizume, *Endocrinol. Jpn.* **24**, 601 (1977).

191. G. W. Bennett, J. A. Edwardson, D. Marcano de Cotte, M. Berelowitz, B. L. Pimstone, and S. Kronheim, *J. Neurochem.* **32**, 1127 (1979).

192. R. Gamse, D. Vaccaro, G. Gamse, M. DuPage, T. O. Fox, and S. F. Leeman, *Proc. Natl. Acad. Sci. USA* **77**, 5552 (1980).

193. R. J. Robbins, R. E. Sutton, and S. Reichlin, *Brain Res.* **234**, 377 (1982).
194. S. R. Ojeda, A. Negro-Vilar, A. Arimura, and S. M. McCann, *Neuroendocrinology* **31**, 7 (1980).
195. L. C. Terry, O. P. Rorstad, and J. B. Martin, *Endocrinology* **107**, 794 (1980).
196. F. Mårki, L. Schenkel, B. Petrack, A. J. Czernik, J. Ansell, M. Allen, D. E. Brundish, J. R. Martin, C. McMartin, G. E. Peters, and R. Wade, *FEBS Lett.* **127**, 22 (1981).
197. J. Conlon, J. Whittaker, V. Hammond, and K. G. Alberti, *Biochim. Biophys. Acta* **677**, 234 (1981).
198. A. Dupont, Y. Merand, and N. Barden, *Life Sci.* **23**, 2007 (1978).
199. L. P. Renaud, in A. M. Gotto Jr., E. J. Peck Jr., and A. E. Boyd III., *Brain Peptides: A New Endocrinology*, Elsevier/North Holland Biomedical, Amsterdam, 1979, p. 119–138.
200. M. Randic and V. Miletic, *Brain Res.* **152**, 196 (1978).
201. Q. J. Pittman and G. R. Siggins, *Brain Res.* **221**, 402 (1981).
202. H. R. Olpe, V. J. Balcar, H. Bittiger, H. Rink, and P. Sieber, *Eur. J. Pharmacol.* **63**, 127 (1980).
203. J. W. Phillips and J. R. Kirkpatrick, *Can. J. Physiol. Pharmacol.* **58**, 612 (1980).
204. S. Ioffe, V. Havlicek, H. Friesen, and V. Chernick, *Brain Res.* **153**, 414 (1978).
205. J. Dodd and S. Kelly, *Nature* **273**, 674 (1978).
206. R. L. Macdonald and L. M. Nowak, *Adv. Biochem. Psychopharmacol.* **28**, 159 (1981).
207. M. A. Dichter and J. R. Delfs, *Adv. Biochem. Psychopharmacol.* **28**, 145 (1981).
208. J. R. Delfs and M. A. Dichter, *Soc. Neurosci. Abstr. (1)* **7**, 429 (1981).
209. R. Guillemin, *Endocrinology* **99**, 1643 (1976).
210. M. Cohen, E. Rosing, K. Wiley, and I. Slater, *Life Sci.* **23**, 1659 (1978).
211. M. Göthert, *Nature* **288**, 86 (1980).
212. L. W. Role, S. E. Leeman, and R. L. Perlman, *Neuroscience* **6**, 1813 (1981).
213. Y. Hirooka, C. S. Hollander, S. Suzuki, P. Ferdinand, and S. I. Juan, *Proc. Natl. Acad. Sci. USA* **75**, 4509 (1978).
214. E. Nemeth and J. Cooper, *Brain Res.* **165**, 166 (1979).
215. A. Tsujimoto and S. Tanaka, *Life Sci.* **28**, 903 (1981).
216. S. Tanaka and A. Tsujimoto, *Brain Res.* **208**, 219 (1981).
217. J. Garcia-Sevilla, T. Magnusson, and A. Carlsson, *Brain Res.* **155**, 159 (1978).
218. D. Malthe-Sørenssen, P. L. Wood, D. L. Cheney, and E. Costa, *J. Neurochem.* **31**, 685 (1978).
219. M. Rezek, V. Havlicek, K. R. Hughes, and H. Friesen, *Pharmacol. Biochem. Behav.* **5**, 73 (1976).
220. M. Rezek, V. Havlicek, K. R. Hughes, and H. Friesen, *Neuropharmacology* **16**, 157 (1977).
221. A. J. Kastin, D. H. Coy, Y. Jacquet, A. V. Schally, and N. P. Plotnikoff, *Metabolism* **27**, 1247 (1978).
222. V. Havlicek and H. G. Friesen, in R. Collu, A. Barbeau, J. R. Ducharme, and J.-G. Rochefort, Eds., *Central Nervous System Effects of Hypothalamic Hormones and Other Peptides*, Raven Press, New York, 1979, p. 381–402.
223. K. Chihara, A. Arimura, M. Chihara, and A. V. Schally, *Endocrinology* **103**, 912 (1978).
224. Y. C. Patel, K. Rao, and S. Reichlin, *N. Engl. J. Med.* **296**, 529 (1977).
225. D. R. Rubinow, P. W. Gold, R. M. Post, J. C. Ballenger, R. Cowdry, J. Bollinger, S. Reichlin *Arch. Gen. Psychiatry* **40**: 409–412, 1983.
226. S. Kronheim, M. Berelowitz, and B. Pimstone, *Clin. Endocrinol.* **6**, 411 (1977).
227. J. A. H. Wass, E. Penman, S. Medbak, L. H. Rees, and G. M. Besser, *Clin. Endocrinol.* **13**, 235 (1980).
228. K. V. Sorensen, S. E. Christensen, A. P. Hansen, J. Ingerslev, E. Pedersen, and H. Orskov, *Neuroendocrinology* **32**, 335 (1981).
229. M. Berelowitz, M. J. Perlow, H. J. Hoffman, and L. A. Frohman, **109**, 2102 (1981).

230. S. Reichlin, R. J. Robbins, and R. Lechan, in S. Raptis, Ed., *2nd International Somatostatin Symposium*, in press (1982).

231. P. Davies, R. Katzman, and R. D. Terry, *Nature* **288**, 279 (1980).

232. M. N. Rossor, P. C. Emson, C. Q. Mountjoy, M. Roth, and L. L. Iversen, *Neurosci. Lett.* **20**, 373 (1980).

233. P. E. Cooper, M. Fernstrom, O. P. Rorstad, S. E. Leeman, and J. B. Martin, *Brain Res.* **218**, 219 (1981).

234. E. D. Bird, *Adv. Biochem. Psychopharmacol.* **28**, 657 (1981).

234a. N. Aronin, P. E. Cooper, L. J. Lorenz, E. D. Bird, S. M. Sagar, S. E. Leeman, and J. B. Martin, *Ann. Neurol*, **13**, 519 [1983].

235. H. I. Hochman, D. M. Judge, and S. Reichlin, *Pediatrics* **67**, 236 (1981).

236. K. V. Sørensen, S. E. Christensen, E. Dupont, A. P. Hansen, E. Pedersen, and H. Orskov, *Acta Neurol. Scand.* **61**, 186 (1980).

237. E. Dupont, A. Prange Hansen, P. Juul-Jensen, K. Lundbaek, I. Magnussen, and B. de Fine Olivarius, *Acta Neurol. Scand.* **488**, (1978).

238. V. Schusdziarra, V. Harris, J. Conlon, A. Arimura, and R. Unger, *J. Clin. Invest.* **62**, 509 (1978).

239. J. A. Chayvialle, M. Miyata, P. L. Rayford, and J. C. Thompson, *Gastroenterology* **79**, 844 (1980).

240. Y. C. Patel, *Life Sci.* **24**, 1589 (1979).

241. M. Molitch and L. Hlivyak, *Horm. Metab. Res.* **12**, 559 (1980).

242. P. Gillioz, P. Geraud, B. Conte-Devolox, P. Jaquet, J. L. Codaccioni, and C. Oliver, *Endocrinology* **104**, 1407 (1979).

243. C. M. Turkelson, K. Chihara, C. Kubli-Garfias, and A. Arimura, Program of the 61st Annual Meeting of the Endocrine Society, Anaheim, Calif., 1979, Abstr. 285.

244. A. Negro-Vilar, S. Ojeda, A. Arimura, and S. McCann, *Life Sci.* **23**, 1493 (1978).

245. K. Chihara, A. Arimura, and A. V. Schally, *Endocrinology* **104**, 1656 (1979).

246. K. Maeda and L. A. Frohman, *Endocrinology* **106**, 1837 (1980).

247. S. B. Richardson, C. S. Hollander, J. A. Prasad, and Y. Hirooka, *Endocrinology* **109**, 602 (1981).

248. S. B. Richardson, C. S. Hollander, R. D'Eletto, P. W. Greenleaf, and C. Thaw, *Endocrinology* **107**, 122 (1980).

249. H. Abe, Y. Kato, T. Chiba, T. Taminato, and T. Fujita, *Life Sci.* **23**, 1647 (1978).

250. J. Epelbaum, L. Tapia-Arancibia, J. Besson, W. H. Rotsztejn, and C. Kordon, *Eur. J. Pharmacol.* **58**, 493 (1979).

251. A. Shimatsu, Y. Kato, N. Matsushita, H. Katakami, and N. Yanaihara, Program of the 63rd Annual Meeting of the Endocrine Society, 1981, Abstr. 198.

252. J. Epelbaum, S. V. Drouva, L. Tapia-Arancibia, E. Laplante, and C. Kordon, *Ann. Endocrinol.* **41**, 478 (1980).

253. K. Hermansen, *Endocrinology* **107**, 256 (1980).

254. H. Abe, K. Chihara, T. Chiba, S. Matsukura, and T. Fujita, *Endocrinology* **108**, 1939 (1981).

255. M. C. Sheppard, S. Kronheim, B. L. Pimstone, *J. Neurochem.* **32**, 647 (1979).

256. S. V. Drouva, J. Epelbaum, L. Tapia-Arancibia, E. Laplante, and C. Kordon, *Neuroendocrinology* **32**, 163 (1981).

257. M. Berelowitz, S. L. Firestone, and L. A. Frohman, *Endocrinology* **109**, 714 (1981).

258. H. Abe, K. Chihara, N. Minamitani, J. Iwasaki, T. Chiba, S. Matsukura, and T. Fujita, *Endocrinology* **109**, 229 (1981).

259. A. Negro-Villar and S. R. Ojeda, *Soc. Neurosci. Abstr.* **6**, Abstr. 180.3 (1980).

30

Neurotensin

NEIL ARONIN

Departments of Medicine and Physiology
University of Massachusetts Medical School
Worcester, Massachusetts

ROBERT E. CARRAWAY

Department of Physiology
University of Massachusetts Medical School
Worcester, Massachusetts

MARIAN DIFIGLIA

Department of Neurology
Massachusetts General Hospital
Harvard Medical School
Boston, Massachusetts

SUSAN E. LEEMAN

Department of Physiology
University of Massachusetts Medical School
Worcester, Massachusetts

1 INTRODUCTION

During the course of work directed towards the purification of the peptide substance P from bovine hypothalamic extracts, another vasoactive
peptide was discovered that caused a characteristic vasodilatation of
exposed cutaneous areas when injected intravenously into anesthetized
rats. This biological property was used to monitor purification procedures. The causal peptide was isolated and named neurotensin (NT) after the tissue from which it was purified and for its hypotensive
property. The isolation (1), sequencing (Figure 1), (2) solid phase synthesis (3), and development of the first radioimmunoassays (4) have been
reviewed in detail (5, 6).

Neurotensin is widely, albeit unevenly, distributed throughout the
central and peripheral nervous systems and the gastrointestinal tract.
At each site, NT no doubt subserves a different physiological function.

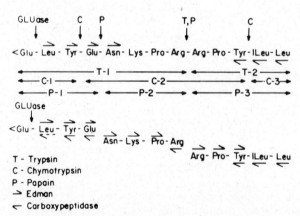

Figure 1. The complete amino acid sequence of NT and the alignment of the fragments
obtained by enzymic cleavage (2). <GLUase, pyrrolidonecarboxylyl peptidase; T-1,2, tryptic peptides; C-1–3, chymotryptic peptides; P-1–3, papain peptides.

In neural tissue, NT has been found in axon terminals (7–9), from which it can be released upon depolarization (10) and can alter the firing pattern of certain neurons following its iontophoresis onto these cells (11). These observations lend support for NT as a neurotransmitter. In the gastrointestinal tract, NT is also present in endocrine-like cells and may subserve endocrine or paracrine functions, or both. This chapter focuses mainly on NT in the central nervous system, the gastrointestinal system, and the recent work on the isolation and characterization of NT-related peptides.

2 CENTRAL NERVOUS SYSTEM: DISTRIBUTION AND FUNCTION

2.1 Localization in Brain

The mapping of neurotensin-like immunoreactivity (NTLI) in the central nervous system (CNS) has been reported in the rat (12, 13), calf (14), monkey (15), and human (16) (Table 1). It is apparent that both the absolute concentrations of NTLI and its distribution vary among the mammalian species studied. For example, the highest levels of NTLI in the rat are located within the limbic system, including the hypothalamus, septal nuclei, nucleus accumbens, and amygdala. In contrast, in postmortem human tissue, the highest content of NTLI has been measured in the substantia nigra, periaqueductal gray, and locus coeruleus, in addition to the hypothalamus. There are several possible explanations for these differences, aside from actual interspecies variations of distribution. These various studies have used different methods to extract the tissues as well as antisera with different specificities. Furthermore, there may also be a loss of immunoreactivity in the postmortem tissue before enzyme inactivation and extraction. Preliminary observations in our laboratory in monkey spinal cord have shown that several fragments of NT can be identified by reverse phase high pressure liquid chromatography and subsequent measurement by radioimmunoassay with an amino-(N)-terminally-directed antiserum. Since these fragments can be generated by trypsin-like and carboxypeptidase A-like activities, it is possible that these smaller peptides represent metabolites of NT that are measurable with N-terminally-directed but not carboxyl-(C)-terminally-directed antisera. To date, no study of the distribution of NTLI in the CNS by radioimmunoassay has dealt adequately with these problems.

Immunohistochemical observations of NTLI in the brain have been made primarily in the rat, where labeled cell bodies are found in the hypothalamus, interstitial nucleus of the stria terminalis, amygdala, midbrain tegmentum, and brain stem regions (17, 18). An NT projection

TABLE 1 Regional Distribution of NTLI in the Central Nervous System of Several Mammalian Species

NTLI:	Rat[a] pmol/gww	Rat[b] pmol/mg protein	Calf[c] pmol/gww	Monkey[d] pmol/gww	Human[e] pmol/gww
Cerebral Cortex					
Area 3-1-2	2.0 ± 0.6			4.1 ± 4.1	
Area 4				10.3 ± 3.8	
Area 5				6.1 ± 0.46	
Area 6				2.5 ± 5.1	
Area 7				3.6 ± 0.63	
Area 17				2.3 ± 0.86	
supplementary motor area				4.7, 6.1	
frontal			1.80 ± 0.11		0.8 ± 0.1
parietal			2.36 ± 0.07		0.8 ± 0.1
uncal					4.9 ± 1.2
entorhinal		0.03 ± 0.1			2.3 ± 0.7
hippocampal formation		<0.01	2.99 ± 0.39	7.6 ± 1.2	4.4 ± 0.6
cingulate		<0.01	3.84 ± 0.24	9.0, 3.8	2.1 ± 0.4
striate					0.7 ± 0.1
occipital pole			2.53 ± 0.30		
precentral gyrus			2.44 ± 0.15		
parahippocampal gyrus			6.56 ± 0.67		
Basal Ganglia					
Caudate (head)		0.017 ± 0.001	11.05 ± 0.13	4.86 ± 0.5	2.9 ± 0.4
Putamen				7.5 ± 3.1	2.5 ± 0.3
Globus pallidus					
internal			9.34 ± 0.66	5.9 ± 1.6	9.8 ± 1.1
external					9.7 ± 1.3
Subthalamic nucleus				27.3, 18.5	9.7 ± 3.7
Substantia nigra		0.18 ± 0.05			
pars compacta				3.5 ± 1.4	23.4 ± 2.0
pars reticulata				9.3 ± 2.9	

	C1	C2	C3	C4	C5
Locus coeruleus				14.5	20.5 ± 2.7
Raphe nucleus					12.8 ± 1.7
Area postrema					11.7 ± 2.4
Inferior olive				8.74, 7.37	2.6 ± 0.2
Reticular formation of medulla				3.3	
Cerebellum					
Cortex	0.82 ± 0.26	<0.011			0.8 ± 0.1
Dentate n.					0.6 ± 0.1
Cortex of lemisphere			<0.32	2.6 ± 0.5	
Cortex of vermis				4.6, 8.7	
Fatigeal n.				13.4, 10.2	
Interpostus n.				15.3 ± 2.1	
Dentate n.				15.5 ± 2.1	
Hypothalamus	60.0 ± 4.0				
Preoptic area		0.97 ± 0.25			
Anterior hypothalamus		0.21 ± 0.086	17.32 ± 3.33		33.4 ± 5.0
Medial basal hypothalamus		0.53 ± 0.69	19.14 ± 3.12		31.2 ± 5.0
Posterior hypothalamus		0.19 ± 0.09			
Median eminence		1.93 ± 0.27		48.9, 52.5	
Arcuate n.		0.56 ± 0.18		40.5 ± 4.1	
Ventromedial n.		0.99 ± 0.18		48.4 ± 7.1	
Retrochiasnatic area		0.47 ± 0.13			
Suprachiasmatic PO[e]		0.73 ± 0.45			
Periventricular PO		0.96 ± 0.19			
Medial PO		1.33 ± 0.13		29.4 ± 6.5	
Lateral PO		1.46 ± 0.13		25.4 ± 9.2	
Dorsomedial nucleus				48.5 ± 5.2	
Lateral area				32.6 ± 3.9	

TABLE 1 *(Continued)*

NTLI	Rat[a] pmol/gww	Rat[b] pmol/mg protein	Calf[c] pmol/gww	Monkey[d] pmol/gww	Human[e] pmol/gww
Mammillary body			11.11 ± 0.88	14.9 ± 12.6	23.6 ± 2.6
Cervical cord		0.080 ± 0.04	1.06 ± 0.008		
Anterior column				15.0 ± 2.3	
Posterior/lateral				10.21 ± 1.5/ 2.9, 6.3	
Gray Matter					
Amygdala		0.37 ± 0.03	1.94 ± 0.38		5.4 ± 1.1
Medial				10.7 ± 3.0	
Central				11.0 ± 3.2	
Thalamus	16.1 ± 5.8				
Anterior n.			4.32 ± 0.66	16.0 ± 2.7	
Ventral n.			1.27 ± 0.22	9.0 ± 1.3	
Dorsomedial n.			2.47 ± 0.09	15.7 ± 3.7	6.0 ± 1.4
Midline n.				26.7 ± 3.6	
Pulvinar complex			1.42 ± 0.03	14.6 ± 1.1	
Centre median				16.3 ± 20.0	
Lateral dorsal					3.1 ± 0.5
Lateral posterior					2.7 ± 0.6
Lateral geniculate				4.6 ± 1.1	1.9 ± 0.3
Medial geniculate				4.86	
Zona incerta				24.8, 16.9	
Nucleus accumbens		0.78 ± 0.15			
Septal area		0.39 ± 0.05			
Brainstem	12.9 ± 3.3				
Interpedunclar nucleus		0.46 ± 0.08		45.1 ± 9.9	
Mesencephalon		0.08 ± 0.05			
Central grey of mesencephalon			0.42 ± 0.05	42.3	

Pons	0.057 ± 0.03	1.25 ± 0.23	2.2 ± 1.1
Medulla	0.10	1.62 ± 0.05	
Ventral tegmental area			27.8
Red nucleus		2.74 ± 0.27	16.7 ± 2.8
Colliculi			
Colliculus superior			3.2, 5.6
Colliculus inferior			8.6 ± 3.3

[a] Carraway and Leeman (12).
[b] Kobayashi et al. (13).
[c] Uhl and Snyder (14).
[d] Kataoka et al. (15).
[e] Cooper et al. (16).
[e] PO =

that originates in the amygdala and enters the stria terminalis has been reported (19).

In the hypothalamus of the rat, a detailed immunohistochemical examination has demonstrated NTLI in somata of the medial preoptic area, periventricular region, parvocellular divisions of the paraventricular nucleus, arcuate nucleus, and lateral hypothalamus (Figure 2) (20). These same regions also contained labeled fibers. In addition, immunostained processes were identified in the posterior mammillary nucleus and the lateral aspect of the external layer of the median eminence.

2.2   Possible Physiological Roles in the Brain

Intracisternal injection of NT in mice has been associated with the development of hypothermia in a dose-dependent manner (21, 22). This phenomenon has been found in rats following both intracisternal (23) and intrathecal (24) administration. Dopamine depletion or blockade (23) has been reported to potentiate the hypothermia. Intracerebroventricular or intracisternal injection of thyrotropin releasing hormone (TRH) at 30 μg (23) and prostaglandin E_2 (PGE_2) at 10 μg (25) has been found to antagonize the NT-related hypothermia, but this effect was not observed with a dose of 10 μg of TRH or with somatostatin or naloxone (25). It remains unclear whether these findings are related to a physiological role of NT, but such observations may be the initial evidence for revealing another regulatory effect of NT in the central nervous system.

2.3   Regulation of Secretion of Anterior Pituitary Hormones

Immunoreactive NT is present in the median eminence, and investigations in numerous laboratories provide preliminary evidence that NT has effects on the secretion of several anterior pituitary hormones. NT has been reported to decrease prolactin secretion following intraventricular injection in rats (26, 27) and to increase levels of this hormone after peripheral injection (26–28). Incubation of rat hemipituitaries with 50 ng/mL (27) and 10^{-8} M (29) of NT has been found to increase prolactin release. This effect has been found to be additive to the effects of TRH, dopamine, or gamma-aminobutyric acid (GABA). However, since the concentrations of NT in these studies are much greater than the peripheral plasma concentration, it seems necessary to determine the level of NT in the pituitary portal circulation before establishing that this may represent a hormonal effect of NT.

Intraventricular injection of NT reduces plasma levels of luteinizing hormone; peripheral administration causes an increase or no change in such concentrations (27). In preliminary observations in this laboratory (30), Ferris and coworkers found that injection of synthetic NT into the

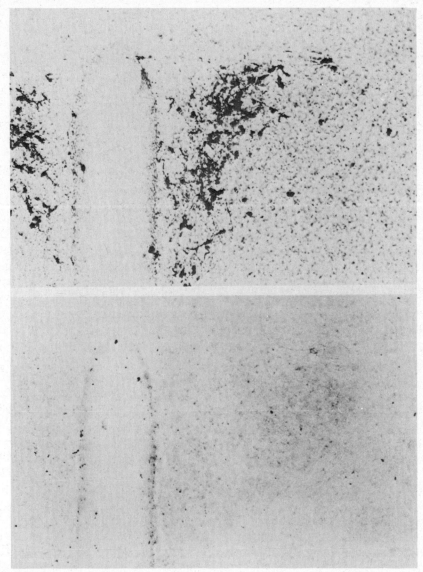

Figure 2. Immunohistochemical labeling of cell bodies containing NTLI in the paraventricular nucleus of the rat (20) is shown in the top panel. Incubation of the NT antiserum with excess synthetic NT markedly reduced staining (bottom panel).

medial preoptic area of the ovariectomized rat is followed by an increase in plasma concentrations of luteinizing hormone. The reasons for the apparently discrepant findings between intracerebroventricular and intracerebral injections are unclear. It is possible that when administered by different central routes NT interacts with different neurons, some of which may not normally have access to the peptide. Since NT fibers have been observed in the rat medial preoptic area, it is possible that the discrete intracerebral injections are more likely to elucidate a physiological role.

The effects of NT on growth hormone secretion have been reported to vary with the route of administration of neurotensin, its dose, and the sex of the animal studied. An increase in growth hormone secretion was found following intravenous administration of 20 μg of NT in urethane-anesthetized rats (28), but growth hormone levels remained unchanged in conscious, ovariectomized rats after 1 μg NT intravenously (31). Intraventricular administration of NT in the anesthetized male rat resulted in a reduction in growth hormone levels (26, 32), in contrast to the increase seen in conscious, ovariectomized rats (31). Incubation of pituitary tissue from ovariectomized animals with NT did not induce growth hormone release (31). It has been suggested that central administration of NT may decrease growth hormone secretion by an increase in somatostatin release into the rat hypophyseal portal blood (33). The release of somatostatin from the pancreas after peripheral NT injection (34) has been postulated to contribute to an increase in hypophyseal portal concentration of somatostatin.

The role of NT in the regulation of thyrotropin secretion has been studied. In anesthetized male rats, NT is reported to inhibit thyrotropin release after intraventricular administration but to stimulate its release after intravenous injection (26). In thyroidectomized rats, intracisternal administration of NT was associated with a decrease in the elevated levels of circulating thyrotropin (23). In conscious, ovariectomized rats, NT failed to alter thyrotropin secretion after administration into the third ventricle, but intravenous injection of NT and its incubation with hemipituitaries did not result in an increase in thyrotropin release. These studies may be interpreted to suggest that one action of neurotensin modulation on thyrotropin release may occur via the pituitary portal vein. In humans, infusion of NT until concentrations of NTLI of 104 $\pm$ 10 pmol/L were obtained was not found to alter plasma levels of thyrotropin, growth hormone, prolactin, luteinizing stimulating hormone, or follicle stimulating hormone (35). However, these results do not necessarily prove that NT lacks effects on the release of these hormones, since it is still possible that higher concentrations of NT are found in the hypothalamic-pituitary portal system than in the peripheral circulation.

2.4   Distribution and Localization in Spinal Cord

Light microscopic localization of NT has been demonstrated in the spinal cord, where it is found almost exclusively within the dorsal horn (7, 9, 36–39). In the rat, immunoreactive NT fibers appear mostly in two discrete bands, a narrow one that lies at the border of laminae I and II and a wider region within inner lamina II. Fibers are also seen in the tract of Lissauer and the dorsal-lateral funiculus.

Following colchicine injection, NT cell bodies are visible primarily in the areas bordering laminae II and III (37, 38) and are found mainly in a rostral-caudal axis (39). Axons from NT neurons were shown to extend long distances in a rostral-caudal direction in cultured explants (300 μm) of lumbar spinal cord from rat embryo (40). The localization of NTLI in somata in the dorsal horn and the persistence of NTLI following dorsal rhizotomy (8) suggest that NT neurons in the dorsal horn are interneurons.

In our laboratory, immunoperoxidase staining of NT was examined in the monkey dorsal horn (7, 9) and showed a different pattern of localization from that found in the rat. Reaction product was contained primarily within small punctate elements extending throughout laminae I–III, with the greatest density appearing in lamina I and then decreasing more ventrally (Figure 3). No discrete bands of labeled fibers were visible. Most labeled terminals ranged in size from 0.5 to 1.5 μm, and some larger 2–3 μm profiles also were seen. Fibers with NTLI were also observed in the central gray area.

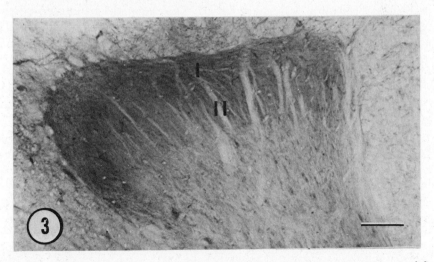

Figure 3. Neurotensin in the monkey spinal cord. Most NTLI was present in animal fibers and terminals within laminae I and II of the dorsal horn. Scale bar, 200 μm.

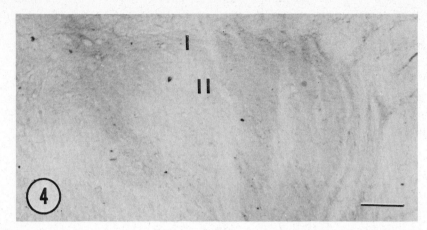

Figure 4. Preabsorption control. A spinal cord section incubated in NT antisera, which had been exposed to synthetic NT, fails to exhibit the specific staining shown in Figure 3. Scale bar, 200 μm.

Although colchicine was not used, some immunoreactive NT cell bodies 12–18 μm in size were found in laminae II and III. Tissue sections exposed to NT antiserum preabsorbed with synthetic NT did not show the specific staining described above (Figure 4).

At the electron microscopic level, NTLI was present within fine caliber unmyelinated and thinly myelinated axons, 0.2–0.5 μm in diameter. Labeled axon terminals contained numerous clear round vesicles and large granular vesicles (LGV) and formed synapses with small and large dendrites throughout laminae I and II. The dendrites of lamina I neurons frequently were postsynaptic to numerous immunoreactive NT axons (Figure 5).

2.5   Possible Role in the Spinal Cord

A possible function of NT in the modulation of peripheral stimuli has been suggested, in part based upon the overlap of the distribution of NTLI-labeled neuronal elements with those that contain immunoreactive enkephalins, which are likely modulators of incoming nociceptive inputs (37, 38, 41) and in part on behavioral neurophysiological studies. Intracisternal administration of NT in mice (42) and rats (21) has been shown to diminish the time of onset and the amount of response to painful stimuli; that is, NT has an antinocisponsive property.* This effect has been found to persist with previous administration of naloxone and cyproheptadine (43) but is antagonized by TRH in mice (44). The in-

*The term nocisponsive is used to describe the response of the test animals to painful stimuli in order to avoid the difficulties inherent in measuring nociception (43).

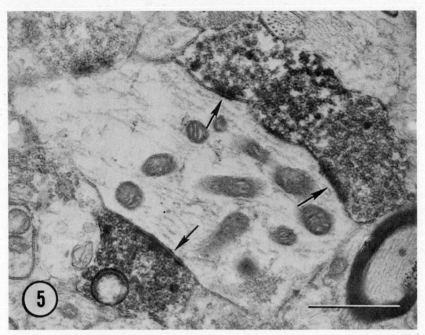

Figure 5. Ultrastructural localization of NTLI in axon terminals in lamina I. Four labeled boutons, containing numerous small round vesicles and some large granular vesicles, are in contact with the same dendrite. At least three of the NT-positive terminals make synaptic contacts (arrows), and one unlabeled bouton (top left) may also synapse with the same dendrite. Scale bar, 1 μm.

trathecal injection of 1 to 80 μg of NT in the rat, unlike morphine, showed no antinocisponsive effect (24). In the cat, however intrathecal injection of 100 μg of NT caused a dose-dependent elevation in the hotplate response that was diminished by pretreatment with naloxone, with little change in the tail flick test (45). Application of NT onto dorsal horn neurons has produced both stimulatory and inhibitory effects. Excitatory responses were reported in the cat in cells located in laminae I–III (46). In the spinal cord of the newborn rat *in vitro*, NT was found to depolarize motoneurons, probably via interneurons since tetrodotoxin markedly diminished this effect (47). In the frog, NT was also found to produce a stimulatory, tetrodotoxin-sensitive effect on motoneurons (48, 49). However, Henry (50) has observed that NT applied to dorsal horn neurons in the cat is associated with both excitation and inhibition and he has cautioned that NT may have multiple effects on nociception. It appears that although there is evidence to support a transsynaptic excitatory role for NT in the ventral horn, the role and site of action of NT as an antinocisponsive or antinociceptive agent in the dorsal horn remains unclear.

3 ADRENAL MEDULLA AND AUTONOMIC NERVOUS SYSTEM

Neurotensin-like immunoreactivity was found in the cat adrenal medulla (51, 52) in a population of norepinephrine-containing chromaffin cells (53). Immunoreactive NT was not observed in the adrenal medulla in guinea pig, dog, monkey, or human (54). Extracts of adrenal medulla applied to gel permeation chromatography on Sephadex G-50 have shown the presence of NTLI eluting in the region of synthetic NT following measurement with a C-terminus antiserum (53). On gel permeation chromatography on Sephadex G-25 and subsequent radioimmunoassay with an N-terminal antiserum, extracts of adrenal medulla resolved into three peaks; with the void volume, prior to synthetic NT, and with synthetic NT (54). Following left splanchnic nerve stimulation, increased concentrations of NTLI were found in the left adrenal vein. This apparent release was diminished by hexamethonium. Neurotensin-like immunoreactivity has also been identified in rat pheochromocytoma cells in monolayer culture (55). Addition of both nerve growth factor and dexamethasone to the culture was found to result in increased concentrations of NTLI in extracts of the pheochromocytoma and medium. Minimal increases in NTLI were associated with incubation of the cultured cells with dexamethasone or nerve growth factors individually. It was suggested that glucocorticoids and nerve growth factor may exert cooperative regulation of the synthesis and release of NTLI in this *in vitro* system. It appears that study of the role of NT in the function of the adrenal medulla and the autonomic nervous system will be a fruitful area of research in the next few years.

4 PLASMA: PRESENCE AND METABOLISM

Neurotensin-like immunoreactivity in plasma includes multiple immunoreactive moieties (56). After extraction of bovine, rat, rabbit, and human plasma by the addition of acid/acetone (56), four antisera with different specificities vs. NT were used to measure concentrations of NTLI. Higher values were found with the antisera directed against the C-terminus than with the N-terminally-directed antisera. Submission of bovine plasma extract to gel permeation chromatography on Sephadex G-25 (Figure 6) and ion exchange chromatography on sulfopropyl-Sephadex G-25 followed by radioimmunoassay with several antisera showed the presence of multiple forms of NTLI. Approximately 30–50% of the NTLI, as measured by a C-terminal-directed antiserum, coeluted with NT on gel permeation chromatography, and it was estimated that 15–25 fmol/mL of NT is found in acid-acetone extracted plasma. Much of the remaining NTLI consisted of smaller-molecular-weight material, some of which was recognized primarily by C-terminal-directed antisera

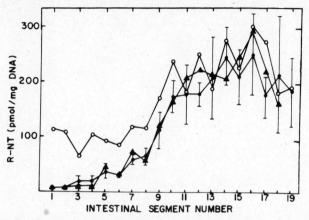

Figure 6. Average measurements of radioimmunoassayable NT (R-NT) at segments sampled in the small intestine of four subjects, as determined with antisera HC-8 (○), TG-1 (▲), and PGL-4 (●). Standard deviation of HC-8 values are indicated by the error bars. Mucosal scrapings from 12-cm-long segments of small intestine at 30-cm intervals were extracted in cold (−10°C) acetone and 0.6 M acetic acid, 7:3 (v/v), prior to assay (63).

or by N-terminal-directed antisera, but not by both. The use of the site-specific antisera not only confirms the presence of NT in plasma but also shows that plasma extracts contain structurally related variants and breakdown products of NT.

The metabolism of intravenously administered NT has been studied in the human and the rat. The half-life of total NTLI in the human after intravenous infusion of NT has been estimated to be 3.5 min (35). The form of the NTLI was not further examined, and the possibility exists that the measured NTLI included metabolic products of NT. In our laboratory, studies have been undertaken to determine whether some of the multiple forms of NTLI are circulating metabolites of NT. The stability of intravenously administered NT and the immunochemical properties of the NTLI following this injection were examined in rats (57). It was observed that NTLI measured by a C-directed radioimmunoassay has a halflife of less than 1 min while that of NTLI measured by an N-terminally-directed antiserum is about tenfold longer (Figure 7). Results of gel-permeation chromatography on Sephadex G-25 and high pressure liquid chromatography have suggested that NT is rapidly metabolized to fragments with physicochemical properties of NT^{1-12}, NT^{1-11} and NT^{1-8}, which then disappear from the circulation at a slower rate than NT. The C-terminal fragment, NT^{9-13}, was found to be cleared rapidly. It is suggested, then, that responses of NTLI to various stimuli should be evaluated with companion studies that identify more precisely the nature of the elevated circulating forms in order to separate immunoreac-

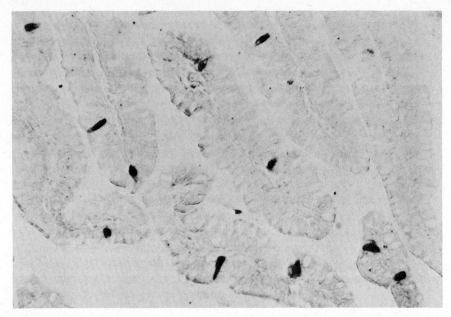

Figure 7. Immunohistochemical labeling by the peroxidase-antiperoxidase method of cells with NTLI in the human ileum. The HC-8 antiserum was used for the histochemistry (see ref. 68 for details).

tivity of metabolites from NT itself. Several of the antisera presently used by others to determine NTLI in human plasma (58, 59) are N-terminally-directed and it has been postulated that some may measure N-terminal metabolites of NT (59).

5 GASTROINTESTINAL TISSUES: DISTRIBUTION AND FUNCTION

The presence of a substance with the same chromatographic and hypotensive characteristics and amino acid composition as NT has been shown in acid-acetone extracts of bovine (60–62) and fresh postmortem human intestinal tissue (63).

5.1 Distribution by Radioimmunoassay

The highest concentrations of radioimmunoassayable NT with use of amino- and carboxyl-terminus-directed antisera have been measured in the distal jejunum and ileum, with lesser concentrations in the stomach, duodenum, and colon (Figure 8) (60, 63). Substances smaller than NT, with cross-reactivity to a carboxyl-terminus antiserum, have been found in extracts of stomach and proximal duodenum.

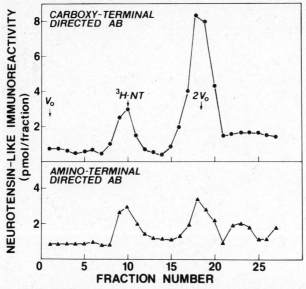

Figure 8. Gel chromatography of extracted bovine plasma on Sephadex G-25. An acid-acetone extract of 1.2 L of bovine plasma was dissolved in 200 mL of column buffer (0.2 M acetic acid) and submitted to a Sephadex G-25 column of (14 × 123 cm; 18.5 L bed volume). Fractions of 500 mL were collected. V_0 indicates void volume. The top panel shows the NTLI determined with the HC-8 antiserum (C-terminal). The bottom panel shows the NTLI measured with the TG-1 antiserum (N-terminal). (See ref. 56 for details.)

5.2 Cellular Localization

The localization by immunohistochemistry of NTLI within the gastrointestinal epithelium has been reported in several species (64–67). In primates, NTLI has been observed histochemically in mucosal cells, named N-cells, which have an endocrine-like morphology (Figure 9) (65, 66). The N-cell contains granules mainly at its base, in the direction of the lamina propria (68). In addition, fibers but not neuronal cell bodies with NTLI have been reported in the esophagus, stomach, duodenum, and cecum (51). These anatomical observations are consistent with the possibility that NT or another immunoreactive form may participate in a variety of roles in the intestine, including endocrine, paracrine, or neurotransmitter.

5.3 Multiple Biological Activities in the Gastrointestinal Tract

Neurotensin has been shown to be capable of affecting numerous functions in the gastrointestinal tract. Intravenous infusion of synthetic NT in dogs at a rate of 4–60 pmol/kg/min has resulted in increased intestinal blood flow with dilation of the mesenteric vascular bed (69), inhibi-

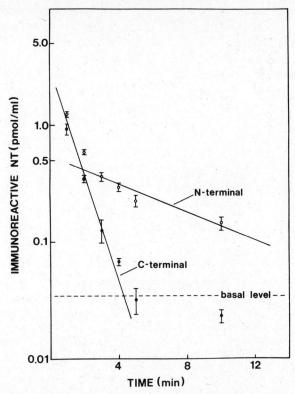

Figure 9. Disappearance curves following intravenous administration of synthetic NT in the rat. NT-like activity measured by TG-1 (○N-terminal antiserum) is more slowly cleared from the circulation than is NTLI by HC-8 (●C-terminal antiserum). Values are indicated as m ± SEM (ref. 57).

tion of gastric acid secretion (70), and suppression of gastric motility (71). The inhibition of acid secretion may be mediated by the vagal nerve, since vagal denervation abolished the NT effect (72). Intravenous infusion of synthetic (Gln⁴)-NT in human volunteers was associated with a marked decrease in lower esophageal sphincter pressure at plasma levels comparable with those found after meals or fat ingestion but one-tenth of that needed for cardiovascular effects or hyperglycemia (73). A net increase in intraluminal fluid volume in the small bowel of the rat has been found during intravenous administration of synthetic NT (74). In this study the circulating levels of NTLI were approximately tenfold higher than the basal concentration.

5.4   Release from Intestine

Immunoreactive NT can be released from the small intestine, and the regulation of this release seems to be closely related to the ingestion of lipids. In dogs an arterial–venous gradient (40 vs. 91 pmol/L) of NTLI has been measured across the small intestine (58). In normal human subjects, an increase in circulating plasma NTLI has been shown to follow ingestion of meals high in fats (58) but not after glucose and amino acids. In gastrectomized patients, ingestion of 50 g glucose has been reported to increase plasma concentrations of NTLI (75). Recently, Hammer and coworkers have used high pressure liquid chromatography and region-specific radioimmunoassay to demonstrate elevated peripheral levels of the NT-metabolites NT^{1-8} and NT^{1-11} after ingestion of a high-fat meal in human subjects (76). Perfusion of lipid into the small intestine of the rat has been found to elevate NTLI and NT itself when collected from the superior mesenteric vein (77); perfusion with amino acids, glucose, hyperosmotic saline, acidified bile salts, and diluted rat bile did not alter plasma NTLI concentrations. Finally, there appears to be a correlation between the ingestion of oleic acid, gastric acid secretion, and NTLI concentrations in the plasma (78). In normal subjects who received oleic acid in the duodenum, the inhibition of the gastric acid secretory response following pentagastrin stimulation was directly correlated with the plasma NTLI concentrations. In patients with duodenal ulcers, oleic acid infusion was associated with both a lesser inhibition of acid secretion and lower concentrations of plasma NTLI.

5.5 Effects on Intestinal Smooth Muscle and Myenteric Neurons

Since the original observations that application of NT is followed by contraction of the guinea pig ileum and relaxation of the rat duodenum (1), many of the effects of NT on gastrointestinal motility have been elucidated. Kitabgi and Freychet (79) have shown in *in vitro* preparations that NT induced relaxation of the rat ileum and contraction of the guinea pig taenia (cecum). A biphasic response, relaxation followed by contraction, was observed in the guinea pig ileum. Tetrodotoxin, which blocks neuronal action potentials without effects on smooth muscle, was found to abolish the contraction phase in the guinea pig ileum but did not alter the relaxation in any of the preparations. This result has been interpreted to suggest that NT has direct effects on intestinal smooth muscle (relaxation) and that its effect on contraction is mediated in part by the nervous system. The cholinergic antagonist atropine partially blocked the NT-induced contraction of guinea pig ileum. Some of the neurally mediated effects of NT are therefore likely to be cholinergic.

Further studies have shown that the NT effects on smooth muscle membranes of the guinea pig taenia-coli include both an induction of depolarization and an increase in spike frequency of a spontaneously discharging preparation. The depolarization was associated with an increase in membrane conductance through enhanced Na^+ and Ca^{2+} conductances (80). In the guinea pig longitudinal ileal smooth muscle system, the anticholinesterase inhibitor neostigmine enhanced the NT-

induced contractility, while atropine blocked this effect (81). Hexamethonium did not alter the NT-related contraction. These findings indicate that part of the neurally mediated activity of NT occurs via the
cholinergic system and that this NT effect occurs at a postganglionic
level. A noncholinergic component, possibly mediated by substance P
and estimated to be about 50% of the NT effect on the contraction of
the guinea-pig ileum, has been shown to be abolished by the opioid
peptides, β-endorphin and Met-enkephalin (82).

Excitation of about 50% of single myenteric neurons has been observed following application of NT. This response was dose-dependent
and persisted in Ca^{2+} free solutions, suggesting that much of the action
is directly onto the cell (83). It appears, therefore, that the effects of NT
on contractility can vary with each subdivision of the intestine and involve direct action onto smooth muscle and onto both the cholinergic
and noncholinergic nervous systems. The origin of the NT that participates in these processes, whether from the circulation, the N-cells, or local or autonomic fibers, is unclear.

In summary, the release of NT from the intestine seems to be linked
to lipid ingestion, and the NT may have a variety of roles in gastrointestinal processes. Some of these presumed functions occur proximal to
a potential release site in the intestine; for example, the inhibition of
gastric acid secretion and gastric motor activity. It has been suggested,
therefore, that NT may function as an enterogastrone (59). Effects on
the mesenteric vascularity and intestinal fluid flux may implicate a local site of action, and in this sense NT may act as a paracrine agent.
These possible distinctions are important if only to indicate that the
same peptide may subserve different roles within the same organ system. Additionally, effects of NT on gastrointestinal motility may be mediated not only by direct actions onto smooth muscle but also by
modulation of its innervation.

5.6   Pancreas: Effects on Secretion of Pancreatic Hormones

A role for NT in the regulation of the endocrine pancreas was first
suggested in several studies in which the intravenous administration of
synthetic NT results in hyperglycemia in the rat and dog (84–87). Most
of the increase in plasma glucose level observed in rat appears not to
result from an alteration in the clearance of glucose (85). An increase in
plasma glucagon levels (84, 86) and a decrease in insulin concentrations
(84) have been observed following the intravenous injection of NT in
rats. In other studies, injection of NT into the pancreaticoduodenal artery in the dog was associated with an increase in both immunoreactive
insulin and glucagon concentrations in the pancreaticoduodenal vein,
concomitant with increases in mean blood flow and plasma glucose levels (88). These responses were attenuated with prior administration of
propranolol. The reasons for these differences are unclear.

In isolated pancreatic islets *in vitro*, NT has been reported to inhibit insulin but stimulate glucagon release (89). However, in another study with use of preparations of isolated pancreatic islets, the effect of NT on the release of pancreatic hormones was found to depend largely upon the glucose concentration in the medium (90). When islets were incubated with synthetic NT for 20 min at 3 mM glucose, increased levels of insulin, glucagon, and somatostatin were measured in the medium. In contrast, incubation of islets with NT at higher glucose levels, 23 mM, for 60 min was associated with a decreased release of insulin, glucagon, and somatostatin in the medium.

In human subjects, following infusion of synthetic NT to reach a level of 104$+$10 pmol NTLI/liter, neither the blood glucose nor plasma concentrations of insulin or glucagon were found to change (35). To date, however, the concentration of basal or stimulated NT in the human pancreaticoduodenal artery is unknown, and in a study in the mouse the localization of NT in pancreatic cells could not be demonstrated by immunohistochemistry (91). Although NT seems to be a candidate regulator of insulin and glucagon release, the origin of NT in the pancreas and its mode of action need further investigation.

Neurotensin concentrations appear to be altered in some laboratory animals made diabetic. In pancreatic extracts of streptozotocin-diabetic rats and genetically diabetic mice, NTLI has been shown to be increased (92). Restoration of euglycemia by insulin administration to the diabetic animals resulted in concentrations of NTLI comparable with those of controls. These findings have been confirmed recently (93) and a possible role of NT in the hormonal changes in diabetes has been suggested.

6 RECEPTORS

The presence of specific receptors for NT using radiolabeled NT has been demonstrated in rat brain membranes (94–96), in a human colon carcinoma cell line (97), and in rat peritoneal mast cells (98, 99). Some of the characteristics of these receptor binding assays are summarized in Table 2. In general, binding to these various preparations was found to be saturable, reversible, selective, and of high affinity. Binding to rat brain membranes has been studied using both ^{3}H-labeled-NT and ^{125}I-labeled-NT, and although these ligands are chemically different, similar properties were derived for the binding reaction (Table 2).

The distribution of NT binding sites in rat and calf brain has been examined by dissection and assay of selected areas (95, 96) as well as by light microscopic autoradiography (100). When the results are compared with those for NTLI determined immunohistochemically and by radioimmunoassay, the distributions overlap although some disparities are evident. The hypothalamus has high amounts of both binding activi-

TABLE 2 Summary of Conditions Employed for and Properties Derived from Receptor Binding Assays for Neurotensin

	(96)	(95)	(94)	(97)	(98)
Reference:					
Labeled Ligand:	^{125}I-NT	^{125}I-NT	^{3}H-NT	^{3}H-NT	^{125}I-NT
Membrane or Cells:	Rat brain, P2 pellet membranes	Rat brain, membranes	Rat brain, synaptic	Human colon carinoma cell-line	Rat mast cells
Buffer:	25 mM Tris acetate pH 7.0 1 BSA	20 mM Tris pH 7.5 0.5 BSA	50 mM Tris pH 7.5 1 BSA	Krebs-Ringer Hepes pH 7.4 1 BSA	10 mM Tris acetate pH 7.0 80 mM sucrose 1 BSA
Incubation Conditions:	10 min 0°C	30 min 4°C	30 min 24°C	30 min 24°C	15 min 0°C
Separation Method:	Whatman GF/C filter	centrifugation 8 min 17,500 × g	Millipore filtration	Millipore filtration	Whatman GF/C filter
Characteristics:	pH sensitive; inhibited by divalent cations	Inhibited by ions	Single population of binding sites	37 fmol/10^6 cells	1270 fmol/10^6 cells
K_d:	8 nM	3 nM	2 nM	1.5 nM	154. nM
$k1$:	4.1 × 10^5 M^{-1} sec^{-1}	9 × 10^5 M^{-1} sec^{-1}	4.3 × 10^5 M^{-1} sec^{-1}		
$K-1$:	1.54 × 10^{-3} sec^{-1}	0.8 × 10^{-3} sec^{-1}	0.67 × 10^{-3} sec^{-1}		
$t_{1/2}$:	0.25 min, 0°C	7.5 min, 4°C	40 min, 24°C		1.5 min, 0°C

ty and NTLI, and the cerebellum has the lowest levels of receptor and NTLI. The rat cerebral cortex is reported to have a receptor-site concentration equal to that of hypothalamus (95, 96) but it contains one-tenth the NTLI by radioimmunoassay (12). Young and Kuhar (100), using light microscopic autoradiography, have observed that the rhinal sulcus and laminae I and II of the cerebral cortex have high densities of NT receptors with little NTLI. Interestingly, they also identified areas known to contain large amounts of NTLI that did not appear to have high concentrations of receptors, such as the parabrachial nuclei, the dorsal raphe nucleus, and the central nucleus of the amygdala.

If NT is released from nerves in the brain to act as a neurotransmitter or modulator on nearby targets, then one would expect its receptor distribution to parallel that of the peptide content. Outside of assay artifacts one explanation for the disparity observed is that some of the putative receptors *in situ* bind peptides closely related to NT, rather than NT itself. Another suggestion is that in some areas of brain, NT is not stored and released in its active form but instead is generated as needed from a stored precursor (or precursors) unrecognized in currently available radioimmunoassays. This arrangement would be reminiscent of the peripheral renin-angiotensin system. At present, however, there is no precedent for such extracellular generation of messenger-peptides in the brain.

In rat brain and human colon carcinoma preparations, the structural requirements for binding have been compared with the requirements for biological activity, as detected by the contraction of guinea pig ileum *in vitro* (97). Binding affinity was found to correlate well with biological potency for NT and for 18 of its synthetic analogs, and both were shown to depend highly upon the integrity of the six C-terminal residues of NT. The positive charges on Arg^8 and Arg^9, the negative charge on the terminal carboxyl group, and the aromatic and hydrophobic side chains on Tyr^{11}, Ile^{12} and Leu^{13} were all found to be important determinants of binding and biological activity. Although all the biological effects of NT examined to date depend primarily upon groups within the C-terminal half of NT, the requirements for each activity were not identical (101). Thus, it may be important when relating binding to biological activity to employ the same tissue (and if possible the same preparation) for the two measurements.

There has been relatively little work concerning the cellular localizations of receptors for NT. Palacios and Kuhar have demonstrated that injection of 6-hydroxydopamine into the substantia nigra zona compacta of rats, causing a specific destruction of dopamine-containing cell bodies in this area, was associated with a 90% loss of NT receptors (102). These results indicate that at least some of the dopamine-containing neurons in the ventral midbrain of the rat have high densities of NT receptors, and the results fit well with other lines of evidence supporting the idea that in some areas of brain NT may interact with the dopaminergic system. Binding of NT to isolated rat peritoneal mast cells has also been demonstrated (98); although the binding appeared to be rather weak (K_d, *ca* 154 nM), it was shown to be sequence-specific and highly dependent upon functional groups located in the C-terminal part of the molecule (99). Furthermore, recent studies indicate that NT stimulates the release of histamine from mast cells both *in vitro* and *in vivo* (103). Perfused preparations of rat skin have been found to be highly sensitive to NT, responding to concentrations near 10^{-11} M (104). It is likely that the mast cell receptors do not display the identical structural selectivity as the CNS receptors, since a number of analogs of NT exhibited strikingly different affinities in the two systems. For example, D-Arg[9]-NT was reported to display 0.5% and 640% potencies relative to NT in binding to CNS receptors (97) and to mast cells (99), respectively. If the differences are not due to differing stabilities of these analogs in the assay systems, then these findings suggest that there exist multiple types of binding sites for NT (and possibly related peptides) within the body.

7 NEUROTENSIN-RELATED PEPTIDES

The generation of region-specific antisera in our laboratory (Figure 10) has facilitated the immunochemical identification of peptides that have close structural similarities to NT (Table 3; see ref. 105 for a detailed review). Antiserum TG-1, which is directed towards the amino- terminal region of NT, cross-reacts approximately 20% with NT[1-8], 60% with NT[1-11] and 100% with NT[1-12] (106). Antisera that recognize the carboxyl-terminal of NT were also generated: PGL-4 cross-reacts about 100% with NT[10-13]; HC-8 requires the NT[6-13] portion for full recognition and cross-reacts <0.05% with NT[10-13] (4). The antiserum Xen-6 against xenopsin (XP; see below), was raised by Dr. Gerhard Feurle, University of Heidelberg, Germany. Xen-6 cross-reacts only 4% with NT and <0.001% with NT1-12.

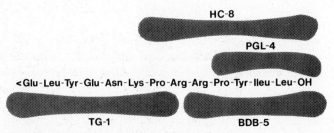

Figure 10. Orientation of proposed antigenic sites for site-specific antisera vs. NT. Cross-reactivities to NT fragments are reviewed in the text and in ref. 105.

In a series of phylogenetic studies, it has become clear that NT-related substances are present in lower animals and that many of these peptides cross-react preferentially with C-terminal directed antisera (107, 108). This conservation of the C-terminal region has been shown for extracts of unicellular organisms, porifera and protozoa, as well as for representatives of all animal classes using both radioimmunoassay and immunocytochemistry (109–111). The N-terminal region of the NT-related material is sufficiently different in submammalian species that antiserum TG-1 gives measurements which are usually less than 1% those obtained with antiserum PGL-4. It appears that NT-like peptides are phylogenetically old and peptides with a structurally unchanged C-terminal region have been co-opted for a variety of different roles in many unrelated species. It therefore may not be surprising that within mammalian species, NT has been reported to participate in the regulation of many different systems.

It is likely that within the same species there exist multiple, biologically-active variants of peptides with conserved C-terminal segments. In the skin of the African frog *Xenopus laevis* (112), a peptide similar to NT, XP has been isolated (Table 3). Extracts of the nervous and gastrointestinal tissues of several amphibia have been found to contain peptides relating to the C-terminal regions of XP and NT, as indicated by gel permeation chromatography, high-pressure liquid chromatography and radioimmunoassay with multiple region-specific antisera (113). Furthermore, NT-like peptides were found to have different distributions: those recognized by HC-8 were concentrated in brain and small intestine, while the PGL-4 immunoreactivity was found mostly in stomach, liver and pancreas. The highest level of XP-like material was measured in stomach, pancreas and *Xenopus* skin. Intravenous injection of purified extracts of these related peptides were all found to increase hemat-

TABLE 3   Comparison of the Structures of NT and Three NT-Related Peptides

Peptide[a]	Structure[b]
NT (bovine)	< Glu-Leu-Tyr-Glu-Asn-Lys-Pro-Arg-Arg-Pro-Tyr-lle-Leu-OH
NT-I (*Gassus demesticus*)[c]	< Glu-Leu-His-Val-Asn-Lys-Ala-Arg-Arg-Pro-Tyr-lle-Leu-OH
NT-II (*G. demesticus*)[c]	H-Lys-Asn-Pro-Tyr-lle-Leu-OH
Xenopsin (*Xenopus laevis*)	< Glu-Gly-Lys-Arg-Pro-Trp-lle-Leu-OH

[a] The animal source for each peptide is shown in parentheses. *Xenopus laevis* is an African frog. (See ref. 105 for details).
[b] The underlined residues denote differences when compared with the corresponding positions in bovine NT.
[c] NT-I refers to the peptide isolated from the first peak of immunoreactivity after gel permeation chromatography (Sephadex G-25) of extract of chick small intestine, NT-II refers to the peptide from the second peak.

ocrit in rats, but not all produced cyanosis. It may be speculated that the N-terminal segments have undergone changes so that peptides immunochemically similar to NT and XP have diverged and subserve different roles within the same animal.

Neurotensin-related material has been found in high concentration in birds (five to ten times higher than mammals). Extracts of chicken small intestine have been shown to include three separate groups of immunoreactivities, as identified on gel permeation chromatography and measured by the PGL-4 antiserum in radioimmunoassay (105). The first peak of activity was found to display the biologic activities characteristic of NT and to contain three amino acid differences from NT, with the identical NT[8-13] fragment (113). The PGL-4 and HC-8 antisera recognized this material on an approximately equimolar basis; however in contrast, the N-directed, TG-1, showed no recognition. The second peak identified immunochemically was detected far better by PGL-4 than by HC-8 (approximately 500 times) in the radioimmunoassay. This substance was shown to be a hexapeptide sharing four C-terminal amino acids with NT (R. E. Carraway, and C. F. Ferris, unpublished results). Biologically, this peptide appeared to be a variant of NT with a different spectrum of activity. Peak three has been shown to be quite heterogeneous and its relationship to NT is presently unclear. The first and second peaks of NT-like peptides are differently distributed in the chicken by radioimmunoassay and appear to be localized in different endocrine-like cells in the intestine as visualized immunohistochemically (R. E. Carraway, M. Reineke, and W. G. Forssmann, unpublished results). In addition, both have been shown to be present in synaptosomal preparations and to be released from chicken brain slices following 60 mM potassium-stimulation in the presence of calcium.

ACKNOWLEDGMENTS

We gratefully thank Ms. Linda Carreaux for her assistance in the preparation of this manuscript. Some of the work presented here was supported by NIH Grants AM 01126-01 (N.A.), AM 28557 and AM 28565 (R.E.C.), NS 16367 (M.D.), and AM 29876-03 (S.E.L.).

REFERENCES

1. R. Carraway and S. E. Leeman, *J. Biol. Chem.* **248**, 6854 (1973).
2. R. Carraway and S. E. Leeman, *J. Biol. Chem.* **250**, 1907 (1975).
3. R. Carraway and S. E. Leeman, *J. Biol. Chem.* **250**, 1912 (1975).
4. R. Carraway and S. E. Leeman, *J. Biol. Chem.* **251**, 7035 (1976).
5. S. E. Leeman, E. A. Mroz, and R. E. Carraway, in H. Gainer, Ed., *Peptides in Neurobiology*, Plenum Press, New York, 1977, pp. 99–144.

6. S. E. Leeman, N. Aronin, and C. F. Ferris, *Recent Prog. Horm. Res.* **38**, 93 (1982).
7. S. E. Leeman, M. DiFiglia, and N. Aronin, *Soc. Neurosci. Abstr.* **6**, 354 (1980).
8. M. Ninkovic, S. P. Hunt, and J. S. Kelly, *Brain Res.* **230**, 111 (1981).
9. M. DiFiglia, N. Aronin, and S. E. Leeman, *Ann. N.Y. Acad. Sci.* **400**, 405 (1982).
10. L. L. Iversen, S. D. Iversen, F. Bloom, C. Douglas, M. Brown, and W. Vale, *Nature* **273**, 161 (1978).
11. W. S. Young, G. R. Uhl, and M. J. Kuhar, *Brain Res.* **150**, 431 (1978).
12. R. Carraway and S. E. Leeman, *J. Biol. Chem.* **251**, 7045 (1976).
13. R. M. Kobayashi, M. Brown, and W. Vale, *Brain Res.* **126**, 584 (1977).
14. G. R. Uhl and S. H. Snyder, *Life Sci.* **19**, 1827 (1976).
15. K. Kataoka, N. Mizuno, and L. A. Frohman, *Brain Res. Bull.* **4**, 57 (1979).
16. P. E. Cooper, M. H. Fernstrom, P. P. Rorstad, S. E. Leeman, and J. B. Martin, *Brain Res.* **218**, 219 (1981).
17. G. R. Uhl, M. J. Kuhar, and S. H. Snyder, *Proc. Natl. Acad. Sci. USA* **74**, 4059 (1977).
18. G. R. Uhl, R. R. Goodman, and S. H. Snyder, *Brain Res.* **167**, 77 (1979).
19. G. R. Uhl and S. H. Snyder, *Brain Res.* **161**, 522 (1979).
20. D. Kahn, G. M. Abrams, E. A. Zimmerman, R. Carraway, and S. E. Leeman, *Endocrinology* **107**, 47 (1980).
21. C. B. Nemeroff, A. J. Osbahr III, P. J. Manberg, G. N. Ervin, and A. J. Prange Jr., *Proc. Natl. Acad. Sci. USA* **76**, 5368 (1979).
22. G. Bissette, C. B. Nemeroff, P. T. Loosen, A. J. Prange Jr., and M. A. Lipton, *Nature (London)* **262**, 607 (1976).
23. C. B. Nemeroff, G. Bissette, P. J. Manberg, A. J. Osbahr III, G. R. Breese, and A. J. Prange Jr., *Brain Res.* **195**, 69 (1980).
24. G. E. Martin and T. Naruse, *Regul. Peptides* **3**, 97 (1982).
25. J. E. Morley, A. S. Levine, M. M. Oken, M. Grace, and J. Kneip, *Peptides* **3**, 1 (1982).
26. K. Maeda and L. A. Frohman, *Endocrinology* **103**, 1903 (1978).
27. E. Vijayan and S. M. McCann, *Endocrinology* **105**, 64 (1979).
28. C. Rivier, M. Brown, and W. Vale, *Endocrinology* **100**, 751 (1977).
29. A. Enjalbert, S. Arancibia, M. Priam, M. T. Bluet-Pajot, and C. Kordan, *Neuroendocrinology* **34**, 95 (1982).
30. C. F. Ferris, J. X. Pan, E. A. Singer, N. Boyd, and S. E. Leeman, *Ann. N.Y. Acad. Sci.* **400**, 379 (1982).
31. E. Vijayan and S. M. McCann, *Life Sci.* **26**, 321 (1980).
32. Y. Taché, M. Brown, and R. Collu, *Endocrinology* **105**, 220 (1979).
33. H. Abe, K. Chihara, T. Chiba, S. Matsukura, and T. Fujita, *Endocrinology* **108**, 1939 (1981).
34. H. Saito and S. Saito, *Endocrinology* **107**, 1600 (1980).
35. A. M. Blackburn, D. R. Fletcher, T. E. Adrian, and S. R. Bloom, *J. Clin. Endocrinol. Metab.* **51**, 1257 (1980).
36. V. Seybold and R. Elde, *J. Histochem. Cytochem.* **28**, 367 (1980).
37. S. J. Gibson, J. M. Polak, S. R. Bloom, and P. D. Wall, *J. Comp. Neurol.* **201**, 65 (1981).
38. S. P. Hunt, J. S. Kelly, P. C. Emson, T. R. Kimmel, R. J. Miller, and J. -Y. Wu, *Neuroscience* **6**, 1883 (1981).
39. V. Seybold and R. Elde, *J. Comp. Neurol.* **205**, 89 (1982).
40. L. W. Haynes, *Neurosci. Lett.* **19**, 185 (1980).
41. N. Aronin, M. DiFiglia, A. S. Liotta, and J. B. Martin, *J. Neurosci.* **1**, 561 (1981).
42. B. V. Clineschmidt and J. C. McGuffin, *Eur. J. Pharmacol.* **46**, 395 (1977).
43. B. V. Clineschmidt, J. C. McGuffin, and P. B. Bunting, *Eur. J. Pharmacol.* **54**, 129 (1979).
44. A. J. Osbahr III, C. B. Nemeroff, D. Luttinger, G. A. Mason, and A. J. Prange, Jr., *J. Pharmacol. Exp. Ther.* **217**, 645 (1981).
45. T. L. Yaksh, C. Schmauss, P. E. Micevych, E. D. Abay, and V. L. W. Go, *Ann. N.Y. Acad. Sci.* **400**, 228 (1982).

46. V. Miletić and M. Randić, *Brain Res.* **169**, 600 (1979).
47. T. Suzue, N. Yanaihara, and M. Otsuka, *Neurosci. Lett.* **26**, 137 (1981).
48. R. A. Nicoll, *J. Pharmacol. Exp. Ther.* **207**, 817 (1978).
49. J. W. Phillis and J. R. Kirkpatrick, *Can. J. Physiol. Pharmacol.* **57**, 887 (1979).
50. J. L. Henry, *Ann. N.Y. Acad. Sci.* **400**, 216 (1982).
51. J. M. Lundberg, T. Hökfelt, A. Änggård, K. Uvnäs-Wallensten, S. Brimijoin, E. Brodin, and J. Fahrenkrug, in E. Costa and M. Trabucchi, Ed., *Neural Peptides and Neuronal Communications*, Raven Press, New York, 1980, pp. 25–36.
52. J. M. Lundberg, Å. Rökaeus, T. Hökfelt, S. Rosell, M. Brown, and M. Goldstein, *Acta Physiol. Scand.* **114**, 153 (1982).
53. Y. C. Lee, G. Terenghi, J. M. Polak, and S. R. Bloom, *Acta Endocrinol.* **97**, Suppl. 243, 84 (1981), Abstract.
54. A. Rokaeus and J. M. Lundberg, *Ann. N.Y. Acad. Sci.*, in press (1982).
55. A. S. Tischler, Y. C. Lee, V. W. Slayton, and S. R. Bloom, *Regul. Peptides* **3**:415 (1982).
56. R. Carraway, R. A. Hammer, and S. E. Leeman, *Endocrinology* **107**, 400 (1980).
57. N. Aronin, R. E. Carraway, C. F. Ferris, R. A. Hammer, and S. E. Leeman, *Peptides* **3**:632 (1982).
58. M. L. Mashford, G. Nilsson, Å. Rökaeus, and S. Rosell, *Acta Physiol. Scand.* **104**, 244 (1978).
59. S. Rosell, Å. Rökaeus, M. L. Mashford, K. Thor, D. Chang, and K. Folkers, in E. Costa and M. Trabucchi, Ed., *Neural Peptides and Neuronal Communication*, Raven Press, New York, 1980, pp. 181–189.
60. R. E. Carraway and S. E. Leeman, *J. Biol. Chem.* **251**, 7045 (1976).
61. P. Kitabgi, R. E. Carraway, and S. E. Leeman, *J. Biol. Chem.* **251**, 7053 (1976).
62. R. Carraway, P. Kitabgi, and S. E. Leeman, *J. Biol. Chem.* **253**, 7996 (1978).
63. R. A. Hammer, S. E. Leeman, R. E. Carraway, and R. H. Williams, *J. Biol. Chem.* **255**, 2476 (1980).
64. L. Orci, O. Baetens, C. Rufener, M. Brown, W. Vale, and R. Guillemin, *Life Sci.* **19**, 559 (1976).
65. V. Helmstaedter, C. Taugner, G. E. Feurle, and W. G. Forssmann, *Histochemistry* **53**, 35 (1977).
66. J. M. Polak, S. N. Sullivan, S. R. Bloom, A. M. J. Buchan, P. Facer, M. R. Brown, and A. G. E. Pearse, *Nature (London)* **262**, 92 (1977).
67. F. Sundler, R. Håkansson, R. A. Hammer, J. Alumets, R. Carraway, S. E. Leeman, and E. A. Zimmerman, *Cell Tissue Res.* **178**, 313 (1977).
68. V. Helmstaedter, G. E. Feurle, and W. G. Forssmann, *Cell Tissue Res.* **184**, 445 (1977).
69. S. Rosell and Å. Rökaeus, *Acta Physiol. Scand.* **107**, 263 (1979).
70. S. Andersson, D. Chang, K. Folkers, and S. Rosell, *Life Sci.* **19**, 367 (1976).
71. S. Andersson, S. Rosell, U. Hjelmquist, D. Chang, and K. Folkers, *Acta Physiol. Scand.* **100**, 231 (1977).
72. S. Andersson, S. Rosell, L. Sjodin, and K. Folkers, *Scand. J. Gastroenterol.* **15**, 253 (1980).
73. S. Rosell, K. Thor, Å. Rökaeus, O. Nyquist, A. Lewenhaupt, L. Kager, and K. Folkers, *Acta Physiol. Scand.* **109**, 369 (1980).
74. P. Mitchenere, T. E. Adrian, R. M. Kirk, and S. R. Bloom, *Life Sci.* **29**, 1563 (1981).
75. S. Ito, Y. Matsubara, Y. Iwaski, T. Momotsu, A. Shibata, and T. Muto, *Horm. Metab. Res.* **12**, 551 (1980).
76. R. A. Hammer, R. E. Carraway, and S. E. Leeman, *J. Clin. Invest.* **70**, 74 (1982).
77. C. Ferris, R. A. Hammer, and S. E. Leeman, *Peptides* **2**, Suppl. 2, 263 (1981).
78. B. Kihl, Å. Rökaeus, S. Rosell, and L. Olbe, *Scand. J. Gastroenterol.* **16**, 513 (1981).
79. P. Kitabgi and P. Freychet, *Eur. J. Pharmacol.* **50**, 349 (1978).

80. P. Kitabgi, G. Hamon, and M. Worcel, *Eur. J. Pharmacol.* **56**, 87 (1979).
81. P. Kitabgi and P. Freychet, *Eur. J. Pharmacol.* **56**, 403 (1979).
82. S. Momer and P. Kitabgi, *Regul. Peptides* **2**, 31 (1981).
83. J. T. Williams, Y. Katayama, and R. A. North, *Eur. J. Pharmacol.* **59**, 181 (1979).
84. M. Brown and W. Vale, *Endocrinology* **98**, 819 (1976).
85. R. Carraway, L. M. Demers, and S. E. Leeman, *Endocrinology* **99**, 1452 (1976).
86. K. Nagai and L. A. Frohman, *Life Sci.* **19**, 273 (1976).
87. R. R. Wolfe, J. R. Allsop, and J. F. Burke, *Life Sci.* **22**, 1043 (1978).
88. A. Kaneto, T. Kaneko, H. Kajinuma, and K. Kosaka, *Endocrinology* **102**, 393 (1978).
89. J. H. Moltz, R. E. Dobbs, S. M. McCann, and C. P. Fawcett, *Endocrinology* **101**, 196 (1977).
90. J. Dolais-Kitabgi, P. Kitabgi, P. Brazeau, and P. Freychet, *Endocrinology* **105**, 256 (1979).
91. I. Lundquist, F. Sundler, B. Ahrin, J. Alumets, and R. Håkanson, *Endocrinology* **104**, 832 (1979).
92. M. H. Fernstrom, M. A. Z. Mirski, R. E. Carraway, and S. E. Leeman, *Metabolism* **30**, 853 (1981).
93. M. Berelowitz and L. A. Frohman, *Ann. N.Y. Acad. Sci.* **400**, 150 (1982).
94. P. Kitabgi, R. Carraway, J. VanRietschoten, C. Granier, J. L. Morgat, A. Menez, S. E. Leeman, and P. Freychet, *Proc. Natl. Acad. Sci. USA* **74**, 1846 (1977).
95. G. R. Uhl, J. P. Bennett, Jr., and S. H. Snyder, *Brain Res.* **130**, 299 (1977).
96. L. H. Lazarus, M. R. Brown, and M. H. Perrin, *Neuropharmacology* **16**, 625 (1977).
97. P. Kitabgi, C. Poustis, C. Granier, J. VanRietschoten, J. Rivier, J. L. Morgat, and P. Freychet, *Mol. Pharmacol.* **18**, 11 (1980).
98. L. H. Lazarus, M. H. Perrin, and M. R. Brown, *J. Biol. Chem.* **252**, 7174 (1977).
99. L. H. Lazarus, M. H. Perrin, M. R. Brown, and J. E. Rivier, *J. Biol. Chem.* **252**, 7180 (1977).
100. W. S. Young and M. J. Kuhar, *Brain Res.* **206**, 273 (1981).
101. G. Bissette, P. Manberg, C. B. Nemeroff, and A. J. Prange, Jr., *Life Sci.* **23**, 2173 (1978).
102. J. M. Palacios and M. J. Kuhar, *Nature* **294**, 587 (1981).
103. R. Carraway, D. E. Cochrane, J. B. Lansman, S. E. Leeman, B. M. Paterson, and H. J. Welch, *J. Physiol.* **323**, 403 (1982).
104. D. E. Cochrane, C. Emigh, G. Levine, R. E. Carraway, and S. E. Leeman, *Ann. N.Y. Acad. Sci.* **400**, 396 (1982).
105. R. E. Carraway, *Ann. N.Y. Acad. Sci.,* **400**, 17 (1982).
106. R. Carraway and Y. M. Bhatnagar, *Peptides* **1**, 159 (1980).
107. R. Carraway, S. Ruane, and H. R. Kim, *Peptides* **1**, 115 (1982).
108. Y. M. Bhatnagar and R. Carraway, *Peptides* **2**, 51 (1981).
109. M. Reineke, K. Almasan, R. Carraway, V. Helmstaeder, and W. G. Forssmann, *Cell Tissue Res.* **205**, 383 (1980).
110. M. Reineke, R. Carraway, S. Falkmer, G. E. Feurle, and W. G. Forssman, *Cell Tissue Res.* **212**, 173 (1980).
111. C. J. P. Grimmelikhuijzen, R. Carraway, A. Rokaeus, and F. Sundler, *Histochemistry* **72**, 199 (1981).
112. K. Araki, S. Tachibana, M. Uchigama, T. Nakajima, and T. Yasuhara, *Chem. Pharmacol. Bull. (Tokyo)* **21**, 2801 (1973).
113. R. Carraway, S. E. Ruane, G. E. Feurle, and S. Taylor, *Endocrinology* **110**, 1094 (1982).
114. R. Carraway and Y. M. Bhatnagar, *Peptides* **1**, 167 (1980).

31

Substance P

NEIL ARONIN
Departments of Medicine and Psysiology
University of Massachusetts Medical School
Worcester, Massachusetts

MARIAN DIFIGLIA
Department of Neurology
Massachusetts General Hospital and Harvard Medical School
Boston, Massachusetts

SUSAN E. LEEMAN
Department of Physiology
University of Massachusetts Medical School
Worcester, Massachusetts

1 INTRODUCTION

During work directed towards the purification of a corticotropin releasing factor, a sialogogic peptide (1) was discovered and characterized by multiple chemical and biological criteria to be the substance responsible for the biological activities described by von Euler and Gaddum (2); it was termed substance P. This chapter emphasizes studies on the cellular localization, distribution, and possible physiological roles of substance P. For details of the discovery and isolation of substance P, the reader is referred to recent reviews (4, 5).

2 SUBSTANCE P: CHEMICAL CHARACTERIZATION

Purification of substance P (SP) was initially accomplished by a series of gel permeation, ion-exchange chromatographic procedures and high voltage paper electrophoresis (6). The amino acid sequence of the sialogogic peptide was determined to be Arg-Pro-Lys-Pro-Gln-Gln-Phe-Phe-Gly-Leu-Met-NH$_2$ (7). In further studies by Studer et al. (8) and Carraway and Leeman (9), the chemical identity of SP from equine intestine, bovine colliculi, and hypothalami was confirmed. The solid phase synthesis of SP, first accomplished by Tregear et al. (10), led to the development of antisera for radioimmunoassay (11, 12) and immunohistochemistry (see below), as well as studies to determine possible biological activities of this peptide.

The bioactive region of SP for its sialogogic activity and spasmogenic activity on guinea pig ileum contraction resides in its carboxyl terminus (for a review, see ref. 13). A loss of sialogogic activity follows oxidation of the terminal methionine (14). Recent studies have reported the presence of SP-related peptides in extracts of the dorsal root ganglia and spinal cord (15) and the terminal octapeptide in extracts of the amygdala (16). It is unclear whether these fragments are physiologically active or are principally metabolites.

Substance P belongs to a family of related peptides that shares its hypotensive properties (Table 1). Among these peptides are eledoisin (17), isolated from the cephalopod salivary glands and physalaemin (18), isolated from the skin of a South American amphibian. The carboxyl-terminus of these peptides is similar to the terminal sequence of

TABLE 1 Structures of Substance P and Related Peptides

Substance P	Arg-Pro-Lys-Pro-Gln-Gln-Phe-Phe-Gly-Leu-Met-NH$_2$
Physalaemin	< Glu-Ala-Asp-Pro-Asn-Lys-Phe-Tyr-Gly-Leu-Met-NH$_2$
Eledoisin	< Glu-Pro-Ser-Lys-Asp-Ala-Phe-Ile-Gly-Leu-Met-NH$_2$
Uperolein	< Glu-Pro-Asp-Pro-Asn-Ala-Phe-Tyr-Gly-Leu-Met-NH$_2$

SP (for a review, see ref. 13). Although SP seems to be the principal member of this group found in the mammalian central nervous system, there is now evidence that immunoreactive physalaemin-like peptides are also present in mammalian tissue (19).

3 DISTRIBUTION: SUBSTANCE P IN THE CENTRAL NERVOUS SYSTEM AND PERIPHERAL NERVOUS TISSUE

The widespread distribution of SP-like peptides has been mapped by both radioimmunoassay and immunohistochemistry. Since several SP fragments or structurally related peptides may be found in brain extracts, the cross-reactivity of each antiserum to these and other peptides should be evaluated for proper interpretation of both radioimmunoassay and immunohistochemistry data. In that line, the term SP-like immunoreactivity (SPLI) is used here to describe results for both of these methods.

SPLI has been measured by radioimmunoassay in the central nervous system of the rat (20, 21) and human (22–24), and a similar distribution has been found in both species (Table 2). The substantia nigra contains the highest concentrations of SPLI in the brain. In the human, the inner globus pallidus, which is also in the extrapyramidal system, has high concentrations of SPLI. The hypothalamus and the ascending afferent sensory systems, the dorsal horn of the spinal cord, and the trigeminal nucleus of the medulla are particularly rich in SPLI. The presence of SPLI in such functionally diverse systems as the endocrine-limbic, extrapyramidal, and somatosensory indicates that this peptide subserves multiple physiological roles in the central nervous system.

Immunohistochemical studies (25, 26) have shown a similar pattern of distribution of SPLI as determined by radioimmunoassay. The densest concentration of fiber staining by immunofluorescence corresponds closely to those areas with the highest levels of radioimmunoassay. Accordingly, the labeling of processes is most abundant in the substantia nigra, the inner aspect of the globus pallidus in the primate (27), the dorsal horn of the spinal cord, and the trigeminal nucleus of the medulla. This correlation is consistent with the likelihood that most of the SPLI is found within axon terminals in the central nervous system. Colchicine treatment frequently is necessary to locate SPLI within cell bodies, presumably by impairing axonal transport of the peptide. At the light microscopic level in the rat, somata with SPLI have been shown in the neostriatum, globus pallidus, nucleus habenulae medialis, nucleus interpeduncularis, septal nuclei, and in numerous regions of the hypothalamus and brainstem. The dorsal root ganglia (28, 29) and the dorsal horn of the spinal cord also contain cell bodies with SPLI (see below).

TABLE 2 Regional Distribution of Substance P in the CNS[a]

Region	Rat[b] pmol/10 mg (wet weight)	Rat[c] pmol/mg protein	Human[d] pmol/10 mg (wet weight)	Human[e] pmol/mg protein
Somatosensory System and Cortex				
Dorsal root ganglia	0.6			
Dorsal horn	9.4			
Trigeminal nucleus	12.1			
Dorsal column	1.1			
Dorsal column nucleus	1.5			
Thalamic nucleus	0.2			
lateral dorsal			0.115	
lateral posterior			0.03	
dorsal medial			0.354	
Somatosensory cortex	0.2			
Cerebral cortex				
frontal			0.08	
parietal			0.07	
uncal			0.12	
entorhinal			0.15	
			0.336	
cingulate			0.11	
striate			0.046	
Visual system				
optic nerve			0.06	
lateral geniculate body	0.7	0.9	0.36	
superior colliculus			1.25	
visual cortex	0.2			
Basal Ganglia				
Striatum		0.9		
Caudate	2.2		1.13	3.7
Putamen			0.81	3.3
Globus pallidus	2.9			18.0
internal			5.18	
external			1.24	
Subthalamic nucleus	2.0		0.21	
Substantia nigra	15.1		9.22	
pars compacta		2.9		47.2
pars reticulata		11.38		47.9
pars lateralis		3.0		
Hypothalamus		2.1		5.2
Anterior			1.22	
Posterior			1.35	
Medial	5.5			
Middle	4.5			
Lateral	4.3			
Medial preoptic nucleus	4.4			
Lateral preoptic nucleus	3.3			
Periventricular nucleus	3.3			
Suprachiasmatic nucleus	1.6			
Supraoptic nucleus		1.6		

TABLE 2 (*Continued*)

Region	Rat[b] pmol/10 mg (wet weight)	Rat[c] pmol/mg protein	Human[d] pmol/10 mg (wet weight)	Human[e] pmol/mg protein
Anterior hypothalamic nucleus	3.2			
Paraventricular nucleus	3.1			
Arcuate nucleus		2.5		
Ventromedial nucleus		2.5		
Dorsomedial nucleus		3.5		
Perifornical nucleus		2.9		
Mammillary bodies	1.8		0.83	
Ventral premammillary nucleus	3.3			
Dorsal premammillary nucleus	1.7			
Posterior premammillary nucleus	2.8			
Medial forebrain bundle, anterior	3.1			
Medial forebrain bundle, posterior	2.3			
Median eminence		1.0	1.34	
Limbic System				
Olfactory bulb	0.5	0.2	0.41	
Olfactory tubercle	2.6			
Olfactory cortex	0.4			
Amygdala	3.3	3.4	0.26	
Hippocampus	0.3			
Habenula	3.3			
Interpeduncular nucleus	5.2	5.9		
Septum	3.5	1.2		
dorsal septal nucleus	2.8			
lateral septal nucleus	3.6			
Interstitial nucleus of stria terminalis		3.3		
Nucleus accumbens	2.4			
Anterior thalamic nucleus	1.9			
Other Regions				
Locus coeruleus			1.99	
Raphe nuclei			0.71	
Area postrema			1.14	
Inferior olive			0.078	
Red nucleus		1.3	0.76	
Medial geniculate		0.8		
Inferior collicalus		1.2	2.34	
Central gray		2.9		
periaqueductal gray			1.30	
Cerebellum	<0.1	<0.1		0.2

TABLE 2   (*Continued*)

Region	Rat[b] pmol/10 mg (wet weight)	Rat[c] pmol/mg protein	Human[d] pmol/10 mg (wet weight)	Human[e] pmol/mg protein
cortex			0.003	
dentate nucleus			0.014	
Pineal	< 0.1f		0.01	0.5

[a] Values measured by radioimmunoassay. No standard errors are presented. All values have been converted to either a mol/10 mg wet weight or pmol/ml protein. These values may be comparable, since nervous tissue contains approximately 10% protein.
[b] Kanazawa and Jessell (21).
[c] Brownstein et al. (20).
[d] Cooper et al. (24).
[e] Gale et al. (22).
[f] M.H. Fernstrom and S.E Leeman, unpublished.

Both neurochemical and electron microscopic data are consistent with the possibility that SP is a candidate neurotransmitter (for a review of this broad topic, see ref. 30). In synaptosomal preparations from rat brain stem, SPLI is releasable upon depolarization with high potassium with calcium ion dependence (31) and there is recent evidence that SPLI is released from vesicles of approximately 117 nm diameter (32). Vesicles of this size range have been found to contain a high density of reaction products by electron microscopic immunocytochemistry with SP antiserum (33, 34).

The vesicles within the rat brain stem that contain SPLI have some properties of vesicles that release transmitters (32). For example, depolarization of the vesicles might be expected to reduce their SPLI level. Incubation of the vesicles with veratridine, which depolarizes rat brain synaptosomes, results in a depletion of SPLI in the vesicle fraction. Furthermore, this depletion was found to be tetrodotoxin-sensitive and calcium-dependent, also features of vesicles that contain neurotransmitters.

4   BIOSYNTHESIS OF SUBSTANCE P

To date, the identification of an SP precursor has remained elusive. There is, however, *in vitro* evidence in the dorsal root ganglia that the incorporation of ^{35}S-methionine into SP is blocked by cyclohexamide, which suggests that a ribosomal dependence is involved in the synthesis of this peptide (35). Further studies in dorsal root ganglia (36) have shown that both ^{35}S-methionine and ^{3}H-proline are incorporated into a peptide that is immunoprecipitated by both N- and C-terminally-directed SP antisera; that this labeled peptide coeluted with SP on high pressure liquid chromatography and that its oxidation formed a derivative with physicochemical properties of substance P-sulfoxide (14). The appearance of the labeled SPLI occurred after 1-2 h of incubation with the labeled amino acids and is consistent with the presence of a larger-molecular-weight precursor. The *in vivo* incorporation of ^{35}S-methionine into SP has been demonstrated following injection of the labeled amino acid into the rat striatum (37). The detection of labeled SP in the substantia nigra, which is diminished by colchicine treatment, is consistent with lesion studies, which show a striatal-nigral SP pathway (see below).

5   SUBSTANCE P ANTAGONISTS

Clarification of the possible functions of SP as a candidate neurotransmitter or modulator has been made difficult by the lack of reliable, specific antagonists. Baclofen, first used as a gamma aminobutyric acid (GABA) antagonist, has been tested as an SP antagonist (38) and also diminishes acetylcholine and glutamate-induced excitation of locus coeruleus nerons. There are now several reports of synthetic peptides, in which D-amino acids are substituted for L-amino (39–41). One of these analogs, SP, D-Pro^2, D-Trp,^{7,9} appears to show particular promise in blocking specifically SP effects in several tissues, despite its weak agonist property. Following local application of this analog, the activity of SP has been blocked in locus coeruleus neurons in anesthesized rats (41) without affecting the excitatory response to acetylcholine or glutamate. In like fashion, this synthetic peptide has been reported to antagonize the SP-mediated inflammatory response in the eye of the rabbit (42), the antidromic vasodilation (which is presumably via a SP effect) following activation of pain fibers in the cat dental pulp (43), and the stimulatory effect of SP on the smooth muscle of the guinea pig ileum (44). Intrathecal injection of this antagonist blunts the scratching and biting behavior elicited by SP administered intrathecally and capsaicin applied to the skin (45). This finding provides additional evidence that SP is a neurotransmitter of primary nociceptive afferents. The influence of this antagonist in other systems where SP has been proposed to have neurotransmitter properties, namely in the striatonigral projection and in the autonomic nervous system, will be followed with great interest.

6   SUBSTANCE P IN THE SUBSTANTIA NIGRA

As noted above, high concentrations of immunoreactive SP are present within the basal ganglia. In the rat, fibers are found by immunofluorescence, in the caudate, putamen, entopenduncular nucleus, and in the substantia nigra, where they appear to be most numerous (26, 46). It is interesting that while SPLI concentrations in the rat substantia nigra are considerably higher in the pars reticulata as measured by radioimmuno-assay (47), immunofluorescence studies show considerable fiber stain-ing in both the compacta and reticulata. In contrast, immunofluorescent SP fibers appear to be more numerous in the inner than the outer palli-dal segment (27). Fluorescent fibers have also been reported in the sub-thalamic nucleus (26). Substance P positive cell bodies have been demonstrated in the neostriatum and globus pallidus (25, 46).

We have examined the distribution of immunoreactive SP in the monkey substantia nigra using the immunoperoxidase method (48). La-beled fibers were observed in both the pars compacta and pars reticulata (Figure 1A). This finding is consistent with the nearly equiva-lent concentrations of radioimmunoassayable SPLI measured in both subdivisions of the human substantia nigra (24). Numerous immunoreac-tive SP axons were observed to course from the cerebral peduncle into the nigra, where they gave rise to branches and terminal swellings. At the electron microscopic level, SPLI was contained within both myeli-nated (Figure 1C) and unmyelinated fibers and in axon terminals that ranged from 0.5 to 1.5 μm and contained clear round and large granular vesicles (LGV) in the range of 100 nm (Figure 1B). Most of the peroxi-dase reaction product was confined to LGV, which were distributed throughout the labeled boutons. Immunoreactive SP terminals formed asymmetric synapses with small and large dendrites and cell bodies within the nigra.

Lesion studies suggest that descending pathways from the neostria-tum and globus pallidus are the source of SP in the substantia nigra (46, 47, 49–51). Application of potassium to the caudate nucleus causes a re-lease of SPLI in the substantia nigra (52). In Huntington's disease, char-acterized by degeneration of neurons in the caudate nucleus and the globus pallidus, there is a marked reduction in SPLI levels within the substantia nigra (53–55).

The anatomical relationships between neuronal elements, which con-tain SP and other peptides and transmitters that are highly concentrated in the basal ganglia, are still unclear. The substantia nigra contains nu-merous enkephalin (56, 57) and glutamic acid decarboxylase immunore-active fibers and terminals (58) that are also thought to originate from cell bodies in the neostriatum (57, 59, 60). While there appears to be lit-tle overlap between gamma-aminobutyric acid (GABA) and SP within the neostriatum (49, 51), it is likely that different striatonigral pathways (including those containing enkephalin-like peptides) interact by con-verging on the same nigral neurons, which in turn can affect activity in the neostriatum and other target structures of nigral efferent pathways. Within the substantia nigra, GABA has been shown to inhibit the potas-sium-evoked release of SP under conditions where dopamine and

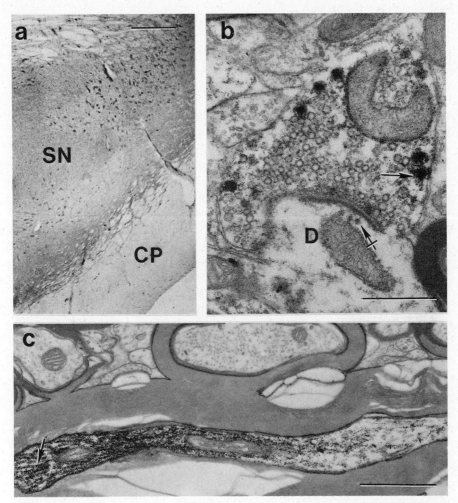

Figure 1. Immunoreactive SP in the monkey substantia nigra (*SN*). (A) Numerous labeled fibers are present throughout the pars compacta and the pars reticulata; some are seen to enter from the adjacent cerebral peduncle (*CP*). The cells of the compacta are visible because of their content of pigment granules. Scale bar, 500 μm. From Mroz et al. (47). (B) Axon terminal with SPLI contains clear round vesicles and large granular vesicles (arrow), in which most of the peroxidase reaction product is heavily deposited. The bouton makes an asymmetric synapse with dendrite D, which contains postjunctional bodies (crossed arrow). Scale bar, 0.5 μm. From Mroz et al. (47). (C) An immunoreactive SP axon is thickly myelinated and exhibits peroxidase reaction product along microtubules (arrow). Note the presence of nearby unlabeled fibers. Scale bar, 1 μm.

enkephalins have no effect (52, 61). Application of SP in the nigra, which causes a marked excitation of nigra neurons (62, 63), has been found to stimulate the release of dopamine in the ipsilateral caudate nucleus (52).

7 SUBSTANCE P IN THE SPINAL CORD

Light microscopic immunocytochemical studies have localized SPLI to widespread areas of the spinal cord gray matter. The densest distribution of immunoreactive SP fibers and terminals has been observed in the superficial laminae (laminae I and outer II) of the posterior horn in both the rat (26, 64) and cat (28). Immunoreactive SP terminals have also been observed in the central (lamina X), intermediate (lamina VII), and ventral gray (laminae VII and IX) areas. Labeled fibers also have been seen in close association with alpha motor neurons (64). In the white matter, immunoreactive SP axons have been noted in the dorsal root entry zone, the tract of Lissauer, and the lateral funiculus.

Following colchicine treatment, some immunoreactive SP neurons have been observed in all laminae of the rat posterior horn (26, 65–67), with the greatest numbers reported in laminae II, III and IV. In addition, SP-positive cell bodies have been found in laminae VII, VIII, and X of the cat (68, 69).

Electron microscopic studies (29, 33, 64) have demonstrated that in the rat dorsal horn SPLI is present within axon terminals that contain small clear and large granular vesicles. The latter, about 100 nm, are usually heavily laden with peroxidase reaction product. Labeled terminals form synapses predominantly with dendritic profiles. Other types of contacts have also been described, including membrane appositions with other axons and with capillaries (64).

Recent work in our laboratory (34) has focused on the distribution of SPLI in the spinal cord of monkeys. Our results using the immunoperoxidase method show a heavy distribution of SPLI fibers and terminals in the dorsal laminae of the spinal cord (Figure 2A), which is similar to that observed in the rat and cat and most recently in the human dorsal horn (70). In addition, the monkey spinal cord exhibits a significant number of SPLI axons in the lateral aspect of the lamina V at the base of the dorsal horn and within the adjacent white matter of the lateral funiculus.

Figure 2. (A,B,C) Immunoreactive substance P in the dorsal horn of the monkey spinal cord. (A) A high density of SPLI fibers appears in the most dorsal aspect, which includes layer I and the outer part of layer II. The lateral aspect of lamina V also exhibits numerous SP positive fibers. Scale bar, 500 mm. From DiFiglia et al. (34). (B) An SPLI axon synapses at multiple sites (arrows) with a neuron in lamina I. Scale bar, 1 mm. (C) A large immunoreactive SP terminal contains clear round and large granular vesicles and forms the central element of a glomerulus in which it is presynaptic to dendrite D and spines.

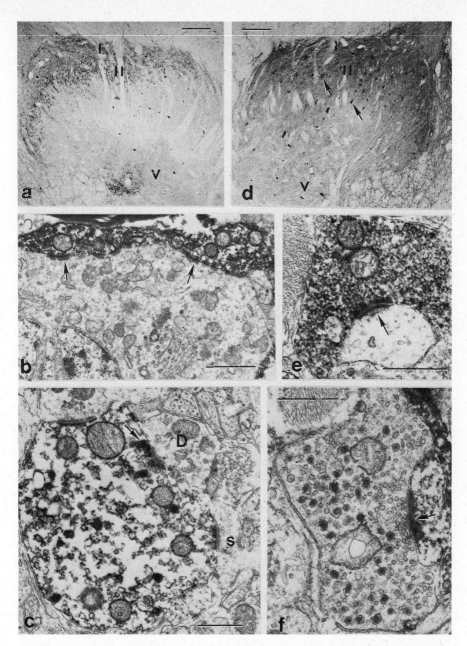

Note that some large granular vesicles are present in presynaptic positions (arrow). Scale bar, 0.5 μm. From DiFiglia et al. (34). (D,E,F) Immunoreactive Leu-enkephalin in the monkey dorsal horn. (D) Labeled cell bodies and fibers are distributed throughout layers I and II. Lamina V also contained some immunoreactive Leu-enkephalin cell bodies and axons. Scale bar, 200 μm. From Jessell and Iverson (81). (E) Immunoreactive Leu-enkephalin axon makes an asymmetric synapse at arrow with small dendrite in lamina I. Scale: 0.5 μm. (F) Immunoreactive Leu-enkephalin dendrite is postsynaptic at arrow to large unlabeled bouton which contains clear round and large granular vesicles. Note the similarity of the latter profile to SPLI terminal in (c). Scale bar, 0.5 μm. From Jessell and Iverson (81).

At the ultrastructural level, SPLI is present mostly in small-diameter unmyelinated and some thinly myelinated fibers. Substance P-positive terminals range from 1 to 4 μm in size and form numerous axodendritic synapses in laminae I and outer II. In addition, the largest boutons form the central elements of the synaptic glomerulus (71), where they participate in synapses with numerous small dendrites and spines (Figure 2C). Some unlabeled neurons in lamina I receive synapses from numerous immunoreactive SP boutons (Figure 2B). Axoaxonic synapses between labeled SP terminals and other axons were observed only rarely in the primate.

As previously observed in the rat dorsal horn, SP reaction product was associated mostly with LGV, which were numerous in the larger axon profiles of the monkey. Labeled LGV were distributed throughout all parts of a bouton and also appeared in close association with both the nonsynaptic and presynaptic portions of the axoplasma membrane (Figure 2C). It is possible that these LGV contain a releasable pool of SP. As previously discussed, immunoreactive SP released by veratridine stimulation in synaptosomal preparations of the rat brainstem is contained within a population of large vesicles in the range of 100 nm (32).

The origin of most immunoreactive SP terminals in the dorsal horn is probably the dorsal root ganglia. Immunoreactive SP cell bodies have been identified in dorsal root ganglia (28, 29) and the distribution of immunoreactive SP fibers within the posterior horn coincides with the known terminations of small diameter dorsal root sensory fibers (72, 73). In addition, the presence of SP within central axons of synaptic glomeruli is consistent with the afferent origin of many of these profiles in the monkey (74). Following dorsal root section there is a marked decrease in the content of SPLI peptides in the spinal cord (75–77) and in the staining of SPLI fibers in the dorsal horn (28, 64).

Substance P is thought to be contained in sensory afferent fibers that mediate pain sensation (67; see also T. M. Jessell, Chapter 13 in this volume). This view is based morphologically in part upon the close correspondence between the distribution in the dorsal horn of SPLI and that of nociceptive fibers identified physiologically and by intracellular HRP injections (78). The localization of SPLI within mostly unmyelinated fibers is consistent with this view, since pain sensory fibers are thought to be primarily without myelin. Moreover, chronic administration of capsaicin, a noxious irritant known to cause release of SP in adult rats, has been shown to elevate pain thresholds (79). Lumbar cisternal injections of capsaicin cause degeneration of central axons of synaptic glomeruli (80), which in the monkey have been observed to contain SPLI (see above).

The opioid pentapeptides, enkephalins, are highly concentrated in the dorsal horn and are thought to modulate nociception in part by direct synapses with SP-containing primary afferent terminals (81). Studies in our laboratory (82) show that, like SPLI terminals, immunoreactive Leu-enkephalin axons are distributed to regions of the dorsal horn that contain spinothalamic projecting cells (Figure 2D) and that they form predominantly axodendritic synapses (Figure 2E). It is likely that enkephalin-containing axon terminals and SP primary afferents converge upon the same nociceptive relay neurons. It has been reported that application of Met-enkephalin causes a hyperpolarization of dorsal horn neurons when studied intracellularly *in vitro* (83). Moreover, we have observed that immunoreactive enkephalin cell bodies (Figure 2D) are distributed throughout laminae I and II and their dendrites are postsynaptic to many types of axons including large central terminals that resemble those containing SPLI (compare Figures 2F and 1C). This would suggest that some SP primary afferents may synapse directly upon enkephalin interneurons.

Most of the SP present within the intermediate and central gray areas is thought to arise from intrinsic cell bodies since SP content (75) and immunocytochemical staining (28, 64) in these regions is unaltered by dorsal rhyzotomy. The synaptic organization of intrinsic SP-containing neurons and their terminals has not as yet been examined at the electron microscopic level. There is some light microscopic evidence, however, that SPLI afferent axons appear in close association with SPLI-containing cell bodies in laminae III–IV of the posterior horn (67).

Immunoreactive SP terminals in the ventral horn may largely originate from supraspinal levels since there is a marked decrease in immunocytochemical staining following spinal cord transection (68, 84). There is also evidence that SPLI terminals in the ventral horn coexist with serotonin (85) or thyrotropin releasing hormone or both (86). The physiological role of descending SP containing fibers on alpha motor neuron output is unsettled, although it is of interest that intrathecal injection of an SP antagonist has been observed to result in limb paralysis (45).

8   SUBSTANCE P IN THE AUTONOMIC NERVOUS SYSTEM AND THE ADRENAL MEDULLA

A wide distribution of SP in the autonomic nervous system has been found by bioassay (87), immunocytochemistry (88), and radioimmunoassay (89). It is likely that at least some of the SP is contained within autonomic sensory neuronal elements, as demonstrated by its depletion following capsaicin (90), which reduces SPLI content only in primary afferent neurons (91). Some of the SPLI has been localized within cell bodies in cultures of the superior cervical sympathetic ganglia in the neonatal rat (92). In adult rats, surgical interruption of preganglionic afferents to the superior cervical sympathetic ganglia and blockage of nicotinic ganglionic transmission have been found to increase the content of SPLI in the ganglia (93). Substance P content was reduced following an increase in sympathetic activity. These results have been interpreted to suggest that neuronal elements in the ganglia that contain SP are affected by preganglionic nerves through a transsynaptic process (93). Insofar as immunoreactive SP has been reported to be transported in the splanchnic nerve towards the celiac ganglion (94) and horseradish peroxidase applied to the inferior mesenteric ganglion has been observed to retrogradely label small somata in dorsal root ganglia (95), it has also been suggested that the inferior mesenteric ganglia may have their cell bodies in the dorsal root ganglia. Interruption of the afferent input to the inferior mesenteric ganglia has been shown to result in a marked reduction in SPLI content (96).

Recent studies suggest that SP may have an excitatory role in the sympathetic ganglia. *In vitro* depolarization of prevertebral sympathetic ganglia following application of K^+ has resulted in release of SP (96), and application of SP to mesenteric ganglia was followed by a slow excitatory postsynaptic potential measured in the ganglion cells (96, 97). The depolarization induced by SP may result from an increase in membrane permeability to Na^+ and a decrease to K^+ (98). Enkephalins have been found to inhibit the slow excitatory potential at a presynaptic site (99, 100). At the ultrastructural level, immunoreactive SP has been observed in axon terminals in the guinea pig celiac ganglion (101, 102). The labeled terminals formed axodendritic synapses and the postsynaptic dendrites occasionally were observed to receive axonic input from an unstained bouton. This synaptic arrangement involving SP fibers is similar to that found in the dorsal horn of the spinal cord (see above).

In contrast with its proposed excitatory role in the sympathetic ganglia, SP may have an inhibitory role in adrenal paraneurons and medullary cells in addition to its possible inhibition of acetylcholine-induced excitation in Renshaw cells (103–105). Substance P has been shown to diminish the nicotinic activation of catecholamine secretion in adrenal paraneurons in culture (106, 107) via inhibition of the acetylcholine- or nicotine-induced calcium-dependent release of ^{3}H-norepinephrine. However, application of SP to this culture does not affect release of ^{3}H-norepinephrine in response to high K^+. Since the adrenal paraneurons do not respond to muscarinic agents, these results suggest that the inhibition by SP acts through a nicotinic receptor channel complex.

Additional support for an inhibitory role of SP on catecholamine release is provided by the experiments of Role et al. (108) with freshly isolated guinea pig adrenal medullary cells. This organ is known to contain immunoreactive SP that coelutes with synthetic SP on gel permeation chromatography. While the adrenal medullary cells responded to both nicotinic and muscarinic agonists, the nicotine-induced catecholamine release was inhibited by SP. The stimulation of catecholamine secretion by pilocarpine-induced (muscarinic), veratridine or high K^+ concentrations was unaffected by SP. These data further indicate that SP inhibition of catecholamine release in the adrenal medulla may result from interactions with nicotinic receptors.

9 SUBSTANCE P IN THE GASTROINTESTINAL TRACT

The bioassay that became the standard for the measurement of SP activity prior to the work of Leeman and colleagues and aided in the discovery of SP from extracts of horse intestine was the spasmogenic effect of this substance on the rabbit ileum (2). Using this bioassay in both guinea pig ileum and rabbit jejunum, Pernow (87) measured SP activity in the intestines of numerous mammalian species and found high amounts of bioactivity present in the small and large intestine, particularly in the muscularis mucosae. An association between SP and the ganglion cells in Meissner's plexus (myenteric) was considered likely. Furthermore, it was postulated that SP has a direct influence on the smooth muscle contraction of the guinea pig ileum, because several ganglionic blockers failed to alter the SP effect. In more recent studies, many of these initial observations have been confirmed and extended.

By radioimmunoassay, SPLI has been reported to be highest in the duodenum and jejunum, although the relative and absolute concentrations vary among the several mammalian species examined (109). With use of immunohistochemistry, SPLI was observed initially in cell bodies and processes of the Auerbach and Meissner plexuses (110) in the small and large intestines of human, dog, pig, and baboon, and myenteric plexus of the proximal colon in the mouse (111). Additionally, SPLI was found in "endocrine-like" cells throughout the small intestine (110, 111).

The origin of the fibers with SPLI is likely to be both intrinsic and extrinsic. Schultzberg et al. (112) have reported that in the large intestine somata with SPLI are more numerous in the myenteric plexus than in the submucous plexus, in contrast to the small intestine where more labeled cells were found in the latter plexus. In the ileum of the guinea pig, Costa et al. (113) found that cell bodies with SPLI comprised 3.6% of the total in the myenteric plexus and 11.3% in the submucous plexus. In both studies, fibers with SPLI were observed in all layers of the gastrointestinal tract and appeared to be closely associated with blood vessels. A detailed analysis of the extrinsic and intrinsic SPLI projections has been provided by Costa et al. (114). In the guinea pig small intestine, extrinsic pathways were found to be related to submucosal blood vessels and ganglia. Intrinsic fibers originating within the myenteric plexus both remained within that plexus and were associated with the circular muscle or submucous nerve somata. The villi were found to receive inputs from both the myenteric and submucous plexuses. It is not known, however, whether these projections originate from individual cells or represent collaterals. Furthermore, evidence has also been presented that in the guinea pig cecum the submucous plexus lacks cell bodies with SPLI and the myenteric plexus supplies pathways with SPLI to the submucous ganglia (115). The extrinsic input of SP to the gastrointestinal tract is likely to be vagal, in part, since this nerve has been shown to contain SPLI by radioimmunoassay (6, 116) and immunohistochemistry.

SPLI has been identified by immunofluorescence in fibers of cultured small intestine of the mouse (117) and has been found to be released in denervated ileal segments after electrical stimulation (118).

To date, the possible function of SP in the gastrointestinal tract is unknown. There is physiological evidence that SP may act directly on the neurons in the enteric nervous system. It has been shown from intracellular recordings of neurons in ganglia of the guinea pig myenteric plexus that iontophoretic application of SP results in depolarization of the neurons studied (119). This depolarization was characterized by slow excitation and was not altered by hexamethonium, atropine, naloxone, or enkephalin. Substance P may also have a direct effect on intestinal muscle. Synthetic SP has been reported to be more potent than acetylcholine on a molar basis in the *in vitro* stimulation of the longitudinal muscle of the guinea pig intestine (120). In addition, material with SPLI has been measured in the cat antral lumen following perfusion with acid, electrical stimulation of the vagus nerve, and intravenous acetylcholine and adrenaline (121).

10 SUBSTANCE P INTERACTIONS WITH ANTERIOR PITUITARY HORMONE RELEASE

Since SP has been found in high concentrations in the hypothalamus, it is understandable that there are a number of reports on its involvement in the regulation of the hypothalamic-pituitary axis. From studies in which this peptide was administered intravenously or intracerebroventricularly, the possible role of SP in the release of anterior pituitary hormones has been postulated. In rats, intravenous and intracerebroventricular injection of SP has been reported to stimulate prolactin release (122, 123). *In vitro* incubation of hemipituitaries with SP has been shown to produce an increase in prolactin release (123). These results suggest that SP has an overall stimulatory effect on prolactin release, although the actual site of action remains unclear.

Both inhibitory and stimulatory effects upon growth hormone release have been found. Following intravenous injection of 5-50 μg/100 g (122) or 20 μg (124) of synthetic SP, an increase in plasma growth hormone concentrations has been shown; at lower doses of 0.5 μg and 2.0 μg, no change has been found (125). Unchanged or reduced levels of growth hormone have been reported after administration of SP in urethane-anesthetized males into the lateral ventricle (126) in contrast to the increase found following injection into the third ventricle in conscious or ovariectomized rats (125). The possibility that the SP effects on growth hormone secretion are mediated via somatostatin has been investigated but to date such modulations remain unclear. Chihara et al. (126) proposed that the effects of intraventricularly applied SP on growth hormone release acted via somatostatin, since pretreatment with somatostatin antiserum abolished this SP modulation. However, in *in vitro* studies on rat hypothalamic fragments, SP has been reported either to result in no change (127) or in an increase (128) in somatostatin concentrations, and recently Abe et al. (129) have reported that intracerebroventricularly injected SP does not change somatostatin concentrations in hypophyseal portal blood in urethane-anesthetized rats. It is interesting that the intravenous injection of 10 μg/100 g of SP into rats has been found to result in a decrease in pancreatic somatostatin simultaneously with the measured increase in hypophyseal portal plasma (130).

As with growth hormone, the effects of SP on the regulation of luteinizing hormone in rats appear to be dependent on the route of administration. Intracerebroventricular injection of SP has resulted in an increase in plasma luteinizing hormone concentrations, while levels of this gonadotropin were reduced following intravenous administration (123). Since there was no change in luteinizing hormone levels after incubation of SP with pituitaries *in vitro*, it has been suggested that the hypothalamic effects of SP are mediated via luteinizing hormone releasing hormone (123). Neither the intravenous nor the intracerebroventricular injection of SP has been shown to modulate the release of thyrotropin stimulating hormone in unanesthetized, ovariectomized rats (125).

Although it appears that SP may be involved in the regulation of some anterior pituitary hormones, possibly via modulation of releasing factors, it is not yet possible to define more precisely the roles of SP in the hypothalamic-pituitary axis. Studies in which SP is administered peripherally are difficult to interpret, since peptides of similar molecular weight have been shown to cross the blood-brain barrier only to a limited extent (131). The injection of microgram quantities of SP by an intracerebroventricular route may possibly result in a nonphysiological effect on hypothalamic and extrahypothalamic nuclear groups that normally receive input from SP neurons. In addition, it is possible that SP via this route may interact with neurons that do not normally have access to this peptide. There is currently available little information on the anatomical associations of SP neuronal elements with cell bodies, dendrites, or axons that contain conventional neurotransmitters or releasing hormones. Ultrastructural studies are needed to help provide a basis for the interpretation of physiologic experiments. Finally, since the distribution of SP in the hypothalamus may vary, as is evidenced by the low density of SP fibers in the median eminence of the rat as opposed to the monkey (132), it is possible that this peptide subserves different roles not only between males and females but also among various mammalian species.

ACKNOWLEDGMENTS

We gratefully thank Ms. Linda Carreaux for her assistance in the preparation of this manuscript. Some of the work presented here was supported by NIH Grants AM 01126-01 (N.A.), AM 28557 and AM 28565 (R.E.C.), NS 16367 (M.D.), and AM 29876-03 (S.E.L.).

REFERENCES

1. S. E. Leeman and R. Hammerschlag, *Endocrinology* **81**, 803 (1967).
2. U. S. von Euler and J. H. Gaddum, *J. Physiol. (London)* **72**, 74 (1931).
3. J. H. Gaddum and H. Schild, *J. Physiol. (London)* **82**, 1 (1934).
4. U. S. von Euler and B. Pernow, Eds., *Substance P*, Raven Press, New York, 1977.
5. S. E. Leeman, N. Aronin, and C. Ferris, *Recent Prog. Horm. Res.* **38**, 93 (1982).
6. M. M. Chang and S. E. Leeman, *J. Biol. Chem.* **245**, 4784 (1970).
7. M. M. Chang, S. E. Leeman, and H. D. Niall, *Nature (London) New Biol.* **232**, 86 (1971).
8. R. O. Studer, H. Trzeciak, and W. Lergier, *Helv. Chim. Acta.* **56**, 860 (1973).
9. R. E. Carraway and S. E. Leeman, *J. Biol. Chem.* **254**, 2944 (1979).
10. G. W. Tregear, H. D. Niall, J. T. Potts, Jr., S. E. Leeman, and M. M. Chang, *Nature (London) New Biol.* **232**, 87 (1971).
11. D. Powell, S. E. Leeman, G. W. Tregear, H. D. Niall, and J. T. Potts, Jr., *Nature (London) New Biol.* **241**, 252 (1973).
12. E. Mroz and S. E. Leeman, in B. M. Jaffe and H. R. Behrman, Eds., *Methods in Radioimmunoassay*, Academic Press, New York, 1979, pp. 121–138.
13. S. E. Leeman, E. A. Mroz, and R. E. Carraway, in H. Gainer, Ed., *Peptides in Neurobiology*, Plenum Press, New York, 1977, pp. 99–144.
14. E. Floor and S. E. Leeman, *Anal. Bioch.* **101**, 498 (1980).
15. V. A. Harmer and P. Keen, *Brain Res.* **220**, 203 (1981).
16. Y. Ben-Ari, P. Pradelles, C. Gros, and F. Dray, *Brain Res.* **173**, 360 (1979).
17. V. Erspamer and A. Anastasi, *Experientia* **18**, 58 (1962).
18. V. Erspamer, A. Anastasi, B. Bertaccini, and J. M. Cei, *Experientia*, **20**, 489 (1964).
19. L. H. Lazarus, R. I. Linnoila, O. Hernandez, and R. P. DiAugustine, *Nature (London)* **287**, 555 (1980).
20. M. J. Brownstein, E. A. Mroz, J. S. Kizer, M. Palkouits, and S. E. Leeman, *Brain Res.* **116**, 299 (1976).
21. I. Kanazawa and T. Jessell, *Brain Res.* **117**, 362 (1976).
22. J. S. Gale, E. D. Bird, E. G. Spokes, L. L. Iverson, and T. M. Jessell, *J. Neurochem.* **30**, 633 (1978).

23. P. C. Emson, A. Arrequi, V. Clement-Jones, B. E. B. Sandberg, and M. Rossor, *Brain Res.* **199**, 147 (1980).

24. P. E. Cooper, M. H. Fernstrom, P. P. Rorstad, S. E. Leeman, and J. B. Martin, *Brain Res.* **218**, 219 (1981).

25. A. Ljungdahl, T. Hokfelt, and G. Nilsson, *Neuroscience* **3**, 861 (1978).

26. A. C. Cuello and I. Kanazawa, *J. Comp. Neurol.* **178**, 129 (1978).

27. S. Haber and R. Elde, *Neuroscience* **6**, 1291 (1981).

28. T. Hökfelt, J. O. Kellerth, G. Nilsson, and B. Pernow, *Brain Res.* **100**, 235 (1975).

29. V. Chan-Palay and S. L. Palay, *Proc. Natl. Acad. Sci. USA* **74**, 4050 (1977).

30. R. A. Nicoll, C. Schenker, and S. E. Leeman, *Ann. Rev. Neurosci.* **3**, 227 (1980).

31. C. Schenker, E. A. Mroz, and S. E. Leeman, *Nature (London)* **264**, 790 (1976).

32. E. Floor, O. Grad, and S. E. Leeman, *Neuroscience* **7**, 1647 (1982).

33. V. M. Pickel, D. J. Reis, and S. E. Leeman, *Brain Res.* **122**, 534 (1977).

34. M. DiFiglia, N. Aronin, and S. E. Leeman, *Neuroscience* **7**, 1127 (1982).

35. A. Harmar, J. G. Schofield, and P. Keen, *Nature* **284**, 267 (1980).

36. A. Harmar, J. G. Schofield, and P. Keen, *Neuroscience* **6**, 1917 (1981).

37. G. Sperk and E. A. Singer, *Brain Res.* **238**, 127 (1981).

38. P. G. Guyenet and G. K. Aghajanian, *Eur. J. Pharmacol.* **53**, 319 (1979).

39. I. Yamaguchi, G. Rackur, J. Leban, U. Bjorkroth, S. Rosell, and K. Folkers, *Acta Chem. Scan. B* **33**, 63 (1979).

40. J. Leban, G. Rackur, I. Yamaguchi, K. Folkers, U. Bjorkroth, S. Rosell, and N. Yanaihara, *Acta Chem. Scand. B* **33**, 664 (1979).

41. G. Engberg, T. H. Svensson, S. Rosell, and K. Folkers, *Nature* **293**, 222 (1981).

42. G. Holmdahl, R. Hakanson, S. Leander, S. Rosell, K. Folkers, and F. Sundler, *Science* **214**, 1029 (1981).

43. S. Rosell, L. Olgart, B. Gazelius, P. Panopoulous, K. Folkers, and J. Horig, *Acta Physiol. Scand.* **111**, 381 (1981).

44. K. Folkers, J. Horig, S. Rosell, and U. Bjorkroth, *Acta Physiol. Scand.* **111**, 505 (1981).

45. M. F. Piercey, L. A. Schroeder, K. Folkers, J.-C. Xu, and J. Horig, *Science* **214**, 1361 (1981).

46. I. Kanazawa, P. C. Emson, and A. C. Cuello, *Brain Res.* **119**, 447 (1977).

47. E. A. Mroz, M. J. Brownstein, and S. E. Leeman, *Brain Res.* **125**, 305 (1977).

48. M. DiFiglia, N. Aronin, and S. E. Leeman, *Brain Res.* **233**, 381 (1982).

49. K. Gale, J.-S. Hong, and A. Guidotti, *Brain Res.* **136**, 371 (1977).

50. J. S. Hong, H.-Y. Yang, G. Racagni, and E. Costa, *Brain Res.* **122**, 541 (1977).

51. T. M. Jessell, P. C. Emson, G. Paxinos, and A. C. Cuello, *Brain Res.* **152**, 487 (1978).

52. J. Glowinski, R. Michelot, and A. Cheramy, *Adv. Biochem. Psychopharmacol.* **22**, 51 (1980).

53. I. Kanazawa, E. Bird, R. O'Connell, and D. Powell, *Brain Res.* **120**, 387 (1977).

54. P. C. Emson, A. Arrequi, V. Clemont-Jones, B. E. B. Sandberg, and M. Rossor, *Brain Res.* **199**, 147 (1980).

55. S. H. Buck, T. F. Burks, M. R. Brown, and H. I. Yamamura, *Brain Res.* **209**, 464 (1981).

56. R. P. Johnson, M. Sar, and W. E. Stumpf, *Brain Res.* **194**, 566 (1980).

57. M. DiFiglia, N. Aronin, and J. B. Martin, *J. Neurosci.* **2**, 303 (1982).

58. C. E. Ribak, J. E. Vaughn, K. Saito, R. Barber, and E. Roberts, *Brain Res.* **116**, 287 (1976).

59. F. Fonnum, I. Grofova, E. Rinvik, J. Storm-Mathisen, and F. Walsberg, *Brain Res.* **71**, 77 (1974).

60. V. M. Pickel, K. K. Sumal, S. C. Beckley, R. J. Miller, and D. J. Reis, *J. Comp. Neurol.* **189**, 721 (1980).

61. T. M. Jessell, *Brain Res.* **151**, 469 (1978).

62. R. J. Walker, J. A. Kemp, H. Yajima, K. Katagawa, and G. N. Woodruff, *Experientia* **32**, 214 (1976).

63. J. Daires and A. Dray, *Brain Res.* **107**, 623 (1976).

64. R. P. Barber, J. E. Vaughn, J. R. Stemmon, P. M. Salvaterra, E. Roberts, and S. E. Leeman, *J. Comp. Neurol.* **184**, 331 (1979).

65. S. J. Gibson, J. M. Polak, S. R. Bloom, and P. D. Wall, *J. Comp. Neurol.* **201**, 65 (1981).

66. S. P. Hunt, J. S. Kelly, P. C. Emson, J. R. Kimmel, R. V. Miller, and J. -Y. Wu, *Neuroscience* **6**, 1883 (1981).

67. J. I. Nagy, S. P. Hunt, L. L. Iverson, and P. C. Emson, *Neuroscience* **6**, 1923 (1981).

68. T. Hökfelt, A. Ljungdahl, L. Terenius, R. Elde, and G. Nilsson, *Proc. Natl. Acad. Sci. USA* **74**, 3081 (1977). Goldberger, *Brain Res.* **191**, 459 (1980).

69. A Tessler, E. Glazer, R. Artymyskyn, M. Murray, and M. E. Goldberger, *Brain Res.* **191**, 459 (1980).

70. C. C. LaMotte and N. C. deLanerolle, *Neuroscience* **6**, 713 (1981).

71. H. J. Ralston III, *J. Comp. Neurol.* **184**, 619 (1979).

72. F. W. L. Kerr, *Pain* **1**, 325 (1975).

73. A. R. Light and E. R. Perl, *J. Comp. Neurol.* **186**, 117 (1979).

74. H. J. Ralston III and D. D. Ralston, *J. Comp. Neurol.* **184**, 643 (1979).

75. T. Takahashi and M. Otsuka, *Brain Res.* **87**, 1 (1975).

76. T. Jessell, A. Tsunoo, I. Kanazawa, and M. Otsuka, *Brain Res.* **168**, 247 (1979).

77. D. Barbut, J. M. Polak, and P. D. Wall, *Brain Res.* **205**, 289 (1981).

78. A. R. Light and E. R. Perl, *J. Comp. Neurol.* **186**, 133 (1979).

79. P. Holzer, I. Jurna, R. Gamse, and F. Lembeck, *Eur. J. Pharmacol.* **58**, 511 (1979).

80. N. N. Palermo, H. Keith Brown, and D. L. Smith, *Brain Res.* **208**, 506 (1981).

81. T. M. Jessell and L. L. Iverson, *Nature* **268**, 549 (1977).

82. N. Aronin, M. DiFiglia, A. S. Liotta, and J. B. Martin, *J. Neurosci.* **1**, 561 (1981).

83. K. Murase, J. Nedeljkov, and M. Randic, *Brain Res.* **234**, 170 (1982).

84. I. Kanazawa, D. Sutoo, I. Oshima, and S. Saite, *Neurosci. Lett.* **1**, 325 (1979).

85. G. Pelletier, H. W. M. Steinbusch, and A. A. J. Verhofstad, *Nature* **293**, 71 (1981).

86. O. Johansson, T. Hokfelt, B. Pernow, S. L. Heffcoate, H. White, H. W. M. Steinbusch, A. A. J. Verhofstad, P. C. Emson, and E. Spindel, *Neurosci.* **6**, 1857 (1981).

87. B. Pernow, *Acta Physiol. Scand. Suppl.* **105**, 1 (1953).

88. T. Hökfelt, L. -G. Elfvin, M. Schultzberg, M. Goldstein, and G. Nilsson, *Brain Res.* **132**, 29 (1977).

89. R. Gamse, A. Wax, R. E. Zigmond, and S. E. Leeman, *Neurosci.* **6**, 437 (1981).

90. R. Gamse, P. Holzer, and F. Lembeck, *Br. J. Pharmacol.* **68**, 207 (1980).

91. T. M. Jessell, L. L. Iverson, and A. C. Cuello, *Brain Res.* **152**, 183 (1978).

92. J. A. Kessler, J. E. Adler, M. C. Bohn, and I. B. Black, *Science* **214**, 335 (1981).

93. J. A. Kessler and I. B. Black, *Brain Res.* **234**, 182 (1982).

94. J. M. Lundberg, T. Hokfelt, G. Nilsson, L. Terenius, J. Rehfield, R. Elde, and S. Said, *Acta Physiol. Scand.* **104**, 499 (1978).

95. L. -G. Elfvin and C. J. Dalsgaard, *Brain Res.* **126**, 149 (1977).

96. S. Konishi, A. Tsumoo, and M. Otsuka, *Proc. Jpn. Acad.* **55B**, 525 (1979).

97. N. J. Dun and A. G. Karczmar, *Neuropharmacol.* **18**, 215 (1979).

98. N. J. Dun and S. Minota, *J. Physiol.* **321**, 259 (1981).

99. S. Konishi, A. Tsunoo, and M. Otsuka, *Nature (London)* **282**, 515 (1979).

100. Z. Jiang, M. A. Simmons, and N. J. Dun, *Brain Res.* **235**, 185 (1982).

101. H. Kondo and R. Yui, *Brain Res.* **222**, 134 (1981).

102. M. R. Matthews and A. C. Cuello, *Proc. Natl. Acad. Sci. USA* **79**, 1668 (1982).

103. K. Krnjevic and D. Lekic, *Can. J. Physiol. Pharmacol.* **55**, 958 (1977).

104. G. Belcher and W. W. Ryall, *J. Physiol. (London)* **272**, 105 (1977).

105. R. W. Ryall and G. Belcker, *Brain Res.* **137**, 376 (1977).
106. B. G. Livett, V. Kozousek, F. Mitzobe, and D. M. Dean, *Nature (London)* **278**, 256 (1979).
107. F. Mitzobe, V. Kozousek, D. M. Dean, and B. G. Livett, *Brain Res.* **178**, 555 (1979).
108. L. W. Role, S. E. Leeman, and R. L. Perlman, *Neuroscience* **6**, 1813 (1981).
109. G. Nilsson and E. Bordin, in U. S. von Euler and B. Pernow, Eds., *Substance P*, Raven Press, New York, 1977, pp. 49–54.
110. A. G. E. Pearse and J. M. Polak, *Histochemistry* **41**, 373 (1975).
111. G. Nilsson, L. -I. Larsson, E. Brodin, B. Pernow, and F. Sundler, *Histochemistry* **43**, 97 (1975).
112. M. Schultzberg, T. Hokfelt, G. Nilsson, L. Terenius, J. F. Rehfield, M. Brown, R. Elde, M. Goldstein, and S. Said, *Neuroscience* **5**, 689 (1980).
113. M. Costa, A. C. Cuello, J. B. Furmers, and R. Franco, *Neuroscience* **5**, 323 (1980).
114. M. Costa, J. B. Furmers, I. J. Llewellyn-Smith, and A. C. Cuello, *Neuroscience* **6**, 411 (1981).
115. K. R. Jessen, M. J. Saffrey, S. Van Noorden, S. R. Bloom, J. M. Polak, and G. Burnstock, *Neuroscience* **5**, 1717 (1980).
116. R. Gamse, F. Lembeck, and A. C. Cuello, *Naunyn-Schmiedebergs Arch. Pharmacol.* **306**, 37 (1979).
117. M. Schultzberg, C. F. Dreyfus, M. D. Gershon, T. Hokfelt, R. Elde, G. Nilsson, S. Said, and M. Goldstein, *Brain Res.* **155**, 239 (1978).
118. R. Franco, M. Costa, and B. Furmers, *Naunyn-Schmiedebergs Arch. Pharmacol.* **306**, 195 (1979).
119. Y. Katayama and R. A. North, *Nature (London)* **274**, 387 (1978).
120. W. M. Yau, *Gastroenterology* **74**, 228 (1978).
121. K. Uvnas-Wallensten, *Acta Physiol. Scand.* **104**, 464 (1978).
122. Y. Kato, K. Chihara, S. Ongo, Y. Iwasaki, H. Abe, and H. Imura, *Life Sci.* **19**, 441 (1976).
123. E. Vijayan and S. M. McCann, *Endocrinology* **105**, 64 (1979).
124. C. Rivier, M. Brown, and W. Vale, *Endocrinology* **100**, 751 (1977).
125. E. Vijayan and S. M. McCann, *Life Sci.* **26**, 321 (1980).
126. K. Chihara, A. Arimura, D. H. Coy, and A. V. Schally, *Endocrinology* **102**, 281 (1978).
127. K. Maeda and L. A. Frohman, *Endocrinology* **106**, 1837 (1980).
128. M. C. Sheppard, S. Kronheim, and B. L. Pimstone, *J. Neurochem.* **32**, 647 (1978).
129. H. Abe, K. Chihara, T. Chiba, S. Matsukura, and T. Fujita, *Endocrinology* **108**, 1939 (1981).
130. H. Saito and S. Saito, *Endocrinology* **107**, 1600 (1980).
131. W. M. Pardridge, H. J. L. Frank, E. M. Cornford, L. D. Braun, P. D. Crane, and W. H. Oldenforf, *Adv. Biochem. Psychopharmacol.* **28**, 321 (1981).
132. T. Hökfelt, B. Pernow, G. Nilsson, L. Wetterberg, M. Goldstein, and S. L. Jeffcoate, *Proc. Natl. Acad. Sci. USA* **75**, 1013 (1978).

32

The Brain Renin-Angiotensin System

WILLIAM F. GANONG

Department of Physiology
University of California
San Francisco, California

Research in the author's laboratory, some of which is reported in this chapter, is supported by USPHS Grant AM06704.

1   INTRODUCTION

The renin-angiotensin system was first described in terms of a renal system that generated circulating angiotensin II (AII), and it is still generally thought of in those terms. The essential components of the system are shown in Figure 1. However, it now appears that there are additional separate renin-angiotensin systems in the uterus, salivary glands, and blood vessels, and possibly in the adrenals and other organs as well (1). In addition, all the components of the renin-angiotensin system have been reported to be present in the brain. The possibility that a separate functional renin-angiotensin system exists in the brain is particularly intriguing, but there is controversy about the nature of some of the components and the degree to which they interact. The present chapter is a review of the current evidence for a brain renin-angiotensin system and a consideration of its possible functions.

2   RELATION TO THE RENAL RENIN-ANGIOTENSIN SYSTEM

2.1   Failure of Circulating Components to Enter the Brain

An obvious question is whether the components of the renin-angiotensin found in the brain are of peripheral origin. Most of the available evidence indicates they are not.

Circulating renin has a molecular weight of approximately 40,000, and is larger than most molecules that penetrate the blood-brain barrier to any significant degree (2, 3). There is no renin in cerebrospinal fluid

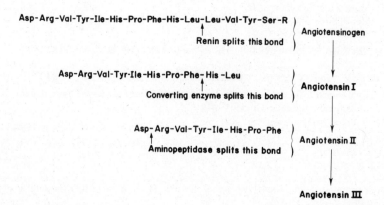

Figure 1.   The renin-angiotensin system. R, remainder of protein. From W. F. Ganong (2).

(CSF), indicating that circulating renin does not cross the blood-CSF barrier. The renin in brain tissue is unevenly distributed in a pattern that does not parallel the vascularity (see below), has a different chemical composition than renal and plasma renin (4), and is still present after bilateral nephrectomy. This last statement is true whether one measures total angiotensin-generating activity (5) or only the renin that cross-reacts with antibodies to renal renin (6).

The substrate in CSF resembles the substrate produced in liver, but the carbohydrate composition of these glycoproteins differs (7, 8). In addition, dexamethasone treatment and nephrectomy both increase plasma angiotensinogen concentration but neither has any effect on the concentration of angiotensinogen in CSF (9).

Converting enzyme in the brain, like renin, is unevenly distributed (10–12), with a pattern that is independent of vascularity, at least when the enzyme is measured biochemically, and it seems unlikely that circulating converting enzyme enters the brain.

It also seems clear that the smaller AI and AII molecules do not cross the blood-brain barrier (13). Hemorrhage, furosemide, insulin-induced hypoglycemia, and β-adrenergic blockade, which produce marked changes in plasma AII, have been reported to have no effect on the AII content of CSF or brain (14–16). In early radioautographic studies using labeled AII, the possibility of diffusion artifact was not ruled out, and there is general agreement today that systemically administered radioactive AI and AII do not appear in measurable amounts in cerebrospinal fluid or brain tissue (see 16, 17). There appears to be one exception to this general statement; when blood pressure is rapidly raised to high levels, the blood-brain barrier is transiently disrupted and small amounts of AII enter brain tissue. However, the blood pressure rise must be rapid and large, and a rise with these characteristics is unlikely to occur except under unusual circumstances.

2.2   Effects of Circulating Angiotensins on the Brain

Although AII does not penetrate the blood-brain barrier, it enters the circumventricular organs with ease (18). AI presumably enters them as well. These small areas of brain tissue are located near the third and fourth ventricles, have fenestrated highly permeable capillaries that are different from the impermeable nonfenestrated capillaries in the rest of the brain (19), and are readily penetrated by circulating molecules of relatively large size. Circulating angiotensins act on one or another of these organs to produce thirst, increase blood pressure, increase vasopressin secretion, and increase ACTH secretion (9). The decrease in renin secretion produced by intracarotid AII is probably also brought about in this manner (20). The actions of circulating angiotensins on the brain are discussed in detail by Reid in Chapter 15.

3 COMPONENTS IN THE BRAIN

Some of the components of the renin-angiotensin system have been reported to be present in CSF, and others have been reported in brain tissue (Table 1). In the paragraphs that follow, each component is considered in terms of evidence for its existence in CSF and brain tissue, and for those reported in brain tissue, localization within the brain is described.

3.1 Angiotensin Receptors

AII receptors, as defined by saturable and specifically inhibitable binding to appropriate preparations of brain tissue, have been found in the brains of various mammalian species (21–24). Their localization varies from species to species. In calves, the highest concentration of receptors is in the cerebellum (21). In rats, the highest concentration is in the thalamus and hypothalamus, followed in descending order by the midbrain, brainstem, cerebellum, striatum, cerebral cortex, and hippocampus (21, 22, 24, 25). Other species of rodents have different patterns of distribution (24).

It is difficult to prove that these receptors are not on blood vessels in the extracted tissue. However, receptor density does not parallel the vascularity of the various areas. In addition, vascular receptors would presumably be located on the blood side of the blood-brain barrier. Baxter et al. (23) infused rats with saralasin intravenously and demonstrated that after 6 weeks of age, the saturable binding of AII was unaf-

TABLE 1   Components of the Renin-Angiotensin System in Cerebrospinal Fluid (CSF) and Brain Tissue[a]

Component	CSF	Brain Tissue
Angiotensin receptors	(0)	Diencephalon, midbrain, brain stem, cerebellum (rat)
Angiotensinase	0	Circumventricular organs
Angiotensin II	+	Hippocampus, striatum, cerebellum, diencephalon, supraoptic and, paraventricular neurons, midbrain
Angiotensin III	+	—
Angiotensin I	+	—
Converting enzyme	+	Choroid plexus, subfornical organ, area postrema, locus ceruleus, substantia nigra, hypothalamus, neurohypophysis
Renin substrate	+	Circumventricular organs, periventricular thalamus and hypothalamus
Renin	0	Choroid plexus, hypothalamus, supraoptic and paraventricular neurons, cerebellar cortex

[a] For brain tissue, the regions or cells reported to contain the highest concentrations are listed.

fected. Since the saralasin in the systemic circulation would inhibit binding to any AII receptors in blood vessels (25), the data provide evidence that the AII receptors in brain tissue are inside the blood-brain barrier.

3.2 Angiotensinase

Brain tissue, and in particular the circumventricular organs, contains appreciable quantities of peptidases that rapidly break down and hence inactivate AII (15, 26). These peptidases appear to be located in cells because there is little or no angiotensinase activity in CSF (15) and CSF is in free communication with brain extracellular fluid. The removal of injected AII from CSF *in vivo* is slower than from blood, but it is removed at an appreciable rate, possibly because it is in contact with the circumventricular organs.

3.3 Angiotensin II and Angiotensin III

Some of the most spirited debate in the brain renin-angiotensin field has revolved around the question whether the central nervous system contains AII or possibly angiotensin III (AIII). In discussing this question, it is appropriate to consider CSF and brain tissue separately, and to analyze both the biochemical and the immunocytochemical evidence.

3.3.1 Cerebrospinal Fluid

AI and AII concentrations that have been reported in CSF are summarized in Table 2. Reid and his associates report undetectable values in

TABLE 2   Reported Concentrations of Angiotensin I and II in Cerebrospinal Fluid[a]

Substance	Species	Concentration (pg/mL)	Reference
Angiotensin I	Human	4, 14, 28	28, 93, 94
	Dog	12	15
	Rat	17.6	15
Angiotensin II	Human	37, 189	95, 93
	Human	0–15	28
	Sheep	30–120	16
	Dog	<6.25, 40	42, 13
	Dog	24	15
	Rat	11, 36, 169	96, 15, 97
		<25	42

[a] Values reported in moles converted to pg. References are cited in the same order as concentration values. All values were obtained by radioimmunoassay, and consequently the material reported as angiotensin II could be angiotensin III or other C-terminal fragments of angiotensin II (see text).

dogs and rats, but in these species as well as sheep and humans, other investigators find values that although low are readily detectable. Most of the values are similar to or slightly lower than values reported for plasma. All the reported values, however, were determined by radioimmunoassay, and chemical identification of the material as AII has not been reported. Indeed, Hutchinson et al. (27) reported that in one group of dogs most of the "AII" measured by radioimmunoassay in CSF had the chromatographic characteristics of AIII. Most antibodies to AII crossreact with Des-Asp^1-angiotensin II (AIII) and with Des-Asp^1-Arg^2-angiotensin II and Des-Asp^1-Arg^2-Val^3-angiotensin II (see ref. 27), so all the material reported as AII in Table 2 could be AIII or one of the other fragments. However, the total amounts of material that reacted with the antibody in the study by Hutchinson et al. (27) were 1000 times the values obtained by the same authors in dogs anesthetized for a longer period. Consequently, the study needs to be repeated. Semple et al. (28) have also studied the chromatographic characteristics of the immunoreactive material in human CSF, and their data suggest the presence of AIII and Des-Asp^1-Arg^2-angiotensin II rather than AII.

3.3.2 Brain Tissue

Reported values for AI and AII in brain tissue are summarized in Table 3. Bioassays, which measure AI and AII together, and radioimmunoas-

TABLE 3　Angiotensins in Brain Tissue[a]

Species	Concentration (ng/g)[b]	Substance	Assay	Reference
Dog	2.7	AI and AII	B	5
	4.9	AI and AII	B	100
	6.8	AI and AII	B	29
	47.7[c]	AI	I	30
	<0.1	AI	I	29
	2.8[c]	AII	I	30
	0.03	AII	I	29
Rabbit	20.2	AI and AII	B	29
	<0.1	AI	I	29
	<0.02	AII	I	29
Rat	21.6	AI and AII	B	29
	78.0	AI	I	99
	8–82	AI	I	92
	<0.1	AI	I	29
	<0.02	AII	I	29
	0	AII	I	98
	0.1	AII	I	26

[a] Abbreviations: AI, angiotensin I; AII, angiotensin II; B, bioassay; I, immunoassay.
[b] Note that the values are in ng/g, whereas the values in Table 2 are in pg/mL.
[c] Reported as an artifact because the tracer was degraded by angiotensinase.

says, which measure AI and AII separately, have both been used. As noted above, most antibodies to AII cross-react with several C-terminal fragments of AII. It has been argued that the bioassay results are non-specific and that the material being measured is not neutralized by AII antibodies (29). An additional problem is the presence of peptidases in brain tissue that rapidly destroy angiotensins. This tends to lower values. However, if there are no angiotensins in the extracted tissue and angiotensinase destroys some of the tracer, angiotensins will be reported to be present when they are not (30). Sirett and her associates (26), circumvented the peptidase problem by extracting the brain in cold ethanol containing a peptidase inhibitor and boiling the extract. With these precautions, the recovery rate of AII added to brain was 40–78%. The value for whole rat brain was 108 ± 16 pg/g, compared with 306 ± 16 pg/g for kidney and 133 ± 15 pg/g for plasma. The highest concentration of AII (about 360 pg/g) was in the hippocampus, followed in descending order by the striatum, cerebellum, diencephalon and midbrain, medulla, and cortex. The concentration in the cortex was about 45 pg/g. These data are an important addition to the accumulating evidence that the brain does contain AII or some of its C-terminal fragments. However, the endpoint was still radioimmunoassay. What is needed is extraction and chemical identification of AI, AII, and AIII in brain tissue to finally settle the matter.

3.3.3 Immunocytochemical Evidence

AII antibodies stain material located in neurons in various parts of the brain (14, 31–34). The reports of angiotensin-like immunoreactivity using antibodies generated in Ganten's laboratory (see ref. 14) led my associates and me to investigate the problem in our laboratory. We initially tested nine antibodies to AII, all of which were active in radioimmunoassays, and none stained brain tissue. However, we subsequently exchanged antibodies with Ganten. He confirmed that our antibodies did not stain brain tissue, and we confirmed the reports from his laboratory that his antibodies CE, DE, and G1 stain neurons (12). Staining was obtained with both the fluorescent and the peroxidase-antiperoxidase techniques. For some time, all the published reports of angiotensin-like immunoreactivity in the brain were based on experiments using the Ganten antibodies. The one unique feature about the positive antibodies is that they were prepared using a glutaraldehyde conjugate of AII, but the significance of this fact is presently unknown. Kilcoyne et al. (32) subsequently developed another antibody that produced staining, and this antibody was not conjugated with glutaraldehyde. One other antibody has been reported to produce staining (33), but other studies do not confirm this report (12).

Is AII the material that stains with these antibodies? The antibodies that gave positive results do not cross-react with a variety of different brain peptides (12) and were most active against AII and AIII, with less activity against AI and the synthetic tetradecapeptide (TDP) that consists of the 14-amino-acid residues at the amino terminal of angiotensinogen (Figure 1). This was true not only in radioimmunoassay but in preabsorption experiments in which it was demonstrated that the ability of the antibodies to stain brain tissue was inhibited by lower concentrations of AII and AIII than AI and TDP. Thus it seems likely that the material being studied is AII or AIII. However, staining of AI, substrate, or an unknown cross-reacting peptide cannot be excluded, and more definitive identification must await chemical characterization.

Most of the angiotensin-like immunoreactivity in the brain that is demonstrated with the use of CE and DE antibodies is in nerve endings with relatively little material in nerve cell bodies (14). None is found in glia or ependyma. The most intense staining is located in the median eminence, posterior lobe of the pituitary, central nucleus of the amygdala, spinal nucleus of the trigeminal nerve, substantia gelatinosa, and intermediolateral column of the spinal cord. A pathway can be followed from the paraventricular nucleus to the median eminence. Immunoreactivity is also found in the cell bodies of neurons in the magnocellular nuclei of the hypothalamus (12, 32), but in our experiments, the staining was not intense unless the animals were treated with colchicine. Because angiotensin-like immunoreactivity and vasopressin occur in the same cells, and because angiotensin-like immunoreactivity as well as vasopressin is reduced in Brattleboro rats, Kilcoyne et al. (32) speculated that AII and vasopressin arose from the same precursor molecule. However, the positively staining neurons that end in the amygdala arise in the magnocellular nuclei, and these neurons do not contain vasopressin.

3.4 Angiotensin I

AI has been reported to be present in human, dog, and rat CSF in quantities ranging from 4 to 28 pg/mL (Table 2), that is, in amounts equal to or less than the reported values for AII. This is in contrast with plasma, where there is considerably more AI than AII (15). The antibodies to AI crossreact with AII and AIII to a very limited degree. The AI content of brain tissue was originally reported to be relatively high (Table 3), but some of these values may be artifactual. Horvarth et al. (29) claim that there is no measurable AI in brain tissue.

3.5 Converting Enzyme

There is a small but measurable amount of converting enzyme in CSF (15, 35). In addition, brain tissue contains converting enzyme activity as measured by the formation of His-Leu from Hip-His-Leu or related synthetic substrates when the latter are incubated with brain tissue. The converting enzyme is unevenly distributed, with very high concentrations in the choroid plexus, subfornical organ, and area postrema. Moderate concentrations are found in the locus ceruleus, substantia nigra, and hypothalamus (Table 1), and lower concentrations in other areas (10, 11, 36, 37).

Immunocytochemical localization of converting enzyme has been carried out with antibodies to rabbit lung converting enzyme (12, 35). In these studies, converting enzyme-like immunoreactivity was found in endothelial cells throughout the brain. Large quantities of converting enzyme-like immunoreactivity were found in the brush border of the choroid epithelial cells facing the spinal fluid. Little staining occurred in the rest of the choroid plexus, including the endothelial cells of its blood vessels. In the subfornical organ and to a lesser extent the organum vasculosum of the lamina terminalis, there was staining in the neuropil. However, no definite staining occurred outside of endothelial cells in the median eminence, the area postrema, and the rest of the brain. It is possible that the converting enzyme measured by hydrolysis of Hip-His-Leu and similar substrates in pieces of brain tissue is due to the converting enzyme in the endothelial cells in the tissue. However, chemical lesions of the striatum that are believed to destroy only nerve cells have been reported to reduce the converting enzyme activity in the substantia nigra (38) and the striatum (39) on the injected side. This is good evidence for converting enzyme in neurons. The reason that converting enzyme is not seen in neurons in the immunocytochemical studies is unknown. One possibility is that the biochemical method is more sensitive than the immunocytochemical technique. Alternatively, there may be enough difference between the enzyme in brain and the enzyme in lung tissue that the brain enzyme does not fully cross-react with antibodies to lung converting enzyme. Evidence against this latter possibility is the observation that in the rat brain converting enzyme is neutralized by antibodies to lung converting enzyme (40). A third possibility, for which there is some evidence (see ref. 12), is that the biochemical method is less specific than the immunocytochemical method.

3.6 Renin Substrate

3.6.1 Cerebrospinal Fluid

Unlike AII and converting enzyme, angiotensinogen is present in CSF in relatively large amounts (41). The concentration of the substrate is about 20% of the concentration in plasma, but the total protein concentration in CSF is only 6% of the concentration in peripheral blood. Consequently, the ratio of substrate to total protein in CSF is more than three times that in plasma. The substrate in spinal fluid appears to be a ready potential source of AI *in vivo*, since intraventricular injection of renin causes formation of abundant AII (42).

3.6.2 Brain Tissue

Substrate is also present in brain tissue (5, 43, 44). High concentrations were found in the area postrema, the organum vasculosum of the lamina terminalis, the periventricular thalamus and hypothalamus, and the median eminence (43). However, this substrate may be principally in brain extracellular fluid. Morris and Reid (44) found that the substrate in brain tissue was primarily located in the supernatant in fractionated brain tissue, and they argued that the small amount in granule fractions was probably due to contamination with extracellular fluid.

The source of the substrate in brain is still unsettled. Like the circulating substrate formed in the liver, it is a glycoprotein. Its molecular weight and amino acid composition are similar to the substrate formed in the liver. However, its carbohydrate structure is different (45), and there are two reports that in dogs and humans, it is immunologically different (7, 8). In addition, when the concentration of substrate in peripheral plasma was increased by nephrectomy and dexamethasone treatment, there was no change in CSF substrate concentration (9). Consequently, it seems unlikely that brain substrate is of peripheral origin.

Another observation that suggests a brain origin of substrate is the release of this material from brain slices *in vitro* (46, 47). However, the release is unaffected by inhibitors of protein synthesis, which prevent the release of substrate from liver slices. In pilot immunocytochemical studies with an antibody to circulating rat substrate, generously provided by Corvol and associates, we have found staining in glial cells (Brownfield, Reid, and Ganong, unpublished data). However, the specificity of this staining has not been determined, and additional research is needed to settle the question of the origin, synthesis, and secretion of substrate in the brain.

3.7 Renin

3.7.1 Angiotensin-Generating Activity in the Central Nervous System

There is general agreement that with the possible exception of conditions that break down the blood-brain barrier (3), there is no renin in spinal fluid (15, 28).

The brain itself is another matter. Ganten and his associates (5) were the first to report the presence of appreciable amounts of angiotensin-generating activity in brain tissue, activity they ascribed to an enzyme they called isorenin. However, the maximum activity in their extracts was present at a more acid pH than the maximum activity of renal renin, and on this basis plus copurification data, Day and Reid (48) argued that the brain renin activity was actually due to the lysosomal protease cathepsin D. Much of the angiotensin-generating activity in unfractionated whole brain is certainly due to cathepsin D, but it now seems clear that the brain also contains small amounts of an enzyme that has a pH optimum resembling that of renal renin and that cross-reacts with antibodies to renal renin (4). The brain enzyme needs to be isolated and characterized chemically, but since the curve of its activity at different pH's is similar to that of renal renin and since it cross-reacts with antibodies to renal renin, it is called brain renin, or simply renin, in this review.

The distribution of the brain renin described above has been studied in hog brain (4). Within the brain, the mean activity ranged from 0.017 ng AI/mg protein/h in the neurohypophysis to 0.482 ng AI/mg protein/h in the hypothalamus. This was in contrast to 18400 ng AI/mg protein/h in renal cortex and 0.714 ng AI/mL/h in normal plasma. However, the activity in choroid plexus was 21.6 ng AI/mg protein/h, and in the adenohypophysis and pineal, it was 32.4 and 325 respectively. A somewhat similar distribution has been reported in rat brains and related organs by Schelling et al. (49). The significance of the high concentrations in the anterior pituitary and pineal glands is unknown, and deserves to be explored.

Antibodies to highly purified renal and salivary renin have been used to determine the distribution of renin in the central nervous system by immunocytochemical techniques. Using antibodies to salivary renin, Fuxe et al. (50) reported the presence of renin-like immunoreactivity in supraoptic and paraventricular neurons and in the cerebellar cortex in rats and mice. Similar findings were reported by Inagami et al. (51) using antibodies to salivary and renal renin. We have observed staining in the supraoptic and paraventricular nuclei of rats with one antibody to hog renal renin, generously provided by Inagami, but not with two others (Brownfield and Ganong, unpublished data). Using antibodies to human renin, Slater et al. (52) found renin-like immunoreactivity in neurons in most parts of the human brain. Staining was also found in glial cells and cells of the anterior pituitary gland. More detailed research needs to be done with immunocytochemical methods and the specificity of the staining needs to be proved, but at least the data provide presumptive evidence that renin is present in neurons in the brain. Additional evidence is the presence of renin in synaptosomes (53). The immunocytochemical studies also rule out the possibility that the renin extracted from brain tissue is actually in arteries rather than neural tissues. Other arteries contain a renin-like enzyme (1), but specific staining of brain arteries was not found in the immunocytochemical investigations.

3.7.2   Prorenin

A large, relatively inactive form of renin, commonly called prorenin, is present in blood and renal tissue (54). Hirose et al. (4) have presented evidence that the brain also contains a prorenin that can be activated by trypsin. The ratio of inactive prorenin to active renin varied from 0.14 in the neurohypophysis to 1.53 in the intracranial portion of the spinal cord. It was zero in the choroid plexus and 2.75 in the adenohypophysis. The renin in cultured neuroblastoma X glioma cells (see below), tumor-derived cells that resemble neurons, is entirely in the inactive, trypsin-activatable form (55).

3.7.3   Renin Activity of Nerve Growth Factor

Intraventricular injection of nerve growth factor causes a prompt increase in water intake and a delayed increase in salt intake (56), as well as an increase in blood pressure and ornithine decarboxylase activity in the brain and liver and increased plasma vasopressin and ACTH (Ramsay et al., unpublished data). These reactions are also produced by injecting renin or AII in the ventricular system (see below), and the nerve growth factor effects are blocked by saralasin, by converting enzyme inhibitors (57), and by the renin-inhibiting peptide pepstatin (Ramsay et al., unpublished data). Thus, they are due to nerve growth factor acting like or activating renin in the brain.

Naturally occurring nerve growth factor is a protein containing three subunits, designated alpha, beta, and gamma. The function of the alpha subunit is unknown. The beta subunit is responsible for stimulation of neural growth, and the gamma subunit is a serine protease (58). Serine proteases are known to activate prorenin (53), and Morris et al. (59) have demonstrated that the gamma subunit of nerve growth factor can activate prorenin. Consequently, the nerve growth factor may exert its renin-mediated effects by activating the prorenin in the brain. However, most nerve growth factor preparations have been extracted from salivary glands, and in salivary glands, nerve growth factor is closely associated with salivary renin and epidermal growth factor. Indeed, it has been suggested that all three are formed as parts of a single common precursor molecule (60). Consequently, the effects produced by intraventricular injection could be caused by renin contaminating the nerve growth factor preparations. Evidence for contamination and against the prorenin hypothesis is the finding that phenylmethylsulfonylfluoride (PMSF), an inhibitor of serine proteases, did not block the formation of AI when nerve growth factor was added to purified CSF in vitro. In addition, generation was prevented by antibodies to salivary renin, and the purified gamma subunit did not generate AI (Ramsay and Reid, unpublished data). However, it is not certain that the salivary renin preparation used to raise the antibodies was free of nerve growth factor, and the antibodies could have been neutralizing activated brain renin rather than renin in the NGF preparation. It has also been reported that antibodies to nerve growth factor block its effects on water and salt intake *in vivo* (61), whereas the antibodies had no effect on the responses to intraventricular renin. Thus, more work needs to be done to determine whether the nerve growth factor effects are due to contamination with renin or activation of prorenin by the serine protease in the gamma subunit.

4 POSSIBLE INTERACTIONS OF THE RENIN-ANGIOTENSIN COMPONENTS IN THE BRAIN

The data presented in the preceding sections show that the various components of the renin-angiotensin system are present in brain but do not prove that they interact. Is there a functional renin-angiotensin system in the brain? Renin and angiotensin-like immunoreactivity are generally localized in the same areas, and possibly in the same neurons. However, the pattern of distribution of converting enzyme-like immunoreactivity is entirely different; moderate amounts are found in the subfornical organ but most of the converting enzyme is located in the choroid plexus. This raises two possibilities: AII could be formed in the brain by some sort of shuttle mechanism from renin in cells to converting enzyme in the choroid plexus back to AII in the cells, or AII could be formed directly from substrate by an intracellular pathway that does not involve converting enzyme.

It is clear that although there is no renin in CSF, the other components interact with ease; abundant AII is formed when renin is placed in the ventricles *in vivo* (42). Does the renin in brain tissue have access to the substrate in CSF? One way to approach this question is to inject extra substrate intraventricularly and monitor the production of AII by its actions or by radioimmunoassay of spinal fluid. Substrate is rate-limiting in the production of AII in blood (54), and one might expect it to be rate-limiting in the brain as well. Intraventricular TDP (see above) produced a prompt increase in water intake, blood pressure, and vasopressin and ACTH secretion in dogs and rats (62, 63), suggesting that it was indeed being exposed to renin. However, Reid and associates (42, 62, 63) were unable to block the drinking response with the renin inhibitors pepstatin and *N*-acetyl-pepstatin. Furthermore, they reported that injection of natural substrate from arterial plasma or CSF failed to produce the effects produced by TDP or to increase CSF AII concentration. This led them to conclude that TDP was not being hydrolyzed by renin but instead by repeated action of converting enzyme with the serial removal of three dipeptides to produce AII. However, others have reported that intraventricular injection of natural substrate does cause drinking (64). In addition, two groups have reported that they can inhibit the drinking response to TDP with renin inhibitors; one employed *N*-acetyl-pepstatin (65) and the other employed isovaleryl-pepstatin (66). Consequently, it remains unsettled whether the renin in brain has access to the substrate in CSF.

On the other hand, the possibility that AII can be formed directly from substrate by an intracellular pathway in neurons that bypasses AI deserves serious consideration. Three different types of cells that contain both renin-like and angiotensin-like immunoreactivity have now been described: juxtaglomerular cells in the kidneys, gonadotrops in the anterior pituitary gland, and neurons in the supraoptic and paraventricular nuclei (Table 4). These cells do not contain immunocytochemically detectable converting enzyme. However, at least two enzymes have been described that can catalyze the direct formation of AII. One is tonin, a serine protease isolated from salivary glands (67), and the other is a protease found in neutrophils (68). This raises the exciting possibility that a totally intracellular pathway leads to the formation of AII within cells. Tonin is present in the brain, and intraventricular tonin raises blood pressure and increases water intake (67).

Renin-like and angiotensin-like immunoreactivity are also found in neuroblastoma X glioma cells (55) and in rat salivary gland duct cells (Brownfield et al., unpublished data). However, converting enzyme-like immunoreactivity is also present in these cells, unlike juxtaglomerular cells, gonadotrops, or supraoptic and paraventricular neurons. In addition, there is evidence for the presence of substrate (Table 4).

An alternative explanation for the presence of renin-like immunoreactivity and angiotensin-like immunoreactivity in juxtaglomerular cells, gonadotrops, and some neurons is that the cells take up AII and internalize it as part of a feedback mechanism that controls renin synthesis

TABLE 4   Cells that Appear to Contain More than One Component of the Renin-Angiotensin System[a]

	Juxtaglomerular Cells	Gonadotrops	Neurons	Salivary Duct Cells	Neuroblastoma Cells
Renin	+	+	+	+	+
Renin substrate	−	−	−	+	+
Converting enzyme	−	−	−	+	+
Angiotensin II	+	+	+	+	+

[a] Data based on immunocytochemical and other observations. Symbols: +, present; −, absent. From W. F. Ganong (101).

or release. AII is known to act directly on juxtaglomerular cells to inhibit renin secretion (69). Of course, there is no evidence for secretion of renin by gonadotropic cells or neurons. However, intraventricular AII stimulates LH secretion (70) and angiotensin-like immunoreactivity is present in the external layer of the median eminence (14), so the peptide could be transported to the gonadotrops via the portal hypophyseal vessels. Research to distinguish between binding and internalization of AII as opposed to intracellular production would seem to be in order in all three types of cells.

5 POSSIBLE FUNCTIONS OF A BRAIN RENIN-ANGIOTENSIN SYSTEM

5.1 Relation to Effects Also Produced by the Action of Systemic Angiotensin on Circumventricular Organs

One obvious way to study the possible function of the brain renin-angiotensin system is to inject AII into the ventricular system and observe the effects that are produced. Five of the effects of intraventricular AII are the same as those produced by the action of circulating AII on the brain: increased water intake, increased blood pressure, increased vasopressin secretion, increased ACTH secretion, and decreased renin secretion (see Chapter 15). Most and probably all these effects of circulating AII are produced via the circumventricular organs. Is intraventricular AII also acting by way of the circumventricular organs? Two types of experiments can help settle this question. One is comparison of the effects of intravenous and intraventricular AII in animals with lesions of the various circumventricular organs. Another is determination whether intraventricular injection of saralasin blocks responses produced by circulating AII. The occurrence of blockade suggests that the saralasin molecules in the ventricle and the AII molecules in the plasma are reaching the same receptors. It is relevant in this regard that labeled AII has been shown to be taken up by the organum vasculosum of the lamina terminalis after intraventricular administration (71). Alternatively, an AII blocker can be injected intravenously and the AII administered intraventricularly. However, it is difficult to be sure that the dose of saralasin injected systemically is adequate to provide complete blockade of the relevant receptors in the circumventricular organs.

5.1.1 Increased Water Intake

Simpson and associates (see ref. 72) initially reported that lesions of the subfornical organ blocked the dipsogenic response to intraventricular and intravenous AII. The view that lesions of the subfornical organ block responses to intraventricular AII has subsequently been challenged (72). However, intraventricular saralasin has been found to abolish the dipsogenic response to intravenous AII (73, 74), and to an increase in circulating renin (75). It may be that AII acts on more than one circumventricular organ to increase water intake, and that a relatively high concentration of AII in CSF can override the effect of subfornical organ lesions by acting on the organum vasculosum of the lamina terminalis or other circumventricular organs whereas circulating AII does not reach a high enough concentration to produce an effect via these backup circumventricular organs.

5.1.2 Pressor Responses

Circulating AII acts on the brain to increase blood pressure by increasing sympathetic discharge and vasopressin secretion. The circumventricular organ that is primarily involved is the area postrema in dogs, rabbits, and cats, but in rats, the pressor effect is mediated by more rostral circumventricular organs (see Chapter 15). Lesions of the area postrema in dogs have been reported to block the response to injection of AII into the vertebral arteries without affecting the response to intraventricular AII (76), and there is evidence that the pressor response to intraventricular AII in cats is due to an action of the peptide on a nucleus in the midbrain rather than a circumventricular organ (77). However, intraventricular saralasin blocks the pressor response to intravertebral AII in dogs (73) and in rats, it lowers blood pressure in animals with hypertension due to increased renin secretion (78), and it reduces the pressor response to intravenous AII (74). Thus, once again the evidence is not conclusive, but it is consistent with the hypothesis that in raising blood pressure, intraventricular AII and intravenous AII both act on circumventricular organs.

5.1.3 Vasopressin, ACTH, and Renin Secretion

It has not been settled as to which circumventricular organs are responsible for the increase in vasopressin secretion produced by intravenous AII, and there are as yet no published experiments comparing the effect of intraventricular and intravenous AII on vasopressin secretion in animals with lesions in these organs. However, intraventricular saralasin abolishes the renin-mediated increase in vasopressin secretion produced by isoproterenol (75) and it abolishes the increase in vasopressin secretion produced by intravenous AII (Ramsay, unpublished data).

There is evidence that the stimulation of ACTH secretion and the inhibition of renin secretion produced by the action of AII in the brain are due in part to increased vasopressin secretion (79, 80), but there are as yet no data on the effects of lesions of circumventricular organs other than the median eminence or the effects of intraventricular saralasin on the ACTH and renin responses to systemic AII.

5.1.4 Resume

Although the data in the preceding paragraphs leave many unanswered questions, it seems reasonable to conclude that the effects of intraventricular AII that are also produced by systemically administered AII are probably due to penetration of AII from CSF into the circumventricular organs. Consequently, it does not seem necessary to postulate the existence of a brain renin-angiotensin system to explain these effects of intraventricular AII. Of course, this does not exclude the possibility that endogenous AII is produced in the brain and passes via the CSF to act in this fashion, but the low level of AII in CSF and the failure as yet to demonstrate increases with dehydration and other related stimuli make this possibility unlikely.

5.2 Relation to Brain Amines

It is well established that AII facilitates noradrenergic transmission in the autonomic nervous system (81). This effect is partly postsynaptic but mainly presynaptic, with the production of increased amounts of catecholamines when sympathetic nerves are stimulated. The possibility of a similar action in the brain deserved serious consideration in view of the extensive systems of noradrenergic, dopaminergic, and adrenergic neurons in the brain (2).

Evidence is now beginning to accumulate that AII can affect catecholamine turnover in the central nervous system. AII has been reported to increase release of norepinephrine from the perfused hypothalamus (82) and to potentiate potassium-evoked release of norepinephrine from the hypothalamus (83). Evidence has also been presented that intraventricular injections of renin increase dopamine turnover in the median eminence and decrease norepinephrine turnover in the magnocellular portion of the paraventricular nuclei (84). The change in dopamine metabolism may be related to the regulation of prolactin secretion, since intraventricular AII inhibits secretion of this pituitary hormone (70) and the effect is blocked by dopamine receptor blocking drugs (Steele et al., unpublished data). Changes in hypothalamic norepinephrine metabolism could be related to the observed effects of intraventricular AII on the secretion of other anterior pituitary hormones (70), via changes in the release of the appropriate hypothalamic hypophysiotropic hormones. Of course, brain catecholamines have many other functions (2), and by affecting these functions a brain renin-angiotensin system could have very widespread effects.

An additional possibility is an effect of centrally produced AII on serotonin metabolism, since AII has been reported to have a stimulating effect on the release of serotonin from synaptosomes and a complex, biphasic effect on serotonin synthesis (85). The serotoninergic systems in the brain, like the catecholamine-secreting systems, have widespread effects on brain function.

5.3 Additional Possibilities

Several investigators have claimed that there is increased activity of a brain renin-angiotensin system in rats with spontaneous hypertension, particularly in stroke-prone spontaneously hypertensive rats (14). However, this evidence is controversial, and although a role for brain AII in the regulation of cardiovascular function remains a possibility, it has not been established.

Another possibility is a role in brain processes related to memory. Amnesia has been reported following injections of AII into the neostriatum (86), and increases in spinal fluid AII produced by intraventricular renin were associated with disruption of conditioned avoidance responses (87). It has been reported that there is a high concentration of AII receptors in the hippocampus (22), that angiotensin-like immunoreactivity can be demonstrated in this structure even though its AII content is low, and that AII excites hippocampal CA I pyramidal cells (88). However, no definite effects of angiotensin II on memory mechanisms have been established. There have been various other reports of direct effects of AII on neurons in the peripheral and central nervous system (89–91).

Another speculative possibility is that AII plays a role in regulating fluid and electrolyte balance within the brain. This possibility is raised by evidence (92) that intraventricular AII may affect the permeability of cerebral capillaries in monkeys.

6 CONCLUSIONS

The data reviewed in the preceding sections make it clear that much remains to be done if we are to understand the nature and function of the components of the renin-angiotensin system found in the brain. However, it seems possible to draw certain tentative conclusions that can at least be presented as working hypotheses.

1. All the components of the renin-angiotensin system—or at least substances that closely resemble them—are present in the central nervous system.

2. These components are not normally of peripheral origin and are presumably manufactured in the brain.

3. An important immediate goal in research should be isolation and chemical identification of the material in the brain that reacts with antibodies to AII. The material could be AII, AIII, a smaller carboxy terminal fragment of AII, or some other cross-reacting substance.

4. CSF contains converting enzyme and substrate and appears to be in contact with converting enzyme in locations such as the choroid plexus and circumventricular organs. Consequently, when renin is added to CSF, there is prompt formation of AII.

5. Brain renin and AII, or the material that cross-reacts with antibodies to AII, are located in cells. This is probably why the concentration of AII in CSF is normally low.

6. The intracellular location of AII and renin and the very different distribution of converting enzyme in the brain raise the possibility that there is direct formation of AII in neurons without formation of AI and conversion.

7. The function of the brain renin-angiotensin system is unsettled. Intraventricular AII produces increased drinking, increased blood pressure, and increased secretion of vasopressin and ACTH, but so does intravenous AII, and it seems probable that intraventricular AII, like circulating AII, is acting on the circumventricular organs.

8. A major function of the brain renin-angiotensin system may be selective adjustment of the output of monoamines from the various endings of the noradrenergic, the dopaminergic, and possibly the serotonergic neurons in the brain, thus playing a role in the regulation of their multiple, widespread functions.

9. Other possibilities include a role in cardiovascular control, memory processing, and other effects produced by direct actions of AII on neurons.

REFERENCES

1. D. Ganten, J. S. Hutchinson, P. Schelling, U. Ganten, and H. Fischer, *Clin. Exp. Pharmacol. Physiol.* **3**, 103–126 (1976).

2. W. F. Ganong, *Review of Medical Physiology*, 10th ed., Lange Medical Publications, Los Altos, Calif., 1981.

3. S. I. Rappaport, *Blood Brain Barrier in Physiology and Medicine*, Raven Press, New York, 1976.

4. S. Hirose, H. Yokosawa, T. Inagami, and R. J. Workman, *Brain Res.* **191**, 489–499 (1980).

5. D. Ganten, A. Marquez-Julio, P. Granger, K. Hayduk, K. P. Karsunky, R. Boucher, and J. Genest, *Am. J. Physiol.* **221**, 1733–1737 (1971).

6. V. J. Dzau, A. Brenner, N. Emmett, and E. Haber, *Clin. Sci.* **59**, Suppl. 6, 45S–48S (1980).

7. T. Ito, P. Eggenn, J. D. Barnett, D. Katz, J. Metter, and M. P. Sambhi, *Hypertension* **2**, 432–436 (1980).

8. B. J. Morris and I. A. Reid, *IRCS Med. Sci.* **7**, 194 (1979).

9. I. A. Reid and R. P. Day, in J. P. Buckley and C. M. Ferrario, Eds., *Central Actions of Angiotensin and Related Hormones*, Pergamon Press, New York, 1977, pp. 267–282.

10. H.-Y. T. Yang and N. H. Neff, *J. Neurochem.* **19**, 2443–2450 (1972).

11. R. P. Igic, C. J. G. Robinson, and E. G. Erdös, in J. P. Buckley and C. M. Ferrario, Eds., *Central Actions of Angiotensin and Related Hormones*, Pergamon Press, New York, 1977, pp. 23–27.

12. M. S. Brownfield, I. A. Reid, D. Ganten, and W. F. Ganong, *Neuroscience*, **7**, 1759–1769 (1982).

13. M. G. Nicholls, *Hypertension* **1**, 228–234 (1979).

14. D. Ganten, K. Fuxe, M. I. Phillips, J. F. E. Mann, and U. Ganten, in W. F. Ganong and L. Martini, Eds., *Frontiers in Neuroendocrinology*, Vol. 5, Raven Press, New York, 1978, pp. 61–100.

15. P. Schelling, U. Ganten, G. Spiner, T. Unger and D. Ganten, *Neuroendocrinology* **31**, 297–308 (1980).

16. S. F. Abraham, J. P. Coghlan, D. A. Denton, D. T. W. Fei, M. J. McKinley, and B. A. Scoggins, Program 6th International Congress of Endocrinology, Melbourne, Australia, 1980, p. 725.

17. M. I. Phillips, *Neuroendocrinology* **25**, 354–377 (1978).

18. M. Van Houten, E. L. Schiffrin, J. F. E. Mann, B. I. Posner, and R. Boucher, *Brain Res.* **186**, 480–485 (1980).

19. A. Weindl, in W. F. Ganong and L. Martini, Eds., *Frontiers in Neuroendocrinology*, Oxford University Press, New York, 1973, pp. 3–32.

20. I. A. Reid, V. L. Brooks, C. D. Rudolph, and L. C. Keil, *Am. J. Physiol.*, **243**, R82–R91 (1982).

21. J. P. Bennett Jr. and S. H. Snyder, *J. Biol. Chem.* **251**, 7423–7430 (1976).

22. N. E. Sirett, A. S. McLean, J. J. Bray, and J. R. Hubbard, *Brain Res.* **122**, 299–312 (1977).

23. C. R. Baxter, J. S. Horvarth, C. G. Duggin, and D. J. Tiller, *Endocrinology* **106**, 995–999 (1980).

24. J. W. Harding, L. P. Stone, and J. W. Wright, *Brain Res.* **205**, 265–274 (1981).

25. J. P. Bennett Jr. and S. H. Snyder, *Eur. J. Pharmacol.* **67**, 11–25 (1980).

26. N. E. Sirett, J. J. Bray, and J. I. Hubbard, *Brain Res.* **217**, 405–411 (1981).

27. J. S. Hutchinson, J. Csicsmann, P. I. Karter, C. I. Johnston, *Clin. Sci. Mol. Med.* **54**, 147–151 (1978).

28. P. F. Semple, W. A. Macrae, and J. J. Norton, *Clin. Sci.* **59**, Suppl. 6, 61S–64S (1980).

29. J. S. Horvarth, C. Baxter, F. Furby, and D. J. Tiller, *Prog. Brain Res.* **47**, 161–165 (1977).

30. I. A. Reid, R. P. Day, B. Moffat, and H. G. Hughes, *J. Neurochem.* **28**, 435–438 (1977).

31. K. Fuxe, D. Ganten, T. Hökfelt, and P. Bolme, *Neurosci. Lett.* **2**, 229–234 (1976).

32. M. M. Kilcoyne, D. L. Hoffman, and E. A. Zimmerman, *Clin. Sci.* **59**, Suppl. 6, 57S–60S (1980).

33. D. G. Changaris, L. C. Keil, and W. B. Severs, *Neuroendocrinology* **25**, 257–274 (1978).

34. J. T. Quinlan and M. I. Phillips, *Brain Res.* **205**, 212–218 (1981).

35. E. Rix, D. Ganten, B. Schull, Th. Unger, and R. Taughner, *Neurosci. Lett.* **22**, 125–130 (1981).

36. A. Weindl, H. Schweisfurth, M. V. Sofroniew, and H. Dahlheim, *Acta Endocrinol.* **85**, Suppl. 212, 158 (1977), abstract.
37. A. Arregui, J. P. Bennett Jr., E. D. Bird, H. I. Yamamura, L. L. Iversen, and S. H. Snyder, *Ann. Neurol.* **2**, 294–298 (1977).
38. A. Arregui, P. C. Emson, and E. G. Spokes, *Eur. J. Pharmacol.* **52**, 121–124 (1978).
39. K. Fuxe, D. Ganten, C. Köhler, B. Schüll, and G. Speck, *Acta Physiol. Scand.* **110**, 321–323 (1980).
40. R. Polsky-Cynkin and B. Fanburg, *Int. J. Biochem.* **10**, 669–674 (1979).
41. I. A. Reid and D. J. Ramsay, *Endocrinology* **97**, 536–542 (1975).
42. I. A. Reid and B. Moffat, *Endocrinology* **103**, 1494–1498 (1978).
43. J. A. Lewicki, J. H. Fallon, and M. P. Printz, *Brain Res.* **158**, 359–371 (1978).
44. B. J. Morris and I. A. Reid, *Endocrinology* **103**, 492–500 (1978).
45. I. A. Reid, B. Moffat, and B. J. Morris, *IRCS Med. Sci.* **6**, 383 (1978).
46. C. Sernia and I. A. Reid, *Brain Res.* **192**, 217–225 (1980).
47. I. A. Reid and M. S. Brownfield, *Exp. Brain Res. Suppl.* **4**, 284–293 (1982).
48. R. P. Day and I. A. Reid, *Endocrinology* **99**, 93–100 (1976).
49. P. Schelling, D. Meyer, H.-E. Loos, G. Speck, A. K. Johnson, M. I. Phillips, and D. Ganten, in J. P. Buckley and C. M. Ferrario, Eds., *Central Nervous System Mechanisms in Hypertension*, Raven Press, New York, 1981, pp. 397–406.
50. K. Fuxe, D. Ganten, T. Hökfelt, V. Locatelli, K. Poulsen, G. Stuck, E. Rix, and R. Taugner, *Neurosci. Lett.* **18**, 245–250 (1980).
51. T. Inagami, M. R. Celio, D. L. Clemens, D. Lan, Y. Takii, A. G. Kasselberg, and S. Hirose, *Clin. Sci.* **59**, 495–515 (1982).
52. E. E. Slater, R. Defendini, and E. Zimmerman, *Proc. Natl. Acad. Sci. USA* **77**, 5458–5460 (1980).
53. A. Husain, R. R. Soneby, J. Krontiris-Litowitz, and R. C. Speth, *Brain Res.* **222**, 182–186 (1981).
54. I. A. Reid, B. J. Morris, and W. F. Ganong, *Ann. Rev. Physiol.* **40**, 377–410 (1978).
55. M. C. Fishman, E. A. Zimmerman, and E. E. Slater, *Science* **214**, 921–923 (1981).
56. M. E. Lewis, D. B. Avrith, and J. T. Fitzsimons, *Nature* **279**, 440–442 (1979).
57. D. B. Avrith, M. E. Lewis, and J. T. Fitzsimons, *Nature* **285**, 248–250 (1980).
58. R. W. Bradshaw, *Ann. Rev. Biochem.* **47**, 191–216 (1978).
59. B. J. Morris, D. F. Catanzaro, and R. T. De Zwart, *Neurosci. Lett.* **24**, 87–92 (1981).
60. Y. Hirata and D. N. Orth, *Endocrinology* **104**, 244A (1979), abstract.
61. J. T. Fitzsimons, D. B. Avrith, and M. E. Lewis, *Neurosci. Lett. Suppl.* **3**, S327 (1979), abstract.
62. J. B. Simpson, I. A. Reid, D. J. Ramsay, and H. Kipen, *Brain Res.* **157**, 63–72 (1978).
63. D. J. Ramsay, I. A. Reid, and C. Brown, *Endocrinology* **105**, 947–951 (1979).
64. W. E. Hoffman, P. Schelling, M. I. Phillips, and D. Ganten, *Neurosci. Lett.* **3**, 299–303 (1976).
65. J. A. D. M. Tonnaer, V. M. Wiegant, and W. de Jong, *Brain Res.* **223**, 343–353 (1981).
66. J. T. Fitzsimons, A. N. Epstein, and A. K. Johnson, *Brain Res.* **153**, 139–331 (1978).
67. K. Kondo, R. Garcia, R. Boucher, and J. Genest, *Brain Res.* **200**, 437–441 (1980).
68. B. V. Wintraub, L. B. Klickstein, C. E. Kaempfer, and K. F. Austen, *Proc. Nat. Acad. Sci. USA* **78**, 1204–1208 (1981).
69. J. O. Davis and R. H. Freeman, *Physiol. Rev.* **56**, 1–56 (1976).
70. M. K. Steele, A. Negro-Vilar, S. M. McCann, *Endocrinology* **109**, 893–899 (1981).
71. S. Landas, M. I. Phillips, J. F. Stamler, and M. K. Raizada, *Science* **210**, 791–793 (1980).
72. J. Simpson, *Neuroendocrinology* **33**, 248–256 (1981).
73. M. C. Lee, I. A. Reid, and D. J. Ramsay, *Fed. Proc.* **40**, 488 (1981), abstract.
74. M. J. Brody and A. K. Johnson, in L. Martini and W. F. Ganong, Eds., *Frontiers in Neuroendocrinology*, Raven Press, New York, 1980, Vol. 6, pp. 249–292.
75. D. J. Ramsay, I. A. Reid, L. C. Keil, and W. F. Ganong, *Endocrinology* **103**, 54–59 (1978).

76. P. L. Gildenberg and C. M. Ferrario, in J. P. Buckley and C. M. Ferrario, Eds., *Central Actions of Angiotensin and Related Hormones*, Pergamon Press, New York, 1977, pp. 157–164.

77. J. P. Buckley, H. H. Smookler, W. B. Severs, and R. R. Deuben, in J. P. Buckley and C. M. Ferrario, Eds., *Central Actions of Angiotensin and Related Hormones*, Pergamon Press, New York, 1977, pp. 149–155.

78. C. S. Sweet, J. M. Columbo, and S. L. Gaul, *Am. J. Physiol.* **231**, 1794–1799 (1976).

79. S. A. Malayan, L. C. Keil, D. J. Ramsay, and I. A. Reid, *Endocrinology* **104**, 672–675 (1979).

80. W. F. Ganong, J. Shinsako, I. A. Reid, L. C, Keil, D. L. Hoffman, and E. A. Zimmerman, *Ann. N.Y. Acad. Sci.*, in press, (1982).

81. S. Z. Langer, *Pharm. Rev.* **32**, 337–362 (1981).

82. C. Chevillard, N. Duchene, R. Pasquier, and J.-M. Alexandre, *J. Pharmacol.* **58**, 203–206 (1979).

83. A. J. Garcia-Sevilla, M. L. Dubocovich, and S. L. Langer, *Eur. J. Pharmacol.* **56**, 173–176 (1979).

84. K. Fuxe, K. Andersson, D. Ganten, T. Hökfelt, and P. Enroth, in F. Gross and G. Vagel, Eds., *Enzymatic Release of Vasoactive Peptides*, Raven Press, New York, 1980, pp. 161–170.

85. V. E. Nahmod, S. Finkielman, E. E. Benarroch, and C. J. Pirola, *Science* **202**, 1091–1093 (1978).

86. J. M. Morgan and A. Routtenberg, *Science* **196**, 87–89 (1977).

87. M. Koller, H. P. Krause, F. Hoffmeister, and D. Ganten, *Neurosci. Lett.* Suppl. **3**, S327 (1979), abstract.

88. H. L. Haas, D. Felix, M. R. Celio, and T. Inagami, *Experientia* **36**, 1394–1395 (1980).

89. D. A. Brown, A. Constanti, and S. Marsh, *Brain Res.* **193**, 614–620 (1980).

90. R. A. Nicoll, in J. A. Ferrendelli, B. S. McEwen, S. H. Snyder, Eds., *Neurosci. Symposia*, Vol. 1, Society for Neuroscience, Bethesda, Md., 1976, pp. 99–122.

91. T. Huwyler and D. Felix, *Brain Res.* **195**, 187–195 (1980).

92. R. L. Grubb Jr. and M. E. Raichle, *Brain Res.* **210**, 426–430 (1981).

93. S. Finkielman, C. Fischer-Ferraro, A. Diaz, D. J. Goldstein, and V. E. Nahmod, *Proc. Natl. Acad. Sci. USA* **69**, 353 (1971).

94. D. G. Changaris, L. M. Demins, L. C. Keil, and W. B. Severs, in J. P. Buckley and C. M. Ferrario, Eds., *Central Actions of Angiotensin and Related Hormones*, Pergamon Press, New York, 1977, pp. 233–243.

95. W. B. Severs, D. G. Changaris, J. M. Kapsha, L. C. Keil, D. J. Petro, I. A. Reid, and J. Y. Summy-Long, in J. P. Buckley and C. M. Ferrario, Eds., *Central Actions of Angiotensin and Related Hormones*, Pergamon Press, New York, 1977, pp. 225–232.

96. A. N. Epstein and D. Ganten, *Fed. Proc.* **36**, 481 (1977), abstract.

97. D. Ganten, J. S. Hutchinson, and P. Schelling, *Clin. Sci. Mol. Med.* **48**, Suppl. 2, 265s–268s (1975).

98. C. J. Wallis and M. P. Printz, *Endocrinology* **106**, 337–342 (1980).

99. B. Slaven, *J. Pharm. Pharmacol.* **27**, 782–783 (1975).

100. C. Fischer-Ferraro, V. E. Nahmod, A. Diaz, D. J. Goldstein, and S. Finkielman, *J. Exp. Med.* **133**, 353–361 (1971).

101. W. F. Ganong, *Life Sci.*, **30**, 561–569 (1982).

33

Enkephalins

ROBERT R. GOODMAN

LLOYD D. FRICKER

SOLOMON H. SNYDER

Departments of Neuroscience, Pharmacology, and Experimental Therapeutics
Psychiatry and Behavioral Sciences
Johns Hopkins University School of Medicine
Baltimore, Maryland

Supported by USPHS grant DA-00264, RSA Award DA-00074 to S.H.S., training grant GM-07309 to R.R.G., and a grant of The McKnight Foundation.

1   INTRODUCTION: THE DISCOVERY OF OPIOID PEPTIDES

The discovery of opioid peptides is intimately linked to the identification of opiate receptors by molecular binding techniques. As with many other drugs, the pharmacological specificity of opiate actions has long indicated that they presumably act at specific receptor sites in mediating their pharmacological effects. The first well-known generally successful approach to labeling neurotransmitter receptors, carried out by several laboratories in 1970–1971, dealt with binding of radioactive toxins to the nicotinic cholinergic receptor in the electric organ of various invertebrates. It appeared improbable that techniques employed in these studies could be readily applied to neurotransmitter receptors in the brain, because in these electric organs the density of cholinergic receptors was as high as 20% of membrane protein, whereas one could calculate that a typical neurotransmitter receptor in the brain might be no more than one millionth by weight of brain tissue. In addition, the cholinergic receptor-specific toxins were extraordinarily potent and acted virtually irreversibly, providing highly efficient tools that were lacking for most central nervous system receptors. However, utilizing ^{3}H-opiates labeled to fairly high specific activity and rapid but thorough washing techniques in filtration assays, it was possible to label opiate receptors (1–3). Many dramatic properties of these receptors were rapidly apparent, such as a heterogeneous distribution in the brain with high densities of receptors concentrated in areas associated with pharmacological actions of opiates (4). Also, sodium was shown to selectively differentiate receptor interactions of agonists, antagonists, and mixed agonists-antagonists, affording a powerful tool for identifying drugs with desired therapeutic actions and emphasizing the functional importance of opiate receptors (5). All these factors suggested that opiate receptors were no evolutionary vestige but might serve to interact with some normally occurring neurotransmitter-like substance. The reversal of brain stimulation analgesia by naloxone also suggested that a morphine-like substance could be released from brain tissue (6).

Two approaches were taken to isolating the morphine-like substance. Hughes examined brain extracts for their ability to mimic the effects of morphine on smooth muscle and in naloxone-reversible fashion, while we showed that brain extracts contained a substance that competed for opiate receptor binding and that had a regional distribution like that of opiate receptors (7, 8). Hughes et al. (9) completely isolated and determined the structures of the two enkephalins, [Met]-enkephalin and [Leu]-enkephalin, while using a different assay, isolation procedure and species, Simantov and Snyder soon afterwards isolated and identified the same two pentapeptides (10).

In exploring the opiate-like activity of pituitary extracts on smooth muscle, first reported by Teschemacher and collaborators (11), several groups identified the 31-amino-acid peptide beta-endorphin, which forms part of the 91-amino-acid peptide beta-lipotropin, which in turn is part of the much larger peptide that also incorporates the adrenocortico-trophic hormone (ACTH) sequence and is referred to as pro-opio-melanocortin or "big ACTH." The localization in pituitary and brain and biosynthetic processes for beta-endorphin differ markedly from those aspects of enkephalin. Additionally, the localizations of enkeph-alin and opiate receptor are closely similar and differ from that of beta-endorphin, whose functions accordingly probably have very little to do with the known pharmacological actions of opiates. For want of space, we will not review the literature of beta-endorphin.

Besides the enkephalins and beta-endorphin, numerous peptide frag-ments incorporating the enkephalin sequence have been described (12–14). Since several of these, especially dynorphin, possess opiate-like ac-tivity, it has been suggested that these also might be opiate-like neuro-transmitters. These peptides generally contain two or three basic amino acids linked directly to the C- or N-terminus of the enkephalin se-quence. It is well established that the biosynthesis of biologically active peptides involves cleavage at such pairs of basic amino acids. Accord-ingly, it is likely that many such fragments are enkephalin precursors, though they may also serve opiate-like functions.

2   ENKEPHALIN AS A NEUROTRANSMITTER

Not only was enkephalin discovered as the endogenous ligand of the opiate receptor, but subsequent studies comparing the localization of opiate receptors by autoradiography and that of enkephalin by immuno-histochemistry (15) indicated a close coincidence (Figure 1). The very fact that enkephalin is contained in nerve terminals and that these are associated with opiate receptors would suggest that enkephalin may be a neurotransmitter of neurons that interact with opiate receptors. How-ever, a long history of transmitter research has suggested that a com-pound must satisfy a large number of criteria before it is considered to be a neurotransmitter. The most stringent criteria require that a sub-stance contained in the nerve terminal at a specific synapse be shown to be released upon depolarization and, at that synapse, the action of the firing of that neuron upon the postsynaptic neuron must be identical with results following application of the compound in question. By these criteria, one would not accept any compound in the central nervous system as a neurotransmitter. Many of the criteria for neurotransmitters were established on the basis of studies of acetylcholine at the neuro-muscular junction and may not be relevant to other neurotransmitters. Thus, the existence of acetylcholinesterase resulted in a criterion that there must exist a specific enzyme to inactivate each neurotransmitter.

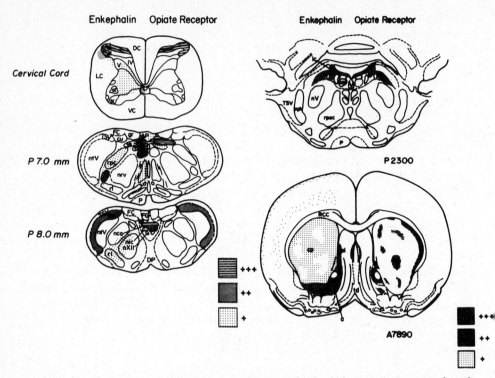

Figure 1. Distribution of opiate receptors (30–32) and enkephalin (15) in rat cervical cord, medulla (P7.0, P8.0), pons (P2300), and forebrain (A7890). Abbreviations: *a*, nucleus accumbens; *amb*, nucleus ambiguus; *AP*, area postrema; *cp*, nucleus caudatus-putamen; *cu*, nucleus cuneatus; *DC*, dorsal column; *DP*, decussatio pyramidis; *FC*, fasciculus cuneatus; *FG*, fasciculus gracilis; *gr*, nucleus gracilis; *io*, nucleus olivaris inferior; *lc*, locus ceruleus; *LC*, lateral column; *nco*, nucleus commissuralis; *nic*, nucleus intercalatus; *npV*, nucleus principalis nervi trigemini; *nrv*, nucleus reticularis medullae oblongatae pars ventralis; *ntd*, nucleus tegmenti dorsalis Gudden; *nts*, nucleus tractus solitarius; *ntV*, nucleus tractus spinalis nervi trigemini; *nV*, nucleus originis nervi trigemini; *nX*, nucleus originis dorsalis vagi; *nXII*, nucleus originis nervi hypoglossi; *P*, tractus corticospinalis; *RCC*, radiatio corporis callosi; *rl*, nucleus reticularis lateralis; *rpc*, nucleus reticularis parvocellularis; *rpoc*, nucleus reticularis pontis caudalis; *sgV*, substantia gelatinosa trigemini; *sl*, nucleus septi lateralis; *td*, nucleus tractus diagnolis (Broca); *ts*, tractus solitarius; *TSV*, tractus spinalis nervi trigemini; *VC*, ventral column. Reproduced from Simantov et al. (15).

Of course, we now know that most biogenic amine and amino acid neurotransmitters are not inactivated by an enzyme but largely by reuptake into the nerve endings that had released them. A number of properties of neurotransmitters have been demonstrated for enkephalin.

One criterion is that the compound should be localized in nerve endings. Radioreceptor assays (16) showed an enrichment of enkephalin in synaptosomal fractions of brain tissue before immunohistochemical studies were carried out which, of course, well demonstrated the existence of enkephalin in cells, axons, and terminals (vide infra). Recently Wilson and colleagues were able to demonstrate enkephalin concentrated in purified vesicles from bovine splenic nerve together with norepinephrine and dopamine-beta-hydroxylase. The occurrence of enkephalin not only in nerve terminals but within synaptic vesicles has been demonstrated by immunohistochemical studies at the electron microscopic level (18–20).

Depolarization-induced release is an important transmitter criterion. In very early studies Smith et al. (21) showed a calcium-dependent release of enkephalin from rat brain synaptosomes depolarized by potassium. Several more recent studies have directly demonstrated calcium-dependent depolarization-induced enkephalin release (22–27).

Demonstrating that enkephalin has synaptic actions has been fairly easy, considering that enkephalins generally mimic all the effects of opiates, which for many years have been observed in numerous systems. The discovery of opiate receptors and enkephalins greatly stimulated research on the synaptic influences of these substances. The multiplicity of effects that have been observed, described below, certainly fits with various effects of physiological nervous activity, but establishing identity of action with influences of physiological neuronal activity at a particular synapse is extraordinarily difficult and debatable for any transmitter.

To sum up, deciding whether a given substance is a neurotransmitter or "neuromodulator" is as much a question of semantics as of experimental evidence. Suffice it to say that enkephalins have satisfied as many criteria as almost any other chemical substance in the central nervous system.

2.1 Neuronal Localizations of Enkephalin

For enkephalins as for most neuropeptides, knowing the localization of their neuronal pathways has been one of the most powerful tools in understanding their functions. In the enkephalin system researchers had a head start; well before the isolation of the enkephalins, light microscopic autoradiography had shown dramatically selective localizations of opiate receptors. These initial studies were conducted *in vivo* because it could be shown that opiate receptors were labeled in the brain even after intravenous injection of low doses of ^{3}H-opiates. The first *in vivo* receptor labeling techniques were conducted in our laboratory with ^{3}H-naloxone (28). About 30% of all the radioactive drug in the brain was associated with opiate receptors. Since autoradiographic analysis visualizes all radioactive grains, ^{3}H-naloxone would not be suitable for autoradiographic studies as the nonspecific grains would provide an unacceptably high blank. The more potent opiate antagonist ^{3}H-diprenorphine proved to be a better candidate as 85% or more of the ra-

dioactivity in the brain following intravenous administration was bound
to opiate receptors (29). With the use of ^{3}H-diprenorphine, opiate receptors were found to be very highly concentrated in certain areas of the
brain and spinal cord, which meshed well with pharmacological actions
of opiates (29–32). For instance, receptors were concentrated in a narrow band in the substantia gelatinosa of the spinal cord, the first way-
station for integrated information about pain in the central nervous system. Similar high densities occurred in the substantia gelatinosa of the
trigeminal nucleus, which carries information about pain sensation in
the face. The locus ceruleus, the major norepinephrine-containing nucleus in the brain, has a high density of opiate receptors, which conceivably could relate to the affective influences of opiates. The medial
thalamus and periaqueductal gray matter, areas in the brain associated
with pain perception, are also enriched in opiate receptors. The first
histochemical localizations of enkephalin showed closely parallel localization of opiate receptors and enkephalin immunoreactivity (15, 33).
These findings indicated that enkephalin indeed is the neurotransmitter
normally associated with opiate receptors. By contrast, when it was
subsequently possible to localize beta-endorphin by immunohistochemistry, it was found that the parts of the brain that had the very
highest concentrations of enkephalin and opiate receptors—such as the
substantia gelatinosa of the spinal cord and trigeminal nucleus, the locus ceruleus, and the corpus striatum—had no beta-endorphin at all, indicating that the beta-endorphin system was not likely to play any
major role in brain functions normally associated with opiate activities
(34–36).

One must be very careful in making assertions about the localization
of a substance by immunohistochemistry, since one may often stain a
substance that reacts with the antibody but is not the same as the substance to which the antibody was raised. The only test of specificity in
immunohistochemical work is to assess whether staining vanishes when
the antibody is adsorbed with the substance being stained, in this case
enkephalin, a control experiment that does not in fact rule out staining
of cross-reacting substances. By contrast, in radioimmunoassay studies
one can fractionate tissue extracts by procedures with high resolving
capacities, such as high performance liquid chromatography, and determine whether the material that interacts with the antibody possesses
physical and chemical properties identical with those of authentic substance. Since detailed regional distribution studies of enkephalin localization with appropriate chemical controls show essentially the same
distribution as immunohistochemical localizations, it is likely that most
if not all of the immunohistochemical data represents staining of
enkephalin (37–39). Since some of the precursor fragments of enkephalin, especially with basic amino acids linked to the carboxyl terminus,
also react with many enkephalin antibodies, it is possible that some
staining reflects such precursors.

The first immunohistochemical studies of enkephalin largely visualized terminal distribution with very few cell bodies apparent (15, 33). Intraventricular injections of colchicine to block axonal flow facilitated a visualization of enkephalin-containing cell bodies, as the enkephalin would accumulate in proximal axons and cell bodies after colchicine treatment (40). Such studies, combined with lesioning experiments, have made it possible to identify some enkephalin-containing pathways. The enkephalins are localized both in small interneurons and in long pathways.

The substantia gelatinosa of the spinal cord has been one of the most carefully studied areas where enkephalin appears to be concentrated in small interneurons. Both enkephalin cells and axon terminals are observed in the narrow band representing layers I and II. Since enkephalin is not depleted from this area following lesions of the dorsal root or spinal cord section, it has been concluded that enkephalin is contained in small interneurons (41). This contrasts with substance P, which occurs in the substantia gelatinosa in terminals but not in cells. Substance P-containing cells are observed in the dorsal root ganglia, which do not contain enkephalin cells. Moreover, dorsal root lesions deplete substance P from the substantia gelatinosa (42). Because the distributions of enkephalin and substance P are quite similar throughout the central nervous system and because of interactions between them—which are discussed below—detailed electron microscopic immunohistochemical studies have explored a possible relationship between nerve terminals of the two peptides in the spinal cord. In the substantia gelatinosa of both the spinal cord and the spinal trigeminal nucleus, enkephalin terminals make axo-dendritic and axo-somatic contacts, whereas no axo-axonic contacts can be demonstrated (43–45). To determine whether enkephalin terminals interact with sensory terminals, dorsal root lesions have been performed; no direct interactions of enkephalin terminals with the degenerating sensory terminals have been observed. Glazer and Basbaum (45) did note enkephalin-containing terminals associated with synaptic glomeruli that contain primary afferent terminals, though there were no direct contacts between the two entities. Some contacts have been observed between enkephalin terminals and gamma-aminobutyric acid (GABA) cells, which in turn contact substance P terminals, suggesting a possible indirect interaction (46).

The reason for seeking evidence of axo-axonic interactions between enkephalin and substance P-containing neurons derives from suggestions that enkephalins regulate pain perception at the spinal cord level by inhibiting the release of pain transmitters such as substance P. Such an interaction was first tested when we found that dorsal root lesions would deplete opiate receptors from the dorsal portion of the monkey spinal cord despite their failure to deplete enkephalin. This suggested that enkephalin in the small interneurons of the spinal cord synapsed upon opiate receptors located on nerve terminals of sensory afferents. If these sensory afferents included unmyelinated pain fibers, then one could propose that enkephalins would act to inhibit the release of a pain neurotransmitter (47). Subsequently, enkephalins and opiates were observed to inhibit substance P release from potassium-depolarized slices of the substantia gelatinosa of the spinal trigeminal (48, 49). Though direct axo-axonic synapses to explain this effect have not been observed, the other close interactions between enkephalin and substance P neurons might account for the observed effects.

Although the major enkephalin system in the spinal cord appears to be in small interneurons, there is a long descending system arising from the pars alpha of the gigantocellular nucleus of the medulla oblongata and descending into the spinal cord to the dorsal root entry zone where these neurons might influence pain transmission (50).

Several enkephalin pathways have been described. The highest concentration of enkephalin in the brain occurs in the globus pallidus (37–39), where only terminals have been observed even after colchicine treatment. A variety of knife cuts separating the caudate and the globus pallidus produced a decline in pallidal enkephalin, suggesting that the caudate might provide cells that have terminals in the globus pallidus (51). However, some workers have found few enkephalin-containing cells in the caudate (40), and even those who report that up to 15% of the caudate cells contain enkephalin observe only faint to moderate staining of these cells (20). More extensive lesion studies do establish that the caudate provides the enkephalin input into the globus pallidus (52). This input is diffuse and overlapping, since with multiple small caudate lesions we were unable to affect pallidal enkephalin. Enkephalin cells, which were the source of pallidal enkephalin, seem to be widespread throughout the caudate and converge upon the smaller globus pallidus, accounting for the lack of any dense clustering of enkephalin cells within the caudate despite the very dense network of enkephalin terminals in the globus pallidus. Despite the diffuse nature of the enkephalin source within the caudate, there is some topographical correspondence with the inferior caudate projecting into the inferior globus pallidus (52).

Because of its role in affective behavior, there has been concern about the disposition of enkephalin neurons within the limbic system. One of the longest and most prominent enkephalin pathways occurs in the limbic system with cell bodies in the central nucleus of the amygdala and terminals in the bed nucleus of the stria terminalis and possibly in other zones of the hypothalamus (53). The central nucleus of the amygdala contains one of the highest concentrations of enkephalin cells, and direct lesions of the stria terminalis cause a buildup of enkephalin immunofluoresence within the central amygdala and some depletion from the bed nucleus of the stria terminalis. Since the bed nucleus of the stria terminalis also contains enkephalin cells, it is conceivable that there might even be a reciprocal enkephalin pathway, but there is no direct evidence for this. Conventional anatomical studies have shown that the central amygdala projects via the stria terminalis to several areas of the hypothalamus as well as to the bed nucleus of the stria terminalis, and it is conceivable that the enkephalin pathway may also reach these hypothalamic regions.

The pathway for which functional roles have been well explored contains enkephalin cells in the supraoptic and paraventricular nuclei of the hypothalamus with terminals in the posterior pituitary (54–57). Earlier radioreceptor and radioimmunoassay studies had failed to detect enkephalin within the pituitary, since the concentrations are not extremely high and the posterior pituitary represents only a small portion of the total pituitary gland. A role for opiate-like substances had been suggested by our finding (58) that the posterior pituitary contains abundant opiate receptor binding, whereas none could be demonstrated in the anterior pituitary. This is in keeping with findings of relatively low beta-endorphin concentrations in the anterior pituitary (59). Enkephalins and opiates inhibit depolarization-induced release of vasopressin from the posterior pituitary, presumably via opiate receptors located on nerve terminals of the neurosecretory vasopressin neurons (60). The course of this enkephalin pathway is the same as that of the oxytocin- and vasopressin-containing neurons, but they are thought to represent distinct neuronal systems (54)—although there have been some suggestions that enkephalin may be co-stored with vasopressin or oxytocin (61). The influence of enkephalin on vasopressin release thus may represent another example of a presumed axo-axonic influence, although no such synaptic interaction has been directly demonstrated and influences on peptide release might be obtained by other synaptic mechanisms.

Despite the considerable mapping efforts already accomplished, much remains to be done in tracing enkephalin-containing pathways. In addition to the areas already cited, fairly strong enkephalin-like immunofluorescent cell bodies have been demonstrated by a typical study (62) in the perifornical area of the hypothalamus, the interpeduncular nucleus, the dorsal cochlear nucleus, the medial and spinal vestibular nuclei, the central gray and reticular formation, the nucleus of the solitary tract, and even Golgi type II cells in the cerebellum. A more recent study (63) has added other enkephalin-containing cell groups in the olfactory bulb and olfactory tubercle; the lateral preoptic nucleus; the suprachiasmatic nucleus; the periventricular nucleus of the hypothalamus; the lateral, cortical, basal, and medial nuclei of the amygdala; pyramidal areas of the hippocampus (especially CA1); the neocortex; the cingulate cortex; the posterior mammillary nucleus; the medial nucleus of the optic tract; the brachium of the inferior colliculus; the ventral tegmental nucleus; the lateral reticular nucleus, and layers II, III, and VII of the cervical spinal cord.

In considering enkephalin–neuronal interactions, conventional synaptic relationships with other neurons may not suffice to explain all neuronal interactions. It is now known that numerous neuropeptides can be colocalized in the same neurons with other transmitters such that their joint release might cause more complex effects than would take place if a neuron released only a single neurotransmitter. Enkephalin has been shown to be contained in the same neurons as somatostatin in the median eminence (64). It is contained in the same neurons as serotonin in the dorsal raphe nucleus (65–67), and in the sacral spinal cord it is stored together with avian pancreatic polypeptide, a 36-amino-acid peptide first identified in the pancreas but now known to be contained in numerous neuronal systems (68). The possible coexistence of enkephalin, oxytocin, and vasopressin has been mentioned above.

It should be borne in mind that most enkephalin neuronal localizations have been studied in the rat, and there is evidence for species variations. There are fairly substantial differences in opiate receptor localization in monkey and rat, which might be mirrored by differences in enkephalin neuronal localization.

2.2   Differential Localizations of [Met]-Enkephalin and [Leu]-Enkephalin

One of the mysteries of enkephalin is why there are two different enkephalins. Interestingly, the genetic codes for methionine and leucine differ by only a single base, suggesting that a simple base substitution accounts for the two enkephalins. For several years following their discovery, researchers asked whether individual neurons contained only one of the two enkephalins or a mixture. Very few antisera to the two enkephalins differentiated them sufficiently to permit such distinctions, since in immunohistochemical studies one utilizes antisera at low dilutions in which even an antisera with tenfold selectivity for one enkephalin would still recognize the other. Recently, in a study that Larsson conducted in association with our laboratory (69), such a distinction was accomplished. The [Met]-enkephalin and [Leu]-enkephalin antisera could be made almost absolutely selective by preabsorption with individual enkephalins. Additionally, [Met]-enkephalin in tissue sections could be destroyed by mono-oxidative treatment with acidic permanganate or cyanogen bromide. It was found that [Met]-enkephalin and [Leu]-enkephalin are stored in distinct neuronal populations in both the brain and intestine (69). Subsequent studies showed that some neurons contain both enkephalins (70). These findings relate to studies of enkephalin biosynthesis to be discussed below, which report an enkephalin precursor that contains six [Met]-enkephalins and one [Leu]-

enkephalin in the sequence and another precursor with only leu-enkephalin sequences.

Though some areas of the brain contain similar densities of [Met]- and [Leu]-enkephalin-containing neurons, others are enriched in one or the other (70). For instance, the hippocampus and thalamus possess more [Met]- than [Leu]-enkephalin neurons, while the central amygdala contains more [Leu]- than [Met]-enkephalin and the substantia gelatinosa of the spinal cord, the caudate, and the cerebral cortex have similar densities of the two types of neurons.

These anatomical distinctions may have functional correlates. Several different apparent subtypes of opiate receptors have been described. The strongest evidence exists for distinct mu and delta opiate receptors. Using ligands selective for the two receptor subtypes, we were able to map them differentially by light microscopic autoradiography (71). The distribution of mu receptors in general parallels that of [Met]-enkephalin neurons; delta receptors fit more with [Leu]-enkephalin localization (Table 1). Mu receptors tend to be more concentrated in areas associated with the integration of pain information, and the limbic system is relatively rich in delta receptors. We have suggested that mu and delta receptors might serve respectively as physiological receptor sites for synaptic actions of [Met]- and [Leu]-enkephalin neurons. It follows that the different pharmacological effects associated with mu and delta receptors might reflect differential physiological actions of the two types of enkephalin neurons.

3 SYNAPTIC ACTIONS OF ENKEPHALINS

Neurophysiologically, most investigators have found enkephalins to inhibit neuronal firing (72). In the hippocampus where enkephalins en-

TABLE 1 Localizations of Mu and Delta Opiate Receptors and Corresponding Localizations of [Met]- and [Leu]-Enkephalin Neurons[a]

Mu > Delta Met > Leu	Mu ∾ Delta Met ∾ Leu	Delta > Mu Leu > Met
Hippocampus	Cerebral cortex	Central amygdaloid nucleus
Paraventricular nucleus	Caudate/putamen	
Periaqueductal gray	Globus pallidus	
Thalamus	Spinal cord	

[a] Exceptions to these similarities are noted in the lateral septum, nucleus accumbens, and supraoptic nucleus. Localizations of mu and delta opiate receptors are from Goodman et al. (71); localizations of [Met]- and [Leu]-enkephalin neurons are from Stengaard-Pedersen and Larsson (70).

hance firing, there is evidence that this is due to inhibition of inhibitory neuronal firing so that the excitation is only indirect (73). A similar disinhibition phenomenon occurs at dendro-dendritic synapses in the olfactory bulb mitral cells (74, 75). Some workers disagree with this disinhibition mechanism and suggested instead that opiates by presynaptic mechanisms facilitate the release of excitatory transmitters (76, 77).

Biochemically, enkephalins inhibit the release of transmitters in several instances, such as substance P (48, 49), vasopressin (61, 79), dopamine (80), acetylcholine in the myenteric plexus (81), and somatostatin (82). One of the tasks of the neurophysiologists is to identify an ionic mechanism that could account for transmitter release inhibition. The difficulty in this task is that one does not know whether inhibition of transmitter release involves axo-axonic synapses or some other synaptic interaction. The ability to demonstrate inhibition of substance P release in isolated cultures of dorsal root ganglia suggests that in this instance enkephalin directly affects substance P terminals (82).

One action that fits with inhibition of transmitter release is the influence of enkephalin on calcium ion flux, which is necessary for transmitter release (82). Another possible mechanism relates to the finding that enkephalins and opiates act directly on intestinal myenteric plexus neurons to cause a naloxone-reversible decrease in firing rate (83–85). There is evidence that this may be due to a naloxone-reversible hyperpolarization of the membrane (83, 85), and it has been proposed that this hyperpolarization may prevent action potential propagation into nerve terminal varicosities (86). While this review deals predominantly with the central nervous system, the myenteric plexus affords a model with some relevance to the central nervous system (vide infra).

The inhibition of transmitter release can be regarded as a presynaptic effect. Opiates also have postsynaptic actions. There is direct evidence that in the locus ceruleus enkephalin terminals make axo-somatic or axo-dendritic synapses upon the norepinephrine cells in this nucleus (19). Opiates and enkephalins inhibit locus ceruleus neuronal firing in a stereospecific naloxone-reversible fashion (87). There are also direct postsynaptic inhibitory effects measured by intracellular recording of enkephalins and opiates on spinal neurons (88–90). Here careful studies have suggested a synaptic mechanism. Enkephalins have been reported to directly hyperpolarize these cells, possibly due to an agonist-induced increase in chloride or potassium ion permeability and thus may act as in the myenteric plexus (87). Another possible mechanism relates to the observation that opioid agonists reduce the response to several excitatory transmitters such as acetylcholine and glutamate. Since both of these transmitters act by enhancing sodium permeability, Zieglgansberger and Bayerl (89) have suggested that enkephalin somehow "paralyzes" the sodium conductance mechanism. Such a concept fits well with the dramatic effects of sodium on opiate receptor binding (5). Physiological concentrations of sodium decrease the affinity of agonists but not antagonists for opiate receptors, an effect highly selective for sodium and not manifested by other monovalent cations such as potassium, rubidium, or cesium.

4 ENKEPHALIN BIOSYNTHESIS

4.1 Enkephalin Precursor Fragments

Most biologically active peptides are synthesized from large precursors by at least two enzymatic steps. First, a trypsin-like enzyme cleaves the precursor at "signaling" pairs of basic amino acids. The immediate precursor of the biologically active peptide frequently consists of the active peptide with one basic amino acid attached to the carboxyl terminus. This is removed by a carboxypeptidase B type of enzyme.

In the enkephalin system, several precursor fragments have been isolated, indicating that the above pattern applies to enkephalin. The earliest such fragment isolated is termed alpha-neo-endorphin and consists of 15 amino acids with a group of three basic amino acids at the carboxyl terminus of a [Leu]-enkephalin sequence (12). Several groups have detected enkephalin with arginine or lysine attached to the carboxyl terminus (91–94).

Dynorphin is a 17-amino-acid peptide detected in fairly substantial concentrations in the pituitary and in very low concentrations in the brain (14, 95). It consists of the [Leu]-enkephalin sequence followed by 2 arginines at the carboxyl terminus and then another 10 amino acids. The fact that dynorphin has important opiate-like activity suggests that it might have a physiological role of its own. However, the immuno-histochemical demonstration of dynorphin in cell bodies in the hypothalamus but much less in terminals in the brain fits also with a precursor role, since peptide precursors are synthesized in cell bodies and then cleaved to the physiological peptide before reaching terminals (96).

One approach that we and others first utilized to identify biosynthetic precursors of enkephalins was to fractionate brain or adrenal extracts and then determine whether substances reacting with enkephalin antibodies or possessing opiate activity in radioreceptor assays were released (13, 39, 93, 97–104). High-molecular-weight precursors ranging from 10,000 to 100,000 daltons have been thus identified in the brain and adrenal. The greatest success in studies of enkephalin precursors has come from Udenfriend's laboratory. They made use of the adrenal gland in which enkephalin is stored in chromaffin granules together with catecholamines, providing a biochemically more homogeneous preparation than brain tissue. A direct precursor-product relationship to enkephalins was demonstrated in adrenal cells in cultures in which ^{35}S-methionine was first incorporated into a 22,000 dalton precursor that could be "chased" into the pentapeptide [Met]-enkephalin (105). These workers initially isolated several large enkephalin-containing peptides, which were sequenced (13). Recently these peptides have been shown to be fragments of the same 50,000 dalton protein, proenkephalin A. Molecular cloning and DNA sequencing have established the primary structure of proenkephalin A, which contains six copies of [Met]-enkephalin and one of [Leu]-enkephalin (106, 107) (Figure 2). All of the enkephalin sequences are preceded by two basic amino acid residues, but only five of the enkephalin sequences are immediately followed by two basic amino acids. The other two enkephalin-containing fragments contain additional amino acids between the C-terminus of enkephalin and the dibasic amino acid signal. Interestingly, these two fragments, [Met]-enkephalin-Arg^6-Phe^7 and [Met]-enkephalin-Arg^6-Gly^7-Leu^8, had been isolated from the adrenal medulla, suggesting that these peptides may be end-products and not enkephalin precursors (94, 108).

The proenkephalin A molecule probably generates most of the [Met]-enkephalin-containing molecules that have been studied, but not the [Leu]-enkephalin-containing peptides, dynorphin and alpha-neo-endorphin. The very recently discovered proenkephalin B or prodynorphin

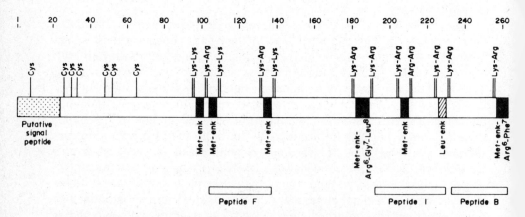

Figure 2. Schematic representation of the structure of bovine preproenkephalin. The sequences of [Met]-enkephalin, [Met]-enkephalin-Arg^6-Gly^7-Leu^8, and [Met]-enkephalin-Arg^6-Phe^7 are indicated by closed boxes, the sequence of Leu-enkephalin by a shaded box, and the putative signal peptide by a stippled box. All the paired basic amino acid residues and cysteine residues are shown. Amino acid numbers are given at top. The known peptide structures, peptide F (residues 104–137), peptide I (residues 192–230), and peptide B (residues 233–263) are displayed underneath by open bars. Not shown are the known peptides representing partial sequences of peptide I–peptide E (residues 206–230), BAM–22P (residues 206–227), BAM–20P (residues 206–225), and BAM–12P (residues 206–217). From Noda et al. (107).

contains only [Leu]-enkephalin sequences and the dynorphin sequene (108a).

4.2 "Enkephalin Convertase"

One of the puzzles of peptide biosynthesis research is whether there exist selective enzymes for processing the precursors or whether general trypsin-like and carboxypeptidase B-like enzymes generate all of the biologically active peptides. No one has yet identified a selective trypsin-like enzyme for processing a biopeptide, even in the case of the best-studied peptide hormone insulin.

Numerous carboxypeptidase enzymes have been described during the past 50 years. Carboxypeptidase B is a generic term referring to an enzyme that removes a basic amino acid from the carboxyl terminus of a peptide. Several carboxypeptidase B-like enzymes are well known. Recently we obtained evidence for a carboxypeptidase B type enzyme that may be selective for enkephalin biosynthesis; we refer to it as "enkephalin convertase" (Table 2).

One of the difficulties in characterizing peptide processing enzymes lies in assay techniques. To evaluate directly the conversion of enkephalin with a basic amino acid at the C-terminus usually requires separating the precursor and product with identification of the released enkephalin by a technique such as radioimmunoassays followed by high performance liquid chromatography. Two of us (L.F. and S.S.) developed a new assay that permits the simple and rapid detection of carboxypeptidase activity with high sensitivity (109). A fluorescent dansyl group is attached to the N-terminus of model substrates resembling enkephalin, such as dansyl-Phe-Leu-Arg. The basic arginine makes the water-soluble substrate insoluble in organic solvents. Enzymatic removal of the arginine forms the water-insoluble dansyl-Phe-Leu which partitions freely into chloroform, allowing rapid separation of product from substrate. In brain, pituitary, and adrenal we detected several different enzymes acting on these substrates. In the adrenal, only one of these carboxypeptidases was found to be localized to the chromaffin granules that contain the major adrenal enkephalin. An enzyme with identical properties also shows a brain regional localization that correlates fairly well with enkephalin levels.

"Enkephalin convertase" has been purified extensively from the adrenal gland and shown to be distinct from any known carboxypeptidase B type of enzyme. It is inhibited by thiol blocking reagents as well as by chelating agents and certain divalent cations (e.g., Ca^{2+} and Cd^{2+}). Unlike the lysosomal carboxypeptidase, "enkephalin convertase" is activated severalfold by cobalt (Co^{2+}). It displays higher affinity (in the micromolar range) for enkephalin hexapeptide precursor than for other peptides and thus could be an enzyme selectively associated with

TABLE 2 Comparison of Enkephalin Convertase with Other Carboxypeptidases

Enzyme	Predominant Localization	Molecular Weight	pH Optimum	Inhibitors	Activators
Carboxypeptidase B	Pancreas	34,000	7–8	Chelating agents	Co^{2+}
Carboxypeptidase N	Plasma	280,000	7–8	Chelating agents, Zn^{2+}	Co^{2+}
Lysosomal carboxypeptidase B (Cathepsin B_2)	Lysosomes	50,000	5–6	Thiol blocking reagents	Thiols Chelating Agents
Enkephalin convertase	Adrenal chromaffin granules; brain; pituitary	60,000	5–6	Chelating agents, Thiol blocking reagents, Zn^{2+}, Cd^{2+}	Co^{2+}

enkephalin biosynthesis. Evidence in favor of its selectivity comes from the very recent purification of enkephalin convertase to homogeneity (109a) and development of inhibitors with nanomolar affinity for enkephalin convertase but only micromolar potency at other carboxy-peptidases (109b).

The ability to identify an enzyme selective for enkephalin synthesis suggests that other such enzymes exist for other biologically active pep-tides and should be actively explored. Whether or not "enkephalin convertase" acts only on enkephalin precursors physiologically is unclear. Conceivably it is the sole enzyme that physiologically converts enkephalin precursors to enkephalin, but it may also have other func-tions. For instance, of the many amino acid decarboxylases known, only a single enzyme serves to decarboxylate dopa to dopamine. How-ever, in serotonin neurons, essentially the same enzyme molecule is concentrated and serves to convert 5-hydroxytryptophan to serotonin. Similarly, acetylcholinesterase is the only one of numerous biologically occurring esterases that inactivates acetylcholine. In the brain, howev-er, besides being localized to areas of cholinergic neurons, acetylcholin-esterase has other localizations indicating other functions not related to acetylcholine. Our observation that the anterior pituitary, which does not contain much enkephalin, is highly enriched in a carboxypeptidase with similar properties to "enkephalin convertase" suggests that in the anterior pituitary it may be associated with the biosynthesis of some other peptide (109).

5   ENKEPHALIN DEGRADATION

As with peptide biosynthesis, the question of selective enzymes associ-ated with the synaptic inactivation of neurotransmitter neuropeptides is a complex one. The extreme selectivity and high affinity of a recently described substance P–degrading enzyme suggests that, at least for sub-stance P, there exists a specific inactivating enzyme (110). Amino acid transmitters and biogenic amines are inactivated by uptake mecha-nisms, but such uptake systems have not been detected for any neuropeptides. Clearly, numerous enzymes can cleave and inactivate enkephalin (Table 3). After administration into the brain or incubation of brain slices or homogenates, enkephalin is largely acted on initially by aminopeptidase, which removes tyrosine. Aminopeptidase activity is distributed homogeneously throughout the brain, suggesting that it is not selectively involved in enkephalin degradation—although there may be several subtypes of aminopeptidase, one of which could be concentrat-ed in enkephalin-rich areas (111–113).

Enkephalin can be degraded by removal of Tyr-Gly dipeptide, an ac-tivity we earlier designated enkephalinase B (114). Recently we have

TABLE 3 Properties of Enkephalin-Degrading Enzymes

Enzyme	Source	Cleavage	Km or K_i (μM)	Reference
Enkephalinase A (A$_1$ and A$_2$)	Rat brain membrane	Tyr-Gly-Gly-Phe-↓Leu — Met	20–30	115; 117, 118
Enkephalinase B	Rat brain membrane	Tyr-Gly-Gly-Phe-↓Leu — Met		115
Aminopeptidases (M I/M II)	Rat brain membrane	↑Tyr-Gly-Gly-Phe-Met	M I 490 M II 18	114
		↑Tyr-Gly-Gly-Phe-↑Leu — Met	2600 23	
Aminopeptidase	Rat brain cytosol	↑Tyr-Gly-Gly-Phe-Leu	20–30	112
	Bovine brain cytosol			113
Peptidyl-dipeptidase B	Rabbit kidney	Tyr-Gly-Gly-Phe-↓Leu — Leu	80	119
Angiotensin-converting enzyme	Brain/kidney membrane	Tyr-Gly-Gly-↓Phe-Met		120
	Rat brain cytosol	Tyr-Gly-Gly-↓Phe-Met — Leu	100	121
			7	
Dipeptidyl aminopeptidase III	Rat brain cytosol	Tyr-Gly-Gly-Phe-Met	9	116

partially purified from brain tissue a dipeptidylaminopeptidase that appears to be the same as the DAP III enzyme earlier purified from pituitary extracts (115). This enzyme cleaves enkephalin similarly to enkephalinase B. The inhibitor specificity of DAP III in brain tissue is closely similar to that of enkephalinase B, so that the two enzymes may be identical. Of many peptides examined, enkephalin and angiotensin display the lowest K_i's among many neuropeptides tested (in the micromolar range) for DAP III. This suggests that this enzyme is a candidate to be the physiological enkephalinase, but the relatively homogeneous distribution of DAP III throughout the brain argues against this possibility.

One enzyme with a regional distribution that does parallel that of endogenous enkephalin and is a dipeptidylcarboxypeptidase has been designated enkephalinase A (114, 116, 117). This enzyme is distinct from two other enzymes that can cleave enkephalin at the same site, peptidyl-dipeptidase B (118) and angiotensin-converting enzyme (119, 120) (Table 3). Enkephalinase A is concentrated in brain membranes, from which it can be readily solubilized by detergents. We were able to physically separate two distinct subtypes, designated enkephalinase A_1 and A_2, and have purified enkephalinase A_1 to apparent homogeneity (114). The two enkephalinase A enzymes differ somewhat in their sensitivity to inhibitors. Like angiotensin-converting enzyme, enkephalinases are metal-requiring enzymes. Accordingly, it was possible to design an inhibitor , thiorphan, whose sulfhydryl group would attack the metal of enkephalinase A just as captopril does for angiotensin-converting enzyme (121). Thiorphan has nanomolar potency as an inhibitor of enkephalin in degradation. In theory, it should provide a powerful tool to determine whether this enzyme (because of its selectivity) is the physiological enkephalinase. If thiorphan itself were to have analgesic effects that were naloxone reversible, one might assert that enkephalinase A was involved in the physiological inactivation of enkephalin. However, owing to its poor penetration into the brain and the difficulty of interpreting studies in which drugs are injected directly into the brain, explorations of this question have provided only ambiguous results. Perhaps the question can be addressed by studies of whether thiorphan or related agents have opiate-like actions in *in vitro* physiological systems such as the guinea pig ileum contraction, ileal mucosal chloride transport, or neuroblastoma adenylate cyclase assays. Alternatively, one must wait for the development of enzyme inhibitors for this and other enzymes that penetrate more readily into the brain.

6 SUMMARY

A vast amount of information on the enkephalins has accumulated in the relatively brief period of six years since their isolation and structure elucidation. Besides elucidating opiate mechanisms, studies of enkephalins have shed considerable light on many basic aspects of neuropeptide physiology and biochemistry and on fundamental ways in which the brain processes information about pain perception, emotional regulation, and other functions. Enkephalin research has not yet resulted in the development of new therapeutic tools, but there is progress in the pharmaceutical industry in using enkephalin as a basis for agents as diverse as antidiarrheal drugs, analgesics, antidepressants, and anti-schizophrenic substances. Finally, the great interest evinced by the entire scientific community and general public in opiate receptor mechanisms and the enkephalins has provided an important stimulus toward research on neuropeptides as transmitters along with stimulating an even broader range of interest in the neurosciences.

REFERENCES

1. C. B. Pert and S. H. Snyder, *Science* **179**, 1011 (1973).
2. L. Terenius, *Acta Pharmacol. Toxicol.* **33**, 377 (1973).
3. E. J. Simon, J. M. Hiller, and I. Edelman, *Proc. Natl. Acad. Sci. USA* **70**, 1947 (1973).
4. M. J. Kuhar, C. B. Pert, and S. H. Snyder, *Nature* **245**, 447 (1973).
5. C. B. Pert and S. H. Snyder, *Mol. Pharmacol.* **10**, 868 (1974).
6. H. Akil, D. J. Mayer, and J. C. Liebeskind, *Science* **191**, 961 (1976).
7. J. Hughes, *Brain Res.* **88**, 295 (1975).
8. G. W. Pasternak, R. Goodman, and S. H. Snyder, *Life Sci.* **16**, 1765 (1975).
9. J. Hughes, T. W. Smith, H. W. Kosterlitz, L. H. Fothergill, B. A. Morgan, and H. Morris, *Nature* **255**, 577 (1975).
10. R. Simantov and S. H. Snyder, *Proc. Natl. Acad. Sci. USA* **73**, 2515 (1976).
11. H. J. Teschemacher, K. E. Opheim, B. M. Cox, and A. Goldstein, *Life Sci.* **16**, 1771 (1975).
12. K. Kanagawa, H. Matsuo, and M. Igarashi, *Biochem. Biophys. Res. Comm.* **86**, 153 (1979).
13. A. S. Stern, B. N. Jones, J. E. Shively, S. Stein, and S. Udenfriend, *Proc. Natl. Acad. Sci. USA* **78**, 1962 (1981).
14. A. Goldstein, S. Tachibana, L. I. Lowney, M. Hunkapillar, and L. Hood, *Proc. Natl. Acad. Sci. USA* **73**, 2156 (1979).
15. R. Simantov, M. J. Kuhar, G. R. Uhl, and S. H. Snyder, *Proc. Natl. Acad. Sci. USA* **74**, 2167 (1977).
16. R. Simantov, A. M. Snowman, and S. H. Snyder, *Brain Res.* **107**, 650 (1976).
17. S. P. Wilson, R. L. Klein, K.-J. Chang, M. S. Gasparis, O. H. Viveros, and W.-H. Yang, *Nature* **288**, 707 (1980).
18. G. Pelletier and R. LeClerc, *Neurosci. Lett.* **12**, 159 (1979).
19. V. M. Pickel, T. H. Joh, D. J. Reis, S. E. Leeman, and R. J. Miller, *Brain Res.* **160**, 387 (1979).
20. V. M. Pickel, K. K. Sumal, S. C. Bechley, R. J. Miller, and D. J. Reis, *J. Comp. Neurol.* **189**, 721 (1980).
21. T. W. Smith, J. Hughes, H. W. Kosterlitz, and R. P. Sosa, in H. W. Kosterlitz, Ed. *Opiates and Endogenous Opioid Peptides*, Elsevier/North-Holland, New York, 1976, pp. 57.
22. I. Lindberg and J. C. Dahl, *Neurochem.* **36**, 506 (1981).
23. A. Bayon, J. Rossier, A. Mauss, F. E. Bloom, L. L. Iversen, W. Ling, and K. Guillemin, *Proc. Natl. Acad. Sci. USA* **75**, 3503 (1978).

24. G. Henderson, J. Hughes, and H. W. Kosterlitz, *Nature* **271**, 677 (1978).
25. L. L. Iversen, S. D. Iversen, F. E. Bloom, T. Vargo, and R. Guillemin, *Nature* **271**, 679 (1978).
26. L. L. Iversen, C. M. Lee, R. F. Gilbert, S. Hunt, and P. C. Emson, *Proc. R. Soc. Ser. B.*, **210**, 91 (1980).
27. H. Osborne, V. Hollt, and A. Herz, *Eur. J. Pharm.* bf 48, 219 (1978).
28. C. B. Pert and S. H. Snyder, *Proc. Natl. Acad. Sci. USA* **73**, 3729 (1979).
29. C. B. Pert, M. J. Kuhar, and S. H. Snyder, *Life Sci.* **16**, 1849 (1975).
30. S. F. Atweh and M. J. Kuhar, *Brain Res.* **124**, 53 (1977).
31. S. F. Atweh and M. J. Kuhar, *Brain Res.* **129**, 1 (1977).
32. S. F. Atweh and M. J. Kuhar, *Brain Res.* **134**, 393 (1977).
33. R. Elde, T. Hokfelt, O. Johansson, and L. Terenius, *Neurosci. Lett.* **1**, 349 (1976).
34. F. E. Bloom, E. Battenberg, J. Rossier, N. Ling, and R. Guillemin, *Proc. Natl. Acad. Sci. USA* **75**, 1591 (1978).
35. S. J. Watson, H. Akil, C. W. Richards, and J. D. Barchas, *Nature* **275**, 226 (1978).
36. S. J. Watson and J. D. Barchas, in R. F. Beers and E. G. Bassett, Eds, *Mechanisms of Pain and Analgesic Compounds*, Raven Press, New York, 1979, p. 227.
37. J. Rossier, T. M. Vargo, S. Minick, N. Ling, F. E. Bloom, and R. Guillemin, *Proc. Natl. Acad. Sci. USA* **74**, 5162 (1977).
38. H.-Y. Yang, J. S. Hong, and E. Costa, *Neuropharmacol.* **16**, 303 (1977).
39. J. Hughes, H. W. Kosterlitz, and T. W. Smith, *Brit. J. Pharmacol.* **63**, 397 (1977).
40. T. Hokfelt, R. Elde, O. Johansson, L. Terenius, and L. Stein, *Neurosci. Lett.* **5**, 25 (1977).
41. T. Hokfelt, A. Ljungdahl, L. Terenius, R. P. Elde, and G. Nilsson, *Proc. Natl. Acad. Sci. USA* **74**, 3081 (1977).
42. T. Takahashi and M. Otsuka, *Brain Res.* **87**, 1 (1975).
43. K. Sumal, V. M. Pickel, R. J. Miller, and D. J. Reis, *Soc. Neurosci.* **6**, 353 (1980).
44. S. P. Hunt, J. S. Kelly, and P. C. Emson, *Neuroscience* **6**, 1871 (1980).
45. E. J. Glazer and A. Basbaum, *Soc. Neurosci.* **6**, 523 (1980).
46. K. K. Sumal, V. M. Pickel, R. J. Miller, and D. J. Reis, *J. Comp. Neurol.*, in press.
47. C. LaMotte, C. B. Pert, and S. H. Snyder, *Brain Res.* **112**, 407 (1976).
48. T. M. Jessell and L. L. Iversen, *Nature* **268**, 549 (1977).
49. H. L. Fields, P. C. Emson, D. K. Leigh, R. Gilbert, and L. L. Iversen, *Nature* **284**, 351 (1980).
50. T. Hokfelt, L. Terenius, H. G. J. M. Kuypers, and O. Dahn, *Neurosci. Lett.* **14**, 55 (1979).
51. A. C. Cuello and G. Paxinos, *Nature* **277**, 178 (1978).
52. F. M. A. Correa, R. B. Innis, L. D. Hester, and S. H. Snyder, *Neurosci. Lett.* **25**, 63 (1981).
53. G. Uhl, M. J. Kuhar, and S. H. Snyder, *Brain Res.* **149**, 223 (1978).
54. P. Micevych and R. Elde, *J. Comp. Neurol.* **190**, 135 (1980).
55. T. A. Reaves and J. N. Hayward, *Proc. Natl. Acad. Sci. USA* **76**, 6009 (1979).
56. T. A. Reaves and J. N. Hayward, *J. Comp. Neurol.* **193**, 777 (1980).
57. J. Rossier, E. Battenberg, Q. Pittman, A. Bayon, L. Koda, R. J. Miller, R. Guillemin, and F. E. Bloom, *Nature* **277**, 653 (1979).
58. R. Simantov and S. H. Snyder, *Brain Res.* **124**, 178 (1977).
59. A. S. Liotta, T. Suda, and D. T. Krieger, *Proc. Natl. Acad. Sci. USA* **75**, 2950 (1978).
60. L. L. Iversen, S. D. Iversen, and F. E. Bloom, *Nature* **284**, 350 (1980).
61. R. Martin and K. H. Voigt, *Nature* **289**, 502 (1981).
62. M. Sar, W. E. Stumpf, R. J. Miller, K.-J. Chang, and P. Cuatrecasas, *J. Comp. Neurol.* **182**, 17 (1978).
63. J. C. W. Finley, J. L. Maderdrut, and P. Petrusz, *J. Comp. Neurol.*, in press (1981).
64. G. Tramu and J. Leonardelli, *Brain Res.* **168**, 457 (1979).
65. A. I. Basbaum, E. J., Glazer, H. Steinbusch, and A. Verhofstad, *Soc. Neurosci.* **6**, 540 (1980).

66.   M. S. Moss, E. J. Glazer, and A. I. Basbaum, *Anat. Rec.* **196**, 131 (1980).
67.   M. S. Moss, E. J. Glazer, and A. I. Basbaum, *Neurosci. Lett.* **2**, 33 (1981).
68.   S. P. Hunt, P. C. Emson, P. Gilbert, M. Goldstein, and J. R. Kimmell, *Neurosci. Lett.* **21**, 125 (1981).
69.   L.-I. Larsson, S. R. Childers, and S. H. Snyder, *Nature* **282**, 407 (1979).
70.   K. Stengaard-Pedersen and L.-I. Larsson, *J. Neurosci.*, in press (1982).
71.   R. R. Goodman, S. H. Snyder, M. J. Kuhar, and W. S. Young III, *Proc. Natl. Acad. Sci. USA* **77**, 6239 (1980).
72.   F. E. Bloom and J. F. McGinty, in J. Martinez and J. McGaugh, Eds., *Endogenous Peptides in Learning and Memory*, in press (1981).
73.   W. Zieglgansberger, E. D. French, G. R. Siggins, and F. E. Bloom, *Science* **205**, 415 (1979).
74.   R. A. Nicoll, B. E. Alger, and C. E. Jahr, *Nature* **287**, 22 (1980).
75.   R. A. Nicoll, B. E. Alger, and C. E. Jahr, *Proc. R. Soc., Ser. B.* **210**, 132 (1980).
76.   H. L. Haas and R. W. Ryall, *J. Physiol.* **301**, 37 (1979).
77.   H. L. Haas and R. W. Ryall, *J. Physiol.* **308**, 315 (1980).
78.   G. P. Clark, P. Wood, L. Merrick, and D. W. Lincoln, *Nature* **282**, 746 (1979).
79.   G. A. Gudelsky and J. C. Porter, *Life Sci.* **25**, 1697 (1979).
80.   R. A. North and M. Tonini, *Brit. J. Pharm.*
81.   M. C. Sheppard, S. Kronheim, and B. C. Pimstone, *J. Neurochem.* **32**, 647 (1979).
82.   A. W. Mudge, S. E. Leeman, and G. D. Fischbach, *Proc. Natl. Acad. Sci. USA* **76**, 527 (1979).
83.   R. Dingledine and A. Goldstein, *J. Pharm. Exp. Ther.* **196**, 97 (1976).
84.   R. A. North and J. T. Williams, *Eur. J. Pharm.* **45**, 22 (1979).
85.   J. T. Williams, Y. Katayama, and R. A. North, *Brain Res.* **165**, 57 (1979).
86.   R. A. North, Y. Katayama, and J. T. Williams, *Brain Res.* **165**, 67 (1979).
87.   C. M. Pepper and G. Henderson, *Science* **209**, 394 (1980).
88.   W. Zieglgansberger and E. A. Puil, *Exp. Brain Res.* **17**, 35 (1972).
89.   W. Zieglgansberger and H. Bayerl, *Brain Res.* **115**, 111 (1976).
90.   W. Zieglgansberger and J. P. Fry, in H. W. Kosterlitz, Eds., *Opiates and Endogenous Opiate Peptides*, Elsevier/North Amsterdam, Holland, 1976, pp. 213.
91.   J. Rossier, Y. Audigier, N. Ling, J. Cros, and S. Udenfriend, *Nature* **288**, 88 (1980).
92.   W.-Y. Huang, R. C. Chang, A. J. Kastin, D. H. Coy, and A. V. Schally, *Proc. Natl. Acad. Sci. USA* **76**, 6177 (1979).
93.   R. V. Lewis, A. S. Stern S. Kimura, J. Rossier, S. Stein, and S. Udenfriend, *Science* **208**, 1459 (1980).
94.   A. S. Stern, R. V. Lewis, S. Kimura, J. Rossier, L. D. Gerber, L. Brink, S. Stern, and S. Udenfriend, *Proc. Natl. Acad. Sci.*
95.   A. Goldstein and V. E. Ghazarossian, *Proc. Natl. Acad. Sci. USA* **77**, 6207 (1980).
96.   V. Hollt, I. Haarmann, K. Bovermann, M. Jerlicz, and A. Herz, *Neurosci. Lett.* **18**, 149 (1980).
97.   S. J. Watson, H. Akil, V. E. Ghazarossian, and A. Goldstein, *Proc. Natl. Acad. Sci. USA* **78**, 1260 (1981).
98.   S. R. Childers and S. H. Snyder, in E. Wei, Ed., *Endogenous and Exogenous Opiate Agonists and Antagonists*, Pergamon Press, New York, 1980, p. 217.
99.   R. V. Lewis, S. Stein, L. D. Gerber, M. Rubinstein, and S. Udenfriend, *Proc. Natl. Acad. Sci. USA* **75**, 4021 (1978).
100. A. Beaumont, J. A. Fuentes, J. Hughes, and K. M. Meters, *FEBS Lett.* **22**, 135 (1980).
101. J. Hughes, A. Beaumont, J. A. Fuentes, B. Malfroy, and C. Unsworth, *J. Exp. Biol.* **89**, 239 (1980).
102. R. V. Lewis, A. S. Stern, J. Rossier, S. Stein, and S. Udenfriend, *Biochem. Biophys. Res. Comm.* **89**, 822 (1979).
103. R. V. Lewis, A. S. Stern, S. Kimura, S. Stein, and S. Udenfriend, *Proc. Natl. Acad. Sci. USA* **77**, 5018 (1980).

104. S. Kimura, R. V. Lewis, A. S. Stern, J. Rossier, S. Stein, and S. Udenfriend, *Proc. Natl. Acad. Sci. USA* **77**, 1681 (1980).

105. S. Stein and S. Udenfriend, *Proc. Natl. Acad. Sci. USA* **77**, 6889 (1980).

106. U. Gubler, P. Seeburg, B. J. Hoffman, L. P. Gage, and S. Udenfriend, *Nature* **295**, 206 (1982).

107. M. Noda, Y. Furutani, H. Takahashi, M. Toyosato, T. Hirose, S. Inayoma, S. Nakanishi, and S. Numa, *Nature* **295**, 202 (1982).

108. D. L. Kilpatrick, B. N. Jones, K. Kojima, and S. Udenfriend, *Biochem. Biophys. Res. Comm.*, in press (1982).

108a. H. Kakidani, Y. Furutani, H. Takahashi, M. Noda, Y. Morimoto, T. Hirose, M. Asai, S. Inayama, S. Nakanishi, and S. Numa, *Nature* **298**, 245 (1982).

109. L. Fricker and S. H. Snyder, *Proc. Natl. Acad. Sci. USA*, **79**, 3886 (1982).

109a. L. D. Fricker and S. H. Snyder, *J. Biol. Chem.*, in press (1983).

109b. L. D. Fricker, T. H. Plummer Jr. and S. H. Snyder, *Biochem. Biophys. Res. Comm.* **111**, 994 (1983).

110. C.-M. Lee, B. E. B. Sandberg, M. R. Hanley, and L. L. Iversen, *Eur. J. Biochem.* **114**, 315 (1981).

111. H. P. Schnebli, M. A. Phillipps, and R. K. Barclay, *Biochim. Biophys. Acta* **569**, 89 (1979).

112. L. B. Hersh and J. F. McKelvy, *J. Neurochem.* **36**, 171 (1981).

113. L. B. Hersh, *Biochemistry* **20**, 2345 (1981).

114. C. Gorenstein and S. H. Snyder, *Proc. R. Soc., Ser. B.* **210**, 123 (1980).

115. C.-M. Lee and S. H. Snyder, *J. Biol. Chem*, **257**, 12043 (1982).

116. B. Malfroy, J. P. Swerts, A. Guyon, B. P. Roques, and J. C. Schwartz, *Nature* **276**, 523 (1978).

117. J. C. Schwartz, S. de la Baume, B. Malfroy, G. Patey, R. Perdrisot, J. P. Swerts, M. C. Fournie-Zaluski, G. Gacel, and B. P. Roques, in E. Costa and M. Trabucchi, Eds., *Neural Peptides and Neuronal Communication*, Raven Press, New York, 1980, p. 219.

118. M. Benuck, M. J. Berg, and N. Marks, *Life Sci.* **28**, 2643 (1981).

119. E. G. Erdos, A. R. Johnson, and N. T. Boyden, *Biochem. Pharmacol.* **27**, 843 (1978).

120. M. Benuck and N. Marks, *Biochem. Biophys. Res. Comm.* **88**, 215 (1979).

121. C. Llorens, G. Gacel, J. P. Swerts, R. Perdrisot, M. C. Fournie-Zaluski, J. C. Schwartz, and B. P. Roques, *Biochem. Biophys. Res. Comm.* **96**, 1710 (1980).

34

Cholecystokinin

G. J. DOCKRAY
Physiological Laboratory
University of Liverpool
Liverpool, England

It is more than 50 years since the role of cholecystokinin (CCK) in the control of digestion was first recognized, but only recently has it become clear that CCK is also likely to have important functions as a neuroregulator in brain. In 1928 Ivy and Oldberg obtained unequivocal evidence for regulation of gallbladder contraction by a hormonal mechanism activated by intestinal luminal stimuli. They called the hormonal factor cholecystokinin. Later and independently Harper and Raper showed that pancreatic enzyme secretion was also controlled by a gut hormone, to which they gave the name pancreozymin. The realization that a single hormonal entity was responsible for both functions came about when Jorpes and Mutt isolated from hog intestine a molecule of 33 residues (CCK33) that had the properties of both hormones (1). Since the late 1960s it has been apparent that the C-terminal octapeptide (CCK8), produced by prolonged tryptic digestion of CCK33, possesses full biological activity. Moreover, the C-terminal pentapeptide is also shared with the antral hormone gastrin. Thus when Vanderhaeghen et al. (2) first described gastrin-like immunoreactivity in brain it was natural to ask whether the material might not also resemble CCK. It soon became clear that the active factor in brain extracts had the properties of CCK8 (3). Recent progress in the elucidation of the neuronal function of CCK is reviewed in this chapter.

1   CHEMISTRY

1.1   Identification

The results of many studies using a variety of analytical methods point to the fact that material with the chromatographic, biological, and immunochemical properties of CCK8 occurs in high concentrations in many areas of the central and peripheral nervous systems of mammals (3–6). The widespread availability of antisera that react with CCK and so may be used in radioimmunoassay (RIA) and immunohistochemistry accounts for much of the rapid progress that has been made in understanding the distribution, release and possible functions of neuronal CCK.

   True gastrin may be found in a limited number of extragastrointestinal sites. In pig pituitary there is evidence from RIA and gel filtration to indicate that the two main forms of gastrin, the peptides of 17- and 34-amino-acid residues (G17 and G34), occur in low concentrations (7). The gastrins are apparently localized to cells of the anterior and intermediate lobes that contain adrenocorticotrophic hormone (ACTH) and alpha melanocyte stimulating hormone (α-MSH), as well as to fibers of the posterior lobe (7). In contrast, in the rat pituitary CCK8 occurs but not gastrin (8). The factors governing the relative distribution of these two substances in the pituitary of different species are unknown. Material with the immunochemical and gel filtration properties of G17 has also been identified in the vagal nerve of dog and cat (9); our experience suggests that in vagus of about 25% of dogs and cats there are low concentrations of G17-like immunoreactivity (1–2 pmol/g) and in the remainder G17 is unmeasurable (<0.3 pmol/g). However, in nearly all animals studied we found CCK8-like immunoreactivity in vagal nerve extracts in concentrations up to about 5 pmol/g (10).

1.2 Extraction

Studies of CCK are complicated by the occurrence of multiple molecular forms that have different tissue distributions and for which there are different optimal extraction conditions. The larger and more basic forms of 33 and 39 residues (CCK39) isolated by Mutt from hog intestine are poorly soluble at neutral or alkaline pH but readily extracted in acid. In contrast, the smaller acidic forms like CCK8 are poorly extracted in acid but are well recovered in neutral or, better still, alkaline conditions (11, 12). Optimal extraction of the main forms is readily achieved by boiling tissues (to inactivate proteases) at neutral or alkaline pH to recover CCK8 and then re-extracting the residue in acid, for example, 0.5 *M* acetic acid, to recover CCK33. The molecular forms can be separated by gel filtration, ion exchange, HPLC, or starch gel electrophoresis, although it must be emphasized that the relative recoveries of different molecular forms frequently vary in different chromatographic systems.

1.3 Estimation

Cholecystokinin and related peptides can be measured by RIA or by bioassay. Radioimmunoassays are frequently sensitive enough to detect femtomole quantities. Many workers make use of C-terminal-specific antisera, which have the advantage of reacting with the biologically active part of the molecule and with all the chemically characterized forms. Many C-terminally directed antisera also show affinity for gastrin, and where samples contain both gastrin and CCK some form of chromatographic separation of the two substances is needed. Antisera with mid- or N-terminal specificity for CCK33 do not react with gastrin, but these antisera suffer from the disadvantage that they may react with biologically inactive fragments; they may also show varying degrees of species specificity (13).

Cholecystokinin is readily estimated by bioassay on guinea pig gallbladder *in vivo*, rabbit gallbladder *in vitro*, or enzyme secretion from rat or guinea pig pancreas *in vitro* (6, 14). It is often possible to detect less than 1 pmol of CCK8 using bioassay systems. There is good agreement between the data from bioassay and RIA for estimation of CCK in brain, but a recent study suggests that CCK8-like factors in rat intestine might not be biologically active (14).

1.4   Chemically Characterized Cholecystokinins

CCK has been isolated from hog duodenum as CCK33 and as an N-terminally extended variant of 39 residues (CCK39) (1). The C-terminal octapeptide of these molecules has been isolated from sheep brain (Figure 1) (15). In addition to a molecule with the chemical, biological, and immunochemical properties of CCK8, we have also isolated from sheep brain a closely related octapeptide variant that appeared slightly less acidic but was otherwise indistinguishable from CCK8 in its chemical and biological properties. The possibility cannot yet be discounted that this material is an artifact generated by internal rearrangements within CCK8, perhaps an alpha-beta shift on the N-terminal aspartic acid residue. During the isolation of CCK8 from sheep brain, purification was monitored by RIA using an antiserum that reacted equally with sulfated and unsulfated forms. The final products had the properties of sulfated CCK peptides, and no evidence was found to suggest that significant quantities of desulfated CCK8 occurred in sheep brain (15). Subsequent studies on rat brain CCK have pointed to a similar conclusion (16).

1.5   Other CCKs in Brain

In addition to CCK8 several other immunoreactive forms of CCK have been found in brain. One of these occurs in apparently low concentrations and elutes in or just after the void volume on Sephadex G-50 and G-25, and could be a large precursor (3). Other minor variants that have been described show the properties of CCK33, and of its C-terminal dodecapeptide, that is, CCK12 (5). Muller et al. (4) originally reported that CCK33-like material identified by a midregion CCK33 antiserum occurred in concentrations comparable with those of CCK8, whereas other workers using C-terminal antisera found only small amounts of CCK33 (3, 5, 6). It now seems that there are relatively high concentrations of

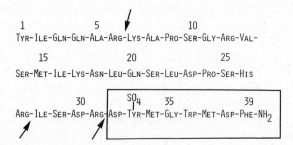

Figure 1.   Amino acid sequence of porcine CCK39. The arrows indicate cleavage points that would liberate the C-terminal 33-residue fragment (CCK33), the C-terminal 12-residue fragment (CCK12), and the C-terminal octapeptide (CCK8). The CCK8 fragment has been isolated from brain (indicated by box).

material in pig brain that react with mid-N-terminal antisera but not C-terminal antisera, and which could correspond to either a C-terminally extended variant or an N-terminal fragment of CCK33 (17). Initial radio-immunoassay studies of the brains of rat, dog, and pig revealed a minor component that eluted after CCK8 on gel filtration and which, it was thought, could correspond to a smaller fragment (3). Rehfeld et al. later reported that material corresponding to the C-terminal tetrapeptide (designated G4, or CCK4) occurred in brain, as well as in gut and pancreas, in concentrations that exceeded those of the other forms of gastrin and CCK (18, 19). These studies were based on RIA using C-terminal antisera with relatively low affinity for G4 compared with CCK8. In further studies we have made use of two antisera with different specifities: one shows equal affinity for G4 and longer fragments of gastrin and CCK, and the other is specific for the N-terminus of G4 and does not react with other forms of CCK and gastrin. The results obtained with the former antiserum confirm CCK8 as the main immuno-reactive form (Figure 2); neither antiserum reveals significant quantities of G4 (20). In the absence of more detailed chemical information, the identity of smaller fragments of CCK-like peptides in brain must remain uncertain.

1.6 Biosynthesis

It is generally thought that CCK8 is generated in its cell of origin by controlled proteolytic cleavage of a large precursor, and that CCK33 or CCK39 might be intermediates in this process (Figure 1). Many active peptides are liberated from their precursors by the action of trypsin- and carboxypeptidase B-like enzymes cleaving at a site of two basic amino acids. However, the cleavage that releases CCK8 from CCK33 is between Arg and Asp, and this bond is relatively resistant to trypsin. Recently Mutt (21) reported that enterokinase readily digests CCK33 to CCK8 and also yields some CCK12. Perhaps, then, an enterokinase-like enzyme has a physiological role in CCK8 biosynthesis. Gel filtration and ultracentrifugation of bovine brain extracts have been shown to separate two fractions, one capable of cleaving Arg-Ile and the other both Arg-Ile and Arg-Asp. These fractions are able to produce both CCK8 and CCK12 from CCK33, but the identity and physiological signif-icance of the enzymes involved are otherwise unknown (22).

Following intracisternal administration of ^{35}S methionine into rats, Goltermann et al. (23) observed incorporation into CCK8 within 15 min. Kinetic evidence was obtained to suggest a product–precursor relation-ship between larger immunoreactive forms and CCK8. The rate of syn-thesis of CCK8 described by Goltermann et al. exceeds that of other neuropeptides for which comparable data is available. Further studies from this group have suggested that radiolabeled CCK8 appears in the

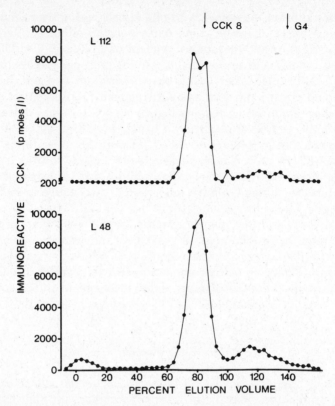

Figure 2. Separation on Sephadex G-25 (1 × 100 cm eluted with 0.25 M ammonium bicarbonate) of a boiling water extract of rat brain. Upper panel shows results obtained with radioimmunoassay (RIA) using an antiserum that reacts well with both CCK8 and G4. Lower panel shows results of RIA with an antiserum that reacts weakly (0.02) with G4 compared with CCK8. Note that both antisera show a major peak coeluting with synthetic sulfated CCK8; minor peaks are shown by both antisera eluting after CCK8, but there is no major peak corresponding to G4. Reproduced from Dockray et al. (20) with permission.

synaptosomal fraction of brain homogenates within 1 h; since synaptosomes generally do not have the capacity for protein synthesis, it would seem that CCK8 is rapidly synthesized in cell bodies and transported to terminal areas.

2   DISTRIBUTION

2.1   Quantitative Studies

There is general agreement from RIA studies that high concentrations of CCK8-like immunoreactivity occur in cerebral cortex (24–26). In the rat, concentrations are 300–500 pmol/g; slightly higher concentrations may occur in hog (24). Other regions in which high concentrations are found include the amygdala and striatum (Figure 3). Concentrations in brain stem and spinal cord are about 20% of those in cortex, and concentrations in cerebellum are about 1% those in cortex. Little work has been done to elucidate the factors determining the quantitative distribution of CCK in brain, but Lamers et al. (27) have reported that tryptophan lowers concentrations of CCK33-like activity in thalamus and hypothalamus, and that morphine lowers concentrations in hypothalamus; no changes were found in cortex. These authors contend that measurement of CCK33-like activity in brain extracts gives a more precise indication of the rate of turnover, and they conclude that serotonergic and opioid systems modulate CCK production. Relatively little is known of the possible changes in brain CCK in disease of the central nervous system. However, preliminary findings suggest that in Alzheimer's disease concentrations of CCK8 in the cerebral cortex are normal (28); whereas in Huntington's disease, Emson et al. (29) have found diminished CCK8-like immunoreactivity in pallidum and substantia nigra but normal concentrations in caudate, putamen, and cortex.

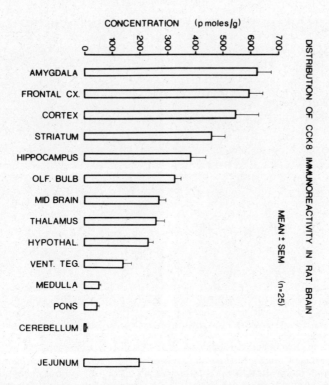

Figure 3. Concentrations of CCK8-like immunoreactivity in various regions of rat brain. The brains were extracted in boiling water and CCK-like immunoreactivity estimated with antiserum L48 (see Figure 2). Reproduced from G. J. Dockray et al., in G. Fink and L. Whalley, Eds., *Neuropeptides: Basic and Clinical Aspects*, Churchill Livingston, 1981.

2.2   Immunohistochemical Studies

C-terminal-specific antisera have been used to map the distribution of
CCK-like peptides in rat and guinea pig brain (25, 30–32). Antisera specific for other regions of CCK give weak or negative staining for reasons that are still uncertain (25). Although localization of CCK8-like
immunoreactivity is said to be "specific" in that it is abolished by
preincubation of antisera with C-terminal fragments of CCK or gastrin,
considerable caution must still be exercised in the interpretation of
these data. The importance of this point is amply demonstrated by recent studies on CCK-like peptides in spinal cord (33). In control rats
CCK8-like immunoreactivity can be localized to fibers of the dorsal
horn; by radioimmunoassay, concentrations (about 100 pmol/g) are two
to three times higher in the dorsal spinal cord than in the ventral cord.
Administration of capsaicin, the active ingredient of red peppers, produces a marked depletion of CCK8-like immunoreactivity visualized by
immunohistochemistry but has no effect on CCK8-like activity identified
and estimated by RIA (Figure 4). In the same rats, substance P detected

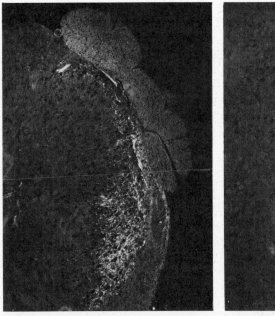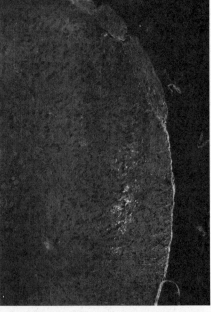

Figure 4.   Immunohistochemical localization of CCK-like immunoreactivity in spinal cord
of a normal rat (left) and a rat treated neonatally with capsaicin (right). Immunofluorescent nerve endings are demonstrated in the dorsal horn of the control animal but are depleted after capsaicin. Extracts of dorsal spinal cord of control and capsaicin rats
contained similar amounts of immunoreactive CCK8 measured by RIA (100 $\pm$ 9 pmol/g,
means $\pm$ S.E., $n = 10$, and 101 $\pm$ 6 pmol/g, $n = 8$, respectively).

by both RIA and immunohistochemistry is depleted. Evidently extractable CCK8 is not visualized by immunohistochemistry; the nature of the material demonstrated by immunohistochemistry remains to be established. Conceivably this material might correspond to a peptide with low affinity for the antiserum in RIA.

Using conventional immunofluorescence and immunoperoxidase methods, extensive systems of nerve fibers, endings, and cell bodies with CCK-like immunoreactivity can be found in many regions of rat brain. Cell bodies occur throughout the cerebral cortex and are particularly numerous in the pyriform cortex (30–32). These cells occur in layers II to VI and are virtually absent from layer I. They tend to be spindle shaped or bipolar and to be oriented radially with respect to the cortical surface. Abundant CCK fibers occur in the amygdala, and reports of cell bodies in this region vary from dense (in the central amygdaloid nucleus) (32) to absent (31). Cell bodies and fibers are also numerous in the hippocampus and in the basal ganglia, particularly caudate.

CCK-like peptides have been localized to numerous cell bodies in the hypothalamus; it is of particular interest that certain magnocellular neurons appear to contain both oxytocin and CCK-like immunoreactivity (32). Moreover, Beinfeld et al. (8) have shown depletion of CCK8 in neural lobe of rats stimulated release both oxytocin and vasopressin by lactation and salt treatment, respectively. Extensive systems of nerve fibers and cell bodies containing CCK-like immunoreactivity occur in several other hypothalamic regions, including periventricular, paraventricular, and dorsomedial nuclei.

In two important midbrain regions immunoreactive CCK has been co-localized with other neuroactive substances. First, in the ventral tegmental region Hökfelt et al. (34) have shown by means of restaining and retrograde tracing experiments that a population of mesolimbic dopaminergic neurons (identified by antibodies to their marker enzyme tyrosine hydroxylase) also contain CCK-like immunoreactivity. Lesions of the medial forebrain bundle, by which the mesolimbic dopaminergic neurons project to the forebrain, caused a highly significant 14-fold increase in concentrations of CCK8-like material in the ventral tegmentum measured by RIA of micropunch samples (35). After administration of 6-hydroxydopamine, or lesions of the medial forebrain bundle, there was depletion of CCK8-like immunoreactivity identified by radioimmunoassay or by immunohistochemistry in limbic terminal areas, namely tuberculum olfactorium, bed nucleus of the stria terminalis, and nucleus accumbens (34, 35). Second, in the periaqueductal gray region, which is known to contain a particularly rich population of CCK-reactive nerve cell bodies (31, 32), there has recently been discovered coexistence of substance P-like and CCK-like peptides (36). The nerve cell bodies that exhibit coexistence appear to be particularly common in the ventral rostral region. It is noteworthy that in addition to cells demonstrating coexistence of CCK and dopamine, and of CCK and substance P immunoreactivity, there are in the regions mentioned other neurons that apparently contain CCK8-, dopamine-, or substance P-like immunoreactivity alone.

CCK8-immunoreactive nerve cell bodies have been identified in the dorsal raphe nucleus in the hindbrain and in both fibers and cell bodies in the parabrachial nucleus (31, 32). A dense population of fibers occurs in dorsal horn of the spinal cord and there is also evidence of cell bodies in the lateral horn, but as already mentioned there are difficulties with the localization of CCK-like peptides in spinal cord.

In the retina of various species, including amphibia, there is CCK-like immunoreactivity in nerve fibers of the inner plexiform layer and in a subpopulation of amacrine cells (37). In the peripheral nervous system, CCK-8-like material occurs in fibers of the prevertebral ganglia and also in the gastrointestinal tract (25, 38). Concentrations in the myenteric plexus of the guinea pig ileum and associated longitudinal muscle are 10 15% those in the mucosa, so that neuronal CCK is a small pool of total gastrointestinal CCK, most of which occurs in endocrine cells. CCK-reactive nerve cell bodies occur in the submucous plexus of the guinea pig proximal colon, and in at least some of these cells there is evidence for coexistence with a somatostatin-like peptide (38). The result of ligation and lesion studies of the vagal nerve indicate that a small amount of neuronal CCK8 in the gut is probably delivered in afferent vagal fibers; these results are of interest in that they also provide direct evidence for axonal transport of CCK (10).

2.3 Phylogeny

Peptides that react with C-terminal-specific antisera to CCK and gastrin can be found in a wide variety of nervous systems, including those of the most primitive multicellular animals, the coelenterates such as *Hydra* (39) as well as advanced invertebrates such as molluscs (40) and insects (41). In the snail, *Helix*, a CCK-like peptide has been localized to a defined neuron, the giant serotonin-containing cell (40). The dual existence of CCK-like material and serotonin in this cell provides an ideal opportunity to study the cellular and molecular implications of the coexistence of neuroregulatory molecules. The occurrence of CCK in both nerves and endocrine cells appears to be a chordate feature that was established in primitive vertebrates such as the cyclostomes, and has since been well conserved (42). Taken as a whole the phylogenetic evidence suggests that CCK established a neuronal function early in the emergence of nervous systems and that its hormonal role is a relatively recent addition.

3 SUBCELLULAR ORIGINS, RELEASE, AND DEGRADATION

Immunoreactive CCK8 has been identified in the synaptosomal fraction of homogenates of various regions of rat brain, such as the cortex, striatum, hypothalamus and brain stem (43, 44). CCK8-like activity can be released from synaptosomes and from brain slices by depolarizing stimuli such as high potassium concentrations in the presence of calcium. When synaptosomes are suspended at low concentration there is a relatively high fractional rate of basal release, which can present difficulties for *in vitro* release studies (43). There is rapid degradation of CCK8 by synaptosomal preparations (43, 45). By following the appearance of tryptophan when CCK-related peptides were incubated with rat brain synaptosomes, Deschodt-Lanckman et al. (45) were able to demonstrate marked differences in the rates of degradation of different analogs; the half-time for degradation of sulfated CCK8 was 52 min, compared with 3 min for G4 and more than 3 h for N-terminally blocked analogs and caerulein. The results suggest that aminopeptidases play an important part in CCK8 degradation.

4 RECEPTORS

Binding of radiolabeled CCK to membrane preparations from pancreas and brain has been reported by several groups. It is well established that a sulfated tyrosine residue in position 7 from the C-terminus is essential for full biological potency on pancreas and gallbladder; desulfation, or shifting the sulfated tyrosine toward (as in gastrin) or away from the C-terminus reduces potency at least a thousandfold (1). Oxidation of the methionines also markedly reduces bioactivity (21). Because sulfated tyrosines are not readily substituted with iodine, the preferred radiolabeled form of CCK for receptor binding studies in pancreas has been CCK33 substituted with ^{125}I by the Bolton-Hunter method. The same label preparations have also been used for brain (46–48). However, evidence discussed below suggests that the specificity of brain receptors might differ from those on pancreatic acinar cells, and it is not yet certain that other labeled preparations, such as desulfated CCK iodinated on the tyrosine residue or even radiolabeled gastrin, might not prove adequate for brain receptor studies.

Binding of ^{125}I-CCK33 to the particulate fraction of rat and guinea pig brain homogenates is saturable, reversible, specific, and high affinity, $K_d 0.4 - 1.7 \times 10^{-9} M$ (46–48). The structural requirements for binding appear to be less stringent than in pancreas. The binding sites in brain show virtually equal affinity for CCK33 and sulfated CCK8; estimates of the affinity for desulfated CCK8 vary from equal to that for sulfated

CCK8 (48) to about 50 times lower (47). Strangely, in two studies desulfated gastrin was reported to have higher affinity than desulfated CCK8 (46, 47). The tetra- and pentapeptides have affinity for brain binding sites similar to that of desulfated CCK8. Zarbin et al. (49) have mapped the distribution of binding sites in guinea pig brain by autoradiography. In the cerebral cortex there are dense populations of binding sites in layers IV and VI, but few in layer I; they are also abundant in mammillary bodies, hippocampus, retina and colliculi. Complementary results have been obtained for distribution of binding sites in particulate fractions of guinea pig brain homogenates (47). CCK receptors also occur on peripheral neurons. Thus CCK8 contracts the longitudinal muscle of the guinea pig ileum by stimulating acetylcholine and substance P release from myenteric plexus neurons (50, 51). Sulfated CCK8 is about a thousand times more potent than desulfated CCK8, gastrins, or G4. On this evidence it seems that the specificity of peripheral neuron receptors resembles that of pancreatic acinar cells and gallbladder more closely than that of brain receptors. It is noteworthy that in addition to different classes of CCK receptor there are also specific receptors for gastrin on gastric parietal cells that show lower affinity for CCK8 than for the gastrins. There may also exist yet a further class of receptor for the CCK–gastrin group of peptides. Thus, stimulation of insulin release from the isolated perfused pig pancreas is strongly stimulated by G4, but longer forms of gastrin and CCK produced by extension of the N-terminus of G4 have markedly reduced potency (19).

Peikin et al. (52) found that the dibutyryl analog of cyclic guanosine monophosphate (Bt_2cGMP) is a potent antagonist of CCK-induced stimulation of pancreatic amylase release, and subsequently it has been shown that Bt_2cGMP acts as a competitive, reversible inhibitor of CCK binding to pancreatic receptors (53, 54). This property is specific to Bt_2cGMP and appears to be attributable to structural similarities with the C-terminal region of gastrin/CCK. The effects of CCK8 on the guinea pig ileum are antagonized by Bt_2cGMP in a competitive manner, suggesting that at least some neuronal CCK receptors have similar specificity to those on pancreas (55). Recently, however, Saito et al. (56) failed to find antagonism of CCK binding to brain receptors by Bt_2cGMP; taken with the previous data, these results provide further evidence for differences between central and peripheral CCK receptors.

5 ACTIONS

5.1 Single Cells: Electrophysiological Studies

Even before the discovery of CCK in brain it had been shown that peripheral administration of CCK8 produced an enhancement of acoustically evoked potentials in several regions of the rat brain (57). Since then electrophysiological methods have been used to study the actions of CCK on a variety of cells in the cortex, hypothalamus, midbrain, and spinal cord (58–62). Dodd and Kelly (60) found that sulfated CCK8 delivered by pressure ejection onto CA1 pyramidal cells in rat hippocampal slices produced a rapid reversible depolarization and a decrease in input resistance (Figure 5). Fragments of gastrin from the tetra- to the tetradecapeptide also had excitatory effects, but desulfated CCK8 was

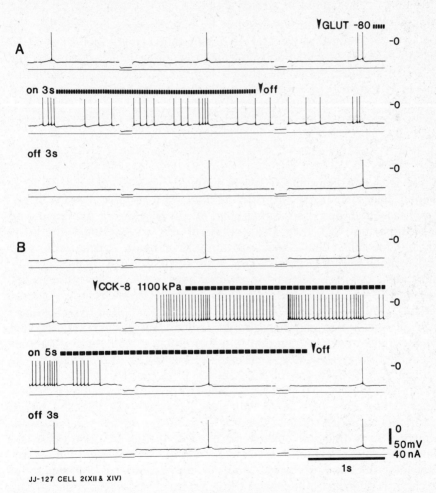

JJ-127 CELL 2(XII & XIV)

Figure 5. Intracellular recording from a CA1 pyramidal cell in a rat hippocampal slice showing the excitatory action of CCK8 (B) and glutamate (A) administered by pressure ejection (started at arrow). Membrane resistance was monitored by intracellular injection of rectangular hyperpolarizing pulses, and excitability was monitored by depolarizing ramps. In traces (A) and (B), the upper trace shows the voltage response of the membrane and lower trace current injected intracellularly. Reproduced with permission from J. Dodd and J. S. Kelly (60).

inactive. The responses were rapid in onset but frequently faded in spite of continued application. Excitatory effects have also been observed in about 50% of cells in laminae I-VII of the cat spinal cord *in vivo* and rat spinal cord *in vitro* (61). The units of the cat spinal cord that responded to CCK8 were activated by nociceptive, mechanosensitive, and both mechanosensitive and nociceptive stimuli. It is not yet possible to relate precisely to electrophysiological data to possible physiological actions of CCK. It is of interest, however, that Skirboll et al. (62) have noted that sulfated CCK7 (i.e., C-terminal heptapeptide) administered either intravenously or by iontophoresis increased the firing rate of ventral tegmental and substantia nigra neurons. CCK7 tended to excite neurons only in those regions in which dopamine and CCK-like peptides could be shown to coexist. The authors speculate that in this system CCK8 might play a role in the coordination of functionally related subpopulations of neurons.

5.2   CCK and Satiety

There is a considerable literature on the inhibitory effect of CCK on feeding behavior. In the rat, CCK administered peripherally (i.v. or i.p.) produces inhibition of feeding; the effect is blocked by vagotomy, suggesting that CCK acts at a peripheral site (63, 64). Since the doses needed for this effect almost certainly give blood concentrations far above those normally encountered after feeding, it seems unlikely that this effect is physiological. In normal rats, CCK given intracerebroventricularly has little or no effect on feeding. However, stress-induced feeding produced by tail-pinching is apparently inhibited by large doses of CCK given into the third ventricle, and by peripheral CCK (65). Levine and Morley (66) suggest that this effect is mediated by adrenal-dependent hyperglycemia. The idea that CCK in brain might be involved in the regulation of food intake is supported by the report of Straus and Yalow (67) that CCK concentrations were reduced in acid extracts of cortex from mice with genetic obesity (ob/ob), and by the report that numbers of CCK-binding sites in the rat hypothalamus and olfactory bulb (but not cortex) increase in fasting (68). However, the data on tissue concentrations must for the present be regarded as controversial since an exhaustive study by Schneider et al. (69) has failed to confirm differences in central CCK in normal and obese rodents.

In sheep, administration of low doses of CCK8 intracerebroventricularly inhibited feeding (70); conversely, feeding is said to be stimulated by administration of CCK antiserum (71), and by Bt_2cGMP (72), into the third ventricle. In both instances the effects could be attributed to blockade of endogenous CCK. Because it seems unlikely that immunoglobulins would freely penetrate the neuropil, it is reasonable to postulate that the effects of immunoblockade are exerted on CCK8 in cerebrospinal fluid. Taken as a whole these data indicate that the satiety effects of CCK administered peripherally are likely to be pharmacological, and they encourage, but by no means prove, the idea that in species such as sheep (although not in rat) central CCK might control feeding behavior.

5.3   CCK and Analgesia

The presence of CCK or a related peptide in several areas known to be involved in nociception—for example, in periaqueductal gray and dorsal horn of the spinal cord—has provided the basis for studies on the possible analgesic actions of CCK. Subcutaneous CCK8 and its amphibian decapeptide analog, caerulein, produced analgesic effects in mice in the hot-plate and writhing tests but not in the tail flick test (73). Administration of CCK8 into several regions of the rat brain, including the periaqueductal gray and subarachnoid space of the spinal cord, has been shown to effect long-lasting inhibition in both tail flick and hot-plate tests (74). These actions are produced by doses 4000–7000 times lower than morphine given at the same sites; CCK8 was about 10 times less potent than caerulein. The effects of CCK8 were abolished by administration of naloxone, suggesting a possible mediation by endogenous opioid peptides.

5.4   CCK and the Pituitary

The presence of high concentrations of CCK in the hypothalamus and its localization to the median eminence has provided the basis for studies of a possible role as a releasing factor. Administration of sulfated CCK8 (40 μg) into the third ventricle in conscious, female, ovariectomized rats stimulated prolactin and growth hormone release, and inhibited luteinizing hormone (LH) and thyroid stimulating hormone (TSH) release (75). In the same experiments intravenous CCK8 stimulated prolactin but had no effect on other anterior pituitary hormones; *in vitro* CCK failed to stimulate hormone release from hemipituitaries. Other investigators, however, have demonstrated that high concentrations of CCK33 (10^{-6} M) will release prolactin from rat, but not human, pituitary monolayer cultures (76). Given that high concentrations of CCK8 are needed to evoke these effects, it seems unlikely that CCK8 has a physiological role as a hypothalamic releasing factor; it would, however, be premature to exclude a physiological role at the level of the hypothalamus in mediating the secretion of other releasing factors.

5.5 Other Actions After Peripheral Administration

Peripheral administration of CCK and its analogs evokes a number of central nervous system responses in addition to those already mentioned. Among these are depression of exploratory behavior in mice (77), inhibition of spontaneous rearing, prolongation of hexobarbital sleeping time (78), and increases in latency in passive avoidance behavior tests (79). The effect on exploratory behavior is very probably mediated by a peripheral site of action since it is abolished after vagotomy (77). As already noted, vagotomy abolishes the satiety effect of peripheral CCK in rats, and it is now plainly important to establish whether other central nervous system responses to peripheral CCK are mediated by the vagus or whether they can be attributed to small amounts of CCK passing through the blood-brain barrier from plasma to CNS. In this context it is worth emphasizing that various CNS responses can be elicited by stimulation of the gastrointestinal tract and are dependent on vagal or splanchnic afferent fibers (80). Thus it may well be that the actions of peripheral CCK are secondary to changes in gastrointestinal motility or secretion.

6 PERSPECTIVES

The accumulated evidence reviewed here indicates that CCK8 occurs in high concentrations in neurons of the brain. Other CCK-related peptides may also be found in brain, but these await complete chemical identification. There is evidence to indicate that CCK8 is synthesized in neurons and transported axonally to nerve endings, where it is stored and released by depolarizing stimuli. There are specific membrane binding sites associated with brain regions containing CCK, and administration of CCK to single neurons in a number of areas evokes excitatory responses. These data are compatible with a neuroregulatory role for CCK8 in brain, although the precise functions are still uncertain. Nevertheless, the time is now obviously ripe to explore certain specific questions. such as the possibility that CCK8 is an excitatory transmitter of interneurons in the cerebral cortex.

Because in a number of cases CCK8-related molecules appear to coexist in nerve cells with other biologically active substances, it is obvious that a full understanding of the physiological role of CCK in the nervous system will need to take account of possible interactions with other substances. A start has already been made in the development of antagonists for CCK8, and the vigorous pursuit of this line of study is of crucial importance in elucidating the functions of CCK8 in brain. Although the central nervous system can be shown to respond in a variety of ways when CCK8 is given peripherally it is by no means certain that these responses are physiological. Indeed, with further study it may well emerge that these effects are secondary to changes in gut function of the type that are evoked by CCK in pharmacological doses.

REFERENCES

1. V. Mutt, in G. B. J. Glass, Eds., *Gastrointestinal Hormones*, Raven Press, New York, 1980, p. 169.
2. J. J. Vanderhaeghen, J. C. Signeau, and W. Gepts, *Nature* **257**, 604 (1975).
3. G. J. Dockray, *Nature* **264**, 568 (1976).
4. J. E. Muller, E. Straus, and R. S. Yalow, *Proc. Natl. Acad. Sci. USA* **74**, 3035 (1977).
5. J. F. Rehfeld, *J. Biol. Chem.* **253**, 4022 (1978).
6. P. Robberecht, M. Deschodt-Lanckman, and J. J. Vanderhaeghen, *Proc. Natl. Acad. Sci. USA* **75**, 524 (1978).
7. L.-I. Larsson and J. F. Rehfeld, *Science* **213**, 768 (1981).
8. M. C. Beinfeld, D. K. Meyer, and M. J. Brownstein, *Nature* **288**, 376 (1980).
9. K. Uvnäs-Wallensten, J. F. Rehfeld, L.-I. Larsson, and B. Uvnäs, *Proc. Natl. Acad. Sci. USA* **74**, 5707 (1977).
10. G. J. Dockray, R. A. Gregory, H. J. Tracy, and W.-Y. Zhu, *J. Physiol.* **314**, 501 (1981).
11. G. J. Dockray, *Nature* **270**, 359 (1977).
12. S. W. Ryder, J. Eng, E. Straus, and R. S. Yalow, *Biochem. Biophys. Res. Comm.* **94**, 704 (1980).
13. E. Straus and R. S. Yalow, *Proc. Natl. Acad. Sci. USA* **75**, 486 (1978).
14. S. J. Brand and R. G. H. Morgan, *J. Physiol.* **319**, 325 (1981).
15. G. J. Dockray, R. A. Gregory, J. B. Hutchinson, J. I. Harris, and M. R. Runswick, *Nature* **274**, 711 (1978).
16. G. J. Dockray, *Brain Res.* **188**, 155 (1980).
17. S. W. Ryder, J. Eng, E. Straus, and R. S. Yalow, *Proc. Natl. Acad. Sci. USA* **78**, 3892 (1981).
18. J. F. Rehfeld and N. R. Goltermann, *J. Neurochem.* **32**, 1339 (1979).
19. J. F. Rehfeld, L.-I. Larsson, N. R. Goltermann, T. W. Schwartz, J. J. Holst, S. L. Jensen, and J. S. Morley, *Nature* **284**, 33 (1980).
20. G. J. Dockray, R. G. Williams, and W.-Y. Zhu, *Neurochem. Int.*, **3**, 281 (1981).
21. V. Mutt, *Peptides*, **2**, Suppl. 2, 209 (1981).
22. S. W. Ryder, E. Straus, and R. S. Yalow, *Proc. Natl. Acad. Sci. USA.* **77**, 3669 (1980).
23. N. R. Goltermann, J. F. Rehfeld, and H. Roigaard-Petersen, *J. Biol. Chem.* **255**, 6181 (1980).
24. J. F. Rehfeld, *J. Biol. Chem.* **253**, 4022 (1978).
25. L.-I. Larsson and J. F. Rehfeld, *Brain Res.* **65**, 201 (1979).
26. N. Barden, Y. Merand, D. Rouleau, S. Moore, G. J. Dockray, and A. Dupont. *Peptides* **2**, 299 (1981).
27. C. B. Lamers, J. E. Morley, P. Poitras, B. Sharp, H. E. Carlson, J. M. Hershman, and J. H. Walsh, *Am. J. Physiol.* **239**, E232 (1980).
28. R. H. Perry, G. J. Dockray, R. Dimaline, E. K. Perry, G. Blessed, and B. E. Tomlinson, *J. Neurol. Sci.* **51**, 465 (1981).
29. P. C. Emson, J. F. Rehfeld, H. Langevin, and M. Rossor, *Brain Res.* **198**, 497 (1980).
30. I. Lorén, J. Alumets, R. Håkanson, and F. Sundler, *Histochemistry* **59**, 249 (1979).
31. R. B. Innis, F. M. A. Correa, G. R. Uhl, B. Schneider, and S. H. Snyder, *Proc. Natl. Acad. Sci. USA.* **76**, 521 (1979).
32. J. J. Vanderhaeghen, F. Lotstra, J. DeMay, and C. Gilles, *Proc. Natl. Acad. Sci. USA.* **77**, 1190 (1980).

33. M. Schultzberg, R. G. Williams, and G. J. Dockray, *Brain Res.*, **235**, 198 (1982).
34. T. Hökfelt, L. Skirboll, J. F. Rehfeld, M. Goldstein, K. Markey, and O. Dann, *Neuroscience* **5**, 2093 (1980).
35. R. G. Williams, R. J. Gayton, W.-Y. Zhu, and G. J. Dockray, *Brain Res.* **213**, 227 (1981).
36. L. Skirboll, T. Hökfelt, J. Rehfeld, C. Cuello, and G. J. Dockray, *Neurosci. Lett.*, **28**, 35 (1982).
37. N. N. Osborne, D. A. Nicholas, A. C. Cuello, and G. J. Dockray, *Neurosci. Lett.* **26**, 31 (1981).
38. M. Schultzberg, T. Hökfelt, G. Nilsson, L. Terenius, J. F. Rehfeld, M. Brown, R. Elde, M. Goldstein, and S. Said, *Neuroscience* **5**, 689 (1980).
39. C. J. P. Grimmelikhuijzen, F. Sundler, and J. F. Rehfeld, *Histochemistry* **69**, 61 (1980).
40. N. N. Osborne, A. C. Cuello, and G. J. Dockray, *Science*, **216**, 409 (1982).
41. G. J. Dockray, H. Duve, and A. Thorpe, *Gen. Comp. Endocrinol.*, **65**, 491 (1981).
42. G. J. Dockray, *Fed. Proc.* **38**, 2295 (1979).
43. P. Dodd, J. A. Edwardson, and G. J. Dockray, *Regul. Peptides* **1**, 17 (1980).
44. P. C. Emson, C. M. Lee, and J. F. Rehfeld, *Life Sci.* **26**, 2157 (1980).
45. M. Deschodt-Lanckman, N. D. Bui, M. Noyer, and J. Christophe, *Regul. Peptides* **2**, 15 (1981).
46. A. Saito, H. Sankaran, I. D. Golfine, and J. A. Williams, *Science* **208**, 1155 (1980).
47. R. B. Innis and S. H. Snyder, *Proc. Natl. Acad. Sci. USA.* **77**, 6917 (1980).
48. S. E. Hays, M. C. Beinfeld, R. T. Jensen, F. K. Goodwin, and S. M. Paul, *Neuropeptides* **1**, 53 (1980).
49. M. A. Zarbin, R. B. Innis, J. K. Wamsley, S. H. Snyder, and M. J. Kuhar, *Eur. J. Pharmacol.* **71**, 349 (1981).
50. E. S. Vizi, G. Bertaccini, M. Impicciatore, and J. Knoll, *Gastroenterology* **64**, 268 (1973).
51. J. B. Hutchison and G. J. Dockray, *Eur. J. Pharmacol.* **69**, 87 (1981).
52. S. R. Peikin, C. L. Costenbader, and J. D. Gardner, *J. Biol. Chem.* **254**, 5321 (1979).
53. R. T. Jensen, G. F. Lemp, and J. D. Gardner, *Proc. Natl. Acad. Sci. USA* **77**, 2079 (1980).
54. P. Robberecht, N. Deschodt-Lanckman, M.-C. Woussen-Colle, P. De Neef, J. C. Camus, and J. Christophe, *Mol. Pharmacol.* **17**, 268 (1980).
55. J. B. Hutchison and G. J. Dockray, *Brain Res.* **202**, 501 (1980).
56. A. Saito, I. D. Goldfine, and J. A. Williams, *J. Neurochem.* **37**, 483 (1981).
57. N. Dafny, R. H. Jacob, and E. D. Jacobson, *Experientia* **31**, 658 (1975).
58. S. Ishibashi, Y. Oomura, T. Okajima, and S. Shibata, *Physiol. Behav.* **23**, 401 (1979).
59. J. W. Phillis and J. R. Kirkpatrick, *Can. J. Physiol. Pharmacol.* **58**, 612 (1980).
60. J. Dodd and J. S. Kelly, *Brain Res.* **205**, 337 (1981).
61. S. Jeftinija, V. Moletic, and M. Randic, *Brain Res.* **213**, 231 (1981).
62. L. R. Skirboll, A. A. Grace, D. W. Hommer, J. Rehfeld, M. Goldstein, T. Hökfelt and B. S. Bunney, *Neuroscience* **6**, 2111, (1981).
63. J. Gibbs, R. C. Young, and G. P. Smith, *Nature* **245**, 323 (1973).
64. G. P. Smith, C. Jerome, B. J. Cushin, R. Eterno, and K. J. Simansky, *Science* **213**, 1036 (1981).
65. C. B. Nemeroff, A. J. Osbahr, G. Bissette, G. Jahnka, M. A. Lipton, and M. A. Prange, *Science* **200**, 793 (1978).
66. A. S. Levine and J. E. Morley, *Regul. Peptides* **2**, 353 (1981).
67. E. Straus and R. S. Yalow, *Science* **203**, 68 (1979).
68. A. Saito, J. A. Williams, and I. D. Goldfine, *Nature* **289**, 599 (1981).
69. B. S. Schneider, J. W. Monahan, J. Hirsch, *J. Clin. Invest.* **64**, 1348 (1979).
70. M. A. Della-Fera and C. A. Baile, *Science* **206**, 471 (1979).
71. M. A. Della-Fera, C. A. Baile, B. S. Schneider, and J. A. Grinker, *Science* **212**, 688 (1981).

72. M. A. Della-Fera, C. A. Baile, and S. R. Peikin, *Physiol. Behav.* **26**, 799 (1981).
73. G. Zetler, *Neuropharmacology* **19**, 415 (1980).
74. I. Jurna and G. Zetler, *Eur. J. Pharmacol.* **73**, 323 (1981).
75. E. Vijayan, W. K. Samson, and S. M. McCann, *Brain Res.* **172**, 295 (1979).
76. W. B. Malarkey, T. M. O'Dorisio, M. Kennedy, and S. Cataland, *Life Sci.* **28**, 2489 (1981).
77. J. N. Crawley, S. E. Hays, and S. M. Paul, *Eur. J. Pharmacol.* **73**, 379 (1981).
78. G. Zetler, *Eur. J. Pharmacol.* **66**, 137 (1980).
79. M. Fekete, T. Kafar, B. Penke, and G. Telegdy, *Neuropeptides* **1**, 301 (1981).
80. P. P. Newman, *Visceral Afferent Functions of the Nervous System*, Edward Arnold, London, 1974.

35

VIP, Motilin, and Secretin

VIKTOR MUTT

Department of Biochemistry II
Karolinska Institute
Stockholm, Sweden

Some of the investigations described in this chapter were supported by the Swedish Medical Council through Grant 13X-01010.

1 DISCOVERY

As early as in 1825, Leuret and Lassaigne (1) showed that in the dog, acidification of the upper intestine led to secretion of pancreatic juice. Their observation did not attract much attention and seems to have been soon forgotten. The effect of intestinal acidification on pancreatic secretion was rediscovered by Pavlov and his coworkers and extensively studied by them (2, 3). Pavlov and others took it for granted that the effect was transmitted by nerves, and extensive investigations were carried out to identify the nerves involved. No such nerves were found, though, and the story took an unexpected turn with the demonstration by Bayliss and Starling in 1902 that an extract of dog intestinal mucosa could, on intravenous injection into the dog, cause intense pancreatic secretion (4, 5). Bayliss and Starling gave the name secretin to the agent in the extract that caused the pancreas to secrete. Since they realized that in all probability not only the intestine sent a chemical messenger to the pancreas to stimulate its activity, but that similar messengers would be found to regulate the activities of other organs, they considered it expedient to create a new word to describe such messengers. On the advice of W. H. Hardy they chose the name hormone, from a Greek word meaning "I arouse to activity" (6).

Bayliss and Starling (4, 5) discussed at some length the presence in acid extracts of intestinal tissue of a substance, distinct from secretin, with vasodepressor properties. They found that whereas secretin could be extracted from epithelial cells, the vasopressor substance occurred in more deeply lying structures, possibly the muscularis mucosa. This would seem to suggest that the depressor substance may have been VIP but other information given by Bayliss and Starling makes this unlikely. Its solubility properties, for instance, resembled those of histamine rather than those of VIP. Ivy and coworkers (7) mentioned, however, that in some preparations of cholecystokinin, obtained by salting out with NaCl from acid extracts of intestinal tissue, they had observed a substance that on intravenous injection into anesthetized dogs caused a fall in blood pressure and, in some cases, stimulated respiration. Since histamine is not salted out by NaCl it is possible that they had VIP in their preparation. Again, other information, such as the high degree of tachyphylaxis, makes this uncertain and the discovery of VIP must be regarded to be a consequence of observations made by S. I. Said on the presence of vasoactive peptides in lung tissue. He came to work on such peptides at the Department of Biochemistry of the Karolinska Institute. Since peptide side-fractions from the isolation of secretin and cholecystokinin had been stored in the laboratory in the hope of finding some unknown interesting peptides in them, it was decided to find out whether they contained vasoactive peptides similar to those found in extracts of lung tissue. Several peptide fractions were indeed shown to have vasoactive properties but one fraction in particular was, on injection into the femoral artery of anesthetized dogs, found to cause a profound increase in blood flow through the artery, and also hypotension (8). The peptide responsible for these actions was isolated and has come to be known as the vasoactive intestinal polypeptide (VIP) (9, 10) although later work has shown that it is not confined to intestinal tissue and has other actions besides vasoactivity.

The name motilin seems first to have been used by Enriquez and Hallion (11) to describe a hypothetical hormone-stimulating intestinal peristalsis. The name did not at that time find its way into textbooks or reviews, and the motilin of today was discovered by J. C. Brown. It was known that acidification of the upper intestine would inhibit gastric emptying and motility, partly presumably by the release of secretin. Brown and coworkers (12) investigated what the opposite would do and found that mild alkalinization of the duodenal contents in dogs with denervated and transplanted pouches of the body of the stomach led to increased motor activity of the pouches. They postulated that alkalinization either inhibited the release of a gastric motor activity-inhibiting substance or released a stimulatory one. Brown then compared two commercially available preparations of pancreozymin and found that one of them, but not the other, stimulated fundic pouch motility (13); in further work together with C. O. Parkes (14) he succeeded in separating the motility-stimulating activity from pancreozymin. Brown, too, then came to the Karolinska Institute and soon succeeded in purifying a gastric motor activity-stimulating peptide from a side-fraction from the isolation of secretin, a different one from the one that yields VIP. This peptide was named motilin (15). Although later work seems to have shown that in humans duodenal alkalinization does not release but instead inhibits immunoreactive motilin (16) and that it is released by duodenal acidification (16, 17), it was the finding that duodenal alkalinization stimulated gastric motor activity that led to the discovery of motilin. In the dog, duodenal alkalinization has been found to release immunoreactive motilin (18).

2 ISOLATION

Numerous attempts were made to isolate secretin during the 1902–1960 period, and important information was obtained on its chemical and physiological properties and its clinical usefulness. But none of this work led to its isolation, and in retrospect it seems highly improbable that any method or combination of methods known before approximately the early 1950s could have done so. In addition, the specific activity of secretin was grossly underestimated and consequently its concentration in intestinal tissue was correspondingly overestimated, resulting in unreasonably small amounts of tissue being processed in many of the attempts at its isolation. When new efficient methods, developed in other areas of biochemistry, for the fractionation of complex peptide mixtures were applied to secretin, several groups of workers obtained highly active preparations of it in the late 1950s. The early work on secretin has been reviewed by many authors, (see, e.g., refs 19–21). The method that finally led to the isolation of (porcine) secretin in a state of purity high enough for the determination of its amino acid sequence was as follows:

Pig upper small intestines were briefly heated in boiling water to inactivate proteolytic enzymes and coagulate the bulk of the structural proteins. Peptides were then extracted from the tissue material with cold dilute acetic acid, adsorbed from the extract to alginic acid, eluted with dilute HCl, and precipitated from the eluate with NaCl at saturation. This precipitate, CTIP (concentrate of thermostable intestinal peptides), was dissolved in 66% ethanol and a precipitate obtained on neutralization of the solution removed. The soluble peptides were recovered in aqueous solution and precipitated at pH 4 with NaCl. The precipitate was extracted with methanol and a precipitate formed on neutralization of the solution was removed. The soluble peptides were precipitated with ether and this precipitate was chromatographed in 0.2 M acetic acid on Sephadex G-25. The fraction containing secretin, and also motilin and VIP, was chromatographed on carboxymethyl cellulose at pH 8, resulting in three fractions: "presecretin," "secretin," and "postsecretin." Secretin was isolated from the "secretin" fraction by means of countercurrent distribution in the system 1-butanol/0.1 M phosphate buffer of pH 7 (22). Motilin was isolated from the "presecretin" fraction by sequential chromatography on carboxymethyl cellulose at pH 6.5, Sephadex G-25 in 0.2 M acetic acid, triethylaminoethyl (or diethylaminoethyl) cellulose at pH 7.8 (15), and two additional chromatographies in 0.2 M acetic acid on Sephadex G-25 (23). VIP was isolated from the "postsecretin" fraction by sequential chromatography on Sephadex G-25 in 0.2 M acetic acid, carboxymethylcellulose in 0.1 M NH_4HCO_3 at pH 8, and countercurrent distribution in the system 1-butanol/0.1 M NH_4HCO_3 (10).

3   AMINO ACID SEQUENCES: INTERSPECIES AND INTRASPECIES VARIATIONS

Porcine secretin is composed of 27 amino acid residues (24):

His-Ser-Asp-Gly-Thr-Phe-Thr-Ser-Glu-Leu-Ser-Arg-Leu-Arg-Asp-Ser-Ala-
Arg-Leu-Gln-Arg-Leu-Leu-Gln-Gly-Leu-Val-NH$_2$

Notable features are the C-terminal alpha amide structure and the absence of no fewer than eight of the amino acid residues that often occur in proteins, that is, the residues of asparagine, cysteine, isoleucine, lysine, methionine, proline, tryptophan and tryosine. Bovine secretin is identical with porcine secretin (25), but chicken secretin (26) is surprisingly different:

His-Ser-Asp-Gly-Leu-Phe-Thr-Ser-Glu-Tyr-Ser-Lys-Met-Arg-Gly-Asn-
Ala-Gln-Val-Glu-Lys-Phe-Ile-Gln-Asn-Leu-Met-NH$_2$

It has the same number of amino acid residues as the porcine but in addition to the types of residues that occur in the latter, residues of asparagine, isoleucine, lycine, methionine, and tyrosine are present. The amino acid sequence of human secretin is not yet known. No fragment of secretin or extended precursor form of it has yet been isolated from natural sources but a variant form with some kind of yet uncharacterized modification in its N-terminal part has been isolated from porcine intestine (27) and evidence has been presented for the occurrence in human plasma during starvation of peptides with secretin-like immunoreactivity of both smaller and larger molecular sizes than the heptacosapeptide (28).

Porcine VIP has the amino acid sequence (29):

His-Ser-Asp-Ala-Val-Phe-Thr-Asp-Asn-Tyr-Thr-Arg-Leu-Arg-Lys-Gln-
Met-Ala-Val-Lys-Lys-Tyr-Leu-Asn-Ser-Ile-Leu-Asn-NH$_2$

Bovine VIP is identical with porcine (30), and VIP isolated from human colonic tissue has the same amino acid composition as porcine-bovine VIP (31) and presumably therefore the same sequence, although this has not yet been directly determined. Chicken VIP has the sequence:

His-Ser-Asp-Ala-Val-Phe-Thr-Asp-Asn-Tyr-Ser-Arg-Phe-Arg-Lys-Gln-
Met-Ala-Val-Lys-Lys-Tyr-Leu-Asn-Ser-Val-Leu-Thr-NH$_2$

It differs from the porcine by having in positions 11, 13, 26, and 28 residues of serine, phenylalanine, valine, and threonine amide instead of residues of threonine, leucine, isoleucine, and asparagine amide, respectively (32). No variant intraspecies form of VIP has yet been isolated, but Dockray and coworkers have presented evidence for the presence in human colonic tissue, besides the known form of VIP, of a peptide showing VIP-like immunoreactivity but of smaller size than the octacosapeptide, and the presence of two peptides of the same size as VIP but apparently less basic (33). A VIP variant, apparently less basic than "ordinary" VIP, has also been found in extracts of rat brain (34);

Yamaguchi et al. (35) have described the occurrence in extracts of certain pancreatic tumors of a peptide (or peptides) showing VIP-like immunoreactivity but evidently of several times larger size than the known VIP; and Obata et al. (36) have found that the mRNA for VIP from human neuroblastoma cells is translated in a cell-free rabbit reticulocyte lysate system to a "preproVIP" of $M_r \sim 20,000$.

The only species for which the amino acid sequence of motilin is yet known is the porcine. This sequence was originally (37) stated to be

Phe-Val-Pro-Ile-Phe-Thr-Tyr-Gly-Glu-Leu-Gln-Arg-Met-Glu-Glu-Lys-Glu-
Arg-Asn-Lys-Gly-Gln

but when checked, using another preparation of the natural peptide, it was found to have a residue of glutamine instead of glutamic acid in position 14 (38). The discrepancy was attributed to a possible artifactual deamidation of the peptide in the material first used for the sequence determination. But later work by Brown and Dryburgh (18) seems not quite to exclude the possibility that both forms of motilin are actually biosynthesized. Christofides et al. (39) have recently provided immunochemical evidence for the existence of a form of motilin larger than the docosapeptide, in addition to the latter, in both porcine and human small intestinal tissue extracts and in human plasma. O'Donohue et al. (40) found that rat motilin could be distinguished from porcine motilin, both on reversed phase liquid chromatography and through its reactivity with certain antisera. They, too, made observations suggesting the occurrence in rat duodenal and brain (*vide infra*) tissues of a larger form of motilin than the docosapeptide, in addition to the latter.

4 CELLULAR ORIGINS: TISSUE DISTRIBUTION

In 1970 and 1971 two groups of workers provided evidence by indirect immunofluorescence methods that secretin in the dog is biosynthesized or stored, or both, in the so-called S-cells of the Wiesbaden classification (41) and that these cells are confined to the upper small intestine (42, 43). This localization of both cells and tissue has been found in humans and in all of the several other mammals investigated, and the finding has not led to any controversy (44). In which cells secretin occurs in the brain (45, 46) and in the pituitary gland (46) is not known. Motilin was first found, in several mammalian species, to occur in enterochromaffin (EC) cells, but only in EC cells of the small intestine, mainly the duodenal and upper jejunal, and not in those of the stomach or colon (47). This was an early example of the coexistence of a hormonal polypeptide and a biogenic amine. There was evidence, however, for the occurrence of motilin not only in the argentaffin but also, to a smaller extent, in argyrophil cells, indicating that the picture of the motilin cell might be complicated. Further investigations suggested that not only motilin but also substance P occurred in EC cells, but in distinct populations (48). These cells have been referred to as EC_2 cells (49). Recently one group of workers have found motilin to occur, at least mainly, in a special group of cells that do not contain 5-hydroxytryptamine (50). Obviously more work is necessary to clarify these discrepant findings (51). An investigation of the ontogeny of motilin and secretin cells in humans has recently been done (52). Both secretin and motilin cells appeared at a gestational age of 16 weeks, and in the same anatomical area as they are found in the adult. The finding of motilin in central and peripheral neurons (40, 53, 54) and in the pituitary and the pineal glands (55) further complicates the picture. VIP-like immunoreactive material was first found to be present in endocrine cells of the upper intestine of several mammalian species and the quail (56). These cells could be reproducibly demonstrated only with the use of some antisera and not with others (57). The reason for this is not clear. The problem has been discussed by Larsson (58) in a recent review article. Obviously there are several possibilities. The antiserum may have reacted with some VIP-like peptide rather than with VIP itself, or possibly with some precursor form of VIP. In contrast, various workers have had no difficulty demonstrating the presence of VIP in a wide variety of peripheral and central neuronal elements. This is discussed in greater detail in the article by Larsson. Of considerable interest is the already mentioned coexistence of VIP and acetylcholine in certain neurons (59).

5 EVIDENCE FOR OCCURRENCE IN BRAIN

Soon after the discovery of VIP it was found that a VIP-like immunoreactive material was present in endocrine cells in the intestines of three mammalian and one avian species (dog, pig, baboon, and quail) (56). Later, such material was also found to be widely distributed in neural tissue, both peripheral and central (60–62). Much work has been carried out in different laboratories to delineate, by means of radioimmunoassay of tissue extracts and by immunocytochemistry, the distribution of this type of material in the brain. There are several recent reviews of this work (63–65), and it would be redundant to provide such a review here. It is evident that the material is unevenly distributed among the different structures of the brain. In the dog and the rat, and also in humans, it has been found in high concentrations in the cortex, certain areas of the hypothalamus, amygdala, hippocampus, and corpus striatum. In humans, but not in the rat, the highest concentrations were found in the median eminence (66). In the cerebellum, the concentrations were low in all species investigated.

To find, in a tissue or tissue extract, material reacting with antibodies to a certain peptide suggests that the tissue may contain this peptide but does not prove it. The finding might be explained by cross-reactivity with some other material or, unless the immunochemical analysis has been carried out with the use of region-specific antibodies (67), the peptide may be part of a precursor protein or a fragment of the molecule against which the antibody was raised. However, we have recently isolated VIP from porcine whole brain (with exclusion for technical reasons of the cerebellum and the pituitary) and found it to be identical in amino-acid sequence with the octacosapeptide amide originally isolated from porcine intestine (68). The isolation procedure was similar to although not identical with that used for intestinal VIP. We obtained 2 mg of essentially pure VIP from 400 kg of heat-coagulated brain (wet weight). With the customary 5–10% overall yield this would mean that the tissue contained, on the average, some 50–100 ngs of VIP per g (wet weight).

The presence of identical peptides in brain and intestine had seemed probable ever since von Euler in 1936 (69) presented evidence for the peptide nature of "substance P," and substance P from bovine collicular tissue (70, 71) and horse intestine (72) were indeed shown to be identical, as was neurotensin from bovine hypothalamus and intestine (73). The interest in identical peptides occurring in brain and intestine increased greatly when Vanderhaeghen et al. (74) found that material reacting with antibodies to the classical gastrointestinal hormone gastrin was present in the central nervous system (CNS) of all of several species investigated. The gastrin-like immunoreactivity was later shown to be from predominantly cholecystokinin-like rather than gastrin-like peptides (see G. J. Dockray Chapter 34 in this volume). The finding of VIP in brain and intestine contributed, of course, to the increase in interest in cerebrogastrointestinal peptides. Oddly, secretin was left out of the discussion. In an early attempt to isolate VIP from porcine brain we observed (45) that the dose-response curve for the stimulatory action on pancreatic bicarbonate secretion of a concentrate of brain peptides was more secretin-like than VIP-like. This led us to attempt the isolation of secretin from porcine brain and we did indeed find that the material with secretin-like bioactivity chromatographed indistinguishably from secretin in several chromatographic systems. The peptide fractions containing this type of bioactivity were also shown to contain a peptide with C-terminal valine amide, like intestinal secretin. Unfortunately, the amount of material was too small for complete isolation of the secretin or secretin-like peptide. Currently we are attempting to isolate it from the relevant side-fraction that we obtained during the isolation of brain

VIP. Quite recently O'Donohue et al. (46) have found and quantitated secretin-like immunoreactivity in extracts of pig and rat brain. On reversed phase high performance liquid chromatography the material with secretin-like immunoreactive material migrated identically whether extracted from porcine brain or intestine, and identically with synthetic porcine secretin. The corresponding material from rat intestine migrated identically with that isolated from rat brain but differed from the porcine material by having a slightly higher speed of migration. The distribution of secretin-like immunoreactive material in rat brain was found to be somewhat different from the distribution of VIP. In particular, the concentrations of secretin in the cortex were low, whereas high concentrations were found in the pituitary and the pineal glands. In addition to the small-sized secretin or secretin-like material, O'Donohue et al. (46) found evidence for the presence in rat brain extracts of a second species with larger molecular size than heptacosapeptide amide secretin.

Evidence for the existence of motilin in brain is accumulating. Yanaihara et al. (55) found that extracts of dog brain contained material with motilin-like immunoreactivity and that its concentration varied among different brain regions. In the hypothalamus, the posterior pituitary, the anterior pituitary, and the pineal gland, its concentration was reported to be 2, 20, 40, and 250 times higher, respectively, than in duodenal tissue. In the cortex, the concentration was only one-fourth of that of the duodenum. Gel chromatographic analyses indicated that the hypothalamic motilin-immunoreactive material was heterogeneous and mainly of larger size than intestinal motilin. Chey and coworkers found motilin-like immunoreactive material to occur widely in both central and peripheral neurons in the human, dog, and monkey (53). Recently, Track and coworkers (75) found motilin-like immunoreactive material to be present in the CNS in several other mammalian and nonmammalian species.

Motilin has a unique distribution in the rat brain. The highest concentrations are in the cerebellum. High concentrations were also observed in the hypothalamic nuclei and the organum vasculosum lamina terminalis (OVLT). Lowest motilin concentrations in the rat brain were in the pons and medulla (40). Motilin-containing neurons were visualized immunocytochemically in the cerebellum (Nilaver, personal communication), medial basal hypothalamus, and OVLT. A rich plexus of motilin-positive fibers was seen in the median eminence and OVLT, and less dense collections of neuronal processes were found in the preoptic area, nucleus interstitialis stria terminalis, hypothalamus, amygdala, mammillary body, and central gray (54). Chan-Palay and coworkers described the occurrence of motilin in some, but not all, Purkinje cells of the cerebellar cortex of mice, rats, and a monkey. In some of these cells both motilin and gamma-aminobutyric acid (GABA) could be demonstrated (76).

6 PHARMACOLOGICAL ACTIONS: PHYSIOLOGICAL ACTIONS, KNOWN AND SPECULATIVE

6.1 Gastrointestinal Actions

Originally, two actions were ascribed to secretin: stimulation of pancreatic secretion and stimulation of hepatic bile secretion (5). The action on the pancreas was soon found to be restricted to stimulation of secretion of water and inorganic electrolytes (bicarbonate mainly) but not of enzymes (77). This varies from species to species, but on the whole secretin acts on the ductule cells and not on the enzyme-secreting acinar cells, which are stimulated by pancreozymin (cholecystokinin, CCK) instead. Before secretin was isolated in essentially pure form, there had—reasonably enough—been speculation whether stimulation of bile secretion was really a property of secretin itself or of some other hormonal substance contaminating the early secretin preparations. With the use of essentially pure, natural and synthetic secretin preparations it was confirmed that secretin not only stimulates bile secretion but also exhibits a surprising number of other actions. A multiplicity of actions had already earlier been found for gastrin (78). In a review written some eight years ago, Gregory (79) listed the following eleven actions for secretin, in certain species at least, in addition to the two already mentioned: inhibition of (i) lower esophageal sphincter pressure, (ii) gastric emptying, (iii) gastric acid secretion, and (iv) duodenal motility; stimulation of (v) pepsin secretion, (vi) insulin release, (vii) Brunner's gland secretion, (viii) renal secretion of water, sodium, and potassium, (ix) lipolysis in fat cells, (x) cardiac output, and (xi) splanchnic blood flow. The list has grown longer since then. For instance, secretin has been found to (xii) stimulate gastric mucus secretion (80, 81); (xiii) release histamine from skin mast cells in certain patients with duodenal ulcers (82); (xiv) increase hepatic bilirubin UDP-glucuronyltransferase activity and cytochrome P-450 concentrations (83); (xv) counteract trophic effects of gastrin (84) but exhibit, in conjunction with CCK, trophic actions of its own (85); and (xvi) stimulate the secretion of parathyroid hormone as well as calcitonin (86).

There has been much discussion concerning which of the actions associated with secretin and other gastrointestinal hormones are physiological and which are seen only under experimental conditions with doses of exogenous hormone giving plasma concentrations far higher than ever seen naturally. A further distinction can be made between important and unimportant physiological effects. When radioimmunoassays for secretin became available it was found that the increases in plasma concentrations in conjunction with meals were, in humans and dogs, very small compared with the concentrations of exogenously administered secretin necessary for briskly stimulating pancreatic flow. This led several workers to question whether secretin actually was important in what had always been considered to be its main action, stimulation of pancreatic secretion. Further work seems nevertheless to have established that, in concert with CCK which potentiates it, secretin does indeed normally play a physiologically important, though not unique, role in stimulating pancreatic secretion (87). It is quite possible that secretin may have other important but yet unrecognized physiological actions. Buchanan and coworkers have found high plasma concentrations of material showing secretin-like immunoreactivity in the plasma of starved persons (88), suggesting some metabolic role for secretin. Further, Dockray and coworkers have shown that in birds, as opposed to mammals, VIP is much stronger than secretin as a stimulant of pancreatic secretion (89). This raises the question what the real function of secretin is in birds. Perhaps it has some unrecognized function in both birds and mammals.

Many different actions have been described for VIP. A newly published multiauthored book of some 500 pages is largely concerned with them (90). Our knowledge concerning which of these actions are of any importance is, however, still quite limited. In this chapter only some of VIP's actions are discussed, and references are mainly, although not exclusively, to review articles. No attempt has been made to assess priorities or to mention all the investigators who have made important observations in the field.

Ever since the work of Mellanby (77), physiologists held the view that secretin stimulated the pancreas to a copious secretion of a juice of low enzyme content whereas the juice secreted in response to vagal stimulation was scanty but of high enzyme content. In 1970, however, Hickson (91) showed that although this picture is undoubtedly true in the common laboratory animals, vagal stimulation in the cat, the dog, and the pig results in a brisk flow of pancreatic juice accompanied by vasodilation. Neither secretion nor vasodilation is inhibited by atropine. Fahrenkrug et al. (92) showed that vagal stimulation of the pig pancreas leads to increased concentrations of VIP in the venous effluent from the gland and suggested that the atropine-resistant effect of the vagus on secretion and blood flow is due to release of VIP from the nerve termini. Intravenously administered VIP is known to stimulate pancreatic secretion, and it may be that VIP released from the intestine into the bloodstream in connection with a meal has a stimulatory action on pancreatic secretion. But the swift disappearance of VIP from the circulation, the small amounts normally released into the blood, and the relative weakness of VIP as a pancreatic stimulant compared with secretin make it unlikely that blood-borne VIP plays any significant role in the stimulation of pancreatic secretion (93) but do not rule out a paracrine action.

A common feature of secretin family peptides is their ability to inhibit gastric secretion. VIP has been considered an enterogastrone because it has a broader spectrum of inhibitory effects on canine acid and pep-

sin secretion than does secretin (94). But recent studies have shown that
VIP increases acid secretion provoked by some stimulants in the cat
(95) and has no effect at all in humans (96).

Long before the discovery of either secretin or VIP, Heidenhain had
shown that nerve stimulation caused secretion and vasodilation in the
submandibular gland and that the secretion, but not the vasodilation,
could be inhibited by atropine (97). Recently, Bloom and Edwards (98)
and Uddman et al. (99), working with cats, and Shimizu and Taira with
dogs (100) have shown that the agent causing this atropine-resistant
vasodilation very probably is VIP released from the parasympathetic
vasodilator nerves. Uddman et al. (99), however, also found marked
variations in the concentrations of VIP in different salivary glands and
species. The concentration in the submandibular gland, for instance,
was 220 pmol/g in the cat but only 45 pmol/g in humans. In the sublin-
gual gland the cat had 150 pmol/g, but none at all was detectable in humans. Lundberg and coworkers have found that VIP-immunoreactive
neurons supplying the salivary glands, the pancreas, the sweat glands,
and the nasal mucosa also contain acetylcholinesterase, suggesting the
coexistence of VIP and acetylcholine in these secretomotor nerves.
They point out that such coexistence is by no means a general phenomenon; many types of nerves contain acetylcholine and no VIP, and others VIP but no acetylcholine (59). Lundberg et al. (101) found that in the
cat submandibular salivary gland, VIP enhances the binding of muscarinic ligands to their receptors.

VIP is present in the genitourinary tract (102) and administration of
exogenous VIP has in rabbits been shown to strongly stimulate myome-
trial blood flow (103).

VIP relaxes tone in the isolated guinea pig trachea *in vitro* and counteracts the spasmogenic effects on it of histamine and carbachol. Chick-
en VIP is about 10 times as strong as porcine VIP in this action (104).
Similarly in dogs *in vivo*, VIP counteracts the bronchoconstrictory effects of histamine and prostaglandin $F_2\alpha$ (105). Exogenous VIP has been
shown in dogs to have strong dilatory actions on coronary blood vessels (106).

Many of the actions of VIP are obviously due to its relaxant action
on vascular and nonvascular smooth muscle. VIP does not always relax
smooth muscle, however. In the intestine it relaxes circular muscle but
may contract logitudinal muscle (107, 108). Following the implication of
VIP as a causative agent in certain diarrheogenic tumors (109), many investigations have been carried out on its effects on intestinal fluid and
electrolyte transport. In humans, infusion of VIP abolished absorption of
water in the jejunum, ileum, and colon. In the jejunum, sodium and potassium absorption were abolished and secretion of chloride induced. In
the ileum absorption of sodium, potassium, and chloride was abolished,
and in the colon sodium absorption was abolished, chloride absorption

decreased, and secretion of potassium and bicarbonate enhanced (110). Similar results had earlier been found in animal experiments *in vivo* (111) and *in vitro* (112). Intravenous injection of VIP led in dogs to *increases* in concentrations of blood sugar and insulin. The raised insulin concentration was not only an effect of the blood sugar concentration since other experiments, such as those with the isolated vascularly perfused pancreas, have shown that VIP may in several species release glucagon, insulin, "pancreatic polypeptide," and somatostatin from the endocrine pancreas—the effects on glucagon and insulin secretion being influenced by the glucose concentration of the perfusing fluid (108).

Compared with secretin and VIP, much less is known about the actions of motilin. As its name implies, it acts on motility in the gastrointestinal tract, but it has been shown to have other actions as well. Thus pepsin secretion was found to be stimulated by porcine motilin in vagally and sympathetically denervated fundic pouches in dogs (15). The 13-norleucine analog of motilin likewise stimulated pepsin secretion in such pouches and also from innervated fundic mucosa (113), as well as in humans (114). Basal gastric acid secretion was found to be slightly stimulated in dogs by 13-norleucine motilin; secretion stimulated by pentagastrin, histamine, or a peptone meal was inhibited (113). Other workers found, also in dogs, that acid secretion stimulated by gastrin was augmented rather than inhibited by motilin (115). In dogs, basal pancreatic secretion of both fluid and protein, was slightly stimulated by 13-norleucine motilin, and the pancreatic secretory effects of secretin were partially inhibited (113), but in humans no such effects of the motilin analog on pancreatic secretion were seen (114).

Investigating the effects of motilin on gastrointestinal muscle *in vitro*, Strunz et al. (116) noted that the norleucine analog of porcine motilin strongly stimulated contractions of human and rabbit antral and upper intestinal muscle but not at all the corresponding guinea pig or rat muscle. Such a high degree of species specificity has not been demonstrated for the classical gastrointestinal hormones secretin, gastrin, and cholecystokinin. Rabbit circular muscle of the colon was also stimulated but not the taenia coli, whereas the opposite was true for the corresponding human muscles.

It is known that in animals who eat at intervals, cyclic waves of motor activity start in the stomach and move down the length of the jejunum into the ileum (117). Such waves of activity, often called interdigestive myoelectric complexes (IMC), are believed to be of physiological importance for cleaning the mucosal surface from desquamated cells, excess mucus, and so on. They also occur in humans, accompanied by the expulsion of small amounts of gastric and pancreatic enzymes into the lumen of the gastrointestinal canal, in keeping with a cleaning function for the IMC (118). It has been shown that exogenous motilin can initiate IMC in experimental animals (119, 120) suggesting a role of "interdigestive hormone" for motilin. Such a role is supported by the finding that plasma concentrations of motilin-like immunoreactivity show cyclic variations with maxima at the start of the IMC (121) and that endogenous increases in plasma motilin or exogenous motilin in dogs with autotransplanted stomach pouches initiate contractile activity in the pouches simultaneously with IMC in the remaining part of the stomach (122). Poitras et al. (123) have found that the action of motilin on the IMC seems to be confined to the stomach and the duodenum, since when motilin release and activity were inhibited with somatostatin, the cyclic motor activity was abolished in the stomach and duodenum but waves of activity continued to start in the jejunum and run toward the cecum.

6.2   CNS Actions

What functions motilin, secretin, and VIP may have specifically in the CNS is not yet known with any degree of certainty. Obviously, they may act in or on neurons or non-neural structures like glial cells and blood vessels. As yet, most investigations have been on VIP, and there are suggestions that this peptide might act in neural transmission, interact with catecholamine systems, influence the release of certain pituitary hormones, regulate the glucose metabolism of cortical cells, and regulate blood flow. Secretin and motilin may be involved in at least some such activities. As mentioned, motilin has been found in neurons (40, 53–55, 75) but in what structures secretin occurs in the CNS is yet unknown. In favor of a role for VIP in neural transmission—apart from its immunocytochemically demonstrated, extensive presence in central and in peripheral (90) neurons are its occurrence in vesicular structures of the type known to contain the classical neurotransmitters acetylcholine and noradrenaline (124, 125) and its axonal transport (126). Application of VIP to ganglia of the myenteric plexus of the guinea pig ileum *in vitro* resulted in excitation of intrinsic neurons in many but not all cases (127).

Phillis and Kirkpatrick (128) have studied the effects of 18 different hormonal peptides on the isolated hemisected toad spinal cord and found various effects. Motilin, secretin, and VIP all had potent depolarizing actions on dorsal and ventral root terminals and motoneurons. The effects of motilin were strongly inhibited by tetrodotoxin, whereas those of VIP and secretin were largely resistant to it, suggesting that motilin might be acting on interneurons in the spinal cord and VIP and secretin might have a direct action on the motoneurons. In further investigations they found (129) that motilin had strong excitatory actions on most of the corticospinal and other neurons in the rat cerebral cortex on which it was tested. VIP too had excitatory effects, but on a smaller number of neurons, and secretin had no effect on most neurons tested but nevertheless did, weakly, excite some neurons and inhibit others.

Chan-Palay et al. (130) found in rabbits that motilin, and also somatostatin, Leu-enkephalin, and Met-enkephalin, inhibited the firing of neurons of the lateral vestibular nucleus. Such inhibitory activity was additive to that of GABA for motilin, somatostatin, and Met-enkephalin whereas the interaction in this respect between Leu-enkephalin and GABA was of a more complex nature.

Intracerebroventricularly injected secretin increased dopamine concentrations in the medial and lateral palisade zones of the median eminence but did not affect norepinephrine concentrations in the hypothalamus of rats. The increased dopamine concentration was accompanied by reduced prolactin secretion. In turnover experiments in which the disappearance rate of catecholamines was recorded following inhibition of tyrosine hydroxylase, it was found that secretin strongly increased dopamine turnover in the above-mentioned zones of the median eminence. There was also some stimulation of norepinephrine turnover in the parvocellular paraventricular hypothalamic nucleus but not in the other hypothalamic nuclei.

VIP, similarly injected, did not significantly influence dopamine concentrations in the median eminence but did reduce them in the anterior periventricular hypothalamic region and in the parvocellular paraventricular hypothalamic nucleus. Norepinephrine turnover was increased in these hypothalamic areas and also in the magnocellular paraventricular hypothalamic nucleus, the posterior periventricular hypothalamic region, and in the subependymal layer of the median eminence. In parallel with the increased norepinephrine turnover there was increased secretion of prolactin and somatotropin, but whether or not there was any causal relationship between these phenomena was not determined by these experiments (131, 132).

Kato et al. (133) found that intracerebroventricular or intravenous injection of VIP in rats led to rises in plasma concentrations of prolactin but that VIP had no prolactin-releasing effect on rat anterior pituitary cells cultured *in vitro*. Said and Porter (134) found that in rats the concentrations of immunoreactive VIP were some twenty times higher in hypophyseal portal than in systemic arterial blood. Vijayan et al. (135) found that intracerebroventricular injections of VIP in rats resulted in release of not only prolactin but also of lutropin and somatotropin. Since no such release effects were found on rat hemipituitaries *in vitro* these workers suggested that in the intact animal, VIP was influencing some hypothalamic mechanism or mechanisms for release of the three pituitary hormones. Ruberg et al. (136) and Shaar et al. (137) found, however, that VIP did release prolactin from rat hemipituitaries *in vitro*, suggesting a direct effect on the prolactin cell. In further work with rat hemipituitaries *in vitro*, Enjalbert et al. (138) confirmed that VIP released prolactin but found in addition that neither somatotropin, lutropin, or follitropin were released. Like VIP, secretin released prolactin, but much higher doses of secretin than of VIP were necessary for this effect to be seen. The findings suggested that although VIP acted directly to release prolactin it acted indirectly to increase lutropin and somatotropin secretion. For somatotropin release, one possible mechanism was suggested to be inhibition of somatostatin release. Indeed, Epelbaum et al. (139) found that release of somatostatin was inhibited by VIP from slices of the hypothalamic area of the rat brain *in vitro*, but not from slices of other somatostatin-containing areas. It may be remembered that somatostatin release from the endocrine pancreas is not inhibited but rather stimulated by VIP (108). As to release of lutropin, Samson et al. have found that VIP releases lutropin from synaptosomes prepared from rat median eminence (140).

There is evidence that release of prolactin from the human pituitary by VIP also occurs. Nicosia et al. (141) found that VIP stimulated prolactin secretion *in vitro* from fragments of human prolactin secreting adenomas. Malarkey et al. (142) found that VIP stimulated prolactin release from monolayer cultures of cells from human normal as well as tumor-bearing pituitary tissue. Unexpectedly, no stimulation was obtained from monolayers of corresponding rodent pituitary cells. Finally, intravenous injections of VIP have been shown to increase plasma prolactin concentrations (143). Apart from anterior pituitary and endocrine pancreatic hormones, VIP, albeit only in large doses, has been shown to stimulate the synthesis and secretion of steroids in monolayer cultures of murine adrenal tumors (144) and the secretion of thyroid hormones in mice (145). VIP is also present in the posterior pituitary, whence it has been suggested that it might stimulate vasopressin release (146). Conversely, exogenous oxytocin has been found to release VIP in the dog (147, 148). In cultures of mouse brain cells consisting mainly of glioblasts, exogenous secretin—and to a lesser degree VIP—stimulated accumulation of cyclic adenosine 3',5'-monophosphate (cyclic AMP). This could be inhibited by somatostatin. The effect of secretin, but not of VIP, could also be inhibited by the C-terminal tricosapeptide amide of secretin, S_{5-27} (149).

Magistretti et al. (150) found that glycogenolysis in mouse brain cortical slices was stimulated by VIP, and by secretin in large doses, but not by glucagon. It was already known to be stimulated by norepinephrine. They suggested that VIP might be of importance for local control of energy metabolism in the cerebral cortex, the more so as the VIP-containing and the norepinephrine-containing nerves have a different type of distribution in the cortex and may complement each other in their actions. Nerve fibers containing VIP, or at least VIP-like immunoreactive material, are found around pial vessels, but whether or not VIP, because of its vasodilatory action is of any physiological importance for cerebral blood flow is not yet known. There seem for pial vessels to be considerable species differences both in densities of VIP-containing nerves (151) and in sensitivity to (porcine) VIP (152).

7 THE ROLE OF CYCLIC NUCLEOTIDES IN MEDIATING THE EFFECTS OF GASTROINTESTINAL PEPTIDES

Case and coworkers found that addition of dibutyryl cAMP to the perfusion fluid causes a saline-perfused preparation of the cat pancreas to secrete a juice of low enzyme concentration, just as it does in response to secretin (153). In the cat pancreas, *in vivo* stimulation of secretion by exogenous secretin leads to a swift increase in pancreatic cAMP concentration (154). The pancreas is a heterogenous organ and the rise in cAMP might of course have been due to the action of secretin on some other cells than those that secrete bicarbonate. However, much subsequent work in different laboratories has not refuted the possibility that rises in cellular cAMP are indeed involved, somehow, in the stimulation of bicarbonate secretion by secretin. Recently, secretin has been shown to stimulate cAMP release from fragments of pancreatic ducts, the area where pancreatic bicarbonate secretion primarily occurs (155). Nevertheless, until it is clearly shown how increases in ductule cell cAMP concentrations result in bicarbonate secretion the possibility, however improbable, cannot be completely ignored that stimulation by secretin of cAMP production and bicarbonate secretion might be parallel unrelated phenomena. The way in which cAMP acts as a second messenger for glucagon has been known, at least in outline, for more than 20 years (156). The differences in the abilities of three synthetic secretin analogs to stimulate adenylate cyclase in cat pancreatic plasma membranes were found to be much smaller than the differences in their abilities to stimulate secretion in the isolated perfused cat pancreas (157). As already mentioned, secretin has been shown to activate adenylate cyclase not only in the pancreatic ductule but also in the acinar cells, at any rate in the guinea pig (158), and outside of the pancreas in the mouse brain (149). It has further been found to have such an action on rat gastric, antral and fundic glands (159), but not on homogenates of human gastric mucosa (160).

VIP has been shown to increase, in several species, cAMP levels in several different organs, such as the liver, the gallbladder, the pancreas, the small and large intestine, the stomach, the pituitary gland, and the brain. References may be found in a recent review article by Amiranoff and Rosselin (161).

Deschodt-Lanckman et al. (162) found that VIP increased cAMP concentrations in a synaptosomal fraction from guinea pig brain. Several workers have studied the effects of VIP on rat brain *in vitro*. Their findings are in general agreement on the existence of great regional differences in brain in the amounts of basal cAMP and in the percentage increases on stimulation with VIP. Nevertheless, there are discrepancies among their findings, presumably due to differences in experimental techniques. Thus, Kaneko et al. (163) found that VIP stimulated *in vitro* cAMP production in the anterior pituitary, hypothalamus, pons, and cerebral medulla but not in the posterior pituitary, cerebellum, or cerebral cortex.

Quik et al. (164) found, using both tissue homogenates and slices, that it stimulated adenylate cyclase but not guanylate cyclase in the cerebral cortex, the hypothalamus, and the striatum, but not in the cerebellum. Borghi et al. (165), using homogenates, found that cAMP concentrations were increased by VIP in both the cerebral and the cerebellar cortex, as well as in the hypothalamus and hippocampus, but not in the brain stem.

The specificities of the binding sites of VIP have been characterized in guinea pig (166) and in rat (167) brain. VIP has been found to increase cAMP concentrations in fat cells from children but not from adults (168).

An obvious but important question is to what extent the rises in cellular concentrations of cAMP caused by VIP in different systems are causally involved in the various known pharmacological actions of VIP. It is possible that cAMP is indeed so involved in some cases and not in others.

Thus in stimulating glycogenolysis in brain cortex (150) it is probable that VIP, in analogy with glucagon in the liver, acts via cAMP. The evidence for a direct involvement of cAMP in the stimulation by VIP of intestinal secretion is also becoming rather convincing (161). On the other hand, the importance of cAMP for its actions on smooth muscle is less clear. Bodanszky and coworkers found that certain component peptides of VIP had definite relaxant actions on guinea pig tracheal and rat stomach muscle *in vitro* (169) whereas the same peptides had no effect at all on cAMP accumulation, admittedly in another biological system, in which VIP itself, however, had strong activity (158). In its stimulating effect on intestinal longitudinal muscle, VIP appears to act via release of acetylcholine (170).

Burnstock et al. (171) described experiments suggesting that adenosine 5'-triphosphate (ATP) might be an inhibitory neurotransmitter in the rat and rabbit anococcygeus muscle.

Gibson and Tucker (172) pointed out that the mechanisms underlying nonadrenergic, noncholinergic autonomic transmission may vary among tissues. They found that VIP produced dose-related relaxations of the mouse anococcygeus similar to those produced by ATP, at much higher concentrations, and suggested that VIP and ATP might either be acting as cotransmitters or else that VIP might be acting to release the actual inhibitory transmitter; both of which possibilities had been suggested earlier for the action of VIP on other tissues (173, 174).

Recently, evidence has been presented that the effects of VIP on the release of anterior pituitary hormones may in some way be regulated by corticosteroid hormones (175). It has been suggested that the vasodilatory effect of VIP on cerebral blood vessels is at least in part mediated by prostaglandins (152). An important question is how the effects of VIP are terminated. A VIP-degrading proteolytic enzyme has been demonstrated to be present in liver, kidney, and brain of the rabbit (176). Motilin by itself evidently does not stimulate smooth muscle contraction by changing muscle cAMP levels. Possibly its action may be inhibited by cAMP concentrations increased by some other agent (177).

8 STRUCTURE–ACTIVITY STUDIES

A peptide hormone has its own amino acid sequence but other peptides will probably always be found with similar sequences. Such peptides may, for instance, be homologous hormones in other species, or other peptides, hormonal or not, in the same species.

Work in different laboratories has led to the conclusion that the amino acid residues in a peptide hormone are not as a rule of equal importance for activity. Some residues may be replaced by a variety of others without drastic effects on activity, while even minor changes in other residues cause significant effects. This is not related to type of amino acid. In the same peptide a certain type of residue may have vastly different importance for activity depending on which position it occupies (178). Charged residues may prove more often important than non-charged residues since ion pair formation between hormone and receptor may be a common mechanism for hormone receptor interaction (179), but empirically it is known that in many peptides a charged group may be less important than a noncharged one. In short, there is at present no way of knowing by looking at the primary structure of a peptide which residues are important for activity and which are irrelevant. Perhaps this will change when the structures of the corresponding receptors eventually become known, but maybe not. In the meantime, the only way to estimate the importance of a certain residue is by synthesizing analogs of the hormone with the residue in question replaced by different amino acids. An enormous amount of such work has been carried out and has given much useful information. Nevertheless, the systematic investigation of the importance of each and every residue in a peptide of only 10 to 30 amino acid residues is so arduous as to be almost impossible, the more so as it often is important to investigate the effects of simultaneous changes in more than one position. Because of this, synthesis of analogs is usually based on guesswork or past experience. One way of making such guesses is to look at the sequences of closely related peptide hormones. For instance it may be reasonable to assume that residues that are identical in the different peptides may be of some special importance for activity. On the other hand correlation of differences in sequences with differences in activities may also give valuable information. VIP and secretin are chemically rather closely related and to some extent this is reflected in their biological activities. Both are related to glucagon, PHI (180), and the "gastric inhibitory" or "glucose dependent insulinotropic polypeptide" (GIP) (181, 182). These similarities may be seen in Table 1, where the sequences of the known secretins, VIPs, glucagons (183), and of porcine PHI are given in one-letter notation (184). The sequence of porcine motilin is also included in the table, and it may be seen that there is some slight similarity between it and the other peptide hormones listed. Motilin, however, seems to be structurally somewhat more closely related to gastrin (185) than to any of these peptides. Leaving motilin and GIP out of the discussion, it may be seen that the other eight peptides in Table 1 all have an N-terminal histidine, residues of phenylalanine in position 6, and threonine in position 7. These three identities are not very impressive, but if instead of looking at identities one focuses on amino acid residues of similar type it is seen that all the peptides have a residue of a hydroxy amino acid in position 11, a basic amino acid in position 12, and hydrophobic aliphatic amino acids in positions 19, 23, and 26.

If subgroups are examined, both identities and other similarities are much more pronounced. Except for PHI, all the peptides have serine in position 2 and either asparagine or glutamine in position 24. Comparing porcine glucagon with porcine secretin, there are 14 identities of 27 possible and four additional similarities, in positions 9, 12, 19, and 23. Such comparisons are not merely of academic interest. The identical N-terminal amino acid in all these peptides suggests that this histidine might be of some functional importance, and indeed it has been shown for both secretin (186, 187) and for glucagon (188) that its removal results in a marked decrease in hormonal activity. Nevertheless, the deshistidine hormones do exhibit some, about 1%, of the potencies of secretin and glucagon respectively and their efficacies are similar to those of the latter. It is often found that some particular amino acid residue is important for the action of a peptide hormone, but not essential. This seems to add weight to the suggestion that peptide hormones act by allosteric mechanisms (189) rather than by participating in reaction schemes. The common phenylalanine residue in position 6 has also been found to be quite important for the action of secretin since even substituting tyrosine for it results in a great decrease in potency (158, 190).

When the sequence of VIP was determined it was pointed out that since VIP and secretin both stimulate pancreatic secretion whereas glucagon does not, it could be of interest to investigate the importance of

TABLE 1 Amino Acid Sequences of VIP, Motilin, and Secretin[a]

Position markers: 1 ... 5 ... 10 ... 15 ... 20 ... 25 ... 30 ... 35 ... 40

	Sequence
1.	F V P I F T Y G E L Q R M Q E K E R N K G Q
2.	H S D G T F T S E L S R L R D S A R L Q R L L Q G L V
3.	H S D G L F T S E Y S K M R G N A Q V Q K F I Q N L M ■
4.	H S D A V F T D N Y T R L R K Q M A V K K Y L N S I L N ■
5.	H S D A V F T D N Y S R F R K Q M A V K K Y L N S V L T ■
6.	H S Q G T F T S D Y S K Y L D S R R A Q D F V Q W L M N T ■
7.	H S Q G T F T S D Y S K Y L D S R R A Q D F V Q W L M S T ■
8.	H S Q G T F T S D Y S K Y L D T R R A Q D F V Q W L M S T ■
9.	H A D G V F T S D F S R L L G Q L S A K K Y L E S L I ■
10.	Y A E G T F I S D Y S I A M D K I R Q Q D F V N W L L A Q K G K K S D W K H N I T Q

[a] 1, porcine motilin; 2, porcine/bovine secretin; 3, chicken secretin; 4, porcine/bovine VIP; 5, Chicken VIP; 6, mammalian glucagon; 7, turkey/chicken glucagon; 8, duck glucagon; 9, porcine PHI; 10, porcine GIP. Residues are given in one-letter notation (136). ■ indicates that the C-terminal residue is in alpha amide form. References to sequences are given in the text.

amino acid residues that are identical in secretin and VIP but different
in glucagon (29). The first such residue is found in position 3 where secretin and VIP both have aspartic acid but glucagon has glutamine. Synthetic work on secretin analogs has shown that residue number 3 is
indeed important for the bioactivity of secretin (157), as it is for the immunoreactivity of glucagon (191). On the other hand, it is quite clear
from the activities of natural substances isolated to date, that having, in
a heptacosapeptide amide, an N-terminal histidine, aspartic acid in position 3 and phenylalanine in position 6, as in secretin and VIP, is not
by itself enough to produce a substance with strong secretin-like activity. All these factors are present in PHI but PHI has only weak secretin-
like activity in the cat, although it does, like VIP, strongly stimulate avian pancreatic secretion (192). Clearly the synthesis of PHI analogs on
the basis of differences in activity between PHI and secretin may lead
to increased understanding of the structural requirements for secretin
activity. It might, for instance, be of interest to find out what effect the
replacement of Ala-2 in PHI with serine (as in secretin, glucagon, and
VIP) might have for the secretin-like activity of PHI or of Glu-24 by
Gln-24 (180).

Frandsen and Moody (193) found that VIP, like glucagon and secretin, has a lipolytic action on rat fat cells and that VIP does not interfere
with the action of glucagon. Desbuquois et al. found that VIP stimulates
adenylate cyclase in rat liver, and fat, cell membranes via receptors
distinct from glucagon receptors but possibly, although not necessarily,
identical to secretin receptors (194). Bataille et al. (195) came to the
same conclusion. Although pancreatic secretion of water and inorganic
electrolytes is mainly by the ductule cells and it is these cells that are
considered to be the main target for the action of secretin (155), it has
been shown that, in the guinea pig at least, the pancreatic acinar cells
too have receptors that react with secretin and with VIP but not with
glucagon. Moreover, these receptors most probably are of two distinct
types: one with a high affinity for VIP but a low affinity for secretin,
and another with a high affinity for secretin but a low affinity for VIP.
The high-affinity VIP receptors apparently differentiate between VIP
and secretin on the basis of structures in the N-terminal parts of the latter, since the C-terminal halves of VIP and of secretin were found to be
equipotent in inhibiting ^{125}I-VIP binding whereas the whole molecule of
VIP was 10,000 times more effective in this respect than the whole molecule of secretin (196). Further work suggested that VIP could stimulate
cAMP production by interacting with both the VIP-preferring and the
secretin-preferring receptors, whereas secretin, although interacting
with both types of receptors, could stimulate cAMP production only via
the secretin-preferring receptors (158). It was also found that secretin$_{5\text{-}27}$
antagonized the stimulation of cAMP production by secretin and by VIP
acting on the secretin-preferring receptor. Several component peptides
of VIP were also investigated for inhibitory effects but none were

found. Both halves of secretin and the N-terminal, but not the C-terminal half of VIP, were found to interact with the secretin receptor, cAMP production being slightly stimulated by the N-terminal half of secretin but not at all by the other two peptides. Further work in different laboratories has shown that VIP-preferring and secretin-preferring receptors are heterogeneously distributed among different tissues; some tissues have both types of receptors, others only the one or the other. The picture is further complicated by evidence suggesting that each receptor type may be heterogeneous in structure. An important finding for further work is the observation that the C-terminal uncosapeptide amide of porcine secretin, secretin$_{7-27}$, seems to be a specific antagonist of the secretin-preferring receptor and does not react at all with the VIP-preferring receptor, while the 5-valine analog of porcine secretin has a greater affinity than secretin for the VIP-preferring receptors (197). Interestingly, Val-5 secretin was found to be as strong as secretin in stimulating water secretion from the rat pancreas but distinctly weaker in stimulating potassium secretion (198). Clearly comparative detailed analyses in different biological systems of secretin and the various analogs of it that have recently been synthesized (198, 199) may be expected to give much interesting information.

Position 15 is interesting since porcine secretin, like glucagon, has an acidic residue here whereas VIP has a basic residue. Gardner et al. (200) found that replacing the Asp-15 in secretin by lysine rendered it more VIP-like in its reaction with pancreatic acinar cell receptors without making it less secretin-like. Using the Asn-15 analog of the peptide, it was found unexpectedly that it was sufficient to eliminate the negative charge on residue 15 for this change towards VIP-like activity to occur. It was not necessary to change the charge from minus to plus. It has also been shown that replacing Asp-15 by Asn-15 or Lys-15 in secretin$_{5-27}$ does not abolish the modest stimulatory activity of the peptide on the rat or guinea pig pancreatic secretion (201). Two experiments of nature may help to further elucidate the effects of changes in position 15. In both PHI and in chicken secretin there is a residue of the small neutral amino acid glycine instead of the aspartic acid residue found in porcine secretin, and chicken secretin has indeed been found to be somewhat VIP-like in its effect on the cat pancreas (26).

In the case of motilin, it was found that removal of its N-terminal pentapeptide decreased activity, measured as stimulation of rabbit duodenal motility *in vitro*, to about 2% of that of the intact molecule, and that removal of three additional amino acids abolished activity completely (202). Replacement of the glycine residue in position 8 by L-alanine decreased activity to 30% of that of motilin, whereas replacement with D-alanine increased it slightly above that of motilin (203).

The amino acid sequence does not describe all that may be of interest about a peptide's structure. Or perhaps it does, but we do not yet know how to interpret the information. Neither secretin, VIP, nor

motilin have been crystallized, at least not reproducibly, and consequently X-ray crystallographic analyses of them have not been carried
out; little indeed is known about their secondary or tertiary structures.
Nevertheless, measurements of optical rotatory dispersion and cyclic di-
chroism spectra indicate that porcine secretin is not wholly random coil
in aqueous solution; it has a modest but definite degree of ordered
structure. There seem to be two helical turns in the molecule, and since
there is no helical structure in the separated halves of secretin it has
been suggested that these two turns are in one-half of the chain and are
stabilized by a hydrophobic sequence in the other half, which bends
onto them. It is, however, not quite clear in which half of the molecule
the helices reside (204). It is tempting to speculate that such tertiary
structure is of importance for secretin activity since the isolated N-terminal half of secretin with its N-terminal histidine, aspartic acid in position 3, and phenylalanine in position 6, all known to be important for
activity, has only very weak activity. In VIP too, some degree of ordered structure seems to exist (205). Unlike secretin, VIP, and motilin,
glucagon crystallizes easily and the tertiary structure of crystalline glucagon has been determined by X-ray crystallography. Although this
structure evidently does not exist in aqueous solution it is believed to
form on interaction of the hormone with its receptor. Blundell et al.
(206) have suggested that such interaction might take place between
two hydrophobic areas located in the helical 6-27 sequence of glucagon
and corresponding hydrophobic areas on the receptor, leaving the flexible nonhelical 1–5 sequence of glucagon to the function of the hormone,
and that because of the similarities in the structures of glucagon, secretin, and VIP the interaction of secretin and VIP with their receptors
might take place in similar fashion.

9 SUMMARY AND CONCLUSIONS

Secretin has now been isolated from three species, two mammalian and
one avian. Of these, the porcine and bovine secretins are identical
open-chain heptacosapeptide amides. Chicken secretin is also a
heptacosapeptide amide but shows a marked degree of sequence dis-
similarity to the mammalian form. The immunochemical and chemical
evidence for the occurrence of secretin in the mammalian CNS is fairly
convincing, but it remains to be isolated from this source and sequenced. This applies also to precursor forms of secretin, the existence
of which is supported by immunochemical evidence. The main physiological action of secretin is still believed to be stimulation of pancreatic
secretion. There is, however, reason to believe that it may have other
important unidentified functions.

Motilin has been isolated and sequenced from only one species, the pig. It is a docosapeptide. Its presence in the brain, pituitary, and pineal gland is also based on immunochemical and suggestive chromatographical evidence only, as are the indications of its variability between mammalian species. There is no reason, however, to doubt this evidence. The extent to which interdigestive motility is regulated by motilin remains to be established.

VIP has been isolated from porcine and bovine upper intestine, chicken intestine, human colon, and porcine brain. The porcine (cerebral and intestinal) and the bovine peptides are octacosapeptide amides of identical sequence. The human material has the same amino acid composition as these and presumably the same sequence but this remains to be proved. Chicken VIP differs from the others by four conservative amino acid replacements.

More work is necessary to define which of the many actions of VIP are physiologically important and whether these or others of its actions may find useful pharmacological applications.

REFERENCES

1. F. Leuret and J.-L. Lassaigne, *Recherches Physiologiques et Chimiques pour Servir a l'Histoire de la Digestion*, Madame Huzard, Paris, 1825.
2. N. M. Becker, *Arch. Sci. Biol. St. Petersburg* **II**, 433 (1893).
3. M. J. Dolinsky, *Arch. Sci. Biol. St. Petersburg* **III**, 399 (1894).
4. W. M. Bayliss and E. H. Starling, *Proc. R. Soc.* **69**, 352 (1902).
5. W. M. Bayliss and E. H. Starling, *J. Physiol.* **28**, 325 (1902).
6. W. M. Bayliss, *Principles of General Physiology*, Longmans, Green, London, 1915.
7. A. C. Ivy, H. C. Lueth, and G. Kloster, *Proc. Soc. Exp. Biol. Med.* **26**, 309 (1929).
8. S. I. Said and V. Mutt, *Nature* **225**, 863 (1970).
9. S. I. Said and V. Mutt, *Science* **169**, 1217 (1970).
10. S. I. Said and V. Mutt, *Eur. J. Biochem.* **28**, 199 (1972).
11. L. Popielski, *Pflügers Arch. Physiol.* **128**, 191 (1909).
12. J. C. Brown, L. P. Johnson, and D. F. Magee, *Gastroenterology* **50**, 333 (1966).
13. J. C. Brown, *Gastroenterology* **52**, 225 (1967).
14. J. C. Brown and C. O. Parkes, *Gastroenterology* **53**, 731 (1967).
15. J. C. Brown, V. Mutt, and J. R. Dryburgh, *Can. J. Physiol. Pharmacol.* **49**, 399 (1971).
16. P. Mitznegg, S. R. Bloom, N. Christofides, H. Besterman, W. Domschke, S. Domschke, E. Wünsch, and L. Demling, *Scand. J. Gastroenterol.* **11**, Suppl. 39, 53 (1976).
17. U. Strunz, P. Mitznegg, W. Domschke, N. Subramanian, S. Domschke, and E. Wünsch, *Acta Hepato-Gastroenterol.* **24**, 456 (1977).
18. J. C. Brown and J. R. Dryburgh, in S. R. Bloom, Ed., *Gut Hormones*, Churchill Livingstone, Edinburgh, 1978, p. 327.
19. E. U. Still, *Physiol. Rev.* **11**, 328 (1931).
20. H. Greengard, in G. Pincus and K. V. Thimann, Eds., *The Hormones*, Vol. 1, Academic Press, New York, 1948, p. 201.
21. V. Mutt, *Arkiv Kemi* **15**, 75 (1959).

22. J. E. Jorpes, V. Mutt, S. Magnusson, and B. B. Steele, *Biochem. Biophys. Res. Comm.* **9**, 275 (1962).
23. J. C. Brown, M. A. Cook, and J. R. Dryburgh, *Gastroenterology* **62**, 401 (1972).
24. V. Mutt, J. E. Jorpes, and S. Magnusson, *Eur. J. Biochem.* **15**, 513 (1970).
25. M. Carlquist, H. Jörnvall, and V. Mutt, *FEBS Lett.* **127**, 71 (1981).
26. A. Nilsson, M. Carlquist, H. Jörnvall, and V. Mutt, *Eur. J. Biochem.* **112**, 383 (1980).
27. K. Tatemoto, in G. B. Glass, Ed., *Gastrointestinal Hormones*, Raven Press, New York, 1980, p. 975.
28. J. C. Mason, R. F. Murphy, R. W. Henry, and K. D. Buchanan, *Biochim. Biophys. Acta* **582**, 322 (1979).
29. V. Mutt and S. I. Said, *Eur. J. Biochem.* **42**, 581 (1974).
30. M. Carlquist, V. Mutt, and H. Jörnvall, *FEBS Lett.* **108**, 457 (1979).
31. M. Carlquist, T. J. McDonald, V. L. W. Go, D. Bataille, C. Johansson, and V. Mutt, *Horm. Metab. Res.* **14**, 28 (1982).
32. A. Nilsson, *FEBS Lett.* **60**, 322 (1975).
33. R. Dimaline and G. J. Dockray, *Gastroenterology* **75**, 387 (1978).
34. M. Maletti, J. Besson, D. Bataille, M. Laburthe, and G. Rosselin, *Acta Endocrinol.* **93**, 479 (1980).
35. K. Yamaguchi, K. Abe, S. Miyakawa, S. Ohnami, M. Sakagami, and N. Yanaihara, *Gastroenterology* **79**, 687 (1980).
36. K. Obata, N. Itoh, H. Okamoto, C. Yanaihara, N. Yanaihara, and T. Suzuki, *FEBS Lett.* **136**, 123 (1981).
37. J. C. Brown, M. A. Cook, and J. R. Dryburgh, *Can. J. Biochem.* **51**, 533 (1973).
38. H. Schubert and J. C. Brown, *Can. J. Biochem.* **52**, 7 (1974).
39. N. D. Christofides, M. G. Bryant, M. A. Ghatei, S. Kishimoto, A. M. J. Buchan, J. M. Polak, and S. R. Bloom, *Gastroenterology* **80**, 292 (1981).
40. T. L. O'Donohue, M. C. Beinfeld, W. Y. Chey, T.-M. Chang, G. Nilaver, E. A. Zimmerman, H. Yajima, H. Adachi, M. Poth, R. P. McDevitt, and D. M. Jacobowitz, *Peptides* **2**, 467 (1981).
41. E. Solcia, G. Vassallo, and C. Capella, in W. Creutzfeldt, Ed., *Origin, Chemistry, Physiology and Pathophysiology of Gastrointestinal Hormones*, F. K. Schattauer Verlag, Stuttgart, 1970, p. 3.
42. G. Bussolati, C. Capella, E. Solcia, G. Vassallo, and P. Vezzadini, *Histochemie* **26**, 218 (1971).
43. J. M. Polak, S. Bloom, I. Coulling, and A. G. E. Pearse, *Gut* **12**, 605 (1971).
44. L.-I. Larsson, F. Sundler, J. Alumets, R. Håkanson, O. B. Schaffalitzky de Muckadell, and J. Fahrenkrug, *Cell Tissue Res.* **181**, 361 (1977).
45. V. Mutt, M. Carlquist, and K. Tatemoto, *Life Sci.* **25**, 1703 (1979).
46. T. L. O'Donohue, C. G. Charlton, R. L. Miller, G. Boden, and D. M. Jacobowitz, *Proc. Natl. Acad. Sci. USA* **78**, 5221 (1981).
47. A. G. E. Pearse, J. M. Polak, S. R. Bloom, C. Adams, J. R. Dryburgh, and J. C. Brown, *Virchows Arch. B, Cell. Path.* **16**, 111 (1974).
48. J. M. Polak, P. Heitz, and A. G. E. Pearse, *Scand. J. Gastroenterol.* **11**, Suppl. 39, 39 (1976).
49. P. Heitz, J. M. Polak, and A. G. E. Pearse, in S. R. Bloom, Ed., *Gut Hormones*, Churchill Livingstone, Edinburgh, 1978, p. 332.
50. V. Helmstaedter, W. Kreppein, W. Domschke, P. Mitznegg, N. Yanaihara, E. Wünsch, and W. G. Forssmann, *Gastroenterology* **76**, 897 (1979).
51. J. M. Polak and A. M. J. Buchan, *Gastroenterology* **76**, 1065 (1979).
52. P. Leduque, C. Paulin, J. A. Chayvialle, and P. M. Dubois, *Cell Tissue Res.* **218**, 519 (1981).
53. W. Y. Chey, R. Escoffery, F. Roth, T. M. Chang, C. H. You, and H. Yajima, *Regul. Pept.* **1** Suppl. 1, S19 (1980).

54. D. M. Jacobowitz, T. L. O'Donohue, W. Y. Chey, and T.-M. Chang, *Peptides* **2**, 479 (1981).

55. C. Yanaihara, H. Sato, N. Yanaihara, S. Naruse, W. G. Forssmann, V. Helmstaedter, T. Fujita, K. Yamaguchi, and K. Abe, *Adv. Exp. Med. Biol.* **106**, 269 (1977).

56. J. M. Polak, A. G. E. Pearse, J.-C. Garaud, and S. R. Bloom, *Gut* **15**, 720 (1974).

57. L.-I. Larsson, J. M. Polak, R. Buffa, F. Sundler, and E. Solcia, *J. Histochem. Cytochem.* **27**, 936 (1979).

58. L.-I. Larsson, in S. I. Said, Ed., *Vasoactive Intestinal Peptide*, Raven Press, New York, 1982, p. 51.

59. J. M. Lundberg, A. Änggård, J. Fahrenkrug, O. Johansson, and T. Hökfelt, in S. I. Said, Ed., *Vasoactive Intestinal Peptide*, Raven Press, New York, 1982, p. 373.

60. M. G. Bryant, J. M. Polak, F. Modlin, S. R. Bloom, R. H. Albuquerque, and A. G. E. Pearse, *Lancet* **1**, 991 (1976).

61. L.-I. Larsson, J. Fahrenkrug, O. B. Schaffalitzky de Muckadell, F. Sundler, R. Håkanson, and J. F. Rehfeld, *Proc. Natl. Acad. Sci. USA* **73**, 3197 (1976).

62. S. I. Said and R. N. Rosenberg, *Science* **192**, 907 (1976).

63. S. I. Said, in G. B. J. Glass, Ed., *Gastrointestinal Hormones*, Raven Press, New York, 1980, p. 245.

64. S. I. Said, S. R. Bloom and J. M. Polak, Eds., in *Gut Hormones*, 2nd ed., Churchill Livingstone, Edinburgh, 1981, p. 379.

65. P. C. Emson, S. P. Hunt, J. F. Rehfeld, N. Golterman, and J. Fahrenkrug, in E. Costa and M. Trabucchi, Eds., *Neural Peptides and Neuronal Communication*, Raven Press, New York, 1980, p. 63.

66. W. K. Samson, S. I. Said, J. W. Graham, and S. M. McCann, *Lancet* **2**, 901 (1978).

67. R. Dimaline, C. Vaillant, and G. J. Dockray, *Regul. Pept.* **1**, 1 (1980).

68. M. Carlquist, H. Jörnvall, K. Tatemoto, and V. Mutt, *Gastroenterology* **83**, 245 (1982).

69. U.S. v. Euler, *Arch. Exp. Pathol. Pharmakol.* **181**, 181 (1936).

70. M. M. Chang, S. E. Leeman, and H. D. Niall, *Nature New Biol.* **232**, 86 (1971).

71. R. Carraway and S. E. Leeman, *J. Biol. Chem.* **254**, 2944 (1979).

72. R. O. Studer, A. Trzeciak, and W. Lergier, *Helv. Chim. Acta* **56**, 860 (1973).

73. R. Carraway, P. Kitabgi, and S. E. Leeman, *J. Biol. Chem.* **253**, 7996 (1978).

74. J. J. Vanderhaeghen, J. C. Signeau, and W. Gepts, *Nature* **257**, 604 (1975).

75. N. S. Track, J. E. T. Fox, E. E. Daniel, and S. Falkmer in N. Basso, E. Lezoche, V. Speranza, and J. H. Walsh, Eds., *Abstracts, International Symposium on Brain-Gut Axis*, 1981, p. 187.

76. V. Chan-Palay, G. Nilaver, S. L. Palay, M. C. Beinfeld, E. A. Zimmerman, J.-Y. Wu, and T. L. O'Donohue, *Proc. Natl. Acad. Sci. USA* **78**, 7787 (1981).

77. J. Mellanby, *J. Physiol.* **61**, 419 (1926).

78. R. A. Gregory and H. J. Tracy, *Gut* **5**, 103 (1964).

79. R. A. Gregory, *J. Physiol.* **241**, 1 (1974).

80. M. Vagne and M.-C. Fargier, *Gastroenterology* **65**, 757 (1973).

81. K. Kowalewski, T. Pachkowski, and A. Kolodej, *Pharamacology*, **16**, 78 (1978).

82. H. W. Baenkler, P. Mitznegg, S. Domschke, E. Wunsch, N. Subramanian, W. Domschke, R. Bötticher, W. Sprügel, and L. Demling, *Lancet* **1**, 928 (1977).

83. G. L. Ricci and J. Fevery, *Biochem. J.* **182**, 881 (1979).

84. L. R. Johnson and P. D. Guthrie, *Proc. Soc. Exp. Biol. Med.* **158**, 521 (1978).

85. H. Petersen, T. E. Solomon, and M. I. Grossman, *Gastroenterology* **76**, 790 (1979).

86. R. Sethi, S. C. Kukreja, E. N. Bowser, G. K. Hargis, and G. A. Williams, *J. Clin. Endocrinol. Metab.* **53**, 153 (1981).

87. M. I. Grossman, *Fed. Proc.* **36**, 1930 (1977).

88. R. W. Henry, R. W. J. Flanagan, and K. D. Buchanan, *Lancet* **2**, 202 (1975).

89.   R. Dimaline and G. J. Dockray, *J. Physiol.* **294**, 153 (1979).
90.   S. I. Said, Ed., *Vasoactive Intestinal Peptide*, Raven Press, New York, 1982.
91.   J. C. D. Hickson, *J. Physiol.* **206**, 299 (1970).
92.   J. Fahrenkrug, O. B. Schaffalitzky de Muckadell, J. J. Holst, and S. L. Jensen, *Am. J. Physiol.* **237**, E535 (1979).
93.   S. Domschke and W. Domschke, in S. I. Said, Ed., *Vasoactive Intestinal Peptide*, Raven Press, New York, 1982, p. 201.
94.   S. J. Konturek, A. Dembiński, P. Thor, and R. Król. *Pflügers Arch.* **361**, 175 (1976).
95.   M. Vagne, S. J. Konturek, and J. A. Chayvialle, *Gastroenterology* **83**, 250 (1982).
96.   M. Holm-Bentzen, J. Christiansen, B. Petersen, J. Fahrenkrug, A. Schultz, and P. Kirkegaard. *Scand. J. Gastroenterol.* **16**, 429 (1981).
97.   R. Heidenhain, *Pflügers* Arch. **5**, 309 (1872).
98.   S. R. Bloom and A. V. Edwards, *J. Physiol.* **295**, 35P (1979).
99.   R. Uddman, J. Fahrenkrug, L. Malm, J. Alumets, R. Håkanson, and F. Sundler, *Acta Physiol. Scand.* **110**, 31 (1980).
100. T. Shimizu and N. Taira, *Br. J. Pharmacol.* **65**, 683 (1979).
101. J. M. Lundberg, B. Hedlund, and T. Bartfai, *Nature* **295**, 147 (1982).
102. J. Fahrenkrug, in S. I. Said, Ed., *Vasoactive Intestinal Peptide*, Raven Press, New York, 1982, p. 361.
103. B. Ottesen and J. Fahrenkrug, *Acta Physiol. Scand.* **112**, 195 (1981).
104. M. A. Wasserman, R. L. Griffin, and P. E. Malo, in S. I. Said, Ed., *Vasoactive Intestinal Peptide*, Raven Press, New York, 1982, p. 177.
105. S. I. Said, A. Geumei, and N. Hara, in S. I. Said, Ed., *Vasoactive Intestinal Peptide*, Raven Press, New York, 1982, p. 185.
106. T. C. Smitherman, H. Sakio, A. M. Geumei, T. Yoshida, M. Oyamada, and S. I. Said, in S. I. Said, Ed., *Vasoactive Intestinal Peptide*, Raven Press, New York, 1982, p. 169.
107. J. B. Furness and M. Costa, in S. I. Said, Ed., *Vasoactive Intestinal Peptide*, Raven Press, New York, 1982, p. 391.
108. G. M. Makhlouf, in S. I. Said, Ed., *Vasoactive Intestinal Peptide*, Raven Press, New York, 1982, p. 425.
109. S. R. Bloom and J. M. Polak, in S. I. Said, Ed., *Vasoactive Intestinal Peptide*, Raven Press, New York, 1982, p. 457.
110. G. J. Krejs, in S. I. Said, Ed., *Vasoactive Intestinal Peptide*, Raven Press, New York, 1982, p. 193.
111. Z. C. Wu, T. M. O'Dorisio, S. Cataland, H. S. Mekhjian, and T. S. Gaginella, *Dig. Dis. Sci.* **24**, 625 (1979).
112. D. B. Waldman, J. D. Gardner, A. M. Zfass, and G. M. Makhlouf, *Gastroenterology* **73**, 518 (1977).
113. S. J. Konturek, A. Dembinski, R. Król, and E. Wünsch, *Scand. J. Gastroenterol.* **11**, Suppl. 39, 57 (1976).
114. S. Domschke, W. Domschke, B. Schmack, F. Tympner, O. Junge, E. Wunsch, E. Jaeger, and L. Demling, *Am. J. Dig. Dis.* **21**, 789 (1976).
115. C. H. S. McIntosh and J. C. Brown, in G. B. J. Glass, Ed., *Gastrointestinal Hormones*, Raven Press, New York, 1980, p. 233.
116. U. Strunz, W. Domschke, P. Mitznegg, S. Domschke, E. Schubert, E. Wunsch, E. Jaeger, and L. Demling, *Gastroenterology* **68**, 1485 (1975).
117. J. H. Szurszewski, *Am. J. Physiol.* **217**, 1757 (1969).
118. G. R. Vantrappen, T. L. Peeters, and J. Janssens, *Scand. J. Gastroenterol.* **14**, 663 (1979).
119. H. Ruppin, H. H. Thompson, D. L. Wingate, and E. Wünsch, *J. Physiol.* **263**, 225P (1976).
120. Z. Itoh, R. Honda, K. Hiwatashi, S. Takeuchi, I. Aizawa, R. Takayanagi, and E. F. Couch, *Scand. J. Gastroenterol.* **11**, Suppl. 39, 93 (1976).

121. C. H. You, W. Y. Chey, and K. Y. Lee, *Gastroenterology* **79**, 62 (1980).
122. P. A. Thomas, K. A. Kelly, and V. L. W. Go, *Dig. Dis. Sci.* **24**, 577 (1979).
123. P. Poitras, J. H. Steinbach, G. VanDeventer, C. F. Code, and J. H. Walsh, *Am. J. Physiol.* **239**, G215 (1980).
124. L. I. Larsson, *Histochemistry* **54**, 173 (1977).
125. P. C. Emson, J. Fahrenkrug, O. B. Schaffalitzky de Muckadell, T. M. Jessell, and L. L. Iversen, *Brain Res.* **143**, 174 (1978).
126. J. M. Lundberg, J. Fahrenkrug, and S. Brimijoin, *Acta Physiol. Scand.* **112**, 427 (1981).
127. J. T. Williams and R. A. North, *Brain Res.* **175**, 174 (1979).
128. J. W. Phillis and J. R. Kirkpatrick, *Can. J. Physiol. Pharmacol.* **57**, 887 (1979).
129. J. W. Phillis and J. R. Kirkpatrick, *Can. J. Physiol. Pharmacol.* **58**, 612 (1980).
130. V. Chan-Palay, M. Ito, P. Tongroach, M. Sakurai, and S. Palay. *Proc. Natl. Acad. Sci. USA* **79**, 3355 (1982).
131. K. Fuxe, K. Andersson, T. Hökfelt, V. Mutt, L. Ferland, L. F. Agnati, D. Ganten, S. Said, P. Eneroth, and J.-Å. Gustafsson, *Fed. Proc.* **38**, 2333 (1979).
132. K. Fuxe, K. Andersson, V. Locatelli, L. F. Agnati, V. Mutt, and P. Eneroth, in E. E. Müller, Ed., *Neuroactive Drugs in Endocrinology*, Elsevier/North-Holland Biomedical Press, Amsterdam, 1980, p. 149.
133. Y. Kato, Y. Iwasaki, J. Iwasaki, H. Abe, N. Yanaihara, and H. Imura, *Endocrinology* **103**, 554 (1978).
134. S. I. Said and J. C. Porter, *Life Sci.* **24**, 227 (1979).
135. E. Vijayan, W. K. Samson, S. I. Said, and S. M. McCann, *Endocrinology* **104**, 53 (1979).
136. M. Ruberg, W. H. Rotsztejn, S. Arancibia, J. Besson, and A. Enjalbert, *Eur. J. Pharmacol.* **51**, 319 (1978).
137. C. J. Shaar, J. A. Clemens, and N. B. Dininger, *Life Sci.* **25**, 2071 (1979).
138. A. Enjalbert, S. Arancibia, M. Ruberg, M. Priam, M. T. Bluet-Pajot, W. H. Rotsztejn, and C. Kordon, *Neuroendocrinology* **31**, 200 (1980).
139. J. Epelbaum, L. Tapia-Arancibia, J. Besson, W. H. Rotsztejn, and C. Kordon, *Eur. J. Pharmacol.* **58**, 493 (1979).
140. W. K. Samson, K. P. Burton, J. P. Reeves, and S. M. McCann, *Regul. Pept.* **2** 253 (1981).
141. S. Nicosia, A. Spada, C. Borghi, L. Cortelazzi, and G. Giannattasio, *FEBS Lett.* **112**, 159 (1980).
142. W. B. Malarkey, T. M. O'Dorisio, M. Kennedy, and S. Cataland, *Life Sci.* **28**, 2489 (1981).
143. D. Bataille, J.-N. Talbot, G. Milhaud, V. Mutt, and G. Rosselin, *C.R. Acad. Sci. Paris, Ser. III* **292**, 511 (1981).
144. R. S. Birnbaum, M. Alfonzo, and J. Kowal, *Endocrinology* **106**, 1270 (1980).
145. B. Ahrén, J. Alumets, M. Ericsson, J. Fahrenkrug, L. Fahrenkrug, R. Håkanson, P. Hedner, I. Loren, A. Melander, C. Rerup, and F. Sundler, *Nature* **287**, 343 (1980).
146. S. Van Noorden, J. M. Polak, S. R. Bloom, and M. G. Bryant, *Neuropathol. Appl. Neurobiol.* **5**, 149 (1979).
147. A. M. Ebeid, J. Escourrou, P. Murray, and J. E. Fischer, in S. R. Bloom, Ed., *Gut Hormones*, Churchill Livingstone, Edinburgh, 1978, p. 479.
148. K. N. Bitar, S. I. Said, G. C. Weir, B. Saffouri, and G. M. Makhlouf, *Gastroenterology* **79**, 1288 (1980).
149. D. Van Calker, M. Müller, and B. Hamprecht, *Proc. Natl. Acad. Sci. USA* **77**, 6907 (1980).
150. P. J. Magistretti, J. H. Morrison, W. J. Shoemaker, V. Sapin, and F. E. Bloom, *Proc. Natl. Acad. Sci. USA* **78**, 6535 (1981).
151. L. Edvinsson, in S. I. Said, Ed., *Vasoactive Intestinal Peptide*, Raven Press, New York, 1982, p. 149.

152. R. J. Traystman, H. A. Kontos, and D. D. Heistad, in S. I. Said, Ed., *Vasoactive Intestinal Peptide*, Raven Press, New York, 1982, p. 161.
153. R. M. Case, T. J. Laundy, and T. Scratcherd, *J. Physiol.* **204**, 45P (1969).
154. R. M. Case, M. Johnson, T. Scratcherd, and H. S. A. Sherratt, *J. Physiol.* **223**, 669 (1972).
155. U. R. Fölsch, H. Fischer, H.-D. Söling, and W. Creutzfeldt, *Digestion* **20**, 277 (1980).
156. E. W. Sutherland and T. W. Rall, *Pharmacol. Rev.* **12**, 265 (1960).
157. E. Wünsch, E. Jaeger, L. Moroder, and I. Schulz, in S. Bonfils, P. Fromageot, and G. Rosselin, Eds., *Hormonal Receptors in Digestive Tract Physiology*, Elsevier/North-Holland Biomedical Press, Amsterdam, 1977, p. 19.
158. P. Robberecht, T. P. Conlon, and J. D. Gardner, *J. Biol. Chem.* **251**, 4635 (1976).
159. C. Gespach, D. Bataille, C. Dupont, G. Rosselin, E. Wünsch, and E. Jaeger, *Biochim. Biophys. Acta* **630**, 433 (1980).
160. B. Simon and H. Kather, *Gastroenterology* **74**, 722 (1978).
161. B. Amiranoff and G. Rosselin, in S. I. Said, Ed., *Vasoactive Intestinal Peptide*, Raven Press, New York, 1982, p. 307.
162. M. Deschodt-Lanckman, P. Robberecht, and J. Christophe, *FEBS Lett.* **83**, 76 (1977).
163. T. Kaneko, S. Nakaya, S. Saito, N. Yanaihara, and H. Oka, *Endocrinol. Jpn.* **27**, Suppl., 7 (1980).
164. M. Quik, L. L. Iversen, and S. R. Bloom, *Biochem. Pharmacol* **27**, 2209 (1978).
165. C. Borghi, S. Nicosia, A. Giachetti, and S. I. Said, *Life Sci.* **24**, 65 (1979).
166. P. Robberecht, P. De Neef, M. Lammens, M. Deschodt-Lanckman, and J.-P. Christophe, *Eur. J. Biochem.* **90**, 147 (1978).
167. D. P. Taylor and C. B. Pert, *Proc. Natl. Acad. Sci. USA* **76**, 660 (1979).
168. H. Kather and B. Simon, *FEBS Lett.* **100**, 145 (1979).
169. M. Bodanszky, Y.S. Klausner, and S. I. Said, *Proc. Natl. Acad. Sci. USA* **70**, 382 (1973).
170. M. L. Cohen and A. S. Landry, *Life Sci.* **26**, 811 (1980).
171. G. Burnstock, T. Cocks, and R. Crowe, *Br. J. Pharmacol.* **64**, 13 (1978).
172. A. Gibson and J. F. Tucker, *Br. J. Pharmacol.* **77**, 97 (1982).
173. I. MacKenzie and G. Burnstock, *Eur. J. Pharmacol.* **67**, 255 (1980).
174. J. T. Williams and R. A. North, *Brain Res.* **175**, 174 (1979).
175. W. H. Rotsztejn, J. Besson, B. Briaud, L. Gagnant, G. Rosselin, and C. Kordon, *Neuroendocrinology* **31**, 287 (1980).
176. T. N. Keltz, E. Straus, and R. S. Yalow, *Biochem. Biophys. Res. Commun.* **92**, 669 (1980).
177. E. Schubert, P. Mitznegg, U. Strunz, W. Domschke, S. Domschke, E. Wünsch, E. Jaeger, L. Demling, and F. Heim, *Life Sci.* **16**, 263 (1974).
178. J. Rudinger, in *Endocrinology 1971*, W. Heinemann, London, 1972, p. 12.
179. M. Bodanszky, in W. Y. Chey and F. P. Brooks, Eds., *Endocrinology of the Gut*, Charles B. Slack, Thorofare, N.J., 1974, p. 3.
180. K. Tatemoto and V. Mutt, *Proc. Natl. Acad. Sci. USA* **78**, 6603 (1981).
181. J. C. Brown, J. L. Frost, S. Kwauk, S. C. Otte, and C. H. S. McIntosh, in G. B. J. Glass, Ed., *Gastrointestinal Hormones*, Raven Press, New York, 1980, p. 223.
182. H. Jörnvall, M. Carlquist, S. Kwauk, S. C. Otte, C. H. S. McIntosh, J. C. Brown, and V. Mutt, *FEBS Lett.* **123**, 205 (1981).
183. H. G. Pollock and J. R. Kimmel, *J. Biol. Chem.* **250**, 9377 (1975).
184. IUPAC-IUB Commission on Biochemical Nomenclature (CBN), *Eur. J. Biochem.* **5**, 151 (1968).
185. N. S. Track, in N. S. Track, Ed., *Endocrinology of the Gut*, McMaster University Symposium, Hamilton, Canada, 1976, p. 126.
186. V. Mutt and J. E. Jorpes, *Rec. Prog. Horm. Res.* **23**, 483 (1967).
187. T. E. Solomon, H. C. Beyerman, and M. I. Grossman, *Clin. Res.* **25**, A574 (1977).
188. M. C. Lin, D. E. Wright, V. J. Hruby, and M. Rodbell, *Biochemistry* **14**, 1559 (1975).

189. J. Monod, J.-P. Changeux, and F. Jacob, *J. Mol. Biol.* **6**, 306 (1963).
190. W. Y. Chey and J. Hendricks, in W. Y. Chey and F. P. Brooks, Eds., *Endocrinology of the Gut*, Charles B. Slack, Thorofare, N.J., 1974, p. 107.
191. D. E. Wright and M. Rodbell, *J. Biol. Chem.* **254**, 268 (1979).
192. R. Dimaline and G. J. Dockray, *Regul. Pept.* Suppl. 1, S27 (1980).
193. E. K. Frandsen and A. J. Moody, *Horm. Metab. Res.* **5**, 196 (1973).
194. B. Desbuquois, M. H. Laudat, and P. Laudat, *Biochem. Biophys. Res. Commun.* **53**, 1187 (1973).
195. D. Bataille, P. Freychet, and G. Rosselin, *Endocrinology* **95**, 713 (1974).
196. J. P. Christophe, T. P. Conlon, and J. D. Gardner, *J. Biol. Chem.* **251**, 4629 (1976).
197. P. Robberecht, P. Chatelain, M. Waelbroeck, and J. Christophe, in S. I. Said, Ed., *Vasoactive Intestinal Peptide*, Raven Press, New York, 1982, p. 323.
198. M. Adler, M. Mestdagh, P. De Neef, W. König, J. Christophe, and P. Robberecht, *Life Sci.* **26**, 1175 (1980).
199. L. Moroder, E. Jaeger, F. Drees, M. Gemeiner, S. Knof, H.-P. Stelzel, P. Thamm, D. Bataille, S. Domschke, W. Schlegel, I. Schulz, and E. Wünsch, *Bioorg. Chem.* **9**, 27 (1980).
200. J. D. Gardner, A. J. Rottman, M. L. Fink, S. Natarajan, and M. Bodanszky, *Endocrinol. Jpn.* **27**, Suppl. 1 (1980).
201. G. M. Makhlouf, M. Bodanszky, M. L. Fink, and M. Schebalin, *Gastroenterology* **75**, 244 (1978).
202. H. Yajima, Y. Kai, H. Ogawa, M. Kubota, Y. Mori, and K. Koyama, *Gastroenterology* **72**, 793 (1977).
203. S. Shinagawa, M. Fujino, H. Yajima, T. Segawa, and Y. Okuma, *Chem. Pharm. Bull.* **26**, 880 (1978).
204. M. Bodanszky, M. L. Fink, K. W. Funk, and S. I. Said, *Clin. Endocrin.* **5**, Suppl., 195s (1976).
205. M. Bodanszky, A. Bodanszky, Y. S. Klausner, and S. I. Said, *Bioorg. Chem.* **3**, 133 (1974).
206. T. L. Blundell, S. Dockerill, K. Sasaki, I. J. Tickle, and S. P. Wood, *Metabolism* **25**, Suppl. 1, 1331 (1976).

36

Insulin in the Nervous System

S. ANNE HENDRICKS

JESSE ROTH

Diabetes Branch
NIADDK, National Institutes of Health
Bethesda, Maryland

SURENDRA RISHI

KENNETH L. BECKER

Department of Medicine
Veterans Administration Hospital and George Washington University
Washington, D.C.

There has been considerable recent interest in the relationships of insulin to the nervous system, although many details are still lacking. In this chapter, to clarify the current work in this area and to provide a framework for future work, we recurrently compare the insulin-related components in the nervous system to their counterparts elsewhere. The chapter will cover (i) an introduction to classical insulin; (ii) evolutionary origins of insulin, especially the neurobiology of insulin in insects; (iii) insulin in the peripheral nerves and brain of mammals in comparison with other extrapancreatic tissues; (iv) insulin in cerebrospinal fluid and other fluid compartments; (v) possible extrapancreatic synthesis of insulin; (vi) insulin receptors in brain and elsewhere; (vii) insulin action on target cells in general with applications to events in the central nervous system.

1   AN INTRODUCTION TO INSULIN

It has been widely believed that insulin is produced solely in the β-cells of vertebrate pancreas, but the current state of affairs is not so simple. Over the last decade, evidence has accumulated that insulin may be produced by organisms that lack pancreatic islet cells (1–8) and, in vertebrates, by extra-pancreatic tissues including nerve cells (9–13, 39–41). To begin, it might be instructive to ask, what is insulin? While all readers intuitively know what insulin is, operationally insulin is a peptide of relatively low molecular weight that causes hypoglycemia *in vivo* (or related metabolic events in insulin-sensitive tissues *in vitro*) and is present in very large amounts in the pancreas of any vertebrate. The structures of insulins from 40 different vertebrate species have been determined (14). All of them have molecular weights of about 6000 daltons and typically consist of an A chain with 21 amino acids connected by two disulfide bridges to a B chain of approximately 30 amino acids (Figure 1). Among species, insulins may differ by 0–40% in amino acid sequence (14, 15).

1.1 Insulin Bioactivity

All insulins are bioactive in all species in which they have been tested but differ by up to 100-fold in biological potencies (16–21). The differences in biopotency are due to differences in affinity for the insulin receptor (20). The insulin receptors are the same in all tissues of one organism and are much more highly conserved over the course of vertebrate evolution than are the insulins—the insulin receptors of all species tested bind chicken insulin > pork insulin > guinea pig insulin (17, 18). Thus in most species the affinity of the endogenous insulin for the endogenous insulin receptor is less than that of another known insulin, for example chicken insulin.

1.2 Insulin Immunoactivity

The most remarkable feature of an insulin immunoassay is its exceptional specificity. The typical immunoassay uses antibodies produced in guinea pigs against a common mammalian insulin such as porcine insulin (19). The antiporcine insulin antibodies react strongly with insulin and insulin precursors from the pig or with structurally similar insulins but react much less strongly with insulins that differ in a number of amino acids. Some insulins are totally unreactive in this immunoassay, most notably the insulins of guinea pigs and their relatives. To be reactive, a molecule must have an A chain and a B chain linked by disulfide bonds; the A chain and B chain alone or together have little, if any, reactivity (20). Furthermore, homologies in amino acid sequence must be 70% or more; guinea pig insulin with a 65% homology has negligible reactivity (15, 20, 21). Thus, reactivity in the immunoassay for insulin is dependent on structural homology and integrity and is largely independent of bioactivity.

1.3 Biosynthetic Precursors of Insulin

Insulin is synthesized as a 12,000 dalton molecular weight precursor (preproinsulin) that is converted very quickly to an intermediate-sized precursor (proinsulin) by removal of a signal sequence at the N-terminus (22). Preproinsulin has such an evanescent existence that it need not be considered further in our discussion. Proinsulin is cleaved at two sites to produce insulin (Figure 1). The conversion of proinsulin to insulin results in a 20-fold increase in biological activity and a fewfold increase

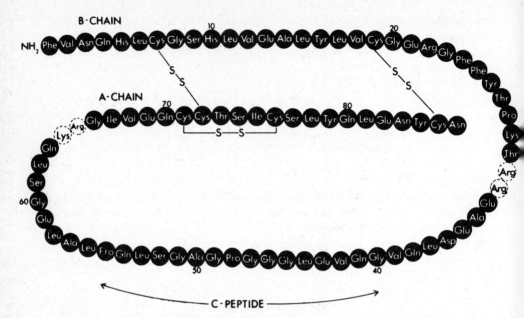

Figure 1. Structure of human proinsulin. The length of both the A chain (21 amino acids) and the B chain (30 amino acids) are the same in nearly all known insulins. Of the 51 amino acids in the insulin portion of the molecule, 19 are invariant in all species sequenced to date.

in immunological activity (4). Proinsulin and proinsulin intermediates (i.e., cleaved at either one of the two sites) represent a minority of the total insulin-related materials that are found in biological fluids and in pancreas (22).

1.4   Plasma Insulin and Tissue Insulin

When we and others discuss "insulin" in situations in which we do not have a purified protein and a defined amino acid sequence, such as in plasma and other biological fluids as well as in extracts of brain and other extrapancreatic tissues, we intend to indicate materials that have properties that closely resemble those of purified pancreatic insulins of common vertebrates. As a minimum this represents specific reactivity in the radioimmunoassay (19). In our work, "insulin" indicates material that has activity in standard insulin immunoassays, that migrates on gel chromatography in the region typical of genuine insulin (Figure 2A inset), that reacts with insulin receptors and produces appropriate metabolic responses when interacted with fat cells of young rats (Figure 2, B and C), and that has its biological activity neutralized or removed by interaction with anti-insulin antibodies, indicating that the immunological and biological recognition sites are harbored on a single molecular

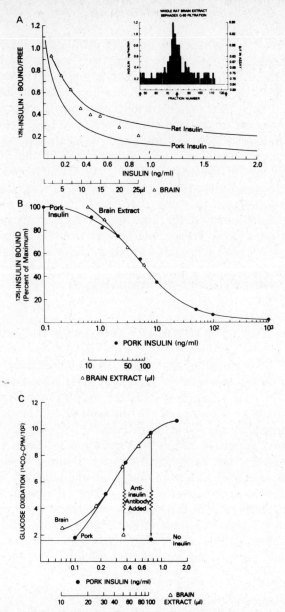

Figure 2. Characterization of brain insulin. (A) Acid ethanol extracts of rat brain ($\triangle$), on serial dilution in the radioimmunoassay, yielded results similar to (but not identical with) purified rat and pork insulin, designated by smooth curves. When the brain extract was gel filtered (A, inset), the immunoactive insulin (solid bars) was largely recovered as a peak in the region typical of insulin (marked by the middle arrow; the other two arrows mark the location of the void and iodide peaks). The effluent fractions corresponding to the insulin region were pooled and lyophilized. (B) This rat brain material ($\triangle$) was indistinguishable from purified pork insulin ($\bigcirc$) in the radioreceptor assay (^{125}I-insulin binding to insulin receptors of IM-9 lymphocytes) or (C) bioassay (stimulation of glucose oxidation in rat adipocytes). In (C), note also that antibodies to insulin neutralized the bioactivity of both the brain insulin and purified pork insulin. From Havrankova, et al. (9).

species (Figure 2C). Furthermore, possible artifacts in each of the methods are systematically excluded. While this "insulin" is indistinguishable from purified insulins by the methods employed, we have not yet defined precisely the resemblance of these materials to the purified insulins isolated from pancreas. However, the specific reactivity of these materials in the immunoassay distinguishes them from noninsulins such as the insulin-like growth factors,* and their elution position on gel chromatography distinguishes them from proinsulin and other high-molecular-weight insulin precursors. The similarity of these materials to the insulins of vertebrates is heightened by the finding that their reactivity with insulin receptors and their bioactivity are reasonably predicted by their immunoactivity, and their bioactivity is neutralized by anti-insulin antibodies. If these materials are not insulin (or insulin with one or two additional amino acids at one end of the A chain or B chain or both), they more closely resemble the purified and sequenced insulins than any other molecules yet described.

2   THE EVOLUTIONARY ORIGIN OF INSULIN

Beta cells, islets, and pancreas make their evolutionary debut in the earliest vertebrates. Neurons first appear in early multicellular invertebrates. Yet material exceedingly similar to vertebrate-type insulins is present in bacteria (*Escherichia coli*) as well as in unicellular protozoa (*Tetrahymena pyriformis*) and unicellular fungi (*Aspergillus* and *Neurospora*); when grown in totally synthetic media, both the organisms and the conditioned culture medium contain the insulin-related material (2, 3). Similar material has been found in annelids, molluscs, insects, and other multicellular invertebrates (4–8). The best characterized chemically is the insulin of the blowfly, which has been purified extensively in multiple systems and for which the amino acid composition has been determined (31). The amino acid composition of another insulin of an insect, the tobacco hornworm, has also been determined (32).

---

*The insulin-like growth factors, or somatomedins, have by definition, insulin-like biological properties and are devoid of reactivity with anti-insulin antibodies. Because they have a reduced affinity for the insulin receptor and are largely bound to plasma proteins, the insulin-like metabolic effects that they exert *in vivo* are slight despite their high concentrations (23–25). Two of these, designated human IGF-1 and IGF-2, and an equivalent murine peptide, MSA, have been purified to homogeneity (26–29). They are exceedingly similar in overall structure to insulin with A chains and B chains that have 50% identity of amino acid sequence with human insulin; they have a much shorter connecting piece than does proinsulin and a small unique addition at the end of the A chain. These peptides are believed to be produced by many tissues throughout the body, with no single site that clearly predominates. The circulating levels of somatomedins or insulin-like growth factors are often increased by the action of growth hormone, insulin or both (23–25, 30).

2.1 Neurobiology of Insulin in Insects

Although a biological role for insulin in nearly all of these nonverte-brates is as yet unknown, the importance of insulin in some molluscs and insects has been established. Immunoreactive insulin has been found in both the brain and the peripheral neurosecretory organs (corpus cardiacum and corpus allatum) of several species of insects (33–37). Using immunocytochemical techniques, investigators have localized insulin, along with several other vertebrate type peptide hormones, in the median neurosecretory cells of the brain and demonstrated insulin in the nerve fibers connecting these cells to the peripheral neurosecretory organs (35). As noted earlier, the insulin in the head of the blowfly has been extensively purified and characterized and is quite similar to vertebrate insulins (7, 8, 36).

The brain appears to be an essential source of insulin in insects, since decapitation, selective extirpation of the median neurosecretory cells, or ligation of the nerves connecting these cells to the peripheral neurosecretory organs results in decidedly elevated concentrations of both glucose and trehalose, the major circulating carbohydrates in insects (8, 36–38). Moreover, administration of extracts from the median neurosecretory cells corrects both the hyperglycemia and hypertrehalosemia (Figure 3).

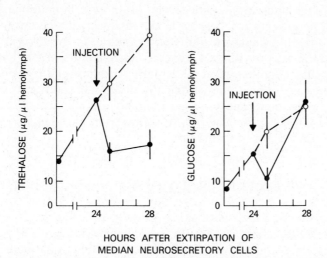

HOURS AFTER EXTIRPATION OF
MEDIAN NEUROSECRETORY CELLS

Figure 3. Biology of insulin in insects. The median neurosecretory cells of the brain of blowflies were extirpated at time 0. Twenty-four hours later both glucose and trehalose concentrations had risen markedly; flies were then injected with a purified extract from the extirpated cells (●) or an equivalent volume of saline (○). Administration of the extract normalized the concentrations of both carbohydrates, while levels in the saline-treated controls continued to rise. The effect on trehalose was evident for at least four hours; the effect of glucose was more transient. Adapted from Duve, et al. (8).

2.2 Biology of Insulin in Molluscs

In contrast with the insects, where insulin's regulation of carbohydrate metabolism is brain-related, the molluscs more closely resemble the vertebrates. Under basal conditions, insulin in molluscs is present in cells of the gastrointestinal tract and in the hemolymph. The administration of glucose results in a reduction of the insulin-related material in the mucosal cells of the gut and a rise in the insulin immunoactivity in the hemolymph (6). Administration of (mammalian or salmon) insulin causes a decrease in the level of circulating glucose and a concomitant activation of glycogen synthase, and the combination of insulin with glucose produces a significant rise in muscle glycogen. Most strikingly, the administration of anti-insulin antibodies to the mollusc results in a state resembling diabetes with hyperglycemia, reduced activity of glycogen synthase, and reduction of muscle glycogen to subnormal levels.

2.3 Summary and Implications of Insulin in Nonvertebrates

Materials very similar to vertebrate-type insulins have been detected in prokaryotes and eukaryotes, both unicellular and multicellular. In the mollusc and the insect the insulin-related material has been shown to play a physiological role, that is, regulates carbohydrate metabolism. In the mollusc, intestinal cells produce and release insulin, whereas in the insect this function is exercised by brain cells in collaboration with peripheral neurosecretory organs. In the mollusc, administration of anti-insulin antibody produces a diabetes-like state. In the blowfly removal of the brain insulin results in a hyperglycemic condition that can be corrected by the administration of insulin or appropriate brain extract. Thus, while insulin has been classically defined in relation to the vertebrate pancreas, materials that share specific immunochemical, physiological, and other properties with mammalian insulins are produced outside of the vertebrate pancreas.

3 INSULIN IN NEURAL TISSUES OF VERTEBRATES

In turning from nonvertebrates to vertebrates, the focus of inquiry undergoes a substantial change. In the nonvertebrates (all of which lack beta cells, islets, and pancreas), the major question about insulin is how closely are these insulins related in structure and in function to pancreatic insulins of vertebrates. In any cell, the amount of insulin is modest, and the site of its actual biosynthesis, while interesting, is not critical. In the vertebrates, the amount of insulin in the islet is extraordinary, and the hormone is essential for health; with regard to the insulin that has been demonstrated in the brain (or other extrapancreatic sites), a major question is whether all of it is of pancreatic origin. Is some or all of it of local origin? Irrespective of its biosynthetic site, does brain insulin (or other extrapancreatic tissue insulin) have a discernible function, in the nervous system or elsewhere? These questions cannot be answered fully at this time, but these issues, because of their importance, are covered in detail later. We begin our discussion with insulin in the peripheral nervous system because it provides a unified set of studies from a single laboratory. This is followed by consideration of insulin in the brain—its regional distribution and characterization. The concentrations of insulin in the brain are then compared with those in other extrapancreatic tissues. Particularly noteworthy will be the reproducibility of data between different laboratories* and the failure of the brain insulin to change concentrations in response to hyper- and hypoinsulinemia. Later in the chapter we devote individual sections to a discussion of the possible biosynthetic sites and functions of nervous system insulin. It should be emphasized that the only situation in which the function of nervous system insulin is truly clear is in the blowfly, where it regulates systemic carbohydrate metabolism, analogous to the role of pancreatic insulin in vertebrates.

3.1   Insulin in the Peripheral Nervous System of Mammals

Immunoactive insulin has been identified in acid ethanol extracts from a number of peripheral nerves of the cat (Figure 4). On HPLC (high performance liquid chromatography) this material elutes in the same position as purified mammalian insulin (39, 40). A distinct pattern of distribution is found. Levels are higher in the radial nerve than in the

---

*Upon examining Figure 6 and Table 1 and seeing the reproducibility of data produced by four different laboratories the reader may well be puzzled by our recurrent emphasis on reproducibility. In fact, one laboratory has concluded that their results differ from those of another and that insulin levels in the brain are actually much lower that those previously described (12, 47, 48, 176, 177). They have suggested that the concentrations found may depend on the size of the animal, with smaller aminals having higher concentrations, or, alternatively, that exogenous contamination might account for some of the results. These interpretations are not borne out by critical examination of all the extant data, as shown in Figure 6 and summarized in Table I. However, such examination does reveal the sources of the apparent discrepancy: (i) organs from different species were compared inappropriately (for example, only 12 of the 100 or more extractions published by Yalow et al. (12) in their initial criticism were of the same organ or species as our previously published work (9–11); (ii) extractions done by two distinctly different methods were assumed to be equivalent (see Section 3.7); (iii) no distinction was made between results that had been recalculated to account for estimated losses in processing and those that had not. As noted in the text, reproducibility is excellent provided that (i) the same method is applied to (ii) the same tissue from (iii) the same species, and (iv) data are expressed as ng of insulin actually measured in the immunoassay per g weight of tissue without any attempt to account for estimated losses in processing. For further discussion, see Ref. 190.

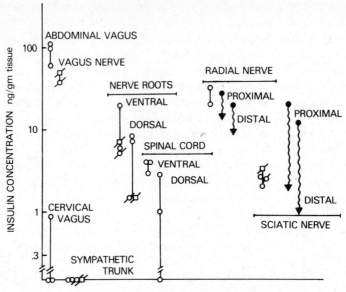

Figure 4. Insulin in peripheral nerves of the cat. Insulin concentrations in individual acid ethanol extracts (○) and in extracts before (◌) and after (▱) HPLC purification show distinct patterns, with levels higher in the abdominal than in the cervical vagus and higher in the radial than in the sciatic nerve. Also shown are the results of clamping the radial and sciatic nerves in two cats for 24 hours. Biopsies taken proximal (●) and distal (▼) to the site of the ligature in the radial nerve show concentrations twofold higher proximal to the clamp. Similar samples from the sciatic nerve reveal a tenfold accumulation of insulin proximal to the clamp. Adapted from Uvnäs-Moberg, et al. (39).

sciatic; in the vagus nerve, levels are markedly higher in the abdominal segment than in the cervical. (Insulin has also been found in extracts of human vagus). In contrast with the high levels found in the parasympathetic vagus, no insulin immunoactivity at all has been found in the sympathetic trunk (39, 40).

Clamping of the sciatic or radial nerve (39) results in the accumulation of insulin proximal to the clamp (Figure 4) suggesting that at least some of the insulin in the nerves may be produced by the neurons themselves. Additionally, in isolated perfused limb preparations, electrical stimulation of the brachial and sciatic nerves causes release of immunoreactive insulin and gastrin (40, 41); appropriate selection of the duration and strength of the stimulus yields distinctive patterns of peptide release (Figure 5).

3.2 Distribution of Insulin in the Brain

Insulin has been found within the brain of a number of vertebrate species. Studies of the distribution of insulin within the central nervous system (CNS) of vertebrates are most remarkable for their scarcity. In

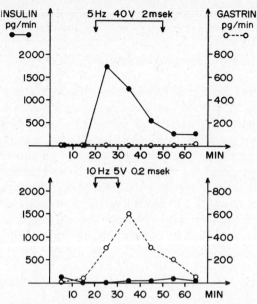

Figure 5. Release of insulin and gastrin from sciatic nerve of the cat. Extirpated hind legs were perfused with Tyrode's solution and the perfusate assayed for hormone levels. Release of gastrin ○ or insulin ● appeared to be dependent on the specific stimulus applied. From Uvnäs and Uvnäs-Wallensten (41).

very limited studies in rats, insulin was present in acid ethanol extracts of all regions studied, with concentrations in hypothalamus > olfactory bulb > cerebellum > brain stem = cerebral cortex = whole brain (9).

Immunocytochemical techniques have also been applied (9, 42–46). Baetans and Orci recently, in extensive studies, have been unable to detect the insulin in brain by immunocytochemical techniques, even with our antiserum and our experimental conditions. (With guinea pig serum at very high concentrations—both control and anti-insulin, with and without absorption—they find widespread "staining" of neurons). Given their expertise and the very preliminary scope of our own studies, we accept their findings as the current state of the art. (For recent work by others, see note added in proof.)

Although excellent for localization, immunocytochemistry is a relatively insensitive technique and is not fully quantitative. Therefore, given the small amounts of insulin in brain, further success in definitely localizing brain insulin by immunocytochemistry may well depend on how highly concentrated the insulin is at both a cellular and subcellular level. When antisera are used at very high concentrations or with magnification techniques, in order to detect small amounts of material, many precautions and extensive studies are needed to confirm the specificity of the findings. At this time the acid ethanol extraction method is superior for identification and characterization of CNS insulin, since it provides excellent sensitivity, specificity, and control of artifacts, while the direct visualization approach is best for localization.

3.3   Characterization of Brain Insulin

The immunoactive insulin in the brain of the rat has been characterized in detail (Figure 2). It behaves like insulin on serial dilution in the immunoassay (Figure 2A) and in its elution pattern on gel filtration on Sephadex G-50 (Figure 2A inset). The gel-filtered material is also indistinguishable from purified insulin in binding to insulin receptors on cultured human lymphocytes (Figure 2B) and in stimulation of glucose oxidation in rat adipocytes *in vitro* (Figure 2C). Further, the biological activity is neutralized by anti-insulin antibodies, suggesting that the biological and immunochemical determinants are present on the same molecule (see later for studies characterizing the insulin in guinea pig brain).

3.4   Insulin Concentrations in Whole Brain

Immunoactive insulin has been found in acid ethanol extracts of whole brain as well as in other extra pancreatic tissues from a variety of mammalian species by several different laboratories. In general, levels found in these tissues are all much lower than the levels found in pancreas and are roughly the same order of magnitude as insulin levels in plasma. There appear to be marked differences in levels between different species, smaller differences in levels between different organs of the same species, and virtually no systematic differences between laboratories (see footnote on page 911).

The concentrations of radioimmunoactive (RIA) insulin in extracts of whole brain are shown in the far right panel of Figure 6 (9–12, 47–49). The impression that species differences may be important—rat (designated *G* in the figure) and mouse (*H*) appear to be higher than dog (*D*), rabbit (*E*), and human (*I*)—is verified by the findings in other

---

Figure 6.   Insulin concentrations in brain and other tissues. *Brain insulin:* At far right are acid ethanol extracts of whole brain (or cerebral cortex); appropriately prepared aliquots were tested in standard radioimmunoassays and results are expressed as ng insulin per g wet weight of tissue, uncorrected for any losses in the processing of the samples. Notice that levels appear to be lower in dogs (*D*), rabbits (*E*), and humans (*I*) than in rats (*G*) and mice (*H*). In rats (*G*), notice that results of Roth and coworkers ● (9–11) are in close agreement with those of Sakamoto and coworkers ○ (49) and Eng and Yalow ▲ (12) which overlap those done by Rosenzweig and Eng △ as quoted in (48) and (72). *Other tissues:* For comparison are shown results of seven other extrapancreatic tissues and, on a different scale, pancreas and human insulinomas. Distinct differences are apparent between species: *A*, beef; *B*, pig; *C*, sheep; *D*, dog; *E*, rabbit; *F*, cat; *G*, rat; *H*, mouse; *I*, human. In general, levels are lowest in rabbits (*E*) and humans (*I*); tissues from rats (*G*) and

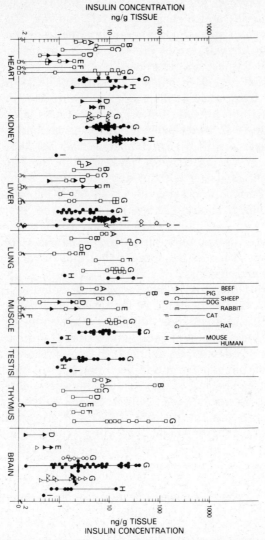

INSULIN CONCENTRATION
ng/g TISSUE

ng/g TISSUE
INSULIN CONCENTRATION

pigs (*B*) show highest levels. Notice that levels in brain are comparable to those in other extrapancreatic tissues and that levels of 25 mg/g or more (equivalent to tissue/plasma ratios of $\geq$ 25) have been noted by multiple groups for several tissues and species (e.g., heart of rat; liver of humans; lung, muscle, and thymus of several species). Also apparent is the overlap in results reported by different investigators (see heart, kidney, liver, and muscle): □ Rishi and Becker (56); △ Abassi and Power (52); ◆ Unger and coworkers (53); ☑ Shames and coworkers (54); ◇ Rees and coworkers (55). Data of Rishi and Becker, previously published only in abstract form (56), represent the mean of duplicate aliquots from individual acid ethanol extracts of tissues assayed for insulin with standard radioimmunoassay techniques. Results are expressed in terms of a human standard for beef, pig, sheep, and dog and in terms of a human standard for rat, cat, and rabbit; as expected, incubation of extracts with cysteine abolished all assayable insulin activity, and progressive dilution of extracts yielded appropriately reduced insulin concentrations.

extrapancreatic tissues shown in the figure. In general, tissue insulin is lowest in rabbit (E) and highest in rat (G) and pig (B), but individual tissues in individual species may be exceptionally high or low. Overall, levels of insulin in brain are of the same order as those found in other extrapancreatic tissues; no difference is apparent between tissues that have very limited access to plasma constituents (e.g., brain and testis) and those with free access to plasma components (e.g., liver and lung).

The reproducibility of data between laboratories is excellent despite separation of up to 15 years when (i) the same method is applied to (ii) the same tissue from (iii) the same species and (iv) data are expressed as nanograms of insulin actually measured in the immunoassay per gram wet weight of tissue without any attempt to recalculate for estimated losses during processing (9–12, 47–56). The widespread agreement is particularly remarkable since there was no attempt to exclude small variations in extraction methodology, differences in the animals (such as age, sex, diet, activity, strain, and anesthesia), or differences in the immunoassay (such as the form of the final extract or the antibody or insulin standards used).

With rat brain, four studies have been contributed to by three laboratories (9, 12, 48, 49). While some of the differences between the studies may be statistically significant, they are remarkably slight given the variables that have not been adequately fixed. Further, there are 13 more examples of other extrapancreatic tissues where two or more laboratories studied the same organ in the same species by the same method—heart in three species, kidney in two, muscle in three, and liver in five. In general, agreement is excellent. In our opinion, the differences in results between laboratories are trivial and are probably less than differences obtained by a single laboratory with single specimens examined with two different insulin standards with two different antibodies (see table 2 in reference 48).

3.5 Failure of Changes in Plasma Insulin Concentrations to Alter Brain Insulin

With systematic changes in plasma insulin concentrations, the insulin in most tissues, including brain, shows little or no variation (Table 1). Three laboratories have shown that two hypoinsulinemic states and three hyperinsulinemic states in three species, which include very large changes in plasma insulin (and blood glucose), cause trivial changes in the insulin content of tissues (10, 12, 49). (The only exception is the kidney, where insulin levels do seem to reflect those in plasma, as shown in Table 1). Again, the insulin content of brain is remarkably similar to the insulin content of the other tissues; this is particularly notable since the insulin receptors in brain do not change with chronic alterations in plasma insulin levels, whereas the receptor concentrations in liver and

TABLE 1 Tissue Insulin in Hypo and Hyper Insulinemic States

	Plasma Insulin	Kidney Insulin	Liver Insulin	Brain Insulin	References
A. Hypoinsulinemic states[a]					
Prolonged fast (rat)					
Rosenzweig et al.	Decreased	Decreased	Unchanged	Unchanged	11
Sakamoto et al.	Decreased	—	—	Unchanged	49
Streptozotocin diabetes (rat)					
Rosenzweig et al.	Decreased	Decreased	Unchanged[b]	Unchanged	11
Sakamoto et al.	Decreased	—	—	Unchanged	49
B. Hyperinsulinemic states[c]					
Dexamethasone (dog)					
Eng and Yalow	Elevated	Elevated	Unchanged	Unchanged	12
Genetic obesity (ob/ob mouse)					
Rosenzweig et al.	Elevated	—	Unchanged	Unchanged	11
Eng and Yalow	Elevated	Elevated	Unchanged	—	12

[a] Rats were fasted 2–3 days to reduce the chronic level of circulating insulin and blood glucose. Another group of rats were treated with streptozotocin to destroy beta cells of the pancreas, which results in hypoinsulinemia, hyperglycemia, and glycosuria. With the decrease in plasma insulin, there was a decrease in the insulin content of the kidney, but the insulin levels in the brain and liver were unchanged.

[b] Values in these animals were slightly lower than the mean values obtained in normal rats, but were not significantly different from those obtained in simultaneously assayed control animals.

[c] Hyperinsulinemia was induced in a normal dog by the administration of dexamethasone. In the mouse with a genetic disorder, hyperinsulinemia is associated with hyperphagia and obesity. Elevations in the plasma insulin up to 20-fold were associated with elevations in the kidney content of insulin, but the insulin concentrations in brain and other organs were unchanged. In a study of the genetically obese Zucker rat, Eng (12) found higher insulin levels in liver than those generally found in our laboratory in normal rats; however, control values in thin littermates are not available.

other organs often change substantially. That tissue content of insulin is largely independent of concentrations of plasma hormone and of cell receptors is consistent with the data in Figure 6; there the large systematic variations of tissue insulin between species (and tissues) are in contrast with the narrow differences among species in plasma insulin concentrations and in tissue receptor content (not shown).

3.6 Recovery of RIA Insulin with Further Purification

How much of the immunoactive insulin measured in acid ethanol extracts shows up as "insulin" following further purification? This varies widely among systems but appears to be predictable for a given system. Virtually all of the immunoactive insulin in extracts of peripheral nerves is recovered as insulin following HPLC. Likewise, nearly all of the RIA insulin in acid ethanol extracts of early chick embryos is recovered in the regions characteristic of insulin (and proinsulin) with gel filtration on Sephadex G-50. With rat brain and some other tissues, about 50% of RIA insulin in the original extract is recovered in the insulin regions on gel filtration, while with the rat-pork type of insulin of guinea pigs, 10% recovery is typical. In each case, the interpretations of the data in any given system need to take this into account.

3.7 Sep-Pak Extractions: Effects on Results

As noted above, the concentrations of tissue insulin reported by four laboratories were quite similar when an individual tissue from an individual species was studied by a single approach; apparent discrepancies arose when different tissues from different species were compared inappropriately (see 12, 48; footnote on page 911). Another cause for apparent discrepancy was the comparison of results obtained by two different extraction methods (47, 48). In contrast with the classical approach employed by most investigators over the last two decades, Eng and Yalow introduced a Sep-Pak extraction technique (47, 48, 57), and although the new method offers many advantages, it typically gives values for endogenous tissue insulin that are substantially lower than those obtained with the classical acid ethanol extraction. In the four examples where Eng and Yalow studied the same tissues from the same species by both methods (rat brain and rabbit brain, kidney, and liver), the results with Sep-Pak were sevenfold to ninefold lower than with the classical approach (12, 47). The Sep-Pak method gives excellent recoveries of insulin added to tissues (and to solutions) but it gives distinctly lower recoveries for endogenous tissue insulin. In our hands, in preliminary experiments, the Sep-Pak technique was particularly poor in recovering immunoactive insulin components of molecular weights higher than insulin.

4 INSULIN IN CEREBROSPINAL FLUID

Insulin is present in cerebrospinal fluid (CSF) and in most other body fluids (58–65). The levels in CSF are lower than those in plasma (58, 64), whereas in lymph and semen they are approximately equal to plasma (63, 65) and in bile they are much higher (64, 65). In most body fluids, the concentrations of insulin appear to vary directly with plasma levels. Thus, insulin concentrations in both lymph and bile are higher in fed than in fasted animals (64, 65), and the intravenous administration of insulin to rats results in a prompt sharp rise in lymphatic insulin concentrations (65).

The situation is more complex in CSF. In the basal state, insulin levels in the CSF of dogs (60, 61), rats (65), and humans (58, 59) average 25–30% of plasma levels (Figure 7 and Table 2). Acute elevations of plasma insulin in dogs, produced either by endogenous secretion following glucose administration (61) or by intravenous insulin injection (60, 61) provoked remarkably limited elevations in CSF insulin concentrations. Thus during a prolonged intravenous insulin infusion, insulin levels in CSF rose gradually, did not appear to reach steady state for at least 3–4 h, and at that time were still 10% or less those in plasma (Table 2). The limited rise in CSF insulin was particularly apparent when plasma insulin was raised to very high levels.

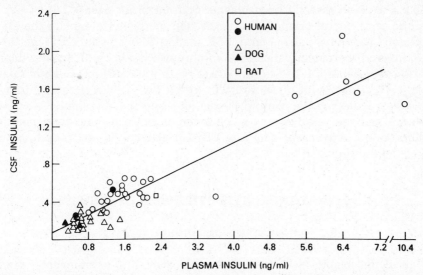

Figure 7. Relationship between plasma and cerebrospinal fluid (CSF) insulin concentrations in the basal state in humans [● Greco, 1970 (58); ○ Owen, 1974 (59)]; dogs [△ Woods, 1977 (61); ▲ Margolis, 1967 (60)], and rats [□ Razio and Conard, 1969 (65)]. The line, drawn by eye, represents a plasma/CSF about 4 to 1. The five patients with plasma insulin concentrations of greater than 5 ng/mL are unusual (for unexplained reasons) in that patients with these conditions typically do not have elevations in plasma insulin to this degree.

TABLE 2   Effects of Intravenous Infusions of Insulin

	Low Dose Insulin[a] (0.2 U/kg/h)			High Dose Insulin[a] (1.0 U/kg/h)		
	Plasma Insulin (x Basal)	CSF Insulin (x Basal)	[CSF] [Plasma]	Plasma Insulin (x Basal)	CSF Insulin (x Basal)	[CSF] [Plasma]
Basal	1	1.0	0.27	1	1.0	0.27
1 h	27	2.4	0.05	100	2.8	0.006
4 h	27	4.0	0.10	100	14.0	0.03

[a] Anesthetized dogs were infused intravenously with insulin (and glucose to prevent hypoglycemia). The delayed and blunted rise in CSF insulin concentrations in the face of marked hyperinsulinemia is compatible with limited passage of insulin from blood to CSF. Adapted from Margolis and Altszuler (60).

Studies of CSF insulin concentrations in states of chronic hypo- or hyperinsulinemia, although rare, tend to indicate better concordance between plasma and CSF levels. In five patients with chronically elevated plasma insulin levels, concentrations of CSF insulin were also elevated (58), and in eight obese patients subjected to a 21-day fast, a 60% reduction in plasma insulin was accompanied by a 45% decrease in CSF insulin (59).

It is as yet quite uncertain whether any or all of the insulin in spinal fluid is derived directly from plasma or from brain tissue (i.e., of pancreatic or of neural origin). We suggest the following to explain the discordance between plasma and CSF insulin levels with acute perturbations and the concordance seen in chronic situations: (i) insulin does not cross the intact blood-brain barrier readily (62, 66); (ii) there is relatively direct access of plasma insulin to the CNS in the circumventricular areas, including the choroid plexus (66); and (iii) this limited area of contact and the relatively slow turnover of cerebrospinal fluid permit equilibration between plasma and CSF but it takes a very long time to reach equilibrium.

5   EXTRAPANCREATIC SYNTHESIS OF INSULIN

5.1   Evidence to Support the Hypothesis

Is all of the insulin in brain, peripheral nerves, and cerebrospinal fluid derived totally from plasma insulin? Is plasma insulin derived solely from pancreas? While the pancreas is the essential and overwhelmingly largest contributor to total body insulin, we believe it may not be the sole supplier of insulin to extrapancreatic sites such as neural tissues and CSF. What is the evidence to support the idea of insulin synthesis by tissues other than pancreatic beta cells? The data from unicellular organisms and from the multicellular invertebrates indicate that neural and non-neural tissues are capable of producing materials that are very similar to mammalian insulins. Did extrapancreatic and neural synthesis of insulin simply cease with the emergence in vertebrates of the endocrine pancreas? We think not. Evidence in favor of extrapancreatic synthesis of insulin in vertebrates is summarized in Table 3; we think the data on the peripheral nerves and the data that show unchanging tissue levels in the face of very wide changes in concentrations of ambient insulin provide substantial, though not incontrovertible, evidence

TABLE 3   Extrapancreatic Production of Insulin

I. Arguments in Favor

1. Unicellular organisms (bacteria, fungi, protozoa) grown in synthetic media produce material very similar to vertebrate insulin (2, 3).

2. Multicellular invertebrates (which lack pancreas, islets, and beta cells) have insulin in brain, peripheral neural organs, and other extrapancreatic sites; anti-insulin serum or extirpation of insulin-containing neurons produces "diabetes" (4–8, 31–38).

3. Vertebrates:
   (a) Particular peripheral nerves differ widely in insulin content, release insulin on stimulation, and accumulate insulin proximal to an axonal clamp (39–41).
   (b) In a given species, insulin concentrations in brain and other extrapancreatic tissues (except kidney) are unchanged by (i) 20-fold increase or twofold decrease in plasma insulin concentrations; or (ii) a twofold increase or fourfold decrease in insulin receptor concentrations (10, 12, 49).
   (c) The insulin content of some tissues in individual animals in some species is multifold higher (25 fold or more) than other tissues in the same or other animal or species, despite very similar or identical levels of plasma insulin and very similar concentrations of surface receptors (9–12, 48–56).
   (d) Insulin content of cells grown in culture can be multifold higher and independent of the concentration of insulin in the medium (11); the cellular insulin is recognized by a monoclonal antibody as different from the insulin that is added with the culture medium (unpublished observation).
   (e) Immunoreactive insulin persists in the circulation of eviscerated rodents far beyond the predicted time of clearance (67, 68).
   (f) Aplastic mammary carcinomas from mice secrete insulin in culture for up to 25 days (69).
   (g) Slices of parotid gland incorporate amino acids into material that closely resembles insulin (13).
   (h) Guinea pigs have a distinctive insulin in brain and other extrapancreatic tissues that is not abundant in its pancreas and which is not detected in its plasma (71–73).

II. Arguments Against

1. Tradition.
2. Failure to detect proinsulin.
3. Failure to detect mRNA for insulin (74).
4. Tissue insulin/plasma insulin ratios less than or equal to 1 in some tissues in some species.

in favor of our hypothesis. Also relevant are the data with parotid tissue *in vitro* which show incorporation of amino acids into material that is similar to insulin. This material coelutes with standard mammalian insulin on gel chromatography and interacts specifically with anti-insulin antibodies; further, the interaction is abolished by the addition of an excess of purified insulin (13).

5.2 Two Insulins in the Guinea Pig

One of the strongest pieces of evidence in favor of extrapancreatic synthesis of insulin by vertebrates comes from studies of the guinea pig. The guinea pig is known to have a unique type of insulin that is present in large amounts in its pancreas (15, 21) and also present in its extrapancreatic tissues and in the circulation (71, 73). This insulin regulates carbohydrate metabolism (70). In addition, extracts of brain and other extrapancreatic tissues of the guinea pig yield a rat-pork type insulin that is clearly distinct from the insulin present in abundance in its pancreas (71–73). In guinea pigs this rat-pork type of insulin has been detected only in tissues, not in plasma.

The failure of others to find the rat-pork type of insulin in the guinea pig is largely due to their use of the Sep-Pak extraction method (47, 57); in our hands this method gives substantially lower amounts than the classical acid ethanol extraction method. We find that when larger amounts of guinea pig tissue are extracted with the Sep-Pak method, the rat-pork type of insulin is found (72). Our finding of the rat-pork type of insulin in the guinea pig has been confirmed by four other laboratories (72). A fifth laboratory has confirmed that there are two types of insulin in the guinea pig and that changes in the extraction method cause marked differences in the concentrations found (73); (they found larger amounts of rat-pork type of insulin using the Sep-Pak technique than with the classical method).

5.3 Arguments Against Extrapancreatic Synthesis

The evidence against extrapancreatic synthesis of insulin is quite limited at the moment. In contrast with others (12, 47, 48) we believe that the absence or presence of proinsulin in tissues would provide little support for either side of the argument; proinsulin is present in the plasma and other biological fluids that bathe the tissues (22) and therefore its presence would not indicate the source of the insulin. In the pancreas, proinsulin typically constitutes only a few percent of the insulin; the techniques that have been used thus far would not have detected proinsulin in tissues unless it constituted a very substantial fraction of the total insulin-related immunoactivity (i.e., 20% or more). Furthermore, the fraction of proinsulin that one might expect would depend on the physical location of the converting enzymes relative to the proinsulin and the duration of their contact with one another. Thus, one could predict from 0 to 100% proinsulin depending on the assumptions one chose.

5.4 Ratio of Tissue Insulin to Plasma Insulin

Since plasma insulin in the basal state is about 1 ng/mL (range 0.1–2.0), the ratio of tissue insulin to plasma insulin ranges from less than one to greater than or equal to 25 depending on the tissue and species (see Figure 6). In fact, ratios may need to be multiplied by two since the values for plasma insulin are generally reduced by that amount when plasma is treated like tissue, that is, when it is extracted with acid ethanol and purified. Since insulin accumulation on surface receptors and in compartments that exchange with the surface is limited, very high tissue/plasma ratios suggest the possibility, but surely do not prove, that some of the insulin is provided by local synthesis. On the other hand, low ratios do not exclude synthesis since many organs tend to make but not store exported proteins and therefore have very low tissue/plasma ratios. In summary, while tissue/plasma ratios of any level do not prove or exclude local synthesis, very high ratios are suggestive of some local synthesis; much more impressive evidence is provided by finding tissue levels of insulin that are unchanged despite wide fluctuations in the plasma concentrations of plasma hormone and tissue receptors.

Another argument raised against extrapancreatic insulin synthesis has been a failure to detect messenger RNA for insulin in the tissues (74). However, if one assumes that the fraction of total mRNA represented by insulin mRNA is the same as the fraction of cellular protein represented by insulin, then for the negative experiments to be meaningful the investigators must demonstrate their capability of detecting insulin mRNA when it is present in only one out of every 10^6 mRNA molecules. Therefore, conclusions should be deferred until further data are available.

A related problem is that the insulin found in vertebrate tissues may or may not represent the product of the same gene that is being expressed in the animal's pancreas. It is quite possible that variable proportions of tissue insulin represent products of another gene or genes, proteins that are similar enough in size and homologous enough to react well with anti-insulin antibodies and with insulin receptors. The rat and the mouse, as well as some fish, have two pairs of insulin genes that are similar to but not identical with one another, both of which are expressed in the pancreas (15, 75). Do other species have analogous pairs or families of insulin genes, one of which is expressed primarily in the pancreas, while others are predominantly expressed in the peripheral tissues? Studies thus far would surely not distinguish these two possibilities.

In summary, increasingly strong evidence from studies in mammals, in multiple classes of invertebrates, and in unicellular organisms supports the idea that cells other than the beta cells of the pancreas can and do synthesize insulin. However, it is not yet certain whether nerve cells of mammals are to be included in this group.

6 INSULIN RECEPTORS IN BRAIN

The essential first step in the action of insulin as a hormone is binding to specific cell surface receptors. Insulin receptors are found on nearly all cells, irrespective of whether they are typical target cells for insulin action (76). The binding properties of the receptors are quite uniform (Figure 8) and largely independent of the tissue or species in which they are found (16–18, 20). The affinity of the receptors for different insulins in absolute terms is quite highly conserved and corresponds closely with the relative biological potencies of these insulins (16–18, 20). Among the other characteristic features of these receptors are the unusually marked effects of both pH and temperature on hormone binding and the regulation of both the affinity ("negative cooperativity") and the concentration ("down regulation") of receptors by the homologous hormone (76–79). Chronic elevations of plasma insulin (as occur in insulin resistant conditions in rodents and man) are often associated with decreases in the concentration of receptors, and chronic hypoinsulinemia (as with starvation or destruction of islet beta-cells by streptozotocin) is associated with elevations in receptor number (76, 78).

Insulin also binds (but with lower affinity) to one or more types of receptors for the insulin-like growth factors (76). These receptors generally bind the insulin-like growth factors better than they do insulin (24–26, 29, 76). Interpretation of insulin-binding studies requires that a distinction be made between the insulin receptors and those of the insulin like growth factors.

6.1 Insulin Receptors in Nervous Tissue

Insulin receptors were identified initially in whole brain preparations of the pigeon, monkey, and rat (80) and later in hypothalamus of the monkey (81). Subsequent studies showed that insulin receptors are widely but unevenly distributed throughout the CNS of the rat (82), with the highest level in the olfactory bulb (Figure 9). These receptors, by multiple criteria, are very similar to the insulin receptors found in classical target cells (reference 76 and Figure 8). In contrast to the receptors on liver and other cells, where concentrations of receptors are inversely related to the resting level of circulating insulin (76, 78, 83), the levels of insulin receptors in the brain (10, 84) are unchanged under conditions of

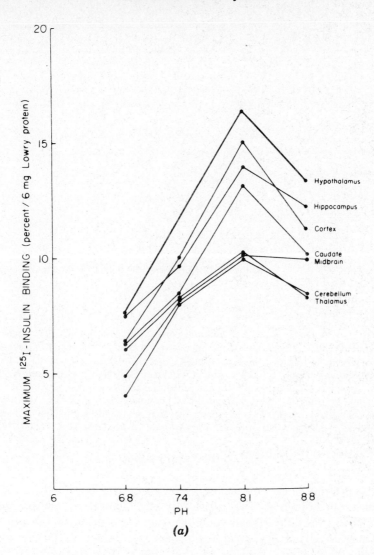

Figure 8. Specificity of insulin binding to brain receptors. (a) ^{125}I-insulin binding to receptors in different regions of brain showed the characteristic pH dependence with a distinct maximum at around pH 8, which is typical of insulin receptors in all tissues and is distinct from the receptors for the insulin-like growth factors. From Pacold and Blackard (84). (b) on p. 926.

hypoinsulinemia (prolonged fasting or streptozotocin-induced diabetes in the rat) or extreme hyperinsulinemia (genetic obesity in the mouse), as shown in Figure 10. It is not clear whether this failure of the insulin receptors in the brain to "up" and "down" regulate is due to a failure of circulating insulin to reach the receptors or is a characteristic of brain tissue, as has been shown occasionally in other tissues (85–87).

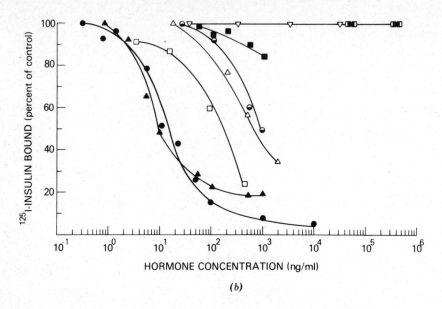

HORMONE CONCENTRATION (ng/ml)

(b)

Figure 8 (*b*). ^{125}I-insulin binding to cerebral cortex was measured in the absence and presence of ▲ unlabeled chicken insulin; ● porcine insulin; □ fish insulin; △ desalanine desasparagine (DAA) insulin; ◓ proinsulin; ■ melanocyte stimulating activity (MSA), an insulin-like growth factor; ▽ human growth hormone; ◨ insulin A-chain; and ◧ insulin B-chain. Nonspecific binding has been subtracted and results are expressed as a percent of ^{125}I-insulin bound in the absence of unlabeled hormone. The findings here are typical of all insulin receptors, except for the failure of chicken insulin to be effective at displacing all of ^{125}I-insulin at high concentrations. Adapted from Havrankova, et al. (82).

6.2   Other Approaches

Autoradiography is an alternative semiquantitative approach to localize receptors more distinctly (88). With this semiquantative method, insulin receptors are broadly distributed throughout the brain of the adult rat with an unusually high concentration in a distinctive pattern in the olfactory bulb; the latter closely parallels the pattern of binding of catecholamines to their receptors in this area (89). The pattern in fetal rat brain is definitely different from that in adults and changes over time between days 13 and 18 of gestation. Thus the failure of brain receptors to be regulated by ambient insulin concentrations contrasts with the substantial changes associated with development.

An *in vivo* approach to the study of insulin receptors in the central nervous system has utilized intravenously injected labeled insulin (in the absence and presence of unlabeled insulins) with autoradiography to measure ^{125}I-insulin binding to rat brain at early time points. With this route of administration, specific binding of ^{125}I-insulin is restricted to regions of the brain that have ready access to the systemic circula-

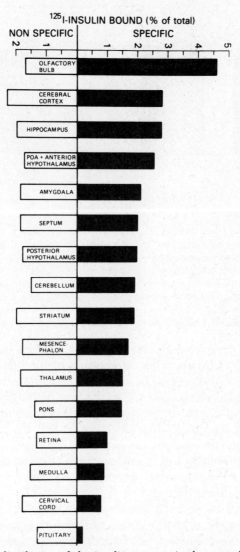

Figure 9. Regional distribution of the insulin receptor in the central nervous system of the rat. ^{125}I-insulin binding to comparable membrane preparations from different regions of the rat brain are shown. Specific binding is represented by the solid bar above the line and nonspecific binding by the open bar below the line. Unlabeled insulin at 20 ng/mL displaced more than 50% of labeled insulin in all cases except for medulla, cervical cord, and pituitary. Adapted from Havrankova, et al. (82).

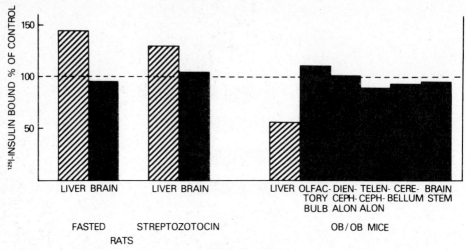

Figure 10. Failure of brain insulin receptors to "up" and "down" regulate. In rats rendered hypoinsulinemic by prolonged fasting or destruction of the pancreatic beta cells by streptozotocin, receptor concentrations (compared with controls) in liver membranes are increased while those in the brain remain unchanged. Adapted from Sakamoto, et al. (49). In the ob/ob mouse, where plasma insulin levels are 20-fold to 50-fold higher than in their thin littermates, insulin receptors in liver and other tissues show a marked diminution in concentration. Under similar conditions, insulin receptors in five regions of the brain are not different from those in control littermates. Adapted from Havrankova, et al. (10).

tion, that is, the circumventricular organs (90). While this method is less precise in quantitation and characterization of binding, it provides specific localization of receptors. In all areas studied, most of the specific binding is to neural elements (91). In the median eminence most of the binding is to axon terminals, while in the arcuate nucleus it is to preterminal axons (92). Recent studies have shown that the receptor-rich axonal processes in the median eminence are connected to cell bodies within the arcuate nucleus (93). In the area postrema, on the other hand, most of the bound radioactivity appears to be associated with intracellular vacuoles of dendrites (94).

Insulin binding to neurons has been supported by studies showing significant binding to preparations of purified synaptosomes (95–97). In addition, preliminary studies with rhodamine-labeled insulin in tissue culture preparations of fetal rat brain localize binding to neurons (98). Insulin receptors have also been demonstrated on the vascular endothelial cells of the microcirculation throughout the brain, both by *in vivo* autoradiographic studies (99) and by more classical studies of purified microvascular elements (100), similar to results with endothelium from other areas (101, 102).

In summary, insulin receptors are widely distributed on neural and vascular elements throughout the brain of the rat. The distribution shows characteristic features, including changes during fetal develop-

ment, but little or no change in association with hyperinsulinemic or
hypoinsulinemic states that regulate insulin receptors in the periphery.
Recognition that insulin receptors represent diverse compartments, only
some of which are accessible to plasma insulin, may permit better localization of specific changes.

7   INSULIN ACTION IN THE CENTRAL NERVOUS SYSTEM

Irrespective of whether insulin in neural structures is of neural or
extraneural origin, a fundamental question remains: What is the physiological role of insulin in or on neural tissue? Except in insects, the question is unanswered at present. To give perspective, we will first review
insulin action in general. Although insulin has a broad range of effects
in non-neural tissues, studies of insulin in the CNS have concentrated
on effects related to fuel metabolism. An appreciation of the broader
possibilities for insulin action should provide a better approach to the
exploration of the roles of insulin in the CNS.

7.1   Perspective on Insulin Action

We first survey the many biological effects of insulin outside of the nervous system to provide a framework for studies of insulin action on
neural tissue. The classical effects of insulin relate to regulation of fuel
metabolism including the distribution, utilization, and storage of carbohydrates, lipids, and amino acids (103, 104). Related processes are conservation of amino acids and cellular proteins as well as stimulation of
protein synthesis, cell growth, and cell division (105–108). Another
group of insulin effects of particular relevance to excitable tissues are
diverse effects on the movement and distribution of sodium and potassium ions (109–112); especially interesting are effects on skeletal muscle,
where insulin produces hyperpolarization (111, 112).

In addition to the effects of insulin common to many tissues, insulin
exerts effects on specialized processes that we associate with unique
cell types (113–115). For example, insulin has effects on the ability of
macrophages to kill antibody-sensitized cells (114), and insulin plays an
essential role in the differentiation of the unique properties of mammary
tissue, including the synthesis of casein and lactalbumin (115).

7.2   Cellular Mechanisms Related to Insulin Action

As noted earlier, the first step in the cellular action of insulin is its recognition by and specific binding to receptors on the cell surface. Insulin
bound to receptor causes the receptor to express the program of activities that is intrinsic to the receptor (76). An early event is the genera-

tion of soluble intracellular "second messengers" (116–122), probably small peptides, possibly generated by endogenous proteases acting on membrane proteins. It is yet unclear what fraction of insulin-mediated cellular events is accounted for by these second messengers. More distally, insulin stimulates and inhibits the phosphorylation and dephosphorylation of enzymes and other macromolecules (116, 123–126). Some of insulin's effects are opposite to (and occasionally the same as) effects produced by cyclic AMP and its associated hormones and kinases (124–126, 133).

A very early event following insulin binding to its receptor is stimulation of the phosphorylation of the insulin receptor itself (127, 128); the biological or biochemical implications of this are not yet known. Three other features of insulin action should be mentioned. First, insulin, in addition to regulating enzyme activity, can regulate the synthesis of enzymes (129, 130). Secondly, in tissues like fat, where insulin stimulation of glucose transport is the rate-limiting step in glucose utilization, insulin acts to cause preformed glucose transporting units to be transferred from intracellular sites to loci on the cell surface (130, 132). A similar mechanism may account for effects of other hormones in other tissues, including hormone-mediated stimulation of water and ion transport (131). (Do insulin-stimulated effects on ionic events utilize this type of mechanism of recruitment of intracellular transporters to the cell surface?) Finally, insulin, in common with other messenger molecules (76), frequently regulates the sensitivity of target cells to its own action (homologous effects) both at receptor and post-receptor levels, as well as modulating the sensitivity of the target cell to other hormones (heterologous effects).

7.3   Insulin Action Within the Central Nervous System

Although the presence of both insulin and insulin receptors within the central nervous system is well documented, the effects of insulin on nervous tissue remain difficult to define. Studies in this area are fragmentary and employ a wide variety of experimental approaches so that results often appear to be conflicting. The difficulty in defining insulin effects on nervous tissue is further compounded by the fact that a specific cellular mediator of insulin action in general has not been identified; therefore a single parameter cannot be uniformly studied. Although results in several areas are promising, the story is far from complete at this time.

In general, studies of "classical" effects of insulin on glucose metabolism (134) within the central nervous system have produced diverse results (134–146; Table 4 Part I). Potential effects of insulin on neurons, comparable to effects on enzyme modulation or ion transport in extraneural tissues, have yet to be fully explored. The results of recent stud-

TABLE 4   Insulin Effects on Central Nervous System

Preparation	Insulin Effect	Reference
	I. Effects on Glucose Uptake and Metabolism	
A. *In vitro* Studies		
Anterior pituitary (calf; rat)	25% increase in glucose uptake and utilization	135
Spinal cord (rat)	Glucose uptake increased; no effect on CO_2 generation or glycogen formation	136, 137
Brain slice (rat)	10% increase in glucose uptake in "first slice" only	138
Isolated perfused brain (dog)	No change in glucose uptake	139
Brain slice (rat)	40% increase in 2-deoxyglucose uptake	140
Microdissected brain regions (rat)	No change in glucose uptake, oxidation, or lipogenesis in anterior or posterior hypothalamus or cerebral cortex	141
B. *In vivo* Studies		
Brain perfusion with ^{14}C-oxymethylglucose (rat)	No effect in euglycemia; prolongation of increased cerebral glucose gain in hyperglycemia	142
Brain perfusion with 2-deoxy-glucose frozen section biopsy (rat)	Minimal change in whole brain uptake after acute injection; no difference in hypothalamus vs. other areas	143
Cerebral glucose anteriovenous difference (human)	Increased cerebral uptake	144
	Lowered threshold for glucose; increased transport across blood brain barrier; no change in net brain uptake	145, 146
	II. Effects on Cell Growth and Enzyme Activity	
A. *In vitro* Studies		
Fetal brain in culture (rat)	Time-dependent increase in AIB uptake; incorporation of valine, leucine, thymidine and uridine into protein	98, 147
Brain slices (rat)	Increase in acetylcholinesterase activity	148
B. *In vivo* Studies		
Brain homogenate (rat)	Increase in ornithine decarboxylase activity after single injection in 2-day-old rats and rats aged 17–60 days; no change in rats aged 5, 9, or 80 days	149

ies on insulin effects on brain growth and development (Table 4 Part II) are promising. Further definition of the specificity of these effects (vis-à-vis the insulin analogs and growth factors as well as the effects of lower concentrations of insulin) should clarify the role of insulin in this important area.

Studies of the interaction of insulin with discrete hypothalamic areas to regulate peripheral fuel homeostasis have provided some intriguing hypotheses. The first of these, that insulin might serve as a signal of body adiposity to modulate feeding behavior (150–153) is reviewed elsewhere in this volume. In addition, there is some evidence that insulin within the hypothalamus may modulate pancreatic insulin secretion and peripheral glucose metabolism. Intraventricular injections of high doses of insulin in both dogs and fowl stimulate pancreatic insulin secretion and the latter causes hypoglycemia (154–157). These effects are decreased by simultaneous intraventricular infusion of glucose (158) and are essentially abolished by vagotomy (155, 156). A similar hypoglycemia occurs after infusion of high doses of insulin into the carotid artery of dogs (159, 160). This effect appears to be mediated by the liver since the reduction in blood glucose is most marked in the hepatic vein (161), and the effect is obliterated by "functional hepatectomy" but not by vagotomy or by pancreatectomy (159, 160).

These data appear particularly interesting in light of recent evidence that neurons within the ventral medial hypothalamus and lateral hypothalamic areas are insulin-sensitive (161–167). Both the firing rate of individual neurons in these areas (168, 169) and the local release of norepinephrine (170) can be modulated by local application of insulin. In addition, electrical stimulation of these areas appears to modulate hepatic glucose metabolism through enzyme activation in the liver (171–175). Since both hypothalamic areas possess high concentrations of insulin receptors and multiple connections with the autonomic nervous system, it is tempting to speculate that circulating insulin may act as a neuromodulator in these areas to affect peripheral metabolism. Again, the evidence to support this hypothesis is not conclusive and firm conclusions must await further studies.

8   SUMMARY

Both unicellular and multicellular nonvertebrates have material that is very similar to vertebrate insulins in their tissues (and extracellular fluids), although they lack pancreatic cells. In the insect, localized areas of brain contain insulin, which appears to regulate the organism's carbohydrate metabolism in a manner analogous to pancreatic insulin in the vertebrate.

In mammals, insulin is found in brain, peripheral nerves, and other extrapancreatic tissues. Results from multiple laboratories are very similar provided that the same organs from the same species are extracted by the same method and the results are expressed as nanograms of immunoactive insulin per gram (wet weight) of tissue without accounting for losses in the extraction. On the other hand, the same organ from different species or studied by different extraction methods can give divergent results.

The insulin concentrations in brain and other extrapancreatic tissues (except kidney) show only trivial changes or no changes in the face of very wide changes in the steady-state concentration of circulating insulin. The independence of tissue insulin from plasma insulin is further demonstrated by studies in the guinea pig, which has an insulin in brain and other extrapancreatic tissues that is clearly different from the insulin found in its blood and pancreas.

Insulin concentrations in cerebrospinal fluid (CSF) are lower than in plasma. The levels of insulin in plasma appears to influence the insulin concentrations in CSF, albeit slowly.

Receptors for insulin are widely but unevenly distributed throughout the central nervous system (CNS) of the rat, including the circumventricular organs and the blood vessels that supply the central nervous system. The receptors in the CNS are very similar to comparable receptors on all other tissues. An unusual feature of the CNS insulin receptors is their unchanging concentration despite wide fluctuations in the chronic level of circulating insulin; most cells show an inverse correlation between their concentration of insulin receptors and the level of ambient insulin. During fetal life, the pattern of distribution of insulin receptors in the brain undergoes major changes.

Except in insects, the function of insulin in the nervous system is unclear. Although insulin influences a very broad range of biological and biochemical events in many types of cells, applications of such studies to neural tissue have been very narrow and limited. The recent elucidation of cellular events in insulin action (phosphorylation of receptors; second messengers) should provide new approaches to study the effects of insulin in the central nervous system.

ACKNOWLEDGMENTS

We thank Maxine A. Lesniak who provided invaluable technical and critical assistance, Drs. Derek Le Roith, James L. Rosenzweig, and Jana Havrankova who provided data and critical suggestions, and Violet Katz and Carol Culwell for their usual expert and patient secretarial assistance.

Note Added in Proof: The following recent articles extend those referred to in the text: insulin in the honey bee (1978); insulin in early chick embryo (179); immunocytochemical localization of insulin in the central nervous system (180–185); two insulins in the guinea pig (186); insulin receptors in hypothalamus (187); insulin effects on enzyme mRNA in liver (188), and Na+–K+ATPase in brain (189); as well as a critical review of insulin in brain extracts (190).

REFERENCES

1. J. Roth, D. Le Roith, J. Shiloach, J. L. Rosenzweig, M. A. Lesniak, and J. Havrankova, *N. Engl. J. Med.* **306**, 523 (1982).
2. D. Le Roith, J. Shiloach, J. Roth, and M. A. Lesniak, *J. Biol. Chem.* **256**, 6533 (1981).
3. D. Le Roith, J. Shiloach, J. Roth, and M. A. Lesniak, *Proc. Natl. Acad. Sci. USA* **77**, 6184 (1980).
4. D. Le Roith, M. A. Lesniak, and J. Roth, *Diabetes* **30**, 70 (1981).
5. S. O. Emdin and S. Falkmer, *Acta Paediatr. Scand.* **270**, Suppl. 15 (1978).
6. E. M. Plisetskaya, V. K. Kazakov, L. Sottitskaya, and L. G. Leibson, *Gen. Comp. Endocrinol.* **35**, 133 (1978).
7. H. Duve, *Gen. Comp. Endocrinol.* **36**, 102 (1978).
8. H. Duve, A. Thorpe, and N. R. Lazarus, *Biochem. J.* **184**, 221 (1979).
9. J. Havrankova, D. Schmechel, J. Roth, and M. Brownstein, *Proc. Natl. Acad. Sci. USA* **75**, 5737 (1978).
10. J. Havrankova, J. Roth, and M. J. Brownstein, *J. Clin. Invest.* **64**, 636 (1979).
11. J. L. Rosenzweig, J. Havrankova, M. A. Lesniak, M. J. Brownstein, and J. Roth, *Proc. Natl. Acad. Sci. USA* **77**, 572 (1980).
12. J. Eng and R. S. Yalow, *Diabetes* **29**, 105 (1980).
13. K. Murakami, H. Taniguchi, and S. Baba, *Diabetologia* **22**, 358 (1982).
14. M. O. Dayhoff, Ed., *Atlas of Protein Sequence and Structure*, National Biomedical Research Foundation, Vol. 5, Suppl. 3, Washington, D.C., 1978.
15. L. F. Smith, *Am. J. Med.* **40**, 662 (1966).
16. P. Freychet, *Diabetologia* **12**, 83 (1976).
17. M. Muggeo, B. H. Ginsberg, J. Roth, D. M. Neville Jr., P. De Meyts, and C. R. Kahn, *Endocrinology* **104**, 1393 (1979).
18. M. Muggeo, E. Van Obberghen, C. R. Kahn, J. Roth, B. H. Ginsberg, P. De Meyts, S. O. Emdin, and S. Falkmer, *Diabetes* **28**, 175 (1979).
19. S. A. Berson and R. S. Yalow, *J. Clin. Invest.* **39**, 1157 (1960).
20. P. Freychet, J. Roth, and D. M. Neville Jr., *Proc. Natl. Acad. Sci. USA* **68**, 1833 (1971).
21. T. H. Jukes, *Can. J. Biochem.* **57**, 455 (1979).
22. D. Porte Jr. and J. B. Halter, in R. H. Williams, Ed., *Textbook of Endocrinology*, 6th ed., W. B. Saunders, Philadelphia, 1981, p. 720*ff*.
23. T. L. Blundell and R. E. Humbel, *Nature* **287**, 781 (1980).
24. K. Megyesi, C. R. Kahn, J. Roth, and P. Gorden, *J. Clin. Endocrinol. Metab.* **41**, 475 (1975).
25. L. S. Phillips and R. Vasselopoulou-Sellin, *N. Engl. J. Med.* **302**, 371 (1980).
26. T. L. Blundell, S. Bedarkar, E. Rinderknecht, and R. E. Humbel, *Proc. Natl. Acad. Sci. USA* **75**, 180 (1978).
27. E. Rinderknecht and R. E. Humbel, *J. Biol. Chem.* **253**, 2769 (1978).
28. E. Rinderknecht and R. E. Humbel, *FEBS Lett.* **89**, 283 (1978).

29. M. M. Rechler, J. M. Podskalny, and S. P. Nissley, *J. Biol. Chem.* **252**, 3898 (1977).
30. U. E. Heinrich, D. S. Schalch, J. G. Koch, and C. J. Johnson, *J. Clin. Endocrinol. Metab.* **46**, 672 (1978).
31. H. Duve and A. Thorpe, personal communication.
32. K. J. Kramer, C. N. Childs, R. D. Spiers, and R. M. Jacobs, *Insect Biochem.*, **12**, 91 (1982).
33. H. S. Tager, J. Markese, K. J. Kramer, R. D. Speirs, and C. N. Childs, *Biochem. J.* **156**, 515 (1976).
34. M. El-Salhy, R. Abou-El-Ela, S. Falkmer, L. Grimelius, and E. Wilander, *Regul. Peptides* **1**, 187 (1980).
35. R. Yui, T. Fujita, and S. Ito, *Biomed. Res.* **1**, 42 (1980).
36. H. Duve and A. Thorpe, *Cell Tissue Res.* **200**, 187 (1979).
37. T. C. Normann, *Nature* **254**, 259 (1975).
38. A. C. Chen and S. Friedman, *J. Insect Physiol* **23**, 1223 (1977).
39. K. Uvnäs-Moberg, B. Uvnäs, B. Posloncec, S. Castenssons, M. Hagerman, and B. Rubio, *Acta Physiol. Scand.*, **115**, 471 (1982).
40. K. Uvnäs-Wallensten, *Diabetologia* **20**, 337 (1981).
41. B. Uvnäs and K. Uvnäs-Wallensten, *Acta Physiol. Scand.* **103**, 346 (1978).
42. M. K. Raizada, *Exptl. Cell Res.* **143**, 351 (1983).
43. B. Pansky, J. Hatfield, G. C. Budd, and H. J. Walker, *Anat. Rec.* **193**, 753 (1979).
44. A. Dorn, H.-G. Bernstein, G. Kostmann, H.-J. Hahn, and M. Ziegler, *Acta Histochem.* **66**, 276 (1980).
45. H.-G. Bernstein, A. Dorn, H.-J. Hahn, G. Kostmann, and M. Ziegler, *Acta Histochem. Cytochem.* **13**, 623 (1980).
46. A. Dorn, H.-G. Bernstein, H.-J. Hahn, M. Ziegler, and H. Rummelfanger, *Histochem.* **71**, 609 (1981).
47. J. Eng and R. S. Yalow, *Proc. Natl. Acad. Sci. USA* **78**, 4576 (1981).
48. J. Eng and R. S. Yalow, *Peptides* **2**, 17 (1982).
49. Y. Sakamoto, Y. Oomura, H. Kita, S. Shibata, S. Suzuki, T. Kuzuya, and S. Yoshida, *Biomed. Res.* **1**, 334 (1980).
50. W. Creutzfeldt, R. Arnold, C. Creutzfeldt, U. Deuticke, H. Frerichs, and N. S. Track, *Diabetologia* **9**, 217 (1973).
51. J. C. Floyd Jr., S. S. Fajans, R. F. Knopf, and J. W. Conn, *J. Clin. Endocrinol.* **24**, 747 (1964).
52. A. Abbasi and L. Power, *Diabetes* **22**, 762 (1973).
53. R. H. Unger, J. de V. Lochner, and A. M. Eisentraut, *J. Clin. Endocrinol.* **24**, 823 (1964).
54. J. M. Shames, N. R. Dhurandhar, and W. G. Blackard, *Am. J. Med.* **44**, 632 (1968).
55. L. H. Rees, G. A. Bloomfield, G. M. Rees, B. Corrin, L. M. Franks, and J. G. Ratcliffe, *J. Clin. Endocrinol. Metab.* **38**, 1090 (1974).
56. S. Rishi and K. L. Becker, *Diabetes* **16**, 516 (1967).
57. J. Eng and R. S. Yalow, *Proc. Natl. Acad. Sci. USA* **79**, 2683 (1982).
58. A. V. Greco, G. Ghirlanda, G. Fedeli, and G. Gambassi, *Eur. Neurol.* **3**, 303 (1970).
59. O. E. Owen, G. A. Reichard Jr., G. Boden, and C. Shuman, *Metabolism* **23**, 7 (1974).
60. R. U. Margolis and N. Altszuler, *Nature* **215**, 1375 (1967).
61. S. C. Woods and D. Porte Jr., *Am. J. Physiol.* **233**(4), E331 (1977).
62. W. A. Mahon, J. Steinke, G. M. McKhann, and M. L. Mitchell, *Metabolism* **11**, 416 (1962).
63. G. Paz, Z. T. Homonnai, N. D. Ayal, T. Cordova, and P. F. Kraicer, *Fertil. Steril.* **28**, 836 (1977).
64. P. M. Daniel and J. R. Henderson, *Lancet* **1**, 1256 (1967).
65. E. Rasio and V. Conard, in J. Östman, Ed., *Diabetes*, J. Ostman, Ed., Proceedings of the Sixth Congress of the International Diabetes Federation, Excerpta Medica Foundation, Amsterdam, 1969.

66. W. M. Pardridge, *Diabetologia* **20**, 246 (1981).
67. S. S. Smith, S. J. Bhathena, D. Nompleggi, J. C. Penhos, and L. Recant, *Diabetologia* **14**, 177 (1978).
68. J. C. Penhos, M. Ezzquiel, A. Lepp, and E. R. Ramey, *Diabetes* **24**, 637 (1975).
69. K. Pavelic, A. Ferle-Vidovic, M. Osmak, and S. Vuk-Pavlovic, *J. National Cancer Institute* **67**, 687 (1981).
70. A. E. Zimmerman, M. L. Moule, and C. C. Yip, *J. Biol. Chem.* **249**, 4026 (1974).
71. J. L. Rosenzweig, M. A. Lesniak, B. E. Samuels, C. C. Yip, A. E. Zimmerman, and J. Roth, *Trans. Assoc. Am. Phys.* **93**, 263 (1980).
72. J. L. Rosenzweig, D. Le Roith, M. A. Lesniak, C. C. Yip, D. N. Orth, H. R. Nankin, M. Berelowitz, L. A. Frohman, A. S. Liotta, D. T. Krieger, and J. Roth, submitted.
73. R. W. Stevenson, *Horm. Metab. Res.*, in press (1983).
74. S. Giddings, J. Chirgwin, and M. A. Permutt, *Endocrinology* **108**, Suppl., 238 (1981).
75. G. I. Bell, R. L. Pictet, W. J. Rutter, B. Cordell, E. Tischer, and H. M. Goodman, *Nature* **284**, 26 (1980).
76. J. Roth and C. Grunfeld, in R. H. Williams, Ed., *Textbook of Endocrinology*, 6th ed., Saunders, Philadelphia, 1981, p. 15*ff*.
77. J. R. Gavin III, J. Roth, D. M. Neville Jr., P. De Meyts, and D. N. Buell, *Proc. Natl. Acad. Sci. USA* **71**, 84 (1974).
78. C. R. Kahn, D. M. Neville Jr., and J. Roth, *J. Biol. Chem.* **248**, 244 (1973).
79. P. De Meyts, J. Roth, D. M. Neville Jr., J. R. Gavin III, and M. A. Lesniak, *Biochem. Biophys. Res. Commun.* **55**, 154 (1973).
80. B. I. Posner, P. A. Kelly, R. P. C. Shiu, and H. G. Friesen, *Endocrinology* **95**, 521 (1974).
81. B. R. Landau, M. A. Abrams, R. J. White, Y. Takaoka, N. Taslitz, P. Austin, J. Austin, and C. Chernicky, *Diabetes* **25**, 322 (1976).
82. J. Havrankova, J. Roth, and M. J. Brownstein, *Nature* **272**, 827 (1978).
83. M. B. Davidson and S. A. Kaplan, *J. Clin. Invest.* **59**, 22 (1977).
84. S. T. Pacold and W. G. Blackard, *Endocrinology* **105**, 1452 (1979).
85. F. A. Karlsson, C. Grunfeld, C. R. Kahn, and J. Roth, *Endocrinology* **104**, 1383 (1979).
86. B. C. Reed and M. D. Lane, *Proc. Natl. Acad. Sci. USA* **77**, 285 (1980).
87. N. D. Neufeld, S. A. Kaplan, B. M. Lippe, and M. Scott, *J. Clin. Endocrinol. Metab.* **47**, 590 (1978).
88. W. S. Young III, M. J. Kuhar, J. Roth, and M. J. Brownstein, *Neuropeptides* **1**, 15 (1980).
89. W. S. Young III and M. J. Kuhar, *Proc. Natl. Acad. Sci. USA* **77**, 1696 (1980).
90. M. Van Houten, B. I. Posner, B. M. Kopriwa, and J. R. Brawer, *Endocrinology* **105**, 666 (1979).
91. M. Van Houten and B. I. Posner, *Diabetologia* **20**, 255 (1981).
92. M. Van Houten, B. I. Posner, B. M. Kopriwa, and J. R. Brawer, *Science* **207**, 1081 (1980).
93. M. Van Houten, D. M. Nance, S. Gauthier, and B. I. Posner, *Diabetes* **31**, Suppl. 2, 43A (1982).
94. M. Van Houten and B. I. Posner, *Endocrinology* **109**, 853 (1981).
95. S. Gammeltoft, P. Staun-Olsen, J. Fahrenkrug, and B. Ottesen, in H. Peeters, Ed., *Receptors*, Proceedings of the 29th Colloquium on Protides of Biological Fluids, Pergamon Press, Oxford, 1981.
96. S. Gammeltoft, P. Staun-Olsen, J. Fahrenkrug, and B. Ottesen, in D. Andreani, R. dePirro, R. Lauro, J. Olefsky, and J. Roth, Eds., *Current Views on Insulin Receptors*, Serono Symposium No. 41, Academic Press, New York, 1981.
97. N. Potau, E. Riudar, and A. Ballabriga, in D. Andreani, R. dePirro, R. Lauro, J. Olefsky, and J. Roth, Eds., *Current Views on Insulin Receptors*, Serono Symposium No. 41, Academic Press, New York, 1981.
98. M. K. Raizada, J. W. Yang, and R. E. Fellows, *Brain Res.* **200**, 389 (1980).

99. M. Van Houten and B. I. Posner, *Nature* **282**, 623 (1979b).
100. H. J. L. Frank and W. M. Pardridge, *Diabetes* **30**, 757 (1981).
101. R. S. Bar, J. C. Hoak, and M. L. Peacock, *J. Clin. Endocrinol. Metab.* **47**, 699 (1978).
102. R. S. Bar, M. L. Peacock, R. G. Spanheimer, R. Veenstra, and J. C. Hoak, *Diabetes* **29**, 991 (1980).
103. R. M. Denton, R. W. Brownsey, and G. J. Belsham, *Diabetologia* **21**, 347 (1981).
104. L. J. Elsas, I. Albrecht, and L. E. Rosenberg, *J. Biol. Chem.* **243**, 1846 (1968).
105. L. S. Jefferson, *Diabetes* **29**, 487 (1980).
106. R. L. Clark and R. J. Hansen, *Biochem. J.* **190**, 615 (1980).
107. J. L. Maller and J. W. Koontz, *Dev. Biol.* **85**, 309 (1981).
108. I. R. Sosenko, J. R. Kitzmiller, S. W. Loo, P. Blix, A. H. Rubenstein, and K. H. Gabbay, *N. Engl. J. Med.* **301**, 859 (1979).
109. R. Creese and D. J. Jenden, *J. Physiol. (London)*, **197**, 255 (1968).
110. K. Zierler, *Am. J. Med.* **40**, 735 (1966).
111. K. Zierler and E. M. Rogus, *Biochem. Biophys. Acta.* **640**, 687 (1981).
112. J. A. Flatman and T. Clausen, *Nature* **281**, 580 (1979).
113. N. D. Neufeld, A. Sevanian, C. T. Barrett, and S. A. Kaplan, *Pediatr. Res.* **13**, 752 (1979).
114. R. S. Bar, C. R. Kahn, and H. S. Koren, *Nature* **265**, 632 (1977).
115. F. F. Bolander, K. R. Nicholas, J. J. Van Wyk, and Y. J. Topper, *Proc. Nat. Acad. Sci. USA* **78**, 5682 (1981).
116. J. Larner, G. Galasko, K. Chen, A. A. De Paoli-Roach, L. Huang, P. Daggy, and J. Kellogg, *Science* **206**, 1408 (1979).
117. L. Jarett, F. L. Kiechle, D. A. Popp, N. Kotagal, and J. R. Gavin III, *Biochem. Biophys. Res. Commun.* **96**, 735 (1980).
118. J. R. Seals and L. Jarett, *Proc. Natl. Acad. Sci. USA* **77**, 77 (1980).
119. J. R. Seals and M. P. Czech, *J. Biol. Chem.* **255**, 6529 (1980).
120. J. R. Seals and M. P. Czech, *J. Biol. Chem.* **256**, 2894 (1981).
121. F. L. Kiechle, L. Jarett, N. Kotagal, and D. A. Popp, *J. Biol. Chem.* **256**, 2945 (1981).
122. A. R. Saltiel, M. I. Siegel, S. Jacobs, and P. Cuatrecasas, *Proc. Natl. Acad. Sci. USA* **79**, 3513 (1982).
123. J. C. Lawrence Jr. and J. Larner, *J. Biol. Chem.* **253**, 2104 (1978).
124. J. C. Lawrence Jr. and J. Larner, *Biochim. Biophys. Acta* **582**, 402 (1979).
125. H. Makino and T. Kono, *J. Biol. Chem.* **255**, 7850 (1980).
126. P. Greengard, *Science* **199**, 146 (1978).
127. M. Kasuga, F. A. Karlsson, and C. R. Kahn, *Science* **215**, 185 (1982).
128. M. Kasuga, Y. Zick, D. L. Blithe, M. Crettaz, and C. R. Kahn, *Nature* **298**, 667 (1982).
129. R. E. Hill, K.-L. Lee, and F. T. Kenney, *J. Biol. Chem.* **256**, 1510 (1981).
130. S. W. Cushman and L. J. Wardzala, *J. Biol. Chem.* **255**, 4758 (1980).
131. S. Gluck, C. Cannon, and Q. Al-Awqati, *Proc. Natl. Acad. Sci. USA* **79**, 4327 (1982).
132. K. Susuki and T. Kono, *Proc. Nat. Acad. Sci. USA* **77**, 2542 (1980).
133. K. J. Catt, J. P. Harwood, R. N. Clayton, T. F. Davies, V. Chan, M. Katikineni, K. Nozu, and M. L. Dufau, *Recent Prog. Horm. Res.* **36**, 557 (1980).
134. H. Lund-Anderson, *Physiol. Rev.* **59**, 305 (1979).
135. C. J. Goodner and N. Freinkel, *J. Clin. Invest.* **40**, 261 (1961).
136. O. Rafaelson, *J. Neurochem.* **7**, 33 (1961).
137. O. Rafaelson and T. Clausen, *J. Neurochem.* **7**, 52 (1961).
138. O. Rafaelson, *J. Neurochem.* **7**, 45 (1961).
139. A. L. Betz, D. D. Gilboe, D. L. Yudilevich, and L. R. Drewes, *Am. J. Physiol.* **225**, 586 (1973).
140. M. E. Phillips and R. V. Coxon, *J. Neurochem.* **27**, 643 (1976).
141. C. J. Goodner and M. A. Berrie, *Endocrinology* **101**, 605 (1977).
142. P. M. Daniel, E. R. Love, and O. E. Pratt, *Proc. R. Soc. Lond. Ser. B.* **196**, 85 (1977).
143. C. J. Goodner, F. G. Hom, and M. A. Berrie, *Endocrinology* **107**, 1827 (1980).

144. U. Gottstein, K. Held, H. Sebening, and G. Walpurger, *Klin. Wsch.* **43**, 965 (1965).
145. W. J. H. Butterfield, M. E. Abrams, R. A. Sills, G. Sterky, and M. J. Whichelow, *Lancet* **1**, 557 (1966).
146. M. M. Hertz, O. B. Paulson, D. I. Barry, J. S. Christiansen, and P. A. Svendsen, *J. Clin. Invest.* **67**, 597 (1981).
147. J. W. Yang and R. E. Fellows, *Endocrinology* **107**, 1717 (1980).
148. R. E. Catalan, A. M. Martinez, F. Mata, and M. D. Aragones, *Biochem. Biophys. Res. Commun.* **101**, 1216 (1981).
149. L. J. Roger and R. E. Fellows, *Endocrinology* **106**, 619 (1980).
150. J. S. Hatfield, W. J. Millard, and C. J. V. Smith, *Pharm. Biochem. Behav.* **2**, 223 (1973).
151. S. C. Woods and D. Porte Jr., *Adv. Metab. Dis.* **9**, 283 (1978).
152. S. C. Woods, E. C. Lotter, L. D. McKay, and D. M. Porte Jr., *Nature* **282**, 503 (1979).
153. D. Porte Jr. and S. C. Woods, *Diabetologia* **20**, 274 (1981).
154. I. Chowers, S. Lavy, and L. Halpern, *Exp. Neurol.* **14**, 383 (1966).
155. S. C. Woods and D. Porte Jr., *Diabetes* **24**, 905 (1975).
156. R. U. Margolis and N. Altszuler, *Proc. Soc. Exp. Biol. Med.* **127**, 1122 (1968).
157. D. K. Anderson and R. L. Hazelwood, *J. Physiol.* **202**, 83 (1969).
158. G. J. Taborsky and R. N. Bergman, *Diabetes* **29**, 278 (1980).
159. A. J. Szabo and O. Szabo, *J. Physiol.* **253**, 121 (1975).
160. O. Szabo and A. J. Szabo, *Diabetes* **24**, 328 (1975).
161. A. Iguchi, P. D. Burleson, and A. J. Szabo, *Am. J. Physiol.* **240**, E95 (1981).
162. A. F. Debons, I. Krimsky, A. From, and R. J. Cloutier, *Am. J. Physiol.* **217** (4) 1114 (1969).
163. A. F. Debons, I. Krimsky, and A. From, *Am. J. Physiol.* **219**, 938 (1970).
164. L. A. Frohman and L. L. Bernardis, *Am. J. Physiol.* **221** (6), 1596 (1971).
165. L. H. Storlien, W. P. Bellingham, and G. M. Martin, *Brain Res.* **96**, 156 (1975).
166. A. B Steffens, *Diabetologia* **20**, 411 (1981).
167. D. A. Bereiter, F. Rohner-Jeanrenaud, H.-R. Bethoud, and B. Jeanrenaud, *Diabetologia* **20**, 417 (1981).
168. Y. Oomura and H. Kita, *Diabetologia* **20**, 290 (1981).
169. H. Kita, A. Niijima, Y. Oomura, S. Ishizuka, S. Aou, K. Yamabe, and H. Yoshimatsu, *Brain Res. Bull* **5** Suppl. 4, 163 (1980).
170. M. L. Mc Caleb, R. D. Myers, G. Singer, and G. Willis, *Am. J. Physiol.* **236**(5), R312 (1979).
171. T. Shimazu, A. Fukuda, and T. Ban, *Nature* **210**, 1178 (1966).
172. T. Shimazu and A. Amakawa, *Biochim. Biophys. Acta* **165**, 335 (1968).
173. T. Shimazu and S. Ogasawara, *Am. J. Physiol.* **228**, 1787 (1975).
174. T. Shimazu, H. Matsushita, and K. Ishikaw, *Brain Res.* **144**, 343 (1978).
175. T. Shimazu, *Diabetologia* **20**, 343 (1981).
176. W. A. Bauman, V. B. Hatcher, M. A. Levitt, and R. S. Yalow, *Diabetes* **31**, 182 (1982).
177. J. E. Eng and R. S. Yalow, *Proc. Natl. Acad. Sci. USA* **79**, 2683 (1982).
178. V. Maier, A. Greischel, P. Steiner, B. Pfeifle, and E. F. Pfeiffer, submitted.
179. F. De Pablo, J. Roth, E. Hernandez, and R. M. Pruss, *Endocrinology* **111**, 1909 (1982).
180. A. Dorn, H.-G. Bernstein, H.-J. Hahn, G. Kostmann, and M. Ziegler, *Verh. Anat. Ges.* **75**, 791 (1981).
181. H.-G. Bernstein, H. Aurin, A. Dorn, J. Weiss, and M. Ziegler, *Acta Histochem.* **69**, 57 (1981).
182. A. Dorn, A. Rinne, H.-J. Hahn, H.-G. Bernstein, and M. Ziegler, *Acta Histochem.* **70**, 326 (1982).
183. A. Dorn, H.-G. Bernstein, A. Rinne, H.-J. Hahn, and M. Ziegler, *Acta Histochem.* **71**, 11 (1982).

184. A. Dorn, H.-G. Bernstein, H. Aurin, J. Frohlich, J. Wiess, and M. Ziegler, *Verh. Anat. Ges.* **76**, 435 (1982).

185. A. Dorn, H.-G. Bernstein, A. Rinne, H.-J. Hahn, and M. Ziegler, *Histochemistry* **74**, 293 (1982).

186. J. L. Rosenzweig, D. Le Roith, M. A. Lesniak, I. MacIntyre, W. H. Sawyer, and J. Roth, *Fed. Proc.*, **42**, 2608 (1983).

187. B. R. Landau, Y. Takaoka, M. A. Abrams, S. M. Genuth, M. Van Houten, B. I. Posner, R. J. White S. Ohgaku, A. Horvat, and E. Hemmelgarn, *Diabetes* **32**, 284 (1983).

188. T. L. Andreone, E. G. Beale, R. S. Bar, and D. K. Granner, *J. Biol. Chem.* **257**, 35 (1982).

189. H.-G. Bernstein, G. Poeggel, A. Dorn, H. Luppa, and M. Ziegler, *Experientia* **37**, 435 (1981).

190. D. Le Roith, S. A. Hendricks, M. A. Lesniak, K. L. Becker, S. Rishi, J. Havrankova, J. L. Rosenzweig, M. J. Brownstein, and J. Roth, in A. J. Szabo, R. Levine, and R. Luft, Eds., *Advances in Metabolic Diseases,* Academic Press, New York, 1983 (in press).

37

Bombesin-like Peptides

JOHN H. WALSH
Veterans Administration, Wadsworth Center
Los Angeles, California

1 STRUCTURE

Bombesin is the generic term applied to a group of structurally related peptides isolated initially from amphibian skin (1–4). These peptides have a characteristic pattern of stimulatory effects on gastrointestinal and urinary smooth muscle and stimulate the release of several hormones, notably gastrin. Bombesin-like peptides have been purified from the skin of several amphibian species (Table 1). The major variations in amino acid sequences are found in the amino-terminal portions of these molecules. The carboxyl-terminal nonapeptide sequence, containing the most important determinants of biological activity, is highly conserved. A major exception to this general pattern is found in the sequences of the ranatensin and litorin peptides, where phenylalanine is substituted for leucine in the penultimate position.

A mammalian equivalent of bombesin has been described by Mac-Donald and coworkers (5, 6) and named gastrin-releasing peptide, or GRP. This peptide, isolated from hog intestine and stomach, contains 27 amino acid residues (Table 1). The carboxyl-terminal nonapeptide sequence of GRP is identical with that of bombesin except for the single substitution of a histidine for a glutamine residue. A series of peptides analogous to GRP have been purified from canine intestinal muscle (J. R. Reeve, personal communication). The largest form contains 27 amino acid residues and differs from porcine GRP at four positions in amino terminal portion of the molecule. Two other carboxyl-terminal fragments of this canine peptide, containing 23 and 10 amino acid residues, also have been isolated. The structure of an avian peptide, similar to porcine GRP, also has been reported (7). Bombesin-like peptides have been identified in extracts of brain and spinal cord of mammals but have not yet been sequenced.

2 DISTRIBUTION

2.1 Amphibians and Birds

Bombesin-like peptides have been identified in tissues and tissue extracts by use of bioassay, radioimmunoassay, and immunohistochemistry. The highest concentrations of these peptides are found in the skin of certain amphibians, where concentrations as high as 1000 μg/g have been reported (1, 8). The cellular localization of these peptides in skin has not been reported. Moderately high concentrations of bombesin-like immunoreactivity have been found in the amphibian stomach, where they are localized in characteristic endocrine cells (9, 10). Lower concentrations of bombesin-like and ranatensin-like immunoreactivity are found in amphibian brain (11). These two classes of peptides were

TABLE 1 Structure of Bombesin-like Peptides

Peptide	Length of Sequence	Amino Acid Sequence
Chicken GRP	27	A P L Q P G G S P A L T K I Y P R G S H W A V G H L M #
Canine GRP	27	A P V P G G Q G T V L D K M Y P R G N H W A V G H L M #
Porcine GRP	27	A P V S V G G G T V L A K M Y P R G N H W A V G H L M #
Bombesin	14	pQ Q R L G N Q W A V G H L M #
Alytensin	14	pQ G R L G T Q W A V G H L M #
Litorin	9	pQ Q W A V G H F M #
Ranatensin	11	pQ V P Q W A V G H F M #
Ranatensin-C	11	pQ T P Q W A V G H F M #
Ranatensin-R	17	S D A T L R R Y N Q W A T G H F M #

Underlined residues differ from sequence above.

found to have separate patterns of distribution in the amphibian brain. Their distribution also differed from that of substance P.

Bombesin-like immunoreactivity and bioactivity have been found in high concentrations in the avian proventriculus (12, 13) and in the avian brain (13). In the proventriculus, immunohistochemical studies with bombesin antisera revealed localization in mucosal endocrine cells (13).

2.2 Mammals

Bombesin-like peptides can be extracted from the mucosa and muscle layers of the mammalian stomach and the muscle layers of the small intestine (14–16). The material extracted from mammalian tissues is heterogeneous in size (15, 16) and appears to have closer immunochemical identity to GRP than to bombesin (17, 18). In contrast with the endocrine cell localization found in amphibians, mammalian bombesin-like peptides appear to be located exclusively in nerve cells and fibers in the gut (19, 20). Within the stomach, fine nerve fibers extend through the mucosa; in the intestine, the fibers appear to be confined to muscle layers (19). In addition, bombesin-like immunoreactivity has been found in nerve fibers in the prevertebral sympathetic ganglia. These fibers have been shown by lesion experiments to originate in cell bodies in the gut wall (Schultzberg and Dockray, personal communication). Endocrine type cells that contain bombesin-like immunoreactivity have been identified in fetal lung but appear to be absent in adult lung (21, 22).

In the rat spinal cord, immunoreactive bombesin had chromatographic properties similar to those of bombesin (23). It was about 15 times more concentrated in the dorsal horn than in the ventral horn or white matter. This material could be released from spinal cord slices by KCl or veratridine in a calcium-dependent manner, but was not released by concentrations of capsaicin that simulated release of substance P. Bombesin-like immunoreactivity also has been characterized in human cerebrospinal fluid (24). The average concentration was about 35 pM and the material resembled bombesin C-terminal nonapeptide more closely than the tetradecapeptide by gel filtration analysis.

Crude dissection of rat brain regions revealed highest concentrations of bombesin-like immunoreactivity in the hypothalamus and lowest concentrations in cerebellum (15, 25). The distribution of bombesin receptors was generally parallel to that of extractable peptide except for the hippocampus, which had a high density of receptors and low peptide content (25). Micropunch analysis of discrete rat brain regions revealed 30-fold differences in concentrations, with highest values obtained in the substantia gelatinosa trigemeni, nucleus of the tractus solitarius, interpeduncular nucleus, and arcuate nucleus (26).

The chemical nature of mammalian brain bombesin-like immunoreactivity has not been determined. Evidence for size and charge heterogeneity has been reported (15, 25, 26). One form appears to be similar in size to GRP and can be converted by trypsin to a smaller form (27). However, the smaller forms are more abundant in tissue extracts (15, 26).

Subcellular fractionation of rat brain homogenates revealed that bombesin receptors and bombesin-like immunoreactivity were concentrated in synaptosomal fractions (28). Bombesin-like immunoreactivity was released from hypothalamic slices by potassium and veratridine in a calcium-dependent manner.

In the newborn rat, immunoreactive bombesin can be detected in the stomach but not in the brain (15). Adult concentrations are reached in the gut by 16 days and in the brain by 26 days.

3 EFFECTS OF BOMBESIN ON CENTRAL NERVOUS SYSTEM FUNCTIONS

Although a physiological role for bombesin has not yet been established, bombesin and bombesin-like peptides have a wide range of pharmacologic actions. One group of actions has been described when bombesin is injected into the brain, usually by intracisternal or intracerebroventricular injection. Some of these activities are discussed elsewhere in this book under specific functions, for example, thermoregulation (Chapter 12) and regulation of food intake (Chapter 10). The following is a synopsis of some of the effects of bombesin on central nervous function.

3.1 Direct Electrical Effects

Application of bombesin into the cell body layer of the pyramidal cells of the hippocampus caused excitatory depolarizations (29) in the CA1 region of hippocampal slices. In the isolated, hemisected toad spinal cord, bombesin had a potent depolarizing action on dorsal root terminals and motoneurons (30).

3.2 Thermoregulation

One of the most potent central effects of bombesin is lowering of the core body temperature in rats (31). This effect is accentuated by exposure to a cold environment and is antagonized by thyrotropin-releasing hormone (TRH), prostaglandin E_2, and naloxone (32). Microinjection experiments revealed that the preoptic area of the anterior hypothalamus was one site of action (33). Decreased body temperature caused by lateral ventricular or preoptic injections of bombesin was associated with parallel decreases in oxygen consumption (34). The hypothermic effect may also be caused, in part, by vasodilation (35). At high ambient temperatures, intraventricular injection of bombesin causes hyperthermia (36). Porcine gastrin-releasing peptide has the same hypothermic effect as bombesin but is somewhat less potent (37). Effects of peptides on temperature regulation are discussed in more detail in Chapter 12.

3.3   Hyperglycemia

Intracisternal injection of small doses of bombesin in conscious rats results in significant elevations of plasma glucose that are independent of ambient temperature (38). This hyperglycemic effect is accompanied by a parallel increase in plasma glucagon and a relative decrease in plasma insulin. Similar effects on blood sugar are produced by subcutaneous injection of epinephrine, and the response to central administration of bombesin is prevented by adrenalectomy. Intracisternal bombesin also causes a significant increase in plasma epinephrine but no increase in plasma norepinephrine or dopamine (39). The response is not prevented by hypophysectomy, and plasma corticosterone concentrations are not increased after bombesin administration. These results are consistent with a primary effect of bombesin in the brain to increase sympathetic outflow to the adrenal gland, with hyperglycemia resulting from increased secretion of adrenal medullary epinephrine. The hyperglycemic effect of bombesin is antagonized by peripheral or central administration of somatostatin or somatostatin analogs (35, 40). This central effect of bombesin is not associated with changes in peripheral glucose turnover and does not appear to be due to activation of central cholinergic or adrenergic pathways (41). In conscious dogs, microinjections of bombesin into specific brain sites including anterior hypothalamus and dorsal-medial hypothalamus caused increases in blood sugar, epinephrine, and mean arterial blood pressure (42). However, injection into other sites caused only increases in blood pressure (e.g., lateral hypothalamus), suggesting separate pathways for these effects.

3.4   Behavioral Effects

Intraventricular administration of bombesin in conscious rats produces a dose-related alteration in behavior characterized by facial grooming and extensive scratching of the upper body and face with the hindpaws (43). This behavior differs from the response to opioids and ACTH fragments in that it is not accompanied by yawning and stretching. It is not altered by administration of naloxone or morphine. Intracisternal administration of bombesin in mice enhanced the impairment of the righting reflex caused by peripheral administration of ethanol, but had no effect when given alone (44).

3.5 Effects on Hypothalamic-Pituitary Hormones

Intraventricular administration of bombesin to conscious rats prevented the normal increase in plasma prolactin produced by cold restraint stress but did not modify the increase in plasma corticosterone or decrease in growth hormone (GH) or luteinizing hormone (LH) produced by stress (45). This effect was not altered by naloxone (45). Central administration of bombesin to nonstressed conscious male rats decreased basal plasma prolactin and inhibited the prolactin response to endorphin, but the prolactin response to suckling in lactating rats was increased by bombesin (46).

Intraventricular injection of bombesin caused a dose-related increase in hypophyseal portal immunoreactive somatostatin in urethane anesthetized rats without measurable changes in jugular venous blood (47). This effect appeared to be of biological significance since it was associated with complete suppression of plasma growth hormone responses to intraventricular β-endorphin or intravenous prostaglandin.

Peripheral administration of bombesin in doses up to 600 pmol·kg^{-1}·h^{-1} in normal human subjects produced no alteration in basal concentrations of plasma GH, prolactin (PRL), thyroid stimulating hormone (TSH), LH, or follicle stimulating hormone (FSH) in one study (48), although a similar dose caused increased PRL in six of eight normal subjects in another study (49).

3.6 Feeding Behavior

Bombesin is one of the peptides known to modify feeding behavior. This topic is discussed in detail elsewhere in this book (Chapter 10). Intraperitoneal injections of bombesin caused inhibition of liquid and solid food intake in conscious rats (50). Bombesin was only one-fifth as potent as cholecystokinin octapeptide for inhibition of liquid food intake, but the two peptides had similar potency for inhibition of solid food intake. The effects of both peptides could be measured only in the first hour of injection. Higher doses of intraperitoneal bombesin also were shown to inhibit sham feeding in rats (51). The decrease in feeding behavior was associated with other behavioral signs of satiety including grooming and apparent sleep. Intraventricular administration of bombesin caused significant inhibition of stress-induced eating in rats (52). This effect appeared to be independent of the associated hyperglycemia and was maintained in adrenalectomized rats. There is some controversy about the ability of doses of bombesin that inhibit food intake to produce conditioned taste aversion (53, 54). The structurally related peptides, litorin and GRP, have effects similar to bombesin in inhibiting food intake when given parenterally (55). The possibility that

peripherally administered bombesin acts indirectly to reduce food intake by release of endogenous CCK peptides was rendered unlikely by
the recent observation that truncal vagotomy prevents the satiety effect
of CCK but not of bombesin (55). Peripheral and central effects of
bombesin on food intake also differ in that centrally administered
bombesin produces behavioral effects at doses lower than those required to inhibit food intake and inhibits ingestion of water as well as
of food. The effects of intraventricular bombesin on water intake are
species specific. Bombesin stimulates water intake in birds but inhibits
water intake in mammals (56).

3.7   Gastrointestinal Function

Central administration of bombesin markedly reduces the incidence and
severity of gastric mucosal lesions produced in rats by cold restraint
stress (57). Further evaluation of this phenomenon revealed that
intracerebroventricular administration of bombesin produced potent inhibition of gastric acid secretion in the pylorus-ligated rat (58). Ventricular administration of bombesin antagonized the acid responses to
vagal stimulation with insulin or 2DG. However, inhibition of acid secretion was not due entirely to inhibition of vagal outflow because it
was retained after truncal vagotomy. Adrenalectomy also did not prevent the inhibition of acid secretion. The inhibition of acid secretion
was associated with a marked increase in plasma gastrin concentration.
Intragastric pH increased after central bombesin administration to 7.8–
8.0, implying stimulation of gastric alkaline secretion in addition to inhibition of acid secretion. Similar effects on acid secretion have been
measured after central administration of gastrin-releasing peptide or its
acetylated C-terminal octapeptide (59). Centrally administered bombesin also prevents the increase in acid secretion produced by central administration of TRH. The central site of action has not been determined,
but there is evidence for involvement of endogenous biogenic amines in
the brain in mediation of the acid-inhibitory responses (60, 61). The inhibition of gastric acid secretion produced by central administration of
bombesin peptides in rats stands in marked contrast to the gastric-relat-
ed stimulation of acid secretion produced by intravenous administration
of these compounds in dogs and humans. These peripheral effects on
the stomach are discussed later.

4   EFFECTS OF BOMBESIN ON PERIPHERAL TISSUES

The most commonly recognized actions of bombesin, other structurally
related amphibian peptides, and mammalian GRP have been stimulation
of gastrin release and alterations in smooth muscle contractions in the

gut and elsewhere. Since bombesin-like peptides are found in nerves of the autonomic nervous system throughout the gut, it is possible that some of the pharmacologic properties of bombesin described after *in vivo* and *in vitro* administration of bombesin represent normal physiologic functions of this neuropeptide. However, there is no peripheral action of bombesin peptides for which a physiological role has been shown with any certainty. The following synopsis of peripheral actions is likely to include one or more effects that will be considered physiologic after more sophisticated methods are developed to inhibit the peripheral responses to bombesin.

4.1 Gastric Exocrine and Endocrine Secretion

The effects of bombesin on gastric function have been explored in the rat, a species in which bombesin stimulates release of gastrin but not acid secretion, and in dogs and humans, in which stimulation of gastrin release is associated with stimulation of acid secretion. In amphibians there is some evidence for a direct stimulatory action of bombesin on acid-secreting gastric mucosa (62), but similar effects have not been reported for mammalian gastric mucosa.

Intravenous administration of bombesin to rats does not stimulate gastric acid secretion (63). As described in Section 3.7, central administration of bombesin to rats causes increased plasma gastrin and decreased acid secretion. Chronic administration of gastrin to rats causes an increase in both antral and serum gastrin concentrations, suggesting a stimulatory effect on gastrin synthesis (64). In anesthetized rats, intravenous administration of bombesin or of bombesin-like immunoreactive peptides purified from rat intestine and stomach caused dose-related increases in serum gastrin concentration (15). In the isolated, perfused rat stomach, arterial perfusion with bombesin resulted in a dose-related increase in secretion of both gastrin and somatostatin in the venous effluent (65). The gastrin response was markedly enhanced by prior administration of somatostatin antiserum. Preliminary evidence was obtained that cholinergic stimulation caused release of immunoreactive bombesin. However, another study suggested that stimulation of gastrin release from rat stomach by bombesin was independent of cholinergic stimulation or somatostatin release and more likely represented direct stimulation of gastrin cells by bombesin (66).

In dogs, intravenous infusion of bombesin produces potent stimulation of both gastrin release and gastric acid secretion (67). The gastrin response is resistant to atropine, partially resistant to antral acidification, but is abolished by antrectomy (67, 68). Vagotomy of the acid-secreting stomach led to increased gastrin response but unaltered acid response to bombesin (69). In dogs with intact vagal nerves, bombesin is a potent stimulant of both gastrin and pancreatic polypeptide release

(70). However, the pancreatic polypeptide response is markedly inhibited by the cholinergic antagonist atropine, and the gastrin response is markedly inhibited by the cholinergic agonist bethanechol. Despite the inhibition of gastrin release, gastric acid secretory response to bombesin plus bethanechol is greater than to bombesin alone. If endogenous bombesin is involved in regulation of antral gastrin release by food, inhibition of food-stimulated gastrin by bethanechol might be anticipated. However, no such inhibition could be demonstrated by a dose of bethanechol that inhibited the gastrin response to bombesin (71).

Porcine GRP produces stimulation of gastrin release and acid secretion in dogs with a potency very similar to that of bombesin (6).

Two peptides that are structurally related to bombesin, litorin and ranatensin, appear to be less potent stimulants of gastrin release and acid secretion than bombesin, whereas the slightly related peptide, substance P, has no stimulatory effect (72). The gastrin and acid stimulatory effects of bombesin in dogs are significantly inhibited by concurrent administration of either somatostatin or an analog of prostaglandin E_2 (73). There is some evidence that bombesin may have a secondary inhibitory effect on gastrin-stimulated acid secretion in dogs (74).

Bombesin also stimulates gastrin release and gastric acid secretion in humans (75). Very low doses of bombesin produced parallel increases in acid secretion and gastrin release; higher doses produced further increases in gastrin without further increases in acid secretion (76). Comparison of acid secretory responses with endogenously released gastrin and exogenously administered gastrin led to the conclusion that the acid secretory response to exogenous bombesin can be explained entirely by release of gastrin (77). However, marked inhibition of gastric emptying during bombesin infusion appeared to be independent of serum gastrin. Bombesin appears to be a relatively specific stimulant of release of gastrin from the gastric antrum and not from the duodenum, since antral resection abolishes the response (78). Somatostatin, calcitonin, and secretin are potent inhibitors of bombesin-stimulated acid secretion in humans but are less potent inhibitors of bombesin-stimulated gastrin release (79, 80).

4.2 Pancreatic Exocrine Function

Intravenous infusion of bombesin in dogs produces stimulation of secretion of protein-rich pancreatic juice and of gallbladder contraction, suggesting that bombesin causes release of cholecystokinin (81). Similar effects of bombesin have been reported in human subjects (82). These observations strongly suggested that bombesin stimulates release of cholecystokinin (CCK) from the intestine. Indeed, there is one report of direct measurement of increased concentrations of immunoreactive CCK during bombesin infusion in dogs (83). A similar mechanism may

not account for stimulation of pancreatic enzyme secretion in the rat
and guinea pig, since bombesin has a direct stimulatory effect on acinar
cells in these species. However, direct stimulation of enzyme secretion
by bombesin could not be demonstrated in a preparation of pancreatic
acini from canine pancreas that responded to CCK and cholinergic stimulation (84).

Bombesin was nearly as potent as CCK in stimulation of amylase release from rat pancreatic fragments, and desensitization to bombesin
did not prevent subsequent calcium efflux in response to CCK,
suggesting that bombesin had a direct effect on acinar cells (85). Direct
evidence for separate acinar cell receptors for CCK peptides and for
bombesin peptides has been obtained in preparations of isolated guinea
pig acini (86). Occupation of these receptors caused a pattern of biological responses that included increased amylase secretion, cyclic GMP
accumulation, outflux of cellular calcium, and enhancement of the response to secretin or VIP (87). A labeled bombesin analog demonstrated
specific binding to acinar receptors that was not altered by occupation
of CCK or cholinergic receptors (86). Desensitization of acini by
bombesin markedly reduced the amylase response to bombesin and
structurally related peptides but did not alter the response to CCK or to
other secretagogs (88). Thus there is little doubt that separate receptors
for bombesin are present on acinar cells in some species and are capable of direct modulation of acinar cell function. Further confirmation of
the existence of separate CCK and bombesin receptors also has been
obtained by electrophysiological microelectrode recordings of mouse
acinar cells (89). Exposure of these cells to dbcGMP abolished the depolarization response to ionophoresis with CCK peptides but not
bombesin. The response of acinar cells to bombesin appears to be due
to specific interactions at the cell membrane, since direct intracellular
injection of bombesin failed to produce any electrical response similar
to that produced by extracellular application (90).

4.3   Release of Gut Hormones

Gastrin is not the only gut hormone released by bombesin. In dogs,
bombesin is a potent pancreatic polypeptide releasing agent (70). In humans this effect of bombesin is less prominent (91, 92). Bombesin infusion in humans causes release of neurotensin and enteroglucagon (92).
A comparison of bombesin and gastrin releasing peptide in dogs revealed that both peptides caused release of gastrin, pancreatic polypeptide, enteroglucagon, pancreatic glucagon, and gastric inhibitory polypeptide (93). Both peptides also caused a transient increase in plasma
insulin, associated with a small decrease in blood glucose and significant increase in glucose disappearance rate, but no changes in plasma
motilin were measured. Similar effects of bombesin on insulin, gluca-

gon, enteroglucagon, and blood sugar were reported in another study in dogs (94). The increase in plasma glucagon-like immunoreactivity was maintained after pancreatectomy. Bombesin infusion also caused an increase in basal and food-stimulated plasma somatostatin in dogs, and this response was not altered by chemical sympathectomy (95). This finding was contradicted in another study that failed to demonstrate an increase in plasma somatostatin during bombesin infusion (96). However, the bombesin-induced release of insulin and glucagon, and to a lesser extent the release of gastrin, were inhibited by exogenous somatostatins 14 and 28. Two studies involving isolated perfused dog pancreas have shown that bombesin increased release of insulin and glucagon but not of somatostatin (97, 98). Bombesin-stimulated insulin release may be a species-specific phenomenon, since release of insulin from isolated pancreatic islets of rats was significantly inhibited by bombesin (99).

The stimulation of release of gastrin and somatostatin from the isolated perfused rat stomach and possible trophic effect of bombesin on gastrin synthesis were discussed in an earlier section.

4.4 Effects of Gastrointestinal Motility

The biological properties of bombesin originally described by Erspamer and coworkers included stimulation of several preparations of isolated muscle strips obtained from the gut, uterus, and urinary tract of several species (1). Tissues found to be most useful for bombesin bioassay were rat uterus, kitten small intestine, guinea pig colon, and rat urinary bladder. In these tissues tachphylaxis was not a problem, but severe tachphylaxis was encountered in guinea pig ileum and guinea pig urinary bladder. In tissues that responded well to repeated doses of bombesin, the contractile responses were not blocked by atropine, hexamethonium, or other antagonists of biogenic amines and this was taken as evidence for a direct effect of bombesin on smooth muscle cells. In contrast, the contractile response of guinea pig ileum was strongly inhibited by atropine, implying stimulation of a cholinergic mediator. By use of a battery of smooth muscle preparations the activity of bombesin could be distinguished clearly from that of other biologically active peptides including bradykinin, cerulein, physalaemin, and oxytocin, and from serotonin, histamine, and prostaglandins.

The effects of bombesin on gastrointestinal motility and smooth muscle contraction have been investigated rather thoroughly in several species, including humans. Intravenous infusion of a relatively large dose of bombesin in normal human subjects caused a variety of changes in the radiographic appearance of the stomach and intestine (100). The responses included contraction of the antral and pyloric region of the stomach, relaxation of the proximal stomach, loss of small bowel motility, and contraction of the ileocecal valve with variable loss of colonic activity. Gastric and intestinal hyperperistalsis were noted when the bombesin infusions were discontinued. Bombesin also was a potent stimulant of contraction of smooth muscle strips obtained from human stomach, small intestine, colon, and appendix (100). The *in vitro* stimulation of contractions was characterized by inceased frequency and tone and was not antagonized by known inhibitors of neurotransmitters and nerve conduction, suggesting a direct stimulatory action on smooth muscle.

The effects of bombesin have been characterized on a variety of gastrointestinal motor functions. It is a potent stimulant of lower esophageal sphincter contraction in the opossum. This effect appears to involve direct stimulation of smooth muscle and indirect stimulation by activation of postganglionic alpha adrenergic fibers (101). Bombesin also is a potent inhibitor of gastric emptying in rats (102) and in humans (103, 104). The delayed emptying in humans cannot be explained by release of gastrin into the circulation. In muscle strips of canine stomach, bombesin increased the frequency of spontaneous contractions in circular muscle by a direct myogenic action, but stimulation of longitudinal muscle involved cholinergic neural pathways (105). Intravenous infusions of bombesin caused almost total inhibition of intraluminal duodenal and jejunal pressure in human subjects (106). Bombesin also causes emptying of the human gallbladder (107). Although this effect may be due in part to stimulation of CCK release, bombesin has a direct stimulating action on gallbladder muscle in some species (108). Bombesin also stimulates electrical activity of the rabbit sphincter of Oddi, but is less potent than CCK (109). Morphine and natural opioids also may antagonize the gut contracting activity of bombesin (110).

It is apparent from the above synopsis that bombesin may act on smooth muscle by direct interaction with smooth muscle cells or by a variety of indirect mechanisms involving other mediators. The role of other endogenously released hormones in mediation of *in vivo* responses to bombesin also require further study.

4.5 Other Peripheral Effects

Bombesin also influences blood pressure, renal function, bladder contraction, and bronchiolar muscle in some species. In most animal species bombesin produces moderate increases in blood pressure, but it has a hypotensive effect in monkeys (111). Major effects on blood pressure have not been reported in humans. In the anesthetized dog, bombesin has a potent antidiuretic effect associated with vasoconstriction of afferent renal arterioles and activation of the renin-angiotensin system (112). Bombesin is a potent stimulant of urinary bladder smooth muscle contraction in rat, guinea pig, and cat but not in hamster, mouse, rabbit, dog, or monkey (113). It also has a direct effect on human bladder muscle but is considerably less potent than angiotensin II and substance P-like peptides (114). A potent, apparently direct spasmogenic effect of bombesin was found for bronchiolar muscle of the anesthetized guinea pig (115).

5   STRUCTURE–FUNCTION RELATIONSHIPS

Testing of a series of synthetic bombesin fragments on a battery of *in vitro* smooth muscle systems revealed that the carboxyl-terminal nonapeptide sequence of the parent peptide was required for full biological activity (116). The carboxyl-terminal heptapeptide and octapeptide retained some activity and this activity was enhanced by the presence of an amino-terminal blocking group. Similar results were found for effects of these peptides on gastrin release (117).

The 27-amino-acid gastrin releasing peptide produces a similar pattern of central nervous actions as bombesin but is less potent (118). A large number of synthetic bombesin analogs have been tested for central effects on thermoregulation (119). Several alterations in the C-terminal decapeptide sequence, including removal of the C-terminal amide group, markedly decreased potency for this effect. The structurally related amphibian peptides ranatensin and litorin were 20% and <1% as potent as bombesin but alytesin had full potency. The C-terminal nonapeptide of GRP and the C-terminal tetradecapeptide have weak central effects, but acetylation of the N-terminal residue of the octapeptide or nonapeptide markedly increases potency (120). A comparison of central and peripheral effects suggests that fragments of GRP may be more readily metabolized in the brain than longer fragments but that the C-terminal nonapeptide sequence of bombesin is sufficient for full activity in most peripheral systems. Full comparisons of a spectrum of bombesin and GRP analogs have not been reported for gastrointestinal motor and secretory actions.

6   MEASUREMENT AND RELEASE

Most of the antibodies used for radioimmunoassay of bombesin are directed at the C-terminal portion of the molecule and bind the biologically active portion of bombesin fragments (121, 122). Other antibodies have been described that are specific for the C-terminal portion of ranatensin and litorin (11) or for the midportion of bombesin (17). Antibodies raised against GRP may exhibit full or only partial crossreactivity with bombesin (18). Most of the C-terminally directed antibodies appear to detect mammalian bombesin-like peptides in tissue extracts and by immunocytochemical reactions. However, it has been difficult to demonstrate release of bombesin-like peptides under physiological conditions. This difficulty may be due to the peripheral localization of these peptides in nerve fibers rather than endocrine cells. In the brain and spinal cord, release of bombesin-like immunoreactivity can be stimulated by potassium or veratridine from tissue slices (23, 28). The presence of bombesin-like immunoreactivity in human spinal fluid also implies release from human brain or spinal cord (24). Attempts to measure changes in immunoreactive bombesin in human plasma after ingestion of a meal have been disappointing (16, 76), but small amounts have been detected by use of a new radioimmunoassay (Okubo, unpublished). There is preliminary evidence for cholinergic stimulation of bombesin release from isolated perfused rat stomach (65). At present there is no conclusive evidence for release of physiologically significant concentrations of bombesin peptides into blood or tissue fluids under physiological conditions of stimulation. Until such measurements can be made or suitable bombesin antagonists are developed, a regulatory role for bombesin peptides must remain speculative.

7　BOMBESIN RECEPTORS

The presence of bombesin receptors on many cell types can be inferred from the wide spectrum of biological activities described above and more specifically from the responses of isolated tissues and cells to bombesin. Studies with pharmacologic blocking agents indicate that many of the smooth muscle contractile responses caused by bombesin are due to direct interaction with smooth muscle membranes, although others may involve neural mediation (1, 101, 105, 110). Stimulation of gallbladder contraction *in vitro* does not appear to involve CCK receptors because the response to bombesin is not inhibited by the CCK antagonist dibutyryl cyclic guanosine monophosphate (dbcGMP) (108).

Direct demonstration of bombesin receptors in rat brain membranes has been achieved by use of radioiodinated Tyr[4] bombesin (123). A single class of high-affinity receptors sites ($K_D = 3$ nM) was found. These receptors exhibited specific, saturable binding of biologically active bombesin and bombesin analogs, and there was generally good correlation between potency of analogs to inhibit receptor binding and potency to induce hypothermia. The use of this radioreceptor assay to map the distribution of bombesin receptors in rat brain revealed high concentrations in many areas including limbic forebrain, hippocampus, amygdala, hypothalamus, periaqueductal gray matter, caudate-putamen, and forebrain (124).

Similar studies of bombesin receptors have been performed in isolated pancreatic acini. Binding of radioiodinated Tyr[4] bombesin was temperature-dependent, reversible, and revealed the presence of a single class of high affinity binding sites with $K_D = 4$ nM (86). There was good correlation between inhibition of binding by bombesin-like peptides and stimulation of amylase secretion. Structurally unrelated peptides, including cholecystokinin, did not interact with bombesin receptors. The stimulation of amylase released by bombesin was associated with calcium outflux and cGMP accumulation. Each pancreatic acinar cell contains about 5000 bombesin receptors. The presence of a distinct group of biologically active bombesin receptors on acinar cells is consistent with other findings that include failure of desensitization of acinar cells by bombesin to alter secretory responses to cholinergic agents or to CCK (88) and failure of the competitive CCK antagonist dibutyryl cGMP to alter acinar electrophysiological responses to bombesin (89). Despite the clear demonstration of bombesin receptors in the pancreas, there is no information that indicates a physiological role of these receptors in regulation of pancreatic secretion.

8 CLINICAL RELEVANCE OF BOMBESIN PEPTIDES

The only evidence for abnormal secretion of bombesin-like peptides presently available is demonstration of relatively high concentrations of immunoreactive bombesin in cell lines obtained from small cell carcinomas of the lung (125). Clinical data relating release of bombesin-like peptides into the circulation to peripheral manifestations of bombesin excess have not been reported.

The relative specificity of bombesin to stimulate release of gastrin from the gastric antrum and not from normal extra-antral sources has been used to identify patients with residual antral tissue after attempted surgical antrectomy (78). However, bombesin also causes release of gastrin from gastrinomas, especially from those originating in the duodenum (126).

9 SUMMARY

Bombesin is an amphibian peptide that has a wide spectrum of biological actions on the central nervous system and on peripheral tissues. Peptides of similar structure are found in mammalian brain and in nerve fibers in the mammalian gut as well as in endocrine cells of the fetal lung. The high potency of bombesin and presence of high affinity specific receptors in target tissues suggests that mammalian bombesin-like peptides may have specific physiological functions. Such functions could include central regulation of body temperature, blood glucose, feeding behavior or gastrointestinal function and peripheral nervous regulation of gastrointestinal motility, secretions, and hormone release. Pathological overproduction of bombesin-like peptides may occur in patients with small cell carcinomas of the lung. However, specific physiological and pathophysiological roles for bombesin-like peptides remain to be defined.

REFERENCES

1. V. Erspamer, G. Falconieri Erspamer, M. Inselvini, and L. Negri, *Br. J. Pharm.* **45**, 333–348 (1972).
2. A. Anastasi, V. Erspamer, and M. Bucci, *Arch. Biochem. Biophys.* **148**, 443–446 (1972).
3. T. Nakajima, T. Yasuhara, and O. Ishikawa, in A. Miyoshi, Ed., *Gut Peptides*, Kodansha, Tokyo, and Elsevier North-Holland Biomedical, Amsterdam, 1979, pp. 14–18.
4. P. Melchiorri, in S. R. Bloom, Ed., *Gut Hormones*, Churchill-Livingstone, Edinburgh, 1978, pp. 534–540.
5. T. J. McDonald, G. Nilsson, M. Vagne, M. Ghatei, S. R. Bloom, and NS C. Mutt, *Gut* **19**, 767–774 (1978).
6. T. J. McDonald, H. Jornvall, G. Nilsson, M. Vagne, M. Ghatei, S. R. Bloom, and V. Mutt, *Biochem. Biophys. Res. Comm.* **90**, 227–233 (1979).
7. T. J. McDonald, H. Jornvall, M. Ghatei, S. R. Bloom, and V. Mutt, *FEBS Lett.* **122** (1), 45–48 (1980).
8. V. Erspamer and P. Melchiorri, *Pure Appl. Chem.* **35**, 463–494 (1973).
9. J. Lechago, A. L. Holmquist, G. L. Rosenquist, and J. H. Walsh, *Gen. Comp. Endocrinol.* **36**, 553–558 (1978).
10. J. Lechago, B. G. Crawford, and J. H. Walsh, *Gen. Comp. Endocrinol.* **45**, 1–6 (1981).
11. J. H. Walsh, J. Lechago, H. C. Wong, and G. L. Rosenquist, *Regul. Peptides* **3**, 1–13 (1982).
12. V. Erspamer, G. Falconieri Erspamer, P. Melchiorri, and L. Negri, *Gut* **20**, 1047–1056 (1979).
13. C. Vaillant, G. J. Dockray, and J. H. Walsh, *Histochemistry* **64**, 307–314 (1979).
14. M. Brown, R. Allen, J. Villarreal, J. Rivier, and W. Vale, *Life Sci.* **23**, 2721–2728 (1978).
15. J. H. Walsh, H. C. Wong, and G. J. Dockray, *Fed. Proc.* **38**, 63–67 (1979).
16. J. H. Walsh, J. R. Reeve, Jr., and S. R. Vigna, in S. R. Bloom and J. M. Polak, Eds., *Gut Hormones*, 2nd ed., Churchill Livingstone, Edinburgh, 1981, pp. 413–418.
17. C. Yanahaira, A. Inoue, T. Mochizuki, J. Ozaki, H. Sato, and N. Yanaihara, *Biomed. Res.* **1**, 96–100 (1980).
18. N. Yanaihara, C. Yanaihara, T. Mochizuki, K. Iwahara, T. Fujita, and T. Iwanaga, *Peptides* **2**, Suppl. 2, 185–191 (1981).
19. G. J. Dockray, C. Vaillant, and J. H. Walsh, *Neuroscience* **4**, 1561–1568 (1979).
20. S. R. Bloom and J. M. Polak, in *Brain Peptides: A New Endocrinology*, Elsevier/North-Holland Biomedical, Amsterdam, 1979, pp. 103–117.
21. J. Wharton, J. M. Polak, S. R. Bloom, M. A. Ghatei, E. Solcia, M. R. Brown, and A. G. E. Pearse, *Nature* **273**, 769–770 (1978).
22. E. Cutz, W. Chan, and N. S. Track, *Experientia*, **37**(7), 765–767 (1981).
23. T. W. Moody, N. B. Thoa, T. L. O'Donohue, and D. M. Jacobowitz, *Life Sci.* **29**, 2273–2279 (1981).
24. T. Yamada, M. S. Takami, and R. H. Gerner, *Brain Res.* **223**, 214–217 (1981).
25. T. W. Moody and C. B. Pert, *Biochem. Biophys. Res. Commun.* **90**, 7–14 (1979).
26. T. W. Moody, T. L. O'Donohue, and D. M. Jacobowitz, *Peptides* **2**, 75–79 (1981).

27. J. A. Villarreal and M. R. Brown, *Life Sci.* **23**, 2729–2734 (1978).
28. T. W. Moody, N. B. Thoa, T. L. O'Donohue, and C. B. Pert, *Life Sci.* **26**, 1707–1712 (1980).
29. J. Dodd and J. S. Kelly, *Brain Res.* **205**(2), 337–50 (1981).
30. J. W. Phillis and J. R. Kirkpatrick, *Can. J. Physiol. Pharmacol.* **57**(8), 887–99 (1979).
31. M. Brown, J. Rivier, and W. Vale, *Science* **196**, 998–999 (1977).
32. M. Brown, J. Rivier, and W. Vale, *Life Sci.* **20**, 1681–1688 (1977).
33. Q. J. Pittman, Yvette Tache, and M. R. Brown, *Life Sci.* **26**, 725–730 (1980).
34. B. A. Wunder, M. F. Hawkins, D. D. Avery, and H. Swan, *Neuropharmacology* **19**, 1095–1097 (1980).
35. R. Francesconi and M. Mager, *Brain Res. Bull.* **7**(1), 63–8 (1981).
36. Y. Tache, Q. Pittman, and M. Brown, *Brain Res.* **188**, 525–530 (1980).
37. M. Brown, W. Marki, and J. Rivier, *Life Sci.* **27**, 125–128 (1980).
38. M. Brown, J. Rivier, and W. W. Vale, *Life Sci.* **21**, 1729–1734 (1977).
39. M. Brown, Y. Tache, and D. Fisher, *Endocrinology* **105**, 660–665 (1979).
40. M. Brown, J. Rivier, and W. Vale, *Endocrinology* **104**(6), 1709–1715 (1979).
41. M. Brown, *Diabetologia* **20**, 299–304 (1981).
42. M. Brown, L. Fisher, and V. Webb, *Soc. Neurosci. Abstr.* **7**, 210 (1981).
43. R. Katz, *Neuropharmacology* **19**, 143–146 (1980).
44. G. D. Frye, D. Luttinger, C. B. Nemeroff, R. A. Vogel, A. J. Prange Jr., and G. R. Breese, *Peptides* **2**, Suppl. 1, 99–106 (1981).
45. Y. Tache, M. Brown, and R. Collu, *Endocrinology* **105**, 220–224 (1979).
46. Y. Tache, Q. Pittman, C. Rivier, and M. Brown, Proceedings of the 61st Meeting of the Endocrine Society, Anaheim, Calif., June 13–15, 1979, p. 289.
47. H. Abe, K. Chihara, N. Minamitani, J. Iwasaki, T. Chiba, S. Matsukura, and T. Fujita, *Endocrinology* **109**, 229–234 (1981).
48. J. E. Morley, A. A. Varner, I. M. Modlin, H. E. Carlson, G. D. Braunstein, J. H. Walsh, and J. M. Hershman, *Clin. Endocrinol.* **13**, 369–373 (1980).
49. A. E. Pontiroli, M. Alberetto, L. Restelli, and A. Facchinetti, *J. Clin. Endocrinol. Metab.* **51**(6), 1303–1305 (1980).
50. J. Gibbs, D. J. Fauser, E. A. Rose, B. J. Rolls, and S. P. Maddison, *Nature* **282**, 208–210 (1979).
51. C. F. Martin and J. Gibbs, *Peptides* **1**, 131–134 (1980).
52. J. E. Morley and A. S. Levine, *Pharmacol. Biochem. Behav.* **14**, 149–151 (1980).
53. J. A. Deutsch and S. L. Parsons, *Behav. Neural Biol.* **31**, 110–113 (1981).
54. P. J. Kulkosky, L. Gray, J. Gibbs, and G. P. Smith, *Peptides* **2**(1), 61–4 (1981).
55. J. Gibbs, P. J. Kulkosky, and G. P. Smith, *Peptides* **2**, 179–183 (1981).
56. G. de Caro, M. Mariotti, M. Massi, and L. G. Micossi, *Pharmacol. Biochem. Behav.* **13**(2), 229–233 (1980).
57. Y. Tache, P. Simard, and R. Collu, *Life Sci.* **24**, 1719–1726 (1979).
58. Y. Tache, W. Vale, J. Rivier, and M. Brown, *Proc. Natl. Acad. Sci. USA* **77**, 5515–5519 (1980).
59. Y. Tache, W. Marki, J. Rivier, W. Vale, and M. Brown, *Gastroenterology* **81**, 298–302 (1981).
60. W. Vale, J. Rivier, and M. Brown, *Peptides* **2**, 51–56 (1981).
61. Y. Tache and R. Collu, *Regul. Peptides* **3**, 51–59 (1932).
62. A. Ayalon, R. Yazigi, J. C. Thompson, P. G. Devitt, and P. L. Rayford, *Biochem. Biophys. Res. Commun.* **99**(4), 1390–1397 (1981).
63. G. Bertaccini, V. Erspamer, and M. Impicciatore, *Br. J. Pharmacol.* **49**, 437–444 (1973).
64. A. Andriulli, T. E. Solomon, T. Yamada, and M. I. Grossman, *Gastroenterology* **78**, 1131 (1980).
65. J. W. DuVal, B. Saffouri, G. C. Weir, J. H. Walsh, A. Arimura, and G. M. Makhlouf, *Am. J. Physiol.* **241**, G242–G247 (1981).

66. R. Martindale, G. L. Kauffman, S. Levin, J. H. Walsh, and T. Yamada, *Gastroenterology*, **83**, 240–244 (1982).

67. G. Bertaccini, V. Erspamer, P. Melchiorri, and N. Sopranzi, *Br. J. Pharmacol.* **52**, 219–225 (1974).

68. M. Impicciatore, H. Debas, J. H. Walsh, M. I. Grossman, and G. Bertaccini, *Rend. Gastroenterol.* **6**, 99–101 (1974).

69. B. I. Hirschowitz and R. G. Gibson, *Digestion* **18**, 227–239 (1978).

70. I. L. Taylor, J. H. Walsh, D. Carter, J. Wood, and M. I. Grossman, *Gastroenterology* **77**, 714–718 (1979).

71. I. M. Modlin, C. Lamers, and J. H. Walsh, *J. Surg. Res.* **28**(6), 539–546 (1980).

72. I. M. Modlin, C. B. H. Lamers, and J. H. Walsh, *Regul. Peptides* **1**, 279–288 (1981).

73. A. Materia, I. M. Modlin, D. Albert, A. Sank, R. F. Crochelt, and B. M. Jaffe, *Regul. Peptides* **1**(4), 297–305 (1981).

74. G. Bertaccini, R. De Castiglione, and M. Impicciatore, *Br. J. Pharmacol.* **52**(3), 463 (1974).

75. G. Delle Fave, A. Kohn, L. de Magistris, M. Mancuso, and C. Sparvoli, *Life Sci.* **27** (11), 993–999 (1980).

76. A. A. Varner, I. M. Modlin, and J. H. Walsh, *Regul. Peptides* **1**, 289–296 (1981).

77. J. H. Walsh, V. Maxwell, J. Ferrari, and A. A. Varner, *Peptides* **2**, Suppl. 2, 193–198 (1981).

78. N. Basso, E. Lezoche, A. Materia, S. Giri, and V. Speranza, *Dig. Dis.* **20**, 923–927 (1975).

79. J. B. Jansen and C. B. Lamers, *Digestion* **21**(4), 193–197 (1981).

80. J. B. M. J. Jansen and C. B. H. W. Lamers, *Regul. Peptides*, **1**, 415–421 (1981).

81. V. Erspamer, G. Improta, P. Melchiorri, and N. Sopranzi, *Br. J. Pharmacol.* **52**, 227–232 (1974).

82. N. Basso, S. Giri, G. Improta, E. Lezoche, P. Melchiorri, M. Percoco, and V. Speranza, *Gut* **16**, 994–998 (1975).

83. M. Miyata, P. L. Rayford, and J. C. Thompson, *Surgery* **87**, 209–215 (1980).

84. G. Bommelaer, G. Rozental, C. Bernier, N. Vaysse, and A. Ribet, *Digestion* **21**(5), 248–254 (1981).

85. M. Deschodt-Lanckman, P. Robberecht, P. De Neef, M. Lammens, and J. Christophe, *J. Clin. Invest.* **58**, 891–898 (1976).

86. R. T. Jensen, T. Moody, C. Pert, J. E. Rivier, and J. D. Gardner, *Proc. Natl. Acad. Sci. USA* **75**, 6139–6143 (1978).

87. E. R. Uhlemann, A. J. Rottman, and J. D. Gardner, *Am. J. Physiol.* **236**(5), E571–E576 (1979).

88. P. C. Lee, R. T. Jensen, and J. D. Gardner, *Am. J. Physiol.* **238**, G213–G218 (1980).

89. H. G. Philpott, O. H. Petersen, *Pflügers Arch.* **382**(3), (1979).

90. H. G. Philpott, O. H. Petersen, *Nature* **281**, 684–686 (1979).

91. L. de Magistris, G. Delle Fave, A. Kohn, and T. W. Schwartz, *Life Sci.* **28**(23), 2617–2621 (1981).

92. E. Lezoche, N. Basso, and V. Speranza, in S. R. Bloom and J. M. Polak, Eds., *Gut Hormones*, 2nd ed., Churchill Livingstone, Edinburgh, 1981, pp. 419–424.

93. T. J. McDonald, M. A. Ghatei, S. R. Bloom, N. S. Track, J. Radziuk, J. Dupre, and V. Mutt, *Regul. Peptides* **2**, 293–304 (1981).

94. T. Matsuyama, M. Namba, K. Nonaka, S. Tarui, R. Tanaka, and K. Shima, *Endocrinol. Jpn.* **1**, 115–119 (1980).

95. V. Schusdziarra, D. Rouiller, V. Harris, E. F. Pfeiffer, R. H. Unger, *Regul. Peptides* **1** (2), 89–96 (1980).

96. N. Vaysse, L. Pradayrol, J. A. Chayvialle, F. Pignal, and J. P. Esteve, *Endocrinology* **108**(5), 1843–1847 (1981).

97. K. Hermansen, *Endocrinology* **107**(1), 256–261 (1980).

98. E. Ipp and R. H. Unger, *Endocrin. Res. Commun.* **6**(1), 37–42 (1979).

99. T. Taminato, Y. Seino, Y. Goto, S. Matsukura, H. Imura, N. Sakura, and N. Yanaihara, *Endocrinol. Jpn.* **25**, 305–307 (1978).
100. G. Bertaccini, M. Impicciatore, E. Molina, and L. Zappia, *Rend. Gastroenterol.* **6**, 45–51 (1974).
101. A. K. Mukhopadhyay and M. Kunnemann, *Gastroenterology* **76**(6), 1409–1414 (1979).
102. C. Scarpignato and G. Bertaccini, *Digestion* **21**(2), 104–106 (1981).
103. J. H. Walsh, V. Maxwell, J. Ferrari, and A. A. Varner, *Peptides* **2**, 193–198 (1981).
104. C. Scarpignato, B. Micali, F. Vitulo, G. Zimbaro, and G. Bertaccini, *Peptides* **2**, 199–203 (1981).
105. E. A. Mayer, J. Elashoff, and J. H. Walsh, *Am. J. Physiol.*, **243**(6), G141–G147 (1982).
106. E. Corazziari, A. Torsoli, G. F. Delle Fave, P. Melchiorri, and F. I. Habib, *Rend. Gastroenterol.* **6**, 55–59 (1974).
107. E. Corazziari, A. Torsoli, P. Melchiorri, and G. F. Delle Fave, *Rend. Gastroenterol.* **6**, 52–54 (1974).
108. P. Poitras, D. Iacino, and J. H. Walsh, *Biochem. Biophys. Res. Commun.* **96**, 476–482 (1980).
109. J. C. Sarles, P. Delecourt, H. Castello, L. Gaeta, M. Nacchiero, J. P. Amoros, M. A. Devaux, and R. Awad, *Regul. Peptides* **2**(2), 113–124 (1981).
110. G. Zetler, *Pharmacology* **21**(5) (1980).
111. V. Erspamer, P. Melchiorri, and N. Sopranzi, *Br. J. Pharmacol.* **45**, 442–450 (1972).
112. V. Erspamer, P. Melchiorri, and N. Sopranzi, *Br. J. Pharmacol.* **48**, 438–455 (1973).
113. G. Falconieri Erspamer, L. Negri, and D. Piccinelli, *Naunyn-Schmiedeberg's Arch. Pharmacol.* **279**, 61–74 (1973).
114. V. Erspamer, G. Ronzoni, and G. Falconieri Erspamer, *Invest. Urol.* **18**(4), 302–304 (1981).
115. M. Impicciatore and G. Bertaccini, *J. Pharm. Pharmac.* **25**, 872–875 (1973).
116. V. Erspamer and P. Melchiorri, *Pure Appl. Chem.* **35**, 463–494 (1973).
117. N. Sopranzi and P. Melchiorri, *J. Pharmacol.* **5**(1), 125 (1974).
118. M. Brown, W. Marki, and J. Rivier, *Life Sci.* **27**, 125–128 (1980).
119. R. Rivier and M. R. Brown, *Biochemistry* **17**, 1766–1771 (1978).
120. W. Marki, M. Brown, and J. E. Rivier, *Peptides*, **2** (Suppl. 2), 169–177 (1981).
121. J. H. Walsh and H. C. Wong, in *Methods of Hormone Radioimmunoassay*, 2nd ed., Academic Press, New York, 1979.
122. C. Yanaihara, A. Inoue, T. Mochizuki, N. Sakura, H. Sato, and N. Yanaihara, "Syntheses of Bombesin-Related Peptides and Their Use for Bombesin-Specific Radioimmunoassay," in N. Izumiya, Ed., *Peptide Chemistry*, Osaka, 1979, pp. 183–188.
123. T. W. Moody, C. B. Pert, J. Rivier, and M. R. Brown, *Proc. Natl. Acad. Sci. USA* **75**, 5372–5376 (1978).
124. A. Pert, T. W. Moody, C. B. Pert, L. A. Dewald, and J. Rivier, *Brain Res.* **193**(1), 209–220 (1980).
125. T. W. Moody, C. B. Pert, A. F. Gazdor, D. N. Carney, and J. D. Minna, *Science* **214**, 1246–1248 (1981).
126. N. Basso, E. Lezoche, A. Materia, E. P. Jun, and V. Speranza, *Br. J. Surg.* **68**(2), 97–100 (1981).

38

Corticotropin Releasing Factor

WYLIE W. VALE

CATHERINE RIVIER

JOACHIM SPIESS

JEAN RIVIER

Peptide Biology Laboratory
The Salk Institute
La Jolla, California

The pioneering studies of Geoffry Harris, the Scharrers, and others have led to our current concepts of the neuroregulation of adenohypophysial function (1, 2). Factors produced by hypothalamic neurons terminating in the median eminence are considered to reach adenohypophysial cells via the hypothalamic hypophysial portal system. These factors then act in concert with other neural, peripheral and perhaps local signals to regulate secretion by adenohypophysial cells.

In 1955, Guillemin and Rosenberg (3) and Saffran and Schally (4) independently provided direct evidence for the existence of a factor present in hypothalamus that could stimulate the production of adrenocorticotrophic hormone (ACTH) by pituitary tissue *in vitro*. This substance was termed corticotropin releasing factor (CRF). Since that time biological and chemical studies have confirmed these neuroendocrine concepts and several hypophysiotropic neuropeptides, thyrotropin releasing hormone (TRH), gonadotropin releasing hormone (GnRH), and somatostatin have been characterized. These three peptides, along with the catecholamine dopamine, have been clearly established to play physiological roles in the neuroregulation of pituitary hormone secretion (5).

Several known naturally occurring substances—including vasopressin, oxytocin, norepinephrine, epinephrine, and angiotensin II—have been found to stimulate ACTH secretion (for reviews, see refs. 5–7, 70). Partially purified hypothalamic or neurohypophysial fractions have been reported by numerous workers to possess peptides with ACTH releasing activity. Some have been partially (8, 9) or fully characterized (10, 11). Yet for various reasons, none of the known peptides met the criteria expected of the principal hypothalamic ACTH releasing factor (5, 6).

In 1981 we reported the isolation, sequence, synthesis, and biological activity of the synthetic replicate of a 41-amino-acid ovine hypothalamic CRF (12, 13). It is likely that this peptide is the principal neuroregulator of adenohypophysial ACTH production. The more than 25-year delay in the characterization of CRF since its discovery can be attributed to several factors.

The bioassays were a problem. *In vivo* methods lacked sufficient sensitivity, and some of them were susceptible to responding to any brain-mediated stressor. The development of *in vitro* assays using acutely dissociated pituitary cells by Sayers' group (14) or cell cultures by our group (15, 16) provided the basis of sensitive quantitative, valid bioassays. With antisera first from Felber and Aubert, and later from D. Orth (17), the ACTH radioimmunoassay (RIA) became the other essential ingredient of our bioassay.

Even the best *in vitro* assays could be complicated by numerous substances that could release ACTH on their own (such as vasopressin and epinephrine) and/or strongly potentiate CRF action. Furthermore, most hypothalamic extracts contain ACTH, which could initially be mistaken for CRF. Finally, *in vitro* systems are vulnerable to nonspecific secretagogs, including myelin basic protein, histones, potassium ion, and the components of various buffers and solvents.

CRF turned out to be larger than expected, 41 amino acids. On gel filtration chromatography, ACTH and CRF coelute; the CRF-like activity of those fractions shown to contain ACTH may have been overlooked.

Generally only pmol levels of CRF are present in hypothalamic extracts, necessitating large amounts of starting material, good recoveries during purification, sensitive sequencing, or some combination of the three.

1 CHARACTERIZATION OF CORTICOTROPIN RELEASING FACTOR (CRF)

Almost one-half-million sheep hypothalamic fragments were extracted with ethanol/acetic acid, defatted, and partitioned by bulk shake-out in the Laboratories for Neuroendocrinology (18). The organic phases were then used in the purification of ovine GnRH and somatostatin. This fraction contained the majority of the CRF activity but was no longer available. The aqueous phase also contained some CRF activity and was provided to us by Roger R. Burgus, M. Amoss, and R. Guillemin.

This fraction was ultrafiltered and the activity retained. The retentates were then gel filtered on Sephadex G-50 yielding two zones of activity (6). Zone I eluting at about 1.3 V_e/V_o and zone 2 eluting at about 2.0 V_e/V_o. Multiple ACTH-releasing zones, including "large CRF's," have been described by various workers (40–48). The two zones showed different intrinsic activities in that zone 1 elicited a much higher secretory V_{max} (secretory rate at maximum concentration of added substance) than did zone 2. The activity in zone 2 was similar to that of vasopressin, and expectedly, further purification of the ACTH-releasing activity of this zone yielded an active fraction with the same amino acid composition as [Arg⁸]-vasopressin (12). Because of the high intrinsic activity of zone 1 and encouraging results of a series of *in vitro* studies, we focused on the further purification of the ACTH-releasing substances in this higher molecular weight fraction (6, 12).

The purification of zone 1 was accomplished by a series of traditional steps and ultimately by high pressure liquid chromatography (HPLC) (12, 19). Initially, multiple HPLC steps were required, but with the development of improved columns with large pore size (300–330 Å), small pore size and monolayered end-capped octadecyl silica, purification could be accomplished with 2 HPLC steps. With the various procedures we ended up with approximately 90 µg (ca. 20 nmol) CRF of greater than 80% purity.

The primary structure of the major component was determined by Edman degradation with the use of a Beckman 890C spinning cup sequencer modified according to Wittmann-Liebold. The phenylthiohydantoin derivatives of the amino acids were identified by reverse phase HPLC. Several analyses of 0.6 to 3.6 nmol of peptide were performed. The initial sequencing attempts were carried out at a low level of peptide revealed that most of the sample was not N-terminally blocked and 27 residues of the sequence were determined. Subsequently, the analysis of 3.6 nmol of peptide confirmed the previous run yielded the sequence of residues 28–39. Residue 40 (Ile) was established by spinning-cup sequencing of the tryptic digest of the peptide. The COOH-terminal alaninamide was identified by HPLC after digestion of CRF with thermolysin and carboxypeptidase Y and confirmed by COOH-terminal tritiation experiments (13).

The primary sequence of ovine CRF was thus determined to be a 41-residue straight-chain peptide with a free N-terminal and amidated C-terminus:

H-Ser-Gln-Glu-Pro-Pro-Ile-Ser-Leu-Asp-Leu-Thr-Phe-His-Leu-Leu-Arg-Glu-Val-Leu-Glu-Met-Thr-Lys-Ala-Asp-Gln-Leu-Ala-Gln-Gln-Ala-His-Ser-Asn-Arg-Lys-Leu-Leu-Asp-Ile-Ala-NH$_2$

Ovine CRF is homologous with several known peptides: sauvagine, urotensin I, calmodulin, and angiotensinogen. Sauvagine was isolated from the skin of the frog *Phylomedusa sauvagei* and characterized by Erspamer and colleagues (20, 21). More than 50% of the residues in sauvagine are identical with those in CRF; the majority remaining are conservative substitutions. Sauvagine had been reported to produce hypotension, antidiuresis, and a variety of pituitary effects including the release of ACTH and β-endorphin and the inhibition of growth hormone, thyroid stimulating hormone (TSH), and prolactin secretion (20–22). Both sauvagine and CRF are closely related to a third peptide, urotensin I isolated from the fish urohyphysis (23, 24). All three produce hypotension when injected peripherally by dilating the superior mesenteric bed and increasing blood flow to the GI tract (22, 25, 26). CRF also shows some homology with calmodulin and with angiotensinogen. The tetrapeptide Phe-His-Leu-Leu is common to both angiotensinogen (27) and CRF (12) and is the site in angiotensinogen of renin and converting enzyme cleavage.

Perhaps this homology reflects a distant ancestral relationship between angiotensinogen and CRF, both of which ultimately regulate the adrenal cortex.

This peptide was synthesized (12) by solid phase methodology (28) and established to be a potent stimulator of ACTH secretion in the cell culture assay used throughout its isolation. The minimal effective concentration of CRF in this assay is generally less than 10 pM and the EC$_{50}$ is observed at approximately 100 pM. The plateau response occurs at approximately 1 nM and is equivalent to that seen with high concentrations of 8-Br 3'5' cyclic AMP. As expected from the mode of biosynthesis of ACTH (39) and from earlier studies (38), CRF releases both

ACTH and β-endorphin-like immunoactivity, about one-third of which cochromatographs with synthetic β-endorphin (12, 29).

Synthetic CRF has been shown to be a potent stimulator of ACTH, β-endorphin, and glucocorticoid production *in vivo* in several species, including the rat (30, 58), dog (31), and human (32, 33). In the rat, CRF is effective in releasing ACTH in unanesthetized animals with indwelling venous cannulae or in rats whose response to stress is blocked, either pharmacologically or by hypothalamic knife cuts (12, 30).

A comparison of the biological activities and HPLC behavior of the synthetic CRF and that isolated from the sheep revealed that in the sheep-derived peptide, the methionine residue was oxidized to its sulfoxide form. The oxidation of CRF presumably occurred during the decade between the extraction of the tissues and the characterization of CRF.

One of the questions raised by the size of CRF is the possibility that we had isolated a prohormone. Against this hypothesis is the finding that several shortened analogs of CRF are much less active (12, 34). On the C-terminus, simply deamidating the peptide removes more than a thousandfold activity. Retaining the amide but shortening by 1 or 2 residues again results in drastic reduction of potency. There is more flexibility at the N-terminus, where the first three residues can be removed with no decrease in potency, the first six with retention of 25% activity. The deletion of nine N-terminal amino acids reduces potency by more than one thousand-fold. It is unlikely that a form of CRF that is very much smaller than this one will be found with high activity.

The three closely related peptides CRF, sauvagine, and urotensin I exhibit similar potencies to stimulate ACTH and β-endorphin secretion *in vitro* and *in vivo* (26, 35). It is interesting that CRF appears less potent than the other two to cause hypotension (26). Perhaps it has been adaptive in the higher vertebrates for the extra pituitary actions of CRF to be diminished. The possibility is under investigation that other CRF-like molecules more closely related to sauvagine or urotensin I exist in the gastrointestinal tract or other peripheral sites of mammals.

The existence of the three naturally occurring peptides with similar ACTH releasing potencies has saved a great deal of time for those interested in structure–function relationships. Only 17 residues of 41 are in common. The fact that many others are very conservative substitutions notwithstanding, this provides real insight concerning the residues responsible for biological activities. From the few analogs made and tested in our group, it appears that the double leucine residues at positions 14 and 15 and at 37 and 38 are critical, as are the basic groups at 16 and 35.

Goodman and Pallai and colleagues have applied Chou and Fassman's predictions to CRF's primary sequence and found a high probability for an α helix from residues 5–30 followed by a β-bend encompassing residues 31–35; CD analysis has confirmed the presence of considerable helical content (36). It is possible that conformationally these three peptides are more closely related than is apparent from their primary structures.

2 DEVELOPMENT OF CRF ANTISERA AND RADIOIMMUNOASSAYS

Rabbits were immunized with 3 different immunogens (37). One rabbit immunized with [Tyr^{22},Gly^{23}]-CRF-1-23 coupled by bisdiazotized benzidine to human α globulin produced antibodies directed against the N-terminal region (residues 4–20) of CRF. Radioimmunoassays using this antiserum, called C-24, can be used to detect CRF-like immunoactivity (CRF-LI) in the hypothalamus/median eminence/pituitary of sheep, dog, rat, monkey, and human. Antibodies produced in rabbits immunized with CRF coupled by glutaraldehyde to human α globulin or with CRF polymerized with 1-ethyl-3-(3-dimethylaminopropyl) carbodiimide are directed towards the middle or C-terminal region of CRF. Radioimmunoassays with these sera read sheep well but detect rat and human poorly (37). These immunological results suggested that sheep CRF is different from the CRF of those other species.

In order to provide the tools for studying the role of CRF in the most common laboratory animal, and to evaluate CRF-like molecules in fresh extracts, we decided to purify CRF from rat hypothalamus. As starting material, we have used rat hypothalamic powder provided by Dr. A. Parlow under the aegis of the National Hormone and Pituitary Program.

Acidic, defatted extracts of rat hypothalamic fragments were applied to a Sephadex G-50 fine column. The eluted fractions were bioassayed for ability to release ACTH *in vitro* and radioimmunoassayed with our N-terminally-directed CRF radioimmunoassay using C-24. We detected the major peak of both biological and immunological activity in the 4000–5000 size range. A smaller peak with biological and immunological activities, perhaps representing a CRF precursor, was seen close to the void volume. Additional zones of biological activity without immunological activity were seen only in the smaller-molecular-weight zones. Neither of these exhibited the high intrinsic activity of CRF in subsequent studies.

The major peak of biological and immunological activity has been purified further using preparative, semipreparative, and analytical HPLC steps, yielding about 50% pure rat CRF. We observed that this CRF elutes later than did an ovine CRF marker. Sequence analysis of this fraction is underway. Preliminary findings suggest that there are at least five deviations between rat and ovine CRF. These changes are distributed throughout the peptide, which also appears to be 41 residues in length.

3   DISTRIBUTION OF CRF

CRF-like immunoactivity has been detected by RIA in the stalk median eminence area of several species. In the rat we measure 1–2 ng CRF-LI/medial basal hypothalamus (37). This value increases about twofold in chronically adrenalectomized rats. In collaboration with F. Bloom and associates (49), we have observed CRF staining in the external zone of the median eminence—the staging area for transport of hypophysiotropic substances to the pituitary gland. Cell bodies of these terminals have been identified in the paraventricular nucleus of the sheep, dog, monkey, and colchicine-treated rat (49). In the colchicine-treated rat, CRF-containing cell bodies are primarily distributed in the parvocellular region of the paraventricular nucleus. Of the 10,000 cells in the paraventricular nucleus of the rat, approximately 2000 contain CRF. Some CRF cells are intermixed with the oxytocin-rich area; little intermixing with the vasopressin region is evident in the rat (50). The localization of the paraventricular nucleus as the site of CRF cell bodies is consistent with physiological studies of Makara and Palkovits (for a review, see ref. 51) and others that have emphasized the importance of this region for the regulation of ACTH secretion.

In addition to the median eminence, CRF fibers are found in the posterior lobe of the pituitary and in other hypothalamic regions, including the vicinity of cells containing pro-opiomelanocortin (POMC) derivatives (49). CRF immunostaining is also found in cell bodies in the central nucleus of the amygdala, the periaqueductal central gray, reticular formation nucleus tractus solitarius, and in the cerebral cortex (50). Fibers are widely distributed, particularly in the limbic areas and brain stem (50).

4   CRF IN PORTAL BLOOD

D. Gibbs, of the University of California, San Diego, collected portal blood from the transsected hypophysial stalk of pentobarbital anesthetized rats. We extracted the CRF-like activity by adsorption onto C_{18} Bond Elut cartridges. After elution, the samples were assayed by an RIA that detects 1 fmol ovine CRF. We found that extracted portal plasma was detected by this assay—giving a response parallel to that of either synthetic ovine CRF or highly purified rat CRF (52). Based upon the ovine standard, about 100 pM CRF-LI was found in portal blood. Since we suspect that this RIA underreads rat CRF, the actual concentration of rat CRF is somewhat higher. Because concentrations of 100–500 pM CRF are highly active *in vitro*, these results suggest that physiologically significant levels of CRF are present in the blood supplying the anterior pituitary.

We have also examined CRF-like immunoactivity in the portal blood of a cat provided by P. Plotsky. In this sample, about 1 nM CRF was detected, based upon the ovine standard.

5 PASSIVE IMMUNIZATION

Perhaps the most definitive approach to the question of the role of endogenous CRF in ACTH is provided by passive immunization experiments. We have examined the effects of administration of antiserum against CRF to freely moving catheterized adrenalectomized rats. This anti-CRF serum dramatically reduced plasma ACTH levels to about 10% of that of rats receiving normal rabbit serum. Thus, in adrenalectomized rats the secretion of ACTH appears to be highly dependent upon endogenous CRF (53).

The effect of anti-CRF serum on the secretion of ACTH during ether stress was also studied. The administration of anti-CRF serum to catheterized rats blocked most of the ACTH response to either CRF or to ether stress (53). However, it must be pointed out that significant residual (ca. 15%) release of ACTH owing to stress remained in three experiments. Either we have failed to neutralize all endogenous CRF or other factors contribute to the stress response. Even so, the fact that anti-CRF serum typically prevents 80–90% of the amount of ACTH released because of stress provides strong support for the physiologic role of an immunologically related endogenous peptide.

6 INTERACTION OF VARIOUS SUBSTANCES WITH CRF *IN VITRO*

6.1 Vasopressin and Oxytocin

Vasopressin, which is a weak ACTH secretogog, exhibits an "effect additive" relationship with CRF (29). Even at plateau concentrations of CRF, the coaddition of vasopressin will result in additional increases in ACTH or β-endorphin secretory rates. At lower CRF levels ($\leq$ 1 nM), the effect of cotreatment with vasopressin can be quite dramatic. Enhancement is seen with concentrations of vasopressin as low as 1 nM. Oxytocin, the closely related neurohypophysial peptide, also enhances CRF. These results are in agreement with some of the early findings of Yates and Lowry and their colleagues (2, 54).

6.2 Epinephrine and Norepinephrine

Norepinephrine and epinephrine acting via α-adrenergic receptors exhibit lower potency and intrinsic activity than CRF to elicit ACTH/β-endorphin release (6). Both enhance the response to CRF at concentrations reached in the blood under stressful circumstances (1–10 nM) which can augment the response to all dose levels of CRF (29).

6.3 Angiotensin II

Gaillard et al. (70) have reported that angiotensin II can release ACTH from acutely dispersed pituitary cells. Although we observed a very modest effect of angiotensin II per se, this peptide also can enhance the action of CRF (29).

Thus, the residual ACTH released by stressed rats given anti-CRF serum may be due to catecholamines, neurohypophysial peptides, angiotensin II, or to other substances.

6.4 Glucocorticoids

Of more certain significance in the regulation of ACTH secretion are the glucocorticoids. Experimental evidence has implicated both pituitary and brain sites of action for the well-established negative feedback effects of glucocorticoids on ACTH secretion (for a review, see refs. 6, 57). Hypothalamic CRF levels as monitored by specific RIA or by immunofluorescence has been observed to increase in response to long term adrenalectomy (55, 50). Neither of these results establish CRF production rates, but would support the possibility that part of the action of glucocorticoids on ACTH secretion can be mediated through changes in CRF secretion.

Glucocorticoids can undoubtedly modulate the response of pituitary cells to CRF or other secretagogs in vivo and in vitro (29, 30). When pituitary cells are pretreated with glucocorticoids, the CRF dose response curve is shifted to the right and the release rate at plateau CRF levels is reduced (29). A family of curves is obtained in which alteration of either CRF or steroid results in a new hormonal secretion rate. CRF can be viewed as having altered the set point for glucocorticoid inhibition or vice versa. The glucocorticoid inhibition of CRF's action is noncompetitive in that the plateau response is reduced. It is noteworthy that even at highest doses of dexamethasone, CRF can still elicit some stimulation of hormone secretion. Thus in this system, when CRF is high ACTH production can be elevated even when glucocorticoids are high. These observations are consistent with the possibility that failure of glucocorticoid suppression of ACTH secretion in some clinical conditions, such as Cushing's disease or in affective disorders like depression, could be CRF mediated.

7 MODE OF ACTION OF CRF

The initial step in the action of CRF on pituitary cells probably involves an interaction with plasma membrane receptors. Consistently, ^{125}I-CRF binds to purified bovine membranes with high affinity ($K_D = 1$ nM) (Perrin, Rivier and Vale, unpublished results).

Cyclic AMP derivatives and phosphodiesterase inhibitors which increase intracellular cyclic AMP levels had been shown earlier to stimulate ACTH release. The addition of CRF to cultured pituitary cells is associated with a rapid increase in the production of adenosine 3'5' monophosphate cyclic (cAMP) (59, 60). CRF increases both intracellular and extracellular (medium) levels of cyclic AMP. Glucocorticoid pretreatment inhibits CRF-mediated increases in intracellular and extracellular cAMP (60). These results suggest that CRF and glucocorticoids may act at least in part through modulation of cyclic AMP production. The observation that glucocorticoids can inhibit ACTH secretion due to exogenous 8-Br cAMP (29) suggests that these steroids may act at multiple sites to block hormonal secretion.

The secretion of ACTH due to CRF is calcium dependent as shown by the observation that incubation of pituitary cells with either cobalt or in low-calcium medium strongly attenuates the secretory response to CRF (29).

Prolonged exposure of pituitary cells to CRF results in an increase in total (intracellular plus extracellular) amounts of ACTH in the cultures (29). These results suggest that CRF can stimulate the synthesis as well as the release of POMC products. Using a hybridization assay we have shown that CRF elevates the level of POMC mRNA (61). Glucocorticoids lower total ACTH and POMC-mRNA levels and block the increases in those parameters due to CRF. The effects of CRF and glucocorticoids on ACTH synthesis may be mediated through changes in POMC mRNA concentrations.

8   CRF ON INTERMEDIATE LOBE

The intermediate lobe of the pituitary gland contains primarily corticotropic cells which secrete a variety of peptides derived from POMC. The processing of the POMC precursor in anterior lobe differs from that in the intermediate lobe. In the latter, the bulk of the ACTH is processed to α-melanocyte stimulating hormone (α-MSH) and betalipotropin (β-LPH) is cleavea to β-endorphin and its acetylated forms (for reviews, see refs. 7, 39).

Cultures of dissociated neurointermediate lobe cells secrete large quantities of β-endorphin-like immunoactivity (β-End-LI) spontaneously. CRF can further increase β-End-LI secretion rates although the dose response curve is shifted to the right of that seen with anterior lobe cultures (29). The EC_{50} for CRF mediated β-End-LI secretion by intermediate lobe cells is observed to be between 1 and 10 nM. The β-End-LI secretory rate at plateau concentrations of CRF is less than that induced by 8-Br3'5' cyclic AMP.

Epinephrine and other β-adrenergic agonists such as isoproterenol markedly stimulate intermediate lobe secretion of POMC products (62, 63) and, in contract to CRF, will elicit a secretory response as great as that due to 8-Br3'5' cyclic AMP (29).

The intermediate lobe is innervated by fibers containing dopamine, which is probably a major physiologic regulator of those cells. Dopamine and a variety of dopaminergic agonists—apomorphine, bromocriptine, pergolide—are powerful inhibitors of β-End-LI secretion by cultured intermediate lobe cells (7, 39). Dopamine noncompetitively inhibits the response to CRF; CRF can partially overcome the inhibitory effects of moderate doses of dopamine but has little effect on high concentrations of dopamine (29).

9 BRAIN ACTIONS OF CRF

The finding that CRF is distributed throughout various brain regions (49, 50) suggests that CRF might have effects within the central nervous system. Siggins, Groul, and colleagues, using intracellular recording of hippocampal slices have observed that CRF depolarizes both CA1 and CA3 pyramidal neurons, accompanied by elevations in spontaneous firing rate (71). We have observed that CRF can stimulate the secretion of somatostatin by cultured rat hypothalamic and cerebral cortical cells (66). These studies demonstrate a direct effect of CRF on brain cells.

In considering the possibility that CRF might play a role beyond the activation of the pituitary-adrenal axis, we were led to examine the effects of this new peptide on other visceral mechanisms involved in an animal's responses to stress. The intracerebroventricular administration of CRF to rats or dogs results in an activation of the sympathetic nervous system. Both norepinephrine and adrenal medullary epinephrine are elevated in plasma within minutes of the delivery of CRF into the brain (64, 26). Consequently, plasma glucagon and glucose levels, mean arterial blood pressure, and heart rate are elevated (64, 65, 26).

Appropriate behavioral modifications are of paramount importance in any animal's strategy of adaptation. The intracerebroventricular administration of CRF in freely moving rats housed in a familiar environment is associated with an increase in locomotor activity (72) and with electroencephalographic changes associated with marked arousal (67). In appetitive motivated tests, CRF increases the rate of acquisition (68). In contrast, CRF decreases performance in aversive tests where punishment rather than reward is involved (73). In the open field, a novel environment, rats respond in such a way to be consistent with an increased emotionality or sensitivity to the "stressful aspects" of the situation (72, 69). It appears, therefore, that the behavioral responses to CRF are complex and very dependent upon environmental factors.

10 CONCLUSION

The evidence implicating CRF or closely related peptides in the neuroregulation of the pituitary corticotropic cells is compelling. Broader roles of CRF within the brain as a transsynaptic or paracrine mediator of endocrine and visceral functions and behavior, particularly under stressful circumstances, are suggested and require further investigation. Fundamental and applied studies of this new regulatory peptide may improve our understanding of the brain and endocrine system and lead to improved means of diagnosis and management of human disease.

ACKNOWLEDGMENTS

We wish to acknowledge the contributions of the numerous collaborators cited in this review. Research is supported by NIH grants AM26741, HD13527, AA03504 and by grants from The Rockefeller Foundation and The Texas Salk Institute Foundation. Research is conducted in part by The Clayton Foundation for Research, California Division. W. Vale, C. Rivier, and J. Spiess are Clayton Foundation Investigators.

REFERENCES

1. G. W. Harris, *Physiol. Rev.* **28**, 139 (1948).
2. F. E. Yates and J. W. Maran, in *Handbook of Physiology*, Vol. 4, Section 7, 1974.
3. R. Guillemin and B. Rosenberg, *Endocrinology* **57**, 599 (1955).
4. M. Saffran and A. V. Schally, *Can. J. Biochem. Physiol.* **33**, 408 (1955).
5. W. Vale, C. Rivier, and M. Brown, *Ann. Rev. Physiol.* **29**, 473 (1977).
6. W. Vale and C. Rivier, *Fed. Proc.* **36**, 8 (1977).
7. W. Vale, J. Rivier, and C. Rivier, *The Role of Peptides in Neuronal Function*, Marcel Dekker, 1980, p. 432.
8. R. Guillemin, *Recent Prog. Horm. Res.* **20**, 89 (1964).
9. A. V. Schally, A. Arimura, C. Y. Bowers, A. J. Kastin, S. Sawano, and T. W. Redding, *Recent Prog. Horm. Res.* **24**, 497 (1968).
10. A. V. Schally, W. Y. Huang, T. W. Redding, A. Arimura, D. H. Coy, K. Chihara, V. Raymond, and F. Labrie, *Biochem. Biophys. Res. Commun.* **82**, 582 (1978).
11. J. Knudsen, Y. Lam, W. Frick, G. Daves, D. Barofsky, C. Bowers, and K. Folkers, *Biochem. Biophys. Res. Commun.* **80**, 735 (1978).
12. W. Vale, J. Spiess, C. Rivier, and J. Rivier, *Science* **213**, 1394 (1981).
13. J. Spiess, J. Rivier, C. Rivier, and W. Vale, *Proc. Natl. Acad. Sci. USA* **78**, 6517 (1981).
14. R. Portanova and G. Sayers, *Proc. Soc. Exp. Biol. Med.* **143**, 661 (1973).
15. W. Vale, G. Grant, M. Amoss, R. Blackwell, and R. Guillemin, *Endocrinology* **91**, 562 (1972).
16. W. Vale et al., *Hypothalamus and Endocrine Functions*, Plenum Press, New York, 1976.
17. D. Orth, *Methods of Hormone Radioimmunoassay*, Academic Press, New York, 1979, p. 245.

18. R. Burgus et al. *Hypothalamus and Endocrine Functions*, Plenum Press, New York, 1976.

19. J. Rivier, C. Rivier, D. Branton, R. Millar, J. Spiess, and W. Vale, *Peptides: Synthesis, Structure, Function*, Pierce Chemical Company, 1982, p. 771.

20. P. C. Montecucchi, A. Henschen, V. Erspamer, Hoppe-Seyler's *Z. Phisiol. Chem.* **360**, 1178 (1979).

21. V. Erspamer and P. Melchiorri, *Trends Pharmacol. Sci.* **20**, 391 (1980).

22. V. Erspamer, P. Melchiorri, M. Broccardo, G. F. Erspamer, P. Falaschi, G. Improta, L. Negri, and T. Renda, *Peptides* **2**(2), 7 (1981).

23. K. MacCannell and K. Lederis, *J. Pharmacol. Exp. Ther.* **203**, 38 (1977).

24. K. Lederis, W. Vale, J. Rivier, K. L. MacCannell, D. McMaster, Y. Kobayashi, U. Suess, and J. Lawrence, *Proc. West. Pharmacol. Soc.* **25**, 223–227 (1982).

25. K. L. MacCannell, K. Lederis, P. L. Hamilton, and J. Rivier, *Pharmacology* **25**, 116–120 (1982).

26. M. R. Brown, L. A. Fisher, J. Spiess, J. Rivier, C. Rivier, and W. Vale, *Regul. Peptides* **4**, 107–114 (1982).

27. L. T. Skeggs, J. R. Kahn, K. Lentz, and N. P. Shumway, *J. Exp. Med.* **106**, 439 (1957).

28. W. Marki, J. Spiess, Y. Tache, M. Brown, and J. Rivier, *J. Am. Chem. Soc.* **103**, 3178 (1981).

29. W. Vale, J. Vaughan, M. Smith, G. Yamamoto, J. Rivier, and C. Rivier, *Endocrinology*, in press.

30. C. Rivier, M. Brownstein, J. Spiess, J. Rivier, and W. Vale, *Endocrinology* **110**, 272 (1982).

31. M. Brown, C. Rivier, J. Rivier, and W. Vale, in press.

32. D. N. Orth, C. R. DeBold, G. S. DeCherney, R. V. Jackson, A. N. Alexander, J. Rivier, C. Rivier, J. Spiess, and W. Vale, *J. Clin.Endocrinol. Metabol.*, submitted (1982).

33. A. Grossman, L. Perry, A. V. Schally, A. C. Nieuwenhuyzen-Kruseman, S. Tomlin, D. H. Coy, A. M. Comaru-Schally, and G. M. Besser, *Lancet*, April 24, p. 922 (1982).

34. J. Rivier, J. Spiess, C. Rivier, R. Galyean, and W. Vale, in K. Blaha and P. Malon, Eds., *Peptides 82*, Walter de Gruyter, 1983, pp. 597–602.

35. C. Rivier, J. Rivier, K. Lederis, and W. Vale, *Regul. Peptides* **5**, 139–143 (1983).

36. P. Pallai, M. Mabilia, M. Goodman, W. Vale, and J. Rivier, *Proc. Natl. Acad. Sci., USA*, in press, 1983.

37. W. Vale, J. Vaughan, G. Yamamoto, T. Bruhn, C. Douglas, D. Dalton, C. Rivier, and J. Rivier, in P. M. Conn, Ed., *Methods in Enzymology*, Academic Press, New York, in press, 1983.

38. W. Vale, C. Rivier, L. Yang, S. Minick, and R. Guillemin, *Endocrinology* **103**(5), 1910 (1978).

39. B. Eipper and R. Mains, *Endocr. Rev.* **1**, 1 (1981).

40. J. Porter and H. W. Rumsfeld Jr., *Endocrinology* **64**, 948 (1959).

41. A. V. Schally, R. N. Andersen, H. S. Lipscomb, J. M. Long, and R. Guillemin, *Nature (London)* **188**, 1192 (1960).

42. A. P. S. Dhariwal, J. A. Rodriques, F. Reeser, L. Chowers, and S. M. McCann, *Proc. Soc. Exp. Biol. Med.* **121**, 8 (1966).

43. M. T. Jones, B. Gillham, and E. W. Hillhouse, *Fed. Proc.* **36**, 2104 (1967).

44. L. T. Chan, M. Schaal, and M. Saffran, *Endocrinology* **85**, 644 (1969).

45. D. M. F. Cooper, D. Synetos, R. B. Cristie, and D. Schulster, *J. Endocrinol.* **71**, 171 (1976).

46. G. Gillies and P. Lowry, *Nature (London)* **278**, 463 (1979).

47. G. Sayers, E. Hanzmann, and M. Bodansky, *FEBS Lett.* **116**, 3 (1980).

48. A. V. Schally, R. C. Chang, A. Arimura, T. W. Redding, J. Fishback, and S. Vigh, *Proc. Natl. Acad. Sci. USA* **78**, 5197 (1981).

49. F. E. Bloom, E. L. F. Battenberg, J. Rivier, and W. Vale, *Regul. Peptides* **4**, 43 (1982).

50. L. W. Swanson, P. E. Sawchenko, J. Rivier, and W. W. Vale, *Neuroendocrinology*, **36**: 165 (1983).

51. M. Palkovits, *Ann. N.Y. Acad. Sci.* **297**, 455 (1977).
52. D. M. Gibbs and W. Vale, *Endocrinology*, **111**:1418 (1982).
53. C. Rivier, J. Rivier, and W. Vale, *Science*, **218**, 377–379 (1982).
54. G. Gillies and P. Lowry, Nature **278**, 463 (1979).
55. T. Bruhn and W. Vale, in preparation (1982).
56. N. Yasuda, M. A. Greer, and T. Aizawa, *Endocr. Rev.* **3**, 123 (1982).
57. J. Buckingham, *Pharmacol. Rev.* **31**, 253 (1980).
58. C. M. Turkelson, A. Arimura, M. D. Culler, and M. Shimizu, *Peptides* **2**, 425 (1981).
59. F. Labrie, R. Veilleux, G. LeFerre, D. Coy, J. Sueiras-Diaz, and A. V. Schally, *Science* **216**, 1007 (1982).
60. L Bilezikjian and W. Vale, *Endocrinology*, in press, (1983).
61. R. Sutton, N. Birnberg, R. Evans, G. Rosenfeld, and W. Vale, *J. Biol. Chem.*, submitted, 1983.
62. A. Bower, M. E. Hadley, and V. J. Hruby, *Science* **184**, 70 (1974).
63. F. J. H. Tilders, F. Berkenbosch, and P. G. Smelik, *Catecholamines and Stress: Recent Advances*, North Holland, Amsterdam 1980 p. 125.
64. M. R. Brown, L. A. Fisher, J. Spiess, C. Rivier, J. Rivier, and W. Vale, *Endocrinology*, **111**:928 (1982).
65. L. A. Fisher, J. Rivier, C. Rivier, J. Spiess, W. Vale, and M. Brown, *Endocrinology* **110**, 2222 (1982).
66. R. A. Peterfreund and W. W. Vale, *Endocrinology*, **112**, 1275–1278 (1982).
67. C. H. Ehlers, S. J. Henriksen, F. E. Bloom, J. Rivier, and W. W. Vale, *Soc. Neurosci. Abstr.* **8** (1982).
68. G. F. Koob, M. LeMoal, F. E. Bloom, R. E. Sutton, J. Rivier, and W. Vale, *Soc. Neurosci. Abstr.*, **8**,41 (1982).
69. D. R. Britton, G. F. Koob, J. Rivier, and W. Vale, *Life Sci.* **31**, 363 (1982).
70. R. C. Gaillard, A. Grossman, G. Gillies, L. H. Rees, and G. M. Besser, *Clin. Endocrinol.* **15** (1981).
71. J. B. Aldenhoff, D. Groul, J. Rivier, and W. Vale, G. Siggins, *Science*, in press (1983).
72. R. Sutton, G. F. Kobb, M. LeMoal, J. Rivier, and W. Vale, *Nature* **297**, 331 (1982).
73. R. E. Sutton, G. F. Koob, M. Le Moal, J. Rivier, and W. Vale, *Nature* **297**, 331–333 (1982).

39

Growth Hormone Releasing Factor

JOSEPH B. MARTIN
*Neurology Service Massachusetts General Hospital
Harvard Medical School
Boston, Massachusetts*

Physiological studies have provided compelling evidence that the hypothalamic control of growth hormone (GH) secretion is dependent upon the stimulatory influence of a GH-releasing factor (GRF). In unanesthetized animals, including primates and humans, GH secretion is characterized by dramatic surges of release that may elevate circulating plasma levels of the hormone by tenfold to a thousandfold (1). These surges, which are repetitive throughout the day and night, are obliterated by lesions that destroy the hypothalamic ventromedial and arcuate (infundibular) nuclei (2). Surges of GH secretion are also completely abolished by pharmacological treatments that interfere with α-adrenergic pathways in the brain (2). Blockade of α-adrenergic receptors with phenoxybenzamine, or with yohimbine, or depletion of norepinephrine with FLA-63, an inhibitor of dopamine-β-hydroxylase, abolishes GH secretion (3). Yet these drugs have no direct effect on the pituitary, indicating that they interfere with GRF secretion. These observations, taken as a whole, provide firm physiological evidence for the necessity of a hypothalamic GRF, presumably produced by neurons in the VMN and arcuate nuclei.

The recent discovery of a peptide with specific and unusually potent stimulatory effects on GH secretion has now been reported (4, 5). The source of this peptide was not the hypothalamus, as was the case with the discovery of thyrotropin releasing hormone (TRH), gonadotropin releasing hormone (GnRH), corticotropin releasing hormone (CRH), and somatostatin, but rather from pancreatic tumors obtained from two patients. In both cases, the patient presented clinically with the symptoms and signs of GH excess (acromegaly). In one patient, pituitary enlargement was diagnosed and transsphenoidal surgery undertaken; the pituitary showed hyperplasia of the GH-secreting cells, the symptoms of acromegaly persisted postoperatively, and a pancreatic tumor was subsequently found. The second patient had a normal pituitary and two pancreatic tumors. In both cases extracts of the pancreatic tumors revealed a peptide of similar structure.

In two reports published within a few weeks of each other, Guillemin et al. (4) and Vale and collaborators (5) have revealed the structure of a 44-amino-acid peptide and a 40-amino-acid peptide, respectively, with GH-releasing effects. The structure of the larger molecule is:

Tyr-Ala-Asp-Ala-Ile-Phe-Thr-Asn-Ser-Tyr-Arg-Lys-Val-Leu-Gly-Gln-Leu-Ser-Ala-Arg-Lys-Leu-Leu-Gln-Asp-Ile-Met-Ser-Arg-Gln-Gln-Gly-Glu-Ser-Asn-Gln-Glu-Arg-Gly-Ala-Arg-Ala-Arg-Leu-NH$_2$ (4)

The active substance was given the name human pancreas growth hormone releasing factor (hpGRF). The structure of the second tumor-derived GRF, reported by Vale et al. (5) contains 40-amino-acid residues identical in sequence to the N-terminus of the larger molecule reported by Guillemin's group; it remains to be established whether the difference in length of the two peptides (44 versus 40 residues, respectively) was the result of degradation of the peptide in the tissue extracts or reflects a difference in posttranslational processing by the tumor cells. Whichever is the case, it is remarkable that the two tumors produced an identical biologically active polypeptide, lending strong support to the likelihood that hypothalamic GRF, when characterized, will have the same structure. In both reports, the GH-releasing effects of hpGRF were highly specific both *in vivo* and *in vitro*. There were no effects on the release of the other pituitary hormones, including prolactin, gonadotropins, adrenocorticotropic hormone (ACTH), or thyroid stimulating hormone (TSH). Studies in humans also confirm a specific, potent effect on GH secretion (6) (Figure 1).

The idea that tumor-derived substances can stimulate excessive GH secretion by the pituitary has emerged gradually over the last decade as more than a dozen such patients were reported, each presenting with acromegaly and a carcinoid or other neural crest–derived tumor (7–9). Frohman and collaborators (8, 9) partially purified extracts of such tumors, showed specific GH-releasing activity, and provided evidence that the GRF activity was peptidergic in nature.

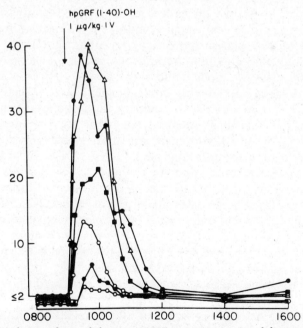

Figure 1. Stimulation of growth hormone (GH) secretion in six adult men by hpGRF (1–40)-OH. The vertical axis shows levels of plasma GH in ng/ml. The horizontal axis shows hours. (From Thorner et al. (6), with permission.

Several of these tumors have produced more than one biologically active peptide, including somatostatin, as was the case in the patient described by Guillemin's group (4). A comparison of tumor-derived GRF-activity with hypothalamic GRF has shown similarities in biological activity with parallel GH-release dose-response curves, similar gel filtration and reverse phase high performance liquid chromatographic characteristics, and inhibition of stimulated GH secretion by somatostatin (4, 5, 7–9).

The biological activity of the hpGRF molecule has been replicated by synthetic peptides; full activity is demonstrated by GRF(1-29)-NH$_2$, GRF(1-32)-NH$_2$, GRF(1-37)-NH$_2$, GRF(1-39)-NH$_2$ as well as by the amidated forms of the 40-amino-acid and 44-amino-acid peptides. Thus a C-terminal amide (-NH$_2$) appears to be important for full biological activity. On the other hand, GRF-(1-27)-NH$_2$ has only 10% of the activity of the full molecule. The carboxyl terminal fragment 28–44 has no biological activity. Moreover, the tyrosine amino terminal is essential for biological activity. Deletion of the amino terminal Tyr, Tyr-Ala, or Tyr-Ala-Asp yields compounds with less than 0.1% of the specific activity of hpGRF. Tissue extracts of the tumor GRF reported by Guillemin et al. also contained two other biologically active peptides corresponding to the (1-37)-OH and (1-40)-OH sequences. Since both the 37–38 and 40–41 peptide bonds are linked to arginine, it is probable that an endopeptidase may exist to cleave the precursor molecule, resulting in multiple forms of active molecules. Such a multiplicity of active fragments is reminiscent of the known processing of other hormones, including somatostatin, cholecystokinin, the enkephalins, and in a somewhat different manner, the pro-opiomelanocortins (10).

With the increasing evidence that biologically active peptides occur in "families," it is of interest to compare the structure of hpGRF with other identified molecules. A survey of other gut peptides reveals a close homology of hpGRF with members of the glucagon-secretin family, in particular to the new intestinal peptide PHI-27, isolated by Tatemoto and Mutt (11). HpGRF-(1-27) and PHI-27 have 12 common residues in an equivalent position, while 12 additional residues could represent single base changes. Strong homologies also are present between hpGRF-(1-27) and vasoactive intestinal polypeptide (VIP), glucagon, secretin, and gastric inhibitory peptide (GIP) (5). From a physiologic standpoint, these peptides, at least in the gut, exert effects opposite to those of somatostatin. Each of these peptides has also been reported to stimulate GH secretion in various species, either *in vivo* or *in vitro*; none, however, has a potency even closely approximating that of hpGRF, and none is effective in pituitary cultures where hpGRF is particularly potent.

HpGRF is active in fmole concentrations in stimulation of GH release when added to pituitary cells in culture (12–15). Its effects are blocked by somatostatin in a noncompetitive fashion; i.e., different receptors appear to be present on the GH cell for mediation of the inhibitory effects of somatostatin and the stimulatory effects of hpGRF. Preliminary studies indicate that GH secretion induced by hpGRF is calcium ion dependent and is accompanied by an increase in intracellular cyclic adenosine 3'5' monophosphate (cAMP). The stimulatory effect is potentiated by pretreatment of cells with glucocorticoids or thyroid hormones, both known to have important regulatory effects on GH secretion (5).

The availability of antibodies to hpGRF has already permitted direct studies of the localization of GRF in the brain. The presence of positively staining neuronal perikarya in the hypothalamic arcuate nucleus and in the VMN of the primate brain has been found (16). A dense network of fibers could be traced to the median eminence in both species. However, staining was not found in the rat or ox brain, suggesting that hypothalamic GRF from those species may not be identical in structure to human GRF. On the other hand, administration of hpGRF antisera to unanesthetized rats abolishes the surges of GH normally present (17), providing additional evidence that GRF is secreted into the blood from the hypothalamus to trigger the surges in pituitary GH release.

Guillemin proposes to replace the acronym GRF by the name *somatocrinin*, from the Greek *somato*, abbreviated from somatotropin, a trivial name for GH, and *crinin*, meaning to secrete. Somatocrinin is thus the endocrine counterpart of somatostatin.

With the discovery of hpGRF, and assuming that a similar, probably identical hypothalamic somatocrinin will be identified, it is tempting to wonder whether the era of discovery that followed Harris's *portal-vessel chemotransmitter hypothesis* can now be formally closed. Have all the hypothalamic factors important for hypothalamic-pituitary regulation been discovered? The answer is probably not. But with the characterization of hpGRF it can now safely be predicted that a fuller appreciation of hypothalamic-pituitary functions will result, and that, as with somatostatin, other unexpected discoveries lie ahead.

REFERENCES

1. J. B. Martin, P. Brazeau, G. S. Tannenbaum, J. O. Willoughby, J. Epelbaum, L. C. Terry, and D. Durand, (1978) in S. Reichlin, R. Baldessarini, and J. B. Martin, Eds., *The Hypothalamus*, Raven Press, New York, pp. 329–355.
2. W. J. Millard, J. B. Martin Jr., J. Audet, S. M. Sagar, and J. B. Martin, *Endocrinology* **110**, 540–550 (1982).
3. L. C. Terry, and J. B. Martin, *Endocrinology* **108**, 1869–1873 (1981).
4. R. Guillemin, P. Brazeau, P. Bohlen, F. Esch, N. Ling, and W. B. Wehrenberg, *Science* **218**, 585–587 (1982).
5. J. Rivier, J. Spiess, M. Thorner, and W. Vale, *Nature* **300**, 276–278 (1982).

6. M. O. Thorner, J. Rivier, J. Spiess, J. L. Borges, M. L. Vance, S. R. Bloom, A. D. Rogol, M. J. Cronin, D. L. Kaiser, W. S. Evans, J. D. Webster, R. M. MacLeod, and W. Vale, *Lancet* 1, 24–28 (1983).

7. M. O. Thorner, R. L. Perryman, M. J. Cronin, A. D. Rogol, M. Draznin, A. Johanson, R. Grindeland, W. Vale, E. Horvath, and K. Kovacs, *J. Clin. Invest.* 70, 965–977 (1982).

8. L. A. Frohman, M. Szabo, M. Berelowitz, and M. E. Stachura, *J. Clin. Invest.* 65, 43–54 (1980).

9. M. Szabo, L. Chu, and L. A. Frohman, *Endocrinology* 111, 1235–1240 (1982).

10. D. T. Krieger, and J. B. Martin, *N. Engl. J. Med.* 304, 876–885, 944–951 (1981).

11. K. Tatemoto, and V. Mutt, *Proc. Natl. Acad. Sci.* 78, 6603–6607 (1981).

12. F. S. Esch, P. Bohlen, N. G. Ling, P. Brazeau, W. B. Wehrenberg, and R. Guillemin, *J. Biol. Chem.*, in press (1983).

13. P. Brazeau, N. Ling, F. Esch, P. Bohlen, C. Mougin, and R. Guillemin, *Biochem. Biophys. Res. Comm.*, 109, 588–594 (1982).

14. J. Spiess, J. Rivier, M. Thorner, and W. Vale, *Biochemistry* 21, 6037–6040 (1982).

15. P. Brazeau, N. Ling, P. Bohlen, F. Esch, S.-Y. Ying, and R. Guillemin, *Proc. Natl. Acad. Sci.*, 79, 7909–7913 (1982).

16. B. Bloch, P. Brazeau, N. Ling, P. Bohlen, F. Esch, W. B. Wehrenberg, R. Benoit, F. Bloom, and R. Guillemin, *Nature* 301, 607–608 (1983).

17. W. B. Wehrenberg, P. Brazeau, R. Luben, P. Bohlen, and R. Guillemin, *Endocrinology* 111, 2147–2148 (1982).

Index